MEDICAL SURGICAL CARE PLANNING

SECOND EDITION

Nancy M. Holloway, RN, MSN
Critical Care Educator
Nancy Holloway & Associates
Orinda, California

Springhouse Corporation
Springhouse, Pennsylvania

Staff

Executive Director, Editorial
Stanley Loeb

Director of Trade and Textbooks
Minnie B. Rose, RN, BSN, MEd

Art Director
John Hubbard

Clinical Consultant
Maryann Foley, RN, BSN

Drug Information Editor
George J. Blake, RPh, MS

Copy Editors
Mary Hohenhaus Hardy, Pamela Wingrod

Designers
Stephanie Peters (associate art director),
StellarVisions, ARC Designs (cover design),
Maryanne Buschini, Lorraine Carbo, Donald
G. Knauss

Typography
David Kosten (director), Diane Paluba (manager), Elizabeth Bergman, Joyce Rossi Biletz, Phyllis Marron, Robin Mayer, Valerie
Rosenberger

Manufacturing
Deborah Meiris (manager), Anna Brindisi,
T.A. Landis

Printed in the United States of America.

MS2E-050596

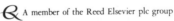 A member of the Reed Elsevier plc group

Library of Congress Cataloging-in-Publication Data
Medical-surgical care planning/ edited by Nancy M. Holloway. — 2nd ed.
p. cm.
Rev. ed. of: Medical-surgical care plans/Nancy M. Holloway. c1988.
Includes bibliographical references and index.
1. Nursing care plans. 2. Nursing. 3. Surgical nursing. 4. Diagnosis-related groups. I. Holloway, Nancy Meyer II. Holloway, Nancy Meyer, Medical-surgical care plans. III. Title: Medical-surgical care planning.
[DNLM: 1. Diagnosis-Related Groups. 2. Nursing Diagnosis. 3. Patient Care Planning. WY 100 M4877]
RT49.M45 1993
610.73—dc20
DNLM/DLC
ISBN 0-87434-489-1
92-20351
CIP

Contents

Section III: Condensed Plans of Care

Consultants and Contributors

Consultants

Susan J. Hricko, RN, MSN
Diabetes Nurse Educator
St. Luke's Episcopal Hospital
Houston

Karen Landis, RN, MS, CCRN
Pulmonary Clinical Nurse Specialist
Allentown (Pa.) Hospital–Lehigh Valley
  Hospital Center

Contributors

Nancy Newell Bell, RN, MN, CCRN, CEN
Critical Care–Trauma Clinical Nurse
  Specialist
Eden Hospital Medical Center
Castro Valley, Calif.;
Assistant Clinical Professor
School of Physiologic Nursing
University of California at San
  Francisco
(Fractured Femur, Multiple Trauma)

Cynthia Bellin, RN,C, MS, CCRN
Metabolic Nutrition Support Nurse
Doctors Hospital
Columbus, Ohio
(Nutritional Deficit, Total Parenteral
  Nutrition)

Audrey J. Berman, MS, RN, OCN
Assistant Professor
Samuel Merritt College
Oakland, Calif.
(Hysterectomy, Lymphoma)

Ruth Brewer, RN, PhD
Coordinator, Graduate Nursing
McNeese State University
College of Nursing
Lake Charles, La.
(Femoral Popliteal Bypass,
  Inflammatory Bowel Disease)

Perla Cardoza, ART
Director of Medical Records
Summit Medical Center
Oakland, Calif.
(Delivering Quality Care in a Cost-
  Conscious Environment)

Cecilia A. Casey, RN, MS, CDE
Diabetes Clinical Nurse Specialist
Department of Medical-Surgical
  Nursing and Division of
  Endocrinology and Metabolism
The Ohio State University Hospitals
Columbus
(Diabetes Mellitus, Diabetic
  Ketoacidosis, Hyperosmolar
  Hyperglycemic Nonketotic
  Syndrome, Hypoglycemia)

Terry Cheney, RN, CETN
Staff Nurse
Skilled Nursing Facility
Summit Medical Center
Oakland, Calif.
(Ileal Conduit Urinary Diversion)

Suzanne Clark, RN, MA, MSN, CS
Clinical Nurse Specialist
Kaiser Permanente, Department of
  Psychiatry
Los Angeles
(Congestive Heart Failure, Ineffective
  Individual Coping)

John M. Clochesy, RN, CS, MS, FCCM
Instructor
Case Western Reserve University
Francis Payne Bolton School of
  Nursing
Cleveland
(Myasthenia Gravis)

Patricia C. Cloud, RN, MSN, OCNS
Associate Professor
McNeese State University
Lake Charles, La.
(Mastectomy)

Laura A. Curtin, RN, MSN
Case Manager
Hospice of Cambridge;
Long Island Shelter Clinic
Cambridge, Mass.
(Geriatric Considerations, Impaired
  Physical Mobility)

Dorothy B. Doughty, RN, MN, CETN
Program Director
ET Nursing Education Program
Emory University
Atlanta
(Colostomy)

Gudrun O. Dybdal, RN, BSN, MA
Manager, Training and Development
Summit Medical Center
Oakland, Calif.
(Cholecystectomy)

Phyllis R. Easterling, RN, EdD
Department Chairperson, Nursing, and
  Associate Professor
Samuel Merritt College
Oakland, Calif.
(Acute Renal Failure, Major Burns,
  Retinal Detachment, Skin Grafts,
  Thoracotomy, Urolithiasis)

Gayle Flo, RN, BSN, MN, CCRN
Critical Care Clinical Specialist
Good Samaritan Hospital
Puyallup, Wash.
(Cerebrovascular Accident)

Patricia C. Hanson, RN
President
Healthcare Management Services
Eagan, Minn.
(Delivering Quality Care in a Cost-
Conscious Environment, Nursing
Discharge Criteria)

Barbara S. Henzel, RN, BSN, CCRN
Clinical Nurse Supervisor
Endoscopy Unit
Hospital of the University of
Pennsylvania
Philadelphia
(Esophagitis and Gastroenteritis)

Mel Herman, RN, CCRN
Assistant Head Nurse, ICU
Summit Medical Center
Oakland, Calif.
(Adult Respiratory Distress Syndrome,
Mechanical Ventilation)

Kathleen Hester, RN, CCRN
Nurse Manager, Critical Care
Mt. Diablo Medical Center
Concord, Calif.
(Acute Myocardial Infarction — Critical
Care Unit Phase, Acute Myocardial
Infarction — Stepdown Unit Phase)

Margaret L. Hodge, RN, MSN
Instructor
California State University
at Sacramento
(Drug Overdose, Seizures)

Nancy M. Holloway, RN, MSN
Critical Care Educator
Nancy Holloway & Associates
Orinda, Calif.
(Acid-Base Appendix, Disseminated
Intravascular Coagulation, Fluid and
Electrolyte Imbalances Appendix,
Knowledge Deficit, Monitoring
Standards Appendix, Nursing
Diagnosis Appendix, Pain, Transfer
Criteria Appendix)

Beth Colvin Huff, RN,C, MSN
Gynecologic Oncology
Clinical Nurse Specialist
Vanderbilt University Medical Center
Nashville, Tenn.
(Radioactive Implant for Cervical
Cancer)

Lauren Marie Isacson, RN,C, BSN, MPA
Clinical Information Systems
Coordinator
Jersey Shore Medical Center
Neptune, N.J.
(Peritoneal Dialysis)

Philip A. John, MRT
Medical Records Consultant
Paradise, Calif.
(DRG Classifications)

Larry E. Lancaster, RN, MSN, EdD
Associate Professor
Vanderbilt University School of Nursing
Nashville, Tenn.
(Chronic Renal Failure)

Robin L. Laurence, RN, BSN, MSN
Psychiatric Nurse
Langley Porter Psychiatric Institute
San Francisco
(Anorexia Nervosa and Bulimia
Nervosa)

Claudia Beverly Leath, RN, MNSc, RNP
Associate Professor
University of Arkansas Medical
Sciences College of Nursing
Little Rock
(Low Back Pain — Conservative
Medical Management, Total Joint
Replacement in a Lower Extremity)

Elizabeth D. MacRae, RN, MS
General Surgery Clinical Nurse
Specialist
Vanderbilt University Medical Center
Nashville, Tenn.
(Abdominal Aortic Aneurysm Repair)

Ruth E. Malone, RN, MSN, CEN
Staff Nurse, Emergency Department
Summit Medical Center
Oakland, Calif.
(Dying)

Wendy M. Mancini, RN, BSN, CCRN, CNA
Critical Care Nurse Clinician
Jersey Shore Medical Center
Neptune, N.J.
(Cardiogenic Shock)

Barbara J. Martin, RN, MS
Unit Leader
Rush–Presbyterian–St. Luke's Medical
Center
Chicago
(Permanent Pacemaker Insertion)

Celestine B. Mason, RN, BSN, MA
Nursing Care Consultant
Good Samaritan Hospital
Puyallup, Wash.
(Alzheimer's Disease, Multiple
Sclerosis, Thrombophlebitis)

Molly J. Moran, RN, OCN, MS
Medical Oncology Clinical Nurse
Specialist
Arthur G. James Cancer Hospital and
Research Institute
The Ohio State University
Columbus
(Anemia)

Scarlott K. Mueller, RN, BSN, MPH
Cancer Center Coordinator and
Assistant Director of Nursing
North Florida Regional Medical Center
Gainesville
(Grieving, Prostatectomy)

Christine Ortiz, RN, BSN
Doctoral Student
University of California at San
    Francisco
(Acquired Immunodeficiency
    Syndrome)

Elizabeth Poulson, RN, MA, MS
Practitioner-Teacher
Rush–Presbyterian–St. Luke's Medical
    Center
Chicago
(Permanent Pacemaker Insertion)

Katherine Purgatorio-Howard, RN,C,
    MSN
Course Coordinator
Ann May School of Nursing
Jersey Shore Medical Center
Neptune, N.J.
(Angina Pectoris, Leukemia)

Ellene Rifas, RN, MSN, EdD
Director, Educational Services
Kaiser Permanente Medical Center
Sacramento, Calif.
(Asthma, Chronic Obstructive
    Pulmonary Disease, Pneumonia)

Dennis Ross, RN, MAE, MSN, PhD
Associate Professor of Nursing
University of Pittsburgh
(Osteomyelitis)

Patricia C. Seifert, RN, CNOR, MSN
Operating Room Coordinator, Cardiac
    Surgery
The Arlington (Va.) Hospital
(Cardiac Surgery, Surgical
    Intervention)

Suzanne Seitz, RN, MS, CCRN
Critical Care Clinical Nurse Specialist
Mt. Diablo Medical Center
Concord, Calif.
(Hypovolemic Shock)

Suzy Temple, RN, MSN
Assistant Professor
Mississippi College School of Nursing
Clinton
(Lung Cancer)

Debra Thelen, RN, BSN, MS
Staff Nurse II
AIDS Unit and Hospice Services
Kaiser Permanente
San Francisco
(Acquired Immunodeficiency
    Syndrome)

M. Susan Theodoropoulos, RN, MSN
Medical-Surgical Clinical Specialist
The Arlington (Va.) Hospital
(Amputation)

Charlene Thomas, RN, MSN
Acting Assistant Chairperson
Rush–Presbyterian–St. Luke's Medical
    Center
Chicago
(Permanent Pacemaker Insertion)

Nancy C. Thomas, RN, BSN
Staff Nurse, Critical Care Center
Good Samaritan Hospital
Puyallup, Wash.
(Cerebrovascular Accident)

Sue L. Thomas, RN
Nurse Manager, Transitional Care Unit
Summit Medical Center
Oakland, Calif.
(Pulmonary Embolism, Sensory-
    Perceptual Alteration)

Susan A. VanDeVelde-Coke, RN, MA,
    MBA
Director of Nursing, Surgery
Health Sciences Centre
Winnipeg, Manitoba, Canada
(Duodenal Ulcer, Gastrointestinal
    Hemorrhage, Liver Failure,
    Pancreatitis)

Carolyn S. Watts, RN, BS, MSN
Associate in Surgery, Clinical Nurse
    Specialist
Vanderbilt University Medical Center
Nashville, Tenn.
(Nephrectomy)

Patricia Harvey Webb, RN, MS
Assistant Professor, Department of
    Nursing
Samuel Merritt College
Oakland, Calif.
(Carotid Endarterectomy, Craniotomy,
    Glaucoma, Guillain-Barré Syndrome,
    Increased Intracranial Pressure,
    Laminectomy)

Alice A. Whittaker, RN, MS
Instructor
Creighton University School of Nursing
Mary Lanning Memorial Hospital
Hastings, Neb.
(Ineffective Family Coping)

Patricia R. Wilson, RN, BSN, MS
Doctoral Candidate
National Research Service Award
Fellow, National Cancer Institute
University of South Carolina College
    of Nursing
Columbia
(Radical Neck Dissection)

Acknowledgments

Publishing a book is never a sole creative endeavor. I extend a special thank you to our contributors and consultants, acknowledged by name in a separate section. In addition, I thank the following people for their extraordinary contributions:

Ruth Malone, a gifted writer who served as consulting editor and contributor for the first edition and contributor to the second. Ruth's perception, sensitivity, and commitment to the vision played a major role in the quality of both editions.

Barbara Scott, administrative assistant, whose flexibility and cheerfulness eased project management immeasurably.

The talented publishing team at Springhouse Corporation, acknowledged on another page.

Michelle Conant, Kathleen Dobkin, Mary Gray, Patricia Hinton-Walker, Jean Lertola, Jean Masunaga, Carla Powell, Julia Quiring, and Cecilia Shaw, contributors to the first edition. Their work helped lay the cornerstones for the current edition.

Dedication
This book is dedicated to D. Michael Holloway, my husband, for championing my dreams, and Jason Holloway, my son, for making it all worthwhile.

Preface

Medical-Surgical Care Planning, Second Edition, is essential. Why? Because it integrates three major factors in nursing—care planning, nursing diagnoses, and diagnosis-related groups (DRGs)—and provides information nurses need to meet the 1992 Joint Commission on the Accreditation of Healthcare Organizations (JCAHO) Nursing Care Standards. Focusing on care of the adult medical-surgical patient, this book:

• distinguishes clearly between nursing's collaborative functions (those shared with medicine) and its independent functions (those uniquely nursing's)
• offers the less experienced bedside nurse, nursing student, and nursing educator comprehensive, realistic clinical plans to meet their educational needs
• offers the experienced bedside nurse a separate section of condensed plans concise enough to be used in today's hectic, cost-conscious practice environment.

Why are plans of care important?

Clinically, plans of care offer a way to plan and communicate appropriate patient care. Legally, they offer a framework for establishing the standard of care for a given situation. Financially, they can validate the appropriateness of care and justify staffing levels and patient-care charges.

If plans of care are so important, why don't more nurses use them?

Most nurses are first exposed to plans of care as students. They soon learn that writing out individual plans can be frustrating and time consuming. After graduation, most nurses practice in a hectic, complex environment that allows little time for thoughtful care planning.

Even nurses who would like to use written plans of care may be at a loss when trying to integrate nursing diagnoses into their planning. Overwhelmed, they may turn to previously published books for guidance only to find the information too general or too theoretical, that common medical problems are renamed, or that nursing diagnoses are not matched to medical disorders.

Yet *clinically relevant* plans of care can help nurses answer many of the questions they ask daily:

• "What are the most important points to cover during a physical assessment when I haven't got time to check everything?"
• "Which laboratory tests and diagnostic procedures should I anticipate, and what do they typically show?"
• "What are this patient's nursing priorities?"
• "Which problems is this patient most likely to experience?"
• "Why are certain interventions important?"
• "Which complications can occur with this disorder?"
• "How long is this patient likely to be in the hospital?"
• "Realistically, how much patient teaching can I accomplish?"
• "From a nursing standpoint, how will I know when this patient is ready for discharge?"

The solution: This book

Medical-Surgical Care Planning, Second Edition provides clinically relevant answers to common questions about patient care because it targets the needs of the "hands-on" nurse clinician through standardized plans of care. Distinguishing features include:

• 11 general plans of care covering conditions nurses encounter daily, such as impaired physical mobility and knowledge deficit
• 70 plans of care, organized by body system, covering various medical-surgical conditions and procedures (including critical care disorders)

• 41 condensed plans of care for the experienced nurse
• nursing diagnoses (using selected terminology from the North American Nursing Diagnosis Association) and collaborative problems (using familiar medical terminology, such as shock) arranged in order of importance.
This approach will help you see the total picture of patient care; differentiate between collaborative and independent nursing responsibilities; apply the latest official nursing diagnoses; and avoid forcing all planning under nursing diagnoses, a process that only renames medical diagnoses and fosters confusion between nursing and medicine.

Each plan presents the latest clinically relevant DRG information, including DRG numbers, principal diagnoses, and mean length of stay, to help you understand the reimbursement system responsible for today's cost-conscious health care environment and to help you anticipate the patient's recovery and plan patient teaching. Common historical and subjective findings are presented according to Gordon's functional health patterns, a widely accepted format that blends both traditional and contemporary methods of nursing assessment; objective findings are listed by body system. This assessment information will help you recognize pertinent signs and symptoms and understand how the nursing diagnoses and collaborative problems were identified.

The plans of care build on a goal-directed, action-oriented approach to care planning that ranks problems and interventions in order of importance and identifies specific outcome criteria. This approach will help you determine the most important patient problems, decide what to do first, and recognize when a problem has been resolved.

But didn't the JCAHO kill the care plan?
No. A close look at the 1992 standards reveals that *although plans of care per se are not required for accreditation, the elements that constitute a plan of care are required,* and *plans of care still may be used* to document patient care. If a plan of care includes assessment, nursing diagnoses, patient care needs, interventions, and outcomes, is it a nursing care plan? Yes, it is.

The new standards' impact on nursing
The 1992 update represents the first major revision of the Nursing Care Standards since 1978. The JCAHO Nursing Standards Task Force, which included 23 representatives from various nursing services and educational programs, adopted the new standards after circulating two drafts and considering feedback from more than 50,000 nurses.

Where the former Nursing Services Standards focused on the process of care to determine if the nursing organization could provide quality care, the new Nursing Care Standards focus more on the patient and the outcomes of care to determine the quality of care provided. In addition, the new standards emphasize patient-family education and discharge planning. Consequently, nurses will play an even more important role in helping hospitals maintain accreditation. Such accountability is likely to *increase* interest in care planning.

The revised standards also place increased emphasis on documentation, requiring that nursing information involving assessment, nursing diagnoses or patient needs, interventions, and outcomes become a permanent part of the medical record. Care may be documented directly in the patient's record or indirectly through references to other documents. However, this documentation does not have to be the handwritten, complex, case-study approach to care planning that educators find helpful, or the routine, repetitive handwritten plan that many hospital nurses rightly dismiss as irrelevant and time consuming. Instead of being required to provide handwritten plans of care for all patients, nursing departments now have more flexibility in documenting care. Nurses may now choose to document care planning through standards of care, clinical practice guidelines, critical paths, or preprinted plans of care.

When individualized as recommended, the standardized plans in this book can help nurses meet all of the JCAHO's new requirements. The plans cover all the elements required for documentation of care planning and also include useful information about patient outcomes, patient-family education, and discharge planning.

Standardized vs. individualized plans

Major differences of opinion exist in nursing concerning standardized and individualized plans of care. Opponents of standardization argue that it equals depersonalization. Advocates argue that standardization promotes efficiency, by limiting planning time without sacrificing quality, and fosters quality assurance. This disagreement cannot be resolved easily; however, this book combines the advantages of standard plans of care with unusual features that help minimize their disadvantages:

• The plans blend standardized and individualized aspects of care. Standardization works better in some areas of care planning than others: problems, priorities, and interventions usually can be standardized, but outcome criteria, timing of interventions, and discharge criteria require significant individualization. This book takes these factors into account and encourages flexibility in areas that vary significantly among patients.

• Space is provided at the end of each problem for the nurse to add additional interventions and rationales specific to the individual patient's needs. These unusual features challenge the nurse to think creatively. Because the resulting plan is pertinent and individualized, its clinical usefulness is ensured.

However, the most important point to remember in the debate over standardized versus individualized plans of care is that *a plan of care does not cause depersonalized care; rather, the nurse's attitude is the culprit.* The nurse who appreciates patients as individuals will use a standard plan as a starting point, staying attuned to the individual patient's responses while applying the art and science of nursing.

Why nurses will continue to use plans of care

Plans of care provide a valuable way to organize care, meet the JCAHO's requirements for documentation, and prepare for site visits. In addition, many institutions have invested substantial time and money to develop systems of care planning appropriate for their patients. Before abandoning such systems, they would need to find a better one and the funds, time, and expertise to implement it — a difficult undertaking in this era of scarce resources. Finally, instructors in schools of nursing will continue to use plans of care as a method for teaching patient care because of the plans' comprehensiveness.

Ultimately, any plan of care is only as good as the nurse who provides the care. Conscientious nurses find plans of care a resource for learning new information quickly, refreshing their knowledge, and focusing their energy on the most important problems their patients may encounter. The contributors to *Medical-Surgical Care Planning, Second Edition* have based their plans on a blend of clinical expertise, nursing diagnosis, and care planning — always keeping in mind the nurse on the front line. This book will provide welcome help for nurses facing the daily challenge of providing quality patient care.

Nancy M. Holloway

Section I

Three professional challenges are covered here: planning and implementing individualized patient care, distinguishing nursing from medical care, and reconciling cost-containment with quality care.

INTRODUCTION

Using the Plans of Care

These plans of care are designed to give you a maximal amount of clinically relevant information within a minimal number of pages. This book is intended as a guide for providing quality "hands-on" nursing care to patients, not as a substitute for the broad clinical knowledge found in more exhaustive nursing references. Every plan of care is divided into sections, each presenting a different type of information. Becoming familiar with the plans' basic format will enable you to use their practical information efficiently. Explanations of each section follow, along with specific recommendations for using the plans of care in practice.

DRG information
Immediately after the title of the clinical plan, abbreviated *DRG information* appears, including:
• relevant DRG numbers (Some clinical disorders always have the same DRG, such as myasthenia gravis. Others, such as circulatory disorders, are divided into several DRGs.)
• mean length of stay (LOS) for treating the disorder
• comments, if appropriate, designed to put the DRG into perspective.

Ideally, each plan of care would include the average LOS for the disorder to guide patient and family teaching and to provide a benchmark against which the nurse could assess the patient's progress toward discharge. Unfortunately, such information is not available. However, this book provides the best substitute: the geometric mean LOS, a statistical measure used in cost accounting (explained in greater detail on page 8). Use this information to anticipate when teaching and discharge planning should be well under way and when maximum hospital benefit usually has been reached. Do not use the mean LOS as a target for discharge; doing so will almost certainly ensure that the hospital loses money. Instead, when the patient's needs permit, plan for a LOS shorter than the mean LOS. Remember that the mean LOS relates to discharge from the hospital, not transfer from one unit to another. Mean LOS information is updated periodically and published in the *Federal Register*.

Introduction
In *Definition and Time Focus*, the disease, surgical procedure, or patient problem on which the plan focuses is briefly discussed within a specific time frame. Surgical plans of care usually cover the immediate preoperative and postoperative phases of care. Medical plans of care focus on the most acute phase of the illness, the period in which the patient is most likely to be hospitalized in an acute-care unit.

Etiology and Precipitating Factors lists factors that directly or indirectly contribute to the condition's development, grouped according to pathophysiologic mechanism when possible.

Focused assessment guidelines
This section is divided into *Nursing History*, *Physical Findings*, *Diagnostic Studies*, and *Potential Complications*.

The assessment guidelines list specific findings common to most patients with the identified condition. The intent is to give you a vivid picture of the typical patient presentation.

The first assessment section, *Nursing History (Functional health pattern findings)*, presents subjective and historical data organized by Gordon's functional health patterns framework (see *Functional health patterns*). The health patterns represent 11 broad categories within the holistic wellness-illness system. Each of the health patterns provides useful parameters for assessing any patient. Because the emphasis here is on definitive or common findings, only those patterns with data relevant to the condition are included.

The second assessment section, *Physical Findings*, presents typical objective findings for a patient with the identified condition. The physical findings are organized by body system, an option familiar to most nurses.

Diagnostic Studies, the next assessment section, provides information regarding laboratory and diagnostic tests usually performed for the diagnosis and treatment of the specified condition. Not all the tests listed may be performed on a particular patient; what actually is ordered depends on individual factors. However, the astute nurse is aware of the significance of studies and tests that may pertain to the patient's condition and, when indicated, collaborates with the doctor to select such studies.

Finally, *Potential Complications* lists the condition's most common complications. Because promoting wellness and preventing illness are now a significant part of nursing practice, the nurse must be aware of potential complications to intervene appropriately on the patient's behalf.

Collaborative problems and nursing diagnoses
This section contains the main body of the plan of care: the predictable patient health problems caused by the pathophysiology. Problems may be actual or high risk. An actual problem is one with identifiable signs and symptoms that are present in all or most patients with the disorder. If the patient does not have signs and symptoms, but is at risk, the problem is labelled high risk (in nursing diagnosis terminology, a high-risk problem was formerly called a potential problem).

Because nursing practice is based on both medical and nursing diagnoses, a patient problem is identified as either a *Collaborative Problem* or *Nursing Diagnosis*.

Collaborative problems are those that require the doctor and nurse to work together to meet desired patient outcomes. Although the doctor is accountable for definitive interventions, the nurse may initiate moni-

FUNCTIONAL HEALTH PATTERNS

1. Health Perception – Health Management Pattern
- perceived pattern of health and well-being
- general level of health care behavior (how health is managed)
- health status related to future planning

2. Nutritional-Metabolic Pattern
- food and fluid consumption relative to metabolic need
- pattern, types, quantity, and preferences of foods and fluids
- skin lesions and healing ability
- indicators of nutritional status (such as skin, hair, and nail condition)

3. Elimination Pattern
- patterns of excretory function
- routines and devices used

4. Activity-Exercise Pattern
- exercise, activity, leisure, and recreation
- activities of daily living
- sports
- factors interfering with activity

5. Sleep-Rest Pattern
- pattern of sleep, rest, and relaxation
- perception of quantity and quality of rest
- energy level
- sleep aids and problems

6. Cognitive-Perceptual Pattern
- adequacy of sensory modes
- pain perception and management
- cognitive functional ability

7. Self-Perception – Self-Concept Pattern
- attitudes about self
- perception of abilities
- body image, identity, and general emotional pattern
- pattern of body posture and speech

8. Role-Relationship Pattern
- role engagements – family, work, social
- perception of responsibilities

9. Sexuality-Reproductive Pattern
- satisfaction or disturbances in sexuality
- reproductive stage
- reproductive pattern

10. Coping – Stress Tolerance Pattern
- general coping pattern and effectiveness
- perceived ability to manage situations
- reserve capacity and resources

11. Value-Belief Pattern
- values, goals, or beliefs that guide choices
- conflicts related to health status

Adapted from: Gordon, M. *Nursing Diagnosis: Process and Application,* 2nd ed. New York: McGraw-Hill Book Co., 1987.

toring, implement medical orders, act under medically approved protocols, or institute measures to prevent complications. Disease-related plans of care are marked with a logo of two boxes joined to form a plus sign, symbolizing collaboration.

Nursing diagnoses are those human responses the nurse can identify and treat independently. The nurse can prescribe nursing interventions that do not require other professionals' approval and can assume accountability for the patient's response. Plans of care that fo-

cus only on nursing diagnoses are marked with a logo of a circle in a box, symbolizing independent action.

In most plans, the most important patient problems are presented first. However, some surgical procedure plans present preoperative problems first to provide logical continuity.

After problem identification, the *Nursing Priority* indicates the focus for the nursing interventions that follow. *Interventions* and *Rationales* are presented in two columns. Interventions are based on clinical experience and the nursing literature and thus represent a blend of practice and theory. The rationales, although purposely brief, incorporate relevant physiologic mechanisms whenever possible, along with other helpful data.

The most important interventions usually appear first. Interventions may be interdependent or independent in nature. Another health care provider, typically a doctor, initiates interdependent functions. However, whether acting under direct or indirect supervision or according to protocol, the nurse must use sound nursing judgment when carrying out an interdependent function. The nurse may initiate independent functions according to the terms of professional licensure and the state's nurse practice act.

Nurses have long recognized that patients respond best to care that takes personal characteristics and preferences into consideration. Consequently, space is provided at the end of each problem section for additional individualized interventions.

Each problem is followed by specific *Target outcome criteria,* defined as ideal expected patient responses to the interventions and grouped according to ideal time periods for achievement. These criteria, based on the clinical expertise of the nurses who contributed to this book, focus on specific, measurable patient responses that can guide the nurse in evaluating care. Such evaluation is particularly important because of the Joint Commission on the Accreditation of Healthcare Organizations (JCAHO) 1991 Nursing Care Standards' emphasis on documenting the patient's response to and outcomes of nursing care. However, these criteria are intended only as a guide; individual variation is to be expected because outcomes depend on many factors.

Discharge planning and documentation
The final section of the plan of care includes three guides for planning discharge and documenting care: *Nursing Discharge Criteria, Patient-Family Teaching Checklist,* and *Documentation Checklist.*

These sections are particularly valuable in light of the JCAHO 1991 Nursing Care Standards' increased emphasis on discharge planning, patient-family education, and documentation as key factors in determining a hospital's accreditation.

Nursing Discharge Criteria, developed by clinical experts and a discharge planning expert, provide specific guidelines for assessing the patient's readiness for discharge from the unit. They are particularly helpful when a rapid discharge or transfer decision must be made, such as when the unit is full and a critically ill patient must be admitted from the emergency department. For critically ill patients, the criteria in this section supplement those in Appendix E, Critical Care Discharge Criteria Guidelines. The criteria are intended as a guide only; if a patient does not meet them, then the health care team must make appropriate arrangements to fulfill any remaining needs.

The *Patient-Family Teaching Checklist* ensures that the patient's and family's learning needs related to the condition have been considered. Ideally, teaching should begin on or before admission and continue throughout the patient's hospital stay and convalescence. Because the plans focus on inpatient care, teaching interventions reflect only what may be reasonable to accomplish on the unit. Interventions related to teaching are interwoven throughout the plans or included in a special "Knowledge deficit" problem. (Refer to the "Knowledge Deficit" plan for general teaching information.) The nurse can expect that various health care professionals, such as dietitians, doctors, clinical specialists, and social workers, will be responsible for different aspects of patient teaching, in addition to what the nurse provides.

Finally, the *Documentation Checklist* provides a summary of items that should appear in the patient record. As has been previously noted, changes in health care payment systems and JCAHO requirements make thorough documentation more essential than ever. Accurate documentation also helps protect the nurse in the event of case-related litigation, although now, as always, the best way to avoid legal problems is to maintain high standards of care, impeccable professionalism, and warm, caring relationships with patients.

Concluding each plan of care is a list of *Associated Plans of Care* found elsewhere in this book and *References,* which may be helpful if you seek further information.

Organization of the book
This book presents three types of plans: "general" plans of care, comprehensive plans of care for specific disorders, and condensed plans. The general plans provide detailed interventions for common patient problems, such as pain, knowledge deficit, grieving, and dying. They are designed to be used with the diagnosis- or procedure-based comprehensive plans that constitute the main portion of the book. The comprehensive plans contain the depth of detail appropriate for education and reference. The nurse already familiar with the care appropriate for a particular condition may prefer the condensed plans of care. These abbreviated plans (arranged alphabetically) address conditions the nurse encounters most frequently.

When using any of these plans of care in clinical practice, you may benefit from closely reading the plan first. Thereafter, you can refer to the plan each shift, addressing problems and documenting interventions in the nurse's notes. Before the patient is discharged, you can review the appropriate sections and evaluate all teaching and documentation, using the checklists as a guide.

INTRODUCTION

Nursing Diagnosis

The American Nurses' Association Social Policy Statement (1980) defines nursing as "the diagnosis and treatment of human responses to actual or potential health problems." The North American Nursing Diagnosis Association (NANDA) defines *nursing diagnosis* as "a clinical judgment about an individual, family, or community response to actual or potential health problems [or] life processes [that] provides the basis for definitive therapy toward achievement of outcomes for which the nurse is accountable." Although nurses have been diagnosing patient problems for years, the term "nursing diagnosis" is relatively recent.

Past diagnostic efforts have been hampered by the lack of a common language for labeling nursing problems. To surmount this barrier, the National Conference Group on the Classification of Nursing Diagnoses began identifying and classifying health problems that nurses treat. That organization, formed at the first National Conference on Classification of Nursing Diagnoses in 1973, became NANDA. Every 2 years, NANDA releases a list of diagnoses accepted for study and clinical testing. The current list appears in Appendix D.

As the nursing diagnosis movement has evolved, nurses have encountered significant difficulty in using the NANDA terminology. Many nurses are frustrated by the categories' complexity, esoteric language, vagueness, wordiness, and differing levels of abstraction. These responses highlight an important problem: Some NANDA diagnostic labels are not useful clinically. Because the clinical experts who wrote the plans of care in this book found some of the NANDA diagnoses functional and others not, the editor made the following decisions:
• This book identifies nursing diagnoses using NANDA-recommended terminology whenever possible. If a contributor could not find a diagnosis on the list to fit a patient problem that nurses treat independently, the contributor generated a new diagnosis. New diagnoses are followed by an asterisk and a footnote identifying them as non-NANDA diagnoses.
• The official list is alphabetized by basic concept first, followed by any modifiers (for example, "airway clearance, ineffective"). In this book, diagnoses are modified to reflect usual conversational sequences.
• Because of its wordiness, "Alteration in nutrition: less than body requirements" has been replaced with "Nutritional deficit."

Two related issues have provoked substantial controversy and major differences of opinion within the nursing diagnosis community—the scope of nursing diagnosis and the possible renaming of medical diagnoses with nursing diagnostic language. In part, this controversy stems from the continued difficulty nurses face in articulating the dimensions of their practice and, particularly, in differentiating it from medical practice.

Many nurses believe that nursing diagnoses should describe only the independent domain of nursing. This domain can be defined as the area of clinical judgment in which the nurse can function in a self-directed manner to prescribe definitive therapy for human responses to health problems, achieving outcomes for which the nurse is accountable. Others believe that nursing diagnoses should address all the areas in which nurses make clinical judgments, including those in which the nurse carries out medical treatments. In this context, Gordon (1987) shed welcome light: "Pathophysiological manifestations of a diseased organ or system, such as impaired gas exchange, are not nursing diagnoses," she asserted. "Judgments related to observations of disease manifestations or to treatments do not have to be labeled as nursing diagnoses. Disease terminology is perfectly adequate. It would seem ridiculous to relabel a disease with a nursing diagnosis when in fact it cannot be treated except under medical protocols. Clearly, not everything a nurse does will be labeled with a nursing diagnosis."

This book supports using nursing diagnoses for only the independent domain of nursing. From this philosophical perspective, several accepted nursing diagnoses, such as "Decreased cardiac output" and "Altered tissue perfusion", do rename medical problems. These phenomena actually are pathophysiologic manifestations of disease.

Renaming problems already defined by other disciplines simply perpetuates the confusion between nursing and medicine. In this book, such problems are clearly identified as *collaborative* problems requiring both medical and nursing interventions. They are named with familiar terminology, such as "cardiogenic shock" instead of "Decreased cardiac output," "ischemia" instead of "Impaired tissue perfusion," and "hypoxemia" instead of "Altered gas exchange."

In some cases, a nursing diagnosis fits a nonacute problem but not a related acute problem, such as "Fluid volume deficit." In a nonacute fluid volume deficit, independent nursing interventions, such as providing preferred fluids and encouraging fluid intake, are paramount. In an acute fluid volume deficit, however, medical interventions, such as ordering the insertion of an intravenous catheter and prescribing specific intravenous solutions, are paramount. In this book, the term "Fluid volume deficit" is used in the first situation and "hypovolemia" in the second for diagnostic clarity. The distinction between acute and nonacute may prove a fruitful path for exploration in further attempts to increase the clinical usefulness of nursing diagnoses.

References

American Nurses' Association, Congress for Nursing Practice. *Nursing: A Social Policy Statement.* Kansas City, Mo.: American Nurses' Association, 1980.

Carroll-Johnson, R. *Classification of Nursing Diagnosis: Proceedings of the Ninth Conference, North American Nursing Diagnosis Association.* Philadelphia: J.B. Lippincott Co., 1991.

Gordon, M. *Nursing Diagnosis: Process and Application,* 2nd ed. New York: McGraw-Hill Book Co., 1987.

INTRODUCTION

Delivering Quality Care in a Cost-Conscious Environment

Medicare's prospective payment system (PPS) has dramatically altered the U.S. health care system. Faced with new restrictions and regulations affecting delivery of care, nurses increasingly have been confronted by twin challenges: sicker patients and shorter hospital stays. Nurses also play a key role in maintaining a hospital's financial viability in this competitive, market-driven health care environment. So, to maintain quality patient care under PPS, they have had to become increasingly sophisticated and innovative.

Evolution of PPS

Charges for hospital care used to be based on a retrospective method of payment. Hospital charges reflected what the market would bear and commonly were arbitrary, unrelated to the actual costs of delivering services. For the most part, nursing was a nonbillable direct service that was bundled under room and board charges in the hospital bill. But in recent years, third-party payers have demanded more explicit accounting for all services and appropriate charges for every area of health care delivery. In response, hospitals have begun to unbundle all units of service, including nursing.

Medicare, as one of the nation's primary insurers, was the first to change its reimbursement method. PPS was a desperate attempt to conserve the rapidly dwindling dollars in the Medicare trust fund set up in the 1960s to ensure that America's elderly citizens would have access to health care.

Under Medicare's PPS, diagnosis-related groups (DRGs) were developed to identify clinically homogeneous groups of diagnoses that use similar tests, treatments, and services and therefore could be reimbursed at similar rates. This federal system is now mandatory for Medicare recipients at all acute-care hospitals. Besides standardizing payment, this classification system was designed to put acute hospitalized patients into groups that could be used to predict resource consumption.

At present, 490 DRGs are grouped into 25 Major Diagnostic Categories (MDCs) based on anatomical organ systems, such as the respiratory system. The predetermined rate of reimbursement for each DRG is based on numerous factors, including the principal diagnosis, the patient's age, the presence of complications or comorbidities, and the occurrence of an operating room procedure. All these factors are taken into account upon the patient's discharge to determine which DRG will be assigned. (See *Ten frequently occurring DRGs.*)

The DRG system is incongruous in many ways, the most important of which is that it does not consider the severity of the patient's illness. Thus, a hospital is reimbursed for a patient who is severely ill and needs more services and a longer length of stay at the same rate as for a patient with the same illness and assigned DRG who is not severely ill. DRGs are, in effect, an averaging system: A hospital loses money on cases whose cost of care exceeds the amount paid for the assigned DRG, and it makes money on cases whose costs are less than the DRG payment. Many patients who would have been hospitalized in the past are now treated as outpatients, and conversely, only patients who meet strict criteria may be admitted to acute-care facilities. Hospitals, therefore, typically have sicker patients to care for than in the past, and patient care must be managed as efficiently as possible for a hospital to remain financially viable.

How DRGs are assigned

After discharge, a patient is assigned a DRG based on the following factors:
• principal diagnosis—the diagnosis that necessitated admission to the hospital
• secondary diagnosis—all secondary conditions that exist at the time of admission or that develop during hospitalization and affect the treatment or length of stay (LOS)
• operative procedures—any surgical procedures performed for definitive treatment rather than for diagnostic or exploratory purposes
• age—for some conditions, a different reimbursement rate applies for patients under and over age 17
• discharge status—whether the patient was discharged home or transferred to another hospital

---

TEN FREQUENTLY OCCURRING DRGs

127	Heart failure and shock
140	Angina pectoris
89	Simple pneumonia and pleurisy with complications
14	Specific cerebrovascular disorders
182	Esophagitis, gastroenteritis, and miscellaneous digestive disorders with complications
96	Bronchitis and asthma with complications
296	Nutritional and miscellaneous metabolic disorders with complications
138	Cardiac arrhythmia and conduction disorders with complications
121	Circulatory disorders with acute myocardial infarction and cardiovascular complications
320	Kidney and urinary tract infections with complications

• complications — any conditions arising during hospitalization that may prolong the LOS at least 1 day in approximately 75% of patients (such as diabetes)
• comorbidity — a preexisting condition that will increase the LOS at least 1 day in approximately 75% of cases.

All these factors need to be considered and the presence or absence of each factor determined to identify the correct DRG.

How DRGs are used

Once the DRG has been determined, the administrator can identify further statistical measures affecting reimbursement:
• geometric mean LOS — each DRG has an assigned geometric mean LOS. The terms "geometric mean LOS" or "mean LOS" in this book refer to specific DRG statistical data for *groups* of patients. (The unqualified term "LOS" is a general abbreviation referring to an *individual* patient's LOS.) The geometric mean LOS is a statistical measure used in cost accounting for the sole purpose of determining when a patient becomes a "day outlier" (discussed in the second bullet below).

The geometric mean LOS is an average derived from data that indicated the mean LOS for patients with specific diagnoses or undergoing specific procedures at the time the DRG system was updated. This has four important implications:
— The geometric mean LOS should be understood as an indicator of when most patients within each DRG *were* discharged during the period of data collection. It was never intended as a guide to determine when a specific patient *should* be discharged.
— Current hospital stays are significantly shorter than the geometric mean LOS. Since 1984, the actual LOS across the country for nearly every DRG has decreased dramatically as more patients receive treatment in outpatient facilities, in doctors' offices, and within a much shorter length of time in the hospital.
— The geometric mean LOS has nothing to do with the point after which a hospital loses money on a case. That point can be determined only after studying each case.
— In most cases, a hospital begins losing money before the geometric mean LOS is reached because actual costs of caring for the patient usually exceed the reimbursement rate before this point. This is partly because hospital costs have continued to increase as the actual LOS has continued to decrease.
• relative weight — a statistical term used in DRG reimbursement that determines the actual dollars a particular hospital is paid for a given DRG. Among other factors, it is based on categorizing the hospital as acute or chronic, teaching or nonteaching, and urban or rural. The weight assigned each DRG is reevaluated and revised regularly. Because relative weights vary greatly from hospital to hospital and area to area, and

because of periodic revisions, they are not specified in this book.
• outlier — a case that uses more than its assigned resources. Two types of outliers exist — day outliers and cost outliers. A day outlier is a case that exceeds the geometric mean LOS by at least 17 days, on average. Although hospitals receive an additional payment for day outliers, payment never covers the costs or charges incurred during an extended LOS.

Day outliers were predicted to account for 5% of all Medicare discharges when PPS was begun. The latest data suggest only 1.5% of discharges become day outliers. In nearly every instance, day outliers are severely ill patients with multisystem failure. Preventing a patient from becoming a day outlier is rarely under the nurse's control.

A cost outlier is a case that does not exceed the allowed number of days but does exceed the expected cost. Cost outliers are even rarer than day outliers. This book does not include information on cost outliers.

Keys to success under DRGs

Several major factors affect a hospital's financial success under DRGs:
• accurate coding of all medical record data upon the patient's discharge. A medical records professional must choose the diagnosis that was chiefly responsible for the admission and take into account all of the factors, such as complications and comorbidities, that will place the diagnosis in the highest-paying category. The coder depends on the documentation in the medical record when assigning the DRG.
• effective and efficient management of the "products" of hospitals, such as hours of nursing care, laboratory tests, medications, supplies, and other services. The more efficiently care is delivered, the greater the hospital's profit.
• an appropriate "case mix" (a hospital's mixture of patients, defined by the severity of illness and assigned DRGs). A hospital must maintain a mixture of patients with various DRGs to plan and manage resource allocation within defined reimbursement parameters.
• using the appropriate site of care and LOS. Care will be reimbursed only if it is provided in the appropriate setting. For example, hospitals will not be reimbursed for care that could have been appropriately provided in an outpatient setting. LOS also must be appropriate. Although patients can be discharged only when medically stable, the hospital must ensure that only necessary costs are incurred.
• preventing complications. Because complications increase the likelihood that care costs will exceed reimbursement, their prevention is a key factor in maintaining fiscal control.

The nurse's role in a PPS

The overall impact of government regulations and third-party payers on the health care delivery system presents the nurse with challenges and opportunities. The nurse is instrumental in ensuring both the quality of care and the hospital's financial success under any PPS. Some of the ways the nurse can maintain quality care and yet dramatically affect a hospital's reimbursement include:

• care planning. The nurse must be able to prioritize and deliver care within the projected LOS—which means establishing and following an explicit plan of care. Care planning is an essential means for determining goals and desired outcomes of care. Only through planning can care be managed effectively and efficiently. This book is designed to help the nurse provide quality care within the constraints of cost containment.

Caring for a patient without a plan of care can be likened to starting out on an unfamiliar trip without a road map. You may eventually reach the desired destination, but most certainly it will involve many unnecessary detours and increased time, effort, and money. This book identifies the "destination" of care — the target outcome criteria—as well as most direct routes for getting there.

• early discharge planning. The nurse must be involved in discharge planning from the moment of patient admission, whenever possible. By beginning early, the nurse can help ensure that the patient is ready for discharge. For example, the nurse can emphasize patient and family education, maximize the patient's self-care abilities, and arrange for continued care when indicated, such as through home care nursing or nursing home placement.

• patient education. Patient and family education is a key element in preventing readmissions. The patient's perception of quality care is also enhanced when the nurse promotes self-care and describes how to manage health problems after discharge.

• documentation. Accurate documentation promotes communication among caregivers, maximizing the benefits of hospitalization while minimizing the LOS. Also, documentation is crucial to receiving appropriate reimbursement for services. Documenting complications and comorbidities is particularly important because they have even greater significance than in the past.

• quality assurance. This mandatory element should include establishing specific nursing standards and monitoring adherence to those standards.

The nurse also needs to be aware of how the new economics of health care affects the professional status of nursing. This is an opportune time to advance the function and image of nurses as independent health care practitioners who can be judged not only on how they benefit patients but also on their contribution to a hospital's economic viability.

Retrospective review

Besides DRGs, other changes in health care delivery continue to increase the pressure to provide care in the most efficient manner possible. Health maintenance organizations (HMOs) and other competitive medical plans, now a major source for health care reimbursement, have been particularly important.

The nurse should be aware of the complexity of reimbursement methods. Most third-party payers (not just Medicare) use a prospective payment mechanism to reimburse hospitals. For example, many HMOs currently pay hospitals on a negotiated rate not unlike DRGs. Also, all third-party payers are negotiating discounted rates for services provided in acute-care facilities in return for guaranteeing that their subscribers will use specific facilities for their acute-care needs. Such arrangements are important for hospitals because they ensure a constant source of admissions. With LOSs much shorter than they were before PPS, hospitals must count on a stable census to ensure maximum efficiency and a constant cash flow.

For patients, incentives from PPSs to hospitals mean shorter stays and possibly fewer services. Because of perceptions of premature patient discharges and underuse of necessary services, state peer review organizations (PROs) were mandated to increase review of care provided in acute-care facilities.

This mandate has led PROs to establish explicit review criteria for medical care. Within the DRG system, however, the Health Care Financing Administration and state PROs are developing and using generic and disease-specific criteria retrospectively to determine the appropriateness of admission and discharge and of the quality of care. Such information could be useful to nurses in care planning. Although PROs are reviewing only Medicare cases now, in the near future all hospital admissions, outpatient procedures, home care services, and care in doctors' offices and long-term facilities will be reviewed in much the same manner.

References

Health Care Financing Administration. "Rules and Regulations," *Federal Register* 55(171):36111-141, September 4, 1990.

Health Systems International. *Diagnosis Related Groups,* 4th revision. New Haven, Conn.: Health Systems International, 1987.

St. Anthony's DRG Working Guidebook. Alexandria, VA: St. Anthony Publications, 1990.

Section II

Comprehensive plans of care, arranged by body system, incorporate DRGs, functional health patterns, nursing diagnoses, collaborative problems, target outcome criteria, patient-family teaching, documentation checklists, and discharge criteria.

Dying

Introduction

DEFINITION AND TIME FOCUS

Death, according to Dr. Elisabeth Kübler-Ross, is "the key to the door of life." An awareness of death's inevitability and the contemplation of our fears and feelings about it can lead to a heightened appreciation for life and a more courageous and thoughtful response to the its challenges. Nurses deal with death daily and thus have repeated opportunities to assist dying patients and their families.

More than any other professional, the nurse has close and continuing contact with patients, direct experience with those who die, and concern for meeting the emotional and physiologic needs of patients and their families. Death remains the "great unknown," but the patient and loved ones have the right to continue sharing life until the end; the nurse can help. This plan focuses on the needs of the dying patient and the bereaved family in the hospital setting.

ETIOLOGY AND PRECIPITATING FACTORS

Death may result from:
• disease (or, occasionally, complications of the treatment of disease)
• injury or accident
• age or debilitation
• suicide or homicide.

Focused assessment guidelines

NURSING HISTORY (Functional health pattern findings)

Note: Because etiologic factors vary so widely in dying persons, no typical findings exist. Thus, this section presents an assessment guide to assist the nurse in planning care for the patient who is admitted with a diagnosis suggesting impending death. However, no such guide is appropriate for all patients. The answers to the following questions may help the nurse intervene effectively on behalf of the dying and their families, but the nurse must use professional judgment in deciding what, when, and how much to ask a patient.

Health perception — health management pattern

• Is the patient aware of the prognosis? If so, for how long? If not, whose decision was it not to tell the patient?
• If not aware of the prognosis, what does the patient believe is the reason for hospitalization?
• What measures were taken to help support or improve the patient's physical or emotional condition before this hospitalization? Does the patient believe they have helped? If so, how?
• What are the patient's expectations about this hospital admission and the proposed treatment?

Nutritional-metabolic pattern

• Does the patient have any dietary preferences or intolerances?
• Has the patient been anorexic, vomiting, or dysphagic?

Elimination pattern

• What is the patient's present elimination status and pattern?
• Are any elimination aids currently used?

Activity-exercise pattern

• What is the patient's current activity level and tolerance?

Sleep-rest pattern

• What are the patient's present sleeping habits?
• Does the patient feel rested? If not, why?

Cognitive-perceptual pattern

• Does the patient have pain? If so, how severe is it?
• Is the patient's pain controlled? If so, by what?

Self-perception — self-concept pattern

• Which events or achievements have brought the patient the most satisfaction?
• What does the patient most want to accomplish before dying?

Role-relationship pattern

• Who are the patient's significant others?
• Among these, has the patient any long-standing, unresolved conflicts or other "unfinished business"?
• Has the patient been able to talk about dying and death with loved ones?
• How are loved ones handling the situation?

Coping — stress tolerance pattern

• If aware of the prognosis, how is the patient coping?
• What resources are available to help the patient cope?

Value-belief pattern

• What is the patient's religious or spiritual orientation?
• What does the patient believe about death?

PHYSICAL FINDINGS

Physical findings in dying patients vary widely, depending on the cause of impending death; see the plan related to the patient's specific disease or condition.

DIAGNOSTIC STUDIES

See the plan related to the patient's specific disease or condition.

Nursing diagnosis: *Fear related to potential pain, loss, emotional upheaval, and the unknowns of dying*

NURSING PRIORITY: Promote identification of and confrontation with specific realistic fears.

Interventions

1. Examine personal fears and feelings about death. Before involvement with the dying patient and the family, identify previous experiences with death, and be aware of personal emotions, religious or spiritual beliefs, and fears. If talking about death is too uncomfortable, refer the patient and family to another professional with the necessary skills.

2. Assess the patient's coping style and previous experience with death of relatives or friends. Observe patient behaviors, and confer with the family and other caregivers as needed.

3. Use role modeling to facilitate expression of feelings, as appropriate: "If I were facing what you face right now, I think I might feel scared (or 'angry' or 'depressed')."

4. Support coping mechanisms. Avoid forcing the patient to confront emotional issues.

5. As indicated by the patient's responsiveness to role modeling, help the patient identify specific fears and prioritize them. Acknowledge the unknowns.

6. Identify the patient's support system and resource base. Coordinate involvement of patient, family, and other members of the health care team in making plans to deal with anticipated problems and needs.

7. Provide appropriate referrals as needed, such as to a psychiatric liaison nurse, social worker, hospice, chaplain, or support group related to the specific disorder.

8. Provide companionship when possible.

9. If the patient is confronting imminent unexpected death (for example, as a result of trauma), provide brief, clear explanations and offer to call a member of the clergy. Provide a support person for the family, and—if at all possible—allow a family member to see the patient before death.

Rationales

1. A caregiver's personal feelings about and experiences with death affect the ability to promote healthy emotional responses. While most health care providers feel some anxiety over discussing dying and death with their patients, nurses who have difficulty with ssues of death are less able to empathize with the patient and family. Appropriate referral allows emotional needs to be addressed.

2. Each person responds differently to the threat of death. When threatened, most people initially revert to familiar coping mechanisms, and caregivers must be aware of these in establishing therapeutic communication. Previous experiences with death do much to shape behavioral responses and may contribute significantly to the patient's overall ability to cope.

3. The patient may need "permission" to discuss fears. Opening discussion by focusing on the caregiver's feelings allows the patient the option of responding with an expression of personal feelings (if ready) and reassures the patient that such feelings are normal and acceptable. For some patients, expression of fears reduces their impact.

4. Each patient moves through various stages, at various times, in coping with death's ultimate threat to individuality. Forcing issues is counterproductive and may damage the therapeutic relationship. Showing respect for the individual promotes trust.

5. Identification of specific fears helps reduce the sense of overwhelming threat. Pain, loss of control, and being a burden to others are common fears of dying patients; identifying fear-causing factors allows a patient to begin making specific plans to cope with them. Acknowledging unknowns reassures the patient that the caregiver recognizes the enormity of the questions faced.

6. Coordination of resources and support for the patient is essential in reducing the sense of isolation, which contributes to fear. The nurse's "in-between" position can help her facilitate teamwork.

7. The patient and family may not be aware of available resources. Even if referrals are not used, knowledge of their availability can be comforting.

8. Simply sitting quietly beside the patient communicates concern and may decrease the sense of isolation.

9. Even in the emergency care setting, patients have the right to caring communication, which may help reduce fear. Survivors of near-death experiences report hearing conversation and being aware of activity around them even when they appeared unresponsive. Surviving spouses of victims of sudden death list their need to see their spouse during resuscitation or before death as the concern that produced the most anguish for them.

10. Additional individualized interventions: _____

10. Rationales: _____

_____

_____

Target outcome criteria
According to individual readiness, the patient will:
• identify specific fears
• express feelings, as desired

• use appropriate resources.

Nursing diagnosis: *Powerlessness related to inevitability of death, lack of control over body functions, and dependence on others for care*

NURSING PRIORITY: Increase the patient's sense of personal power while promoting acceptance of the condition.

Interventions	Rationales
1. Encourage personal decision making whenever possible. Allow maximum flexibility for scheduling activities, treatments, or visitors. Include the dying patient in making care-related decisions, as appropriate.	1. Patients relinquish many freedoms, regardless of the reason for their hospitalization. Allowing as many choices as possible promotes a sense of control and increases the patient's coping ability. "Taking over" by caregivers diminishes the patient's self-esteem and should be avoided unless absolutely necessary.
2. Recognize and support courageous attitudes.	2. Regardless of external circumstances, individuals maintain the freedom to choose their attitude and approach to life and death. Acknowledgment of courageous attitudes reinforces feelings of self-worth.
3. Accept personal powerlessness to alter the fact that the patient is dying.	3. Health care professionals usually are anguished when they cannot save their patients. Realistic self-assessment is essential to prevent caregiver burnout and to maintain the potential for effective intervention in areas that can be altered.
4. Help the patient identify inner strengths. Ask the patient to recall past losses: How did the patient deal with them? What did the patient learn from them?	4. Recalling other losses may help the patient build on previously learned coping skills. Losses throughout life may have uniquely provided the individual with qualities that can be used in facing death.
5. Encourage the patient to establish realistic goals for the remainder of life.	5. Establishing goals provides a focus for energy and reduces helplessness. Realistic evaluation of capabilities helps acceptance.
6. Assist the patient, as needed, to put affairs in order—for example, funeral and memorial planning, writing a will, settling economic affairs, and making arrangements for survivors.	6. Putting affairs in order increases the patient's sense of control and may help soften the anticipated effects of the death on loved ones. "Unfinished business" may interfere with the patient's ability to move through coping stages.
7. Additional individualized interventions: _____	7. Rationales: _____

Target outcome criteria
According to individual readiness, the patient will:
• participate in decisions related to care
• verbalize inner strengths

• set realistic goals
• initiate activity to put affairs in order.

Nursing diagnosis: *Personal identity disturbance related to imminent threat of death*

NURSING PRIORITY: Help the patient maintain and enrich personal identity throughout the remainder of life.

Interventions

1. Use active listening skills, paying special attention to nonverbal or symbolic communication. Use reflective statements and open-ended observations to offer an opportunity for discussion of difficult issues.

2. Accept and respect the patient's right to use denial or avoidance behavior. Whatever the patient's response, try to communicate your understanding.

3. Be honest with the patient in answering questions, but do not force discussion of issues the patient has not introduced or has not responded to. Take care to maintain hope for meaningful experiences.

4. Encourage reminiscence and review of life experiences.

5. Promote creative expression. Encourage family and friends to provide materials the patient can use for drawing, painting, writing or other creative pursuits, or obtain materials from the occupational therapy department.

6. Explore the option of preparing audio- or videotaped messages or mementos for family and friends to share after the patient's death (or earlier, if the patient wishes).

7. Use touch generously when providing care, unless it makes the patient uncomfortable. Encourage family affection, including holding, rocking, and even lying next to the patient.

8. Additional individualized interventions: _____

Rationales

1. A patient facing mortality may use nonverbal or symbolic communication to describe experiences and to test another's willingness to talk about them. Rushed or distracted behavior from caregivers may distance the dying patient and contribute to feelings of alienation. Active listening and sharing show concern and respect for the patient as an individual.

2. The patient may choose to use denial or avoidance to the end; respect this choice. In addition, denial correlates with longer survival, according to research.

3. Honesty, even when truths are painful, reflects respect for the patient as an individual. But the patient has the right to choose which issues to discuss. Research suggests that hopelessness correlates with poorer prognosis.

4. Life experiences have helped to shape the patient's unique identity. Reminiscence helps the patient remain connected to important core experiences and provides the caregiver with additional information that may aid in understanding the patient's behavior and response to family needs.

5. Creative activity gives voice to individual expression, helping the patient maintain a sense of uniqueness. Also, drawings, paintings, or other original work may provide clues to the patient's state of acceptance.

6. The patient may feel more comfortable expressing feelings in this way. The process of recording helps achieve acceptance of impending death. Such mementos may offer the patient comfort in sensing that some aspect of individual identity will endure. These records may also be valued by families in preserving the memory of the loved one.

7. Illness and hospitalization may reduce the frequency of physical contact with others, which normally helps provide body image self-definition. Encouraging family affection helps maintain physical contact. Also, touch provides comfort and communicates genuine caring more effectively than almost any other measure.

8. Rationales: _____

Target outcome criteria
According to individual readiness, the patient will:
• maintain preferred coping behaviors
• recall and review life experiences

• participate in creative activity (as able)
• touch family members freely.

Nursing diagnosis: *High risk for spiritual distress related to confrontation with the unknown*

NURSING PRIORITY: Help the patient savor the remaining period of life and identify meaning in impending death.

Interventions

1. Support the patient's personal spiritual beliefs, even if they seem unusual or unfamiliar.

2. Recognize that facing death and dealing with separation are developmental tasks for all humans. Promote a focus on growth and learning, rather than on disease or injury.

3. Acknowledge what dying patients have to teach others, and express this to the patient and family, when appropriate.

4. Provide privacy according to the patient's wishes.

5. Offer to call the spiritual adviser of the patient's choice—for example, a member of the clergy, counselor, or friend. Obtain and provide religious texts and other inspirational readings if requested.

6. Explore the possibility of organ donation, if appropriate, with the patient and family. Be familiar with hospital and regional policy and procedure for arranging donation of organs. Consider the underlying disease before discussing donation of specific organs.

7. Address the patient while providing care, even if the patient appears unresponsive or comatose. Encourage family members to continue talking to the patient.

8. Worry less about saying the "wrong thing" than about being afraid to communicate caring. In this way, set an example that family members may follow.

Rationales

1. Spiritual beliefs provide comfort based on specific personal meaningfulness to the patient. Attempting to alter such beliefs or supplant them with others shows lack of respect for the patient's choices and may precipitate undue conflict and distress.

2. Because our culture places such emphasis on youth, we lack the societal integration of death as part of life that many primitive cultures take for granted. To help a patient accept impending death, caregivers must acknowledge it as a stage of development and validate its importance. Non-disease-related interventions (discussed throughout this plan) help redirect coping efforts toward positive life closure.

3. Nurses can learn much from dying patients that may help in caring for others. In this way, dying patients may touch the lives of others they will never meet. Recognition of the lessons a dying person may pass on to others can help the patient find meaning in death and a sense of connectedness with life.

4. The hospital environment may allow the patient minimal time to be alone. A patient struggling with spiritual issues may need uninterrupted time for prayer or meditation.

5. A spiritual adviser may provide guidance or perform rituals the patient views as essential. Religious readings may be satisfying to a patient with a traditional religious orientation, although others may find comfort in nonreligious literature that has special personal significance.

6. Patients and families can find meaning and consolation in knowing others may benefit from organ donation. Many programs now have broad interlinking systems for identification of donors and transplantation of donated organs. Underlying disease may make some organs unsatisfactory for donation, but others (such as skin) typically are usable and may not require immediate transplantation.

7. Survivors of near-death experiences and persons who recover from deep or prolonged coma have reported remembering conversation that took place around them while they were apparently unconscious.

8. Because of prolonged close contact with dying patients and interaction with their families, nurses are uniquely suited to help facilitate dialogue about dying between the patient and family. In many cases, patients and families are afraid to raise the subject directly, out of concern that they may cause emotional upset. No cultural prescriptions exist to guide families, but the nurse may be able to act as a liaison to help communication, thereby reducing guilt and anxiety and further preparing the patient and family for separation.

GENERAL PLANS OF CARE

9. Maintain a positive attitude. Promote activities that provide even a few moments of enjoyment. Avoid generalizations that attempt to explain the patient's suffering.

9. The caregiver's positive attitude may help the patient maintain hope and find pleasure in living even while approaching death. Small pleasures may be extremely meaningful when the patient's world view is narrowed by illness. Generalizations or attempts to provide simplistic explanations (for example, "It may be a blessing") indicate shallow appreciation for the patient's situation and may be interpreted as dismissal of real concerns.

10. Additional individualized interventions: _____

10. Rationales: _____

Target outcome criteria
Throughout the remainder of life, the patient will:
• maintain personally meaningful spiritual and religious practices
• find pleasure in some activities.

Nursing diagnosis: *High risk for pain related to underlying disease or injury*

NURSING PRIORITY: Relieve pain while allowing the patient to remain as alert as possible.

Interventions

1. See the "Pain" plan, page 69.

2. Assess the patient's level of discomfort frequently and urge calling for medication before the pain becomes severe.

3. To the extent possible, include the patient in decisions regarding pain medications.

4. When possible, control pain with oral medication rather than with intramuscular injections. If the patient is unable to tolerate oral medications, consider arranging for intravenous or subcutaneous pumps. Investigate analgesic combinations, such as long- and short-acting medications or narcotics and non-steroidal anti-inflammatory drugs (NSAIDS).

5. Recognize that the usual safe dose levels may not apply to the terminally ill patient. Consult the doctor if the ordered dosage no longer seems effective.

6. Assess for psychological factors that may exacerbate pain, and intervene to treat them.

7. If abdominal distention causes pain, consider using return-flow enemas. Ensure that routine laxatives have been prescribed, as indicated by the patient's condition.

8. Additional individualized interventions: _____

Rationales

1. This plan provides interventions useful for any patient in pain.

2. A patient's level of discomfort has a significant impact on the emotional adjustment to limited life expectancy: Patients with poorly controlled pain tend to have more difficulty coping with other issues. Medication given early in the pain cycle is most effective.

3. Ability to control pain allows the patient to use limited energy for other, more rewarding, purposes.

4. Repeated intramuscular injections, particularly in the debilitated patient, traumatize skin and gradually become less effective as areas of scarring develop and inhibit absorption. Analgesic combinations may achieve better control over chronic and acute pain episodes. NSAIDs may be effective for bone pain.

5. A patient maintained on narcotic analgesics for an extended period may develop significant tolerance and require amounts of medication considerably larger than the usual dosage to achieve comparable effects.

6. The pain threshold may be lowered by boredom, anxiety, and loneliness.

7. Lack of activity and resultant slowing of peristalsis may cause painful abdominal distention and constipation. Gentle return-flow enemas may reduce discomfort. Medications can contribute further to constipation, and laxatives may be required regularly.

8. Rationales: _____

Target outcome criteria
Throughout the hospital stay, the patient will:
• participate in decisions regarding pain control (to the extent possible)
• verbalize the effectiveness of pain-control measures.

Nursing diagnosis: High risk for fluid volume deficit related to anorexia and dehydration associated with imminent death

NURSING PRIORITY: Promote patient comfort during the dying process.

Interventions

1. Avoid vigorous fluid replacement for terminally ill patients.

2. Offer frequent mouth care, ice chips, or hard candy, as indicated by the patient's condition.

3. Provide meticulous skin care. Use soap sparingly and lotion generously if dry skin is present. Turn the patient carefully to prevent shearing.

4. Additional individualized interventions: _____

Rationales

1. Dehydration is normal in terminal illnesses. Intravenous fluid replacement may unnecessarily prolong discomfort.

2. These measures may help reduce discomfort related to mouth dryness and minimal oral intake.

3. Dehydration and debilitation contribute to poor skin turgor and increased risk of skin breakdown. Soap dries skin, increasing irritation. Gentle massage with lotion and careful turning demonstrate care and help prevent complications.

4. Rationales: _____

Target outcome criterion
During the final phase of the dying process, the patient will experience minimum discomfort related to dehydration.

Nursing diagnosis: Altered family processes related to imminent death of a family member

NURSING PRIORITY: Promote family integrity by facilitating healthy coping, mutual support, and communication with the dying person.

Interventions

1. See the "Ineffective Family Coping" plan, page 47.

2. Assess the family's level of acceptance and coping by observing behaviors and interactions of individuals with the patient and by providing time for private discussions with family members, as needed. Be alert to differences among individual family members and clues to the family's previous experiences with death, if any.

3. Liberalize visiting policies, as needed. Allow private time for the family to be with the patient. Encourage family members to participate in care, remaining alert for signs of possible anxiety or discomfort.

Rationales

1. This plan provides guidelines for helping families at risk for crisis.

2. Effective intervention must be appropriately correlated with the stage of acceptance. Each member of the family may respond differently to the threat of loss. Previous family deaths may affect members' ability to cope in mutually supportive ways.

3. Family integrity is more likely to be maintained when members are able to continue their usual level of contact with one another. Helping with patient care reduces the family's sense of helplessness and provides special comfort to the patient. However, this should not substitute for the nurse's cultivation of close involvement with the patient and family: The nurse must avoid giving the impression of dismissing or neglecting the patient.

4. When possible, facilitate family dialogue, remaining aware of established family roles and expectations. Offer to introduce topics, as needed; strive to promote face-to-face communication when possible.

4. Discussing issues surrounding death is difficult for most families and may be compounded by unresolved conflicts, guilt, or role demands. The nurse may be able to open up communication about sensitive issues. Family stability is related to long-standing patterns of behavior, so interventions that are at odds with these will be unsuccessful. Direct communication promotes maximum understanding and helps minimize later guilt over things left unsaid.

5. Be aware of cultural attitudes that may affect family response.

5. Different cultures view death in different ways. Some observe specific rituals for the occasion; some emphasize withdrawal from others. Being aware of such differences helps the nurse plan interventions to support the family's cultural heritage.

6. Help the family identify and mobilize external resources, such as friends, clergy, counselors, and financial resources. Provide referrals to a psychiatric clinician or social worker or for pastoral care, as needed.

6. A family coping with death, especially if the dying is prolonged, may require added support to deal with stresses. Other professionals may offer such assistance as spiritual or psychological counseling, temporary housing placement, and guidance in identifying programs to help with the financial burden of care.

7. Encourage family members to maintain their physical and emotional strength. Emphasize the importance of adequate rest, food, and exercise. Suggest that family members take turns at the bedside if they are reluctant to leave the patient unattended.

7. Maintenance of physical and emotional well-being is essential if family members are to continue providing support for the patient and each other. "Break times" help the family maintain contact with external resources and reduce the emotional strain of constant attendance to the dying person's needs.

8. Additional individualized interventions: _____

_____

8. Rationales: _____

_____

Target outcome criteria
Throughout the patient's hospital stay, the family will:
• participate in care
• share concerns with the patient and each other
• appear well rested most of the time.

Throughout the hospital stay, the patient will exhibit minimal anxiety over the family's well-being.

Nursing diagnosis: *Family coping: potential for growth related to bereavement and mourning*

NURSING PRIORITY: Facilitate the initiation of healthy grieving after death.

Interventions

1. See the "Grieving" plan, page 31.

2. If not already acquainted with the family, introduce yourself, identify your relationship as the patient's caregiver, and express sympathy.

3. Allow family members to see and touch the body. If death was sudden and unexpected, prepare them for the appearance of the body in advance, explaining that all measures were tried in an attempt to restore life. Ensure that the body is respectfully covered. Do not remove all indications of emergency intervention before allowing the family into the room, but leave side rails down and face and hands visible.

Rationales

1. This plan contains general interventions helpful in caring for bereaved families.

2. If the family arrives after the patient has died, or if the family does not know caregivers from previous contact, such an introduction serves to reassure them that the patient died with concerned caregivers at hand.

3. Seeing and touching the body of the loved one helps the family accept the reality of death. Advance preparation may help reduce distress. The face and hands invite touch if accessible; if not, the family may be reluctant to disturb coverings. Gross blood or other secretions should be removed before the family enters, but putting away all supplies and cleaning the room before the family sees the body may create doubts that "everything possible was done" for the patient.

4. Use direct, simple sentences, avoiding use of euphemisms, to describe the death. Provide comforting observations when possible—such as, "He died quietly and appeared to have no pain" or "She told me last night about the good times you used to have, and she seemed very happy."

4. Most family members are too anxious at this time to comprehend complex explanations. Euphemisms such as "passed on" may offend some family members and can interfere with reality orientation. Sharing selected, specific observations with family members may help minimize guilt and promote healthy grieving.

5. Acknowledge the family's loss by gently reorienting them to the reality of death with such statements as "It must be hard to accept that he's really dead." Avoid overly sentimental statements.

5. Shock and disbelief are normal initial responses to sudden death and, to a certain degree, even to expected death. Gentle reorientation aids in integrating death into reality. Overly sentimental utterances may be inappropriate to the family's actual relationship with the deceased.

6. Avoid recommending or encouraging sedation of a family member unless severely dysfunctional behavior is present.

6. Sedation may delay initiation of the normal grieving process.

7. Offer to call a friend, member of the clergy, or counselor to help with immediate arrangements. If the family does not designate such a person, offer the services of the hospital chaplain, a liaison nurse, or another in-house professional skilled in dealing with grief.

7. During the initial stages of grieving, family members may exhibit indecision, disorganization, and disorientation. Providing an advocate helps reduce the family's distress while they are making necessary arrangements, such as for disposition of the body.

8. Prepare the family for the work of grieving. Emphasize the normality of a wide range of emotional responses (such as anger, guilt, sadness, frustration, resentment, fear, and depression) and behaviors (such as crying, laughing, withdrawal, and confusion) in response to loss of a loved one.

8. Family members are sometimes unprepared for the various feelings experienced in the grieving process; some may feel they are "going crazy" when unexpected feelings occur. Understanding that such emotional disorganization is a normal and healthy response to loss can help the family deal with these feelings.

9. Listen patiently to retellings of the story of the death, especially if it was unexpected. Avoid statements that might be interpreted as judgmental.

9. Retelling of events by survivors is an essential part of reality acceptance and coping. Judgmental utterances may provoke severe guilt reactions in family members.

10. Reemphasize the need for health-promoting self-care behaviors during the grieving period.

10. Grieving places additional stress on survivors, who are at increased risk for developing physical illness during mourning. Health-promoting behavior, such as exercise, can help release emotional energy and reduce the effects of stress.

11. Ensure that significant others will be available to be with survivors after they leave the hospital.

11. Grieving is facilitated by sharing feelings with others. Few cases of loneliness are as profound as that of a bereaved person, newly alone.

12. If possible, provide a follow-up call to surviving family members 1 to 3 months after the death. Keeping a callback calendar on the unit can help in organizing this task.

12. Follow-up from caregivers to survivors is the final step in care of the dying patient and provides the family with added assurance that their loved one was special and received care accordingly. This call also provides an opportunity to identify dysfunctional grieving and make appropriate referrals, if needed.

13. Additional individualized interventions: _____

13. Rationales: _____

Target outcome criteria
Before survivors leave the hospital, they will:
• view and touch the body, if desired
• express initial grief or disbelief
• make contact with advocacy groups or support persons.

One to three months after death, family members will cope effectively, with adequate support.

GENERAL PLANS OF CARE

Discharge planning

NURSING DISCHARGE CRITERIA

If the patient is discharged home before death, documentation shows evidence of:
• referral to a hospice or to a home health care agency
• adequate support system for family members.

PATIENT-FAMILY TEACHING CHECKLIST

If the patient is discharged home before death, document that the patient and family demonstrate an understanding of:
___ support and resources available
___ what to do when death is imminent
___ what to do after death occurs
___ what to expect in normal mourning and grieving.

DOCUMENTATION CHECKLIST

If the patient is discharged home before death, using outcome criteria as a guide, document:
___ fears
___ feelings expressed
___ goals
___ preferred coping behaviors
___ spiritual or religious practices
___ pain-control measures
___ family members' behaviors
___ patient-family teaching
___ discharge planning.
If death occurs in the hospital, document:
___ time and circumstances of death
___ disposition of body and effects
___ family support measures implemented.

ASSOCIATED PLANS OF CARE

Geriatric Considerations
Grieving
Ineffective Family Coping
Ineffective Individual Coping
Pain
(See also the plan for the specific disease or disorder.)

References

Bishop, A.H., and Scudder, J.R. *The Practical, Moral and Personal Sense of Nursing.* Albany, N.Y.: State University of New York Press, 1990.

Charmaz, K. *The Social Reality of Death.* Menlo Park, Calif.: Addison-Wesley Publishing Co., 1980.

Fanslow, J. "Needs of Grieving Spouses in Sudden Death Situations: A Pilot Study," *Journal of Emergency Nursing* 9(4):213-16, July-August 1983.

Frankl, V.E. *Man's Search for Meaning.* Old Tappan, N.J. Pocket Books, 1984.

Hoff, L.A. *People in Crisis: Understanding and Helping,* 3rd ed. Menlo Park, Calif.: Addison-Wesley Publishing Co., 1989.

Jung, C.G. *Modern Man in Search of a Soul.* New York: Harcourt, Brace, Jovanovich, 1955.

Kalish, R.A., ed. *The Final Transition.* Farmingdale, N.Y.: Baywood Publishing Co., 1987.

Kamerman, J.B. *Death In the Midst of Life.* Englewood Cliffs, N.J.: Prentice Hall, 1988.

Kneisl, C.R., and Ames, S.A. *Adult Health Nursing: A Biopsychosocial Approach.* Menlo Park, Calif.: Addison-Wesley Publishing Co., 1986.

Kübler-Ross, E., ed. *Death: The Final Stage of Growth.* Englewood Cliffs, N.J.: Prentice-Hall, 1975.

Kübler-Ross, E. *Living with Death and Dying.* New York: Macmillan Publishing Co., 1982.

Saunders, C., and Baines, M. *Living with Dying: The Management of Terminal Disease,* 2nd ed. New York: Oxford University Press, 1989.

Tatelbaum, J. *The Courage to Grieve: Creative Living, Recovery, and Growth Through Grief.* New York: Harper & Row Publishers, 1984.

Geriatric Considerations
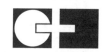

Introduction
DEFINITION AND TIME FOCUS
The geriatric patient is defined as a person age 75 or older who is admitted into an acute care hospital setting. This plan focuses on care needs specific to aging and to the sudden impact of hospitalization.

ETIOLOGY AND PRECIPITATING FACTORS
The geriatric patient is prone to health problems because of the following changes associated with aging:
• increased susceptibility to infection
• decreased muscle strength and generalized debility
• increased potential for chronic disease because of genetic flaws that appear with advancing age
• psychosocial isolation
• limited income and earning ability.

Focused assessment guidelines
NURSING HISTORY (Functional health pattern findings)

Health perception—health management pattern
• may report various presenting problems, depending on the underlying disease

Nutritional-metabolic pattern
• may report decreased appetite resulting from trauma or disease and impact of hospitalization
• when stable, likely to prefer usual dietary pattern of frequent small meals
• appetite may be greatest during morning hours
• may report use of dentures or chewing problems

Elimination pattern
• may report constipation
• may report regular use of laxatives or enemas
• may report urinary incontinence or urine retention related to prostatic hyperplasia (males), relaxation of perineal support (females), immobility, or environmental changes

Activity-exercise pattern
• may identify stiffness resulting from bed rest and decreased activity
• may fear falls because of general weakness

Sleep-rest pattern
• may report shorter sleep cycles and early morning awakening

Cognitive-perceptual pattern
• may report difficulty remembering or comprehending events that led to hospitalization
• may report discomfort from forced confinement and limited physical activity
• may report visual or sensory deficits

Self-perception—self-concept pattern
• may report lack of self-confidence in maintaining independent activities
• may communicate sense of despair because of inability to provide personal self-care (if ability is curtailed by disease or health problem)

Role-relationship pattern
• may report social isolation with hospitalization or may be isolated in usual home setting
• may express fear of uselessness and of becoming a family burden with increased care needs arising from health problem

Coping—stress tolerance pattern
• may evidence anticipatory grief over loss of personal independence caused by chronic disease
• may become dependent and give up interest in living because of helplessness caused by illness

Value-belief pattern
• may mourn loss of meaningful religious practices such as church attendance
• may become angry at God and direct anger toward others or self, reflecting depression
• may see no meaning or purpose in existence
• may possess strong ethnic identity that may conflict with values of hospital and staff

PHYSICAL FINDINGS
Note: General physiologic differences associated with aging are noted here. Specific physical findings related to particular disease or illness are not discussed.

Gastrointestinal
• decreased saliva and ptyalin secretion
• decreased esophageal nerve function
• decreased gastric and intestinal motility
• decreased hydrochloric acid production
• delayed gastric emptying
• decreased fat and calcium absorption

Cardiovascular
• increased systolic pressure
• increased pulse rate
• orthostatic hypotension
• arterial insufficiency
• narrowing of vessels
• decreased blood flow to organs
• thickening of capillary walls

Neurologic
• decreased sense of smell, taste, vision, touch, and hearing
• decreased deep-tendon reflexes
• reduced nerve conduction time

- generally slower responses
- reduced speed of fine motor movements
- alteration in sleep patterns (3- to 4-hour sleep periods)

Integumentary
- increased wrinkles
- loss of skin turgor and elasticity
- thinning skin (from reduced subcutaneous fat)
- reduced sebaceous and sweat gland function
- skin dryness
- changes in nail thickness
- brown or black wartlike areas of skin (seborrheic keratosis)
- red-purple overgrowth of dilated blood vessels (cherry angioma)

Musculoskeletal
- decreased bone mass, possible osteoporosis
- decrease in height
- flexed posture
- calcified cartilage and ligaments
- decreased muscle tone and strength
- gait changes
- decreased range of motion (may be from calcium salt deposits around joints)

Respiratory
- decreased lung tissue compliance (elasticity)
- calcification of vertebral cartilage, with reduced rib mobility and chest expansion
- decreased vital capacity
- decreased coughing efficiency

Genitourinary
- in male, enlarged prostate
- decrease in number of renal nephrons
- decrease in urine concentration ability
- increased nocturia
- in female, reduced vaginal lubrication

Endocrine
- thyroid—increased nodularity
- parathyroid—decreased hormone release
- pancreas—delayed insulin release from beta cells
- adrenals—decreased aldosterone and ketosteroid levels

Eye
- decreased light permeability of lens and cornea (cataracts)
- decreased speed of adaptation to darkness
- decreased accommodation
- increased astigmatism
- less efficient intraocular fluid absorption (can lead to glaucoma)
- white lipid deposit at edge of iris (arcus senilis)
- drying of conjunctivae
- increased nystagmus on lateral gaze

Ear
- pure tone loss
- high-frequency loss
- impacted cerumen

Nose
- increase in coarse hairs

Mouth and throat
- decreased saliva
- increased dryness
- loss of teeth
- receding gums
- atrophy of taste buds
- slowed gag reflex

DIAGNOSTIC STUDIES
Tests ordered depend on the particular disease or on presenting pathophysiology or symptomatology.

POTENTIAL COMPLICATIONS
- mental confusion
- contractures
- fecal impaction
- falls and fractures
- urine retention and cystitis
- pulmonary emboli
- depression
- hopelessness
- loneliness
- grief

Nursing diagnosis: *High risk for altered thought processes: slowed or diminished responsiveness related to cerebral degeneration*

NURSING PRIORITY: Allow ample time for all behaviors and responses.

Interventions

1. Assess mental status: note orientation, remote and recent memory, ability to interpret and abstract, and general rapidity of response.

Rationales

1. Mental status may be altered because of cerebral degeneration or other factors, such as medications, but must be assessed individually. Many elderly patients retain full alertness.

2. Depending on deficits identified, institute appropriate measures:

• Allow increased response time when speaking with an older person.

• Give information concisely and slowly.

• Allow ample time for activities of daily living and care-related procedures.

• Avoid shouting at the patient or using baby talk when communicating.

2. Compensation for any deficits can allow an older person to maintain dignity and active participation in daily activities.

• Thought processing may be slower in an older adult.

• Concise, slowed speech helps prevent information overload and decreases the risk of misunderstanding.

• Slower thinking may be accompanied by slower performance of tasks.

• Slowed responses do not necessarily imply a hearing deficit. Shouting may increase the patient's anxiety, further impairing performance of tasks. Use of baby talk is demeaning and may erode self-esteem already compromised by disability and dependence on others for care.

3. Once hospital activities are established, maintain a routine as much as possible.

3. Adaptation to change may be slower in an older patient. Routines provide security and reassurance. Major environmental alterations, particularly when accompanied by physiologic changes, may precipitate depression, confusion, or psychosis.

4. Additional individualized interventions: _____

_____

4. Rationales: _____

_____

Target outcome criteria
Throughout the hospital stay, the patient will:
• perform self-care activities (to the degree possible) without evidence of feeling rushed
• appear relaxed

• adapt to hospital routine without agitation.

Nursing diagnosis: *High risk for altered thought processes: confusion related to diminished perception of sensory data*

NURSING PRIORITIES: (a) Promote increased clarity of sensory-perceptual stimuli, and (b) decrease agitation related to confusion.

Interventions

1. When confusion is evident, attempt to identify the cause, such as a change in hearing, visual ability, or mental status (see previous diagnosis). Be aware of other factors that can cause confusion, such as metabolic alterations, hypoxemia, electrolyte imbalances, or medications. Plan time to sit with the patient, engage in conversation, and provide reorientation to surroundings. If the patient is amenable, use touch often during communications.

2. Before speaking, alert the patient by touch; speak only when clearly in the patient's line of vision.

3. Speak in a low tone. (If the patient's hearing is greatly impaired and no hearing aid is available, place a stethoscope into the patient's ears, then speak into the bell.)

4. Provide the patient's own glasses for reading, as needed.

5. Allow extra time for adjustment to changes in light levels. Turn on lights slowly if there are several in the room.

Rationales

1. Confusion may be related to misunderstanding because of deafness or to disorientation from visual impairment. Confusion may also be a symptom of more serious problems. Assuming that confusion is the normal mental state of a patient may leave unresolved problems that have physical or physiologic causes. Touching and engaging in conversation can reduce the depersonalizing effects of hospitalization that may increase confusion.

2. If information is not heard clearly, it may be misperceived and increase confusion. Older persons may compensate for hearing deficits by lipreading.

3. Loss of high-frequency hearing ability usually occurs first.

4. Distance accommodation decreases with aging.

5. Light accommodation also decreases with aging.

6. Provide adequate illumination during the day and at night.

6. Sundowning is a condition in which the older patient tends to become confused at the end of the day, when fading light causes loss of visual cues. Often marked by wandering, it is reduced when the available lighting allows clear visualization of persons, objects, and surroundings.

7. Use restraints only as necessary to prevent injury when the patient is unattended. Explain the reasons for using restraints to both patient and family.

7. Confusion may contribute to falls and accidents, but restraints should not be used as a substitute for adequate care and supervision. Use of restraints may damage the patient's self-esteem and promote dependence on others for meeting basic needs. Restraints may actually cause injury, such as falls or decreased circulation if restraints become too tight.

8. Provide environmental cues to orient the patient: for example, a clock, a calendar, or pictures of loved ones.

8. Confusion and disorientation are reduced by familiar objects in the immediate environment.

9. Encourage the use of audio- or videotaped messages from family members if disorientation persists.

9. Taped messages provide the comfort of familiar voices (or voices and faces) when the family is not able to visit and may decrease agitation and restlessness associated with disorientation.

10. Additional individualized interventions: _____

10. Rationales: _____

Target outcome criteria
Within 2 days of admission, the patient will:
• maintain orientation at or above the usual level
• participate appropriately in care activities without agitation.

Collaborative problem: *High risk for renal impairment related to physiologic degeneration of nephrons and glomeruli*

NURSING PRIORITY: Compensate for decreased renal function.

Interventions

1. Monitor all medications for toxic side effects.

2. Administer narcotics and sedatives judiciously.

3. Collaborate with the doctor to adjust fluid intake.

4. Monitor for signs of fluid overload, such as neck vein distention, increased central venous pressure readings, crackles, dependent edema, increased pulse rate, and rapid weight gain.

5. Additional individualized interventions: _____

Rationales

1. Altered and erratic renal function caused by aging may affect the drug excretion rate, causing toxicity at lower doses.

2. Normal doses of these drugs may create an overdose for the older person because of the cumulative effect of reduced renal excretion.

3. Impaired renal function may cause congestive heart failure (CHF). In addition, the aging heart is less efficient, further contributing to the risk of CHF.

4. Impaired renal function may cause fluid retention.

5. Rationales: _____

Target outcome criteria
Throughout the hospital stay, the patient will show:
• no medication-induced confusion or stupor
• no toxic side effects from medications

• no medication overdose from cumulative effect of reduced renal function
• no signs or symptoms of fluid overload.

Nursing diagnosis: *High risk for nutritional deficit related to taste bud atrophy, poor dentition, decreased saliva and ptyalin secretion, economic limitations, or poor dietary habits*

NURSING PRIORITY: Promote optimal nutritional intake.

Interventions

1. With the dietitian, assess the patient's dietary habits and history. Note the adequacy of protein, calorie, vitamin, and mineral intake. Assess the levels of saturated fat and sodium in the usual diet. Note special dietary preferences.

2. Plan, with the patient and dietitian, for meeting therapeutic dietary needs during hospitalization, providing foods according to the patient's usual pattern if the diet is nutritionally adequate. If the diet isn't adequate, teach the patient about dietary recommendations.

3. Ensure that the diet plan is compatible with the patient's chewing capability. Arrange for a dental consultation if poor dentition is a factor.

4. Encourage liberal seasoning of food with herbs and spices, observing dietary limitations required for underlying conditions.

5. Assess for environmental, physical, and emotional factors that may contribute to poor nutritional intake at home. Examples include:
• inadequate income
• lack of transportation for shopping
• lack of space or equipment for food preparation or storage
• lack of energy for preparing food
• loneliness and depression.

6. Before discharge, make appropriate referrals to alleviate or eliminate any identified problems.

7. Additional individualized interventions: _____

Rationales

1. Nutritional deficits place the patient at increased risk for infection, skin breakdown, and other complications. A high intake of saturated fats and salt may contribute to coronary artery disease and hypertension—two factors associated with mortality in elderly patients. Preferences must be considered, however, because an older patient may be reluctant to alter established dietary patterns.

2. Including the patient in diet planning promotes a sense of control and may improve compliance. Familiar foods are more likely to be eaten. Maintaining usual patterns whenever possible helps provide a sense of security—particularly important to the elderly person in an unfamiliar environment.

3. Chewing difficulty may compromise adequate nutritional intake.

4. Since taste bud sensitivity diminishes with age, bland foods may not be eaten.

5. An elderly patient may be reluctant to verbalize reasons for poor nutrition unless questioned specifically.

6. Careful predischarge assessment, problem solving, and referral are essential to prevent exacerbation of nutritional problems after discharge.

7. Rationales: _____

Target outcome criteria
Within 1 day of admission, the patient will:
• verbalize dietary habits and preferences
• identify factors interfering with adequate nutritional intake
• express satisfaction with meals.

By the time of discharge, the patient will:
• list dietary recommendations and specific foods to avoid or increase in diet
• identify resources and referrals for assistance with meals, shopping, or financial needs (if appropriate).

Nursing diagnosis: *High risk for impaired physical mobility related to general weakness, calcification around joints, arthritis, or debilitation from underlying disease*

NURSING PRIORITY: Maintain healthy skin, optimal activity pattern, and bowel functions.

Interventions

1. Skin care
- Omit soap during bathing.

- Apply oil to dry skin areas.

- Maintain the patient's usual bathing pattern — for example, every other day.
- Inspect the patient's skin twice daily for tissue breakdown.

2. Activity
- Take the patient's history to identify activities of daily living and the need for special exercises.

- Institute active or passive exercise, or both, as soon as medical protocol permits.

- Maintain all parts of the patient's body in functional anatomic alignment.
- If the patient is on bed rest, turn from back to side according to nursing protocol or at least every 2 hours during the day and every 4 hours at night.
- Encourage deep-breathing exercises hourly while the patient is awake. Each shift, assess lung sounds. Report decreased breath sounds, crackles, or other abnormal findings promptly.

3. Bowel function
- Identify the patient's typical bowel care regimen. If the patient is dependent on enemas or laxatives, discuss more appropriate alternatives.
- Add bran, prune juice, or other acceptable roughage to meals, as the patient's medical condition allows.
- Maintain adequate fluid intake.

- Administer and document the use of stool softeners or laxatives, as ordered.
- Provide bedpan or commode assistance, following the patient's schedule as closely as possible.

4. Additional individualized interventions: _____

_____

Rationales

1. Skin care
- Soap is drying, and older persons have fewer sebaceous glands.
- Oil may prevent increasing dryness, which can lead to tissue breakdown.
- Increasing the frequency of baths may reduce normal skin flora and increase irritation and dryness.
- Pressure on bony prominences may produce pressure ulcers because older adults have less elastic body tissue and less fatty tissue.

2. Activity
- Maintaining normal activity and exercise patterns is essential for optimal physiologic function. Special exercises may be required to maintain the tone of particular muscle groups.
- Exercise helps prevent thrombophlebitis, contractures, foot drop, and external rotation of the legs — complications associated with impaired mobility.
- Functional alignment prevents contractures and external rotation.
- Regular movement reduces the risk of hypostatic pneumonia and pressure ulcers.

- Decreased elasticity in lung tissue, commonly associated with aging, places these patients at increased risk for stasis of pulmonary secretions and resultant pulmonary infection. In this population, pneumonia is associated with higher mortality.

3. Bowel function
- Individualized care is essential for normal bowel function and a sense of emotional well-being.

- Decreased physical mobility contributes to constipation. Adding roughage to the diet stimulates peristalsis.
- Adequate fluid intake is essential to prevent drying of stool in the rectal vault, which can lead to fecal impaction.
- If unable to assume a normal position on the toilet, the older person may need some medicinal assistance.
- Maintaining routine timing facilitates bowel evacuation.

4. Rationales: _____

_____

Target outcome criteria
Throughout the hospital stay, the patient will:
- show no evidence of reddened skin areas
- show no new dry skin areas
- show no pruritus
- show no skin lesions or infections
- have no crackles, fever, or other evidence of hypostatic pneumonia
- establish regular bowel elimination
- have stool normal in amount, color, and consistency.

Nursing diagnosis: *Sleep pattern disturbance related to reduction in exercise, stress arising from concern with illness, anticipation of personal losses, unfamiliarity of surroundings, or discomfort associated with illness*

NURSING PRIORITY: Minimize sleep disturbance during hospital stay.

Interventions	Rationales
1. Provide frequent rest and sleep periods.	1. Older persons have less stage IV sleep and frequently awaken spontaneously. Shorter, more frequent sleep and rest periods are, in many cases, more appropriate than one long sleep period.
2. Assess for and document factors that may cause sleep disruption. Treat causes appropriately—for example, if pain causes wakefulness, administer analgesics before bedtime or provide other comfort measures. Group procedures to avoid interrupting sleep cycles.	2. Sleep deprivation may result in confusion, irritability, short-term memory loss, or other neuropsychiatric manifestations.
3. Adapt the hospital environment to simulate the patient's home setting whenever possible.	3. Moving the bed into a position similar to that at home or modifying other room details (such as the position of the radio or television) can produce a sense of security and familiarity and promote environmental comfort, inducing rest and sleep.
4. Provide as quiet an environment as possible (for example, turn off the radio or television if this reflects the usual home situation).	4. Similarity of environmental sounds enhances relaxation.
5. "Shorten" the night by arranging activities around late bedtime and checking in early in the morning with food and conversation.	5. Because older people sleep for shorter periods, their night's sleep may be only 4 to 5 hours.
6. Additional individualized interventions: _____	6. Rationales: _____

Target outcome criteria
Within 2 days of admission, the patient will:
• appear rested
• verbalize "I slept well."

Nursing diagnosis: *Self-esteem disturbance related to dependent patient role, anxiety over loss of physical or mental competence, powerlessness to alter the aging process, societal emphasis on youth, or sense of purposelessness* ✓

NURSING PRIORITY: Promote a positive self-image while providing opportunities to demonstrate competence.

Interventions	Rationales
1. Whenever possible, offer choices and include the patient in decision making related to care.	1. Participating in decision making increases the patient's sense of personal competence and promotes independence.
2. Involve the patient in self-care activities as much as possible, paying special attention to grooming and hygiene needs.	2. "Taking over" by caregivers devalues the patient's abilities and may lead to dependence and depression. A neat personal appearance contributes to feelings of self-worth.
3. Affirm positive qualities (for example, "You have a good sense of humor"). Help the patient identify and use coping behaviors learned in dealing successfully with earlier situations.	3. Expressing appreciation of positive attributes helps reinforce associated behaviors. Examining coping skills learned from previous experiences may help the patient build strengths in dealing with the current situation.

GENERAL PLANS OF CARE

4. Move the conversation away from constant repetition of bodily problems.

4. Repetition of negative thoughts only reinforces their impact.

5. Review life activities that reflect accomplishments.

5. Achievements and their recognition bolster a sense of societal usefulness.

6. Allow time for verbalization of feelings, such as sadness and powerlessness. Avoid overoptimistic responses.

6. Aging entails dealing with multiple losses, and feelings of sadness are a part of normal coping. Active listening and acceptance show respect for the patient as an individual and promote a sense of self-worth.

7. Encourage realistic goal setting.

7. Goal achievement fosters feelings of self-mastery.

8. Facilitate behavior that is considerate of others.

8. Focusing on others' needs reduces dependence and increases feelings of usefulness.

9. Provide diversionary activity appropriate to the patient's abilities, allowing opportunities for creative expression whenever possible. Refer the patient to the occupational therapist, as indicated.

9. Emotional well-being is enhanced by diversionary activities. Creative activities allow another avenue for expression of feelings and demonstration of unique abilities. The occupational therapist can help the patient select diversionary activities appropriate to functional capabilities.

10. Additional individualized interventions: ＿＿＿＿＿

10. Rationales: ＿＿＿＿＿＿＿＿＿＿＿＿＿＿＿

Target outcome criteria
Throughout the hospital stay, the patient will:
- participate in decision making
- participate in self-care to the extent possible
- set realistic goals and pursue them
- initiate involvement with others.

Nursing diagnosis: *Social isolation related to decreased physical capacity, effects of illness, fear of burdening others, death or disability of peers, or sense of personal uselessness*

NURSING PRIORITY: Promote social interaction and provide opportunities for positive feedback from others.

Interventions

1. Include ethnicity in initial and ongoing assessment of adaptation to hospitalization.

2. Assess the patient's social resources and the willingness and ability of family, friends, and other caregivers to participate in care.

3. Involve loved ones in care planning and, when possible, in provision of care. Ask family members to identify specific needs or preferences the patient may have.

4. Encourage generous use of touch in care provision and as affectionate gestures, unless the patient appears uncomfortable with physical contact.

5. Encourage family members to help the patient maintain previously established roles and functions in the family as much as possible.

Rationales

1. Culturally sensitive care is essential to prevent social isolation.

2. Social isolation results from numerous factors. For example, the patient may hesitate to verbalize needs because of pride and independence; tactful intervention by the nurse may help link the patient with untapped social contacts.

3. Involvement of loved ones in care helps reduce isolation related to unfamiliar surroundings and prevents a sense of abandonment, which can occur in a hospitalized elderly patient. Participation in care while the patient is hospitalized also allows family members to practice care techniques and ask questions in a "safe" setting. Family members are most attuned to the patient's special needs.

4. Older adults have diminished sensory capacities. Touch reduces "skin hunger" (the desire for human tactile contact) and communicates caring.

5. Maintaining roles—for example, as wise counselor or confidante—helps the older person maintain a sense of belonging and decreases feelings of uselessness.

6. Ensure telephone access. Discuss bedside telephone costs with the family or social worker, explaining the critical need for the patient to maintain communication with family and friends.

6. For many elderly patients with impaired mobility, the telephone provides an essential link to the outside world. Also, elderly friends may be unable to visit, so the telephone may be their only means of offering support to the patient.

7. Initiate a social services referral, as needed, to arrange transportation for visitors — such as a senior citizens' or church group's van.

7. The patient and family may be unaware of available transportation resources.

8. Present socialization concerns and problems to other members of the hospital staff, including the chaplain, dietitian, and housekeepers.

8. Interaction with all members of the hospital staff may serve as a temporary replacement for the patient's normal social contacts.

9. Additional individualized interventions: _____

9. Rationales: _____

Target outcome criteria
Within 3 days of admission, the patient will:
• maintain social contacts
• make no comments reflecting loneliness.

Within 3 days of the patient's admission, family members will approach nurses freely with care suggestions and questions.

Nursing diagnosis: *Spiritual distress related to inability to maintain usual religious and spiritual practices (if any) or loss of sense of life's meaning and purpose*

NURSING PRIORITY: Provide for participation in meaningful religious and spiritual practices, if desired.

Interventions

1. Identify the patient's normal preference and pattern for religious activities, if appropriate. Encourage participation in formal services if available. Arrange for visits by clergy as permitted, or suggest that the family provide a tape of the religious service. See the "Dying" plan, page 11.

2. If the patient wishes to read religious literature but cannot do so, read it, get a volunteer to read it, or obtain it on a cassette tape.

3. Provide privacy for personal prayer time, when desired.

4. Keep religious articles such as rosary beads conveniently available.

5. Additional individualized interventions: _____

Rationales

1. Maintenance of usual spiritual support increases coping ability. The "Dying" plan contains other specific interventions for patients experiencing spiritual distress.

2. Maintaining continuity in religious experience provides special comfort.

3. Encouraging expressions of trust and faith in God or a supreme being provides solace and a sense of providential care during crises.

4. Religious articles may provide reassurance and serve as a reminder of spiritual resources.

5. Rationales: _____

Target outcome criteria
Throughout the hospital stay, the patient will:
• verbalize or display satisfaction with provisions for spiritual needs (if appropriate)
• show a tranquil facial expression

• express an ability to endure crisis (if appropriate).

Discharge planning

NURSING DISCHARGE CRITERIA

Upon the patient's discharge, documentation shows evidence of:
• meeting of discharge criteria for the specific disease or condition
• appropriate referrals made for home care assistance, as needed, or for care facility placement, if indicated
• special attention to age-related needs, such as hearing aid or eyeglasses.

PATIENT-FAMILY TEACHING CHECKLIST

Document evidence that the patient and family demonstrate an understanding of:
__ details specific to the patient's disease or condition
__ all discharge medications' purpose, dosage, administration schedule, and side effects requiring medical attention
__ care needs arising from illness
__ dietary needs
__ feeding assistance needs
__ mental status changes: thought processing, insight, judgment, or confusion
__ toileting needs
__ mobility and transfer needs
__ hygiene needs
__ speech changes
__ social and emotional needs to reduce loneliness and isolation
__ need for relationships with family and friends
__ family and friends' access to care facility, if placement planned
__ resources available for older persons
__ how to contact the doctor.

DOCUMENTATION CHECKLIST

Using outcome criteria as a guide, document:
__ clinical status on admission
__ significant changes in status
__ patient-family teaching
__ discharge planning
__ other data pertinent to specific disease or condition.

ASSOCIATED PLANS OF CARE

Dying
Grieving
Ineffective Family Coping
Ineffective Individual Coping
Knowledge Deficit
Pain
(See also the plan for the patient's specific disease or condition.)

References

Ashervath, J., and Kiza-Kipunner, K. "Achieving Continence in the Confused Eldery," *Advancing Clinical Care* 5(4):37-40, July-August 1990.

Bangs, M. "High-Touch as Valuable as Hi-Tech Nursing," *Geriatric Nursing Home Care* 7(12):14-15, 1990.

Jirovec, M., Brink, C., and Wells, T. "Nursing Assessments of the Inpatient Geriatric Population," *Nursing Clinics of North America* 23(1):219-30, March 1988.

Johnston, L., and Gueldner, S. "Remember When...? Using Mnemonics to Boost Memory in the Elderly," *Journal of Gerontological Nursing* 15(8):22-26, August 1989.

Jones, P., and Millman, A. "Wound Healing and the Aged Patient," *Nursing Clinics of North America* 25(1):263-77, March 1990.

Kain, C., Reilly, N., and Schultz, E. "The Older Adult: A Comparative Assessment," *Nursing Clinics of North America* 25(4):833-48, December 1990.

Kositzke, J. "A Question of Balance: Dehydration in the Elderly," *Journal of Gerontological Nursing* 16(5):4-11, May 1990.

Rempusheski, V. "The Role of Ethnicity in Elder Care," *Nursing Clinics of North America* 24(3):717-24, September 1989.

Rodgers, B. "Loneliness: Easing the Pain of the Hospitalized Elderly," *Journal of Gerontological Nursing* 15(8):16-21, August 1989.

Simon, J. "The Therapeutic Value of Humor in Aging Adults," *Journal of Gerontological Nursing* 14(8):8-13, August 1988.

Witte, M. "Pain Control," *Journal of Gerontological Nursing* 15(3):32-37, March 1989.

GENERAL PLANS OF CARE
Grieving

Introduction
DEFINITION AND TIME FOCUS
Grief is the normal response to an actual or potential
loss. It is a natural, necessary, and dynamic process.
Anticipatory grieving occurs before an actual loss.
Dysfunctional grieving is the ineffective, pathologic,
delayed, or exaggerated response to an actual or potential loss. Theoretical phases of the grieving process
have been outlined by various authors (see *The grieving
process*). As in all theoretical models, the phases are
overlapping and may or may not be sequential; that is,
the patient or family may fluctuate among phases during the process.

THE GRIEVING PROCESS

LINDEMAN (1944)
Shock or disbelief—Acute mourning—Reentry into daily
life—Decreased image of deceased

ENGEL (1964)
Denial—Developing awareness—Restitution

KÜBLER-ROSS (1969)
Denial—Anger—Bargaining—Depression—
Acceptance

RANDO (1981)
Avoidance—Confrontation—Reestablishment

This plan focuses on the patient and family members
coping with impending or actual losses.

ETIOLOGY AND PRECIPITATING FACTORS
• loss of body image or some aspect of self (such as social role or body part by amputation or mastectomy)
• loss of loved one or significant other through separation, divorce, or death
• loss of material objects (such as income or belongings)
• loss through a maturational or developmental process
(such as aging or weaning an infant)

Focused assessment guidelines
NURSING HISTORY (Functional health pattern findings)

Health perception—health management pattern
• loss may be real or imagined

Nutritional-metabolic pattern
• may report nausea and vomiting, weight loss, or anorexia
• may report increased food, drug, or alcohol intake as
means of self-gratification

Elimination pattern
• may report gastrointestinal upset, diarrhea, or constipation

Activity-exercise pattern
• may report shortness of breath
• may report feelings of exhaustion, weakness, inability to maintain organized activity patterns, or restlessness

Sleep-rest pattern
• may report insomnia caused by disruption of normal
sleep pattern or frequent crying episodes

Cognitive-perceptual pattern
• may describe feelings of guilt
• may report feelings of sorrow, emptiness, or "heaviness"

Self-perception—self-concept pattern
• may express feelings of worthlessness
• may report decreased ability to fulfill personal life
expectations

Role-relationship pattern
• may report episodes of withdrawal or social isolation
(especially with dysfunctional grieving)

Sexuality-reproductive pattern
• may report loss of sexual desire or hypersexuality
• if female, may report menstrual irregularity

Coping-stress tolerance pattern
• may have difficulty expressing feelings about the loss
• may rationalize or intellectualize the loss to make it
less painful, especially during bargaining phase
• may be tearful and describe frequent crying episodes,
usually during shock and denial and depression phases
• may be hostile during the anger phase in an attempt
to resist the impact of the loss
• may avoid discussing the loss (especially with dysfunctional grieving)
• may report previous experiences with depression
• may "rehearse" events surrounding the loss
• may be preoccupied with lost object or image

Value-belief pattern
• may express need for increased spiritual or pastoral
support
• may report increased use of prayer or meditation
• may report doubts in religious beliefs

PHYSICAL FINDINGS
Loss is a body stressor that can trigger physiologic as
well as psychological stress and can decrease the immune system's resistance to infection and illness.

Cardiovascular
- palpitations
- hypertension
- arrhythmias

Pulmonary
- increased respirations
- deep sighing

Gastrointestinal
- vomiting
- diarrhea or constipation

Neurologic
- irritability
- anxiety
- agitation
- paresthesias

Integumentary
- diaphoresis

- cold, clammy skin
- flushed skin

Musculoskeletal
- decreased muscle tone
- weakness

DIAGNOSTIC STUDIES
Physical debilitation and illness resulting from grieving may require studies, but these will vary widely, depending on the signs and symptoms exhibited. For example, palpitations and pulse irregularities may indicate the need for an electrocardiogram (ECG) to rule out significant cardiac problems.

POTENTIAL COMPLICATIONS
- crisis state
- major depression with suicidal or homicidal potential
- physical deterioration
- dysfunctional grieving

Nursing diagnosis: *Grieving related to impending or actual physical or functional loss*

NURSING PRIORITY: Facilitate a healthy grieving process.

Interventions

1. Provide the patient with accurate information before any procedure or treatment that may affect appearance, physical or sexual functioning, or role performance.

2. Assess and document the patient's response to information about the disease, implications, and treatment. Include responses to past experiences with loss.

3. Discuss meaning of the loss with the patient.

4. Discuss changes in social roles or relationships that may result from the loss.

5. Provide time to be with the patient and family.

6. Assess and document the patient's current phase of grief . Recognize that fluctuations among phases may occur.

7. Support and facilitate the expression of feelings associated with anger, guilt, sorrow, and sadness during any phase of grieving. Listen nonjudgmentally. Recognize and accept any feelings of anger directed toward the health care team.

Rationales

1. Accurate information prevents misconceptions and may decrease fears related to the loss.

2. Past experiences and values influence the current loss experience.

3. Establishing the significance of the loss enhances the person's ability to identify and release feelings related to the loss.

4. Physical or functional loss may result in social changes associated with income, career, and relationships. Discussion of these changes helps to identify the impact of the loss and alternatives for adjustments in life-style.

5. The nurse's time spent with the patient and family can encourage the necessary review and processing of the loss. Feelings of loneliness or social isolation may also be decreased, reassuring the patient that caregivers perceive the loss as significant.

6. Identifying unresolved issues facilitates the grieving process.

7. Expressing feelings openly may enable the patient to move more easily through the phases of grieving. The nurse's nonjudgmental listening enables the patient to express feelings without fear of rejection.

8. Encourage the release of emotion through crying. If the patient is receptive, hold the patient's hand and use touch liberally.

8. The nurse's encouragement reassures the patient (and family, if indicated) that crying is a normal response to loss. Hand holding and use of touch provide reassurance and help the patient relax.

9. Assess for and promote positive coping mechanisms — for example, building and sharing close relationships, engaging in creative activities and exercise, and openly expressing feelings related to loss and readjustment. See the "Dying" plan, page 11.

9. Coping with loss is a developmental task. Losses increase in occurrence and intensity throughout life. Adaptive coping methods are derived from previous losses. The "Dying" plan contains general interventions helpful to those coping with loss.

10. Provide spiritual support as requested by the patient throughout grieving, or suggest appropriate resources.

10. Spiritual support assists with fostering a sense of meaning, hope, love, and satisfaction with life.

11. Encourage participation in daily self-care activities.

11. Self-care promotes feelings of self-control and independence, increasing self-esteem.

12. Provide positive reinforcement and realistic hope about the patient's progress.

12. Reinforcement and reassurance build self-confidence.

13. Allow the patient to make decisions whenever possible.

13. Decision making enables the person to maintain control.

14. Assess and assist activation of personal support systems.

14. The patient may need gentle guidance to identify resources. Sharing feelings with closest friends or family aids in adjustment to loss.

15. Additional individualized interventions: _____

15. Rationales: _____

GENERAL PLANS OF CARE

Target outcome criteria
According to individual readiness, the patient will:
• identify the meaning of the loss
• communicate feelings of anger, guilt, sorrow
• identify strategies to cope with the loss
• identify role and relationship changes
• identify and use spiritual support and resources
• perform self-care
• make decisions about care.

Nursing diagnosis: *High risk for dysfunctional grieving related to unresolved feelings about physical or functional loss*

NURSING PRIORITY: Identify dysfunctional grieving and make appropriate referrals.

Interventions

1. Assess and document the patient's responses to the loss. Identify feelings of unresolved guilt or anger. Recognize avoidance of discussing the loss. Be alert to possible use of alcohol or recreational drugs as an escape.

Rationales

1. Accurate assessment allows understanding of the dynamics of the grieving process. Unresolved guilt and anger are common symptoms of pathologic grief and may result in major depression. Avoidance of discussing the loss may indicate delayed grief. Drug or alcohol abuse contributes to dysfunctional resolution of loss.

2. Assess and document the patient's daily activity level and ability to perform roles.

2. Withdrawal and social isolation commonly occur with chronic grieving.

3. Assess the patient's physical well-being and initiate a medical referral as indicated. Teach the importance of maintaining physical health.

3. Grieving requires emotional and physical energy. Prolonged grieving may result in physical illness and debilitation. Somatic symptoms may mask a depression resulting from delayed or absent grief.

4. Monitor and document the administration of tranquilizers, antidepressants, or sedatives.

4. Tranquilizers, antidepressants, or sedatives may occasionally be helpful; however, overmedication may result in prolonging the grieving.

ASSESSMENT OF SUICIDE POTENTIAL

The alert nurse is aware of suicide risk factors and specifically assesses patients at risk by asking direct questions:

MAJOR RISK FACTORS

Intent
Contrary to popular myth, asking patients directly about suicide does not cause attempts. Patients tend to answer truthfully and are typically relieved that someone has acknowledged their distress.

Plan
Patients who verbalize clearly defined, detailed plans for suicide are at greater risk than those who vaguely want to die.

Lethality of method
Highly lethal methods (such as firearms, hanging, or jumping from a height) greatly increase risk.

Availability of means
Patients who have the means readily available are at higher risk.

Personal and family history
Most people who succeed at suicide have made previous attempts. If previous attempts used highly lethal means or were unsuccessful only by accident (that is, if the plan did not allow for rescue), risk is increased. Those who have lost loved ones to suicide are at greater risk.

Goals
If the patient is unable to envision or articulate future goals or plans, suicide potential is increased.

QUESTIONS
"Are you thinking about killing yourself?" or "Are you considering suicide?"

"Do you have a plan to do it?"

"How would you do it?"

"Do you have a gun at home?"

"Have you tried to kill yourself before?"
"How? What happened?"
"Has anyone in your family committed suicide?"

"Where do you see yourself next month? In 1 year? In 5 years?"

ADDITIONAL RISK FACTORS

Resources
Lack of social and personal resources to deal with external or internal crises, or a perception by the patient that such resources are unavailable, increases the likelihood of suicide.

Recent loss or life changes
Loss or the threat of loss increases suicide risk. Even other kinds of change (a promotion, household move, or changes in roles or responsibilities) can increase stress and overwhelm the patient's coping abilities.

Physical illness
Physical illness may increase suicide risk, particularly if the illness involves major life changes or a threat to essentials of self-image.

Alcohol or drug abuse
Substance abuse may increase impulsive behavior and contribute to depression, thus increasing suicide risk. Additionally, alcohol or drugs may increase risk by potentiating other drugs or decreasing overall level of awareness.

Sudden behavior change
Any abrupt change in behavior may signal suicidal intent.

Isolation
Physical or emotional isolation greatly increases suicide risk.

Age, sex, marital status
Older males have a higher rate of successful suicide, possibly because they tend to choose more certain means. Risk of suicide may be increased for separated, widowed, or divorced persons. These parameters, however, are less reliable predictors than those above.

5. Observe the patient for signs and symptoms of potential suicide or homicide: increased agitation, insomnia, self-incrimination, and feelings of worthlessness, helplessness, and hopelessness.

6. Assess suicide risk (see *Assessment of suicide potential*) by talking with the patient. Consult with the patient's doctor regarding referral or intervention.

7. Involve other resource persons such as social workers, chaplains, or psychiatrists, as indicated or requested by the patient and family.

8. Provide follow-up referral for the patient after discharge.

5. Anxiety and depression may be exaggerated during chronic grieving states.

6. Frank discussion of suicide potential with the patient helps identify and define stressors and may relieve anxiety; it will not cause a suicide attempt.

7. Interdisciplinary referral helps identify available financial, social, spiritual, and community resources. Psychiatric intervention focuses on understanding unhealthy responses and the reactivation of healthy grieving.

8. Follow-up visits by nurses, chaplains, social workers, and other support persons should be based on individual needs. During early grieving, weekly visits are most likely to be helpful. Support groups may also be helpful.

9. Additional individualized interventions: _____

9. Rationales: _____

Target outcome criteria
According to individual readiness, the patient will:
• acknowledge the loss
• discuss the experience realistically
• use healthy coping strategies
• understand and accept own and other's responses
• express and accept personal feelings
• identify resources within the family and community
• verify the absence of suicidal or homicidal potential.

Discharge planning
NURSING DISCHARGE CRITERIA
Upon the patient's discharge, documentation shows evidence of:
• acknowledgment of the loss and its meaning
• demonstration of positive coping behaviors
• identification of social and community support systems
• no display of suicidal or homicidal potential.

PATIENT-FAMILY TEACHING CHECKLIST
Document evidence that the patient and family demonstrate an understanding of:
___ normal grief responses
___ phases of the grieving process
___ information concerning role changes and physical loss
___ importance of maintaining physical health and well-being of the patient and family
___ information about the patient's illness and medical treatment
___ need to be understanding and accepting of those who are grieving
___ community resources including support groups and interagency referral.

DOCUMENTATION CHECKLIST
Using outcome criteria as a guide, document:
___ past experiences and responses to loss
___ current perception and meaning of loss
___ changes in role relationship, body image, and self-esteem
___ positive or maladaptive coping behaviors
___ support systems
___ level of activity and participation in self-care
___ medication with tranquilizers, antidepressants, or sedatives
___ signs and symptoms of suicidal or homicidal potential
___ interdisciplinary referrals
___ patient-family teaching
___ discharge planning.

ASSOCIATED PLANS OF CARE
Dying
Ineffective Family Coping
Ineffective Individual Coping

References
Archer, D., and Smith, A. "Sorrow Has Many Faces: Helping Families Cope with Grief" *Nursing88* 18(5): 43-45, May 1988.

Grainger, R. "Successful Grieving," *American Journal of Nursing* 90(9):12, 15, September 1990.

Gyulay, J. "Grief Responses," *Issues in Comprehensive Pediatric Nursing* 12(1):1-31, January-February 1989.

Jones, M., and Peacock, M. "Nursing Interventions with Continuing Loss," *Focus on Critical Care* 15(3):26-30, June 1988.

Karl, G. "Janforum: A New Look at Grief," *Journal of Advanced Nursing* 12(5):641-45, September 1987.

Martocchio, B. "Grief and Bereavement: Healing Through Hurt," *Nursing Clinics of North America* 20(2):327-41, June 1985.

McAteer, M. "Some Aspects of Grief in Physiotherapy," *Physiotherapy* 75(1):55-58, January 1989.

McNally, J., et al. *Guidelines for Cancer Nursing Practice,* 2nd ed. Philadelphia: W.B. Saunders Co., 1991.

Rando, T. *Grief, Dying and Death: Clinical Interventions for Caregivers.* Champaign, Ill.: Research Press Co., 1984.

Rando, T. *Loss and Anticipatory Grief.* New York: Free Press, 1986.

Worden, J. *Grief Counseling and Grief Therapy: A Handbook for the Mental Health Practitioner* New York: Springer Publishing Co., 1991.

GENERAL PLANS OF CARE

Impaired Physical Mobility

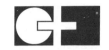

Introduction
DEFINITION AND TIME FOCUS
Impaired physical mobility is a problem for almost every patient in the medical-surgical unit. Acutely ill or injured patients are physically unable to engage in normal activities; physical recovery itself may demand activity limitations. Rest is essential for healing and should be encouraged; however, prolonged bed rest can result in well-documented physical and emotional disabilities that can add to the patient's problems. The effects of decreased mobility must be addressed early in care planning and reviewed frequently throughout the patient's hospital stay. This plan focuses on the care of the patient whose condition causes or requires impaired physical mobility.

ETIOLOGY AND PRECIPITATING FACTORS
• injury that prevents weight bearing (such as trauma)
• illness that causes activity intolerance (such as cardiopulmonary disorders)
• acute injury that causes paralysis or paresis (such as cerebrovascular accident [CVA] or spinal cord injury)
• chronic or acute disabling conditions (such as severe arthritis or Guillain-Barré syndrome)
• sensory-perceptual alterations (as in CVA)
• therapeutic restrictions
• reluctance to attempt movement

Focused assessment guidelines
NURSING HISTORY (Functional health pattern findings)
Because the patient's subjective responses to immobility may vary widely, depending on the underlying condition, this section presents a guide to assessing the patient with a mobility impairment.

Health perception — health management pattern
• Is the patient's mobility problem new, or does it reflect long-standing disability?
• What is the extent of the patient's activity limitation?
• Does the patient normally use any mobility aids at home (such as a walker, cane, or wheelchair)?
• Does the patient have a cast, splint, traction, or other immobilizing device?
• Does the patient have equipment that interferes with normal mobility, such as a ventilator or multiple I.V. lines?
• Does the patient have preexisting conditions that affect mobility, such as CVA or amputation, or a progressive debilitating disease, such as multiple sclerosis or acquired immunodeficiency syndrome?
• Does the patient have a history of blood disorders, integumentary problems, pulmonary disease, or cardiac disease?

Nutritional-metabolic pattern
• What is the patient's baseline nutritional status? (See the "Nutritional Deficit" plan, page 63.)
• Is the patient able or permitted to take oral nourishment?
• Is the patient receiving artificial nutrition such as total parenteral nutrition or nasogastric or gastric tube feedings?

Elimination pattern
• When was the patient's last bowel movement?
• Does the patient normally use elimination aids, such as laxatives or enemas?
• Does the patient have a preexisting condition requiring a bowel regimen that includes removal of impacted feces?
• Does the patient have a history of calculi, renal disease, or recurrent urinary tract infections?
• If the patient has an indwelling urinary catheter, when was it placed?

Activity-exercise pattern
• Is the patient able to perform any self-care activity?
• What was the patient's baseline activity tolerance before hospitalization?
• Are all joints capable of full range of motion?

Cognitive-perceptual pattern
• Is the patient conscious and alert?
• Does the patient have any sensory deficits (such as blindness, deafness, or hemiparesis)?

Self-perception — self-concept pattern
• What is the patient's attitude toward resuming physical activity?

Role-relationship pattern
• Does the patient's occupation require full mobility?
• Does the patient have a supportive social network?
• Are family members involved in care of the patient at home?

Sexuality-reproductive pattern
• Does the patient's mobility impairment potentially affect sexual function?

Coping — stress tolerance pattern
• Has the patient used physical activity as a primary coping behavior or stress-relieving measure?

PHYSICAL FINDINGS
Because physical findings vary widely in patients with reduced mobility, depending on their underlying

condition, this section has been refocused to outline some of the major physiologic effects of immobility on body systems.

Cardiovascular
• orthostatic hypotension (related to reduced autonomic neurovascular reflex response)
• reduced stroke volume
• gradually increasing tachycardia (related to deconditioning effects)
• decreased oxygen uptake
• venous pooling (related to lack of muscle activity)
• plasma volume loss
• blood volume loss
• reduced cardiac reserve

Respiratory
• restricted diaphragmatic and costal excursion
• reduced ciliary activity
• reduced vital capacity
• reduced gas exchange (related to gravitational effects)
• reduced production of surfactant

Gastrointestinal
• decreased peristalsis
• increased sphincter tone
• abdominal distention
• anorexia

Neurologic
• decreased sensorium
• paralysis or paresis related to CVA or spinal cord injury

Integumentary
• reduced skin turgor
• impaired wound healing
• dependent edema

Musculoskeletal
• reduced muscle mass
• decreased strength and endurance
• bone demineralization (at increased rate)
• fibrosis or ankylosis
• calcium deposition in soft tissue

Renal
• hypercalciuria and precipitation of calcium salts (related to bone demineralization)
• increased renal blood flow
• initial diuresis (related to decreased antidiuretic hormone [ADH] release)
• bladder distention
• urinary stasis

Metabolic
• increased rate of catabolism
• decreased basal metabolic rate
• increased excretion of electrolytes

DIAGNOSTIC STUDIES
Because no diagnostic studies are specifically applicable to all patients with impaired mobility, only the usual laboratory test findings related to the physiologic changes described in the preceding section are presented here. Laboratory tests include:
• serum protein level — usually decreased from accelerated catabolism
• serum and urine calcium and phosphate levels — increased from bone demineralization
• arterial blood gas (ABG) measurements — may show reduced PaO_2 and increased $PaCO_2$, indicating hypoventilation and impaired gas exchange
• blood urea nitrogen level — may be elevated from catabolic activity
• urine pH — may be elevated from decreased levels of acid end products released by muscle activity
• hematocrit — may be increased from plasma and blood volume losses and diuresis.

POTENTIAL COMPLICATIONS
• thromboembolic phenomena
• atelectasis
• pneumonia
• infections
• skin breakdown, potential pressure ulcer formation
• constipation
• contractures
• osteoporosis
• muscle wasting
• urinary calculi
• difficulty coping

GENERAL PLANS
OF CARE

Nursing diagnosis: *High risk for ineffective airway clearance related to reduced diaphragmatic and costal excursion, stasis of secretions, decreased ciliary activity, weakness, and underlying disease process*

NURSING PRIORITIES: (a) Maintain a clear airway and (b) prevent pulmonary complications.

Interventions

1. Assess pulmonary capabilities at least every 2 hours while the patient is awake. Evaluate level of alertness, ability to cough and deep breathe, respiratory rate and effort, and lung sounds.

Rationales

1. Initial and ongoing assessments provide direction for care planning. The factors listed are crucial determinants of the patient's capability to counteract the effects of bed rest on pulmonary function.

2. Evaluate for risk factors that affect pulmonary status, such as obesity, lung disease, incisions, abdominal distention, neuromuscular dysfunction, chest wall pathology, and medications that depress respirations.

2. The risk factors listed are associated with increased incidence of serious pulmonary complications.

3. Monitor vital signs, fluid intake and output, hemodynamic pressures, and electrocardiogram (ECG) findings according to Appendix A, "Monitoring Standards," or unit protocol. Report changes or abnormal findings promptly.

3. Bed rest has significant effects on cardiovascular function, including a reduction in stroke volume (which may be compensated by tachycardia), redistribution of blood flow (which may contribute to orthostatic hypotension), and decreased cardiovascular reserve (resulting in reduced exercise tolerance and general deconditioning). Careful monitoring of cardiovascular parameters aids in early detection of preventable complications.

4. Obtain and monitor ABG measurements as ordered. Monitor vital capacity and other pulmonary function studies, as ordered, and report any abnormal findings promptly.

4. ABG measurements provide direct evaluation of ventilatory status. Pulmonary function studies aid further classification and evaluation of the effects of bed rest on the lungs (bed rest is associated with decreased ventilatory capacity).

5. Initiate measures to promote effective breathing:

5. Maintaining an effective breathing pattern reduces the risk of developing pulmonary complications.

• Place the patient in Fowler's or semi-Fowler's position, as condition permits, and change position at least every 2 hours.

• Patients on bed rest commonly assume a slumped position, decreasing the adequacy of chest expansion. Frequent repositioning helps facilitate gravity drainage of secretions.

• Encourage deep breathing at least every 2 hours while awake, and assist the patient using an incentive spirometer, as ordered. Check with the doctor about including coughing with deep breathing.

• Deep breathing and incentive spirometry may increase inspiratory reserve volume, promote maximum alveolar inflation, and improve ventilation-perfusion ratios. Deep breathing may actually reverse microatelectasis related to hypoventilation. The incentive spirometer also provides a goal for the patient. The effectiveness of coughing as an airway clearance measure is controversial because its direct effects on small airways have not been shown, and coughing may increase intrathoracic pressure and lead to alveolar microatelectasis. Some clinicians believe coughing may result in a "milking" effect from smaller to larger airways. If coughing is used, it should always be followed by several deep breaths to help reinflate alveoli.

• Teach or assist the patient to splint incisions, if present.

• Splinting may decrease the fear of pain and promote deeper breathing and fuller chest wall expansion.

• Reduce abdominal distention, when possible, through use of gastric suction, return-flow enema, or other measures, as ordered.

• Abdominal distention exerts upward pressure on the diaphragm, reducing chest excursion.

6. Initiate measures to promote airway clearance:

6. Pulmonary hygiene measures help reduce the risk of developing pulmonary complications.

• Provide humidification of inspired air.

• Humidification may help decrease the viscosity of secretions and helps minimize upper airway irritation if constant supplemental oxygen is required.

• Encourage an adequate fluid intake, typically 8 to 12 8-oz glasses (2,000 to 3,000 ml) a day as condition allows.

• Rehydration of dehydrated patients can promote increased mucociliary clearance.

• Suction, as needed, providing supplemental oxygen before and after the procedure.

• Suctioning may be necessary for airway clearance, especially in persons with weak or absent cough or artificial airways. Supplemental oxygen is essential because suctioning can cause significant reduction in PaO_2.

• Perform chest physiotherapy every 4 hours while the patient is awake (or more frequently, as indicated).

• Chest physiotherapy may help prevent pooling of secretions and loosen mucus plugs. When used in combination with postural drainage, it can help bring secretions into larger airways for easier expectoration.

7. Monitor for pulmonary complications associated with bed rest, as follows:
- pneumonia—crackles, rhonchi, chest pain, fever, productive cough, tachypnea, tachycardia, whispered pectoriloquy, or consolidation or effusion on chest X-ray

- atelectasis—bronchial or decreased breath sounds, dull percussion note over affected side, tachypnea, tachycardia, restlessness, tracheal shift toward affected side on chest X-ray, or cyanosis (in advanced macroatelectasis)

- pulmonary embolus—see the "High risk for thromboembolic phenomena" problem below.

8. Additional individualized interventions: _____

_____

7. Pulmonary insult complicates treatment and increases mortality risk in the acutely ill patient.

- Prompt detection and treatment of pulmonary infections is essential because their presence exacerbates ventilatory compromise. Purulent sputum is more tenacious because it contains viscous leukocyte deoxyribonucleic acid. In addition, proteolytic enzymes released from destroyed leukocytes can increase inflammation, resulting in bronchoconstriction.

- Bed rest aids the development of atelectasis because of reduced chest expansion, ventilatory capacity, and secretion clearance. Microatelectasis is common and may appear on chest X-ray. When atelectasis occurs, ventilatory capacity is reduced because inspired air cannot reach the affected areas.

- Pulmonary embolus is the most immediately life-threatening complication associated with bed rest, with a mortality rate of approximately 38%.

8. Rationales: _____

_____

Target outcome criteria
Throughout the hospital stay, the patient will:
- exhibit an effective breathing pattern
- change position (or be turned) at least every 2 hours
- perform pulmonary hygiene measures at least every 2 hours, as condition permits

- exhibit no evidence of pneumonia, atelectasis, or pulmonary embolus.

Collaborative problem: *High risk for thromboembolic phenomena related to venous pooling, loss of vasomotor tone, lack of skeletal muscle contraction, and increased blood viscosity*

NURSING PRIORITY: Prevent or promptly detect and treat thromboembolic complications.

Interventions

1. Evaluate the patient for factors that increase the risk of thromboembolism, including:
- previous history of deep-vein thrombosis
- abdominal, pelvic, or orthopedic surgery
- trauma
- history of varicosities, cancer, smoking, CVA, or bleeding disorders
- use of oral contraceptives or other medications that affect clotting
- dehydration
- obesity
- hypertension, diabetes mellitus, or renal disease
- paralysis
- decreased alertness
- age (over 40 years).

2. Initiate measures to promote venous return and decrease venous pooling:
- Teach the patient to perform leg exercises every 1 to 2 hours while awake, such as flexion and extension of the feet and quadriceps setting. Elevate legs 15 degrees.
- Avoid use of the knee gatch, leg crossing, or pillows placed directly under the popliteal area.

Rationales

1. Any factor that contributes to venous stasis, hypercoagulability, trauma, or degeneration of blood vessels increases the risk of thromboembolism. Because bed rest can cause thromboembolism complications, noting any additional contributing factors will help identify the highest-risk patients and plan their care.

2. Venous stasis is associated with increased incidence of thromboembolic complications.
- Leg exercises cause muscle contraction, promoting venous return toward the heart. Leg elevation promotes gravity drainage from peripheral vessels.
- These measures may cause venous compression or occlusion, increasing the risk of complications.

• Apply graded antiembolism hose, taking care to remove them at least three times daily for 30 to 60 minutes, or according to unit protocol. Discuss use of pneumatic devices, such as special boots, with the doctor.

• Increase activity to permit ambulation as soon as the patient's condition allows. Use caution when first getting the patient out of bed.

3. For high-risk patients, administer prophylactic anticoagulants, if ordered (typically low-dose heparin or warfarin sodium [Coumadin]). Monitor clotting studies (prothrombin time [PT] or partial thromboplastin time [PTT]) daily for these patients, as ordered. Question anticoagulant orders for trauma patients and others with possible cardiovascular instability or bleeding problems. Monitor for signs and symptoms of occult bleeding, such as positive test for hemoglobin in stool or urine, in patients receiving anticoagulant therapy.

4. Monitor for evidence of thromboembolic complications, including:

• pulmonary embolism—tachypnea, sudden dyspnea, pleuritic chest pain, restlessness, feelings of impending doom, diaphoresis, hypotension, pallor, or cyanosis. If these signs and symptoms occur, elevate the head of the bed, administer oxygen, obtain a specimen for ABG study, and notify the doctor immediately.

• thrombophlebitis—erythema, edema, tenderness, venous patterning or engorgement, positive Homans' sign, cording, or calf pain. Avoid deep palpation of the affected area. If swelling is suspected, initiate daily measurements of leg circumference at a designated point (make an indelible mark on the patient for subsequent measurement). If these signs and symptoms occur, notify the doctor immediately and elevate the affected extremity.

5. Additional individualized interventions: _____

_____

• Antiembolism hose "squeeze" superficial vessels and may promote venous return. Removal permits skin examination and allows drying of accumulated moisture. Pneumatic devices may also promote venous return; their use is particularly desirable if heparin is contraindicated.

• Weight bearing increases muscle contraction and also decreases bone demineralization associated with immobility. Clots from immobility are most likely to embolize when the patient first resumes activity.

3. Heparin inactivates fibrin, thus preventing fibrin clot formation and reducing the risk of enlargement of existing clots. Warfarin interferes with vitamin K production, thus decreasing production of clotting factors. Monitoring PT and PTT permits dosage adjustment as needed. Anticoagulants may induce bleeding in susceptible patients.

4. Early detection and treatment of thromboembolic phenomena may minimize their effects.

• Pulmonary embolism is the blockage of a pulmonary artery by a thrombus. As a result, alveoli are ventilated but not perfused, resulting in increased alveolar dead space in the affected lung tissue. A large embolus may significantly increase pulmonary vascular resistance, which may lead to right-sided heart failure. Pulmonary infarction may also occur if the embolus is large. ABG findings guide intervention.

• Thrombophlebitis may occur in superficial or deep veins; the leg veins are affected most frequently. Superficial thrombophlebitis, although not dangerous, can cause significant discomfort; deep vein thrombophlebitis, however, may lead to life-threatening movement of clots to the lung. Initial erythema, swelling, and tenderness are related to inflammatory changes, while later signs (such as cording and a positive Homans' sign) represent actual thrombus formation. Deep palpation may cause dislodgement clots. Measuring leg circumference provides an objective evaluation of swelling. Elevating the affected extremity helps minimize venous stasis.

5. Rationales: _____

_____

Target outcome criteria
Throughout the hospital stay, the patient will:
• perform leg exercises at least every 2 hours as instructed or receive passive range-of-motion exercises
• increase activity to maximum level permitted

• display no signs of pulmonary embolus or thrombophlebitis.

Nursing diagnosis: *High risk for impaired skin integrity related to impeded capillary flow, possible altered sensation, or venous stasis*

NURSING PRIORITY: Prevent skin breakdown.

Interventions

1. On the patient's admission to the unit, and at least daily thereafter, inspect the skin carefully, evaluating color, texture, turgor, dryness, sensation, and capillary refill.

Rationales

1. Initial and ongoing assessment is the first step in providing individualized care. Abnormal findings may provide clues to problems and can be used to guide care planning.

2. Evaluate for factors that increase the risk of skin breakdown, such as nutritional deficit, obesity, diabetes mellitus (or other conditions affecting vascular status), incontinence, decreased sensation, infection, excessive moisture, old age, decreased alertness, and paralysis.

3. Initiate measures to prevent skin breakdown, including:

• turning and repositioning every 1 to 2 hours, massaging areas of pressure and bony prominences

• careful turning technique

• judicious use of lotion, avoidance of harsh soaps, and careful cleaning, especially for the incontinent patient, followed by gentle but thorough drying

• use of convoluted foam mattress, flotation pad or water bed, sheepskins, air mattress, air-fluidized bead system (Clinitron therapy bed), low-air-loss bed, or kinetic (Roto-Rest) bed, as available and indicated

• adequate nutrition.

4. Monitor for evidence of impending skin breakdown: edema, blanching, coldness, tenderness, redness, or blistering. Brief reactive hyperemia of the skin is normal following relief from pressure. If reactive hyperemia does not resolve after 15 minutes, institute additional protective measures for the affected area.

5. If a pressure ulcer develops, institute a therapeutic regimen immediately, according to the doctor's orders or unit protocol.

6. Additional individualized interventions: _____

_____

2. Bed rest alone places any patient at increased risk for skin problems because pressure areas may develop rapidly if motion is restricted or impossible. The patient with one or more of the conditions listed should be considered at extremely high risk. Early evaluation of such factors allows for preventive measures.

3. Preventing skin breakdown is much easier than treating a problem after it develops.

• Repositioning allows redistribution of pressure. Massage stimulates circulation and promotes comfort; bony prominences are the most common sites of skin breakdown.

• Rapid or overly vigorous turning may cause delicate skin to shear.

• Dry skin is more prone to cracking and peeling, but excessive moisture provides a medium for bacterial growth and may lead to maceration. Soaps may be irritating. Urine and feces, if left in contact with skin, may cause chemical irritation and contribute to rapid breakdown of tissue.

• Special bedding or beds may help improve patient comfort, distribute pressure more evenly, and reduce the deleterious effects of impaired mobility.

• Immobility contributes to increased catabolism and tissue breakdown; also, using stored fats as an energy source may reduce adipose tissue that provides cushioning. Protein is essential for maintaining and rebuilding tissue.

4. Early detection of impending problems permits treatment before skin breakdown occurs. The signs and symptoms listed result when pressure and immobility diminish perfusion. Pressure ulcers can result from as little as 1 hour of pressure and immobility, if the pressure is great enough to impede capillary flow. Additionally, subcutaneous tissue and muscle have usually suffered ischemia before the ulcer becomes apparent on the skin surface, so early detection and treatment are vital.

5. Treatment of pressure ulcers varies among practitioners and institutions. Prompt treatment is essential to avert development of additional complications, such as osteomyelitis.

6. Rationales: _____

_____

Target outcome criteria
Throughout the hospital stay, the patient will:
• maintain clean, intact skin
• exhibit no evidence of skin breakdown

• maintain adequate nutritional intake.

Nursing diagnosis: *High risk for altered urinary elimination related to diuresis, stasis of urine, positioning, or bone demineralization*

NURSING PRIORITIES: (a) Promote normal urinary elimination and (b) prevent urinary system complications.

Interventions

1. Assess the patient's normal urinary elimination pattern, if possible, by noting the following:
• frequency, times, and amounts of voidings
• any change in the usual pattern
• continence
• special measures used to initiate or control voiding, color, odor, and appearance (including inspection for increased sedimentation).

2. Evaluate factors that may increase the risk of urinary complications, such as:
• dehydration
• incontinence
• indwelling catheters
• narcotics, sedatives, diuretics, or other medications that affect renal function or alertness
• diabetes
• neurogenic bladder dysfunction
• pregnancy
• immunosuppression
• shock
• altered acid-base or electrolyte status.

3. Initiate measures to promote normal urinary elimination:

• Have a female patient sit on a bedside commode and allow a male patient to stand to urinate, condition permitting.

• Encourage adequate fluid intake, unless contraindicated, to between 8 and 12 8-oz glasses (2,000 and 3,000 ml) daily.

• Promote as much activity as the condition permits—turning, sitting, leg dangling, standing, walking, or range-of-motion exercises.

• Provide privacy during attempts to void.

• Use measures to promote full emptying of the bladder, as needed, such as running water nearby, pouring warm water over the perineum, and applying manual pressure over the bladder.

• Use urinary catheterization only as needed to prevent distention and stasis. Exercise strict aseptic technique in insertion and care of catheters.

4. Measure urine output hourly and report values less than 60 ml/hour for 2 hours. Assess for bladder distention at least every 8 hours. Measure urine pH every 8 hours and report levels greater than 6. Monitor routine urine cultures, as ordered.

Rationales

1. Assessment of the patient's normal elimination status is the first step in planning individualized care.

2. Immobility has several effects on urinary elimination. Bed rest increases the solute load of the kidneys because tissue breakdown and bone demineralization both occur at an increased rate. The increased thoracic blood volume associated with the supine position triggers decreased ADH release, resulting in diuresis. The supine position also contributes to urinary stasis, because downward urine flow is normally enhanced by gravity. Additionally, complete bladder emptying may be harder to achieve in the supine position. Any additional factors, such as those listed, contribute further to the risk of complications and must be considered in care planning.

3. Measures to promote normal elimination may help reduce the risk of developing urinary system complications.
• The upright position facilitates improved urine flow from the ureters and bladder and usually is more comfortable for the patient. In addition, studies report no significant differences in oxygen consumption and cardiovascular response between in-bed and out-of-bed toileting. Weight-bearing exercise of any kind, including the effort to sit or stand, may also help reduce deleterious orthostasis and bone demineralization.

• Calcium precipitation, and resultant calculi formation, is less likely to occur in dilute urine. In addition, an adequate quantity of dilute urine increases frequency of micturition, reducing the likelihood of infection from stasis.

• Position changes promote urine drainage, minimize stasis, and reduce protein breakdown associated with immobilization.

• The sphincter relaxation necessary for voiding may be difficult to achieve unless privacy is ensured.

• Bladder distention may cause back pressure and eventual nephron damage. Incomplete bladder emptying is also associated with increased risk of infection.

• Urinary catheterization is associated with a high incidence of nosocomial infections. Placement of a catheter in the normally sterile urinary tract exposes the patient to pathogens that may cause infection.

4. Urine output of less than 60 ml/hour may indicate impending renal failure or other complications. Bladder distention and resultant urine stasis may occur even in a catheterized patient if the tube becomes obstructed by sediment, blood clots, or calculi. Alkaline urine contributes to the formation of calcium calculi. Routine urine cultures allow early detection of infection.

5. Monitor for indications of urinary tract complications, as follows:

• infection—burning, frequency, and urgency (if voiding voluntarily); cloudy, foul-smelling urine; hematuria; fever; or low back pain

• calculi—severe flank pain, lower abdominal pain, hematuria, nausea, or altered urine stream (if a calculus lodges in the bladder neck or urethra).

6. If indications of urinary complications are detected, notify the doctor promptly and collaborate in treatment.

7. Additional individualized interventions: _____
_____

5. Urinary tract complications usually result from several interrelated factors.

• Urinary tract infection may be related to stasis, dehydration, bladder distention, or any factor that damages the protective mucosal lining of the bladder, such as calculi or catheterization.

• Calcium excretion is increased in a patient on prolonged bed rest because of increased bone breakdown. Most calculi are composed of calcium salts. Such factors as stasis, infection, and decreased urine volume contribute to calculi formation. Also, because of low levels of muscle contraction, a smaller-than-normal quantity of acid end products is excreted, and the urine becomes increasingly alkaline, a condition that favors calculi formation.

6. Treatment of urinary pathology in acutely ill patients must be carefully coordinated with treatment of the patient's primary condition to avoid further complications.

7. Rationales: _____
_____

GENERAL PLANS OF CARE

Target outcome criteria
Throughout the hospital stay, the patient will:
• maintain urine output of at least 60 ml/hour
• maintain fluid intake of at least 8 8-oz glasses (2,000 ml) daily, unless contraindicated

• exhibit no signs of urinary tract infection or calculi.

Nursing diagnosis: *High risk for constipation related to lack of contraction of abdominal muscles, weakness, loss of defecation reflex, slowed peristalsis, altered nutritional intake, or psychological inhibition*

NURSING PRIORITY: Promote normal bowel elimination.

Interventions

1. Assess the patient's normal bowel elimination pattern, if possible, noting the frequency, times, color, and consistency of stools; any change in the usual pattern; continence; use of laxatives or enemas; date and time of last bowel movement; and bowel sounds. Monitor bowel status daily.

2. Evaluate the patient for factors that may increase the risk of constipation, including dehydration; narcotics, iron intake, anticholinergics, or other medications affecting peristaltic function; paralysis; age (because of reduced colon tone); cachexia; emphysema (because of reduced ability to increase intra-abdominal pressure); abdominal surgery; abdominal tumors; pregnancy; ascites; hemorrhoids; nothing-by-mouth status; and trauma.

3. Initiate measures to promote normal bowel elimination:

• Allow the use of a bedside commode or toilet, if the condition permits. Encourage the patient to attempt defecation at usual times, or whenever the urge arises.

• Encourage the patient to contract abdominal muscles while exhaling during defecation attempts. Instruct the patient to avoid Valsalva's maneuver.

Rationales

1. Assessment of the patient's normal elimination status is the first step in planning individualized care. Daily monitoring helps in early identification of potential problems.

2. Because normal bowel motility depends in part upon abdominal muscle contraction and physical activity, immobility predisposes the patient to constipation. Any additional factors, such as those listed, contribute further to the risk of complications and must be considered in care planning.

3. Maintaining normal bowel elimination reduces the risk of developing bowel complications.

• The normal defecation position facilitates evacuation. If defecation is suppressed despite impulses from rectal distention, colon motility eventually may be inhibited.

• Contraction of abdominal muscles increases intra-abdominal pressure and aids in evacuation. Valsalva's maneuver causes a vagal response and, in susceptible patients, may result in bradycardia, heart block, or other cardiovascular complications.

• As the patient's condition permits, teach exercises to maintain or strengthen abdominal muscles, such as contracting and relaxing abdominal muscles several times per hour and performing leg lifts.

• Encourage an adequate fluid intake, unless contraindicated.

• Encourage natural laxatives and high-fiber foods, as permitted and tolerated.

• Provide privacy and comfort measures during toileting, such as ensuring warmth and providing air freshener.

4. Assess for indications of constipation, such as absence of bowel movements; hard, dry, small stools; rectal pressure sensation; abdominal distention or mass; headache; decreased appetite; hard stool felt in rectal vault on digital examination; or ribbonlike diarrhea.

5. As necessary, collaborate with the doctor to select appropriate elimination aids, such as laxatives, suppositories, enemas, or stool softeners.

6. Additional individualized interventions: _____

_____

• Bed rest results in generalized muscle atrophy. Weakness of the abdominal muscles may render the patient unable to assist with evacuation.

• Inadequate fluid intake may cause dry, hard stools that are more difficult to expel.

• Whole-grain cereals, fruits and vegetables, and prune juice help promote natural elimination.

• Bowel activity may be inhibited if the patient is anxious, embarrassed, or uncomfortable.

4. In the absence of normal bowel elimination, water continues to be reabsorbed from the stool that remains in the bowel, and the stool becomes harder, dryer, and more compacted. As softer stool collects behind it, increasing peristaltic pressure may result in a forceful expulsion of diarrhea past the hard stool mass.

5. Laxatives, suppositories, and enemas may be necessary occasionally, but their frequent use may disrupt normal bowel functioning. Stool softeners may help in the natural expulsion of stool and are not habit-forming.

6. Rationales: _____

_____

Target outcome criteria
Throughout the hospital stay, the patient will:
• maintain normal bowel elimination
• perform abdominal exercises as taught, if the condition permits

• exhibit no signs of constipation.

Nursing diagnosis: *High risk for disuse syndrome: muscle atrophy and joint contractures related to disuse, nonfunctional positioning, and reduced muscle tone*

NURSING PRIORITY: Maintain maximum functional integrity of bone and muscle.

Interventions

1. Evaluate the patient for factors that increase the risk of significant muscle, bone, and joint complications, including preexisting conditions that reduce mobility (such as arthritis, paralysis, paresis, or debilitation), decreased level of alertness, spinal injury or surgery, major burns, and trauma.

2. Initiate measures to preserve motor function and strength:
• weight bearing, as the condition permits, even if only standing at the bedside or on a tilt table several times daily

Rationales

1. Normal bone and muscle function depend on activity, which maintains and increases muscle strength, maintains balanced muscle tone, and promotes normal bone formation. When a muscle is immobilized, 10% to 15% of its strength may be lost in as little as 1 week, and it may atrophy to half its size within a month. Disuse atrophy leads to shortening of muscle fibers and reduces joint motion. Immobilization decreases osteoblastic deposition of bone matrix, but normal osteoclastic destruction continues, depleting calcium and other minerals essential for bone stability. The other factors listed may add to the risk of significant bone- and muscle-related complications.

2. Maintaining healthy bone and muscle function is easier than restoring function after disability.
• Weight-bearing exercise stimulates osteoblastic activity by providing normal stress to bones. Lack of weight bearing is the primary contributor to osteoporosis, a condition in which the bones are so weakened that the patient is prone to fractures.

• active exercise, as the condition permits, including hourly ankle rotation and flexion and extension of the feet and quadriceps

• complete range of motion to all joints at least four times daily, as the condition permits

• careful positioning to maintain functional alignment, using such devices as trochanter rolls, hand rolls, splints, footboards, and padding between thighs (if hip adduction is a problem); alternate flexion and extension of extremities when turning; and repositioning at least every 2 hours.

3. Additional individualized interventions: _____

• Active exercises promote maximum muscle contraction and help maintain strength and endurance.

• Putting the joint through its full range of motion stretches the surrounding muscle fibers and maintains the coordinated function of joint structures.

• Serious joint contractures requiring surgical intervention or prolonged corrective physical therapy may result if functional alignment is not maintained.

3. Rationales: _____

Target outcome criteria
Throughout the hospital stay, the patient will:
• perform exercises as taught, if the condition permits
• maintain functional alignment of all joints.

Nursing diagnosis: *Situational low self-esteem related to dependent patient role*

NURSING PRIORITY: Promote positive self-image.

Interventions

1. Assess the effects of reduced mobility on self-concept. Encourage expression of feelings and identification of primary losses.

2. Encourage the patient's participation in self-care and decision making, as the condition permits.

3. Anticipate such behaviors as regression, withdrawal, aggression, apathy, and crying. Try to help the patient interpret these normal responses to loss.

4. See the "Sensory-Perceptual Alteration" plan, page 75.

5. See the "Ineffective Individual Coping" plan, page 51.

6. Additional individualized interventions: _____

Rationales

1. Identifying what the loss of normal mobility means to the individual is the first step in care planning. A patient's reaction to immobility can vary enormously, depending on baseline activity level and the importance of physical function to identity.

2. Participating in self-care, even in small ways, preserves a patient's sense of identity and integrity.

3. Immobility may cause disorganization of the psyche as the individual attempts to cope with the profound loss of usual roles, stimulation, and independence. Helping the patient to understand the normalcy of his reactions may reduce psychic disequilibrium and facilitate healthy coping strategies.

4. Immobility results in significant reduction in normal sensory stimulation. This can contribute to decreased motivation, reduced ability to learn and solve problems, sleep disturbances, and other problems that may compound the patient's distress. The "Sensory-Perceptual Alteration" plan contains detailed information on preventing, detecting, and treating this problem.

5. The "Ineffective Individual Coping" plan contains further interventions that may be helpful in caring for the patient with low self-esteem.

6. Rationales: _____

> **Target outcome criteria**
> Throughout the hospital stay, the patient will:
> • express feelings related to losses
> • participate in decision making related to care
>
> • exercise healthy coping behaviors.

Discharge planning
NURSING DISCHARGE CRITERIA
Upon the patient's discharge, documentation shows evidence of no life-threatening or disabling complications of immobility.

PATIENT-FAMILY TEACHING CHECKLIST
Document evidence that the patient and family demonstrate an understanding of:
___ activity recommendations, restrictions, and limitations
___ measures to avert orthostatic hypotension and activity intolerance
___ indicators of clinically significant activity intolerance
___ signs of complications related to impaired mobility
___ use of any mobility aids.

DOCUMENTATION CHECKLIST
Using outcome criteria as a guide, document:
___ clinical status on admission
___ significant changes in status
___ pertinent laboratory and diagnostic test findings
___ protective measures initiated
___ response to resumption of activity
___ complications of immobility, if any
___ patient-family teaching
___ discharge planning.

ASSOCIATED PLANS OF CARE
Geriatric Considerations
Ineffective Individual Coping
Nutritional Deficit
Sensory-Perceptual Alteration

References
Alessi, C., and Henderson, C. "Constipation and Fecal Impaction in the Long-Term Care Patient," *Clinics in Geriatric Medicine* 4(3): 571-88, 1988.

Hill, S., Milnes, J., Rowe, J., et al. "Nursing the Immobile: A Preliminary Study," *International Journal of Nursing Studies*, 24(2):123-28, 1987.

Holloway, N. *Nursing the Critically Ill Adult*, 3rd ed. Menlo Park, Calif.: Addison-Wesley Publishing Co., 1988.

Holm, K., and Hedricks, C. "Immobility and Bone Loss in the Aging Adult," *Critical Care Nurse Quarterly* 12(1): 46-51, June 1989.

Kozier, B., and Erb, G. *Fundamentals of Nursing: Concepts, Process and Practice*, 4th ed. Menlo Park, Calif.: Addison-Wesley Publishing Co., 1991.

Lincoln, R., and Roberts, R. "Continence Issues in Acute Care," *Nursing Clinics of North America* 24(3):741-54, September 1989.

Luckmann, J., and Sorensen, K. *Medical-Surgical Nursing: A Psychophysiologic Approach,* 3rd ed. Philadelphia: W.B. Saunders Co., 1987.

Milde, F. "Focus: Impaired Physical Mobility," *Journal of Gerontological Nursing* 14(3):20-24, March 1988.

Olson, E.V., et al. "The Hazards of Immobility," *American Journal of Nursing* 90(3):43-48, March 1990.

Rubin, M. "The Physiology of Bed Rest," *American Journal of Nursing* 88(1):50-56, January 1988.

Selikson, S., Damus, K., and Hamerman, D. "Risk Factors Associated with Immobility," *Journal of the American Geriatrics Society* 36(8):707-12, 1988.

Walsh, M., and Judd, M. "Long-term Immobility and Self-Care: The Orem Nursing Approach," *Nursing Standard* 3(41):34-36, July 8, 1989.

Ineffective Family Coping

Introduction
DEFINITION AND TIME FOCUS
A patient's hospitalization can cause a crisis within the family because their usual coping and support mechanisms may be overwhelmed. This plan focuses on the family's ability to manage the stressors that affect them during the patient's hospital stay.

ETIOLOGY AND PRECIPITATING FACTORS
• illness or injury of family member
• disruption of usual family activities and routines
• family disunity
• loss of control by patient or family
• role changes within the family
• unfamiliar hospital environment, restricted visitation of loved ones
• loss of income, cost of medical care
• poverty

Focused assessment guidelines
NURSING HISTORY (Functional health pattern findings for family system)

Nutritional-metabolic pattern
• may neglect nutritional intake while family member is hospitalized

Sleep-rest pattern
• may not get adequate sleep or rest while family member is hospitalized

Cognitive-perceptual pattern
• may have inaccurate understanding of the patient's condition
• may not request clarification of information about the patient's situation
• may pay attention to only some aspects of the information given
• may lack skills or education to understand complex medical information

Self-perception—self-concept pattern
• may report feeling unable to cope with current situation
• may verbalize anxiety, fear, or anger
• may express unresolved feelings of guilt or hostility
• may lack awareness of each other's feelings or perceptions
• may appear uncomfortable with each other's emotional reactions

Role-relationship pattern
• may not interact with each other
• may have difficulty communicating feelings and perceptions to each other
• may experience difficulty reaching decisions
• may have rigidly established roles within the family structure
• may be unable to provide emotional support for each other

Coping—stress tolerance pattern
• may use inappropriate coping methods in the present situation
• may have used non-growth-promoting methods to handle past crises (denial, depression, violence, or substance abuse)
• may not identify all coping strategies available within the family system
• may exhibit regression or increased dependence by relying on others to solve problems

Value-belief pattern
• may have value conflicts between family members
• may have unrealistic beliefs about health, disease, or roles and abilities of other family members

PHYSICAL FINDINGS
Not applicable

DIAGNOSTIC STUDIES
Not applicable

POTENTIAL COMPLICATIONS
• high anxiety levels among family members
• transfer of anxiety from family to patient
• unrealistic expectations of patient—for example, expecting full recovery of neurologic function in brain-damaged person
• unrealistic expectations of other family members—for example, expecting uncommunicative member to become emotionally supportive in crisis
• inattention to family members' physical and psychosocial needs
• inadequate preparation for the patient's discharge or death
• disintegration of the family unit

Nursing diagnosis: *Ineffective family coping related to illness and hospitalization of family member*

NURSING PRIORITY: Help the family identify, develop, and use healthy coping skills.

Interventions

1. Assess and document the origins of the crisis and the family members' responses to it. Identify factors contributing to vulnerability in a crisis state. Observe nonverbal behaviors, such as eye contact and body posture.

2. Demonstrate interest and concern for the patient's family members. Acknowledge the family's feelings about the situation—for example, "This must be very difficult for you."

3. Take measures to minimize the family members' level of anxiety: provide a quiet, private place for discussion; avoid elaborate information or unnecessary questions; and remain available to the family. Document the family's initial status and response to nursing interventions.

4. Provide accurate, timely information about the patient's treatment and care. Give explanations in lay terms, encourage questions, and introduce topics likely to be of interest. Reinforce information given by the doctor. Document the information given to the family.

5. Clarify family members' perceptions of the information given to them. Document the family's level of understanding.

6. Reduce the stress associated with the hospital environment. Individualize visitation privileges. Orient the family to hospital facilities. Arrange for a quiet place for the family to meet with the doctor. Provide pillows and blankets for family members spending the night at the hospital.

7. Assist family members to care for their own physical and psychosocial needs. Encourage adequate rest periods. Reinforce the need for adequate dietary intake.

8. Encourage family members to express their feelings about the impact of the patient's illness. Ask open-ended questions. Listen carefully to each person. Support communication among family members. Observe how feelings are expressed and how family members behave. Document the family's response and behavior. Identify, when possible, the family member who is the primary health and illness resource for the family, and include that person in all teaching. Also, make sure that person has an adequate support system.

Rationales

1. Consider situational factors (such as illness or death), transitional states (developmental turning point or life-cycle phase), and sociocultural factors. Families in which several of these factors are present are at higher risk for crisis development. Nonverbal behaviors, such as clenched fists or lack of eye contact, provide valuable clues about the family's emotional state.

2. Approaching the family with a warm and respectful attitude lays the groundwork for developing a trusting relationship.

3. In states of heightened anxiety, the ability to think clearly, handle new information, and make appropriate decisions is impaired. Minimizing distractions reduces anxiety and helps family members regain control of their thinking processes.

4. Family members must be well informed to develop an accurate perception of the patient's illness or injury. Medical jargon may increase anxiety in some individuals. Clear, simple explanations will be understood best. Encouraging questions dispels possible discomfort over not knowing answers, while suggesting topics reduces possible discomfort over not knowing what to ask. Anxiety and misunderstanding can be minimized by giving explanations in lay terms and by reinforcing or clarifying information given by the doctor. Family members who understand their own problems as well as the patient's can recognize their needs and identify appropriate solutions.

5. Do not assume that what was said was what the family heard. Asking for feedback and clarification allows the nurse to determine the family members' actual level of understanding.

6. Manipulating the hospital environment decreases the family's physical distress in adjusting to the patient's hospitalization.

7. Development of problem-solving skills and effective coping strategies is impaired when family members are physically exhausted, malnourished, or stressed by unmet emotional or psychosocial needs.

8. Awareness of feelings and the ability to express them clearly and appropriately are important elements of healthy coping behaviors. Help-seeking behaviors are aided by intrafamily communication and realistic discussion of how the patient's illness may affect family functioning. By using open-ended questions, the nurse can guide the family's communication. Listening to the family and helping them clarify their feelings and perceptions will help the nurse identify areas where additional support is needed. Most families have one member who is the informed "health liaison person" who may act as caregiver, teacher, and interpreter. Acknowledgment of this role facilitates therapeutic intervention.

9. Promote awareness of family strengths by identifying areas in which the members work well together. Document identified family strengths and weaknesses. Direct nursing interventions toward encouraging family strengths— for example, support family efforts to learn care techniques or to bring in special items from home, as permitted.

9. Acknowledging family strengths, such as closeness, open communication, or willingness to help each other, helps the family identify their resources for coping with the crisis.

10. Facilitate family communication when dysfunctions are present. Encourage verbalization and recognition of feelings. Provide referrals to other professionals (mental health liaison nurse, social worker, clinical specialist, clinical psychologist, or member of the clergy) when family problems lie outside the role of the staff nurse.

10. The nurse's role is to listen, support, and clarify, not to solve the family's problems. The nurse helps the family to identify available resources and to make informed decisions about using them.

11. Focus on immediate, concrete problems.

11. A primary nursing focus is to decrease the family members' anxiety so they can pull their thinking together and make use of problem-solving skills. In many cases, anxiety can be decreased by attending to easily removed stressors; for example, refer an outof-town family to the social services department to arrange for housing while the patient is hospitalized.

12. Help the family develop a realistic appraisal of the situation and an action plan. Explore coping skills and support systems available to the family. Help them identify resources, such as friends, other family members, self-help groups related to the diagnosis, home health care nurses, or homemaking assistance. Ensure that the plan is appropriate to the family's functional level, dependence needs, and life-style.

12. In establishing an action plan, family members need to match their own needs and the patient's with available resources. By providing such information, the nurse helps the family develop a plan to meet their needs.

13. Encourage independent decision making by family members.

13. The nurse who makes decisions for family members invites their dependence.

14. With the patient and family, follow up and evaluate the action plan's implementation.

14. Evaluation of the action plan reinforces successful strategies and may suggest additional or alternate interventions. Evaluation done with the family is an excellent way to provide positive feedback and acknowledge their new coping skills.

15. Avoid imposing personal values or codes of behavior on family members.

15. In order to intervene effectively with a family in crisis, the nurse must develop an awareness of personal value systems and beliefs related to cultural norms. This allows the nurse to view the family's problems without imposing personal values on the family system.

16. Additional individualized interventions: _____

16. Rationales: _____

Target outcome criteria

Within 2 days of the patient's admission, family members will:
• verbalize feelings to the nurse
• recognize their physical needs for food and rest.

By the time of the patient's discharge, family members will:
• verbalize feelings appropriately to each other
• participate actively in caring for the ill family member
• use healthy coping mechanisms
• demonstrate listening and supportive behaviors to each other
• identify resources within and outside the family
• develop a plan or strategy to provide necessary care and support for the ill family member after discharge.

GENERAL PLANS OF CARE

Discharge planning

NURSING DISCHARGE CRITERIA

Upon the patient's discharge, documentation shows evidence of:
• identification of the impact of the patient's illness on family function
• plan for dealing with changes within the family
• identification of internal and external resources available to family members
• initial contact with selected external resources.

PATIENT-FAMILY TEACHING CHECKLIST

Document evidence that the patient and family demonstrate an understanding of:
___ extent and implication of the patient's illness and limitations
___ changes in family roles and function, such as new responsibilities each member must assume to facilitate care of the patient at home
___ resources and referrals available to the family.

DOCUMENTATION CHECKLIST

Using outcome criteria as a guide, document:
___ family's initial emotional status
___ precipitating factors in crisis and meaning of crisis to family members
___ changes in emotional status related to nursing interventions
___ treatment and care information given to family members
___ family's level of understanding of information provided
___ family members' ability to express feelings
___ identified family strengths and weaknesses
___ referrals to community resources.

ASSOCIATED PLANS OF CARE

Dying
Grieving
Ineffective Individual Coping
Knowledge Deficit

References

Caine, R.M. "Families in Crisis: Making the Critical Difference," *Focus on Critical Care* 16(3):184-89, June 1989.

Carpenito, L. *Nursing Diagnosis: Application to Clinical Practice*, 4th ed. Philadelphia: J.B. Lippincott, 1992.

Heiney, S.P. "Assessing and Intervening with Dysfunctional Families," *Oncology Nursing Forum* 15(5):585-90, September-October 1988.

Hickey, M. "What are the Needs of Families of Critically Ill Patients? A Review of the Literature since 1976," *Heart & Lung* 19(4):401-15, July 1990.

Kleeman, K.M. "Families in Crisis due to Multiple Traumas," *Critical Care Clinics of North America* 1(1):23-31, March 1989.

GENERAL PLANS OF CARE

Ineffective Individual Coping

Introduction
DEFINITION AND TIME FOCUS
Ineffective coping is the inability to use adaptive behaviors in response to a perceived threat, with a resulting disruption in physiologic and psychological balance. The patient is unable to find a solution to whatever is causing feelings of insecurity and uncertainty. This plan focuses on the patient who is hospitalized for an acute illness or an exacerbation of a chronic condition, and whose usual coping mechanisms are not effective in maintaining psychological equilibrium.

ETIOLOGY AND PRECIPITATING FACTORS
• stimuli likely to cause ineffective coping in illness
  —pain and incapacitation
  —lack of sleep
  —stressful hospital environment and treatment procedures
  —loss of control over what is happening to self
  —loss of hope
  —lack of meaningful contact with loved ones
  —uncertain future
• conditions necessary for a stimulus to cause ineffective coping
  —perception of a harmful stimulus, or cues that a harmful stimulus is imminent
  —perception that the harmful stimulus threatens the individual's goals or values
  —perception that the patient's resources are not equal to coping with the threat

Focused assessment guidelines
NURSING HISTORY (Functional health pattern findings)

Health perception — health management pattern
• commonly perceives illness and hospitalization as a loss of control that threatens fulfillment of usual roles or threatens life itself
• may report drastically reduced ability to solve problems effectively
  —may select course of action without weighing alternatives
  —may be overwhelmed by alternatives and unable to select a course of action
• may not follow treatment plan

Nutritional-metabolic pattern
• may report anorexia, nausea, or vomiting
• may report weight loss from anorexia
• may report frequent overeating to deal with stress

Elimination pattern
• may report diarrhea or constipation from dietary changes or stress

Activity-exercise pattern
• may report occasional hyperactivity and inability to rest
• may report occasional withdrawal, listlessness, or fatigue

Sleep-rest pattern
• may report sleep disturbance
  —may sleep more than usual
  —may have difficulty falling asleep
  —may report falling asleep but awakening early, then being unable to return to sleep (early morning insomnia)
  —may report frequent night-time awakening

Cognitive-perceptual pattern
• may show diminished ability to view the world objectively
• may show decreased ability to take in information
• typically expresses lack of information necessary to make decisions
• may begin to suspect intentions of caregivers

Self-perception — self-concept pattern
• may feel the threat is greater than available internal resources to combat it
• may feel unable to control events affecting the situation

Role-relationship pattern
• may report or show decreased ability to communicate needs
• may report feeling isolated and unable to respond to caring from others
• may report occasional inability to control impulsive behavior; may become suicidal or hostile and aggressive

Sexuality-reproductive pattern
• may report loss of libido, impotence, or orgasmic dysfunction

Coping — stress tolerance pattern
• may report experiencing physiologic responses related to sympathetic nervous system stimulation, such as tachycardia
• may report increased number of infections related to alteration in the immune system
• may have denied symptoms and delayed seeking treatment
• may display various negative coping behaviors, depending on individual and environmental factors
  —anger and hostility
  —anxiety and hyperactivity
  —depression and withdrawal
  —suicidal ideation

• may behave in a manner that alienates caregivers and removes a source of support
• may have a history of ineffective coping mechanisms, such as drug or alcohol abuse, nicotine addiction, or overeating

Value-belief pattern
• may have experienced a loss of faith related to feelings of hopelessness and abandonment

PHYSICAL FINDINGS
General appearance
• anxious facial expression
• flat affect
• poor eye contact

Cardiovascular
• elevated blood pressure
• increased heart rate
• occasionally, increased ventricular arrhythmias

Pulmonary
• increased rate and depth of respirations

Gastrointestinal
• vomiting
• diarrhea
• if stress ulcer develops, GI bleeding

Neurologic
• occasionally, dilated pupils (sympathetic nervous system response)
• restlessness
• lethargy

Integumentary
• occasionally, diaphoresis

Musculoskeletal
• increased muscle tension and pain

DIAGNOSTIC STUDIES
In the clinical setting, laboratory tests are not normally done to identify ineffective coping. Remember, however, that physiologic responses to stress can mimic disease.
• arterial blood gas measurements may reveal respiratory alkalosis from an increased rate and depth of respiration (hyperventilation)
• white blood cell count may be increased
• mental status examination:
  —appearance may yield clues about self-perception (patients coping ineffectively may not care about their appearance)
  —behavior (facial expression, posture, body movements, tone of voice) is an indicator of the person's

ability with self-expression, an important coping skill; behavior may vary, depending on the patient's expressive style. The relationship of the patient with caregivers is also important to assess: Is the patient controlling, passive, aggressive, suspicious, uncooperative? May demonstrate inability to solve problems
  —feelings shown indicate which emotions the patient expresses and their appropriateness to the situation; wide variety of feelings possible, ranging from anxiety to anger to depression and typically including feelings of isolation and hopelessness
  —perceptions indicate the patient's view of the situation; perceptions of threat are based on previous experience, values, and beliefs along with perception of inadequate resources in relation to the magnitude of the threat. Which coping mechanisms were used in the past? Which were useful? Which are potentially harmful—for example, smoking, alcohol use, or drug use?
• suicide assessment—a patient who feels hopeless and helpless needs to be asked about presence of suicidal thoughts; this question does not cause a patient to think about suicide but instead provides an opportunity to talk about these disturbing feelings. Factors associated with high risk include:
  —high level of anxiety or panic
  —severe depression
  —minimal ability to perform activities of daily living
  —few or no sources of support or significant others
  —continued abuse of alcohol or drugs, or both
  —negative view of previous psychiatric help (if applicable)
  —one or more previous suicide attempts
  —marked hostility
  —frequent or constant thoughts of suicide
  —suicide plan that is specific in method and timing
  —possession of means to carry out the plan, such as physical capacity and weapon
(See also *Assessment of suicide potential*, page 34, in the "Grieving" plan.)

POTENTIAL COMPLICATIONS
• physiologic
  —increased risk of falls and accidents
  —ventricular arrhythmias
  —increased susceptibility to infections
  —sudden death (possible)
• psychological
  —suicide or homicide
  —major depression
  —reactive psychosis
  —disintegration of family unit

Nursing diagnosis: *Ineffective individual coping related to perception of a harmful stimulus*

NURSING PRIORITIES: (a) Establish rapport and trust, (b) accurately identify threat and coping resources, (c) intervene to optimize coping skills, and (d) evaluate the effectiveness of interventions.

Interventions

1. Form a positive relationship with the patient.
• Convey a sense of caring and concern for what happens to the patient.
• Use appropriate eye contact.
• Convey feelings of comfort and relaxation by approaching the patient calmly, including the patient in all bedside conversations, and speaking in a well-modulated tone.
• Identify personal reactions to the patient's coping style that could interfere with formation of a helping relationship. Avoid judging the patient's behavior.

2. Rule out organic causes for such behavioral changes as decreased alertness, impaired memory, confusion, restlessness, or depression.

3. Provide factual information about the illness and treatment plan. Reinforce information the patient has received from the doctor. Be prepared to repeat information in clear, concise language.

4. With the patient, identify the source of the threat.

5. Help the patient be specific about what seems threatening.

6. With the patient, identify modifiable components of the threat.

7. Help the patient identify personal strengths and external resources, such as family, friends, and economic means.

8. Identify external resources and make appropriate referrals—for example, for social services, spiritual counseling, or psychiatric interventions.

9. Keep pain at a tolerable level.

Rationales

1. Patients report that feelings of being uncared for interfere with their recovery and contribute to feelings of hopelessness. An ineffective relationship with caregivers drains energy that could be better used for healing. Conversely, patients who feel positive about their nurses say this gives them an energy that helps with healing, decreases isolation, and increases coping ability. People express anxiety, pain, and needs for privacy and intimacy in a various ways, depending on their cultural and personal biases. For example, if the patient who feels comfortable expressing pain openly is cared for by a nurse who believes that pain should be tolerated in silence, an ineffective nurse-patient relationship may result. Recognizing one's cultural and personal biases is the first step in avoiding prejudicial responses to the patient's behavior, which is a unique pattern used to decrease anxiety.

2. Behavioral changes that appear to be signs of ineffective coping may actually represent such physiologic problems as hypoxia, electrolyte imbalance, or drug toxicity. Assuming that all behavioral responses are related to psychological mechanisms may delay needed medical treatment.

3. For problem solving to begin, the patient needs accurate information. Patients who are coping ineffectively have a decreased ability to hear and assimilate information.

4. Whether or not a stimulus is felt as threatening depends on values, beliefs, and the perception of available resources. The patient may not perceive an obvious, identifiable threat (such as a diagnosis of cancer) as the primary threat. Conversely, what seems routine to the nurse may be frightening to the patient.

5. Patients may have misconceptions about what is happening to them. If they can specify their fears, the nurse can plan specific actions, such as providing information that helps the patient see the situation realistically.

6. People coping ineffectively are often unable to separate their situation into manageable parts; instead, they view the problem as overwhelming and unmanageable. If they can view the problem in its component parts, their anxiety may be reduced and effective coping behaviors become more possible.

7. People in crisis may not identify their strengths. They will need assistance in assessing resources and identifying ways to activate them.

8. Expansion of the patient's base of support helps decrease the perceived magnitude of the specific threat.

9. Pain is a common source of fear. Uncontrolled pain increases anxiety and decreases the energy available for coping.

GENERAL PLANS OF CARE

10. Ensure adequate nutrition and sleep.

11. Control environmental stimuli that drain adaptive energy needed to maintain psychological equilibrium: Provide privacy for all invasive procedures and for nursing and self-care activities; eliminate conversation around the bedside that does not include the patient; and decrease environmental noise.

12. Offer alternative strategies to counteract the effects of the threat—for example, guided imagery, relaxation techniques, or back rubs.

13. Give choices related to the patient's care and situation whenever possible.

14. Provide opportunities for loved ones to interact with the patient in meaningful ways.

15. Assess responses to nursing interventions, and collaborate with the doctor to determine if pharmacologic intervention would be helpful.

16. Additional individualized interventions:_____

_____

10. Inadequate diet and lack of sleep are stressors themselves and, as such, decrease the amount of energy available for coping and adaptation.

11. Every stimulus in the environment is a potential threat. Stimuli not normally viewed as threatening may, in combination, create more stress and decrease coping ability.

12. The relaxation response is the physiologic opposite of anxiety. Relaxation techniques may help the patient cope with stress and regain control.

13. Maintaining some ability to control one's life helps to combat feelings of helplessness.

14. A positive response from loved ones encourages a more positive response to treatment and decreases the sense of isolation.

15. Antianxiety medications may be helpful in decreasing potentially harmful physiologic and psychological effects of anxiety. Antidepressants may be useful in patients with signs of severe depression.

16. Rationales: _____

_____

Target outcome criteria
Within 2 days of identification of ineffective coping, the patient will:
• express an accurate understanding of the current situation and treatment plan
• state that any pain is within tolerable limits
• participate in developing a plan of care
• use support offered by caregivers.

Discharge planning
NURSING DISCHARGE CRITERIA
Upon the patient's discharge, documentation shows evidence of:
• perception of increased ability to cope with the situation
• ability to name resources appropriate to the situation
• increased ability to manage the current situation by defining the problem and reasonable solutions.

PATIENT-FAMILY TEACHING CHECKLIST
Document evidence that the patient and family demonstrate an understanding of:
___ diagnosis, treatment plan, and prognosis
___ expected physiologic responses during recovery
___ community resources appropriate to perceived problems
___ appropriate alternative coping strategies
___ how to contact the doctor.

DOCUMENTATION CHECKLIST
Using outcome criteria as a guide, document:
___ coping status on admission
___ significant changes in appearance, affect, behavior, and perception
___ psychological responses to hospitalization and interventions
___ significant physiologic stress responses
___ sleep patterns
___ nutritional intake
___ pain control
___ response to caregivers
___ response to interventions designed to increase coping skills
___ suicide risk
___ referrals made
___ patient-family teaching
___ discharge planning.

ASSOCIATED PLANS OF CARE
Dying
Grieving
Ineffective Family Coping
Knowledge Deficit
Pain

References

Clark, S. "Ineffective Coping," in *Cardiac Critical Care Nursing.* Edited by Kern. Frederick, Md.: Aspen Press, 1988.

Clark, S. "Nursing Diagnosis: Ineffective Coping. Part 1: A Theoretical Framework; Part 2: Planning Care," *Heart and Lung* 16(6):670-85, November 1987.

Cronin, S.N., and Harrison, B. "Importance of Nurse Caring Behaviors as Perceived by Patients After Myocardial Infarction," *Heart and Lung* 17(4):374-380, July 1988.

Gorman, L.M., Sultan, D., and Luna-Raines, M. *Psychosocial Nursing Handbook for the Non-psychiatric Nurse.* Baltimore: Williams and Wilkins, 1989.

Larson, P.J. "Comparison of Cancer Patients' and Professional Nurses' Perceptions of Important Nurse Caring Behaviors," *Heart and Lung* 16(2):187-192, 1987.

Lazarus, R. *Psychological Stress and the Coping Process.* New York: McGraw-Hill Book Co., 1966.

Moos, R.H., and Tsu, V.S. "The Crisis of Physical Illness: An Overview," in *Coping with Physical Illness.* Edited by Moos, R. New York: Plenum Medical Book Co., 1977.

Weisman, A.D. "Coping with Illness," in *Massachusetts General Hospital Handbook of General Hospital Psychiatry,* 2nd ed. Edited by Hackett, T.P., and Cassem, N.H. St. Louis: C.V. Mosby, 1987.

GENERAL PLANS OF CARE

Knowledge Deficit

Introduction
DEFINITION AND TIME FOCUS
A lack of knowledge or skills necessary for health recovery or maintenance comprises a knowledge deficit. This teaching plan focuses on the acutely ill patient and family. Although a major teaching program during this period is inappropriate for most patients, you can capitalize on unexpected teaching opportunities to meet immediate learning needs as well as to identify long-range learning needs. The latter are usually addressed after the patient has been discharged or transferred to a more conducive environment.

Through expert teaching, the nurse can provide a context for the patient and family to understand the rationale for therapeutic interventions. Teaching is most effective when it pervades all phases of patient care.

ETIOLOGY AND PRECIPITATING FACTORS
• unfamiliar diagnostic procedure
• new diagnosis
• alteration in existing health problem
• unfamiliar or altered treatment plan
• complex treatment regimen
• denial
• anxiety

Focused assessment guidelines
NURSING HISTORY (Functional health pattern findings)
Note: Because each patient's knowledge deficit will be individual, this section presents an assessment guide of teaching and learning factors.

Health perception — health management pattern
• Did the patient delay seeking needed medical attention?
• Does the patient lack knowledge about the disorder?
• Does the patient express lack of confidence in managing the condition?
• Does the patient express misconceptions about health status?
• Has the patient failed to comply with recommended health practices?
• Does the patient fail to carry out self-care, even though physically able?

Nutritional-metabolic pattern
• Does the patient express concerns about the effects of the disorder on nutrition and eating habits?
• Has the patient had difficulty staying on a prescribed dietary regimen?

Activity-exercise pattern
• Does the patient express concerns about life-changing physical limitations because of the disorder?

Cognitive-perceptual pattern
• Does the patient express concerns about specific details of a diagnostic or therapeutic procedure?
• Does the patient have sensory deficits, such as visual or hearing impairments?
• Does the patient lack psychomotor skills needed to maintain a home treatment regimen?
• Has the patient experienced confusion or changes in thought processes from the disorder?
• Has the patient shown signs of misinterpreting information, such as by asking inappropriate questions?

Self-perception — self-concept pattern
• Does the patient express concerns about an inability to maintain the treatment regimen?
• Does the patient report anxiety about changes in body image from the disorder?

Role-relationship pattern
• Does the patient want a family member present or available during procedures?
• Does the patient express concerns about job, income, or family responsibilities because of the disorder?
• Does the patient express concerns about the family's response to life-style changes because of the disorder?

Sexuality-reproductive pattern
• Does the patient report concern about the disorder's impact on sexual activity?
• Does the patient express concern about the impact of changes in sexual activity on a spouse or partner?

Coping — stress tolerance pattern
• Does the patient display an unusual amount of anxiety?
• Does the patient display denial of the disorder?
• Does the patient report depression because of life-style changes caused by the disorder?
• Does the patient express concerns about coping behaviors and motivation?

PHYSICAL FINDINGS
Not applicable

DIAGNOSTIC STUDIES
Not applicable

POTENTIAL COMPLICATION
• Exacerbation of disorder

Nursing diagnosis: *High risk for knowledge deficit related to lack of readiness to learn**

NURSING PRIORITY: Determine readiness to learn.

Interventions

1. Assess the impact of the patient's disorder on life-style.

2. Determine the patient's stage of adaptation to the disorder: shock and disbelief, developing awareness, or resolution and reorganization. Dovetail teaching objectives and content with psychological issues during each phase.

3. Assess the patient's physical readiness to learn: Is the patient physiologically stable, rested, and pain-free? If not, defer a formal teaching program.

4. Determine the patient's motivation to learn. For example, has the patient asked appropriate questions about status or care? Is the patient preoccupied, distracted, or emotionally labile?

5. Determine the general pattern of health maintenance; for example, has the patient sought regular medical checkups, followed previous health recommendations, eaten a balanced diet, and exercised regularly?

6. Assess the patient's current knowledge of the disorder and its implications, the likelihood of complications, and the likelihood of cure or disease control. Specifically ask about the doctor's explanations, the patient's past experiences, and information received from family, friends, and the media.

7. Ask how much the patient wants to know, if possible. Consider the patient's preference for information in planning teaching.

Rationales

1. The degree of impact determines the extent of teaching necessary. Areas of impact provide foci around which learning experiences should be structured.

2. Different psychological work occurs in each of these phases. Attempting to provide teaching inappropriate for a particular phase results in increased learner anxiety or irritation and inability to absorb information.

3. Teaching is most effective when the patient is ready to learn. Readiness to learn depends on physical as well as psychological factors. Determining readiness to learn requires weighing the interaction of numerous variables. Learning requires energy that will not be available if the patient is unstable, tired, or in pain. Because of shortened hospital stays, few patients reach physical or emotional readiness to learn extensive amounts of information before discharge.

4. Motivation is the crucial variable in learning and may be absent initially because of anxiety or preoccupation with personal needs. Prolonged absence of interest in learning about the condition may be a clue to an underlying emotional disorder requiring treatment before the patient can assume independent selfcare. Motivation may be developed through teaching by linking relevant information to the patient's particular concerns.

5. The general pattern can provide clues to overall acceptance of responsibility for self-care and receptivity to teaching.

6. Adults learn best when teaching builds on previous knowledge or experience. Assessing recall of the doctor's explanations as well as the patient's past experiences and exposure to health information provides an opportunity for evaluating attitudes and the accuracy and completeness of knowledge.

7. Research suggests that the common assumption that teaching reduces anxiety or otherwise helps the patient is not always true; people vary in the degree of detail they find helpful. According to Watkins, Weaver, and Odegaard (1986), learners fall into two groups: those who cope with a threatening experience by avoiding it ("blunters") and those who cope by learning as much as possible about it ("monitors"). Blunters generally want to know relatively little about impending experiences, whereas monitors want to know a great deal. Providing a blunter with detailed information increases anxiety, whereas withholding it from a monitor worsens stress. When possible, match preference and teaching appropriately to respect individual differences and support the patient's preferred learning style.

GENERAL PLANS OF CARE

---

*Because of the importance of knowledge deficit as a patient problem and because of the large number of possible interventions, problems in this plan are subdivided by cause.

8. Determine learning needs. Consider needs expressed by the patient and family; predictable disorder-related concerns and responses; and activities necessary to monitor health status, prevent disease, implement prescribed therapy, and prevent complications or recurrence.

8. Learning needs determine appropriate content. Learning occurs most rapidly when it is relevant to current needs and past experiences. Responding to expressed needs displays sensitivity to the patient's and family's concerns. Identifying predictable concerns and responses and necessary self-care activities helps the nurse fulfill learning needs of which the patient and family may be unaware.

9. Estimate learning capacity. Assess the patient's age; language skills; ability to read, write, and reason; and educational, religious, and cultural background.

9. Sociocultural factors affect the speed and degree of learning. Awareness of the patient's age, background, and general capacity for logical thought and self-expression helps the nurse present material at an appropriate learning level.

10. Additional individualized interventions: _____

10. Rationales: _____

Target outcome criteria
Before initiation of teaching, the patient will:
• be physiologically stable
• discuss current knowledge of the disorder when asked

• identify primary perceived learning needs
• display motivation to learn, such as by asking appropriate questions.

Nursing diagnosis: *High risk for knowledge deficit related to teaching program inappropriate for current needs*

NURSING PRIORITY: Plan an individualized teaching strategy.

Interventions

1. Determine realistic goals for learning while the patient is in the hospital. Work with the patient and family to ensure that goals are mutually acceptable.

2. Determine what to teach by assessing what is essential from the patient's viewpoint. Set priorities for content by dividing it into "need to know now" and "need to know later" categories.

3. Provide a logical sequence to the information presented. In general, teach the acutely ill patient only:
• information about expressed concerns

• high-priority information—specific teaching without which the patient's condition may be seriously jeopardized.

4. Select appropriate teaching methods:
• individual bedside instruction
• discussions
• demonstrations.

Rationales

1. Goals determine content. Goal-directed learning is more efficient than fragmented, unfocused learning. Active participation in goal setting increases the likelihood that the patient and family will understand goals and support them.

2. Because the patient's attention span may be limited and the hospital stay may be short, set priorities for content. Content largely determines the appropriate teaching method.

3. Proper sequencing allows the patient to build upon current knowledge and experience.

• Learning is strongest when it fulfills perceived needs. Dealing with initial concerns displays sensitivity to the patient, helps establish rapport and trust, and frees the patient's energy to focus on further learning. In general, only crucial questions are answered for the acutely ill patient; the remainder are deferred.

• Presenting essential information early in the teaching period helps ensure that all the critical information will have been covered by the time of discharge.

4. Although various teaching methods exist (see *Teaching strategies*), individual instruction, discussion, and demonstration are most appropriate in the hospital because of constraints imposed by the patient's condition and the environment.

TEACHING STRATEGIES

Method	Characteristics	Most appropriate for	Disadvantages
Individual bedside instruction	One-on-one interaction between teacher and patient Immediate feedback Informal	Acute phase Sensitive topics "Private" patient Emotionally labile patient Patient with language difficulties Patient with limited education	Time consuming
Group session	Small or large number of patients Informal Interchange of ideas	General content Patients at similar readiness levels	Lack of individualization
Lecture	Highly structured Efficient	Large amount of factual content Rehabilitation program	Lack of opportunity for teacher-patient interaction Possible failure to engage the patient's interest (Disadvantages may be overcome by alternating lectures with interactive learning opportunities, such as question-and-answer periods or skill demonstrations.)
Discussion	Interchange of ideas More informal than lecture More opportunity to adapt content and evaluate patient comprehension	Acute phase Sensitive topics When attitudinal change is desired Highly verbal patient	Time consuming May be uncomfortable for some patients because of their cultural norms against expression
Demonstration and return demonstration	Observation and supervised practice Immediate feedback	Teaching psychomotor skills	Requires actual equipment

5. Be creative in choosing appropriate teaching materials, such as booklets, instruction sheets, films, videotapes, models or dolls, slides, and audiotapes. Consider the advantages, availability, patient's learning style, and the learning environment.

5. The more senses involved in learning, the more likely the patient will retain the information. Printed materials provide consistency, reinforce orally presented information, and provide a source to which the patient can refer as needed. Models (for example, of the heart and a pacemaker) help the patient visualize how something works. Dolls may be useful adjuncts for teaching children. Slides, audiotapes, films, and videotapes can vividly present an experience—for example, by showing a diagnostic procedure from the patient's viewpoint. These audiovisuals may not be suitable, however, unless the patient is stable enough to focus attention on them and the learning environment is conducive to using them. If used, they should be supplemented by a one-on-one follow-up discussion.

6. Determine how best to teach the content to an individual patient at a particular time. Consider the advantages and disadvantages of various teaching methods, the appropriateness and availability of educational materials, and the patient's personality.

6. In many cases, combinations of teaching methods and educational materials can achieve a desired goal. Selecting the combination most appropriate to this patient makes learning "come alive."

7. Decide who should teach what: Consider the primary nurse, a nurse with special related expertise, and other health care professionals. Mention the availability of visitors from community or self-help groups when the patient is more stable physiologically.

7. Depending on the content and patient preferences, different teachers may be necessary or appropriate to reinforce learning. Support groups may provide especially relevant information based on personal experience with the patient's disorder. In many cases, their credibility makes them invaluable in helping the patient accept the need for long-term education and rehabilitation. Their visits may need to be deferred until after the patient has stabilized and can benefit from their insights and competencies. Knowing that others have coped productively with similar experiences may provide the patient with hope that facilitates the necessary learning.

8. Decide when to teach.

8. Choosing appropriate times to teach capitalizes on learning readiness. Appropriate sequencing builds upon previously presented material and enhances integration of learning.

9. Plan evaluation strategies, such as observation, questions, and having the patient demonstrate new skills, that are based on goals and objectives.

9. Evaluation commonly is interwoven with the presentation. Clear evaluation plans help ensure measurable goals and increase the likelihood that the nurse will recognize spontaneous opportunities for evaluation and respond appropriately to them.

10. Communicate the teaching strategy to other professionals involved in the patient's care.

10. Communication enhances consistency of information provided by caregivers, permits appropriate reinforcement, and minimizes unnecessary repetition.

11. Identify and document long-range learning needs. If the patient is transferred to another unit, communicate learning needs to colleagues on the receiving unit and arrange for continuation of the teaching plan.

11. The patient's condition, extensiveness of learning needs, and the busy unit atmosphere may complicate the patient's learning before transfer. Documentation and communication of long-range learning needs allow personalization of ongoing educational efforts.

12. Additional individualized interventions: _____

12. Rationales: _____

Target outcome criteria
According to individual readiness, the patient will:
• identify priority learning needs
• participate in goal setting.

Nursing diagnosis: *High risk for knowledge deficit related to inadequate or ineffective implementation of the teaching plan*

NURSING PRIORITY: Implement an individualized teaching plan that maximizes learning, retention, and compliance.

Interventions

1. Incorporate teaching into other nursing activities. Be alert for unexpected teaching opportunities; for example, use symptomatic episodes (such as an insulin reaction in a new diabetic) to help the patient and family learn to identify symptoms.

Rationales

1. The hectic pace of most units allows little time for extended teaching sessions. Incorporating teaching into other activities increases the likelihood of accomplishing it and contributes to an atmosphere of naturalness and informality. Activity-related teaching also reinforces learning (for example, teaching stoma care whenever the stoma is visible). The immediacy of a symptomatic episode makes it a powerful teaching tool for establishing the importance of the patient's and family's active involvement in learning.

2. Present yourself as enthusiastic, knowledgeable, and approachable.

2. Enthusiasm is contagious. Presenting yourself as knowledgeable increases credibility, and maintaining approachability allows the patient to feel comfortable capitalizing on your expertise.

3. Present manageable amounts of information at any one time.

3. Too much information at one time causes confusion. The patient may lose sight of key points.

4. Provide simple explanations, using easy-to-understand terminology.

4. Medical and nursing jargon distances the patient and family members. Intricate explanations may confuse or overwhelm them.

5. Use review and repetition judiciously, considering individual factors.

5. Physiologic changes, pain medications, anxiety, the unit environment, and the patient's age may contribute to a short attention span and poor retention. (Elderly persons commonly have difficulty remembering details.)

6. Before planned teaching, assess for physiologic needs (such as thirst or an urge to void) and intense emotions. Meet any physiologic needs first, and encourage the patient to express any strong emotions.

6. Unmet physiologic needs and strong emotions interfere with the ability to concentrate on learning.

7. Provide opportunities for immediate application of learning. For example, after you have taught pulse-taking, have the patient count your radial pulse while you take your carotid pulse for comparison.

7. Immediate application improves retention.

8. Ask for feedback: Were the words understandable? Was the presentation too fast, too slow, too much, or too little? Adjust terminology, pace, and amount of information accordingly.

8. The patient may be reluctant to reveal lack of understanding. Soliciting feedback demonstrates respect for the learner and permits adjustments before the patient becomes lost, overwhelmed, or bored.

9. Be alert for signs of pain, fatigue, confusion, or boredom, such as grimacing, fidgeting, yawning, agitation, or lack of eye contact.

9. These nonverbal signs may provide clues to the need for modification or conclusion of the teaching session.

10. Promote a positive outlook; solicit feelings and convey confidence in the patient's ability to learn.

10. The patient may initially feel overwhelmed and insecure about learning because of the magnitude, urgency, or unfamiliarity of necessary adaptations to illness.

11. Encourage active participation. Use interactive teaching methods.

11. Adults learn best when actively involved. Active participation also facilitates changes needed to allow recovery from or adaptation to the patient's disorder.

12. Document teaching sessions. Communicate progress to appropriate caregivers.

12. Documentation provides a teaching record for legal purposes and enhances continuity of teaching among caregivers.

13. Additional individualized interventions: _____

13. Rationales: _____

Target outcome criteria
According to individual readiness, the patient will:
• indicate interest in learning during care activities
• provide relevant feedback.

Nursing diagnosis: *High risk for knowledge deficit related to lack of needed modification in teaching*

NURSING PRIORITIES: (a) Evaluate learning and (b) modify teaching when appropriate.

Interventions

1. During and after teaching, determine what learning has occurred. For example, observe the patient, ask questions, or have the patient demonstrate a new skill.

Rationales

1. Determining learning accomplishment permits resolution of some learning needs and provides guidance for meeting others.

2. With the patient, compare learning learning to date against previously identified goals.

2. Comparison indicates whether goals have been achieved or whether their appropriateness should be re-evaluated.

3. Modify the teaching plan as indicated by unmet goals or new learning needs.

3. Frequent evaluation and modification of the teaching plan ensures that the teaching is tailored to individual learning capabilities and ongoing learning needs.

4. Refer the patient and family to health care and community agencies, as appropriate, before discharge.

4. Needs not met by the time of discharge require follow-up.

5. If the patient is noncompliant, evaluate why. Refer to the noncompliance problem in the "Congestive Heart Failure" plan, page 329, for further information.

5. The patient has the right of control, including the right to reject treatment or teaching. In many cases, the patient has valid reasons for noncompliance; for example, the need to focus energy on meeting basic needs for food, clothing, and shelter may rule out time-consuming self-care practices. The noncompliance problem in the "Congestive Heart Failure" plan details the assessment of noncompliant behavior and appropriate interventions.

6. Additional individualized interventions: _____

6. Rationales: _____

Target outcome criteria
According to individual readiness, the patient will:
• demonstrate learning
• display minimal anxiety about self-care
• express satisfaction with fulfullment of learning needs
• display realistic appraisal of continuing learning needs
• identify appropriate learning resources.

Discharge planning
NURSING DISCHARGE CRITERIA
Upon the patient's discharge, documentation shows evidence of:
• identification of learning needs
• teaching accomplished during the stay.

PATIENT-FAMILY TEACHING CHECKLIST
Document evidence that the patient and family demonstrate an understanding of:
___ key pathophysiologic aspects of the disorder
___ signs and symptoms requiring medical attention
___ dietary modifications, if appropriate
___ medications
___ other therapies
___ community resources for adjustment to life-style changes.

DOCUMENTATION CHECKLIST
Using outcome criteria as a guide, document:
___ assessment of readiness for learning
___ identification of factors that may inhibit learning
___ identification of learning goals
___ response of the patient and family to the teaching plan
___ problems encountered in teaching
___ evaluation of learning.

ASSOCIATED PLANS OF CARE
Ineffective Family Coping
Ineffective Individual Coping
Pain
(Also see the plan for the specific disorder.)

References
Carpenito, L. *Nursing Diagnosis: Application to Clinical Practice,* 4th ed. Philadelphia: J.B. Lippincott Co., 1992.
Cifani, L., and Vargo, R. "Teaching Strategies for the Transplant Recipient: A Review and Future Directions," *Focus on Critical Care* 17(6): 476-79, December 1990.
Gordon, M. *Nursing Diagnosis: Process and Application,* 2nd ed. New York: McGraw-Hill Book Co., 1987.
Scalzi, C., and Burke, L. "Education of the Patient and Family," in *Cardiac Nursing,* 2nd ed. Edited by Underhill, S., et al. Philadelphia: J.B. Lippincott Co., 1989.
Watkins, L., Weaver, L., and Odegaard, V. "Preparation for Cardiac Catheterization: Tailoring the Content of Instruction to Coping Style," *Heart & Lung* 15(4):382-89, July 1986.

Nutritional Deficit

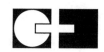

Introduction
DEFINITION AND TIME FOCUS
A nutritional deficit exists when a patient does not ingest or absorb the nutrients necessary to meet metabolic needs. Adequate nutrition is vitally important in recovering from critical illness. Besides glucose needs for cellular metabolism and energy production, many other nutritional needs exist. For example, calories, protein, and potassium are necessary to rebuild injured tissue; proteins, fatty acids, and phosphate are necessary to fight infection; and trace elements are necessary for optimal functioning of enzyme systems. This plan focuses on the acutely ill patient whose survival and recovery may be threatened by inadequate nutrition.

ETIOLOGY AND PRECIPITATING FACTORS
- contraindications to eating, as with peptic ulcer or pancreatitis
- decreased appetite
- inability to chew, as with jaw wiring or poor dentition
- impaired swallowing, as with cerebrovascular accident (CVA), coma, or obstruction
- preexisting malnutrition, as with cancer or anorexia nervosa
- decreased GI motility, as with paralytic ileus
- failure to absorb nutrients, as with malabsorption syndrome or ulcerative colitis
- hypermetabolic state, as with burns or trauma

Focused assessment guidelines
NURSING HISTORY (Functional health pattern findings)

Health perception—health management pattern
- may have history of chronic GI disorder
- may have preexisting debility

Nutritional-metabolic pattern
- may complain of anorexia, indigestion, nausea, or vomiting
- may report difficulty or pain on swallowing
- may refuse to eat

Activity-exercise pattern
- may report weakness or lack of energy

Cognitive-perceptual pattern
- may complain of abdominal pain

Coping—stress tolerance pattern
- may complain of or display depression

PHYSICAL FINDINGS
General appearance
- emaciation (if preexisting malnutrition exists)
- weakness

Gastrointestinal
- weak mastication or swallowing muscles
- inflamed oral cavity or tongue
- vomiting
- absent bowel sounds
- diarrhea

Neurologic
- lethargy
- decreased level of consciousness
- paresthesias
- confusion
- disorientation

Integumentary
- subcutaneous fat loss
- dry, scaly skin
- poor skin turgor
- sparse, lackluster, or easily plucked hair
- dry, cracked lips
- thin, brittle nails

Musculoskeletal
- weakness
- body weight at least 20% below ideal weight for height and frame
- poor muscle tone
- muscle wasting

DIAGNOSTIC STUDIES
See *Diagnostic studies in nutritional deficit,* page 64.

POTENTIAL COMPLICATIONS
- reduced immunocompetence
- electrolyte imbalances
- poor wound healing

DIAGNOSTIC STUDIES IN NUTRITIONAL DEFICIT

To assess muscle protein stores

• *height-weight ratio:* 85% or less of the expected value indicates significant protein-calorie malnutrition. (Height and weight are the most significant factors in determining malnutrition.) In the Harris-Benedict equation, the patient's height-weight ratio predicts calorie expenditure. The creatinine-height ratio predicts skeletal muscle loss. The height-weight ratio is compared with the patient's historical height-weight ratio to determine the severity of malnutrition and the preferred method of feeding the patient.

• *midarm circumference (MAC)* and *midarm muscle circumference (MAMC):* estimate fat and skeletal muscle mass; measurements are compared to a standard table—35% to 40% of normal indicates mild depletion of muscle and fat; 25% to 34%, moderate depletion; and less than 25%, severe depletion. MAMC is calculated using MAC and skin-fold measurements and evaluated in comparison with standard tables.

• *24-hour urine urea nitrogen excretion:* indicates the severity of protein catabolism. 4 to 10 g/day is normal; greater than 10 g/day in a patient with major injuries or sepsis indicates hypermetabolism and a need for increased calories or nitrogen for tissue repair. In a patient who is stable, has no injuries, and is gaining weight, a 24-hour urine urea greater than 10 g/day can indicate overfeeding. (To ensure a positive nitrogen balance in the catabolic patient, approximately 4 to 6 g of nitrogen is given in excess of the amount excreted in the urine.)

• *creatinine height index:* shows relationship between creatinine level and patient's height; indirectly measures depletion of muscle mass; 60% to 80% of normal represents moderate protein depletion; less than 60% indicates severe depletion. (Creatinine excretion varies directly according to loss of skeletal muscle mass; creatinine height index is obtained by comparing creatinine and height-weight ratio with charts listing normal creatinine excretion for height and weight. Increased creatinine excretion indicates skeletal muscle breakdown.)

• *nitrogen balance:* obtained by comparing urinary urea nitrogen excretion with nitrogen intake (calculated from protein intake). In malnutrition, negative nitrogen balance reveals a catabolic state. A positive nitrogen balance of 2 to 3 g is ideal; in severe illness, zero nitrogen balance may be the realistic maximum attainable.

To assess visceral protein stores

(includes plasma proteins, hemoglobin, clotting factors, hormones, antibodies, and enzymes)

• *total lymphocyte count (TLC):* helps evaluate immunocompetence; 1,200 to 2,000/mm³ indicates mild lymphocyter depletion, 800 to 1,199/mm³, moderate depletion, and less than 800/mm³, severe depletion. (Severe depletion indicates inadequate antibody production and an impaired ability to fight infection. Nutritional repletion is indicated to improve the body's defense mechanisms. TLC is not an accurate indicator of nutritional status in patients on immunosuppressive therapy.)

• *albumin:* serum level less than 3 g/dl correlates with increased severity of illness. (2.8 to 3.5 g/dl indicates mild visceral protein depletion, 2.1 to 2.7 g/dl, moderate depletion, and less than 2.1 g/dl, severe depletion. Because the albumin level falls slowly, it is not a reliable early indicator of malnutrition.)

• *transferrin:* measures level of a protein synthesized in the liver. Serum level of 150 to 200 mg/dl indicates mild visceral protein depletion, 100 to 149 mg/dl, moderate depletion, and less than 100 mg/dl, severe. Serum concentration levels fall rapidly with starvation and stress over approximately 8 days. Serial serum transferrin levels indicate response to nutritional therapy.

• *skin-test antigens:* evaluate cell-mediated immunity, which can decrease with severe malnutrition. (This may be assessed using skin-test antigens such as mumps, *Candida,* streptokinase, or streptodornase. If a negative reaction occurs, malnutrition may be the cause, and the body lacks defense mechanisms to fight infection. A positive reaction is induration exceeding 5 mm, in response to at least two antigens, within 24 to 48 hours.)

To estimate body fat reserves

• *skin-fold measurements* (such as triceps skin fold): estimates body fat reserves. Measurements are compared with a standard table of values: 35% to 40% of normal indicates mild fat depletion; 25% to 34%, moderate depletion; and less than 25%, severe depletion. Difficult to evaluate if patient has edema or cannot sit.

Other studies

• *basal energy expenditure:* provides data to estimate the patient's daily caloric needs. Several methods can determine basal energy expenditure (the number of calories required for maintenance of weight at rest), including the Harris-Benedict equation that uses height, weight, sex, and age to determine the required energy expenditure to maintain weight while at rest. The dietitian then adds a factor for the stress the patient is experiencing (sepsis, multiple trauma, surgery) to arrive at the number of calories needed to promote anabolism. Indirect calorimetry determines energy expenditure by measuring carbon dioxide production and oxygen consumption with a gas analyzer connected to a tube into which the patient breathes. The amount of oxygen consumed and the carbon dioxide produced indicate the number of calories being expended at the time—the resting energy expenditure. Measurement of energy expenditure by this method is time consuming, and potential sources of error are numerous. (For example, test results may be inaccurate if the face mask does not fit.)

• *total iron-binding capacity (TIBC):* measures ability of iron to bind with transferrin transported in the blood. Followed serially, TIBC indicates if nutritional support is correcting the nutritional state.

• *serum electrolyte levels:* obtained as baseline values and to guide replacement therapy; in patients with malnutrition, they typically reveal hyponatremia, hypokalemia, hypomagnesemia, and hypophosphatemia.

Nursing diagnosis: *Nutritional deficit related to difficulty chewing or swallowing, sore throat after endotracheal extubation, or dry mouth*

NURSING PRIORITY: Compensate for eating difficulties.

Interventions

1. Assess and document causes. Initiate referrals as appropriate—for example, to dentist or speech pathologist.

Rationales

1. Some eating difficulties call for diagnosis or interventions beyond the scope of nursing. For example, a dentist may be able to diagnose jaw pain or a speech pathologist may be able to teach swallowing techniques.

2. Assess level of consciousness and ability to chew and swallow, and check for gag reflex.

3. In collaboration with the dietitian and as ordered, provide a diet appropriate to the patient's abilities — for example, liquids, soft foods, or food requiring little cutting.

4. If the patient has a sore mouth or throat, obtain an order for viscous lidocaine (Xylocaine). If the patient has been extubated recently, explain that the sore throat usually resolves spontaneously within a few days.

5. Place the patient sitting upright for meals, with the head flexed forward about 45 degrees, unless contraindicated.

6. Have suction equipment available nearby but out of the patient's sight. Suction food, fluids, and accumulated saliva, as needed.

7. Provide assistance, as needed. If the patient has had a CVA, place food in the unaffected side of the mouth.

8. Document feeding technique and food intake.

9. Additional individualized interventions: _____

_____

2. Alertness, ability to chew and swallow, and a gag reflex determine if the patient can safely ingest nutrients orally.

3. An appropriate diet minimizes patient frustration when eating.

4. Use of viscous lidocaine, a topical anesthetic, reduces discomfort. Knowing that the sore throat, common after extubation, will probably disappear after extubation may increase the patient's tolerance of the discomfort.

5. This position maintains esophageal patency, facilitates swallowing, and minimizes the risk of aspiration.

6. If the patient has sudden difficulty swallowing, prompt suctioning prevents aspiration. Keeping the equipment out of sight creates a more pleasant eating environment.

7. Providing assistance increases food intake. Placing the food in the unaffected side facilitates use of the tongue to move food toward the back of the mouth.

8. Documenting the technique provides for continuity of care; records are necessary to monitor the adequacy of food intake.

9. Rationales: _____

_____

GENERAL PLANS OF CARE

Target outcome criteria
According to individual readiness, the patient will:
• eat the prescribed diet
• swallow without choking.

Nursing diagnosis: *Nutritional deficit related to anorexia*

NURSING PRIORITY: Promote appetite.

Interventions

1. Assess possible causes of anorexia, such as nausea and vomiting, unpleasant sights and odors, depression, and medications. Determine food preferences.

2. Provide a pleasant eating environment. For example, place an emesis basin nearby but out of direct sight (if someone will be staying at the bedside); remove tissues containing sputum.

3. Before meals, promote rest; administer analgesics or antiemetics, as needed and ordered; avoid painful procedures; and provide oral hygiene.

4. Emphasize the importance of eating. Use positive terms when presenting food; for example, "Here's a milkshake to help you regain your strength," rather than "Do you think you'll be able to keep this down?"

5. Provide social interaction during meals, preferably with family and friends.

Rationales

1. Accurate identification of anorexia's cause facilitates selection of appropriate interventions.

2. Removal of noxious sights and smells may decrease anorexia, nausea, and vomiting.

3. Adequate rest conserves the energy necessary to eat. Analgesics, antiemetics, and avoidance of painful procedures remove the influences of pain, nausea, and emotional stress. Oral hygiene removes unpleasant tastes.

4. Emphasizing the importance of eating encourages the patient to eat despite anorexia. Positive terms capitalize on the power of suggestion to influence the subconscious mind.

5. Social interaction increases food intake by providing a pleasant distraction from anorexia. Involving family and friends strengthens interpersonal bonds.

6. Offer small, frequent feedings of highly nutritious foods, including the patient's preferences whenever possible.

6. Small meals promote prompt gastric emptying, lessening anorexia and nausea. When food intake is low, every mouthful must count toward meeting nutrient needs.

7. Limit fluid intake at mealtimes.

7. Large amounts of fluid distend the stomach, causing early satiety and promoting nausea.

8. If the patient begins to feel nauseated, encourage slow, deep breathing. If vomiting occurs, document the amount and type of emesis. Provide oral hygiene afterward.

8. Deep breathing helps to diminish the vomiting reflex. Documentation of emesis is necessary to maintain accurate intake and output records and to evaluate the adequacy of oral nutrition. Oral hygiene removes unpleasant tastes.

9. Praise the patient for signs of increased appetite.

9. Praise acknowledges the patient's efforts to overcome anorexia and reinforces desired behavior.

10. Additional individualized interventions: _____

10. Rationales: _____

Target outcome criterion
According to individual readiness, the patient will eat and retain at least three-quarters of the prescribed diet.

Collaborative problem: *Nutritional deficit related to inability to digest nutrients or hypermetabolic state*

NURSING PRIORITY: Provide nutrients in a form that can be assimilated.

Interventions

1. Stay alert for increased nutrient needs, such as from trauma, burns, infection, surgical wounds, and fever. Also observe the patient for indicators of possible inability to absorb nutrients, such as diarrhea.

2. Collaborate with the dietitian, nutritional support service, and doctor to obtain a comprehensive nutritional assessment.

3. Assess and document bowel sounds and abdominal distention every 4 hours.

4. Collaborate with nutritional experts to establish nutrient requirements, depending on whether the following exist:

• starvation

Rationales

1. Early recognition of the patient's decreased absorptive ability or increased needs helps provide adequate nutrition before debilitation occurs.

2. A comprehensive assessment includes anthropometric and laboratory measurements performed by colleagues with special nutritional expertise. These measurements document the type and degree of nutritional deficit and provide guidelines for selecting appropriate nutritional interventions.

3. Bowel sounds indicate whether the patient can tolerate enteral feedings or whether parenteral feedings are necessary. Abdominal distention suggests paralytic ileus.

4. Nutrient requirements vary depending on whether the patient is merely nutritionally depleted or is experiencing a hypermetabolic state.

• Early starvation is characterized by various compensatory mechanisms, including glycogenolysis, lipolysis, proteolysis, and gluconeogenesis. Rapid catabolism produces rapid weight loss, osmotic diuresis, and urinary nitrogen loss. After approximately 10 days, the metabolic rate slows and weight loss continues at a slower rate while the body uses fat as its primary energy source. After several months, exhaustion of fat stores causes the body to use visceral protein for energy.

• hypermetabolism.

• The release of catecholamines, glucocorticoids, and mineralocorticoids in response to stress cause the traumatized or infected patient to develop greater glucose mobilization than the starved patient. Rapid weight loss and osmotic diuresis are delayed for approximately 24 to 48 hours after trauma.

5. Provide the appropriate nutritional replacement, as ordered. Options include the following:

• enteral feeding (via nasogastric, gastrostomy, or jejunostomy tubes), such as:

— meal replacements

— nutrient supplements

— defined-formula diets

• parenteral nutrition

— peripheral parenteral nutrition (PPN)

— central venous nutrition, also known as total parenteral nutrition (TPN).

5. Nutritional replacement methods depend on the patient's needs.

• Enteral feeding is preferred for the patient with a functioning GI tract.

— Meal replacements are nutritionally complete but require digestive and absorptive abilities.

— Supplements, although nutritionally incomplete, can replace one or more specific nutrients.

— Defined-formula diets are nutritionally complete and require little digestion.

• Parenteral nutrition is appropriate for patients who cannot meet nutritional needs through GI absorption. It is administered peripherally or centrally.

— PPN may be prescribed if calorie needs are relatively low, if relatively short-term GI dysfunction is anticipated and if peripheral veins are adequate.

— TPN is appropriate for patients with relatively high calorie needs because TPN solutions have greater calorie and protein content than peripheral venous solutions.

6. If the patient is receiving tube feedings:

• Check tube placement before each feeding.

• Monitor bowel sounds, bowel movements, residual amounts, abdominal girth, intake and output, and weight.
• Keep the head of the bed elevated during and for 1 hour after feedings.
• Begin with small amounts of dilute solution. Increase the amount and concentration as tolerated, within prescribed parameters.
• Use a continuous enteral pump, as ordered.

6. Nursing measures for tube feedings are designed to facilitate absorption and prevent complications.

• Checking tube placement confirms that the tube is in the stomach or jejunum, as appropriate. With a nasogastric tube, checking ensures that it has not migrated upward into the trachea.

• Monitoring promotes early identification of complications, such as ileus or obstruction.

• Elevation prevents reflux of solution into the esophagus.

• Large amounts of concentrated solution may provoke osmotic diarrhea. Gradual increases allow time for the GI system to adapt to the increased volume and solute load.

• Delivery with a continuous enteral pump is less likely to provoke diarrhea.

7. If the patient is receiving TPN, ensure delivery of the prescribed solutions and monitor for complications. Refer to the "Total Parenteral Nutrition" plan, page 411, for details.

7. TPN is a complex therapy with numerous nursing considerations.

8. Additional individualized interventions: _____

8. Rationales: _____

Target outcome criteria
Within 7 days of admission, the patient will:
• tolerate enteral or parenteral feedings without adverse effects
• gain up to 2.5 lb (1 kg) per week.

GENERAL PLANS OF CARE

Discharge planning

NURSING DISCHARGE CRITERIA

Upon the patient's discharge, documentation shows evidence of:
• assessment of nutritional status
• implementation of appropriate nutritional support.

PATIENT-FAMILY TEACHING CHECKLIST

Document evidence that the patient and family demonstrate an understanding of:
__ importance of nutrition to recovery
__ rationale for selection of specific nutritional support method.

DOCUMENTATION CHECKLIST

Using outcome criteria as a guide, document:
__ clinical status on admission
__ significant changes in status
__ pertinent diagnostic test findings
__ specific nutritional support method
__ tolerance of method
__ complications, if any
__ daily nutritional intake
__ medications administered, if any
__ attitude toward eating
__ patient-family teaching
__ discharge planning.

ASSOCIATED PLANS OF CARE

See the plan for the specific disorder.

References

Blackburn, G., Bell, S., and Mullen, J. *Nutritional Medicine.* Philadelphia: W.B. Saunders Co., 1989.

Cerrato, P. "New Answers to 'How Much Should I Weigh?'," *RN* 53(2):83-86, February 1990.

Gibson, R. *Principles of Nutritional Assessment.* New York: Oxford Press University, 1990.

Holloway, N., and Forlaw, L. "Nourishment of the Critically Ill," in *Nursing the Critically Ill Adult,* 3rd ed. Edited by Holloway, N. Menlo Park, Calif.: Addison Wesley Publishing Co., 1988.

Jeejeebhoy, K., Detsky, A., and Baker, J. "Assessment of Nutritional Status," *Journal of Parenteral and Enteral Nutrition* 14(5Suppl.):193S-196S, 1990.

Nutritional Assessment: What Is It? How Is It Used? Columbus, Ohio: Ross Laboratories Publication, 1988.

Pressman, A., and Adams, A. *Clinical Assessment of Nutritional Status,* 2nd ed. Baltimore: Williams and Wilkins, 1990.

Recommended Dietary Allowances, 10th ed. Washington, D.C.: National Research Council, 1990.

Silberman, H. *Parenteral and Enteral Nutrition,* 2nd ed. Norwalk, Conn.: Appleton & Lange, 1989.

Skipper, A. *Dietitian's Handbook of Enteral and Parenteral Nutrition.* Rockville, Md.: Aspen Publishers, 1989.

Taylor, C., and Sparks, S. *Nursing Diagnosis Cards,* 6th ed. Springhouse, Pa.: Springhouse Corp., 1991.

GENERAL PLANS OF CARE
Pain

Introduction
DEFINITION AND TIME FOCUS
Pain represents neurologic or emotional suffering in response to a noxious stimulus. It is best prevented and relieved when the nurse continually anticipates it. Although individuals experience pain differently, pain's symbolic meaning as a danger and threat commonly heightens a patient's perceptions of it. Sophisticated pain management demands patience, sensitivity, compassion, and a repertoire of pain-control techniques. Because of individual factors and the availability of the various pain-control techniques to choose among, the nurse must exercise keen judgment in selecting the best strategy for a particular patient at a particular time. This plan focuses on the care of a patient experiencing acute pain, lasting minutes to days, rather than chronic pain, because acute pain is more common among acutely ill patients.

ETIOLOGY AND PRECIPITATING FACTORS
• surgical or accidental trauma
• inflammation
• musculoskeletal disorders, such as muscle spasm
• neuropathies, such as multiple sclerosis
• visceral disorders, such as myocardial infarction
• vascular disorders, such as sickle cell anemia
• invasive diagnostic procedures
• excessive pressure, such as with immobility
• cancer

Focused assessment guidelines
NURSING HISTORY (Functional health pattern findings)

Health perception – health management pattern
• reports acute physical discomfort, typically described as pain, pressure, tightness, soreness, or a crushing or burning sensation

Nutritional-metabolic pattern
• may describe anorexia, nausea, or vomiting

Activity-exercise pattern
• commonly reports intense fatigue

Sleep-rest pattern
• may report inability to rest or sleep

Cognitive-perceptual pattern
• commonly reports inability to concentrate

Self-perception – self-concept pattern
• may report anxiety or depression

Role-relationship pattern
• may express concern that others discount pain
• may describe decreased desire to interact with others

Coping – stress tolerance pattern
• may report increased stress level
• may report decreased ability to deal with frustration or other stress

Value-belief pattern
• may express belief that suffering is punishment for wrongdoing or bad deeds
• may express reluctance to take medication for pain relief because of religion, belief system, or fear of addiction

PHYSICAL FINDINGS
General appearance
• tense, guarded posture
• facial grimacing
• crying
• moaning

Musculoskeletal
• writhing
• muscle spasms
• unnatural stillness
• increased physical activity (uncommon)

Integumentary
• diaphoresis
• pallor

Neurologic
• impaired concentration
• irritability
• restlessness

Cardiovascular
• hypertension and tachycardia
• hypotension and bradycardia (uncommon)

Respiratory
• tachypnea
• gasping

DIAGNOSTIC STUDIES
No specific studies indicate the presence or degree of pain. Various procedures may be indicated in the differential diagnosis of pain. For example, for chest pain, the patient may undergo a 12-lead electrocardiogram, chest X-ray, creatine phosphokinase level measurements, and pulmonary ventilation scan to differentiate acute myocardial infarction from pulmonary embolism. See plans of care on specific disorders for details.

POTENTIAL COMPLICATIONS
• exhaustion
• intractable pain
• suicide

Nursing diagnosis: *Pain from tissue injury, ischemia, infarction, inflammation, edema, tension, or spasm*

NURSING PRIORITY: Prevent or ameliorate pain.

Interventions

1. Monitor continually for possible indicators of pain, including verbalization, grimacing, diaphoresis, tense posture, splinting, restlessness, irritability, emotional withdrawal, and vital-signs changes.

2. Analyze and document pain characteristics systematically; for example, use the PQRST mnemonic:
• P precipitators
• Q quality
• R region and radiation
• S severity
• T time (frequency and duration).
Promptly report any new or increased pain to the doctor.

3. Prepare the patient for brief, unavoidably painful experiences, such as percutaneous skin puncture for arterial blood gas sampling. State clear expectations for behavior, such as, "If it hurts, squeeze my hand but hold your other arm still."

4. When preparing the patient for a painful experience, try to find out how much the patient wants to know. If possible, tailor the degree of detail to the patient's preference for information and the procedure's extensiveness.

5. During painful procedures, provide ongoing support and positive reinforcement:

• Use brief, simple directions, as needed. Use therapeutic touch, if accepted by the patient.

• When the experience is over, encourage the patient to ventilate feelings, if desired. Convey acceptance for the way the patient handled pain, using praise generously when appropriate.

6. Reduce factors that may increase pain, such as anxiety that reports of pain will not be believed, a sense of isolation, and fatigue. Accept the patient's description of pain. Convey the sense that the patient is not alone. Encourage the patient to rest sufficiently. Control environmental factors, such as noise, temperature, and lighting, when possible.

Rationales

1. The acutely ill patient may not be fully conscious because of the underlying disease process or medications that blunt perception. As a result, verbal reports alone may not adequately indicate the presence and degree of pain. Astute observation may provide ongoing protection against unreported or underreported pain.

2. Careful analysis of pain characteristics aids in the differential diagnosis of pain. Systematic analysis prevents hasty and possibly inaccurate conclusions about the quality or probable cause of pain. New or increased pain requires prompt medical evaluation.

3. The psychological assault of unexpected pain can unnerve even the most stoic person and make coping with the pain needlessly stressful. Brief explanations decrease fear of the unknown and help the patient prepare for the experience. Positive suggestions provide an appropriate way to cope with the pain.

4. Patient teaching does not necessarily reduce anxiety; people vary in the degree of detail they find helpful. According to Watkins, Weaver, and Odegaard (1986), "blunters," who tend to avoid threatening aspects of situations to lessen their psychological impact, usually want to know relatively little about impending experiences, whereas "monitors," who tend to seek information about stressful events to lessen their psychological impact, want to know a great deal. Providing a "blunter" with detailed information increases anxiety, while withholding it from a "monitor" worsens stress. When possible, appropriate matching of preference and preparation respects individual differences and supports the patient's preferred coping style.

5. Providing support and encouragement during the experience increases the patient's sense of security and control.

• Brief, simple directions are necessary because pain reduces comprehension and retention of information. Touch may convey comfort more profoundly than words.

• Discussing the pain experience afterward provides an opportunity for psychological integration and closure of the experience, which is necessary to "let go" of it. Conveying acceptance is particularly important for patients who scream or otherwise lose control because it reassures them and may relieve any residual feelings of shame.

6. Listening to the patient respectfully and implying an alliance against pain help reduce anxiety. Feeling well-rested increases tolerance of pain and the ability to cope with it. Environmental factors may exacerbate the pain: constant, irritating noise, for example, may cause increased muscle tension and irritability.

7. For patients with ongoing pain, explicitly convey the goal of aggressive pain management. State the intent to prevent or "stay on top" of the pain. Explain the rationale for and importance of reporting a painful episode as soon as possible. Encourage the patient to request relief before the pain becomes severe.

8. Work with the patient to identify the most effective ways to control pain. Explore various pain-control methods. Use positive terms and the power of suggestion.

9. Use a repertoire of nonpharmacologic pain-control strategies:

• positioning—Cushion and elevate the painful area, if possible. Avoid pressure or tension on it. Encourage the patient to rest in a comfortable position, but also to change position every hour while awake. Explain the rationale for position changes, provide gentle reminders, and assist with movement, as necessary.

• cutaneous stimulation from massage or applications of heat, cold, or mentholated ointments

• contralateral stimulation, such as scratching or massage, when the injured area is not directly accessible (for example, under a cast).

10. Explore various behavioral pain-control strategies, including:

• distraction techniques, such as talking or listening to lively music

• relaxation techniques, such as rhythmic breathing, progressive muscle relaxation, listening to relaxation tapes or soothing music, or meditation.

7. Explicit goals imply that the situation is manageable, which is reassuring and reduces the fear of being overwhelmed by pain. Pain can be more easily brought under control in its early stages. Giving explicit permission to request relief early reduces stoicism and unnecessary suffering.

8. Involving the patient in pain-control strategies promotes a sense of mastery that reduces fears of helplessness or loss of control. Trying a variety of pain-control measures allows for an individualized, multifaceted approach, which is more likely to be successful than a single strategy. Using positive terms interrupts the cycle of negativity, in which pain worsens negativity and negativity worsens pain. Capitalizing on the power of suggestion creates an expectation that interventions will be successful. It may also help trigger release of endorphins, opiate-like analgesic substances that the body releases in response to certain stimuli.

9. Because various factors may cause or exacerbate pain, various techniques may bring relief. A multifaceted approach is more likely to succeed than a single strategy.

• Cushioning increases comfort, while elevation reduces edema. Avoiding pressure or tension eliminates additional painful stimuli to an already sensitive area. Rest increases pain tolerance. Position changes improve perfusion, helping remove chemical mediators of inflammation and bringing oxygen and other nutrients to healing tissue. Position changes also help prevent complications of immobility. Because moving the painful area may temporarily increase pain, patient education, gentle but firm reminders, and active assistance may be necessary to ensure attention to this important need.

• Pain impulses are believed to be transmitted along peripheral nerve fibers to ascending spinal cord pathways to the brain. Sharp, acute pain is transmitted along small-diameter, type A fibers, whereas dull, chronic pain is transmitted along smaller type C fibers. Stimulation of large sensory (nonpain) fibers inhibits these ascending pain pathways. In addition, massage increases perfusion and reduces muscle tension. Cold-induced vasoconstriction reduces edema and is especially helpful in the first 24 hours after injury. Heat increases circulation, mobility, and muscle relaxation, which is particularly helpful in decreasing painful reflex muscle spasms.

• Stimulation of the area opposite the painful one may provide relief, probably by triggering release of endorphins, opiate-like substances that relieve pain.

10. Behavioral strategies divert attention from the pain, promote a sense of self-control, encourage muscle relaxation, and may stimulate endorphin release.

• Distraction is especially helpful for brief episodes of pain, but may increase pain perception and fatigue after the distracting stimulus is removed.

• These techniques reduce muscle tension, enhance rest, and promote a sense of well-being.

11. If the above methods are inappropriate or ineffective, collaborate with the doctor and clinical pharmacist, as needed, to determine an effective analgesic regimen. Administer and document analgesics, as ordered, which may include:

• potent narcotics, such as morphine and meperidine (Demerol)

• mild narcotics, such as codeine, and narcotic agonists or antagonists, such as butorphanol (Stadol)

• nonnarcotic analgesics, such as aspirin, acetaminophen (Tylenol), and ibuprofen (Motrin)

• analgesic adjuncts, such as hydroxyzine (Vistaril).

11. The above methods require a certain amount of emotional energy and ability to concentrate, which the patient may lack, or pain may be too severe for them to be effective. Personalizing the analgesic regimen recognizes individual differences in pain perception and provides the most effective control for a particular patient.

• Narcotics act centrally to blunt pain perception. Potent narcotics, although effective in relieving severe pain, may cause sedation, respiratory depression, nausea, vomiting, and other adverse effects.

• Used for moderate pain, these agents are less likely to cause respiratory depression.

• Appropriate for mild pain, these agents block synthesis of prostaglandins (inflammatory mediators that increase pain).

• Adjuncts increase the analgesic's effects, lessen muscle spasm, cause sedation, and may diminish pain recall.

12. Minimize discomfort from side effects of narcotic analgesics.

12. Narcotic analgesic use can result in constipation, nausea and vomiting, stomatitis, and injury. (See *Preventing narcotic analgesic side effects.*)

13. Involve the family in pain-relief strategies. Help them understand the patient's behavior in the context of the pain. Explain the rationale for pain-control techniques. Correct misconceptions, if present. When possible, have family members participate in providing the pain relief, such as massage. Explicitly acknowledge the difficulty in observing a loved one's pain, and provide emotional support.

13. Capitalizing on family bonds can provide a level of interpersonal comfort that exceeds what concerned, supportive staff can provide. Understanding pain behaviors may help the family be more patient, and correcting misconceptions (such as the danger of addiction) may relieve unwarranted anxiety. Acknowledgment of family members' emotional suffering conveys respect and concern for them, and nurturing family members increases their coping skills and ability to support the patient.

14. If constant pain is present, collaborate with the patient, family, doctor, and pharmacist to optimize pain relief, through such measures as:

• continuous I.V. or subcutaneous infusion or patient-controlled analgesia devices

• spinal (epidural or intrathecal) narcotic administration

• transcutaneous electrical nerve stimulation (TENS) or acupuncture

• hypnosis, guided imagery, and biofeedback.

14. Persistent pain may demoralize the patient and make suffering seem unbearable. A collaborative approach using several options increases the likelihood of finding the optimal pain-control regimen for a given patient.

• Continuous infusions allow for more effective control by maintaining constant analgesic blood levels. Patient-controlled analgesia devices allow for immediate pain relief, increasing the patient's sense of control over pain.

• These techniques deliver small doses of narcotics directly to endorphin receptor sites, allowing powerful pain control without the usual systemic effects of narcotics.

• TENS transmits an electrical stimulus to the painful area, whereas acupuncture uses needles to stimulate sensitive areas. The techniques are thought to stimulate endorphin and enkephalin release, thus providing analgesia, and to block ascending pain transmission pathways.

• These techniques alter pain perception but require motivation and training, so they may not be appropriate for some patients.

15. Exert particular caution with spinal (epidural or intrathecal) narcotic administration.

• Double-check the dosage.
• Reduce or discontinue the parenteral dosage, as ordered.

15. These techniques are used for long-term pain control in cancer and postoperative patients (such as after thoracotomy, orthopedic surgery, or abdominal surgery). They allow potent pain control with fewer side effects than systemic analgesics by delivering small doses of analgesic agents, such as morphine or meperidine, close to endogenous endorphin receptor sites.

• Narcotic overdoses delivered via this route can be lethal.

• Central narcotic administration is so potent that continuation of normal parenteral dosage will result in narcotic overdose.

PREVENTING NARCOTIC ANALGESIC SIDE EFFECTS

Complication	Interventions	Rationales
Constipation	• Encourage bowel evacuation as soon as the urge to defecate occurs.	• Bowel evacuation can be delayed by voluntary inhibition of the urge to defecate, leading to constipation. Learning to defecate as soon as the urge occurs avoids this problem.
	• Encourage intake of at least 8 8-oz glasses (2,000 ml) of fluids daily and a high-fiber, well-balanced diet.	• A diet high in fiber increases peristalsis; fluids promote optimal stool consistency.
	• Encourage moderate exercise, unless contraindicated, with emphasis on increasing abdominal muscle tone.	• Voluntary contraction of abdominal wall muscles helps expel feces.
	• Administer and document medications for increasing bowel elimination, as ordered.	• Stool softeners retard reabsorption of water and coat the intestinal lining. Laxatives stimulate peristalsis or add bulk.
	• Evaluate and document the frequency of elimination and consistency of stool.	• Monitoring elimination patterns determines the effectiveness of, and need for, continued use of laxatives.
Nausea and vomiting	• Instruct the patient that nausea may decrease after a few doses.	• Information helps reduce anxiety, which can increase nausea.
	• Eliminate noxious sights and smells from the environment.	• Noxious stimuli can stimulate the vomiting center.
	• Encourage the patient to move and change position slowly.	• Movement may stimulate the vomiting center in the medulla.
	• Encourage the patient to deep breathe and swallow.	• Deep breathing and swallowing decrease the strength of the vomiting reflex.
	• Consult with the doctor about changing the narcotic analgesic.	• The patient may have less nausea and vomiting in response to another narcotic.
	• Administer and document an antiemetic, as ordered, using nursing judgment.	• Antiemetics decrease stimulation of the vomiting center and usually potentiate narcotic effects.
	• Evaluate and document the effects of antiemetics in relieving nausea and vomiting.	• Monitoring the response to medication determines its effectiveness and the need for continued antiemetics.
Stomatitis	• Encourage or provide mouth care at frequent intervals, after meals and as needed.	• Narcotic-induced mouth dryness may cause discomfort and contribute to mucous membrane breakdown (stomatitis). Cleanliness and moisture maintain the integrity of the mucous membrane.
	• Encourage the patient to breathe through the nose, if possible.	• Dryness of the oral mucous membrane may cause breakdown.
	• Encourage fluid intake of at least 8 8-oz glasses (2,000 ml) daily.	• Adequate hydration reduces discomfort and helps maintain the integrity of the oral mucous membrane.
	• Instruct the patient not to use mouthwashes or other products that contain alcohol.	• Alcohol has a drying effect on the oral mucous membrane.
Injury	• Orient the patient to time and place, verbally and with touch, and explain the call system.	• Information provides support and relieves anxiety.
	• Instruct the patient to request assistance when getting out of bed.	• Assistance with ambulation will help prevent falls.
	• Secure the side rails and keep the bed at its lowest level.	• These measures prevent injuries and avert the possibility of the patient's falling out of bed.
	• Instruct the patient and family regarding the hazards of sedation when driving, smoking in bed, and so forth.	• Information about specific hazards helps prevent accidents and injury.

• Use preservative-free narcotics, such as morphine, meperidine, or fentanyl (Sublimaze).

• Maintain the catheter as prescribed by unit protocol.

16. Evaluate and document evidence of response to pain-relief measures hourly and as needed. Be alert for "clock watching" for the next analgesic dose.

17. Additional individualized interventions: _____

_____

• The preservative in most commercial preparations causes meningeal irritation.

• Specific catheter care varies but includes maintenance of catheter patency and observation for catheter displacement.

16. Monitoring the effectiveness of pain relief determines the appropriateness of methods used. The main reason for "clock watching" behavior is inadequate pain relief.

17. Rationales:_____

_____

Target outcome criteria
Within 1 hour after the onset of pain, the patient will:
• verbalize increased comfort
• have a relaxed posture and facial expression
• have vital signs within normal limits.

Discharge planning
NURSING DISCHARGE CRITERIA
Upon the patient's discharge, documentation shows evidence of:
• pain-relief measures effective in reducing pain to tolerable level
• vital signs within normal limits.

PATIENT-FAMILY TEACHING CHECKLIST
Document evidence that the patient and family demonstrate an understanding of:
___ anticipated course of pain in relation to the medical condition
___ all discharge medications' purpose, dosage, administration schedule, and side effects requiring medical attention (usual discharge medications are oral analgesics)
___ nonpharmacologic relief strategies
___ symptoms and severity of pain warranting medical care
___ dates, times, and location of follow-up appointments
___ how to contact the doctor.

DOCUMENTATION CHECKLIST
Using outcome criteria as a guide, document:
___ clinical status on admission
___ significant changes in status
___ pertinent laboratory and diagnostic test findings
___ pain characteristics
___ analgesic administration
___ nonpharmacologic strategies
___ behavioral strategies
___ effectiveness of measures
___ patient's and family's response to pain
___ patient-family teaching
___ discharge planning.

ASSOCIATED PLANS OF CARE
Dying
Grieving
Impaired Physical Mobility
Ineffective Family Coping
Ineffective Individual Coping
Sensory-Perceptual Alteration

References
Bragg, C. "Practical Aspects of Epidural and Intrathecal Narcotic Analgesia in the Intensive Care Setting," *Heart & Lung* 18(6):599-608, November 1989.

Copp, L. "The Spectrum of Suffering," *American Journal of Nursing* 90(8):35-39, 1990.

Gregory, C., and Holloway, N. "Pain," in *Nursing the Critically Ill Adult*, 3rd ed. Edited by Holloway, N. Menlo Park, Calif.: Addison-Wesley Publishing Co., 1988.

Guyton, A. *Textbook of Medical Physiology*, 8th ed. Philadelphia: W.B. Saunders Co., 1991.

McCaffry, M., and Beebe, A. "Giving Narcotics for Pain: The Secrets to Giving Equianalgesic Doses," *Nursing89* 19(10):161-68, October 1989.

Puntillo, K. "Pain Experiences of Intensive Care Unit Patients," *Heart & Lung* 19(5):526-33, September 1990.

Puntillo, K., ed. *Pain in the Critically Ill: Assessment and Management* Gaithersburg, Md.: Aspen Publishers, 1991.

Watkins, L., Weaver, L., and Odegaard, V. "Preparation for Cardiac Catheterization: Tailoring the Content of Instruction to Coping Style," *Heart & Lung* 15(4):382-89, July 1986.

Sensory-Perceptual Alteration

Introduction
DEFINITION AND TIME FOCUS
A sensory-perceptual alteration is a change in the patient's experience of the surroundings. Such alterations may affect a patient's overall well-being in numerous ways. The hospital unit environment, the physiologic manifestations of illness, and the psychological stress caused by hospitalization may have a severe cumulative effect unless the nurse initiates astute anticipatory intervention. Most nurses are familiar with the phenomenon of a patient's environmental disorientation. This distressing response may be averted or minimized by careful assessment and attention to modifiable aspects of the patient's environment. Family members may be a particularly helpful resource for nursing care planning for this problem because they can provide information about the patient's usual home environment and sensory-perceptual abilities. Nursing intervention for this problem, perhaps more than for any other nursing diagnosis, must be individually tailored to the patient's subjective view of the situation.

ETIOLOGY AND PRECIPITATING FACTORS
• unfamiliar, complex environment
• monotonous environment
• perceptual deficits, such as uncompensated deafness
• chemical alterations (endogenous or exogenous)
• psychological stress
• bed rest
• medications

Focused assessment guidelines
NURSING HISTORY (Functional health pattern findings)
The patient with a sensory-perceptual alteration may be unable to provide meaningful subjective data for assessment purposes. The patient's family may be especially helpful in providing information about baseline mental status and normal activities and interests. Although findings may vary widely among individuals, the following are common findings associated with sensory-perceptual alteration.

Health perception—health management pattern
• may express unrealistic ideas regarding condition

Nutritional-metabolic pattern
• may display reduced appetite or apathy toward food

Activity-exercise pattern
• may complain of insomnia or fatigue
• may engage in wandering behavior
• may become hyperactive

Cognitive-perceptual pattern
• commonly demonstrates impaired judgment
• may demonstrate loss of time sense
• may demonstrate memory impairment
• is likely to exhibit reduced attention span
• may misidentify familiar persons
• may display increased need for pain medications

Self-perception—self-concept pattern
• may assume all external stimuli have reference to self (ideas of reference)
• commonly verbalizes paranoid ideas
• may express suicidal thoughts

Coping—stress tolerance pattern
• may withdraw from others in response to perceived threat
• may become increasingly demanding or make repeated requests for minor needs
• may exhibit obsessive or compulsive behavior, such as constant rearrangement of familiar items
• may be unable to make decisions
• may exhibit aggressive behavior or make verbal or sexual overtures
• may respond to minor frustration or annoyance by crying or becoming enraged

PHYSICAL FINDINGS
Physical manifestations of sensory-perceptual alteration may vary widely, depending on the patient's underlying condition and other factors. The findings listed below, however, may indicate such an alteration is present, and the astute nurse will be alert to such cues.

General appearance
• nervous mannerisms
• anxious facial expression
• flat affect

Neurologic
• restlessness
• irritability
• combativeness
• confusion or disorientation
• nystagmus
• delusions or hallucinations
• psychosis
• depression

Cardiopulmonary
• cardiac arrhythmias (associated with sleep deprivation)

Respiratory
• hyperventilation or other physiologic manifestations of tension or anxiety
• reduced ventilatory response to hypoxia and hypercapnia (associated with sleep deprivation)

Musculoskeletal
• increased muscle tension
• hand tremors

DIAGNOSTIC STUDIES
No laboratory tests or diagnostic procedures exist specifically for patients with sensory-perceptual alteration; however, any patient with altered mental status for any reason should be evaluated for possible toxic, endocrine, or metabolic causes for symptoms.

POTENTIAL COMPLICATIONS
• acute brain syndrome
• physical injury from confusion
• crisis state

Nursing diagnosis: *Sensory-perceptual alteration related to excessive or insufficient environmental stimuli**

NURSING PRIORITIES: (a) Promote normal processing and integration of environmental cues, and (b) control stimuli for maximum therapeutic effect.

Interventions

1. Assess the unit environment. Evaluate the type, quantity, duration, frequency, and clarity of auditory, visual, olfactory, tactile, and gustatory stimuli. To maintain alertness to the unit environment, the staff might periodically role-play as patients, as unit census permits.

2. Assess the patient's normal routines, including the general home environment, activity, diet, and sleep patterns. Ask the patient or family to provide information regarding specific personal habits or preferences, such as reading before bedtime or leaving the television or radio on during waking hours. Ask the patient or family to describe a typical 24-hour period. As feasible, modify care routines and the unit environment to resemble the patient's home surroundings. If possible, provide food that is familiar.

3. Orient the patient and family to the unit, explaining structure and routines. At the same time each day, review with them the day's activity plan and instruct them regarding special procedures or changes that are anticipated. As much as possible, prepare the patient and family in advance for change of any kind. Attempt to provide continuity in staffing.

4. Provide cues to orientation and reinforce them frequently while providing care. Ensure, for example, that a large clock and calendar are placed within the patient's visual field; wear easily read name tags and introduce yourself to the patient at least once a shift until familiarity is established. For patients with visual deficits, always introduce yourself when approaching the bedside and before touching the patient. For a patient without visual impairment, encourage the family to bring in photographs or other small items from home to place on the wall or at the bedside.

Rationales

1. The patient in the hospital unit is subjected to a dramatic reduction in some types of stimuli (visual, gustatory, tactile) and an increase in other types (auditory). Such changes, particularly when the patient's ability to perceive, integrate, and cope with new information is impaired by physiologic stress, may result in significant mental status alterations. Staff awareness of the environment to which most patients are constantly exposed is essential for effective intervention on the patient's behalf. Nurses may become so habituated to the work environment that their sensitivity to its effects on patients is reduced. Role-playing as a patient may increase awareness.

2. Careful assessment of the patient's usual prehospitalization surroundings is essential to making appropriate adjustments. A description of the customary 24-hour routine provides valuable information about interrelationships and the significance of various aspects of the patient's life. Modification of routines, surroundings, and food may promote a sense of security.

3. Structure and routine aid the patient in interpreting and processing unfamiliar environmental cues. Reviewing plans at the same time each day reinforces the routine and increases security. Advance preparation allows the patient and family to integrate and cope with change more effectively. Continuity of staffing adds to the patient's repertoire of familiar information.

4. Reality testing requires input of familiar, predictable, and meaningful external informational cues. Without such orientation guides, internal and external events may become confused. Studies have shown that even normal, healthy individuals experience sensory-perceptual alterations when subjected to bed rest and its attendant sensory-perceptual deprivation. Even a few familiar items from home, particularly photographs of loved ones, may help the patient maintain orientation and reduce the alienation patients experience in the strange environment of the hospital unit.

---

*The numerous interventions for sensory-perceptual alteration have been grouped into problems according to cause.

5. Control environmental stimuli, as possible, to provide an environment that is secure and meaningful for the patient. Pay particular attention to the type and level of unit noise, ensuring that extraneous conversation is kept to a minimum. Encourage questions and provide interpretation of unfamiliar sensory stimuli as part of the patient's orientation to the unit—for example, "That beeping sound is an alarm on a patient's I.V. monitor," or "The hissing you hear is a machine that helps another patient to breathe."

6. As the patient's condition permits, encourage family participation in care. Explain the potential benefits of family-patient contact even when the patient is unresponsive. Speak to the patient when providing care, using touch generously unless the patient appears uncomfortable with physical contact.

7. Schedule care to provide uninterrupted patient sleep cycles of 2 hours or more by:

• grouping necessary procedures

• using continuous monitoring devices to check routine vital signs and other parameters

• scheduling planned sleep times, as possible, to coincide with usual home pattern

• minimizing noise (especially sudden loud sounds), setting alarms as low as safety allows, and turning off equipment when not in use

• evaluating for possible effects of medications on the sleep pattern and discussing their probable benefits and risks with the doctor, as appropriate

• assessing for pain

• providing eyeshades, earplugs, extra blankets or pillows, and other comfort measures

• teaching relaxation techniques, such as imagery, progressive muscle relaxation, massage, and deep breathing.

8. Assess the patient's mental status daily, noting particularly any alteration in orientation or memory. Be especially observant for indications of sensory-perceptual alteration in elderly patients and in children.

9. When leaving the bedside, always explain to the patient where you are going and approximately when you will return.

5. Studies have shown that ambient noise in hospital units distress the patient, increasing muscle tension and diastolic pressure and contributing to sleep disturbances. Nurse, staff, and visitor conversations may be even more disruptive to normal rest and sleep than the steady noise from equipment. Without normal sensory stimulation, the patient commonly interprets all overheard conversations as self-pertaining. For example, the patient who overhears a staff conversation about a surgical procedure may assume he is to undergo such a procedure. By interpreting unfamiliar stimuli and answering all questions, the nurse can increase the patient's security and promote adaptation to the unit environment.

6. Family contact decreases the strangeness of the environment and promotes orientation. Even patients who appear unconscious may continue to process environmental input, particularly sounds. Familiar verbal and tactile stimuli reduce sensory deprivation and provide reassurance. Touching the patient is one way of acknowledging the human dimension of care, which the patient may otherwise perceive as secondary in the high-technology setting.

7. The function of sleep is unknown, but it may help maintain central nervous system control of various homeostatic mechanisms. Some theories postulate that sleep is essential for normal processing and integrating of information. Studies have shown a decrease in the mental status of sleep-deprived patients. The following procedures help minimize these effects.

• Grouping procedures minimizes interruption of normal sleep cycles, which usually last 90 to 120 minutes.

• Monitoring devices do not require waking the patient.

• Once the patient's usual rhythm is disrupted, an effective sleep pattern may be difficult to reestablish.

• Even sounds that do not cause the patient to awaken completely may disrupt the normal sleep cycle. Abrupt loud sounds are more likely to cause awakening, though even continuous, low-level noise may alter the normal pattern.

• Many medications, including morphine, phenobarbital (Barbita), and diazepam (Valium), may decrease rapid eye movement (REM) sleep. REM sleep is considered essential to normal psychological functioning. The greatest amount of REM sleep occurs toward the end of a sleep period.

• Pain management can prevent restlessness and promote relaxation and sleep.

• Most people find sleeping in lighted areas difficult. Reducing stimulation and providing comfort measures help achieve sleep.

• Relaxation can induce sleep.

8. Early detection allows for preventive intervention. Older and younger patients are most susceptible to the effects of significant sensory-perceptual changes.

9. Knowing what to expect from the nurse decreases the patient's free-floating anxiety and provides a time reference.

GENERAL PLANS
OF CARE

10. Additional individualized interventions: _____

10. Rationales: _____

_____

_____

Target outcome criteria
Within 24 hours of admission, the patient will:
• verbalize understanding of unit routines
• state the names of two nurses, if requested

• experience at least one uninterrupted sleep cycle of 2 hours or more.

Nursing diagnosis: *Sensory-perceptual alteration related to altered sensory reception, transmission, or integration*

NURSING PRIORITY: Minimize or compensate for sensory-perceptual deficits.

Interventions

1. Assess for conditions in which sensory reception, transmission, or integration is likely to be impaired, such as old age, neurologic abnormalities, use of neuromuscular blocking agents, vision or hearing problems, immobilization, endotracheal intubation, tracheostomy and mechanical ventilation, altered level of consciousness, depression, or anxiety. If such conditions are present, identify the type and level of dysfunction, if possible, and note it in the care plan or post a notice near the patient's bed—for example, "Deafness in right ear, full hearing in left" or "Speak slowly."

2. Consult the medical history for additional pertinent data regarding specific deficits, such as anatomic site and physiologic effects of cerebrovascular accident. Tailor care accordingly.

3. Ensure reading glasses or a hearing aid is available to the patient who needs either. Consider using mirrors to expand vision field if immobilization restricts movement.

4. For any patient with altered mentation or consciousness, provide reality orientation at regular, planned intervals (at least every 8 hours). Include the time, day, date and year, location, and a brief explanation of the patient's immediate circumstances. Even if the patient is unresponsive, continue to provide such information regularly until the patient can repeat it on request.

5. Additional individualized interventions: _____

Rationales

1. Evaluation for risk factors permits early intervention to avert severe sensory deprivation and its distressing sequelae.

2. Attempting to implement interventions that are inappropriate to the patient's functional level may increase frustration and reduce the patient's motivation to communicate.

3. Accurate visual and auditory perceptions are the patient's primary connections to the external world and enhance reality orientation.

4. Reality orientation provides an essential anchor and a sense of security for patients recovering from altered consciousness, who commonly are uncertain whether they are dead or alive. Numerous case studies reveal that even unresponsive patients are receptive to auditory stimuli and frequently remember conversations of others even after a prolonged coma.

5. Rationales: _____

Target outcome criterion
Within 8 hours of admission and then daily, the patient will repeat baseline reality orientation information when asked, if physically able.

Nursing diagnosis: *Sensory-perceptual alteration related to endogenous or exogenous chemical alterations*

NURSING PRIORITY: Identify and treat possible causes of biochemical alteration.

Interventions

1. Assess for conditions that may contribute to chemically induced sensory-perceptual alterations, such as the therapeutic medication regimen, drug intoxication, diabetes or other metabolic disorders, or electrolyte and acid-base imbalances. Collaborate with the doctor to treat the underlying cause.

2. Provide appropriate, accurate explanations to the patient and family about the effects of psychotropic medications or other chemical causes of sensory-perceptual alteration.

3. Additional individualized interventions: _____

Rationales

1. Appropriate intervention to decrease the effects of sensory-perceptual changes depends upon accurate identification of their cause.

2. The patient and family may be alarmed or ashamed about chemically induced behavior. Providing explanations and displaying an attitude of acceptance promotes trust and open communication.

3. Rationales: _____

Target outcome criteria
Throughout the hospital stay, the patient will:
• display a clear sensorium
• make verbal statements congruent with reality.

Nursing diagnosis: *Sensory-perceptual alteration related to psychological stress*

NURSING PRIORITY: Promote effective coping.

Interventions

1. Be aware of the patient's needs for personal space. Ask permission and provide explanations before performing procedures. Provide effective screening to protect the patient's privacy.

2. See the "Ineffective Individual Coping" plan, page 51.

3. Additional individualized interventions: _____

Rationales

1. Everyone is protective of unconsciously defined personal boundaries, which help an individual maintain ego integration. For the acutely ill patient, these boundaries are constantly assaulted by invasive tubing, procedures, and noise the patient cannot control. Even small measures to acknowledge these boundaries may reduce stress from loss of control.

2. The "Ineffective Individual Coping" plan contains detailed interventions for the patient experiencing psychological stress.

3. Rationales: _____

Target outcome criteria
Throughout the hospital stay, the patient will:
• express feelings regarding stressors, on request
• display relaxed posture and facial expression.

GENERAL PLANS OF CARE

Discharge planning

NURSING DISCHARGE CRITERIA

Upon the patient's discharge, documentation shows evidence of:
• identification of specific sensory-perceptual alterations, if present
• successful resolution or ongoing treatment of sensory-perceptual problems.

PATIENT-FAMILY TEACHING CHECKLIST

Document evidence that the patient and family demonstrate an understanding of:
__ signs and symptoms of sensory-perceptual alteration
__ causes of sensory-perceptual alterations
__ reality orientation measures
__ stress-reduction measures
__ measures to promote sleep.

DOCUMENTATION CHECKLIST

Using outcome criteria as a guide, document:
__ clinical status on admission
__ significant changes in status
__ pertinent diagnostic test findings
__ reality orientation measures
__ sleep status
__ family participation in care
__ patient-family teaching
__ potential discharge needs
__ safety measures.

ASSOCIATED PLANS OF CARE

Impaired Physical Mobility
Ineffective Individual Coping
Knowledge Deficit
Pain

References

Dootson, S. "Critical Care: Sensory Imbalance and Sleep Loss," *Nursing Times* 86(35):26-29, August 29, 1990.

Gordon, M. *Manual of Nursing Diagnosis 1991-92.* St. Louis: Mosby-Year Book, 1991.

Hahn, K. "Think Twice About Sensory Loss," *Nursing89* 19(2):97-99, February 1989.

Moore, T. "Making Sense of Sensory Deprivation," *Nursing Times* 87(6):36-38, February 6, 1991.

Williams, S. *Decision Making in Critical Care.* St. Louis: Mosby-Year Book, 1990.

GENERAL PLANS OF CARE

Surgical Intervention

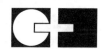

Introduction

DEFINITION AND TIME FOCUS
Surgical intervention is an important mode of medical therapy used for various diagnostic, curative, restorative, palliative, or cosmetic reasons. This plan focuses on care of the patient admitted for any surgery.

ETIOLOGY AND PRECIPITATING FACTORS
Precipitating factors are not applicable in this general plan of care because of the many disorders treated with surgery. For precipitating factors related to particular surgeries, see the plans for specific disorders.

Focused assessment guidelines

Focused assessment guidelines also are not applicable in this general plan of care because of the wide variety of disorders treated with surgery. For focused assessment guidelines related to particular types of surgery, see the plans for specific disorders.

DIAGNOSTIC STUDIES
The following laboratory tests are standard preoperative studies:

- urinalysis
- complete blood count (CBC)
- prothrombin time and partial thromboplastin time
- electrolyte panel
- blood urea nitrogen and creatinine levels
- blood typing and cross-matching.

The following are standard preoperative diagnostic procedures:
- chest X-ray
- 12-lead electrocardiogram (ECG)
- special studies depending on the disorder.

POTENTIAL COMPLICATIONS
- shock
- atelectasis
- pulmonary embolism
- thrombophlebitis
- wound infection, dehiscence, and evisceration
- paralytic ileus
- acute renal failure
- urine retention
- aspiration
- malignant hyperthermia
- hypothermia

Nursing diagnosis: *Knowledge deficit: perioperative routines, related to lack of familiarity with hospital procedures*

NURSING PRIORITY: Prepare the patient for perioperative routines.

Interventions

1. See the "Knowledge Deficit" plan, page 56.

2. Instruct the patient in the various aspects of perioperative routines, such as time of surgery, food or fluid restrictions, type of anesthesia, insertion of intravenous and intra-arterial lines, personnel, the environments of the operating and recovery rooms and surgical intensive care unit, type of wound and dressing, tubes, drains, and postoperative respiratory care. Include demonstrations and return demonstrations of coughing, deep breathing, spirometry, splinting the incision, and leg exercises.

3. Additional individualized interventions: _____

Rationales

1. Generalized interventions regarding patient teaching are included in the "Knowledge Deficit" plan.

2. Patients will be more likely to remember and comply with pre-, intra- and post-operative procedures if they understand the rationale for them, have been instructed before surgery, and have practiced activities where appropriate.

3. Rationales: _____

Target outcome criteria
Before surgery, the patient will:
- verbalize understanding of perioperative routines
- demonstrate ability to cough, deep-breathe, use the incentive spirometer, and perform leg exercises.

Collaborative problem: *High risk for postoperative shock related to hemorrhage or hypovolemia*

NURSING PRIORITY: Detect shock.

Interventions

1. Monitor and document vital signs on admission to the nursing unit and every 4 hours. If vital signs have changed significantly from recovery room findings, monitor every 15 to 30 minutes until stable. Report abnormalities. Estimate intraoperative blood loss from the surgical record and laboratory blood studies.

2. Assess the surgical dressing on admission to the unit, every hour for 4 hours, then every 4 hours. Mark any drainage, and note on the dressing the date and time it occurred. Document and report excessive drainage.

3. Assess the amount and character of drainage from wound-drainage tubes when assessing the surgical dressing. Report bright-red bloody drainage.

4. Reinforce the surgical dressing as needed. Do not change the original surgical dressing unless specifically ordered to do so.

5. Assess the surgical area for swelling or hematoma. Document and report abnormalities.

6. Monitor for changes in mental status. Be alert for restlessness and a sense of impending doom. Document and report such signs.

7. Assess and maintain I.V. line patency. Maintain I.V. fluids at the ordered rate.

8. Monitor urine output every hour for 4 hours, then every 4 hours, during the immediate postoperative period. Report urine output of less than 60 ml/hour and, in such cases, measure urine specific gravity. Administer I.V. fluids and diuretics as ordered, to maintain urine output at greater than 60 ml/hour and specific gravity at 1.010 to 1.025.

9. Monitor hematocrit and hemoglobin level, as ordered. Determine availability of blood and blood products.

10. Monitor fluid intake and output every 8 hours with an accumulated total every 24 hours for at least 3 to 4 days after surgery.

11. Additional individualized interventions: _____

Rationales

1. Hypotension and tachycardia may indicate hemorrhage. Estimated blood loss guides fluid and blood replacement.

2. Hemorrhage typically occurs within the first several hours after surgery. Frequent assessments allow for its prompt detection. Marking the extent of drainage permits objective serial measurements.

3. Bright-red blood from drainage tubes may indicate arterial hemorrhage.

4. Changing the surgical dressing may disrupt the wound edge, cause bleeding, and introduce bacteria.

5. Swelling or hematoma may indicate internal bleeding.

6. Changes in mental status may reflect cerebral hypoxia, indicating decreased cerebral perfusion from hemorrhage or hypovolemia.

7. A patent I.V. line is essential to fluid replacement. Fluids will be ordered according to the surgeon's preference. At times, fluid replacement is the only treatment necessary for hypovolemic shock.

8. Urine output decreases if the patient is bleeding or is hypovolemic. The kidneys retain fluid to maintain intravascular pressure. Urine specific gravity will reveal urine concentration as the body attempts to conserve fluid. Additionally, blood flow to the kidneys is reduced if the patient is in shock, thereby decreasing the glomerular filtration rate and urine output. I.V. fluids and diuretics help maintain the glomerular filtration rate to prevent acute tubular necrosis.

9. Hematocrit and hemoglobin level do not drop immediately with excessive blood loss because plasma is lost along with red blood cells. If bleeding persists, the blood remaining in the vessels will become more dilute as kidneys conserve water and as fluid shifts from interstitial to intravascular spaces; then hematocrit and hemoglobin level will drop. Rapid administration of blood and blood products may be necessary; confirming their availability avoids delays in initiating therapy.

10. For the first 48 hours after surgery, intake may exceed output because of fluid loss (from hemorrhage, vomiting, or diaphoresis) and increased secretion of antidiuretic hormone and aldosterone.

11. Rationales: _____

Target outcome criteria
Within 12 hours after surgery, the patient will:
• have vital signs within normal limits
• display minimal bloody drainage on dressing and in wound drains
• maintain a urine output greater than 60 ml/hour.

Within 2 days after surgery, the patient will display balanced fluid intake and output.

Nursing diagnosis: *Pain related to surgical tissue trauma, positioning, and reflex muscle spasm*

NURSING PRIORITY: Relieve pain.

Interventions

1. See the "Pain" plan, page 69.

2. Additional individualized interventions: _____
_____

Rationales

1. The "Pain" plan contains detailed information on pain assessment and management.

2. Rationales: _____
_____

Target outcome criteria
Within 1 hour of reporting pain, the patient will:
• verbalize adequacy of pain relief measures
• appear relaxed.

Collaborative problem: *High risk for postoperative atelectasis related to immobility and ciliary depression from anesthesia*

NURSING PRIORITY: Prevent atelectasis.

Interventions

1. Assess vital signs according to unit protocol for the first day after surgery, then every 4 hours. Note the characteristics of respirations. Monitor the amount and characteristics of sputum. Document and report abnormalities.

2. Auscultate breath sounds every 4 hours on the first postoperative day, then once per shift. Document and report abnormalities.

3. Instruct and coach the patient in diaphragmatic breathing and chest splinting.

4. Assist the patient in using the incentive spirometer—10 breaths every hour during the day, every 2 hours at night. In the first 24 hours, coach the patient on its use; then, once the patient is alert, encourage independent use and assess its effectiveness.

5. Help the patient turn every 2 hours unless contraindicated.

6. Help the patient progressively increase ambulation.

7. Encourage adequate fluid intake.

Rationales

1. Elevated temperature may indicate atelectasis, which can lead to pneumonia. Respirations may be shallow after anesthesia.

2. Breath sounds may be diminished postoperatively because air exchange is decreased in atelectatic areas.

3. Diaphragmatic breathing increases lung expansion by allowing the diaphragm to descend fully. Chest splinting reduces pain and facilitates breathing.

4. Use of the incentive spirometer promotes sustained maximal inspiration, which inflates alveoli as fully as possible.

5. Position changes provide for better ventilation of all lobes of the lungs and promote drainage of secretions.

6. Ambulation promotes adequate ventilation by increasing the respiratory rate.

7. Respiratory secretions will be thinner and more easily expectorated if the patient is well hydrated.

GENERAL PLANS OF CARE

8. Additional individualized interventions: _____

8. Rationales: _____

_____

_____

Target outcome criteria
Throughout the postoperative period, the patient will:
• display respiratory rate of 12 to 20 breaths/minute
• have nonlabored, deep respirations
• manifest audible, clear breath sounds in all lobes.

Collaborative problem: *High risk for postoperative thromboembolic phenomena related to immobility, dehydration, and possible fat particle escape or aggregation*

NURSING PRIORITY: Prevent thromboembolism.

Interventions

1. Instruct and coach the patient to do leg exercises hourly while awake: flexing and extending the feet, ankle rotation, flexing and extending the knees, and quadriceps setting.

2. Assess twice daily for signs of thromboembolic phenomena. If any of these signs or symptoms are present, alert the doctor promptly:

• thrombophlebitis (redness, swelling, increased warmth along the vein, possibly a positive Homans' sign, and pain)
• pulmonary thromboembolism (sharp, stabbing chest pain, worsening on deep inspiration or coughing; hemoptysis; pleural friction rub; and tachypnea)

• fat embolism (dyspnea, restlessness, and petechiae)

• peripheral vascular thromboembolism (pallor, weak pulse, loss of sensation).

3. Encourage early ambulation after surgery.

4. Avoid using the knee gatch or placing pillows under the patient's knees.

5. Encourage adequate fluid intake (in the initial postoperative period, I.V. fluids will be administered).

6. Apply antiembolism stockings, if ordered. Remove them twice daily for 1 hour.

7. Before discharge, teach the patient and family about guidelines for resuming normal activity.

Rationales

1. Leg exercises promote blood flow in the legs. Muscle contractions compress the veins and help prevent venous stasis, a major cause of clot formation.

2. Systematic observations aid in prompt detection of thromboembolic phenomena. Prompt treatment reduces the risk of clot extension, pulmonary infarction, or pulmonary arrest.
• Vessel wall inflammation and clot formation produce signs and symptoms of thrombophlebitis.

• Pulmonary thromboembolism occurs when a clot detaches from a vessel and lodges in the lungs.

• Fat embolism is a risk after orthopedic trauma or surgery (such as femur fractures or sternum-splitting incisions). It may result from the escape of fat particles from bone marrow or from an aggregation of fat particles in the bloodstream.
• Blood clots and sclerotic plaques can detach and lodge in the peripheral vascular bed.

3. Ambulation promotes blood flow in the legs.

4. Pressure on the popliteal blood vessels can slow blood circulation to and from the legs. Appropriate positioning also decreases venous stasis.

5. Inadequate fluid intake causes dehydration, which leads to increased blood viscosity—another major contributor to clot formation.

6. Antiembolism stockings compress the leg veins and prevent venous stasis. Stockings should be removed periodically to allow for thrombophlebitis assessment and skin inspection.

7. Patients and families probably will have specific questions or concerns about the type and progression of allowable activity after discharge. Providing guidelines promotes the resumption of activity at an appropriate pace, which in turn lessens immobility-related complications and promotes a sense of well-being.

8. Additional individualized interventions: _____

8. Rationales: _____

Target outcome criteria
Throughout the postoperative period, the patient will show no signs of thromboembolic phenomena.

By the time of discharge, the patient will be able to identify an appropriate postdischarge activity schedule.

Nursing diagnosis: *High risk for postoperative injury related to possible changes in mental status caused by anesthesia and analgesia*

NURSING PRIORITY: Prevent injury.

Interventions

1. Assess the patient's level of consciousness, orientation, and ability to follow directions every 30 to 60 minutes in the first 8 to 10 hours postoperatively. Compare to preoperative level of consciousness and mental status.

2. Position the drowsy patient in a side-lying position.

3. Keep side rails up in the initial postoperative period, until the patient is awake and alert.

4. Keep the call cord within the patient's reach.

5. Keep the bed in the low position.

6. Monitor postural vital signs and assist the patient with initial postoperative activity.
• Observe for a pulse rate increase of 20 to 30 beats/minute, a systolic blood pressure decrease of 20 to 30 mm Hg, and dizziness or an unsteady gait. If these signs are present, reposition the patient slowly.
• Observe for a pulse rate increase of more than 30 beats/minute, a systolic blood pressure decrease of more than 30 mm Hg, a decreased level of consciousness, diaphoresis, and cyanosis. If present, discontinue activity and alert the doctor.

7. Additional individualized interventions: _____

Rationales

1. A greater risk of injury exists if the patient is drowsy or disoriented. Frequent observation allows prompt detection of injury risk factors, if present. Preoperative status provides a baseline for comparison.

2. In a side-lying position, the patient has less risk of aspirating secretions or vomitus.

3. Side rails help prevent falls.

4. If the call cord is within reach, the patient is more likely to ask the nurse for assistance.

5. The low bed position is safer for the patient.

6. When first ambulating, the patient may feel dizzy or have an unsteady gait from orthostatic hypotension. This occurs because immobility compromises the ability of peripheral vessels to constrict when the patient assumes an upright position. Orthostatic hypotension can also occur if the patient is hypovolemic, producing the more alarming signs listed and requiring medical evaluation and I.V. fluid replacement.

7. Rationales: _____

GENERAL PLANS OF CARE

Target outcome criteria
Within 36 hours after surgery, the patient will:
• be free from injury
• seek appropriate assistance with activity from the nurse.

Nursing diagnosis: *High risk for infection related to surgical intervention*

NURSING PRIORITY: Promote wound healing.

Interventions

1. Identify risk factors for surgical wound infection:

• obesity
• extremes of age

• immunosuppression
• poor nutritional status
• diabetes mellitus.

2. Assess the surgical wound and other invasive sites once a shift for:
• evidence of normal healing, such as approximation of wound margins and absence of purulent or foul-smelling drainage

• signs of dehiscence, such as poorly approximated wound edges and serous drainage from a previously non-draining wound (if dehiscence occurs, cover with a dry sterile dressing and notify the doctor immediately)

• signs of evisceration, such as disruption of the surgical wound with protrusion of the viscera (if evisceration occurs, cover the viscerated organs with sterile saline-soaked gauze and notify the doctor immediately).

3. Determine wound classification:

• clean—minimal endogenous contamination present (such as with breast biopsy)

• clean-contaminated—possible endogenous bacterial contamination present (such as with appendectomy)

• contaminated—contamination present (such as with trauma)
• dirty—infected tissue present (such as with abscess).

4. Monitor temperature every 4 hours. Document and report elevations.

5. Maintain a clean, dry incision. Perform wound care as ordered.

6. Use strict aseptic technique when performing wound care. Instruct the patient and family in hand washing technique; aseptic technique; and wound care, including dressing change and application, irrigations and cleansing procedures, proper disposal of soiled dressings, and bathing by shower (not tub) until the wound is healed.

7. Instruct the patient and family in signs and symptoms of infection: elevated temperature, abdominal pain, and purulent or foul-smelling wound drainage.

8. Encourage adequate nutritional intake every shift. Document intake every shift.

Rationales

1. Knowledge of risk factors enables the nurse to individualize patient care.
• Adipose tissue is poorly vascularized, retarding healing.
• The very young and the very old have less physiologic reserve.
• A compromised host is at greater risk for infection.
• A catabolic state retards wound repair.
• Impaired glucose metabolism delays healing.

2. Regular assessment promotes early detection of suboptimal healing.
• The normally healing wound is well approximated and without evidence of infection. (The surgical wound, however, may be reddened in the first 3 postoperative days—the normal inflammatory response.)
• Wound dehiscence most commonly occurs 3 to 11 days after surgery. Application of a sterile dressing reduces the risk of infection.

• Eviscerated organs must be kept moist and surgical intervention must be prompt because blood supply to tissues is compromised when organs herniate.

3. Wound classification is a predictor of surgical wound infection.
• In this wound class, the respiratory, alimentary, or genitourinary tract is not entered during surgery so the likelihood of contamination is minimal.
• In this wound class, the respiratory, alimentary, or genitourinary tract is entered under controlled conditions, but infection is not noted and the risk of postoperative infection is increased only slightly.
• In this wound class, gross GI spillage or traumatic wounds place the patient at higher risk for infection.
• In this wound class, retained devitalized tissue or existing infection pose the greatest risk for infection.

4. A low-grade temperature present in the first 3 postoperative days is associated with the normal inflammatory response. Fever that persists may signify infection.

5. A clean, dry incision is at less risk for infection. Moisture can harbor microorganisms.

6. Aseptic technique prevents cross-contamination and transmission of bacterial infections to the surgical wound.

7. Educating the patient and family promotes their sense of control and minimizes anxiety and fear during preparation for discharge.

8. Sufficient intake of protein, calories, vitamins, and minerals is essential to promote tissue healing.

9. Additional individualized interventions: _____

9. Rationales:_____

Target outcome criteria
Within 3 days after surgery, the patient will:
• be afebrile
• show no signs of infection.

Within 7 days after surgery, the patient will have a clean, dry, and well-approximated surgical wound.

Nursing diagnosis: *High risk for postoperative urine retention related to neuroendocrine response to stress, anesthesia, and recumbent position*

NURSING PRIORITY: Prevent urine retention.

Interventions

1. Assess for signs of urine retention. Include subjective complaints of urgency as well as objective signs, such as bladder distention, urine overflow, and marked discrepancy between the fluid intake amount and the time of the last voiding.

2. Initiate interventions to promote voiding as soon as the patient begins to sense bladder pressure.

3. Provide noninvasive measures to promote voiding, such as normal position for voiding, ambulation to the bathroom if possible, running water, relaxation, a warm bedpan if needed, pouring warm water over the perineum, and privacy.

4. Provide a supportive atmosphere: use conscious positive suggestion; reassure the patient that voiding usually occurs eventually; do not threaten catheterization.

5. If the patient complains of bladder discomfort or has not voided within 8 hours after surgery, obtain an order for straight catheterization.

6. If the patient requires catheterization, drain the bladder of no more than 1,000 ml at a time. If urine output reaches 1,000 ml, clamp the catheter, wait 1 hour, then drain the rest of the urine from the bladder.

7. After catheterization, assess for dysuria, hematuria, pyuria, burning, and frequency and urgency of urination as well as for suprapubic discomfort. Assess and document the amount, appearance, odor, and clarity of urine. Report any signs of urinary infection.

8. Additional individualized interventions: _____

Rationales

1. The distended bladder can be palpated above the level of the symphysis pubis. Overflow incontinence occurs when intravesical pressure exceeds the restraining ability of the sphincter and enough urine flows out to decrease the intravesical pressure to a level at which the sphincter can control urine flow. A difference of several hundred milliliters between fluid intake and output, with the passage of several hours since the last voiding, implies retention.

2. Prompt treatment of potential voiding problems may reduce anxiety, which can further impair the ability to void.

3. These measures are designed to promote relaxation of the urinary sphincter and facilitate voiding. Successful use of noninvasive measures prevents unnecessary catheterization and related psychological strain and urethral trauma.

4. Conscious positive suggestion and reassurance promote relaxation and set up expectations for spontaneous voiding.

5. Straight catheterization poses less risk of infection than indwelling catheterization; an indwelling catheter can provide a pathway for bacteria to ascend into the bladder.

6. Draining more than 1,000 ml from the bladder releases pressure on the pelvic vessels. The sudden release of pressure allows subsequent pooling of blood in these vessels. Rapid withdrawal of this blood from the central circulating volume may cause shock.

7. Urine retention (stasis) and the introduction of a urethral catheter increase the risk for lower urinary tract infection.

8. Rationales: _____

Target outcome criterion
Within 1 day after surgery, the patient will void at least 200 ml of clear urine at a time.

Collaborative problem: *High risk for postoperative paralytic ileus, abdominal pain, or constipation related to immobility, surgical manipulation, anesthesia, and analgesia*

NURSING PRIORITIES: (a) Detect paralytic ileus and (b) prevent constipation.

Interventions

1. Assess the abdomen twice daily for bowel sounds and distention. Assess for the presence of flatus or stool. Question the patient about abdominal fullness.

2. If paralytic ileus occurs, implement measures, as ordered, such as instructing the patient not to eat or drink anything, connecting a nasogastric tube to low intermittent suction, using a rectal tube to expel flatus, and administering I.V. fluids.

3. Implement comfort measures if paralytic ileus occurs: provide frequent mouth care, position and tape the nasogastric tube carefully, and administer analgesics.

4. Provide a diet appropriate to peristaltic activity. Ensure that peristalsis has returned before progressing from nothing-bymouth status to liberal fluid and solid food intake.

5. Encourage fluid intake of at least 8 8-oz glasses (2,000 ml) per day unless contraindicated (such as by congestive heart failure). Provide fluids that the patient prefers.

6. Encourage frequent position changes and ambulation.

7. Provide privacy for the patient during defecation. Assist with ambulation to the bathroom if necessary.

8. Consult with the doctor concerning use of laxatives, suppositories, or enemas.

9. Additional individualized interventions: _____

_____

Rationales

1. Bowel sounds will be hypoactive initially but should return to normal within the first 2 days after surgery. The presence of flatus or stool signals the return of peristalsis. Abdominal distention and absence of bowel sounds, flatus, and stool may indicate paralytic ileus.

2. These measures help prevent abdominal distention while promoting return of peristalsis. I.V. fluids maintain fluid and electrolyte balance while the patient has no oral intake.

3. Maintaining patient comfort is important to prevent further anxiety.

4. If peristalsis has not returned, feeding the patient will cause distention.

5. Sufficient fluid intake is required for proper stool consistency. Providing preferred fluids promotes hydration.

6. Activity promotes peristalsis.

7. Providing privacy eliminates possible embarrassment.

8. A laxative, suppository, or enema may be needed to promote bowel evacuation. These supplements should be used judiciously to avoid bowel dependence or possible damage to healing tissues.

9. Rationales: _____

_____

Target outcome criteria
Within 2 days after surgery, the patient will have normal bowel sounds.

Within 4 days after surgery, the patient will:
• have soft, formed bowel movements
• not strain at stool.

Within 7 days after surgery, the patient will establish a regular bowel elimination pattern.

Collaborative problem: *High risk for malignant hyperthermia related to inherited skeletal muscle disorder, anesthetic agents, and abnormal calcium transport*

NURSING PRIORITIES: (a) Detect malignant hyperthermia and (b) initiate treatment.

Interventions

1. Assess the patient's susceptibility to malignant hyperthermia:

Rationales

1. Malignant hyperthermia is an inherited skeletal muscle disorder causing a hypermetabolic state induced by anesthetic agents. Assessment identifies patients at risk for malignant hyperthermia, which can be fatal.

- personal and family history of malignant hyperthermia and response to anesthesia
- history of muscle abnormality: muscular hypertrophy, musculoskeletal problems (club foot, hernia, ptosis)
- young age, male

2. Assess for signs and symptoms of malignant hyperthermia:
- ventricular arrhythmias (tachycardia, fibrillation)
- tachypnea
- hot, diaphoretic, mottled skin with or without cyanosis
- elevated temperature
- excessive muscle rigidity
- oliguria, anuria.

3. Monitor vital signs, arterial blood gases, electrolytes and ECG.

4. Alert anesthesiologist or nurse anesthetist to discontinue anesthesia (intraoperatively).

5. Administer dantrolene sodium (Dantrium), as ordered: initial I.V. dose is 2 to 3 mg/kg, followed by 1 mg/kg every 10 minutes up to 10 mg/kg.

6. Administer 100% oxygen.

7. Administer iced I.V. solutions or iced lavages of stomach, rectum, or bladder; employ hypothermia blanket.

8. Evaluate interventions; repeat regimen as indicated.

9. Before discharge, educate the patient and family about the future risk of malignant hyperthermia.

10. Additional individualized interventions:_____

_____

- A genetic predisposition exists for malignant hyperthermia.
- Musculoskeletal abnormalities may predispose the patient toward malignant hyperthermia.
- The condition occurs more often in children than adults, and more often in males than females.

2. Systematic observations aid in prompt detection of condition.
- Increased circulating catecholamines and hyperkalemia produce cardiac rhythm abnormalities.
- The respiratory rate increases to compensate for increased carbon dioxide production (respiratory acidosis).
- The body reacts to the hypermetabolic state by vasodilating and perspiring.
- Temperature increase reflects increased energy use.
- Anesthetic agents induce rigidity.
- Hypovolemia and decreased cardiac output cause decreased urine production.

3. Monitoring provides information about the extent of respiratory and metabolic acidosis and guides treatment of physiologic derangements.

4. Discontinuation of anesthesia removes a contributing factor.

5. Use of this skeletal muscle relaxant reduces muscular rigidity; this is the definitive pharmacologic treatment.

6. Oxygen administration provides increased oxygen to meet metabolic demands.

7. Cooling the body reduces the metabolic rate and lowers body temperature.

8. Hypermetabolic reaction can recur.

9. Malignant hyperthermia can recur.

10. Rationales:_____

_____

Target outcome criteria
Throughout the postoperative period, the patient will show no signs of malignant hyperthermia

By the time of discharge, the patient will:
- be aware of risks for malignant hyperthermia
- inform health care providers of risk before any future surgery.

Collaborative problem: *Nausea or vomiting related to GI distention, rapid position changes, or cortical stimulation of the vomiting center or chemoreceptor trigger zone*

NURSING PRIORITY: Prevent or relieve nausea or vomiting.

Interventions

1. Prevent GI overdistention: maintain patency of the nasogastric tube; change the patient's diet only as tolerated.

Rationales

1. Overdistention of the GI tract, particularly the duodenum, triggers the vomiting reflex.

2. Limit unpleasant sights, smells, and psychic stimuli, such as intense anxiety and pain.

3. Caution the patient to change position slowly.

4. As soon as possible, advance the patient from narcotics to other analgesics (as ordered), and then to nonpharmacologic pain-control measures.

5. Administer antiemetics, as ordered.

6. Additional individualized interventions: _____

_____

2. These factors stimulate the chemoreceptor trigger zone in the medulla, which causes vomiting.

3. Rapid position changes also stimulate the trigger zone.

4. Medications, especially narcotics, may excite the chemoreceptor trigger zone.

5. Agents that depress the vomiting center or trigger zone responsiveness may be necessary when the measures described above are inappropriate or ineffective.

6. Rationales: _____

_____

Target outcome criteria
Within 1 hour of onset of nausea or vomiting, the patient will:
• verbalize relief of nausea
• be free from vomiting.

Discharge planning

NURSING DISCHARGE CRITERIA
Upon the patient's discharge, documentation shows evidence of:
• return to preoperative level of consciousness
• absence of fever
• absence of pulmonary and cardiovascular complications
• stable vital signs
• healing wound with no signs of infection
• hemoglobin and white blood cell counts within normal ranges
• I.V. lines discontinued for at least 24 hours
• ability to tolerate oral food intake
• ability to perform wound care independently
• ability to void and have bowel movements as before surgery
• ability to ambulate and perform activities of daily living as before surgery
• knowledge of activity restrictions
• ability to control pain using oral medications
• adequate home support, or referral to home care or a nursing home if indicated by lack of home support system or by inability to perform self-care.

PATIENT-FAMILY TEACHING CHECKLIST
Document evidence that the patient and family demonstrate an understanding of:
__ plan for resumption of normal activity
__ wound care
__ signs and symptoms of wound infection or other surgical complications
__ all discharge medications' purpose, dosage, administration, and side effects requiring medical attention (postoperative patients may be discharged with oral analgesics)
__ when and how to contact the doctor
__ date, time, and location of follow-up appointment with the doctor
__ community resources appropriate for surgical intervention performed.

DOCUMENTATION CHECKLIST
Using outcome criteria as a guide, document:
__ clinical status on admission
__ significant changes in preoperative status (level of consciousness, emotional status, baseline physical data)
__ preoperative teaching and its effectiveness
__ preoperative checklist (includes documentation regarding preoperative consent, urinalysis, CBC, 12-lead ECG, chest X-ray, preoperative medication administration, surgical skin preparation, voiding on call from the operating room, and removal of nail polish, jewelry, prostheses, dentures, glasses, and hearing aids)
__ clinical status on admission from the recovery room
__ amount and character of wound drainage (on dressing and through drains)
__ skin condition
__ patency of tubes (I.V., nasogastric, indwelling urinary catheter, drains)
__ pulmonary hygiene measures
__ pain-relief measures
__ activity tolerance
__ nutritional intake
__ elimination status (urinary and bowel)
__ pertinent laboratory test findings
__ patient-family teaching
__ discharge planning.

ASSOCIATED PLANS OF CARE
Grieving
Impaired Physical Mobility
Ineffective Individual Coping
Knowledge Deficit
Pain
Sensory-Perceptual Alteration

References

Brunner, L., and Suddarth, D. *Textbook of Medical-Surgical Nursing,* 6th ed. Philadelphia: J.B. Lippincott Co., 1988.

Carpenito, L. *Nursing Diagnosis: Application to Clincal Practice,* 4th ed. Philadelphia: J.B. Lippincott Co., 1991.

Guyton, A. *Textbook of Medical Physiology,* 8th ed. Philadelphia: W.B. Saunders, 1991.

Meeker, M., and Rothrock, J. *Alexander's Care of the Patient in Surgery,* 9th ed. St. Louis: Mosby-Yearbook, 1991.

Rothrock, J. *Perioperative Nursing Care Planning.* St. Louis: Mosby-Yearbook, 1990.

Sparks, S., and Taylor, C. *Nursing Diagnosis Reference Manual.* Springhouse, Pa.: Springhouse Corp., 1991.

Thompson, J., et al. *Mosby's Manual of Clinical Nursing,* 2nd ed. St. Louis: Mosby-Yearbook, 1989.

GENERAL PLANS
OF CARE

NEUROLOGIC DISORDERS
Alzheimer's Disease

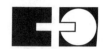

DRG information
DRG 012 Degenerative Nervous System Disorders.
    Mean LOS = 6.9 days

Additional DRG information: Patients are rarely admitted with only Alzheimer's disease (AD); usually, another disorder, such as pneumonia or dehydration, is the primary diagnosis. Because AD as a comorbidity would probably increase the other disorders' LOS and relative weight (depending on the primary diagnosis), a patient with AD is more likely to be assigned that DRG number than DRG 12.

Introduction
DEFINITION AND TIME FOCUS
AD is chronic, irreversible neuronal degeneration of the central nervous system, leading to severe disorders of cognition in the absence of other neurologic manifestations. Senile plaques and neurofibrillary tangles characterize the insidious, relentless progression of structural brain atrophy. This clinical plan focuses on the AD patient admitted at any of the progressively deteriorating stages of the disease.

ETIOLOGY AND PRECIPITATING FACTORS
Etiology is obscure, but ongoing research suggests the following theories:
• neurochemical deficiency of neurotransmitters acetylcholine and somatostatin (important for cognition and memory)
• neurometabolic disorder, causing diminished cellular protein synthesis
• genetic and environmental factors, with autosomal dominant transmission in certain families
• aluminum deposits in senile plaques (a conglomeration of protein) and neurofibrillary tangles (twisted nerve fibers) abundant in the hippocampus of the brain, a cortical area considered necessary for memory
• slow viruses (those that invade the host but remain dormant for years before symptoms develop) whose effects sometimes resemble those of AD
• immune system dysfunctions implicated in the degenerative disease.

Focused assessment guidelines
NURSING HISTORY (Functional health pattern findings)

Health perception — health management pattern
• the patient may perceive memory loss as related to normal aging
• the patient may disguise confusion and disorientation by using learned social skills and fabrication
• significant others may describe mental decline

Nutritional-metabolic pattern
• family may report anorexia because the patient forgets to eat or does not recognize hunger signs
• family may report weight loss
• the patient may report fatigue and malaise
• the patient may report dysphagia (in later stages)

Elimination pattern
• family may report constipation related to forgetfulness and disorientation
• family may report urinary and fecal incontinence (in later stages)

Activity-exercise pattern
• family may describe activity limited to familiar environment as confusion and disorientation increase
• family may describe compromise of activities of daily living as dependence increases because of inability to perform actions sequentially
• the patient may demonstrate incompetence in performing complex tasks, such as shopping, telephoning, and banking
• the patient may jeopardize personal safety through loss of locomotion or wandering behavior

Sleep-rest pattern
• nocturnal restlessness with insomnia
• altered sleep-awake cycle
• arousal more difficult as disease progresses

Cognitive-perceptual pattern
• progressively impaired judgment
• progressively impaired ability to orient self in the environment
• immediate, recent, and remote memory, including episodic (events) and semantic (knowledge) memory, is lost
• affect tends to be incongruent and inconsistent, often depressed
• progressively reduced conceptualization, attention, arousal, concentration, and abstract thinking
• progressively impaired expressive language and increased receptive aphasia

Self-perception — self-concept pattern
• the patient may attempt to sustain internal locus of control, sense of dignity, and self-esteem

Role-relationship pattern
• altered family dynamics from role reversals with increased patient dysfunction
• increased social withdrawal (isolationism)

Sexuality-reproductive pattern
• may reject intimate contact

Coping—stress tolerance pattern
• may demonstrate defense mechanisms of rationalization, denial, and projection
• may demonstrate apathy, depression, and helplessness
• may exhibit primary emotional lability manifested by irritability, anger, fear, agitation
• may exhibit signs of ego disintegration—hallucinations, illusions, and suicidal ideology

Value-belief pattern
• may display altered value system resulting from defective mental faculties

PHYSICAL FINDINGS
Neurologic
• confusion
• disorientation
• memory loss
• language disintegration
• irritability
• cognitive dysfunction
• labile affect
• clinical depression

Integumentary
• poor skin turgor (or other signs of dehydration)

Musculoskeletal
• decreased activity tolerance
• lack of coordination
• immobility
• limited range of motion

Genitourinary
• urine retention
• urinary incontinence

Gastrointestinal
• fecal incontinence

DIAGNOSTIC STUDIES
Note: Postmortem brain biopsy is the only definitive diagnostic test for AD.
• hematologic measurements of neurotransmitters and neurotransmitter metabolites—may be low, implicating a biochemical deficiency as etiologic factor
• complete blood count, Venereal Disease Research Laboratory test, blood chemistries, endocrine studies—performed for differential diagnosis of reversible cognitive impairment
• vitamin B_{12} levels—may be low, indicating nutritional deficit
• computed tomography scan—may indicate cortical atrophy and widening of the ventricles
• lumbar puncture for cerebrospinal fluid examination—may show presence of abnormal protein levels (common)
• positron emission tomography—may reflect diminished brain metabolism
• skull X-rays—may reflect cerebral atrophy
• electroencephalography—may show decreased electrical activity contributing to dysfunction
• magnetic resonance imaging—performed to rule out reversible cognitive impairment
• language ability tests—performed for differential diagnosis
• vision and hearing tests—establish sensory deficits (versus cognitive impairment) as the cause of selected symptoms
• 12-lead electrocardiography—may indicate coronary insufficiency contributing to the symptoms

POTENTIAL COMPLICATIONS
• total loss of mental faculties
• pneumonia
• injury

Collaborative problem: *Impaired cognitive function related to degenerative loss of cerebral tissue*

NURSING PRIORITIES: (a) Provide a safe, structured environment, (b) promote an optimum level of functioning, and (c) establish effective communication patterns.

Interventions

1. Assess the patient's level of cognitive functioning, using functional rating scale for symptoms of dementia or mini-mental status exam (see *Assessing Alzheimer's disease,* page 94). Prepare the patient for psychological testing.

2. Assign the patient to a room close to the nursing station for frequent observation.

3. Minimize hazards in the environment.

Rationales

1. Information gleaned from the patient and family provides a guide for planning care. Psychological testing will provide information necessary to structure a therapeutic regimen.

2. The patient may wander aimlessly or require frequent attention.

3. Confusion and faulty judgment contribute to accidental injury.

ASSESSING ALZHEIMER'S DISEASE

Understanding how Alzheimer's disease progresses helps the nurse plan appropriate care and maximize the patient's functional ability. This chart summarizes the stages of disease progression.

Stage	Approximate duration	Signs and symptoms	Nursing considerations
I	2 to 4 years	• "Fishing" for words • Forgetfulness progressing to inability to recall details of recent events • Irritability or apathy • Occasional episodes of getting lost • Periods of disorientation • Significantly impaired reasoning ability and judgment	• The patient typically can manage most daily activities and does not require institutionalization. • The patient senses a decrease in mental faculties and may use denial to cope with this. Do not force the patient to "face the facts."
II	2 to 12 years	• Reduced vision, hearing, and pain sensation • Hyperorality (chewing or tasting anything within reach) • Inability to recognize familiar things (may not recognize own mirror reflection) • Increased aphasia (language defect) • Increased appetite without weight gain • Preservation (repeating the same word or action over and over) • Seizures • Social inappropriateness, such as poor table manners, personal hygiene, and grooming	• Assist the patient with hygiene and grooming to preserve self-esteem and dignity. • Avoid using puns or jokes because these will confuse the patient. • Call the patient by name rather than "Honey," "Grandma," or another belittling term. • If the patient has trouble walking, accompany the patient on walks several times a day to prevent muscle contractures and other complications of immobility. • Maintain a consistent, calm environment to orient the patient. • Make sure the patient wanders only in safe areas. • Monitor the items the patient places in the mouth. • Maintain the patient on a toileting schedule to minimize incontinence. • Stay with the patient during meals to observe for swallowing problems and assist with table manners.
III	1 year	• Apraxia (inability to perform purposeful movements, even on command) • Bladder and bowel incontinence • Decreased appetite • Disappearance of preservation and hyperorality • Generalized tonic-clonic seizures • Muteness • Unresponsiveness to verbal and physical stimuli	• Maintain a consistent routine. • Monitor the patient's skin for breakdown and pressure ulcers. • Monitor all body systems carefully for physiologic deterioration. • Perform passive range-of-motion exercises at least 4 times a day to prevent contractures, if the patient is bedridden.

Adapted with permission from R. Charles, M. Truesdell, and E. Wood (1982). Alzheimer's disease: Pathology, progression, and nursing process. *Journal of Gerontological Nursing,* 8(2), pp. 69-73.

4. Maintain consistency in nursing routines.

4. Assigning the same nurse, serving meals on time, scheduling rest periods, and so forth provide the patient with structure in an unfamiliar environment.

5. Promote self-care independence within the scope of the patient's abilities; assist when necessary. Identify specific individual needs in the plan of care.

5. Self-esteem is preserved when the patient can provide self-care. As the disease progresses, complete physical care in bathing, dressing, and toileting becomes necessary. Identifying needs in the plan of care promotes appropriate care.

6. Establish and maintain a therapeutic relationship by dealing with the patient in a calm, reassuring, affirming, and nonthreatening manner.

6. Trust must be established to achieve any goal because of the patient's suspicions and increasing paranoia.

7. Capture and retain the patient's attention by giving simple, specific directions for accomplishing tasks; use eye contact and unobtrusive guidance.

7. The effects of memory loss and a reduced attention span can be minimized with clear directions and appropriate guidance.

8. Orient the patient to reality frequently and repetitively.

8. Although disorientation seems to prevail, repetitive reorientation may reduce the patient's anxiety.

9. Administer and document medications, as ordered.

9. Tacrine (THA) for improving memory and bethanechol (Urabeth) for increasing neurotransmission are under study. Anti-anxiety drugs may be helpful. Other drugs may include ergoloid mesylates (Hydergine) or lecithin for cognition and memory; doxepin (Sinequan), nortriptyline (Pamelor), or amitryptyline (Elavil) as antidepressants; and sleep maintenance drugs such as temazepam (Restoril).

10. Use aids to improve language skills and verbal repetition and pictures to improve recall.

10. Both methods may assist the patient with word recall.

11. Minimize communication barriers. Be aware that anxiety, cultural influences, spiritual beliefs, and language difficulties may contribute to paranoia and withdrawal.

11. Knowing and understanding the patient's cultural background and beliefs can further open communication.

12. Encourage social interaction with individuals and groups by including the patient in unit activities when possible, allowing maximum flexibility in visiting hours, and providing occupational therapy referral.

12. Continued social interaction reinforces reality and contributes to a sense of self-worth and identity.

13. Prevent excessive stimulation and promote usual sleep-rest pattern.

13. Moderate stimulation is necessary and important for orientation, but excessive stimulation increases confusion. Sleep deprivation contributes to confusion.

14. Be attentive and consistent in verbal and nonverbal responses to the patient.

14. Nurse-patient dialogue must reflect trust and understanding. Consistency between verbal and nonverbal responses to the patient reduces cognitive dissonance.

15. Encourage reminiscence in patient dialogue.

15. Remembering past events assists the patient in maintaining self-identity. Distant memory may be retained even when recent memory is impaired.

16. Prepare an identity card, a bracelet, or a name tag for the patient. Include name, address, phone number, medical problem, and other pertinent information.

16. Should the patient wander, identification information can facilitate the patient's prompt return.

17. Additional individualized interventions: _____

17. Rationales: _____

Target outcome criteria
Within 1 week of admission, the patient will:
• be free from injury
• perform self-care as much as possible
• communicate needs clearly
• wear some means of identification.

Nursing diagnosis: *Nutritional deficit related to memory loss and inadequate food intake*

NURSING PRIORITY: Stabilize and improve nutritional status.

Interventions

1. Assess present nutritional status: weigh the patient and record customary dietary intake on admission. See the "Nutritional Deficit" plan, page 63, and the "Total Parenteral Nutrition" plan, page 411, for more information on nutritional assessment.

Rationales

1. Assessing the patient's nutritional status provides necessary information for determining actual deficits; an appropriate dietary regimen may then be implemented.

2. Offer a balanced diet consisting of small meals at regular intervals and nutritious snacks in between. Provide finger foods when possible.

2. Regularly scheduled meals are important in maintaining a structured environment. Small quantities may be more appealing and provide the patient with a sense of achievement when all the food is consumed. Finger foods are easier to handle than food that must be eaten with a utensil.

3. Prepare the tray in advance with appropriate portions of food arranged conveniently so that the patient may eat unassisted (cut the meat, provide a spoon, open containers, and so forth).

3. Coordination difficulties may develop, impairing use of utensils. Preparation of food servings avoids the humiliation of being unable to provide self-care and decreases frustration.

4. Provide time and privacy for meals.

4. The patient who has difficulty chewing or swallowing will need more time to eat. Lack of coordination may result in socially unacceptable eating habits.

5. Monitor and record daily weight and the amount and type of food intake. Adjust the dietary plan accordingly.

5. Evaluation of weight and intake provides guidelines for modifying the dietary plan.

6. Provide dietary information to the home caregiver.

6. The patient will probably continue to need assistance in menu selection, cooking, and eating after discharge. The person shopping, cooking, and offering meals to the patient may need to be instructed in individual dietary needs.

7. Additional individualized interventions: _____

7. Rationales: _____

Target outcome criterion
Within 1 week of admission, the patient will gain a pre-determined number of pounds, or maintain a stable weight.

Nursing diagnosis: *High risk for injury related to wandering behavior, aphasia, agnosia, or hyperorality*

NURSING PRIORITY: Prevent injury while maximizing independence.

Interventions

1. Consider using a bell to alert caregivers when the patient is wandering.

Rationales

1. Wandering behavior and restlessness characterize later stages of AD. Unattended, the patient may become lost even in familiar surroundings.

2. Ensure that the patient is dressed appropriately for the temperature. Provide shoes that fit well; avoid loose slippers.

2. The patient may be unable to make appropriate choices about dress and may have a reduced ability to identify or verbalize discomfort. Loose slippers may be lost or may contribute to injuries from falls.

3. Avoid using restraints.

3. Restraints increase the patient's agitation and paranoia and may contribute to injury.

4. Recommend safety measures to the family for home care:
• safely storing knives, medications, matches, firearms, and cleaning solutions and other toxic household chemicals
• using night lights

4. The home environment may contribute to injuries if the family is not prepared.
• The patient may be unable to recognize familiar objects (agnosia) and so may inadvertently cause self-injury or harm to others by using them inappropriately.
• Night lights may decrease falls and help with ongoing reorientation to the environment.

• storing small objects safely

• AD patients may be prone to hyperorality (chewing or tasting anything within reach) and may put small objects in their mouths, swallowing or choking on nonfood items they no longer recognize.

• securing door locks and using bells on the patient's person

• Door locks and bells may help prevent wandering behaviors or alert the family to it.

• using consistency in placement of objects

• Consistency may help expedite environmental reorientation.

• alerting neighbors to the patient's condition.

• If neighbors are aware of the patient's illness, they can alert the family to wandering or other unsafe behaviors they witness.

5. Encourage a regular exercise program, as tolerated.

5. Regular exercise decreases restlessness and agitation, promotes muscle tone, and contributes to a sense of well-being. Overactivity, however, may contribute to fatigue and confusion.

6. Observe for nonverbal cues to injury, such as grimacing, rubbing, panting, or protecting the injured area. Also note repetitive words or seemingly inappropriate statements. Alert the family to cues observed.

6. The patient may be unable to identify or express discomfort but may reveal illness or injury through nonverbal cues. Because aphasia may make expressions of discomfort convoluted, such words as "cold" or "hurt," especially if repeated, may warrant investigation.

7. Additional individualized interventions: _____

7. Rationales: _____

Target outcome criteria
Throughout the hospital stay, the patient will:
• be appropriately dressed for the temperature
• walk about only when attended
• perform daily exercise
• avoid injury.

By the time of the patient's discharge, the family will list five safety measures for the home environment.

Nursing diagnosis: *Constipation related to memory loss about toileting behaviors and to inadequate diet*

NURSING PRIORITY: Establish an effective elimination pattern.

Interventions

1. Identify the bathroom clearly—symbolic signs or color codes may be helpful.

2. Prompt the patient, at regular intervals, to use toileting facilities. With an incontinent patient, use universal precautions.

3. Encourage a therapeutic diet with ample fluid and fiber intake during waking hours.

4. Observe the patient for nonverbal clues signaling the need for elimination.

5. Administer and document use of elimination aids (stool softener, laxative, or cathartic), as ordered.

6. Monitor and document the frequency of elimination.

Rationales

1. An AD patient may develop constipation because of forgetting the location of the bathroom.

2. When memory fails, the patient may neglect toileting. Reminders, with assistance at regular intervals, promote a regular elimination pattern and help prevent accidents.

3. Proper diet promotes effective elimination. Ample fluids and fiber help prevent constipation.

4. The patient may exhibit restlessness, picking at clothing, or clutch the genitals but may be unable to verbalize the need to eliminate.

5. Aids may be necessary to facilitate regular elimination.

6. Noting the frequency of elimination helps to identify a regular bowel pattern and minimize problems.

NEUROLOGIC DISORDERS

7. Additional individualized interventions: _____

7. Rationales: _____

Target outcome criteria
Within 1 week of admission, the patient will:
• demonstrate knowledge of bathroom location
• regularly eliminate soft, formed stools.

Nursing diagnosis: *High risk for ineffective family coping related to progressive mental deterioration of the patient with AD*

NURSING PRIORITY: Facilitate necessary role transitions while maintaining family integrity.

Interventions

1. Involve the family in all teaching. Use teaching as an opportunity to assess family roles, resources, and coping behavior. See the "Ineffective Family Coping" plan, page 47.

2. Offer support, understanding, and reassurance to the family. Support efforts to provide care for the patient in the home setting. Encourage family members to give each other "vacations" from providing care.

3. Involve a social worker or discharge planner in decisions regarding home care or nursing home placement. If appropriate, encourage family members to verbalize feelings regarding the decision to place the patient in a nursing home.

4. Provide information about community resources, such as home care, financial and legal assistance, and an Alzheimer's support group. Encourage use of all available resources.

5. Additional individualized interventions: _____

Rationales

1. Because AD patients require long-term care, the family must be taught how to cope effectively with this chronic, progressive disease. If the patient develops a childlike dependence after holding a strong provider role, others must assume new roles to maintain family stability. Assessment of family status provides a baseline for determining the best approach and needed interventions.

2. Caring for the AD patient is frequently a frustrating and thankless task, involving endless repetition and, often, emotional confrontations that may leave family members drained. However, maintenance of a stable home environment and the presence of familiar caregivers help provide the patient with a sense of worth, reduce isolation, and may minimize disorientation. Frequent breaks from caregiving help increase family cohesiveness and prevent burnout.

3. Patient needs may become unmanageable in the home setting. The social worker or discharge planner may offer special expertise in answering questions about long-term care. Family members may feel guilt, relief, anguish, or other conflicting emotions and will need support if this decision becomes necessary.

4. Community support may help lessen the family's burden and promote healthy family adaptation to change. The AD patient is likely to appear in the emergency department when the family becomes overwhelmed. A social service referral may decrease such inappropriate use of resources and help avert family crises.

5. Rationales: _____

Target outcome criteria
Throughout the hospital stay, the family will become involved in teaching and care provision.

By the time of the patient's discharge, the family will:
• arrange a plan for care and mutual support
• identify community support resources.

Discharge planning

NURSING DISCHARGE CRITERIA
(See also specific nursing discharge criteria for primary diagnosis if other than AD.)
Upon the patient's discharge, documentation shows evidence of:
• vital signs stable and within normal limits for this patient
• adequate nutritional intake
• regular bowel and bladder elimination
• adequate home support system or referral to home care or a nursing home if indicated.

PATIENT-FAMILY TEACHING CHECKLIST
Document evidence that the family demonstrates an understanding of:
___ diagnosis and disease process—for example, through literature from the Alzheimer's Association (70 East Lake Street, Suite 700, Chicago, IL 60601)
___ preparatory plans for adequate supervision and behavior management
___ approaches recommended to minimize environmental hazards
___ instructions for promotion of self-care independence
___ recommended procedure for reorientation to home environment
___ identification bracelet or other medical alert device
___ all discharge medications' purpose, dosage, administration schedule, and adverse effects requiring medical attention
___ techniques for continued improvement of language skills
___ specific suggestions for meeting nutrition and elimination needs
___ available community resources
___ need for restoration of family equilibrium as roles change and patient dependence increases
___ probability of total patient regression
___ how to contact the doctor.

DOCUMENTATION CHECKLIST
Using outcome criteria as a guide, document:
___ clinical status on admission, including level of cognitive function
___ planned approach to maintain patient safety, security, and orientation
___ laboratory data and diagnostic findings
___ any change in the patient's behavioral response
___ level of communication and social interaction
___ dietary intake and elimination patterns
___ patient-family teaching
___ discharge planning.

ASSOCIATED PLANS OF CARE
Geriatric Considerations
Grieving
Ineffective Family Coping
Ineffective Individual Coping
Knowledge Deficit

References
Gwyther, L. *Care of Alzheimer's Patients: A Manual for Nursing Home Staff.* American Health Care Association and Alzheimer's Disease and Related Disorders Association, 1985.
Newbern, V. "Is It Really Alzheimer's?" *American Journal of Nursing* 91(2):50-54, February 1991.
Rakel, R. *Conn's Current Therapy.* Philadelphia: W.B. Saunders Co., 1991.
Wilson, J.D. *Harrison's Principles of Internal Medicine,* 12th ed. New York: McGraw-Hill Book Co., 1990.

NEUROLOGIC DISORDERS

Cerebrovascular Accident

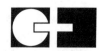

DRG information

DRG 014 Specific Cerebrovascular Disorders. Except transient ischemic attack.
Mean LOS = 7.3 days
Principal diagnoses include:
- cerebral aneurysm
- aphasia
- nontraumatic intracerebral hemorrhage
- nontraumatic intracranial hemorrhage
- nontraumatic subarachnoid hemorrhage
- occlusion of cerebral arteries.

Introduction
DEFINITION AND TIME FOCUS

A cerebrovascular accident (CVA), commonly called a stroke, can take the form of any of several pathophysiologic events that disrupt cerebral circulation. The resulting cerebral ischemia can cause widely varied symptoms or functional deficits, the most classic being hemiplegia.

The most common causes of CVA are thrombosis, embolism, and hemorrhage. Rarely, CVA may be related to arterial spasm or to compression of cerebral blood vessels from tumor growth or other causes. The consistent factor in all CVAs, regardless of etiology, is brain injury resulting from disrupted blood circulation.

Deficits resulting from CVA may be either temporary or permanent, depending on the portion of the brain and the vessels involved, the extent of injury, the patient's preexisting physical and emotional health, and the presence of other diseases or injuries.

This clinical plan focuses on the care of the noncritical patient who is admitted to a medical-surgical unit for diagnosis and nonsurgical treatment of a CVA. Surgical interventions for CVA—such as carotid endarterectomy, extracranial-intracranial bypass, and craniotomy—are not discussed in this plan.

ETIOLOGY AND PRECIPITATING FACTORS
- factors causing occlusion of blood supply to cerebral tissue:
  - cerebral thrombosis, such as from atherosclerosis, inflammation related to infection or other disease process, mechanical constriction as in increased intracranial pressure, prolonged vasoconstriction, systemic hypotension, and hematologic disorders that increase clotting tendencies
  - cerebral embolism, such as from cardiac disease, plaques or clots from elsewhere in circulatory system, substances (such as air, fat, or tumor particles) that enter the bloodstream, and clotting disorders

- factors contributing to intracerebral bleeding:
  - hemorrhage, hypertension, ruptured aneurysm, trauma, ruptured arteriovenous malformations, bleeding related to tumor growth, bleeding disorder associated with a disease (for example, leukemia, anemia, sickle cell disease, hemophilia), anticoagulant therapy, or edema
- factors causing cerebral ischemia:
  - arterial spasm, systemic hypoxemia, and compression of cerebral blood vessels
- factors that increase an individual's risk of CVA:
  - hypertension, heart disease, smoking, diabetes, hypercholesterolemia, use of oral contraceptives, obesity, family history of CVA, and congenital anomalies

Focused assessment guidelines
NURSING HISTORY (Functional health pattern findings)

Health perception—health management pattern
- symptoms may have developed over several days (thrombosis), minutes to hours (hemorrhage), or a few minutes (embolus)
- may have had recent episodes of sudden weakness, vertigo, numbness or tingling sensation of face or limbs, or speech or vision disturbances that resolved within 24 hours (transient ischemic attacks [TIAs]) or resolved in more than 24 hours, but left little or no deficit (reversible ischemic neurologic deficits)
- if young female, may be taking oral contraceptives or may smoke cigarettes
- if older adult, may be under treatment for hypertension, heart disease, diabetes, or other chronic condition
- may be noncompliant with antihypertensive regimen or may have not seen a doctor for many years
- may have long history of smoking

Nutritional-metabolic pattern
- may report difficulty swallowing
- may report nausea and vomiting (most often associated with hemorrhage)

Elimination pattern
- may report incontinence of urine or stool

Activity-exercise pattern
- may be unable to move one side of body (hemiplegia)
- may be afraid of falling
- family may report syncopal episodes

Cognitive-perceptual pattern
• may be unable to understand explanations of what has happened or respond to questions
• may complain of dizziness, drowsiness, headache, burning or aching in extremities, and stiff neck
• may complain of slowed thinking and clumsiness

Sleep-rest pattern
• symptoms — most commonly from thrombosis — may have developed during sleep or shortly after awakening

Self-perception — self-concept pattern
• may show no awareness of affected side of body

Role-relationship pattern
• family may note emotional lability, behavioral changes, altered speech or thinking abilities in patient

PHYSICAL FINDINGS
(May or may not be present depending on the site of the CVA)

General appearance
• facial droop
• lateralized weakness or flaccidity on side opposite brain lesion

Cardiovascular
• hypertension
• hypotension

Pulmonary
• respirations may be increased or decreased

Neurologic
• seizures
• altered level of consciousness
• nuchal rigidity
• memory impairment
• confusion
• retinal hemorrhage
• hemianesthesia
• hemianopia (visual field deficit in one or both eyes)
• apraxia (inability to perform purposeful acts)
• receptive aphasia (inability to understand words) or expressive (inability to say words)
• agnosia (inability to recognize familiar objects)
• disorientation
• unequal pupil size
• diplopia
• dysconjugate gaze
• dysphagia
• dysarthria (lack of muscle control to form words)
• sensory deficits

Integumentary
• flushing
• pallor

Musculoskeletal
• flaccidity
• paralysis

DIAGNOSTIC STUDIES
Initially, the priority in obtaining diagnostic studies is determined by whether the CVA is from hemorrhagic or nonhemorrhagic causes (treatment is significantly different for each). Laboratory data may show no significant abnormalities unless other conditions are present.
• complete blood count — performed to establish a baseline; may reveal blood loss if CVA was caused by significant hemorrhage
• chemistry panel — obtained to establish a baseline; assesses renal function and electrolyte levels, which may be significant in a patient requiring fluid restriction; rules out hypoglycemia and hyperglycemia as contributors to the altered mental state
• prothrombin time (PT) and partial thromboplastin time (PTT) — performed to establish a baseline because the patient with a CVA caused by occlusion may be started on anticoagulants as part of treatment regimen
• urinalysis — baseline study of renal adequacy rules out preexisting urinary tract infection (important because these patients commonly are catheterized)
• computed tomography (CT) scan of the head — may be performed with or without contrast medium; differentiates infarction from hemorrhage and reveals extent of bleeding and brain compression, if present; contrast medium aids in visualizing cerebral vessels; may take several days for infarct to become visible
• cerebral angiography — visualizes cerebral blood vessels and reveals site of bleeding or blockage
• positron emission tomography scan — computer interpretation of gamma ray emissions provides information on cerebral blood flow, volume, and metabolism
• brain scan — cerebral infarction indicated by areas of radioisotope uptake; may not be positive for two weeks after a CVA
• electroencephalography (EEG) — reveals areas of abnormal brain activity and may be helpful in diagnosis; however, a normal EEG does not rule out a pathologic condition
• lumbar puncture — bloody cerebrospinal fluid may indicate intracerebral hemorrhage; used less frequently since CT scan became available
• skull and cervical spine X-rays — may be ordered to rule out fractures, especially if patient suffered a fall with the CVA
• Doppler ultrasonography — identifies abnormalities in blood flow in carotid and intracerebral arteries

NEUROLOGIC DISORDERS

POTENTIAL COMPLICATIONS
- brain stem failure, cardiopulmonary arrest
- brain compression
- brain infarction
- brain abscess
- encephalitis
- pulmonary embolism
- arrhythmias
- congestive heart failure
- thrombophlebitis
- pneumonia
- dysfunctional limb contractures
- pressure ulcers
- malnutrition

Nursing diagnosis: *High risk for ineffective airway clearance related to hemiplegic effects of a CVA*

NURSING PRIORITIES: (a) Maintain a patent airway and (b) prevent pulmonary complications.

Interventions

1. Position the patient with head turned to the side, supporting the trunk with pillows as needed. Elevate the head of the bed slightly. Never leave the patient supine while unattended. Provide a call button within easy reach of the unaffected arm, or provide alternative means of signaling for help, as needed.

2. If hemiplegia is present, position the patient on the affected side for shorter periods (less than 1 hour) than on the unaffected side (2 hours). Avoid positioning a patient's affected arm over the abdomen.

3. Encourage coughing (except in the patient with a hemorrhagic CVA) and deep breathing every 2 hours while awake. Suction accumulated secretions as necessary.

4. Assess lung sounds at least every 4 hours while awake. Also note the adequacy of respiratory effort, the rate and characteristics of respirations, and skin color. Investigate restlessness promptly, especially in the aphasic patient. Report any abnormalities.

5. Allow nothing by mouth until ability to swallow is evaluated. If the patient is able to swallow with minimum difficulty, assist with or observe the patient's eating, as needed. Place small bites of food in the unaffected side of the mouth. (Semisolid foods are usually handled better than thin liquids.)

6. Additional individualized interventions: _____

Rationales

1. Hemiplegia, impaired cough reflex, or dysphagia may render the patient unable to clear the airway. If left supine while unattended, the patient may aspirate; additionally, the supine position increases the risk of airway obstruction from the tongue, especially if the patient is obtunded. Providing the means to call for help is essential when the airway is potentially compromised.

2. Lying on the affected side may cause pooling of secretions, which are ineffectively cleared because of hemiplegia. The weight of an arm over the abdomen may further reduce the adequacy of thoracic expansion.

3. Accumulated secretions may obstruct the airway or predispose the patient to atelectasis or pneumonia. (Respiratory infection is one of the primary causes of death for CVA patients.) Coughing should be avoided in hemorrhagic CVA to prevent increasing intracranial pressure, which can cause further bleeding.

4. Many CVA patients have preexisting hypertension or heart disease, which may predispose them to development of congestive heart failure. Abnormal lung sounds (crackles, gurgles) may be the first indicators of complications related to hypoventilation. Increased respiratory effort, tachypnea, ashen or cyanotic color, or restlessness may indicate hypoxemia. Early detection and reporting facilitate prompt treatment.

5. Hemiplegia and associated dysphagia predispose the patient to aspiration. The patient may be better able to initiate swallowing if food is placed on the unaffected side. Small bites and thicker liquids decrease the risk of choking from aspiration.

6. Rationales: _____

Target outcome criteria

Throughout the hospital stay, the patient will:
• have a clear airway
• cough and perform deep-breathing exercises every 2 hours

• have clear lung sounds or pulmonary problems promptly identified and treated
• take food and fluids (as ordered) without aspirating or choking.

Collaborative problem: *High risk for further cerebral injury related to interrupted blood flow (embolus, thrombus, or hemorrhage)*

NURSING PRIORITY: Improve cerebral tissue perfusion.

Interventions

1. Assess neurologic status, checking level of consciousness, orientation, grips, leg strength, pupillary response, and vital signs every hour until neurologic status is stable and at least every four hours thereafter. Promptly report any abnormalities or changes, especially decreasing alertness, progressing weakness, restlessness, unequal pupil size, widening pulse pressure, flexor or extensor posturing, seizures, severe headache, vertigo, syncope, or epistaxis.

2. Elevate the head of the bed slightly and provide supplemental oxygen as ordered.

3. If the CVA is occlusive:

• Administer anticoagulants, as ordered. Monitor appropriate laboratory findings (PT and PTT), and check current results before giving each dose. Observe carefully for (and advise the patient or family to report) melena, petechiae, epistaxis, hematuria, ecchymosis, oozing from wounds, or any unusual bleeding. Observe for and report any signs of intracranial bleeding (headache, irritability, weakness, decreased level of consciousness, or nuchal rigidity).

• Administer antiplatelet aggregation medications, as ordered. Observe for gastric irritation.

• Administer medications to control blood pressure, as ordered. Be alert for signs of decreased cerebral perfusion (as noted in Intervention 1 above); immediately report any that occur. Check blood pressure at least every 4 hours while the patient is awake.

Rationales

1. When blood flow to and oxygenation of the brain is decreased, cerebral vasodilation and edema occur as the body attempts to compensate for the deficiency. Increasing cerebral edema causes increased intracranial pressure and may have fatal consequences if not treated promptly. Hemorrhage into enclosed intracranial space may also increase pressure. A decline in neurologic signs indicates progressive injury.

2. Elevating the head helps minimize cerebral edema which can contribute to increased ischemia. The brain uses 20% of the oxygen normally available to the body. When a CVA causes cerebral ischemia, supplemental oxygen may help prevent brain tissue death.

3. For an occlusive CVA:

• Use of anticoagulants, although still somewhat controversial, can inhibit stroke progression and possibly reduce the number of thromboembolic events. Heparin inactivates thrombin, thus preventing fibrin clots. Therapeutic PTT should be 2 to 2½ times normal value. Warfarin (Coumadin) interferes with vitamin K production, thus decreasing synthesis of several clotting factors. Therapeutic PT should be 1½ to 2½ times normal value. Anticoagulants predispose the patient to systemic bleeding and may also cause intracranial bleeding.

• Drugs such as aspirin and dipyridamole (Persantine) inhibit platelet aggregation and thus reduce the risk of embolus formation. Undesirable side effects include GI upset and bleeding, so these drugs should not be used if the patient has preexisting GI problems.

• Severe hypertension may further decrease the oxygen supply to the brain or increase the risk of hemorrhage, leading to increased neurologic deficits. Many CVA patients have preexisting hypertension, and their cerebral circulation has accommodated to higher pressures over time. Sudden lowering of blood pressure may cause further ischemia.

NEUROLOGIC DISORDERS

4. If the CVA is hemorrhagic:

• Maintain the patient on complete bed rest for the first 24 hours to 1 week, as ordered. Minimize stress and external stimulation as much as possible. Administer stool softeners or laxatives, as ordered.

• Administer medications to control blood pressure, as ordered. Be alert for signs of neurologic deterioration and immediately report any that occur.

• Administer I.V. aminocaproic acid (Amicar), if ordered. Observe for and report hypotension, bradycardia, or signs of thrombus formation, such as calf pain, sudden chest pain, or shortness of breath.

• Monitor the patient to maintain optimal fluid status, observing fluid restrictions as ordered. Administer osmotic diuretics, as ordered. Monitor intake and output carefully.

4. For a hemorrhagic CVA:

• Minimizing activity and stimulation helps decrease the risk of further intracerebral hemorrhage. Stool softeners or laxatives prevent straining at stool, which can cause bleeding.

• Patients with hemorrhagic CVA commonly have significant vasospasm; lowering blood pressure too much, or too rapidly, may cause cerebral ischemia.

• Normally, a fibrin clot breaks down spontaneously about 7 days after a hemorrhagic episode. Aminocaproic acid inhibits breakdown of the fibrin clot by preventing activation of plasminogen. Because the drug acts systemically to prevent fibrinolysis, thrombus formation and embolic complications may occur elsewhere in the body.

• Fluid overload may cause fatal increases in intracranial pressure or recurrent hemorrhage. Osmotic diuretics, such as mannitol, reduce cerebral edema by drawing fluid into the intravascular space and stimulating diuresis. Mannitol also reduces the volume of circulating cerebrospinal fluid. Patients with other preexisting conditions, such as cardiac or renal disease, may not tolerate the temporary intravascular volume increase. Careful patient monitoring, including an accurate fluid intake and output record, is essential to prevent such complications.

5. Additional individualized interventions: _____

5. Rationales: _____

Target outcome criteria

Within 2 days of admission, the patient will:
• show no further decrease in level of consciousness
• show stable or improving neurologic signs.

Throughout the hospital stay, the patient will:
• maintain fluid balance
• maintain normal electrolyte values.

Nursing diagnosis: *Impaired physical mobility related to damage to motor cortex or motor pathways*

NURSING PRIORITY: Minimize effects of immobility and prevent associated complications.

Interventions

1. Maintain functional alignment in positioning the patient at rest, using a footboard, handroll, or trochanter roll as necessary. Support the affected arm when the patient is out of bed.

2. Provide passive (and active, if appropriate) range-of-motion exercise to all extremities at least four times a day, beginning immediately upon admission. Increase activity levels as permitted and tolerated, depending on the CVA's cause. Collaborate with the physical therapist to plan a rehabilitation schedule with the patient and family.

3. When permitted, encourage the patient to perform as much self-care as possible.

Rationales

1. A functional position prevents contractures and deformities that further complicate recovery. The weight of an unsupported arm may cause shoulder dislocation, joint inflammation, or both.

2. Even passive exercise helps maintain muscle tone and establish new impulse pathways and neuron regeneration. Adjacent brain cells may take up the function of damaged cells, new nerve cell fibers may develop collaterally, or alternative nerve pathways may function to resume activity. Learning and repetition appear to be key factors in the development of new neuronal connections. Establishing a schedule helps the patient set goals, maintain a sense of control, and measure progress.

3. Independence in self-care helps maintain self-respect and may improve motivation to increase mobility.

4. Provide antiembolic stockings, as ordered. Assess for signs of thromboembolic complications. Report immediately any chest pain, shortness of breath, calf pain, or redness or swelling in an extremity.

5. Turn the patient from side to side at least every 2 hours. Keep bedding clean and dry. Massage bony prominences. Be alert to fragile, thin, or excoriated skin, which may shear during turning. Provide special mattresses or foam or other padding. Report any red or broken skin areas immediately.

6. Maintain adequate elimination. If the patient is catheterized, begin bladder retraining as soon as possible, according to an established protocol or medical order. If the patient is not catheterized, offer a bedpan every 2 hours. Observe urine and report cloudiness, excessive sediment, or pyuria. Provide stool softeners and laxatives, as ordered, and monitor the frequency and characteristics of bowel movements. Provide reassurance that bowel and bladder control usually returns as rehabilitation progresses.

7. Additional individualized interventions: _____

_____

4. Antiembolism stockings promote venous return, thus decreasing the risk of thrombus formation from immobility and venous stasis. The signs and symptoms noted may indicate pulmonary embolus or thrombophlebitis.

5. Impeccable skin care can prevent skin breakdown in the immobilized patient. Moisture promotes bacterial growth and increases skin friability. Turning and massage help prevent pressure areas and promote circulation. Older patients are likely to have delicate skin, particularly if they are debilitated. If help did not arrive quickly after the CVA, the skin may be excoriated from urine, pressure, and dehydration effects. Special mattresses and padding help redistribute pressure. Prompt intervention can prevent serious skin problems that can interfere with recovery.

6. When neurosensory pathways are disturbed by injury, the patient may have limited or altered sphincter control related to either actual brain damage or CVA-related memory and inhibitory lapses. Incontinence and urine stasis predispose the patient to infection. Bladder and bowel retraining reestablish patterns and bolster the patient's confidence in resuming activities as permitted. Reassurance that incontinence is usually temporary helps decrease anxiety, embarrassment, and a sense of helplessness.

7. Rationales: _____

_____

Target outcome criteria
Within 24 hours of admission, the patient will:
• begin passive range-of-motion exercises
• have clean and dry skin
• have a patent urinary catheter or use a bedpan every 2 hours with minimal incontinence.

Throughout the hospital stay, the patient will:
• maintain functional alignment
• perform as much self-care as possible
• maintain intact skin
• maintain adequate bowel and bladder elimination, with no signs of infection
• show no thromboembolic complications.

Nursing diagnosis: *High risk for sensory-perceptual alteration related to cerebral injury*

NURSING PRIORITY: Minimize effects of deficits in perception and prevent related complications.

Interventions

1. Establish closeness by using a calm and reassuring manner, eye contact, and touch. Call the patient by a preferred name. Approach the patient's unaffected side.

2. Protect the patient from injury to the affected side. Give regular reminders to look at and touch the affected side.

3. If visual field deficits are present, remind the patient that frequent head-turning will widen the visual field. Always ensure that food and objects at bedside are placed well within the patient's visual field.

Rationales

1. Sensory-perceptual and communication deficits may contribute to profound isolation for the patient who has suffered a CVA. Use of nonverbal communication establishes contact and helps decrease anxiety. The patient may be unable to see or feel on the affected side of the body.

2. Hemiplegia may be accompanied by full or partial hemianesthesia, making the patient unaware of actual or impending injury. Relearning awareness and acceptance of the affected side, by engaging in activities using that side, is a necessary step toward functional recovery.

3. Visual field deficits may prevent the patient from receiving warnings or other cues to prevent injury. Accidents or insufficient nutritional intake may result if visual field defects are not considered in arranging the bedside tray.

NEUROLOGIC DISORDERS

4. Additional individualized interventions:_____

4. Rationales:_____

Target outcome criterion
Throughout the hospital stay, the patient will:
• look at and touch the affected side of the body
• establish protective behavior for affected limbs

• demonstrate use of techniques to compensate for sensory loss.

Nursing diagnosis: *High risk for impaired verbal communication related to cerebral injury*

NURSING PRIORITY: Establish effective means of communication.

Interventions

1. Assess communication ability. Explain to the patient that the CVA may have affected speech. Ask simple questions that evaluate ability to repeat words, interpret, follow directions, and express feelings. Allow ample time for responses.

2. Speak slowly and clearly, using short sentences. Do not shout at the patient. Use simple explanations and gestures. Always include the patient in conversation when others are present. Avoid answering for the patient. Never use baby talk. Provide alternative means of communication (such as a word board or pencil and paper) if needed.

3. If significant speech deficits are present, arrange referral to a speech therapist for more comprehensive evaluation and rehabilitation services.

4. Reassure the patient that functional recovery is possible with patience and consistent rehabilitation efforts. Help with practice and repetition of verbal and physical exercises. Involve family members in practice. If the patient uses inappropriate profanity, counsel the family.

5. Additional individualized interventions: _____

Rationales

1. Identification of speech problems (expressive vs. receptive aphasia, for example) is the first step in planning rehabilitation. A patient with receptive aphasia may still be able to process information, but interpretation of stimuli and formation of responses is slowed.

2. Rapid or complex explanations may cause neurosensory overload and contribute to patient frustration. Hearing is usually not impaired, and shouting may add to the patient's distress over deficits. Answering for the patient, "talking around" the patient, and using baby talk are demeaning and contribute to the patient's sense of helplessness. Alternative means of communication may be needed while the patient relearns verbal skills.

3. A speech therapist can provide expertise in pinpointing and treating specific speech problems.

4. A patient with severe deficits may despair of resuming normal activities, but maintaining hope is essential for the fullest possible recovery. Over time, the brain can develop new pathways for functions: repetition aids this process. Family support helps maintain morale. Family members may be shocked by inappropriate profanity; advise them that this is common in patients whose speech has been affected by CVA.

5. Rationales: _____

Target outcome criterion
Within 1 hour of admission, the conscious patient will establish some form of verbal or nonverbal communication.

Nursing diagnosis: *Knowledge deficit related to disease manifestations, the rehabilitation process, and ongoing home care*

NURSING PRIORITY: Provide thorough patient and family teaching.

Interventions	Rationales
1. See the "Knowledge Deficit" plan, page 56.	1. This plan provides general information for use in patient and family teaching.
2. Explain to the family that some emotional lability is commonly associated with cerebral injury but that such behavior usually decreases over time. Help the family provide the patient with gentle guidance in relearning appropriate emotional and physical responses. Encourage a show of affection and patience, and use of humor.	2. Family members may be confused and distressed by unexpected emotional outbursts, and they may be reassured to know that physiologic factors are at least partially responsible. The family may help the patient reestablish appropriate responses through supportive, gentle reminders. Family understanding and patience, with humor at appropriate moments, may defuse potentially volatile emotional outbursts.
3. Maintain an attitude of acceptance and understanding. Do not exacerbate emotional outbursts by reacting personally to them. Encourage normal expression of feelings related to lost abilities.	3. A patient who has suffered a CVA typically exhibits excessive or inappropriate emotions as a result of brain injury. The profound alteration such deficits as aphasia cause in the patient's relationship with the environment can also cause widely varied emotional reactions ranging from rage to grief; expression of such feelings is part of coping. The patient may be unable to control emotional responses, and excessive reactivity on the part of family members or caregivers may add to the patient's isolation and distress.
4. Instruct the patient and family about all medications to be taken at home, including antihypertensives, anticoagulants, and antiplatelet aggregation medication.	4. Thorough understanding helps minimize the risk of inadvertent errors and noncompliance. Pharmacologic control may decrease the risk of CVA recurrence.
5. If the patient is to be discharged home on anticoagulant therapy, provide thorough instructions about:	5. Because anticoagulant use may cause life-threatening bleeding, the patient and family must understand the regimen completely.
• medications' action, dosage, and schedule	• Anticoagulants should be taken on a regular schedule in the prescribed dosage.
• the need for frequent follow-up laboratory testing to determine dosage requirements	• Tests determine the need for dosage adjustments.
• signs of bleeding problems (melena, petechiae, easy bruising, hematuria, epistaxis) and the need to report them	• Untoward bleeding may indicate the need for a dosage adjustment, a therapeutic antidote, or both.
• measures to control bleeding	• Uncontrolled hemorrhage can be fatal.
• dietary considerations	• Vitamin K intake affects dosage requirements.
• avoidance of aspirin and other over-the-counter medications	• Aspirin and other over-the-counter medications may potentiate anticoagulants' effects.
• avoidance of trauma	• Even minimal trauma may cause serious injury in the patient whose clotting status is altered by anticoagulants.
• the importance of wearing a medical alert tag and of notifying other health professionals (such as the dentist or optometrist) of anticoagulant therapy.	• Other health care providers must be aware of the patient's medication regimen so that their interventions can be altered accordingly to prevent injury.
6. Teach the importance of life-style modifications to minimize the risk of CVA recurrence; these include blood pressure control, weight control, smoking cessation, diabetes control, diet modifications, and stress reduction.	6. These related risk factors may directly or indirectly contribute to CVA recurrence.

NEUROLOGIC DISORDERS

7. Teach the patient and family to recognize and report symptoms associated with TIAs: vertigo, vision disturbances, sudden weakness or falls without loss of consciousness (drop attacks), paresthesias of face or extremities, speech disturbances, and lateralized temporary weakness.

7. TIAs may be precursors of CVA recurrence; prompt reporting allows for preventive intervention, such as medication adjustment for better blood pressure control.

8. Teach the patient and family about rehabilitation plans and arrange home care follow-up or in-home assistance, as needed. Teaching should also address specific individualized information on activity, safety, and positioning recommendations; use of mobility aids (slings, braces, or walkers); airway maintenance and feeding considerations; bowel and bladder control program; signs and symptoms of complications (decreasing neurologic status, infection, bleeding, or thromboembolic events); food and fluid intake recommendations; skin care; communication techniques; and coping with emotional lability.

8. The rehabilitation level at discharge varies from patient to patient and may also depend on the availability of home care resources. Most CVA patients require some assistance at home after discharge, either from motivated and well-taught family members or from professional caregivers. Because of the impact of DRGs, a CVA patient may be discharged from the hospital at an early rehabilitation stage. Discharge planning should always address ongoing rehabilitation.

9. Discuss with the family the advisability of learning cardiopulmonary resuscitation techniques.

9. Many risk factors for CVA—such as hypertension and atherosclerosis—also are risk factors for myocardial infarction and cardiac arrest. Cardiac arrest also can cause further CVA from ischemia.

10. Additional individualized interventions: _____

10. Rationales: _____

Target outcome criteria
By the time of discharge, the patient or family will:
• express understanding of what has happened
• name risk factors associated with a potential recurrence of CVA
• list and discuss all medications for use at home
• list four signs of bleeding (if the patient is taking an anticoagulant)
• list signs of TIA and CVA
• demonstrate understanding of the activity regimen and perform activities
• use mobility aids appropriately, if needed

• name measures to protect the affected side
• verbalize understanding of the bowel and bladder control program
• express understanding of food and fluid intake recommendations
• tolerate frustration over speech deficits and use alternative measures to communicate
• understand the plan for ongoing rehabilitation
• express understanding of normal emotional responses.

Discharge planning
NURSING DISCHARGE CRITERIA
Upon the patient's discharge, documentation shows evidence of:
• absence of fever and pulmonary or cardiovascular complications*
• stable vital signs*
• absence of signs and symptoms indicating progression of neurologic deficit*
• prothrombin level within acceptable parameters*
• absence of skin breakdown and contractures
• ability to tolerate activity within expected parameters
• ability to transfer and ambulate
• ability to perform activities of daily living
• ability to compensate for neurologic deficit, such as paralysis, spasticity, or speech impairment

• ability to control bowel and bladder functions
• ability to tolerate nutritional intake*
• physical and occupational therapy program with maximum benefit attained*
• referral to home care if the patient is progressing toward maximum rehabilitation potential and home support system is adequate, or, if the home support is inadequate or the patient needs continued rehabilitation outside the home:
    — referral to a rehabilitation facility or nursing home for continued rehabilitation
    — referral form reflecting the patient's progress, potential, and goals and containing all other appropriate information necessary to provide continuity of care.

---

*Factors that must be met by the time of discharge. All other factors must be addressed in the medical record but may not be within normal parameters because maximum return of function may not have been achieved by discharge.

PATIENT-FAMILY TEACHING CHECKLIST

Document evidence that the patient and family demonstrate an understanding of:

___ injury or disease process and implications
___ all discharge medications' purpose, dosage, administration schedule, and adverse effects requiring medical attention (discharge medications may include anticoagulants, antiplatelet aggregation medications, and antihypertensives)
___ need for follow-up laboratory tests (if indicated)
___ signs of cerebral impairment
___ signs of infection
___ signs of thromboembolic or other complications
___ activity and positioning recommendations and mobility aids
___ food and fluid intake recommendations
___ bowel and bladder control program
___ risk factors
___ safety measures
___ use of medical alert tag
___ advisability of cardiopulmonary resuscitation classes for the family
___ skin care
___ communication measures
___ verbal practice exercises
___ expected emotional lability and coping methods
___ community resources
___ when and how to use the emergency medical system
___ date, time, and location of follow-up appointment
___ home care arrangements.

DOCUMENTATION CHECKLIST

Using outcome criteria as a guide, document:

___ clinical status on admission
___ significant changes in status
___ neurologic assessments
___ pertinent laboratory and diagnostic test findings
___ medication therapy
___ activity and positioning
___ food intake
___ fluid intake and output
___ bowel and bladder control measures
___ communication measures
___ patient-family teaching
___ discharge planning.

ASSOCIATED PLANS OF CARE

Geriatric Considerations
Grieving
Impaired Physical Mobility
Ineffective Family Coping
Ineffective Individual Coping
Knowledge Deficit
Nutritional Deficit
Seizures
Thrombophlebitis

References

Bronstein, K., Popovich, J., and Stewart-Amidei, C. *Promoting Stroke Recovery: A Research-based Approach for Nurses.* St. Louis: Mosby-Year Book, 1991.

Emergencies. Nurse's Reference Library: Springhouse, Pa.: Springhouse Corp., 1985.

Luckmann, J., and Sorensen, K. *Medical-Surgical Nursing: A Psychophysiologic Approach,* 3rd ed. Philadelphia: W.B. Saunders Co., 1987.

Marshall, S., Marshall, L., Vos, H., and Chesnut, R. *Neuroscience Critical Care: Pathophysiology and Patient Management.* Philadelphia: W.B. Saunders Co., 1990.

Swearingen, P. *Manual of Nursing Therapeutics: Applying Nursing Diagnoses to Medical Disorders,* 2nd ed. St. Louis: Mosby-Year Book, 1990.

NEUROLOGIC DISORDERS

Craniotomy

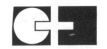

DRG information

DRG 001 Craniotomy. Except for trauma. Age 17 + .
   Mean LOS = 12.9 days
   Principal procedures include:
   • biopsy of brain or cerebral meninges
   • excision of brain or skull lesion
   • clipping or repair of cerebral aneurysm
   • insertion of ventricular shunt
   • repair of arteriovenous fistula
   • incision of brain or cerebral meninges
   • incision or excision of intracranial vessels.
DRG 002 Craniotomy for Trauma. Age 17 + .
   Mean LOS = 12.1 days
   Principal diagnoses include:
   • concussion
   • skull fracture
   • hemorrhage (subarachnoid, subdural, or extradural) following injury
   • cerebral laceration or contusion
   • fracture of vertebral column with spinal cord injury.
Additional DRG information: These diagnoses must be treated surgically; see DRG 001 for examples of procedures.
DRG 003 Craniotomy. Age 0 to 17.
   Mean LOS = 12.7 days
   Principal procedures for DRG 003: see principal procedures listed under DRG 001.

Introduction
DEFINITION AND TIME FOCUS
Craniotomy, the most common neurosurgical procedure, is the surgical opening of the skull to provide access to the brain. It is performed to treat intracranial disease; for example, to remove tissue for biopsy or to remove a mass lesion (a substance occupying the cranial cavity and compromising either the space or the integrity of the brain). The surgery involves making a series of small holes, called burr holes, in the cranium with a special drill, then cutting between the holes to allow removal of a flap of bone and scalp. At the end of the surgery, the flap is replaced and the muscle and scalp are realigned and sutured.

   Although the surgical approach depends on the location of the lesion, surgery is performed in two general areas. In the supratentorial craniotomy, the cranium is incised above the tentorium (the fold of dura mater that separates the cerebral cortex from the cerebellum and brain stem). This approach is used for lesions in the frontal, parietal, temporal, and occipital lobes of the cerebral hemispheres. The infratentorial approach, in which the cranium is incised below the tentorium, is used for lesions in the brain stem (midbrain, pons, and medulla) and cerebellum.

   A craniotomy may be an emergency procedure for removal of a rapidly expanding lesion, such as an epidural hematoma or intracranial abscess, or an elective procedure in situations where the growth rate of the space-occupying lesion has been slow, such as with benign tumors. This clinical plan focuses on the immediate preoperative care and postoperative care (in the critical-care unit) of a patient undergoing an elective craniotomy.

ETIOLOGY AND PRECIPITATING FACTORS
• presence of tumors, abscesses, aneurysms, chronic hematomas, cysts, or arteriovenous malformations
• any condition requiring repair of a cerebral injury

Focused assessment guidelines
NURSING HISTORY (Functional health pattern findings)

Health perception – health management pattern
• may have history of headache that is worse on arising in the morning and is aggravated by movement or straining at stool
• may have experienced personality changes
• may have experienced mental changes or mood swings
• may be at increased risk because of age (adults are at increased risk)
• may be at increased risk because of family or personal history of diabetes mellitus, intolerance to previous operative procedures, history of adrenocortical steroids, or signs and symptoms of endocrine dysfunction

Nutritional-metabolic pattern
• may report vomiting

Activity-exercise pattern
• may have been hospitalized and on bed rest
• may have been restricted in physical activity as a result of motor or sensory deficits

Cognitive-perceptual pattern
• may have experienced changes in vision, hearing, touch, taste, or smell depending on location and duration of the lesion
• may experience language and memory problems with chronic lesion

Self-perception – self-concept pattern
• if undergoing radiation or chemotherapy for chronic lesion, may have negative self-image because of body disfigurement
• may express anger, embarrassment, or denial

Role-relationship pattern
• depending on duration of lesion, may have alteration in role as spouse and breadwinner

Sexuality-reproductive pattern
• depending on location of lesion, may have impaired sexual functioning

Coping—stress tolerance pattern
• may exhibit ineffective coping patterns
• may have anticipatory grieving for loss

Value-belief pattern
• may have delayed seeking medical attention because of fear of the unknown, surgery, and possibility of death
• may feel frustrated with the health care system if diagnosis was delayed because of vague symptoms

PHYSICAL FINDINGS
Note: Signs and symptoms depend on the lesion's site. The following are general findings that would indicate cerebral dysfunction.

Neurologic
• decreased level of consciousness
• mental changes, such as impaired memory, lack of initiative, or mood changes
• visual deficits, such as decreased visual acuity, blurred vision, diplopia, or changes in extraocular eye movements
• sensory deficits
• motor deficits
• seizures
• papilledema
• cranial nerve dysfunction

Gastrointestinal
• vomiting

DIAGNOSTIC STUDIES
• complete blood count—decreased hemoglobin may indicate anemia or blood dyscrasia as well as the need for blood transfusion before surgery to ensure adequate transport for oxygen in the blood; increased white blood cell (WBC) count may signify the beginning of infection or an abscess, which is a contraindication for surgery (unless the abscess is in the brain)
• blood urea nitrogen (BUN), serum creatinine—used to monitor renal function; increased values may indicate an impaired ability to cope with the sodium and water retention that result from the body's stress reaction to surgery
• electrolyte analyses—used to monitor fluid status and detect hypokalemia and hyperkalemia; the patient may develop diabetes insipidus or syndrome of inappropriate antidiuretic hormone secretion

• fasting blood glucose levels—used to detect diabetes mellitus, which would require control before and after surgery
• typing and cross-matching blood—makes blood more readily available if the patient requires blood replacement from surgical loss
• computed tomography (CT) scan—used to diagnose cerebral lesions, such as hematomas, tumors, cysts, hydrocephalus, cerebral atrophy, cerebral infarction, and cerebral edema; serial scanning may be done before and after surgery
• cerebral angiography—used to diagnose cerebrovascular aneurysms, cerebral thrombosis, hematomas, tumors with increased vascularization, vascular plaques or spasm, arteriovenous malformations, cerebral fistulas, or cerebral edema
• radionuclide imaging studies (brain scan)—used to diagnose intracranial masses such as malignant or benign tumors, abscesses, cerebral infarctions, intracranial hemorrhage, arteriovenous malformations, or aneurysms; they have been largely replaced by CT scans
• magnetic resonance imaging—used to assess brain edema, hemorrhage, infarction, blood vessels, and tumors and to measure fluid flow
• chest X-ray—can rule out congestion, pneumonia, atelectasis, or other pulmonary diseases that would compromise respirations
• electrocardiography—can detect cardiac abnormalities, such as arrhythmias, that would be aggravated by the stress of a prolonged surgical procedure and drug therapy

POTENTIAL COMPLICATIONS
• increased intracranial pressure (ICP)
• shock (hemorrhagic, hypovolemic, or from intracranial bleeding)
• hematoma, subdural or epidural
• atelectasis
• pneumonia
• seizures
• neurogenic pulmonary edema
• diabetes insipidus
• meningitis
• wound infection
• neurologic deficits, such as decreased level of consciousness, motor weakness, or paralysis
• loss of corneal, pharyngeal, or palatal reflexes
• cardiac arrhythmias
• thrombophlebitis
• hyperthermia
• postoperative hydrocephalus
• GI ulceration and bleeding
• cranial nerve III damage (eye drop), visual disturbances
• personality changes

NEUROLOGIC DISORDERS

Nursing diagnosis: *Preoperative knowledge deficit related to impending craniotomy*

NURSING PRIORITY: Prepare the patient and family for the craniotomy.

Interventions

1. Implement the measures in the "Knowledge Deficit" plan, page 56, as appropriate.

2. Assess what the patient and family already know about the impending craniotomy and what they want to know. Consider the patient's educational level, level of consciousness, mental changes, and memory loss. As appropriate, ask the patient or family what has been learned from the doctor, other family members, or someone who has had a craniotomy.

3. Describe the preoperative procedure, including neurologic assessment, weight measurement, nothing by mouth after midnight, hair washing, and the possibility that long hair will be braided.

4. Explain that the hair is cut and the scalp shaved in the operating room. Explain the rationale and allow time for the patient to express any feelings. If the operating room personnel are willing to save the patient's hair, ask the patient if this is desired. Explain to the patient that, if desired, all hair can be shaved to promote uniform regrowth. If possible, have the family present during this explanation.

5. Discuss the unit environment and the effects of the craniotomy during the immediate postoperative period. Mention that headaches and altered consciousness may occur.

6. Encourage the patient and family to express fears and concerns about the impending surgery.

7. Additional individualized interventions: _____

_____

Rationales

1. The "Knowledge Deficit" plan contains detailed, general information about teaching. This plan covers only specific information about craniotomy.

2. Level of consciousness, mental changes, and memory loss affect the patient's knowledge base. Although the doctor should have informed the patient and family about the procedure and potential complications, anxiety, memory loss, or limited comprehension may interfere with understanding and retention. Also, the patient and family may have limited or confusing information from various sources. Assessing the knowledge base allows the nurse to reinforce appropriate information, correct misconceptions, and fill in knowledge gaps.

3. Knowing what to expect usually decreases anxiety.

4. Hair is an important component of body image and self-concept. Having the hair cut may be extremely distressing to the patient. Knowing why it must be removed and that it may be saved may alleviate some of the distress and sense of loss. Allowing time for the patient to express feelings conveys sensitivity and validates the patient's emotions. Having the family present may provide the support necessary to cope with this situation and prepare them for how the patient will look after surgery.

5. Knowing in advance about the unit environment may increase the patient's sense of security when awakening after surgery. Knowing that headaches and altered consciousness are common after the operation may help decrease the patient's and family's anxiety.

6. Fear of death, anxiety over other possible outcomes, and anticipatory grieving for the possible loss of body function interfere with learning. Providing an environment where the patient is comfortable discussing these feelings may help facilitate learning and reduce preoperative and postoperative anxiety.

7. Rationales: _____

_____

Target outcome criteria
Before surgery, the patient and family will:
• verbalize understanding of the upcoming surgery and its potential effects and complications
• describe their anxieties and how they are coping with them.

Collaborative problem: *High risk for cerebral ischemia related to increased ICP*

NURSING PRIORITIES: (a) Decrease ICP and (b) minimize fluctuations in cerebral perfusion pressure.

Interventions

1. Implement the measures in the "Increased Intracranial Pressure" plan's "high risk for potential cerebral ischemia" collaborative problem, page 136.

2. Additional individualized interventions: _____

Rationales

1. Numerous problems may raise ICP to dangerous levels after a craniotomy, including surgical trauma, cerebral edema, blood pressure fluctuations, and nursing activities. The plan for "Increased Intracranial Pressure" covers this problem in detail.

2. Rationales: _____

Target outcome criteria
Within 72 hours after surgery, the patient will:
• have an ICP of 0 to 15 mm Hg and a cerebral perfusion pressure geater than 60 mm Hg
• have a mean arterial pressure greater than 60 mm Hg
• display no clinical signs of increased ICP and herniation.

Within 1 week after surgery, the patient will demonstrate improved neurologic status.

Nursing diagnosis: *High risk for infection related to surgery, invasive techniques, continuous intracranial monitoring, ventricular drains, or cerebrospinal fluid (CSF) leakage*

NURSING PRIORITY: Prevent or promptly detect signs of infection.

Interventions

1. Implement the measures in the "Increased Intracranial Pressure" plan's "high-risk for infection" nursing diagosis, page 138.

2. Administer antibiotics as ordered, usually immediately before surgery begins.

3. Assess for respiratory infection:
• auscultate lungs every 2 hours and as necessary for adventitious sounds
• assess sputum for color, consistency, amount, and odor; culture if necessary
• observe for temperature elevation and WBC elevation.

Rationales

1. The "Increased Intracranial Pressure" plan provides general measures for prevention, assessment, and treatment of infection. This plan discusses additional care specific to the craniotomy patient.

2. Wound infection occurs in 0.7% to 5.7% of neurosurgical patients. Prophylactic antibiotic administration helps prevent infection by establishing the optimal tissue concentration of antibiotic before possible contamination. Antibiotic administration also may be repeated during a lengthy procedure. Antibiotics may be discontinued at the completion of surgery.

3. The overall pulmonary infection rate in the neurosurgery patient is 13% to 16%. Impaired mobility, characteristic of the surgical and postoperative periods, compromises the respiratory system by increasing stasis of secretions, promoting atelectasis, and producing generalized hypoxia. To decrease ICP, the patient's fluid balance is maintained at a slight deficit. Dehydration increases the tenacious nature of the sputum, increasing the risk of consolidation and pneumonia. Adventitious lung sounds, purulent or foul-smelling sputum, fever, and WBC elevation strongly suggest the development of pulmonary infection.

4. Observe the surgical wound daily for signs and symptoms of infection, such as redness, edema, suture stretch, pigskin appearance of the epidermis, tenderness, or drainage. Also observe for systemic manifestations, including fever, malaise, leukocytosis, or tachycardia.

4. Scalp margin necrosis, wound dehiscence, CSF leakage, presence of a drain and monitoring device, possible scratching and manipulation by the patient, and environmental factors increase the risk of wound infection in the postcraniotomy patient. A stitch abscess may appear before a major wound infection. A true wound infection rarely occurs before the second day after surgery and usually occurs within the first 2 weeks.

5. Assess constantly for signs and symptoms of meningitis, such as temperature elevation, lethargy, severe headache, nausea and vomiting, nuchal rigidity, positive Kernig's sign, photophobia, irritability, decreased level of consciousness, or generalized seizures. Assist with CT scan and lumbar puncture if necessary.

5. Patients at risk for developing this acute inflammation of the meninges of the brain or spinal cord include those with cranial or spinal wound infections, CSF fistulae following operative procedures on the dura mater, and subarachnoid bolts or ventricular drains. All of these risk factors for meningeal contamination may apply to the postcraniotomy patient. Abnormal lumbar puncture findings typically confirm the diagnosis. These findings include a positive culture, an elevated opening pressure of 200 to 700 mm H_2O, WBC count increased from 10 to 1,000 cells/mm^3, an increased protein count, decreased glucose and chloride levels, and, in purulent bacterial meningitis, a tan or milky appearance of the fluid. A CT scan may be performed before the lumbar puncture to determine the risk of brain herniation from the sudden removal of CSF from the spinal canal.

6. Additional individualized interventions: _____

6. Rationales: _____

Target outcome criteria
By 72 hours after surgery, the patient will:
• have a normal temperature and WBC count
• display negative cultures
• manifest no signs or symptoms of infection.

By the time of discharge, the patient will have no signs or symptoms of wound infection.

Collaborative problem: *High risk for respiratory failure related to decreased level of consciousness, neurologic deficits, effects of anesthesia, immobility, altered respiratory patterns, and tenacious secretions associated with fluid loss and decreased fluid intake*

NURSING PRIORITY: Maintain effective gas exchange.

Interventions

1. Implement the measures discussed in the "Increased Intracranial Pressure" plan's "high risk for respiratory failure" collaborative problem, page 140.

2. Additional individualized interventions: _____

Rationales

1. The neurosurgical patient requires meticulous respiratory assessment, support of oxygenation and ventilation, and pulmonary hygiene.

2. Rationales: _____

Target outcome criteria
Within 24 hours after surgery, the patient will:
• have an airway free from secretions
• have arterial blood gas (ABG) levels within desired limits.

By the time of discharge, the patient will:
• have a normal respiratory rate and pattern
• have normal ABG levels
• have a clear chest X-ray.

Nursing diagnosis: *High risk for injury related to decreased level of consciousness, effect of anesthetics, seizures, or drug therapy*

NURSING PRIORITY: Prevent injury.

Interventions

1. Implement the measures discussed in the "Increased Intracranial Pressure" plan's "high risk for injury" nursing diagnosis, page 144.

2. Additional individualized interventions:_____

_____

Rationales

1. Although the risk factors for injury for the neurosurgical patient differ somewhat from those for the patient with increased ICP, the measures used to prevent them are the same.

2. Rationales: _____

_____

Target outcome criterion
Throughout the hospital stay, the patient will remain free from injury.

Nursing diagnosis: *High risk for fluid volume excess related to physiologic stress response to surgery, steroid therapy, or syndrome of inappropriate secretion of antidiuretic hormone*

NURSING PRIORITY: Maintain the patient in a slightly dehydrated state.

Interventions

1. Implement the measures discussed in the "Increased Intracranial Pressure" plan's "high risk for fluid volume excess" nursing diagnosis, page 142.

2. Additional individualized interventions:_____

_____

Rationales

1. "Increased Intracranial Pressure" discusses potential for fluid volume excess in detail.

2. Rationales: _____

_____

Target outcome criteria
By the time of discharge, the patient will:
• display electrolyte levels, BUN level, hematocrit, and serum osmolality within normal limits
• have a urine output within normal limits

• manifest hemodynamic values within normal limits.

Nursing diagnosis: *High risk for fluid volume deficit related to diuretic therapy, fluid restriction, diabetes insipidus, hyperthermia, or GI suction*

NURSING PRIORITY: Maintain fluid volume within prescribed limits.

Interventions

1. Implement the measures discussed in the "Increased Intracranial Pressure" plan's "high risk for fluid volume deficit" nursing diagnosis, page 141.

2. Additional individualized interventions:_____

_____

Rationales

1. Diabetes insipidus most commonly occurs after neurosurgery. The "Increased Intracranial Pressure" plan discusses this problem in detail.

2. Rationales:_____

_____

NEUROLOGIC DISORDERS

Target outcome criteria
By the type of discharge, the patient will:
• maintain a urine output within normal limits
• have electrolyte levels, hematocrit, BUN level, and serum osmolality within normal limits

• maintain hemodynamic values within normal limits.

Nursing diagnosis: *Body-image disturbance related to hair loss, possible disruption in sensory or motor function, or possible alteration in personality and thought processes*

NURSING PRIORITIES: (a) Promote a healthy body image and (b) minimize damage to self-concept.

Interventions

1. Encourage the patient to express feelings, beliefs, and concerns about changes resulting from the diagnosis and craniotomy. Offer emotional support, as appropriate, based on knowledge of diagnosis and success of surgery.

2. Implement measures to minimize the patient's reaction to loss of hair and to the misshapen skull, if a bone flap was removed.
• Provide a surgical cap or scarf to wear; encourage usual grooming, makeup habits, and wearing a wig; reinforce that hair will regrow.
• Use therapeutic touch and visit frequently.

3. Provide appropriate stimuli:
• Place the patient in a room with a window, if possible.
• Provide a clock and calendar.
• Provide objects of interest to the patient, such as photographs of loved ones.
• Play the radio, tapes, or television, if desired.
• Talk with the patient.
• Encourage the family to interact with the patient.

4. Implement the measures in the "Impaired Physical Mobility" plan, page 36, as appropriate. Encourage participation in self-care, occupational therapy, activities of daily living, and ambulation, as permitted.

5. Additional individualized interventions:_____
_____

Rationales

1. The patient may have fears or misconceptions that can be clarified. Some residual effects of surgery are temporary. Recovery may be slow (months or years).

2. Specific interventions to minimize the body image changes may make the patient feel less self-conscious.

• These measures to improve appearance and become aware of the temporary nature of alterations in body image may encourage greater acceptance of the changes.
• Therapeutic touch and frequent visits convey acceptance, which may facilitate the patient's self-acceptance.

3. The measures listed provide stimulation and reality orientation. Talking with the patient and encouraging family interaction are particularly important because they reinforce a sense of human connection in the unfamiliar hospital environment.

4. The measures in this plan prevent deformities and other complications resulting from the enforced immobility associated with major surgery. Maintaining motor function, muscle strength, and joint mobility are particularly important in preserving the patient's ability to benefit from later rehabilitation programs. Participation in activities fosters the patient's belief that independence can be reestablished.

5. Rationales: _____
_____

Target outcome criteria
Within 5 to 7 days after surgery, the patient will:
• verbalize feelings of self-worth
• participate in self-care
• demonstrate an interest in personal appearance

• demonstrate an interest in occupational therapy, activities of daily living, and a potential rehabilitation program.

Nursing diagnosis: *Postoperative knowledge deficit related to follow-up care*

NURSING PRIORITY: Provide early teaching regarding rehabilitation and follow-up care.

Interventions

1. Implement measures in the "Knowledge Deficit" plan, page 56, as appropriate. Defer formal teaching until the condition stabilizes.

2. Provide informal teaching, as appropriate. Encourage questions, provide brief explanations about the current situation, and clarify misconceptions.

3. Identify and document long-range teaching needs as the patient or family raises or displays them. Upon the patient's discharge, communicate these needs to the receiving staff.

4. Provide information to the patient and family about community agencies and support groups, such as head injury support groups, vocational rehabilitation, and the American Cancer Society.

5. Additional individualized interventions: _____

_____

Rationales

1. In the first days after surgery, the craniotomy patient usually is too ill for a structured teaching program, and the patient's and family's attention is directed toward more immediate needs. Formal teaching is best accomplished after the condition has stabilized and the patient has been transferred to a more conducive teaching environment.

2. Capitalizing on informal opportunities conveys a willingness to meet the patient's and family's immediate learning needs.

3. Planning for discharge teaching is most effective when an awareness of its importance pervades all phases of care. Documentation and colleague-to-colleague communication enhance continuity of care.

4. These organizations provide many forms of support for patients and families. In many cases, their credibility allows them to provide invaluable practical information on long-range education and rehabilitation. Knowing that others have coped with similar experiences may provide a sense of rapport and trust that facilitates the learning necessary to adjust successfully to cranial surgery and possible residual deficits.

5. Rationales: _____

_____

Target outcome criteria
By the time of discharge, the patient and family will:
• verbalize questions
• express satisfaction with the staff's willingness to answer questions
• begin identifying long-range learning needs.

Discharge planning
NURSING DISCHARGE CRITERIA
Upon the patient's discharge, documentation shows evidence of:
• stable vital signs
• stable neurologic function
• ICP within normal limits
• healing incision
• headache controlled by oral analgesics
• absence of pulmonary, cardiovascular, or GI complications
• normal fluid and electrolyte balance
• absence of infection
• absence of fever.

PATIENT-FAMILY TEACHING CHECKLIST
Document evidence that the patient and family demonstrate an understanding of:
___ diagnosis and extent of surgery

___ extent of neurologic deficits, if present
___ extent and demands of the rehabilitation process
___ need for continued family support.

DOCUMENTATION CHECKLIST
Using outcome criteria as a guide, document:
___ clinical status on admission
___ significant changes in status
___ pertinent laboratory and diagnostic test findings
___ fluid intake and output
___ neurologic status
___ neurologic deficits, if present
___ GI bleeding, if any
___ wound condition
___ seizures, if any
___ rehabilitation program needs.

NEUROLOGIC DISORDERS

ASSOCIATED PLANS OF CARE
Impaired Physical Mobility
Ineffective Individual Coping
Knowledge Deficit
Nutritional Deficit
Pain
Sensory-Perceptual Alteration

References

Gordon, M., *Nursing Diagnosis, Process and Application,* 2nd ed. New York: McGraw-Hill Book Co., 1987.

Ignatavicius, D.D., and Bayne, M.V. *Medical-Surgical Nursing, A Nursing Process Approach.* Philadelphia: W.B. Saunders Co., 1991.

Kee, J.L. *Laboratory and Diagnostic Tests with Nursing Implications,* 3rd ed. East Norwalk, Conn.: Appleton and Lange, 1990.

Kinney, M.R., et al. *AACN'S Clinical Reference for Critical-Care Nursing,* 2nd ed. New York: McGraw-Hill Book Co., 1988.

Lewis, S.M., and Collier, I.C. *Medical-Surgical Nursing Assessment and Management of Clinical Problems,* 2nd ed. New York: McGraw-Hill Book Co., 1987.

Thompson, J.M., et al. *Mosby's Manual of Clinical Nursing,* 2nd ed. St. Louis: Mosby-Year Book, 1989.

NEUROLOGIC DISORDERS

Drug Overdose

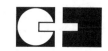

DRG information

DRG 449 Poisoning and Toxic Effects of Drugs.
Age 17+. With Complications or Comorbidities (CC).
Mean LOS = 4.3 days
Principal diagnoses include:
• poisoning by drugs of all varieties, affecting multiple body systems
• toxic effects of alcohol.

DRG 450 Poisoning and Toxic Effects of Drugs.
Age 17+. Without CC.
Mean LOS = 2.6 days
Principal diagnoses include selected principal diagnoses listed under DRG 449. The distinction is that DRG 450 excludes complications or comorbidities.

DRG 451 Poisoning and Toxic Effects of Drugs.
Age 0 to 17.
Mean LOS = 3.8 days
Principal diagnoses include selected principal diagnoses listed under DRG 449. The distinction is that DRG 451 excludes patients age 17+.

Introduction
DEFINITION AND TIME FOCUS

The patient admitted after a drug overdose is a challenge. The patient may be comatose, withdrawn, agitated, somnolent, or otherwise unable to provide clear historical data. The type of drug involved may be unknown, or evidence may suggest multiple drug ingestion. If illegal substances are involved, family members may be reluctant to provide a full history because they fear possible criminal prosecution, even if assured of medical confidentiality.

Even when the patient or family clearly identifies a specific drug that was taken, the possibility of multiple drug ingestion or potential interaction of other medications with the drug must always be considered. For the purposes of this plan, overdose is an intentional act in which the patient ingests, injects, sniffs, inhales, or otherwise self-administers a dose that proves to be toxic.

Using this definition, the plan omits discussion of overdoses from accidental poisoning, toxic reactions to prescribed medications taken at recommended dosages, and industrial or agricultural exposure to toxic substances. This plan focuses on the patient who is admitted to a critical-care unit for treatment of an intentional overdose, commonly associated with a suicide gesture or attempt.

ETIOLOGY AND PRECIPITATING FACTORS

For each patient, different factors may cause the overdose event, but usually one or more of the following are involved:
• drug or alcohol abuse or addiction
• unhealthy coping patterns
• unusually stressful life event or circumstances
• despair, depression, anger, or the desire for revenge.

Focused assessment guidelines
NURSING HISTORY (Functional health pattern findings)

Health perception – health management pattern
• may reveal history of short- or long-term drug or alcohol abuse or addiction
• may reveal intent to commit suicide
• may admit previous suicide attempt

Sleep-rest pattern
• may give history of insomnia or early morning awakening (associated with depression)

Cognitive-perceptual pattern
• may show poor concentration or memory impairment
• may experience difficulty making decisions

Self-perception – self-concept pattern
• may express helpless or hopeless self-perception (common)
• may make self-deprecating statements

Role-relationship pattern
• may lack a significant other
• may describe recent conflict or breakup with significant other
• may reveal recent or chronic job difficulties
• may have experienced the death of a loved one recently

Coping – stress tolerance pattern
• may use unhealthy coping behavior habitually, such as drug abuse

Value-belief pattern
• may express surprise or disbelief about seriousness of overdose

PHYSICAL FINDINGS

Because physical findings vary widely in patients with drug overdoses, depending on the drug taken, this section is omitted. See *Nurse's guide to common drug overdoses,* or consult pharmacologic references for findings associated with specific drug overdoses.

DIAGNOSTIC STUDIES

Appropriate laboratory tests vary widely, depending on the drug taken. The following are commonly performed for toxicity screening and evaluation.
• serum electrolyte levels—may be abnormal; several drugs commonly seen in overdose cases, including salicylates and alcohol, may cause electrolyte abnormalities
• arterial blood gas (ABG) values—essential for monitoring the adequacy of respiratory efforts; salicylates and other drugs cause acid-base abnormalities
• liver enzymes—may reveal liver damage; many medications can cause liver damage at toxic levels, most notably acetaminophen and alcohol
• blood alcohol level—an important screening test in any overdose because alcohol potentiates many drug effects, thus increasing central nervous system (CNS) depression
• toxicology screening assay—checks for various substances, depending on the laboratory, but usually includes barbiturates, narcotics, amphetamines, salicylates, and acetaminophen, among others

• serum salicylate level—may reveal toxicity; time-elapsed nomograms are obtained in acute overdose to assess toxicity level; because salicylates have a prolonged half-life, the sample should be obtained at least 6 hours after ingestion; toxic level is greater than 150 mcg/ml
• urine narcotic levels—determine narcotic presence and concentration; most narcotics are excreted in urine within 48 hours of administration; toxic levels vary depending on the narcotic
• serum barbiturate levels—determine the concentration of barbiturates in the blood. Salicylates may interfere with the test; alcohol ingestion may increase barbiturate levels; toxic levels vary depending on the barbiturate taken
• serum antidepressant levels—identify drug presence and concentration; toxic levels vary, depending on the antidepressant; for most tricyclic antidepressants, toxic level is greater than 1,000 ng/ml
• abdominal X-rays—can reveal a mass of pills in the stomach
• gastroscopy—may be performed to remove substances if X-rays reveal a coalesced mass of material that cannot be removed by lavage

POTENTIAL COMPLICATIONS

See *Nurse's guide to common drug overdoses.*

Nursing diagnosis: *High risk for ineffective airway clearance related to reduced alertness, decreased or absent gag reflex, obstruction by tongue, vomiting, or lavage procedures*

NURSING PRIORITY: Maintain a clear airway.

Interventions

1. Assess the patient's airway status continually by noting the adequacy of spontaneous respiratory effort, chest excursion, breath sounds, gag reflex, skin color, and level of consciousness.

2. Place the patient in a side-lying position. Ensure that suction equipment is at the bedside, ready for use.

3. If lavage is initiated, ensure airway protection by placing the patient in a head-down position or assisting with placement of a cuffed endotracheal tube if the patient is obtunded.

4. If the patient's gag reflex is reduced or absent or if respirations are less than 12 or more than 24 per minute, shallow, or labored, anticipate and assist with endotracheal intubation and mechanical ventilation. See the "Mechanical Ventilation" plan, page 227, for details.

Rationales

1. Initial and ongoing airway evaluation is essential in the patient who has taken a drug overdose because many medications cause CNS depression. If several medications were taken, their combining or potentiating effects may further reduce the patient's ability to clear the airway.

2. The side-lying position facilitates drainage from the mouth and reduces the probability of aspiration. Suctioning may be needed if the patient vomits.

3. Aspiration of gastric contents predisposes the patient to aspiration pneumonitis, a complication associated with increased morbidity and mortality.

4. Toxic CNS effects may interfere with vital functions. Unless promptly corrected, respiratory impairment results in permanent damage to the brain and other organs.

NURSE'S GUIDE TO COMMON DRUG OVERDOSES

Drug	Therapeutic effects	Signs and symptoms of overdose	Treatment	Complications
acetaminophen	Reduces fever and raises pain threshold; exact mechanisms unclear; metabolized in liver	• Anorexia • Nausea and vomiting • Diaphoresis • Right upper quadrant abdominal pain • Hypotension • Altered level of consciousness	• Emesis or lavage • Cathartics • Acetylcysteine (Mucomyst) given orally, if more than 7.5 g ingested within 24 hours and serum level in toxic range 4 hours after ingestion	• Hepatic failure • Coagulation defects • Renal failure • Hepatic encephalopathy • Shock
alcohol (ethanol)	Central nervous system (CNS) depression, peripheral vasodilation	• Ataxia • Reduced comprehension • Vomiting • Respiratory depression • Hypotension • Seizures • Flushing • Coma	• Emesis or lavage, if ingestion within 4 hours • I.V. fluids • Ventilatory support, especially in multiple drug overdose • Observation for withdrawal, including anxiety, tremors, diaphoresis, tachycardia, and hypertension (usually occurs 24 to 48 hours after last alcohol intake) • If withdrawal symptoms are noted, sedation	• Respiratory depression • Aspiration • Hepatic failure • GI tract bleeding • With chronic abuse: —Esophageal varices —Portal hypertension —Hepatic encephalopathy • Additive effects if taken with another CNS depressant
barbiturates	CNS depression	• Cardiopulmonary depression • Hypotension • Tachycardia • Sluggish pupil response • Nystagmus • Bullae • Hypothermia • Confusion • Ataxia • Coma	• Ventilatory support • Emesis or lavage (if ingested) • Activated charcoal • Cathartics • I.V. fluids • Observation for withdrawal, including tremors, vomiting, weakness, and hallucinations • Dialysis possible for large doses	• Arrhythmias • Respiratory arrest • Shock • Seizures • Pulmonary edema • Coma
benzodiazepines	CNS depression	• Lethargy • Hypotension • Tachycardia • Respiratory depression • Confusion • Ataxia • Coma	• Ventilatory support • Emesis or lavage (if ingested) • Activated charcoal • Cathartics • Flumazenil (Mazicon) given I.V. in repeated doses • I.V. fluids • Hemodialysis and forced diuresis *not* effective	• Taken alone, usually not fatal but when taken with other CNS depressants, additive effects can lead to respiratory depression, coma, and death
cocaine	CNS stimulation, local anesthesia	• Hyperexcitability • Anxiety • Hypertension or hypotension • Fever • Tachypnea • Tachycardia • Confusion • Hallucinations • Dilated pupils • Diaphoresis • Seizures, coma	• Sedatives • Anticonvulsants • Cardiac monitoring • Emesis or lavage, if ingested • Activated charcoal, if ingested • Cathartic, if ingested • Fever control measures	• Myocardial infarction • Cerebral hemorrhage • Respiratory arrest • Status epilepticus • Cardiomyopathy • Rhabdomyolysis (rare)

continued

NEUROLOGIC DISORDERS

NURSE'S GUIDE TO COMMON DRUG OVERDOSES *(continued)*

Drug	Therapeutic effects	Signs and symptoms of overdose	Treatment	Complications
opiates	CNS depression, analgesia, peripheral vasodilation	• Respiratory depression • Constricted pupils • Reduced level of consciousness • Hypothermia • Hypotension • Bradycardia	• Ventilatory support • Naloxone (Narcan) I.V. in repeated doses • Close monitoring, because respiratory depression may recur • Cardiac monitoring • Emesis or lavage, if ingested	• Respiratory arrest • Shock • Arrhythmias • Coma
salicylates	Analgesia	• Nausea and vomiting • Hyperthermia • Electrolyte imbalances • Acid-base imbalances (usually respiratory alkalosis and metabolic acidosis) • Hyperglycemia (in children, hypoglycemia) • Hyperpnea • Hyperventilation • Oliguria • Tinnitus • Confusion • Seizures • Petechiae	• Ventilatory support • Cardiac monitoring • I.V. fluids • Cooling measures • Correction of electrolyte and acid-base abnormalities • Emesis or lavage • Activated charcoal • Cathartics • Alkalinization of urine with sodium bicarbonate and potassium chloride (a urine pH between 7.5 and 8.5 promotes increased renal excretion)	• Respiratory failure • Arrhythmias or other life-threatening conditions caused by electrolyte or acid-base abnormalities • Renal tubular necrosis • GI bleeding • Hepatotoxicity • Pulmonary edema • Shock • Interference with normal clotting • Increased gastric motility
tricyclic antidepressants	Relieves symptoms of depression in patients with mood disorders	• Lethargy • Dry mouth • Dilated pupils • Confusion • Tremors • Urine retention • Tachycardia • Hypotension • Respiratory depression • Cardiac conduction delay • Hypothermia • Seizures • Coma	• Ventilatory support • Cardiac monitoring • Emesis or lavage • Activated charcoal • Cathartics • I.V. fluids • Sodium physostigmine 1 to 3 mg I.V., if large amount ingested • Cardiac pacing, if complete heart block • Anticonvulsants • Alkalinization with sodium bicarbonate • Temperature regulation measures • Dialysis *not* effective	• Arrhythmias • Myocardial depression • Complete heart block • Congestive heart failure • Shock • Paralytic ileus • Central and peripheral anticholinergic effects, myocardial depression

5. Monitor ABG levels, as ordered. See Appendix B, "Acid-Base Imbalances."

5. Changes in ABG levels may provide early warning of impaired ventilatory status even before clinical evidence is apparent. Also, toxic levels of many medications cause acid-base abnormalities; ABG studies serve as a guide for corrective intervention.

6. Additional individualized interventions: _____

6. Rationales: _____

Target outcome criteria
Throughout the hospital stay, the patient will:
• maintain a clear airway
• maintain spontaneous respiratory rate of 12 to 24
breaths/minute or receive mechanical ventilatory assistance.

Collaborative problem: *High risk for multi-organ dysfunction related to systemic toxic drug effects*

NURSING PRIORITIES: (a) Support and monitor vital organ functions, and (b) identify and counteract drug effects.

Interventions

1. Collect as much historical data as possible about the overdose by questioning the patient, family, friends, and other caregivers. Determine the following, if possible:
• what was taken
• how much was taken
• when it was taken
• how it was taken (for example, ingested or injected)
• concomitant alcohol use
• underlying health problems
• other medications taken
• what has been done for the patient so far.

2. Monitor vital signs, hemodynamic pressures, and electrocardiogram findings according to Appendix A, "Monitoring Standards," or unit protocol.

3. Collaborate with the doctor and regional poison control center personnel in selecting and initiating measures to reverse or eliminate the drugs from the body (some measures may have already been implemented in the emergency department). Initiate one or more of the following, as appropriate:

• induced emesis with ipecac syrup, 30 ml orally with 10 to 12 oz (300 to 350 ml) of fluids. Observe for onset of vomiting within 15 to 30 minutes. If no emesis, the dose may be repeated once. If still no emesis, consult the doctor and prepare for gastric lavage. Never administer ipecac if the patient has an absent gag reflex, signs of decreasing alertness, a history of seizures, or ingested corrosives. Consult with the poison control center before administering ipecac to a patient who has ingested a hydrocarbon.

Rationales

1. Thorough history-taking may be difficult, but it provides vital clues for effective intervention and ongoing monitoring.

2. At toxic levels, many drugs can interfere with the vasomotor center's control of cardiac function and blood vessel constriction. Baseline and ongoing assessment of these parameters provides early warning of cardiovascular dysfunction.

3. Since the institution of regional poison control centers, with their "hot line" consultative services, mortality from poisonings has fallen significantly. The poison control center provides expert advice on treating all types of drug overdoses.

• Ipecac syrup is thought to act both centrally and locally on the gastrointestinal tract to stimulate vomiting. Fluids are given with ipecac because, without adequate gastric volume, esophageal injury may occur from forceful retching. Doses greater than 60 ml may have cardiotoxic effects. Ipecac administration is contraindicated in the circumstances noted because vomiting under such conditions may result in aspiration. Also, vomiting of corrosives may cause or increase damage to esophageal and oropharyngeal mucosae. Treating hydrocarbon ingestion depends on the specific substance. Ipecac may not be effective if the patient has taken an overdose of antiemetic medication, such as a phenothiazine.

NEUROLOGIC DISORDERS

• gastric lavage, using a large-bore Ewald tube and the irrigant that the doctor prefers, usually normal saline solution. Lavage with 100 to 200 ml fluid boluses and avoid overdistending the stomach. Lavage until return is clear, unless otherwise ordered, usually 1,000 to 1,500 ml total. Monitor inflow and outflow volumes and report discrepancies. Save aspirated fluid for analysis, as needed. Monitor serum electrolyte levels in conjunction with large-volume or prolonged lavage.

• Gastric lavage is used when vomiting is contraindicated (for example, if the patient has a reduced or absent gag reflex). It effectively removes ingested substances from the stomach, but is thought to be somewhat less effective than induced emesis. The choice of fluid is controversial and may depend on the drug ingested. Fluid boluses larger than 200 ml are thought to wash the toxin into the small bowel. A discrepancy between the amounts of instilled irrigant and returned fluid may indicate a need to reposition the patient to promote drainage or may indicate fluid reabsorption and risk of fluid overload. The aspirate may be examined for diagnostic clues. Electrolyte imbalances, and their cardiovascular sequelae, may result from prolonged or large-volume lavage.

• dilution, usually with milk or water, unless the patient is obtunded.

• Dilution is used primarily to treat ingestion of corrosives or other substances that preclude emesis. Distending the abdomen with fluid, if the patient is obtunded, may increase the risk of aspiration.

• gut lavage, using a peristaltic pump to deliver warmed electrolyte solution to the stomach.

• This relatively new therapy may be used to aid clearance of certain herbicides from the bowel.

• activated charcoal, usually 25 to 50 g in a slurry, administered orally or via gastric tube after emesis or lavage is completed. Do not give charcoal with ipecac syrup.

• Activated charcoal is an inert substance that adsorbs toxins. It should not be given at the same time as ipecac syrup because it will inactivate the ipecac and prevent emesis. Clinicians' opinions vary on whether the charcoal should be removed after a given time or allowed to pass through the gut.

• cathartics, as ordered, usually mixed with charcoal. Cathartics ordered include magnesium sulfate and magnesium citrate.

• Saline cathartics stimulate peristaltic activity by drawing fluid into the bowel through osmosis, thus hastening drug excretion and reducing absorption from the gut.

• specific antidotes or antagonists, as ordered.

• A few drugs, notably narcotics and acetaminophen, are effectively treated with antidote-antagonist substances; however, multiple drug ingestion is always a possibility, so the clinician must remain vigilant even if these measures are employed.

• other measures, as recommended by the doctor or poison control center, such as forced diuresis, peritoneal dialysis, hemodialysis, exchange transfusion, or gastroscopy.

• Forced diuresis may be used if the drug involved is excreted primarily through the urinary tract. Dialysis may help remove certain substances, but its effectiveness depends on the drug's pharmacologic properties and its distribution within body tissues. Exchange transfusion may be used for certain drugs if the dosage is massive and recent enough that tissue absorption has not yet taken place. Gastroscopy may be performed if abdominal X-rays reveal a coalesced mass of pills in the stomach.

4. Perform meticulous serial evaluations of level of consciousness, mental status, and gag and corneal reflex status every 1 to 2 hours during the first 24 hours or until the patient's condition stabilizes.

4. Decreasing alertness and diminished or absent protective reflexes indicate CNS impairment and an impending need for airway management or ventilatory support. Serial evaluations allow early detection of subtle changes.

5. Monitor fluid intake and output and promptly report a dropping urine output (less than 60 ml/hour) to the doctor.

5. Because many medications are detoxified or excreted through the renal system, the possibility of renal failure from toxic effects must always be considered. Also, a dropping urine output is a clue to the early development of shock, another potential complication of drug toxicity.

6. Assess and monitor initial or serial laboratory test findings, as ordered, for overdose substances.

6. Specific initial and serial urine or serum studies provide information about the amount of drug taken and the rate of absorption, thus guiding therapeutic treatment.

7. Additional individualized interventions: _____

7. Rationales: _____

Target outcome criteria
Within 1 hour of admission to the hospital, the patient will receive initial treatment for specific drug overdose.

Throughout the hospital stay, the patient will maintain vital organ functions.

Nursing diagnosis: *Hopelessness related to low self-esteem, emotional disorganization, or sense of having inadequate resources to cope with life*

NURSING PRIORITIES: (a) Promote a sense of hope, and (b) foster self-esteem.

Interventions

1. Examine your attitudes toward suicide and drug abuse. Assume a concerned but nonjudgmental attitude and avoid vindictive or punishing behavior when providing care. Seek peer support or consult with a psychiatric liaison nurse if negative attitudes affect patient care.

2. Foster communication.

• Use touch, as appropriate.

• Use active listening skills.

• Note and acknowledge nonverbal cues (body posture and gestures, facial expression, tone of voice, and silences).

• Make eye contact.

3. Encourage the patient to participate in care-related decisions as soon as possible.

4. Arrange referral to psychiatric resources (such as a psychiatric nurse specialist, psychiatrist, or other mental health professional). Place the patient on suicide precautions, if appropriate.

5. See the "Ineffective Individual Coping" plan, page 51, and the "Dying" plan, page 11.

Rationales

1. Many health professionals have difficulty caring for a suicidal or self-abusive patient. Frustration and anger are common when the patient seems to be undermining the efforts of health care providers. Punishing attitudes, however, tend to further decrease the patient's already fragile self-esteem and reduce coping ability. The patient is likely to interpret such behavior as "just one more sign I'm no good for anything," adding to self-directed anger and hopelessness. Peer or psychiatric liaison support can help professionals address and resolve issues raised by abusive or noncompliant responses to care.

2. Commonly, the patient who has overdosed perceives a lack of personal resources or cannot communicate feelings because of emotional disorganization. Opening communication is the first step in identifying more positive responses to the problems that may have led to the overdose.

• Touch can convey profound messages of acceptance and caring and, for some patients, may be less threatening than verbal interaction as a way to initiate the therapeutic relationship.

• Active listening involves an attentive attitude, feedback, and rephrasing or reflection to help the patient clarify feelings and ideas. This reassures the patient of the worth of personal feelings and of the importance of the individual.

• Acknowledging nonverbal communication may help verify expressed feelings or open discussion of unexpressed feelings.

• Making eye contact in a nonthreatening manner is a simple way to express interest and the intent to communicate.

3. Consideration of the patient's stated wishes may, in many cases, be secondary to saving the patient's life. However, as the condition stabilizes, a return to participation in self-care helps bolster self-respect and reduces feelings of powerlessness.

4. Any patient admitted with an intentional overdose warrants psychiatric evaluation and counseling as part of the treatment plan. Careful evaluation of suicide potential is essential. If suicidal ideation is present, suicide precautions are warranted.

5. The "Ineffective Individual Coping" plan contains interventions for patients struggling with emotional adjustments. The "Dying" plan addresses issues that may relate to the care of the patient who has attempted suicide.

NEUROLOGIC DISORDERS

6. Ensure appropriate follow-up care arrangements before discharge from the unit, including continuation of suicide precautions, if appropriate.

6. The patient who has been severely depressed may attempt suicide again once physical energy has been restored and personal appearance seems improved. Careful follow-up, both on the unit to which the patient is transferred and after discharge from the hospital, is vital in assisting the patient's transition to everyday life.

7. Additional individualized interventions: _____

7. Rationales: _____

Target outcome criteria
Before discharge from the unit, the patient will:
• discuss reasons for the overdose and identify precipitating factors
• participate, to the extent possible, in self-care and care planning
• begin to display coping behaviors that are health-promoting
• make contact with follow-up care providers.

Discharge planning

NURSING DISCHARGE CRITERIA
Upon the patient's discharge, documentation shows evidence of:
• spontaneous respirations and airway clearance
• stable vital signs for at least 12 hours
• completion of specific measures to remove or reverse drugs consumed
• drug levels (if applicable) declining since admission
• urine output greater than 60 ml/hour
• ABG values within normal limits
• initial psychiatric evaluation and follow-up arrangements made
• implementation of suicide precautions, if appropriate.

PATIENT-FAMILY TEACHING CHECKLIST
Document evidence that the patient and family demonstrate an understanding of:
___ toxic effects of drugs and possible later complications
___ treatment measures undertaken
___ signs and symptoms of complications, if any anticipated
___ health-promoting coping behaviors
___ resources available for help.

DOCUMENTATION CHECKLIST
Using outcome criteria as a guide, document:
___ clinical status on admission
___ significant changes in status
___ pertinent laboratory and diagnostic test findings
___ effectiveness of measures to promote elimination or reversal of drugs
___ mental health measures
___ suicide precautions, if used
___ follow-up plans
___ patient-family teaching
___ discharge planning.

ASSOCIATED PLANS OF CARE
Acute Renal Failure
Dying
Grieving
Impaired Physical Mobility
Ineffective Individual Coping
Mechanical Ventilation
Sensory-Perceptual Alteration

References
Acee, A., and Smith, D. "Crack," *American Journal of Nursing* 87(5):614-17, May 1987.

Alspach, J. *Core Curriculum for Critical Care Nursing*, 4th ed. Philadelphia: W.B. Saunders Co., 1991.

Kitt, S., and Kaiser, J. *Emergency Nursing, A Physiologic and Clinical Perspective*. Philadelphia: W.B. Saunders, 1990.

Moisan, D. "Poison and Drug Overdose," in *Critical Care Nursing: A Holistic Approach*, 5th ed. Edited by Hudak, C., et al. Philadelphia: J.B. Lippincott Co., 1990.

O'Boyle, C., et al. *Emergency Care: The First 24 Hours*. East Norwalk, Conn.: Appleton-Lange, 1985.

Rea, R., Bourg, P., Parker, J., and Rushing, D. *Emergency Nursing Core Curriculum*, 3rd ed. Philadelphia: W.B. Saunders Co., 1987.

Thurkauf, G. "Acetaminophen Overdose," *Critical Care Nurse* 7(1):20-31, January-February 1987.

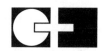

NEUROLOGIC DISORDERS
Guillain-Barré Syndrome

DRG information
DRG 018 Cranial and Peripheral Nerve Disorders.
With Complication or Comorbidity (CC).
Mean LOS = 6.0 days
Principal diagnoses include:
• disorders of cranial or peripheral nerves
• mononeuritis of upper or lower limb
• neuritis or radiculitis of brachial or unspecified nerve
• various types of neuropathy (including Guillain-Barré syndrome)
• various types of polyneuropathy.
DRG 019 Cranial and Peripheral Nerve Disorders.
Without CC.
Mean LOS = 3.9 days
Principal diagnoses include select principal diagnoses listed under DRG 018.

Introduction
DEFINITION AND TIME FOCUS
Guillain-Barré syndrome, also known as acute idiopathic polyneuritis, Landry–Guillain-Barré–Strohl syndrome, and polyradiculoneuritis, is a demyelinating disorder affecting the peripheral nervous system. First described in 1859, it is diagnosed typically when the patient complains of sudden weakness or paralysis of the legs that progresses upward symmetrically. Its cause is unknown; however, the disorder may result from an autoimmune response in which sensitized lymphocytes infiltrate the peripheral nervous system and produce demyelination, edema, and inflammation. The destruction of the myelin sheath, which increases impulse transmission by allowing impulses to jump from node to node along the axon, results in slowed conduction or, if significant edema is present, complete blockage of impulse transmission.

Commonly, the disorder causes progressive loss of function over 2 to 3 weeks, at which time the patient may require ventilatory support because of respiratory paralysis. However, the symptoms are potentially reversible because the myelin sheath can regenerate; full recovery without residual deficits eventually occurs in 75% to 85% of cases. Complete recovery is slow and commonly takes 18 to 24 months from the onset of symptoms. This plan focuses on the patient who is admitted with a diagnosis of Guillain-Barré syndrome.

ETIOLOGY AND PRECIPITATING FACTORS
• idiopathic origins
• possible link to autoimmune factors
• immunizations (vaccinations for smallpox, tetanus, influenza, and measles have been implicated in the syndrome)
• viral illnesses
• immunosuppression (Hodgkin's disease and other lymphomas may increase risk)
• previous surgery

Focused assessment guidelines
NURSING HISTORY (Functional health pattern findings)

Health perception–health management pattern
• typically complains of sudden, symmetric weakness of legs, increasing and ascending over several days, and mild to moderate sensory changes, such as tingling and muscle pain
• usually has experienced self-limiting, mild respiratory or GI illness 2 to 3 weeks before onset of symptoms
• may note frequent paresthesias before onset of weakness, such as a "stocking-and-glove" numbness and tingling
• may have difficulty speaking

Nutritional-metabolic pattern
• may complain of dysphagia

Elimination pattern
• usually retains sphincter control; may become incontinent if autonomic nervous system (ANS) involvement develops

Activity-exercise pattern
• notes leg weakness or paralysis that progresses upward to trunk, arms, and head (common)
• reports that arms were affected first (uncommon)
• may present with injuries from falling
• may complain of shortness of breath
• complains of easy fatigability (uncommon)

Cognitive-perceptual pattern
• may note pain, tingling "pins and needles" sensation, or numbness in arms and legs
• may describe altered sense of position

Coping–stress tolerance pattern
• likely to express extreme anxiety over progression of symptoms

Self-perception–self-concept pattern
• likely to complain of feelings of helplessness
• may express anxiety about role and responsibilities

PHYSICAL FINDINGS

Cardiovascular
- hypotension or, more commonly, hypertension (if ANS involved)
- tachyarrhythmias or bradyarrhythmias (if ANS involved)

Pulmonary
- diminished breath sounds
- difficulty clearing secretions
- shallow respirations
- use of accessory muscles

Neurologic
- diminished or absent deep tendon reflexes
- symmetrical paralysis or paresis
- loss of position and vibration sense
- cranial nerve abnormalities, most commonly cranial nerve VII (facial); others, in order of frequency, include: VI (abducens), III (oculomotor), XII (hypoglossal), V (trigeminal), and IX (glossopharyngeal) — manifested by facial paralysis; dysphagia; ptosis; diplopia; deviated tongue; difficulty chewing, swallowing, or talking; loss of gag and cough reflexes

Gastrointestinal or renal
- occasionally, urine or fecal retention (if ANS involved)

Musculoskeletal
- ascending weakness or flaccid paralysis of arms and legs
- tenderness to deep palpation of leg or arm muscles

Integumentary
- usually, warm, flushed skin
- cold, clammy skin if ANS involved
- occasionally, anhydrosis if ANS involved

DIAGNOSTIC STUDIES
Diagnosis of Guillain-Barré syndrome is based primarily on clinical findings and progression of symptoms; no specific diagnostic tests exist.

- routine blood studies — may reveal no significant abnormalities
- lumbar puncture — reveals classic findings of albuminocytologic dissociation (elevated protein level of more than 45 mg/dl and normal white blood cell count of 5 to 10/mm³); serial punctures commonly are performed to monitor disease course; cerebrospinal fluid protein level may not reveal elevation until 1 to 2 weeks after onset of symptoms
- electromyography studies — reveal denervated areas; recordings show repetitive firing of single units rather than normal sectional activity (may not appear until 2 weeks after onset of symptoms)
- nerve conduction velocity tests — reveal marked reduction in conduction speed
- pulmonary function studies — provide baseline data for evaluating degree of respiratory impairment; usually, decreased vital capacity (less than 20 ml/kg) is revealed

POTENTIAL COMPLICATIONS
- respiratory failure (occurs in about 25% of patients)
- thrombophlebitis
- pulmonary embolus
- ileus
- gastric dilatation
- atelectasis
- pneumonia
- skin breakdown
- urinary tract stones and infection
- GI bleeding
- septicemia
- autonomic dysfunction and arrhythmias
- muscle atrophy
- ineffective coping
- syndrome of inappropriate antidiuretic hormone secretion

Collaborative problem: *High risk for respiratory failure related to weakness or paralysis of respiratory muscles*

NURSING PRIORITY: Maintain adequate ventilatory status.

Interventions

1. Assess airway patency, breath sounds, respiratory rate and effort, ability to count slowly from 1 to 10, skin color, chest excursion, and vital capacity (VC) at least every 2 hours. Immediately report dyspnea, increasing restlessness, increasing use of diaphragmatic and accessory muscles, cyanosis, decreased breath sounds, shallow or irregular respirations, and VC of less than 20 ml/kg or reduced respiratory effort.

Rationales

1. Respiratory failure can occur subtly but rapidly in Guillain-Barré patients, and about 25% develop significant pulmonary problems. As muscular paralysis ascends, the phrenic nerve may become involved, affecting diaphragmatic excursion and impairing the patient's ability to maintain an adequate tidal volume and clear secretions from the airway.

2. Encourage hourly coughing and deep breathing, and assist with pulmonary hygiene measures (postural drainage, percussion, and incentive spirometry). Monitor carefully for development of fever, crackles, or areas of consolidation.

3. Use pulse oximetry to monitor oxygen saturation continuously or as needed. Obtain and monitor arterial blood gas (ABG) values, as ordered. Report changes or abnormal findings promptly.

4. Prepare to assist with endotracheal intubation or tracheotomy if VC falls below 800 ml or if the patient cannot clear secretions.

5. Suction as necessary, hyperinflating and hyperoxygenating with 100% oxygen before and after suctioning. Observe for a vasovagal response during suctioning.

6. Every 1 to 2 hours, monitor vital signs and neurologic status, including level of consciousness, muscle strength, and ability to gag, cough, and swallow. Also monitor hemodynamic parameters and electrocardiography findings according to Appendix A, "Monitoring Standards," or unit protocol. Assess for and immediately report the onset of sweating, flushing, altered vital signs, or arrhythmias. If life-threatening arrhythmias are present, institute appropriate pharmacologic treatment according to unit protocol.

7. When muscles of upper arms, shoulders, or swallowing show reduced function, be particularly vigilant for respiratory changes.

8. If mechanical ventilation is required, maintain ventilator settings and monitor ABG levels. Teach the patient and family about ventilator use and alarm systems. Reassure the patient and family that mechanical ventilation is usually temporary and that independent breathing should return when the patient's condition improves. See the "Mechanical Ventilation" plan, page 227.

9. Additional individualized interventions: _____

---

2. Reduced ventilatory capacity and resultant stasis of secretions may lead to atelectasis or pneumonia. Pulmonary hygiene measures help promote airway clearance. Coughing may lead to microatelectasis from the associated increase in intrathoracic pressure, if not followed by deep breathing to reexpand collapsed alveoli.

3. Ventilatory support is indicated if the patient's PCO_2 increases 10 to 15 mm Hg or if the PO_2 decreases 10 to 15 mm Hg compared with normal ranges. ABG values are a helpful adjunct to clinical observation of respiratory status. Pulse oximetry provides ongoing monitoring without invasive procedures.

4. In many cases, positive-pressure mechanical ventilation is necessary during the acute phase.

5. Careful suctioning, as indicated, helps avert mucus plugs or pulmonary infection from secretion stasis. Also, suctioning may be required because of facial or glossopharyngeal nerve involvement, which may cause drooling and impaired swallowing. Hyperinflation and hyperoxygenation are essential because lower oxygen levels are common with impaired respiratory effort and suctioning further depletes the oxygen supply. ANS dysfunction in Guillain-Barré syndrome is linked to a vagal nerve (cranial nerve X) deficit. Hypoxia and vagal stimulation occurring with suctioning can cause severe bradycardia or cardiac arrest. If oxygenation does not abolish the reflex, treat with intravenous atropine, as ordered.

6. Bradycardia, tachycardia, or blood pressure alterations may indicate hypoxemia or ANS involvement. Reduced cranial reflex responses, lethargy, or drowsiness may indicate increased carbon dioxide retention from respiratory insufficiency. Sweating, flushing, or arrhythmias may indicate ANS involvement. Vagus nerve involvement may be responsible for life-threatening arrhythmias.

7. These muscle groups are commonly affected just before breathing muscles; dysfunction may herald impending respiratory problems.

8. Ventilator settings should be correlated with current ABG levels and status. The patient and family may be extremely anxious over the use of and need for mechanical ventilation. Careful explanations may decrease fear and minimize "fighting" the machine. The "Mechanical Ventilation" plan provides details regarding care of the patient on a ventilator.

9. Rationales: _____

NEUROLOGIC DISORDERS

Target outcome criteria

On admission, the patient will have a clear airway.

Within 4 hours of admission, the patient will have:
• clear breath sounds
• regular respirations
• bilaterally equal chest excursion
• PO_2 greater than 70 mm Hg
• PCO_2 of 35 to 45 mm Hg.

Nursing diagnosis: *Impaired physical mobility related to slowed or absent conduction of motor nerve impulses, resulting in weakness or flaccid paralysis*

NURSING PRIORITY: Prevent complications associated with immobility.

Interventions

1. See the "Impaired Physical Mobility" plan, page 36, for detailed interventions regarding positioning, range-of-motion exercises, skin care, infection prevention and treatment, elimination aids, and promotion of circulation.

2. Caution the patient and family in handling arms and legs; they should be aware of risks of pressure, temperature, and, as function returns, overexertion and fatigue.

3. Administer corticosteroids or corticotropin, if ordered. Monitor closely for signs and symptoms of gastric irritation, edema, hypokalemia, or other untoward effects. Be aware that steroid use may mask signs and symptoms of underlying infection.

4. Prepare the patient for plasmapheresis, if ordered. For the patient undergoing plasmapheresis, monitor for complications: trauma or infection at the site of vascular access; hypovolemia; hypokalemia and hypocalcemia; and temporary circumoral and distal extremity paresthesias, muscle twitching, and nausea and vomiting related to the administration of citrated plasma.

5. Provide eye care, including use of artificial tears and eye protectors, as needed.

6. Early in the hospital stay, provide assistance with physical activities and teach the patient to use splints and assistive devices, as needed. As soon as possible, encourage the patient to resume normal activities, beginning by assuming the upright position with the use of a tilt table or bed adjustment. Arrange referral to a physical therapist and supervise coordination of the activity program.

Rationales

1. The "Impaired Physical Mobility" plan contains interventions for preventing complications associated with prolonged immobility. The patient with Guillain-Barré syndrome is at increased risk for the following immobility-related problems: infections, thromboembolic phenomena, joint contractures, muscle atrophy, skin breakdown, constipation or ileus, and urinary calculi. Preventive and therapeutic measures for these complications are an essential part of caring for the patient with Guillain-Barré syndrome. Frequent changes of position may also help reduce pain caused by the disease or immobility.

2. Reduced sensory capabilities associated with nerve dysfunction may cause the patient to be unaware of impending or actual injury. When function begins to return, the patient must use caution in resuming activity, because overexertion may exacerbate the symptoms.

3. Steroid use is controversial and of questionable value in reducing the inflammatory reaction that impairs mobility. Adverse reactions may negate potential benefits, so if such medication is ordered, monitor carefully. Corticotropin may shorten the syndrome's duration in some cases, but its use is still being investigated.

4. Plasmapheresis has been shown to have possible benefit in chronic relapsing or in progressive Guillain-Barré syndrome. Although the reason for the benefit is unknown, the procedure may remove antimyelin antibodies that are linked to the development of the disorder, possibly shortening the disease course. However, neither this nor any other treatment has been proven to have direct therapeutic effects, so monitoring and support remain the primary interventions.

5. Trigeminal nerve impairment may cause the loss of corneal sensation. Facial nerve involvement commonly affects eyelid function.

6. Early activity and proper positioning prevent contractures and injuries from disuse. Gradually resuming an upright position helps regain vascular tone. Venous pooling associated with bed rest may contribute to initial orthostatic hypotension when the patient resumes the upright position. Function may return asymmetrically, predisposing the patient to falls, back problems, or other injuries. A physical therapist can provide expert guidance in planning rehabilitation.

7. Additional individualized interventions: _____

7. Rationales: _____

Target outcome criteria

On admission and continuously, the patient will:
• have intact skin
• have normal eye lubrication or protective measures instituted.

Within 3 days of admission, the patient will:
• have a bowel movement
• receive regular active or passive range-of-motion exercise, as condition allows.

As function returns, the patient will:
• show no exacerbation of condition
• suffer no accidental injuries.

Nursing diagnosis: *High risk for nutritional deficit related to dysphagia, depression, tracheostomy, or mechanical ventilation*

NURSING PRIORITY: Provide adequate nutrition.

Interventions

1. See the "Nutritional Deficit" plan, page 63.

2. Assess the patient's gag reflex, ability to swallow, presence of facial paralysis, and motor and sensory function of upper extremities before eating.

3. If oral intake is tolerated, use techniques to help minimize choking and aspiration:
• elevate the patient's head and flex the neck while swallowing
• have suction equipment at hand and supervise the patient closely during meals
• provide semisolid foods; avoid liquids initially; allow the patient to make choices about diet when possible.

4. Administer enteral and parenteral feedings as ordered during the acute phase of illness. If enteral feedings are used, check for residual every four hours or before each feeding, and maintain the patient in a sitting position, or with the head of the bed elevated, during and for 1 hour after feeding.

5. Additional individualized interventions: _____

Rationales

1. The "Nutritional Deficit" plan contains interventions for assessment and support of the patient with a potential nutritional deficit.

2. If the disease affects cranial nerves V (trigeminal), VII (facial), IX (glossopharyngeal), X (vagus), or XII (hypoglossal), the patient will have difficulty chewing and swallowing and will not have a gag reflex. Aspiration can occur easily if the patient attempts to eat or is fed orally.

3. Cranial nerve involvement may cause dysphagia; when the patient takes food by mouth before and after acute phase of illness, use care to avoid aspiration. Permitting choices, when possible, helps the patient maintain or regain a sense of self-control.

4. Adequate nutrition is essential to minimize muscle wasting, maintain the body's defenses against infection, and promote healing. During the acute phase, dysphagia may be too severe to safely permit oral intake. Precautions must be taken with enteral feedings to prevent regurgitation and aspiration of feedings.

5. Rationales: _____

Target outcome criteria

By the time of discharge, the patient will:
• be receiving optimum nutritional intake, as reflected by stable weight (plus or minus 2 or 3 lb [0.9 to 1.4 kg] per week)
• eat without aspirating, if able to tolerate oral food intake.

NEUROLOGIC DISORDERS

Nursing diagnosis: *Powerlessness related to rapidly progressing symptoms, altered communication, dependency on others for basic needs, and fear of death*

NURSING PRIORITY: Maintain psychological equilibrium.

Interventions

1. See the "Ineffective Individual Coping" plan, page 51.

2. Provide frequent, factual explanations about the condition, emphasizing the temporary, potentially reversible nature of the disorder. Prepare the patient and family for potential problems of the acute phase. Point out any small improvements in the patient's condition as they occur. Encourage family members to participate in care.

3. If communication ability is impaired, arrange for use of signals (eye blinks or motion-sensor call devices) or use a writing tablet or word board. Anticipate needs; be sensitive to nonverbal cues such as facial expression.

4. Encourage the use of relaxation and stress control techniques. Emphasize that proficient use of such techniques may benefit the patient even after the disorder has resolved. Assist and teach the patient about the following, as appropriate:
• progressive relaxation
• guided imagery
• "thought-stopping" and positive affirmation
• meditation.

5. Whenever possible, encourage the patient to make choices regarding care and involve the family in care planning.

6. Encourage ventilation of feelings. Cultivate an attitude of acceptance. If manipulative or dysfunctional behavior occurs, try to provide the patient with increased control and choices. Encourage family members to talk to the patient, even if the patient cannot respond. Refer the patient to a mental health professional, if appropriate.

7. Provide appropriate referrals to social services staff or other agencies, as needed.

8. Provide pain relief measures, as needed, with nonnarcotic analgesics as ordered, supportive repositioning, and alternative pain control techniques. See the "Pain" plan, page 69, for details.

Rationales

1. The "Ineffective Individual Coping" plan provides interventions helpful in caring for the patient and family experiencing illness-related disorganization.

2. Depression and hopelessness are common emotional responses to the sudden losses caused by Guillain-Barré syndrome. Preparatory teaching may reduce panic as the acute phase progresses. Maintaining hope and providing encouragement throughout the extended course of the illness is an essential part of nursing care, especially because the patient usually remains alert and oriented despite functional deficits. Family participation in care provides tangible support for the patient.

3. Paralysis of the facial nerve (VII), paralysis of the extremities, and intubation alter the patient's ability to communicate. This inability to communicate can be terrifying. Providing the patient with some means of signaling helps reduce anxiety.

4. The patient who cannot do anything physically may still find comfort in psychological self-help. Learning and practicing such techniques helps the patient maintain control and a sense of active participation in recovery. Relaxation techniques have been shown to avoid many stress-related health problems.

5. The debilitating nature of Guillain-Barré syndrome promotes dependency and helplessness. Allowing some choices, even in small matters, increases the patient's sense of self-control and reduces powerlessness.

6. The losses caused by Guillain-Barré syndrome and their long-term effects on the patient's life will cause normal reactions of anger, depression, grieving, and even paranoia. Acceptance of feelings facilitates healthy coping behavior. Manipulative behavior is commonly an attempt to regain a sense of control. Although motor function is impaired, the patient can still hear and understand verbal communication. Mental health referral may be warranted for long-term supportive therapy.

7. The sudden transition from healthy, working adult to hopeless, disabled patient is frightening enough, but the patient may have additional worries about income, child care, or other arrangements. Facilitating early referrals may avoid undue anxiety about such problems.

8. Patients with Guillain-Barré syndrome may experience varying degrees of limb pain or uncomfortable paresthesias. Unrelieved pain decreases coping ability and adds to the patient's physiologic stress. The "Pain" plan contains interventions applicable to any patient in pain.

9. Whenever possible, after the patient is physiologically stable, attempt to create a more normal environment, such as by permitting television, flowers, and personal items from home.

10. Additional individualized interventions: _____

_____

9. Normalization of the patient's environment reinforces improvement and decreases the depersonalizing effects of the hospital setting.

10. Rationales: _____

_____

Target outcome criteria
Within 2 hours of admission, the patient will:
• have an effective communication method
• be pain-free.

Within 24 hours of admission, the patient will:
• participate in making choices about care
• begin expressing feelings
• display reduced anxiety and fear as evidenced by relaxed expression.

Discharge planning
NURSING DISCHARGE CRITERIA
Upon the patient's discharge, documentation shows evidence of:
• spontaneous respiration
• effective airway clearance
• stable vital signs within normal limits for the patient
• ABG measurements within normal limits
• effective communication ability.

PATIENT-FAMILY TEACHING CHECKLIST
Document evidence that the patient and family demonstrate an understanding of:
___ nature and progression of the syndrome; expected prognosis
___ indications of possible exacerbation
___ relaxation and stress-reduction measures
___ activity program and use of assistive devices
___ safety precautions.

DOCUMENTATION CHECKLIST
Using outcome criteria as a guide, document:
___ clinical status on admission
___ significant changes in status
___ pertinent laboratory and diagnostic test findings
___ respiratory support measures
___ nutritional status
___ measures to prevent complications of immobility
___ communication measures
___ relaxation and stress-reduction teaching
___ activity progression
___ patient-family teaching
___ discharge planning.

ASSOCIATED PLANS OF CARE
Impaired Physical Mobility
Ineffective Individual Coping
Knowledge Deficit
Mechanical Ventilation
Nutritional Deficit
Sensory-Perceptual Alteration

References
Alspach, J., ed. *Core Curriculum for Critical Care Nursing,* 4th ed. Philadelphia: W.B. Saunders Co., 1991.
Gulanick, M., et al. *Nursing Care Plans, Nursing Diagnosis and Interventions.* St. Louis: C.V. Mosby Co., 1990.
Hudak, C., et al. *Critical Care Nursing, A Holistic Approach,* 5th ed. Philadelphia: J.B. Lippincott Co., 1990.
Ignatavicius, D., and Bayne, M. *Medical-Surgical Nursing, A Nursing Process Approach.* Philadelphia: W.B. Saunders Co., 1991.
Luckmann, J., and Sorensen, K. *Medical-Surgical Nursing: A Psychophysiologic Approach,* 3rd ed. Philadelphia: W.B. Saunders Co., 1987.
Patrick, M., et al. *Medical-Surgical Nursing: Pathophysiological Concepts,* 2nd ed. Philadelphia: J.B. Lippincott Co., 1991.
Thelan, L., et al. *Textbook of Critical Care Nursing, Diagnosis and Management.* St. Louis: Mosby-Year Book, 1990.

NEUROLOGIC DISORDERS

Increased Intracranial Pressure

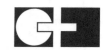

DRG information

Increased intracranial pressure (ICP) is a sign of an underlying problem and not a condition in and of itself in terms of coding guidelines. The DRG assigned for increased ICP depends entirely on the underlying cause that requires hospitalization, such as hemorrhage, hematoma, head trauma, abscess, or radiation. The length of stay depends entirely on the principal diagnosis.

Introduction
DEFINITION AND TIME FOCUS

Increased ICP occurs when the components of the intracranial cavity — brain tissue, cerebral blood, and cerebrospinal fluid (CSF) — exceed the cavity's compensatory capacity. The volume of these three components usually remains relatively constant, with a normal ICP of 0 to 15 mm Hg. Autoregulatory mechanisms in the brain compensate for volume changes of the contents, so an increase in one component is counteracted by a decrease in another.

These mechanisms include displacement of CSF from the cranial cavity to the subarachnoid space surrounding the spinal cord (the primary compensatory mechanism); increased CSF reabsorption; and the reduction of cerebral blood volume by compression of the venous system, displacing venous blood from the intracranial cavity into the systemic circulation. Displacement of brain tissue without concurrent decompensation is extremely limited and occurs primarily with slowly expanding masses, such as tumors or chronic subdural hematomas.

When these autoregulatory mechanisms can no longer compensate for changes in the components of the intracranial cavity, increased ICP results. When ICP is sufficiently elevated to reduce cerebral perfusion pressure, irreversible brain damage may occur. This plan focuses on the critically ill patient with acutely increased ICP.

ETIOLOGY AND PRECIPITATING FACTORS

• increase in brain volume caused by intracranial hemorrhage or hematoma, cerebral edema caused by surgical or head trauma, fast growing tumors, abscess, metabolic coma, radiation, chemotherapeutic agents, infarction, and anoxic events
• increased cerebral blood volume from loss of autoregulation; hyperthermia; vasodilation caused by hypoxemia, hypercapnia, anesthetic agents, or narcotics; venous outflow obstruction caused by compression of the internal jugular veins or intrathoracic or intra-abdominal pressure; fluctuations above a mean arterial pressure (MAP) of 160 mm Hg or below 60 mm Hg

• obstruction of CSF outflow because of hematomas in the posterior fossa; brain shift and herniation; or impaired reabsorption from the subarachnoid space caused by inflammation of the meninges either by subarachnoid hemorrhage or infection, or obstruction of arachnoid villi by blood cells or bacteria

Focused assessment guidelines
NURSING HISTORY (Functional health pattern findings)

Health perception — health management pattern
• exhibits sudden onset of change in the level of consciousness, ranging from flattening of affect to coma; may have loss of consciousness for less than 24 hours
• may have history of head trauma as a result of a motor vehicle accident, fall, assault, gunshot or stab wound, or recreational accident; may be at increased risk if between ages 15 and 24 and male, because of this group's higher incidence of head injury from motor vehicle accidents
• may have history of infection, particularly in the middle ear, mastoid cells, or paranasal sinuses
• may have history of receiving anesthetic agents or narcotics, radiation, or chemotherapeutic agents
• may have history of hypoxia, such as hypoventilation, apnea, chest trauma, pneumonia, or ventilation-perfusion abnormalities

Nutritional-metabolic pattern
• may report vomiting (uncommon); if present, not preceded by nausea

Cognitive-perceptual pattern
• may report a headache (uncommon); if present, worse on arising in the morning; straining or movement may increase the pain.

Self-perception — self-concept pattern
• may have feelings of anxiety or apprehension if the level of consciousness is such that the patient understands something abnormal is happening

PHYSICAL FINDINGS

Note: Many of the classic signs and symptoms of increased ICP now are considered indicators of brain shift and brain stem dysfunction. Clinical signs and symptoms alone are not reliable in determining if ICP is elevated, in detecting early increased ICP, or in determining the severity of increased ICP. Frequent neurologic assessment and ICP monitoring are the most reliable methods for detecting early deterioration.

Neurologic

Early stage of increased ICP:
• decreasing level of consciousness (most sensitive indicator of increased ICP), indicated by such signs as confusion, restlessness, or lethargy
• pupillary abnormalities, with the pupil dilating gradually and becoming slightly ovoid and sluggish, ipsilateral to the cause of increased ICP
• visual deficits, such as decreased visual acuity, blurred vision, diplopia, and changes in extraocular eye movements
• motor weakness (monoparesis or hemiparesis) contralateral to the cause of increased ICP

Later stage of increased ICP:
• coma
• pupillary abnormalities, including dilated and non-reactive (fixed) ipsilateral pupil; with herniation, pupils become bilaterally fixed and dilated
• loss of deep tendon reflexes
• hemiplegia and abnormal posturing (sometimes termed decorticate or decerebrate posturing), which may be unilateral or bilateral; as death approaches, the patient becomes bilaterally flaccid
• Babinski response present
• hyperthermia from hypothalamic injury
• loss of brain stem reflexes, including corneal, oculocephalic (doll's eyes), and oculovestibular reflexes (the oculovestibular reflex is not as readily compromised as the oculocephalic and is a more sensitive indicator of any remaining brain stem function; gag, cough, and swallowing reflexes also are lost)
• papilledema (rarely), more common with chronically increased ICP

Cardiovascular

Later stage of increased ICP:
• Cushing's reflex (rare) — rising systolic blood pressure, widening pulse pressure, and bradycardia; pulse is full and bounding; as death approaches, pulse becomes irregular, rapid, and thready, then stops

Pulmonary

• irregular respirations, commonly in patterns that relate to the level of brain dysfunction; Cheyne-Stokes respirations, central neurogenic hyperventilation, and ataxia are common in later stage of increased ICP; may be difficult to assess with the mechanically ventilated patient

Gastrointestinal

• vomiting (uncommon); if present, not preceded by nausea

DIAGNOSTIC STUDIES

Note: No laboratory test for diagnosing increased ICP exists.
• arterial blood gas measurements — used to monitor the patient's acid-base balance and to detect hypoxemia and hypercapnia, which increase ICP

• complete blood count — may reveal elevated white blood cell count, which may signify the beginning of an infection or abscess
• electrolyte panel — used to monitor the patient's fluid status and potassium and sodium levels. Sodium is retained during stressful events whereas potassium is lost; sodium and potassium levels also are altered in diabetes insipidus (DI) and syndrome of inappropriate antidiuretic hormone secretion (SIADH), two abnormalities that may occur with increased ICP
• serum creatinine, blood urea nitrogen (BUN) levels — used to monitor renal function, particularly if osmotic diuretics are administered
• glucose tolerance test — used to monitor for hyperglycemia if dexamethasone (Decadron) therapy is used
• serum osmolality — used to monitor for hyperosmolality when mannitol therapy is used and aids in establishing diagnosis of DI or SIADH
• urine specific gravity — may indicate DI if low or SIADH if high
• urine glucose and acetone levels — may reveal glucose in the urine, which may be an adverse reaction to dexamethasone therapy
• computed tomography (CT) scan — can differentiate among many conditions that cause increased ICP. Clearly outlines ventricles and assesses size and position in relation to midline structures. CT scan is useful in diagnosing cerebral edema, hematomas caused by intracranial bleeding, abscesses, cerebral infarctions, and tumors. Serial scanning is useful in patients who deteriorate or who do not improve as rapidly as expected. It may show intracranial hematomas in patients whose initial CT scan was negative.
• skull X-rays — useful in detecting linear and depressed skull fractures and may demonstrate intracranial shifts. A high incidence of developing masses and intracranial hemorrhage occurs with linear fractures. Skull X-rays should be considered when the patient has an altered level of consciousness any time after injury, focal neurologic signs, or CSF discharge from the nose or ears.
• cerebral echoencephalography — may be used if a CT scan is not available. It is useful in detecting shifts of normally midline structures, but not reliable in generalized cerebral edema that does not produce a midline shift.
• cerebral angiography — may be used if a CT scan is not available. It will reveal space-occupying lesions, such as subdural hematoma and epidural hematoma, and cerebral edema. Because cerebral angiography is an invasive study, CT scan is preferred.
• magnetic resonance imaging (MRI) — gives clearer images of soft tissues than a CT scan and can detect brain edema, hemorrhage, infarction, and blood vessel disruptions more clearly. At this time, it has limited usefulness for the patient with increased ICP because it cannot be used for patients with metal-containing devices, such as electrocardiogram electrodes, or with mechanical ventilation.

NEUROLOGIC DISORDERS

• ICP monitoring—may reveal values of 15 to 40 mm Hg, indicating moderately elevated ICP, or 40 mm Hg or greater, indicating severely elevated ICP
• electrocardiography (ECG)—useful in assessing changes, such as development of tall T waves in early increased ICP that become progressively flatter or inverted with an ICP greater than 45 mm Hg. ST segment changes occur with transient changes in ICP and return to normal with the return of ICP to previous levels. Low levels of increased ICP produce abnormally shortened QT intervals, whereas prolonged QT intervals occur with ICP greater 65 mm Hg.

POTENTIAL COMPLICATIONS
• brain herniation
• permanent neurologic deficits
• seizures
• pneumonia
• atelectasis
• GI ulceration and hemorrhage
• infection
• DI
• SIADH
• neurogenic pulmonary edema

Collaborative problem: *High risk for cerebral ischemia related to fluctuations in arterial blood pressure, stressful events, nursing activities, hypoxemia, or hypercapnia*

NURSING PRIORITY: Minimize fluctuations in cerebral perfusion pressure.

Interventions

1. Assess the patient's level of consciousness, behavior, motor and sensory function, pupillary reactions (size, position, and reactivity), and respiratory patterns every 1 to 2 hours and as necessary.

2. Monitor ICP (if an ICP monitoring device is in place) and MAP continually and compare readings to a desirable level. Document every hour or as changes occur. Calculate cerebral perfusion pressure (CPP) as changes occur (see Appendix A, "Monitoring Standards").

3. Maintain MAP at a level that will result in a CPP of 60 mm Hg or more.

• If pharmacologic support of blood pressure is needed, administer dopamine hydrochloride (Intropin) or other vasopressors, as ordered.

• If systemic hypertension is present, titrate fluid restriction, vasodilator administration, or other therapies according to CPP, as ordered.

4. Monitor arterial blood gas (ABG) levels as ordered. Maintain ABG levels within prescribed parameters, typically PaO_2 greater than 70 mm Hg and $PaCO_2$ between 25 and 30 mm Hg.

Rationales

1. Changes in any of these parameters may indicate a deterioration in the patient's neurologic condition. The level of consciousness is the most sensitive and reliable indicator of increasing ICP. A change in respiratory patterns, also a sensitive indicator of increased ICP, is an early indicator of hypoxemia or hypercapnia, which also lead to increased ICP.

2. ICP indicates how well the three components of the intracranial cavity are balanced. CPP is the blood pressure gradient across the brain and is calculated as the difference between the incoming MAP and the opposing mean ICP (CPP = MAP − ICP). Alterations in either MAP or intracranial volume affect CPP and the integrity of brain tissue. A CPP of at least 60 mm Hg must be maintained to provide a minimally adequate blood supply to the brain. A CPP of less than 30 mm Hg results in cell death and is fatal.

3. Blood pressure must be maintained to ensure adequate CPP. Between a MAP of 60 to 160 mm Hg, the brain automatically regulates blood vessel diameter to maintain constant cerebral blood flow (CBF) and thus CPP. If the autoregulatory mechanism is lost, CBF and cerebral blood volume are passively dependent on the blood pressure and CPP, so that hypotensive episodes provoke ischemia, whereas hypertensive bursts push fluid into the brain.

• Failure to reverse systemic hypotension results in worsening cerebral ischemia and necrosis.

• Treating hypertension may be difficult because blood pressure already may be elevated as a compensatory mechanism for ischemia. Usually, blood pressure is lowered only after ICP is controlled. CPP is considered the best guide for gauging the effects of therapies to control systemic hypertension in patients with increased ICP.

4. Hypoxemia and hypercapnia are potent vasodilators and increase CBF and ICP. Keeping the patient well-oxygenated and slightly hypocapnic helps limit CBF and therefore helps control ICP.

5. Observe ICP levels with an ICP monitoring device during activities that are known to cause sustained increases in ICP, such as suctioning, moving the patient, emotional upsets, noxious stimuli, arousal from sleep, coughing, sneezing, or Valsalva's maneuver.

5. Clinical symptoms of increased ICP are not always present, even when a substantial increase in pressure occurs. By maintaining an awareness of activities that produce spikes in ICP and by monitoring ICP levels, you can modify or terminate these activities as ICP increases.

6. Instruct the alert patient to avoid the following activities: straining at stool, holding breath while moving or turning in bed, coughing, nose blowing, and extreme hip flexion (90 degrees or more).

6. These activities increase intrathoracic and intra-abdominal pressure, which is transmitted to the jugular veins, impeding cerebral venous return and increasing ICP.

7. Instruct the alert patient to avoid pushing the feet against a footboard or the arms against the bed.

7. These activities produce isometric muscle contractions, which increase muscle tension without lengthening the muscle. These contractions elevate systemic blood pressure and result in increased ICP.

8. Administer pharmacologic agents, as ordered, for shivering and abnormal posturing, typically chlorpromazine hydrochloride (Thorazine) for shivering and pancuronium bromide (Pavulon) for severe abnormal posturing. Document administration and effects.

8. Shivering commonly occurs in response to hypothermia, which may be used to control ICP. Shivering is a form of isometric contraction and thus can increase ICP. Abnormal posturing also produces muscle contractions, which elevate ICP.

9. Structure the environment to reduce unpleasant stimuli:
• avoid unnecessary or unintended emotionally stimulating conversation (for example, about prognosis or condition)
• provide a quiet room
• avoid jarring the patient's bed
• provide soft stimuli, such as a soft voice, soft music, and gentle touch when necessary
• space painful nursing or medical procedures
• when necessary to awaken the patient, use gentle touch and a soft voice
• avoid unnecessary disturbances.

9. Unpleasant or noxious stimuli can increase ICP. They also increase systemic blood pressure, which may increase ICP in the patient with poor or absent autoregulation.

10. Assess the patient's level of comfort and administer ordered medications as needed, documenting administration and effectiveness:
• analgesics when permitted for headache and pain
• antiemetics for nausea and vomiting
• stool softeners for constipation.

10. Pain, nausea, vomiting, and constipation are noxious stimuli that increase ICP. Additionally, vomiting increases intra-abdominal and intrathoracic pressure, impeding venous return from the brain.

11. Use restraints only when absolutely necessary and as ordered.

11. Restraints may cause the patient to struggle. Both the stimulation and the resulting increased activity (producing increased heart rate and increased blood flow to the brain) elevate ICP.

12. Space activities when possible, especially routine care activities, such as baths, mouth care, and bed changes.

12. Closely spaced activities can have a cumulative effect, causing a greater and more prolonged elevation of increased ICP than a single activity.

13. Maintain venous drainage from the brain by proper alignment and positioning: keep the head and neck in a neutral position and the head of the bed elevated 15 to 60 degrees at all times, or as ordered.

13. Because the cerebral venous system has no valves, jugular vein compression causes increased pressure throughout the system, impeding drainage from the brain and increasing ICP. Placing the patient flat or in a Trendelenburg position prevents venous drainage as well; the Trendelenburg position actually increases blood flow to the brain. Elevating the head of the bed improves venous drainage.

14. Implement therapeutic measures, as ordered:

• corticosteroids, usually dexamethasone

14. Interventions help maintain ICP at a level consistent with optimal CPP.
• Although the value of corticosteroids in reducing ICP is controversial, clinicians usually consider them effective in reducing cerebral edema in some clinical problems, such as tumors. Their exact mechanism of action is unknown.

NEUROLOGIC
DISORDERS

• diuretics (see the "High risk for fluid volume excess" nursing diagnosis in this plan)

• CSF drainage, via an intraventricular drain

• barbiturate coma, typically with pentobarbital (Nembutal) or thiopental (Pentothal Sodium), for severe, persistent, refractory increased ICP in adults.

• Diuretics limit cerebral intracellular and extracellular swelling and CSF volume.

• Draining CSF helps control erratic ICP increases and is most helpful when decreased CSF absorption is causing increased ICP.

• Barbiturates induce cerebral vasoconstriction and decrease cerebral metabolism, thus lowering ICP, preserving ischemic cells, and preventing irreversible damage. Because barbiturate coma requires complete life support and extensive nursing supervision, it is used to manage uncontrolled intracranial hypertension unresponsive to conventional treatment.

15. When noninvasive therapeutic interventions do not control ICP, prepare the patient and family for surgical intervention (see the "Craniotomy" plan, page 110).

15. Surgical intervention may be necessary to control the cause, such as intracranial hematoma, or to "buy time" to prevent herniation while slower therapies reduce swelling. The latter is achieved by removing a bone flap to allow brain expansion.

16. Additional individualized interventions: _____

16. Rationales: _____

Target outcome criteria
Within 72 hours of admission, the patient will:
• have an ICP of 0 to 15 mm Hg and a CPP greater than 60 mm Hg
• have an MAP greater than 60 mm Hg
• display no clinical signs of increased ICP and herniation.

Within 1 week of admission, the patient will demonstrate improved neurologic status.

Nursing diagnosis: *High risk for infection related to invasive techniques, immunosuppression, or surgical or other trauma*

NURSING PRIORITIES: (a) Prevent infection and (b) monitor for signs and symptoms of infection.

Interventions

1. Maintain strict sterile or aseptic technique as appropriate for catheterizations, endotracheal tube care, and closed intracranial drainage system care.

2. Change dressings as ordered, using sterile technique. Change the dressing at the intracranial monitoring device site every 24 to 48 hours, or as ordered. Apply gentamicin (Garamycin) or other ointment around the insertion site only if ordered.

3. Maintain ICP monitoring devices as closed systems. Do not flush the system routinely. Instill antibiotic solutions (such as bacitracin or gentamicin) via the ICP monitoring line every 24 to 48 hours, followed by normal saline solution, only if ordered.

Rationales

1. Sepsis is the primary concern with any invasive equipment or procedure. Using the appropriate technique will help prevent infection.

2. Preventing infection and sepsis is of primary importance, particularly at sites with direct access to the brain. Cerebral infection increases the cerebral metabolic rate and CBF, thus increasing ICP. Practices regarding use of antibiotic ointment around the insertion site vary.

3. Maintaining a closed system may be critical in preventing infections in the CSF. Flushing an ICP monitoring line is not a routine procedure and is not considered a safe practice by many clinicians, so do it only on specific orders. Prophylactic instillation of antibiotics may be effective in helping control infection but is highly controversial.

4. Assess periodically for signs and symptoms of infection:
• redness, tenderness, or warmth around all insertion sites or wounds (check daily)
• cloudy or foul-smelling drainage (check daily)
• fever (check every 4 hours)
• elevated white blood cell (WBC) count (monitor as ordered)
• positive urine, sputum, blood, or wound cultures (monitor as ordered)
• infiltrates on chest X-ray (monitor as ordered).

4. Early detection of infection allows for prompt and appropriate intervention. An elevated WBC count may confirm an infection; however, the value may be elevated if the patient is on steroids.

5. Administer antibiotics, as ordered, typically if the patient has an ICP monitoring device or ventricular drainage system, or if signs and symptoms of infection are present. Document administration and monitor for effectiveness and adverse reactions.

5. Broad-spectrum antibiotics may be ordered prophylactically for direct access to the brain. Once infection has been documented, selecting appropriate antibiotics is guided by culture results.

6. Additional individualized interventions: _____

6. Rationales: _____

Target outcome criteria
Within 48 to 72 hours of admission, the patient will:
• have a normal body temperature
• have a WBC count within normal limits.

By the time of discharge, the patient will display no indicators of infection.

Collaborative problem: *High risk for increased cerebral metabolism related to temperature elevations caused by infection and hypothalamic injury*

NURSING PRIORITY: Maintain normal body temperature.

Interventions

1. Monitor and document temperature every 4 hours and as needed.

2. Administer antipyretics, as ordered, typically acetaminophen (Tylenol). Administer tepid sponge baths, as ordered.

3. Apply a cooling (hypothermia) blanket, as ordered, for an elevated temperature that does not respond to more conservative measures.

Rationales

1. In the later stages of increased ICP, pressure on the hypothalamus may cause hypothalamic injury, disrupt normal thermoregulatory mechanisms, and cause extremely elevated temperatures. Because an elevated temperature increases systemic and cerebral blood flow and contributes to increased ICP, it should be controlled as soon as possible.

2. With infection, the temperature will rise because interleukin 1 (IL-1) may act as a pyrogen. Both IL-1 and the fever it triggers activate the body's defense mechanisms. These measures along with antibiotic administration (discussed above) may be sufficient to control an elevated temperature caused by infection.

3. Temperature elevation from hypothalamic injury and loss of autoregulatory control usually requires more aggressive intervention to return the temperature to normal levels.

NEUROLOGIC DISORDERS

4. Maintain appropriate precautions when using the hypothermia blanket:

• Cover the hypothermia blanket with a sheet or bath blanket.

• Check the rectal temperature every 30 minutes (or use a rectal probe).

• Turn the blanket off when the rectal temperature slightly exceeds desired temperature, according to unit protocol.

• Control shivering by administering medication, as ordered, usually chlorpromazine hydrochloride (Thorazine).

5. Remove excess bed clothes, and allow for adequate ventilation in the patient's room.

6. Additional individualized interventions: _____

_____

4. Hypothermia has numerous physiologic effects that may result in injury.

• Direct contact between the patient's skin and the hypothermia blanket can cause skin damage similar to frostbite.

• The degree of hypothermia must be controlled carefully to prevent adverse reactions. A rectal thermometer or probe accurately measures body temperature.

• The patient's temperature will continue to drop and will return to normal gradually because the solution inside the blanket remains cold.

• As mentioned earlier, shivering is a form of isometric contraction that results in increased ICP.

5. Inadequate ventilation and excess bed clothes maintain body temperature and increase the time needed to reduce the patient's temperature to normal.

6. Rationales: _____

_____

Target outcome criterion
By the time of discharge, the patient will maintain a temperature within normal limits without the aid of a hypothermia blanket.

Collaborative problem: *High risk for respiratory failure related to increased ICP, cerebral dysfunction, obstructed airway, absence of spontaneous respirations and gag or cough reflex, aspiration, atelectasis, ventilation-perfusion abnormalities, altered level of consciousness, or neurogenic pulmonary edema*

NURSING PRIORITY: Maintain effective gas exchange.

Interventions

1. Assess and document the respiratory rate, depth, and pattern every 15 to 60 minutes. Notify the doctor of a rate less than 14 or greater than 24 breaths/minute, shallow respirations, or changes in the respiratory pattern. Assist with intubation if the patient cannot maintain adequate airway, respiratory depth, or respiratory pattern.

2. Auscultate breath sounds every 2 hours and as needed to determine adequacy of aeration and presence of adventitious sounds. Observe for restlessness and tachycardia. Assess for cyanosis around the mouth, in nail beds, and in earlobes.

3. Assess the color, amount, and consistency of respiratory secretions. Culture as needed.

4. Monitor ABG levels, as ordered. Keep ABG levels within prescribed parameters, as described under the "High risk for cerebral ischemia" diagnosis above. Obtain chest X-rays, as ordered. Correlate the findings with clinical observations.

Rationales

1. Respiratory status is the result of a complex interplay of factors including airway patency and medullary and pontine control mechanisms. The respiratory rate is a sensitive indicator of airway patency and increasing ICP, whereas respiratory patterns may correlate with the level of brainstem dysfunction. If the patient cannot maintain adequate gas exchange, intubation and mechanical ventilation may be necessary to avert cardiopulmonary arrest.

2. Normal breath sounds indicate proper lung expansion. Adventitious sounds may require therapeutic intervention. Restlessness and tachycardia are key findings in early hypoxemia. Cyanosis indicates inadequate gas exchange, although it is a late finding.

3. Secretions may indicate infection or the need for hydration to facilitate clearance.

4. Objective documentation of pulmonary status is a valuable adjunct to clinical observations.

5. Position the patient with the head of the bed elevated to the prescribed height and the patient's waist at the break in the bed.

5. Proper positioning allows for complete lung expansion.

6. Turn the patient every 2 hours, if ICP levels allow.

6. Dependent lung lobes are not fully expanded, thus compromising gas exchange. Turning allows for full expansion of all lobes and aids in preventing atelectasis and pneumonia, which interfere with gas exchange. However, turning may increase ICP levels, as described above, so its benefits must be weighed against its risks.

7. Suction as needed, hyperventilating with 100% oxygen before and after suctioning and limiting suctioning to no more than 15 seconds. Administer lidocaine (Xylocaine) via endotracheal tube or intravenously, as ordered. Monitor for seizures, depressed respirations, or cardiac arrhythmias. If given I.V., administer 2 minutes before suctioning; endotracheally, administer 5 minutes before suctioning.

7. Suctioning-induced hypoxemia contributes to increased ICP and compromised CPP. Suctioning can raise ICP to levels as high as 100 mm Hg. Used topically, lidocaine limits elevation of ICP in response to suctioning. When given as an I.V. bolus, lidocaine can sustain this effect over time. Lidocaine overdoses may cause seizures, respiratory arrest, or cardiac arrest.

8. Implement care related to mechanical ventilation, if used. See the "Mechanical Ventilation" plan, page 227.

8. Carbon dioxide and oxygen levels are more precisely controlled when the patient is intubated and ventilated mechanically. The "Mechanical Ventilation" plan contains detailed information about this intervention.

9. Additional individualized interventions: _____

_____

9. Rationales: _____

_____

Target outcome criteria
Within 24 hours of admission, the patient will:
• have an airway free from secretions
• have ABG levels within desired limits.

By the time of discharge, the patient will:
• have a normal respiratory rate and pattern
• have normal ABG levels
• have a clear chest X-ray.

Nursing diagnosis: *High risk for fluid volume deficit related to diuretic therapy, fluid restriction, diabetes insipidus, hyperthermia, or GI suction*

NURSING PRIORITY: Maintain fluid volume within prescribed limits.

Interventions

1. See Appendix C, "Fluid and Electrolyte Imbalances."

Rationales

1. The "Fluid and Electrolyte Imbalances" appendix contains general information; this plan focuses on fluid and electrolyte problems specific to increased ICP.

2. Monitor and correlate fluid intake and output, both hourly and cumulatively. Measure and document urine specific gravity. Report the following:

2. Diuretic therapy, hyperthermia, restricted fluid intake, and DI may produce an overwhelming fluid deficit. Hourly and cumulative correlation of values aids in prompt deficit detection.

• urine output greater than 200 ml/hour for 2 hours, with specific gravity 1.001 to 1.005

• Urine output greater than 200 ml/hour usually indicates DI. In patients with increased ICP, DI results from failure of the pituitary gland to secrete antidiuretic hormone (ADH) because of damage to the hypothalamus, the supraopticohypophyseal tract, or the posterior lobe of the pituitary gland. Such damage occurs most commonly after neurosurgery, but it can also occur secondary to vascular lesions or severe head injury. Because ADH is absent, the renal tubules fail to conserve water, resulting in the excretion of large volumes of dilute urine. The low specific gravity reflects the dilute urine. Urine output of this magnitude can rapidly create a fluid volume deficit.

• urine output less than 30 ml/hour for 2 hours, with specific gravity greater than 1.030.

• A urine output less than 30 ml/hour for 2 hours with a high specific gravity indicates that a fluid volume deficit already exists.

3. Monitor laboratory values, as ordered. Report the following:
• urine osmolality, usually less than 200 mOsm/kg
• serum osmolality, usually greater than 300 mOsm/kg
• serum sodium, usually greater than 145 mEq/liter
• hematocrit and BUN, usually elevated.

3. Laboratory values provide objective evidence of an imbalance. The low urine osmolality reflects diuresis, whereas the elevated serum osmolality, serum sodium, and hematocrit reflect hemoconcentration.

4. Monitor the ECG and hemodynamic pressures continually. Report promptly:
• the appearance of U waves, prolonged QT interval, depressed ST segment, and low T waves

• arrhythmias, particularly bradycardia, first and second degree heart block, atrial arrhythmias, and premature ventricular contractions (PVCs)
• low hemodynamic pressures and cardiac output.

4. Continual monitoring provides prompt warning of potentially fatal conditions.
• ECG signs reflect cardiac cells' decreased responsiveness to stimuli, which results from hypokalemia secondary to renal potassium washout.
• Bradycardia, heart blocks, atrial arrhythmias, and PVCs reflect hypokalemia. Prompt treatment is necessary to prevent hypokalemic arrest.
• Low pressures reflect hypovolemia, whereas decreased cardiac output indicates insufficient preload.

5. Administer replacement therapy, as ordered, usually isotonic solution with potassium chloride (KCl) added if serum potassium is low. Monitor the I.V. flow rate closely. Anticipate increased fluid requirements if hyperthermia or infection is present.

5. Isotonic solution is the replacement fluid of choice for lost body fluids. Close monitoring is essential to prevent fluid volume overload. Solutions with potassium should be carefully monitored because potassium is very irritating to the vein and rapid potassium infusion can cause hyperkalemia, possibly leading to complete heart block, ventricular fibrillation, or ventricular standstill. Hyperthermia and infection accelerate fluid loss by increasing metabolic rate and increasing skin and respiratory fluid excretion.

6. Additional individualized interventions: _____

6. Rationales: _____

Target outcome criteria
By the time of discharge, the patient will:
• maintain a urine output within normal limits
• have electrolytes, hematocrit, BUN, and serum osmolality within normal limits

• maintain hemodynamic values within normal limits.

Nursing diagnosis: *High risk for fluid volume excess related to stress, steroid therapy, or syndrome of inappropriate antidiuretic hormone secretion*

NURSING PRIORITY: Maintain fluid volume within prescribed limits.

Interventions

1. See Appendix C, "Fluid and Electrolyte Imbalances."

Rationales

1. The "Fluid and Electrolyte Imbalances" appendix contains general information on fluid and electrolyte problems. This plan focuses on problems specific to increased ICP.

2. Monitor and correlate fluid intake and output hourly. Report a urine output less than 30 ml/hour for 2 hours with a specific gravity greater than 1.030. Insert an indwelling urinary catheter, if necessary and as ordered.

2. Carefully monitoring fluid intake and urine output helps detect potential problems that increase ICP. Decreased urine output may reflect a fluid volume deficit (see the previous diagnosis) or SIADH, whereas high specific gravity reflects increased water reabsorption. SIADH is characterized by abnormally high levels or continuous secretion of ADH, resulting in water being continually reabsorbed from the renal tubules. Increased ADH secretion is caused by several factors related to increased ICP, including hyperthermia, hypotension, trauma, stress response, and administration of drugs, such as chlorpromazine, barbiturates, and acetaminophen. Sodium and water retention also are caused by corticosteroids and the physiologic response to stress. Awareness of water retention may prevent further complications, such as pulmonary edema.

3. Monitor serum electrolyte level, BUN level, creatinine level, osmolality, and hematocrit daily or as ordered. Report the following:
• urine osmolality (usually high)
• serum osmolality (usually less than 280 mOsm/kg)
• serum sodium (usually less than 126 mEq/liter)
• hematocrit and BUN level (usually low).

3. High urine osmolality reflects water retention. Low serum osmolality, sodium level, hematocrit, and BUN level reflect hemodilution.

4. Monitor the ECG and hemodynamic pressures continually. Report promptly:
• the appearance of U waves, prolonged QT interval, depressed ST segment, or low T waves
• arrhythmias, particularly bradycardia, first- and second-degree heart block, atrial arrhythmias, and PVCs
• elevated hemodynamic pressures and decreased cardiac output.

4. Constant monitoring provides early warning of impending problems.
• These ECG findings reflect dilutional hypokalemia.

• The rhythms listed are commonly caused by hypokalemia.

• Hemodynamic pressures indicate fluid overload, whereas decreased cardiac output results from the heart's inability to handle the excessive preload.

5. Institute therapy, as ordered.
• fluid restriction

• diuretics, generally mannitol and furosemide (Lasix).

5. An increase in cerebral blood volume increases ICP.
• Fluid restriction aids in decreasing extracellular fluid. Patients with increased ICP usually are maintained in a slightly dehydrated state.
• Mannitol is an osmotic diuretic that moves water from the brain and CSF into plasma by an osmotic gradient, thus decreasing ICP. Furosemide, a loop diuretic, inhibits distal tubular reabsorption, promoting diuresis. Additionally, furosemide appears to selectively dehydrate injured cerebral tissue, thus reducing cerebral edema and ICP.

6. Additional individualized interventions: _____

6. Rationales: _____

Target outcome criteria
By the time of discharge, the patient will:
• display electrolyte levels, BUN level, hematocrit, and serum osmolality within normal limits
• have a urine output within normal limits

• manifest hemodynamic values within normal limits.

NEUROLOGIC DISORDERS

Nursing diagnosis: *High risk for injury related to decreased level of consciousness, seizures, and drug therapy*

NURSING PRIORITY: Maintain patient safety.

Interventions

1. Observe the patient closely at all times. Keep side rails up at all times, except for periods of direct nursing care.

2. Assess for seizures. Implement seizure precautions, such as padded side rails. Administer and document antiseizure medication, as ordered, typically phenytoin (Dilantin) or phenobarbital.

3. Assess for gastric bleeding. Administer medications as ordered, usually antacids such as aluminum and magnesium hydroxide (Maalox), cimetidine (Tagamet), or ranitidine (Zantac).

4. Assess for an absent corneal reflex and apply artificial tears and eye patches, as needed.

5. Additional individualized interventions: _____

Rationales

1. Decreased level of consciousness is one of the earliest indications of increased ICP. The patient may not be alert and aware of surroundings and possible danger.

2. Seizures may be caused by the altered neuronal function associated with increased ICP. If the patient does have a seizure, padded side rails lessen the potential for such physical injuries as cuts, abrasions, and fractures.

3. Gastric irritation and GI bleeding are major adverse reactions to corticosteroid therapy. Also, gastric bleeding occurs with increased ICP, although the exact mechanism is unknown. Increased ICP hypothetically stimulates the vagal nuclei directly, resulting in hypersecretion of gastric acid and hyperacidity. Patients with increased ICP are usually placed on prophylactic antacid and histamine$_2$-blocker therapy to decrease the risk of bleeding.

4. During the later stages of increased ICP, brain-stem dysfunction results in the loss of the corneal reflex. Artificial tears lubricate the eyes, whereas both the tears and patches prevent injury to the cornea.

5. Rationales: _____

Target outcome criterion
Throughout the hospital stay, the patient will remain free from injury.

Discharge planning
NURSING DISCHARGE CRITERIA
Upon the patient's discharge, documentation shows evidence of:
• stable ICP within normal limits
• stable vital signs
• absence of cardiopulmonary complications
• absence of gastrointestinal bleeding
• normal fluid and electrolyte balance
• ABG levels within normal limits
• stable temperature
• stable neurologic function
• removal of ICP monitoring line.

PATIENT-FAMILY TEACHING CHECKLIST
Document evidence that the patient and family demonstrate an understanding of:
__ causes of increased ICP
__ extent of neurologic deficits, if present
__ need for continued family support
__ requirements for rehabilitation program, if known.

DOCUMENTATION CHECKLIST
Using outcome criteria as a guide, document:
__ clinical status on admission
__ significant changes in status
__ pertinent laboratory and diagnostic test findings
__ fluid intake and output
__ neurologic status
__ neurologic deficits, if present
__ GI bleeding, if any
__ seizures, if any.

ASSOCIATED PLANS OF CARE
Impaired Physical Mobility
Ineffective Individual Coping
Knowledge Deficit
Nutritional Deficit
Pain
Sensory-Perceptual Alteration

References

Bates, B. *A Guide to Physical Examination and History Taking,* 5th ed. Philadelphia: J.B. Lippincott Co., 1991.

Dossey, B.M., et al. *Essentials of Critical Care Nursing: Body, Mind, Spirit.* Philadelphia: J.B. Lippincott Co., 1990.

Drummond, B.L. "Preventing Increased Intracranial Pressure: Nursing Care Can Make the Difference," *Focus on Critical Care*17(2):116-22, April 1990.

Gordon, M. *Nursing Diagnosis, Process and Application,* 2nd ed. New York: McGraw-Hill Book Co., 1987.

Hickey, J.V. *The Clinical Practice of Neurological and Neurosurgical Nursing,* 3rd ed. Philadelphia: J.B. Lippincott Co., 1992.

Hudak, C.M., et al. *Critical Care Nursing, A Holistic Approach,* 5th ed. Philadelphia: J.B. Lippincott Co., 1990.

Ignatavicius, D.D., and Bayne, M.V. *Medical-Surgical Nursing, A Nursing Process Approach.* Philadelphia: W.B. Saunders Co., 1991.

Jess, L.W. "Assessing Your Patient for Increased ICP," *Nursing87* 17(6):34-41, June 1987.

Kee, J.L. *Laboratory and Diagnostic Tests with Nursing Implications,* 3rd ed. East Norwalk, Conn.: Appleton & Lange, 1990.

Kinney, M.R., et al. *AACN'S Clinical Reference for Critical-Care Nursing,* 2nd ed. New York: McGraw-Hill Book Co., 1988.

Lehne, R.A., et al. *Pharmacology for Nursing Care.* Philadelphia: W.B. Saunders Co., 1990.

Lewis, S.M., and Collier, I.C. *Medical-Surgical Nursing Assessment and Management of Clinical Problems,* 2nd ed. New York: McGraw-Hill Book Co., 1987.

Nikas, D.L. "Critical Aspects of Head Trauma," *Critical Care Nursing Quarterly* 10(1):19-44, June 1987.

Pollack-Latham, C.L. "Intracranial Pressure Monitoring: Part I. Physiologic Principles." *Critical Care Nurse* 7(5):40-1, 44-48, 50-52, September-October 1987.

Thelan, L.A., et al. *Textbook of Critical Care Nursing, Diagnosis and Management.* St. Louis: Mosby-Year Book, 1990.

Walleck, C.A. "Intracranial Hypertension: Interventions and Outcomes," *Critical Care Nursing Quarterly* 10(1):45-57, June 1987.

Laminectomy

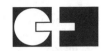

DRG information

DRG 004 Spinal Procedures. (This DRG would be applicable if the laminectomy is performed to excise a lesion of the spinal cord or meninges.)
Mean LOS = 10.8 days

DRG 214 Back and Neck Procedures. With Complication or Comorbidity (CC)
Mean LOS = 10.0 days

DRG 215 Back and Neck Procedures. Without CC.
Mean LOS = 6.6 days

Introduction
DEFINITION AND TIME FOCUS

Laminectomy is a major spinal surgery in which one or more vertebral laminae are removed to expose the spinal cord and nearby structures. Most commonly, it is performed to facilitate removal of part or all of a disk (nucleus pulposus) that has herniated and is pressing on a spinal nerve root. Almost all herniated disks occur in the lumbar spine, 90% to 95% occurring at the level of L4 or L5 to S1.

A laminectomy also may be performed for spinal cord compression from a fracture, dislocation, hematoma, or abscess; spinal nerve surgery; or removal of a spinal cord tumor or vascular malformation. Less often, it may be performed to treat intractable pain by sectioning posterior nerve roots or interrupting spinothalamic tracts.

Lumbar laminectomy is more common than cervical laminectomy. A posterior surgical approach is used most commonly for lumbar laminectomy, an anterior approach for cervical laminectomy.

If the spine is unstable, a spinal fusion may be done at the same time, typically using iliac crest bone fragments. Recovery takes longer with fusion because the bone graft heals slowly.

This plan focuses on the patient undergoing lumbar laminectomy for lumbar disk herniation that has not responded to conservative medical management. Spinal fusion is not discussed.

ETIOLOGY AND PRECIPITATING FACTORS

For herniated disk:
• disk degeneration
• trauma—for example, accidents, strain, or repeated minor stresses
• poor body mechanics (causing low back strain)
• congenital predisposition

Focused assessment guidelines
NURSING HISTORY (Functional health pattern findings)

Health perception—health management pattern
• typically reports pain in the lumbosacral area accompanied by varying degrees of sensory and motor deficit
• may report dull pain in the buttocks followed by unilateral or bilateral leg pain that may extend to the foot, depending on the level of disk herniation
• may report numbness and tingling in the toes and feet
• may report pain usually increased with activities that cause increased intraspinal pressure (such as sitting, sneezing, coughing, straining, and lifting)
• may have natural deformity of the lumbar spine
• may be obese
• may have a history of chronic low back pain
• may have a history of employment involving straining, lifting, or twisting
• if between ages of 20 and 45 and male, at increased risk

Nutritional-metabolic pattern
• may have a dietary history consistent with obesity (high-calorie, high-fat intake)

Activity-exercise pattern
• may report altered mobility because of asymmetrical gait
• may report lack of physical activity because of pain

Sleep-rest pattern
• may report sleep disturbances related to chronic low back pain, aggravated by sleeping on the stomach

Role-relationship pattern
• may report greatest concern about ability to return to work, especially if work involves lifting

PHYSICAL FINDINGS
General appearance
• anxious or pained facial expression

Cardiovascular
• radiating pain elicited by compression of the jugular veins with the patient in a standing position (Naffziger's test) indicates lumbar disk disease

Gastrointestinal
• constipation (related to inactivity or pressure on spinal nerve roots)

Genitourinary
• urine retention (related to pressure on spinal nerve roots)

Neurologic
• increased pain in affected leg with straight-leg raising (positive Lasègue's sign)
• sensory and motor deficit in affected leg and foot
• pain with extension of knee when both hip and knee are at 90-degree flexion (positive Kernig's sign)
• pain with deep palpation over the affected area
• decreased or absent Achilles and patellar reflexes
• deformity of lumbar spine

Musculoskeletal
• muscle spasms
• muscle weakness or atrophy in the affected leg and foot
• asymmetrical gait
• decreased ability to bend forward
• restricted lateral movement
• leaning away from affected side during standing or ambulation
• absence of normal lumbar lordosis and presence of lumbar scoliosis with reflex muscle spasms
• tense posture

DIAGNOSTIC STUDIES
• cerebrospinal fluid (CSF) — protein may be elevated 70 to 100 mg/dl
• hemoglobin and hematocrit — measurement obtained as a prerequisite for surgery and as a baseline for comparison with postoperative values to detect bleeding
• computed tomography scan — may show disk protrusion or prolapse
• spine X-ray — may show narrowed vertebral interspaces at the level of disk degeneration, with flattening of the lumbar curve
• magnetic resonance imaging (MRI) — may reveal disk pressure on the spinal cord or nerve root
• myelogram — may confirm a herniated disk and indicate the precise level of herniation
• electromyogram — may indicate neural and muscle damage as well as the level and site of injury

POTENTIAL COMPLICATIONS
• unrelieved acute pain
• muscle weakness and atrophy
• paralysis
• altered bowel or bladder function

Nursing diagnosis: *Preoperative knowledge deficit related to impending surgery*

NURSING PRIORITY: Prepare the patient to cope with the surgical experience.

Interventions

1. Provide specific preoperative teaching for the patient who will have a lumbar laminectomy. Also provide general preoperative teaching (see the "Surgical Intervention" plan, page 81, for details).

Rationales

1. The patient having a laminectomy usually has undergone a long period, or intermittent periods, of conservative treatment. The surgery is preceded by chronic pain, a decrease in physical activity, and possible absence from work. The patient may view the surgery with relief but also with anxiety about the results. Information about the specific procedure will help to allay anxieties about having spinal surgery.

NEUROLOGIC DISORDERS

2. Provide information about the postoperative routine:
• frequent taking of vital signs and neurovascular observations of the extremities
• turning by logrolling during the first 48 hours
• positioning with pillows to maintain proper body alignment
• coughing and deep breathing with the back firmly against the mattress or with a pillow held against the chest for splinting purposes
• using a urinal or bedpan while flat in bed
• wearing antiembolism stockings and doing ankle and foot exercises
• beginning progressive activity 24 to 48 hours after surgery, depending on the doctor's preference
• avoiding flexing, hyperextending, turning, or twisting the lumbar spine
• using the correct method for moving from the lying to the standing position (for example, maintaining spinal alignment and using arm and leg muscles to change position)
• exercising as ordered to strengthen arm, leg, and abdominal muscles
• using a trapeze as ordered by the doctor.

2. The patient's understanding of the postoperative routine helps avoid complications, such as increased pressure on the operative site or twisting of the spinal column. Perfect alignment of the body should be maintained in all positions to prevent trauma to the surgical site and to decrease discomfort. Other potential complications, such as pneumonia or atelectasis and thromboembolism, also may be prevented by proper postoperative care.

3. Provide instruction about sources of postoperative pain. Explain that preoperative numbness or pain in the affected leg will remain for some time after the surgery because of nerve irritation and edema. Also explain that muscle spasms may occur.

3. This knowledge helps allay the patient's anxiety or fear that the surgery has not been successful when numbness or tingling is experienced or when weakness makes moving the extremities difficult.
    Muscle spasms that typically occur on the third or fourth postoperative day are accompanied by severe pain.

4. Provide information about comfort measures:

• open communication with the staff about the patient's pain (characteristics and tolerance) and anxiety

• availability of analgesics

• avoidance of injections in painful areas

• positioning

4. The patient should know that measures are available to promote postoperative comfort.
• Pain tolerance is individual. Anxiety regarding injury from movement potentiates postoperative discomfort.
• Medicating as needed and encouraging the patient to request medication before the pain becomes severe help maintain comfort.
• Intramuscular injections should be given in the unaffected buttock or in the deltoid muscle if both buttocks are affected.
• Proper body alignment increases patient comfort.

5. Additional individualized interventions: _____

5. Rationales: _____

Target outcome criteria
By the day of surgery, the patient will:
• verbalize understanding of preoperative instruction
• list five measures to prevent postoperative complications.

Collaborative problem: *High risk for sensory and motor deficits related to the surgical procedure, edema, or hematoma at the operative site*

NURSING PRIORITY: Prevent or minimize neurovascular impairment.

Interventions

1. Document the lower extremities' neurovascular status every 2 hours or as needed for 24 to 48 hours: skin color and temperature, sensation and motion, edema, peripheral pulses, capillary refill, ability to flex and extend the foot and toes, muscle strength, numbness or tingling in the extremities, and tone and strength in the quadriceps.

2. Assess pain in the lower extremities. Determine exact location and whether the pain is diminishing or worsening.

3. If signs and symptoms of neurovascular damage occur, notify the doctor immediately.

4. Implement measures to prevent neurovascular damage in the lower extremities:
• Maintain proper body alignment by logrolling (every 2 hours for the first 24 to 48 hours) and positioning with pillows.
• Use a firm mattress and a bedboard.

5. Maintain patency of the wound drainage system if present.

6. Administer corticosteroids, if ordered, and document their use.

7. Implement measures to minimize neurovascular damage if initial signs and symptoms of impairment occur.
• Assess for and correct improper body alignment.
• If footdrop is present, initiate passive range-of-motion exercises every 1 to 2 hours.
• Stabilize the foot with ancillary equipment, such as a footboard, sandbags, pillows, foam boots, or foot positioners.

8. Prepare the patient for surgical intervention if evacuation of a hematoma at the surgical site is indicated. See the "Surgical Intervention" plan, page 81.

9. Additional individualized interventions: _____

_____

Rationales

1. Postoperative deficits may result from pressure on the spinal cord or spinal nerve roots caused by surgical trauma or hematoma. Early detection of altered function facilitates prompt intervention.

2. Although preoperative numbness and pain in the lower back and affected leg will remain for some time after surgery, pain may increase from edema secondary to nerve compression. Early detection of nerve compression facilitates prompt intervention.

3. Prompt intervention may help minimize neurovascular damage.

4. These measures will assist in reducing stress and pressure on the surgical site until healing has taken place.

5. Maintaining drainage decreases pressure on the surgical site. Hematoma development may precipitate serious neurovascular complications.

6. Corticosteroids decrease inflammation in the surgical area.

7. These measures help prevent further damage from uneven or excessive pressure on the operative site. Permanent disability may be prevented by careful attention to the occurrence and prompt treatment of motor and sensory deficits.

8. Prompt evacuation of a hematoma may minimize damage. Adequate preparation of the patient for surgical intervention helps allay anxieties. The "Surgical Intervention" plan provides further details.

9. Rationales: _____

_____

Target outcome criteria
Within 48 hours after surgery, the patient will:
• have normal circulatory, motor, and sensory function in the lower extremities (same as before hospitalization or improved)
• have no signs and symptoms of hematoma

• maintain correct body alignment.

Collaborative problem: *High risk for cerebrospinal fistula associated with incomplete closure of the dura at the surgical site*

NURSING PRIORITY: Detect any CSF leakage promptly.

Interventions

1. Observe the patient carefully every 2 to 4 hours for CSF drainage on the dressing: a clear halo or a watery pink ring around bloody or serosanguineous drainage.

2. Test the dressing with a reagent strip to determine if glucose is present.

3. Determine if the patient has a headache.

4. Document any CSF drainage, and notify the doctor immediately if it occurs.

5. Implement measures to reduce stress on the surgical site. See the "Pain" nursing diagnosis in this section.

6. Change the dressing when damp, using strict aseptic technique. Assess for infection at the incision site.

7. Administer antibiotics, as ordered, and document their use.

8. Monitor temperature every 4 hours for 48 to 72 hours after surgery. Monitor the white blood cell (WBC) count daily, as ordered.

9. Assess for signs and symptoms of meningitis: headache, fever, chills, nuchal rigidity, photophobia, and positive Kernig's and Brudzinski's signs.

10. If a fistula occurs and does not heal spontaneously, prepare the patient for surgical closure. See the "Surgical Intervention" plan, page 81.

11. Additional individualized interventions: _____

Rationales

1. An abnormal opening between the subarachnoid space and the incision causes CSF to drain. Drainage on the dressing is a major sign of a fistula, usually a late postoperative complication occurring about a week after surgery. Early detection of CSF leakage facilitates prompt intervention and treatment.

2. Glucose is a CSF component whose presence indicates a fistula. Glucose is not normally present in serous wound drainage.

3. Headache is a common symptom associated with CSF loss.

4. Untreated CSF leakage may be fatal.

5. Decreasing stress on the surgical site promotes healing of the dura, which is incised during the surgical procedure. The "Pain" diagnosis contains specific details about stress reduction measures.

6. Microorganisms can ascend through the fistula, multiply in the CSF, and infect the central nervous system. Changing a damp dressing immediately, using aseptic technique, helps prevent infection at the site and reduces the risk of meningitis.

7. Antibiotics combat specific causative microorganisms.

8. The temperature may be elevated to 102° F (38.9° C) for the first few postoperative days because of the body's normal response to tissue injury and inflammation. Temperature elevation from infection would normally be accompanied by an increased WBC count.

9. Meningitis is a common complication resulting from contamination of CSF. Undetected, it may be fatal within a short time.

10. Adequate preparation before surgical closure of the dura helps allay patient anxiety.

11. Rationales: _____

Target outcome criteria
Throughout the postoperative period, the patient will have:
• no CSF drainage from a lower back incision
• no signs or symptoms of meningitis.

Nursing diagnosis: *Pain related to immobility, muscle spasm, and paresthesias secondary to surgical trauma and postoperative edema*

NURSING PRIORITY: Relieve discomfort or pain.

Interventions

1. Assess the patient for discomfort or pain—specifically, muscle spasm and pain in the lower back and hips, and pain, numbness, or tingling in the affected leg or legs—every 2 to 4 hours.

2. Assess for associated signs and symptoms: rubbing the lower back and hips, guarding the affected extremity, and showing reluctance to move.

3. Administer muscle relaxants or anti-inflammatory agents, as ordered, and document their effects.

4. Administer analgesics judiciously, as ordered, and document their use. Assess for pain relief 30 minutes after medication is administered, and document findings.

5. Implement measures to reduce discomfort:
• positioning the patient to maintain body alignment with the spine straight
• using a firm mattress or a bedboard under the mattress
• avoiding the prone position
• logrolling for the first 48 hours after surgery to avoid twisting, flexing, or hyperextending the spine
• elevating the head of the bed with the patient's knees slightly flexed or positioned as ordered
• turning the patient every 2 hours
• using a bed cradle over areas of paresthesia
• placing personal items within the patient's reach
• teaching the patient to avoid coughing, sneezing, or straining at stool.

6. Maintain the patient on bed rest for 24 to 48 hours or as ordered.

7. Use a trapeze bar if prescribed.

8. When increased activity is ordered, instruct the patient about getting out of bed using arm and abdominal muscles; limiting initial activity to sitting in a straight-backed chair for short intervals or ambulation; and avoiding slumping or limping.

9. Consult with the doctor for antitussives, decongestants, laxatives, or stool softeners, as needed.

10. Additional individualized interventions: _____

Rationales

1. Preoperative numbness and pain in the lower back and affected leg will remain for some time after surgery. (Some patients experience pain and muscle spasm throughout the hospital stay). Postoperative pain and muscle spasm are usually caused by nerve root and muscle irritation from edema and surgical trauma. Muscle spasms tend to occur on the third or fourth postoperative day.

2. The patient may not report pain, but nonverbal indicators may reveal its presence. Some patients are reluctant to request pain medication.

3. These drugs decrease pain and discomfort. Muscle relaxants (such as diazepam [Valium] or methocarbamol [Carbacot]) decrease muscle spasms; anti-inflammatory agents (such as dexamethasone [Decadron]) reduce edema and inflammation at the operative site.

4. Pain medication is more effective when given before the onset of severe pain. If accustomed to chronic back pain, the patient may wait until the pain is severe to request medication, when it may provide less than optimal relief.

5. These measures help alleviate discomfort by reducing stress and strain on the surgical site and by reducing pressure on the spinal nerve roots.

6. Bed rest promotes healing.

7. This will assist the patient in moving.

8. Activity must be increased gradually and proper body alignment must be maintained at all times to prevent muscle spasm and spinal trauma. Although slumping and limping may be comfortable at first, they cause fatigue.

9. Use of these medications, as indicated, prevents pressure and associated stress on the surgical site.

10. Rationales: _____

> **Target outcome criteria**
> Within 1 day of surgery, the patient will:
> • verbalize decreased pain, numbness, and tingling
> • show relaxed facial expression and body posture.
>
> Within 2 days of surgery, the patient will increase participation in activities (as allowed).
>
> Within 3 days of surgery, the patient will tolerate prescribed activity.
>
> By the time of discharge, the patient will use correct body mechanics and ambulate well.

Collaborative problem: *High risk for paralytic ileus related to anesthesia, medications, retroperitoneal bleeding, or injury to the spinal nerve roots*

NURSING PRIORITY: Prevent or promptly detect paralytic ileus.

Interventions

1. Perform a complete abdominal assessment every 4 hours for at least the first 48 hours after surgery, then as needed. Auscultate for bowel sounds and inspect, palpate, and percuss for abdominal distention. Measure abdominal girth if distention is present.

2. Assess for associated signs of ileus, such as nausea, vomiting, and increased back pain.

3. Document assessment findings and notify the doctor of abdominal distention or absent bowel sounds. See the "Surgical Intervention" plan, page 81, for further management.

4. Allow the patient to sit for bowel movements, condition permitting. Otherwise, logroll the patient onto a fracture bedpan.

5. Additional individualized interventions: _____

Rationales

1. Transient paralytic ileus is a common complication after laminectomy. Parasympathetic nervous system and sympathetic nervous system (SNS) innervation of the bowels originates in the lumbosacral spine. SNS stimulation contributes to loss of peristalsis and to decreased contraction of the internal sphincters, resulting in paralytic ileus. Normal bowel sounds (5 to 30 per minute) and a soft, tympanic, nondistended abdomen indicate normal bowel functioning.

2. If ileus is present, attempts to take fluids orally will cause nausea and vomiting. Back pain may increase from increased pressure on the surgical site.

3. These may indicate ileus has developed. Immediate intervention is required. The "Surgical Intervention" plan provides further details.

4. The sitting position facilitates the patient's ability to expel flatus and stool while allowing for correct spinal alignment.

5. Rationales: _____

> **Target outcome criteria**
> Within 2 days of surgery, the patient will:
> • have bowel sounds
> • expel flatus.
>
> By the time of discharge, the patient will have normal bowel sounds.

Collaborative problem: *High risk for hypovolemia related to blood loss during surgery, vascular injury, hemorrhage at the incision site, or retroperitoneal hemorrhage*

NURSING PRIORITY: Prevent or minimize bleeding.

Interventions

1. Implement standard postoperative care related to potential hypovolemia: monitor vital signs, clinical status, hemoglobin and hematocrit values, and surgical drainage. See the "Surgical Intervention" plan, page 81, for details.

Rationales

1. The "Surgical Intervention" plan contains detailed measures applicable to any postoperative patient. This plan provides additional measures specific to laminectomy.

2. Assess for flank pain, tenderness, and paresthesias every 2 to 4 hours for the first 72 hours, then every 8 hours. Compare findings to previous assessments.

3. Notify the doctor of any unusual bleeding or a change in status.

4. Additional individualized interventions: _____

_____

2. These symptoms may indicate retroperitoneal hemorrhage.

3. Prompt intervention is essential to prevent shock.

4. Rationales: _____

_____

Target outcome criteria
Within 4 hours of surgery, the patient will have no unusual bleeding or change in status.

Within 24 hours of surgery, the patient will have stable vital signs, no signs of bleeding, and normal hemoglobin and hematocrit values.

Nursing diagnosis: *Urine retention related to supine positioning, pain, anxiety, anesthesia, decreased activity, or injury to the spinal nerve roots innervating the bladder*

NURSING PRIORITY: Prevent or minimize urine retention.

Interventions

1. Assess for signs and symptoms of urine retention, such as absence of voiding within 8 hours of surgery, frequent voiding of small amounts (50 ml or less), complaints of bladder fullness or urgency, and suprapubic distention.

2. Implement standard postoperative care related to fluid intake and output monitoring, measures to facilitate voiding, and catheterization. See the "Surgical Intervention" plan, page 81, for details.

3. Additional individualized interventions: _____

_____

Rationales

1. Transient voiding problems caused by temporary loss of bladder tone from cord edema are common after lumbar laminectomy. Autonomic innervation of the bladder smooth muscle is from the thoracolumbar sympathetic outflow and the sacral parasympathetic outflow. The micturition center is located in the lumbosacral area.

2. These measures are the same for any postoperative patient. They are explained further in the "Surgical Intervention" plan.

3. Rationales: _____

_____

Target outcome criteria
Within 3 hours of surgery, the patient will have:
• adequate urine output
• no complaints of urgency, fullness, or suprapubic discomfort
• no suprapubic distention.

Within 2 days of surgery, the patient will:
• show balanced fluid intake and output
• void sufficiently at normal intervals.

Nursing diagnosis: *Knowledge deficit related to home care*

NURSING PRIORITY: Increase knowledge about home care.

Interventions

1. Provide information on signs and symptoms to report to the doctor:
• change in movement, sensation, color, pain, or temperature in the extremities
• increased pain at the incision site
• difficulty standing erect
• persistent or severe headache
• drainage from the incision site
• elevated temperature
• loss of bowel or bladder function.

2. Provide information regarding what postsurgical activity restrictions to observe at home and when the patient can saftely resume activities:
• restricted driving and riding in cars
• avoidance of pulling, bending, pushing, lifting, twisting, or stair climbing
• avoidance of tub bathing
• avoidance of sexual activity
• avoidance of sitting for prolonged periods
• avoidance of heavy work for 6 to 12 weeks after surgery.

3. Provide information about comfort measures, including:
• lying with knees bent
• using stronger muscles, such as arm and leg muscles, to change positions
• shifting weight from one foot to the other when standing for long periods
• sitting with knees higher than hips
• using correct posture when sitting or standing
• sitting forward with knees crossed and with abdominal muscles tightened to flatten the back (if sitting for long periods)
• sleeping in the side-lying position
• sleeping on the back only if the knees are supported with a pillow
• using a heating pad as needed
• using prescribed muscle relaxants or analgesics
• avoiding fatigue and chilling.

4. Provide information about recommended alterations in life-style to reduce back strain:
• sleeping on a firm mattress or a bedboard
• sitting on firm, straight-backed chairs
• using proper body mechanics (for example, bending at the knees rather than at the waist and carrying objects close to the body)
• maintaining correct posture
• wearing supportive shoes with moderate heel height
• avoiding lifting heavy objects
• using thoracic and abdominal muscles when lifting objects
• scheduling adequate rest periods
• reducing or stopping any activity that causes or aggravates discomfort
• reducing weight after a prescribed, progressive exercise program.

5. Additional individualized interventions: _____

Rationales

1. Knowing what to observe for and report will help minimize complications.

2. Patients may hesitate to ask questions about home activities. Providing information about activities that place stress on the spinal column and incision site, before discharge, may prevent complications.

3. Muscle spasms and pain may persist for a time after surgery. Reducing pain, spasms, and stress on the lumbosacral spine will increase comfort.

4. Disk herniation can recur in the same area or at other levels of the lumbosacral spinal cord, particularly if degenerative changes are already present. Reducing back strain lessens the potential for disk herniation.

5. Rationales: _____

Target outcome criteria
By the time of discharge, the patient will:
• list signs and symptoms of complications to report to the doctor
• verbalize understanding of recommended follow-up home care
• list five ways to help prevent recurrent disk herniation.

Discharge planning
NURSING DISCHARGE CRITERIA
Upon the patient's discharge, documentation shows evidence of:
• stable vital signs
• absence of fever
• absence of signs and symptoms of infection
• absence of cardiovascular or pulmonary complications, such as atelectasis and thrombophlebitis
• WBC count and hemoglobin and hematocrit values within normal parameters
• decreasing pain, muscle spasm, numbness, and tingling in lower extremities
• ability to control pain using oral medications
• absence of bowel or bladder dysfunction
• wound drainage within expected parameters
• ability to perform wound care independently or with minimal assistance, using appropriate technique
• ability to tolerate adequate nutritional intake
• knowledge of activity restrictions
• ability to perform activities of daily living and to transfer and ambulate independently or with minimal assistance
• completion of initial physical therapy assessment and instructions
• adequate home support system or referral to home care if indicated by inadequate home support system or inability to perform self-care.

PATIENT-FAMILY TEACHING CHECKLIST
Document evidence that the patient and family demonstrate an understanding of:
___ all discharge medications' purpose, dosage, administration schedule, and adverse effects requiring medical attention (pain medications may be prescribed for continued pain and muscle spasm; laxatives may be prescribed to prevent constipation)
___ infection prevention
___ signs and symptoms of postoperative infection
___ signs and symptoms of CSF drainage
___ when and how to report signs and symptoms of complications
___ recommended alterations in life-style to prevent recurrence of back problems
___ comfort measures
___ correct body mechanics
___ use of pain-relief measures, including prescribed medications
___ postsurgical activity restrictions
___ date, time, and location of follow-up appointments
___ how to contact the doctor.

DOCUMENTATION CHECKLIST
Using outcome criteria as a guide, document:
___ clinical status on admission
___ significant changes in status, especially regarding motor or sensory deficits, headaches, and weakness
___ results of myelography, spinal X-ray, CT scan, electromyography, MRI, and hemoglobin and hematocrit testing
___ episodes of muscle spasms, severe pain at incision site or in extremities
___ pain-relief measures
___ nutritional intake
___ elimination habits
___ preoperative teaching
___ patient-family teaching
___ discharge planning.

ASSOCIATED PLANS OF CARE
Ineffective Individual Coping
Knowledge Deficit
Pain
Surgical Intervention

References
Bates, B. *A Guide to Physical Examination and History Taking,* 5th ed. Philadelphia: J.B. Lippincott Co., 1991.
Cole, H.M., ed. "Diagnostic and Therapeutic Technology Assessment: Laminectomy and Microlaminectomy for Treatment of Lumbar Disk Herniation," *JAMA* 264(11):1469-72, September 19, 1990.
Cyriax, J. *Textbook of Orthopaedic Medicine, Volume 1, Diagnosis of Soft Tissue Lesions,* 8th edition. Philadelphia: Bailliere Tindall, 1989.
Ignatavicius, D.D., and Bayne, M.V. *Medical-Surgical Nursing, A Nursing Process Approach.* Philadelphia: W.B. Saunders Co., 1991.
Kee, J.L. *Laboratory and Diagnostic Tests with Nursing Implications,* 3rd ed. East Norwalk, Conn.: Appleton and Lange, 1990.
Patrick, M.L., et al. *Medical-Surgical Nursing: Pathophysiological Concepts,* 2nd ed. Philadelphia: J.B. Lippincott Co., 1991.
Phipps, W.J., et al. *Medical-Surgical Nursing: Concepts and Clinical Practice,* 4th ed. St. Louis: Mosby-Year Book, Inc., 1991.

NEUROLOGIC DISORDERS

NEUROLOGIC DISORDERS

Multiple Sclerosis

DRG information

DRG 013 Multiple Sclerosis and Cerebellar Ataxia.
   Mean LOS = 7.2 days

Additional DRG information: Patients with multiple sclerosis (MS) are most commonly admitted to an acute care setting for complications, such as pneumonia or bowel or bladder dysfunction. However, in the past 5 years, some neurologists have been admitting MS patients for trials of various I.V. medications used to counteract MS symptoms. Only in these rare circumstances would MS be the principal diagnosis. More commonly, an MS patient would be diagnosed with another illness, and the DRG would be one related to the principal diagnosis.

Introduction
DEFINITION AND TIME FOCUS

MS is a relatively common chronic, degenerative, disease causing demyelinization of the central nervous system (CNS). Approximately 500,000 cases occur in the United States each year. The disease is characterized by recurrent inflammatory reactions and the formation of sclerotic plaques throughout the CNS, interfering with normal impulse conduction and eventually causing irreversible neurologic deficits. Exacerbations and remissions are common, with some symptoms appearing only briefly or intermittently. The prognosis is variable: approximately one-third of patients experience minimal disability and can continue most normal activities; the remaining two-thirds have moderate to severe limitations and are susceptible to complications associated with relative or absolute immobility. MS affects women about five times as frequently as men and typically is diagnosed between ages 20 and 40. This clinical plan focuses on the patient admitted for diagnosis or management during an acute episode of MS.

ETIOLOGY AND PRECIPITATING FACTORS

Theories under study include:
• nutritional deficiencies
• excessive dietary animal fat
• heavy metal poisoning
• vascular disturbances
• acute viral infection
• viruses that invade the host early in life but remain dormant in the body for years before symptoms develop (results of slow-virus research studies bear some resemblance to the effects of MS)
• allergic or CNS hypersensitivity response to a common virus (90% of MS patients have high concentrations of measles antibodies in cerebrospinal fluid [CSF])
• immunologic disorder, particularly of cell-mediated immunity
• autoimmune response (immune cells are found in the demyelinated plaques)
• genetic and environmental predisposition
• stress, trauma, pregnancy, or fever (may induce first episode or exacerbation).

Focused assessment guidelines
NURSING HISTORY (Functional health pattern findings)

Health perception—health management pattern
• onset generally between ages 20 and 40
• typically reports a history of symptom-recovery cycles: mild, transient symptoms occurring in one body part, then subsiding, with the patient continuing to see self as healthy until appearance of symptoms in another part of body
• may report that symptom-recovery cycles have been increasing in frequency and severity
• may report a history of symptom remission-exacerbation cycles

Nutritional-metabolic pattern
• typically describes difficulty chewing food
• may report exhaustion from effort of eating
• may report choking (dysphagia) episodes (from poor muscle control)

Elimination pattern
• may report constipation, impaction, or incontinence (related to weakness or spasticity of anal sphincter)
• may report urgency, frequency, or retention (from loss of bladder sphincter control)

Activity-exercise pattern
• may report spasticity and weakness of limbs
• may report weakness and fatigue with activity

Sleep-rest pattern
• initially, reports that rest reduces symptoms
• later, may report that spasticity interrupts sleep

Cognitive-perceptual pattern
• describes diplopia and eye pain (common)
• may exhibit mentation disorders, such as impaired judgment and failure to comprehend or conceptualize

Self-perception—self-concept pattern
• may discuss feelings of diminished self-worth as job performance becomes impaired (psychosocial disequilibrium)
• family may report emotional lability

Role-relationship pattern
• may relate increased dependence on others as disease progresses

Sexuality-reproductive pattern
• if male, may report occasional impotence
• if female, may report alterations in vaginal sensation

Coping—stress tolerance pattern
• may report difficulty adjusting to the disease if diagnosed in early to middle adult life (prime productive years)
• may report usual coping mechanisms effective, if in remission phase early in the disease, or ineffective, if exacerbation cycles become more frequent and symptoms more disabling

Value-belief pattern
• may have ignored mild, transient symptoms (denial), only to seek medical attention later when recurring symptoms became more severe

PHYSICAL FINDINGS
Gastrointestinal
• impaction or incontinence

Neurologic
• Charcot's triad (classic): nystagmus, intention tremors, and scanning (slow, monotonous, slurred) speech
• loss of coordination
• ataxia
• paralysis
• cranial nerve impairment
 —evidence of optic neuritis with visual field deficits
 —presence of blind spot
 —dysarthria
 —dysphagia
 —loss of facial muscle control
• Lhermitte's sign (sudden "shock wave" down the body on forward neck flexion)
• hyperreflexic deep tendon reflexes
• sensory loss, including paresthesia
• decreased vibratory sensation
• decreased or absent proprioception

Musculoskeletal
• spasticity
• reduced mobility
• contractures (related to immobility)

Genitourinary
• incontinence

Integumentary
• reddened pressure points, skin breakdown (effects of immobility)

DIAGNOSTIC STUDIES
• electrophoresis—elevated oligoclonal banding of immunoglobulin G in 90% of patients (contributes evidence for differential diagnosis of MS)
• hematology—gamma globulin levels abnormally high, reflecting increased immune system activity
• evoked response potentials—delayed response after adequate stimulation of visual, auditory, or somatosensory mechanism suggests MS
• computed tomography (CT) scan—may indicate lesion of CNS white matter, atrophy, or ventricular enlargement
• lumbar puncture—increased protein and white blood cells in CSF
• core hyperthermia—use as a diagnostic procedure is controversial because results may resemble symptoms of other CNS diseases; increasing body core temperature to 102° F (38.9° C) causes marginal conduction to become incomplete or blocked; besides being diagnostically inconclusive, the test presents some risk to the patient
• magnetic resonance imaging—may identify discrete lesion

POTENTIAL COMPLICATIONS
(associated with immobility)
• phlebitis
• urinary tract infection
• respiratory tract infection
• thromboembolic phenomena

NEUROLOGIC DISORDERS

Nursing diagnosis: *Impaired physical mobility related to demyelinization*

NURSING PRIORITIES: (a) Preserve maximum physical functioning and (b) protect from effects of immobility.

Interventions	Rationales
1. Provide rest; prevent fatigue.	1. Rest seems to alleviate symptoms; fatigue may worsen symptoms.

2. Begin a physical therapy program, as ordered:
• active and passive range-of-motion exercises
• limb splints
• gait training
• leg weights and heavy shoes for balance during weight bearing
• swimming.

3. Administer medications, as ordered, to control pain and muscle spasm. Observe precautions and watch for adverse reactions, as follows:
• diazepam (Valium) — observe for increased fatigue, sedation, confusion, or depression
• dantrolene sodium (Dantrium) — monitor liver function studies (serum aspartate aminotransferase and serum alanine aminotransferase), as ordered, and observe for jaundice or other signs of liver damage as well as for drowsiness or increased weakness
• baclofen (Lioresal) — observe for increased fatigue, drowsiness, or dizziness.

4. Assess lung sounds at least every 8 hours. Report crackles, rhonchi, decreased breath sounds, or other abnormal findings promptly. Encourage incentive spirometer use, as ordered, or other pulmonary hygiene measures.

5. Teach the patient the need for specific mobility aids, such as a cane, a walker, crutches, or a wheelchair.

6. Instruct the patient in safety measures to prevent injury related to sensory loss:
• use of a thermometer to test water temperature
• use of gloves in inclement weather
• use of an eye patch to alleviate eye disturbances
• use of kitchen utensils with insulated handles to prevent burns.

7. Frequently assess skin and bony prominences for pressure signs. Reposition the patient to alleviate pressure effects. Teach the patient and family how to assess skin and minimize pressure.

8. Minimize the cardiovascular effects of immobility, using the following measures:
• Use antiembolism stockings.
• Teach leg exercises to increase venous return.
• Check indices of peripheral circulation — pulses, color, temperature, sensation, mobility, and capillary refill time.
• Note dependent edema.

9. Administer the following medications, as ordered, observing for untoward effects and providing appropriate patient teaching:

• corticotropin or corticosteroids — observe for excessive weight gain and signs of bleeding, infection, or gastric distress. Caution the patient not to stop taking the medication abruptly without consulting the doctor.

• immunosuppressant drugs — caution the patient about the increased risk of infection, and review infection signs and symptoms and precautionary measures with the patient.

2. Exercising prevents joint contractures and improves muscle tone. Circulation improves with musculoskeletal activities. A sense of achievement can be attained as exercise endurance increases.

3. Medications (antidepressants, analgesics, and antispasmotics) relax the patient by relieving pain and spasm, promoting comfort, and permitting physical activity. Adverse reactions to these medications may make their benefits of questionable value in some MS patients. Reduced muscle tone may contribute to increased weakness and risk of injury.

4. Immobility contributes to stasis of lung secretions, predisposing the MS patient to infections and other complications related to inadequate chest excursion.

5. Teaching the patient the importance of mobility aids helps facilitate adjustment to using them. Although adjustment to them may be difficult, aids can prevent injury and offer the patient a sense of security while mobile.

6. Impaired sensory perception may cause injury. Especially significant is the effect of temperature changes: increased core temperature has the potential to accentuate MS symptoms by blocking impulse conduction.

7. Frequent assessment and treatment of pressure areas is necessary because immobility predisposes the patient to circulatory impairment and resultant skin breakdown. Frequent position changes redistribute pressure. Teaching the patient and family may avert postdischarge problems.

8. Immobility influences all systems. Increasing venous return may reduce venous stasis and the risk of thromboembolism. Identifying arterial insufficiency helps ensure peripheral oxygenation. Edema suggests decreased peripheral circulation and the need for prompt limb elevation.

9. Numerous medical therapies are under investigation. Medication therapy varies widely, depending on patient status and doctor preference.

• These drugs may reduce the length of exacerbations. Sudden withdrawal from corticosteroids may cause adrenal insufficiency.

• Immunosuppressants are still of questionable value for longterm MS therapy but may offer longer-lasting effects than corticosteroids.

10. Use stress reduction techniques, such as deep breathing, progressive relaxation, or visualization, when appropriate.

10. Stress may induce an acute episode.

11. Additional individualized interventions: _____

11. Rationales: _____

Target outcome criteria
Within 3 days of admission, the patient will:
• recognize need for rest
• determine need for medication
• show no evidence of skin breakdown or other effects of immobility.

Within 5 days of admission, the patient will:
• recognize the need for mobility assistance
• list three safety measures
• function at or above admission level.

Nursing diagnosis: *Constipation and altered urinary elimination related to demyelinization*

NURSING PRIORITY: Maintain bowel and bladder function.

Interventions

1. Assess and record the patient's pattern of bowel and bladder function. Identify any dysfunctional pattern.

2. Evaluate dietary habits. Determine the need for high-fiber, high-bulk foods and foods low in saturated fat.

3. Increase and record fluid intake as appropriate.

4. Initiate a bowel or bladder program, as appropriate—for example, manual extraction, stimulation, Credé's maneuver, or an indwelling urinary catheter. Consult rehabilitation protocols for bowel or bladder retraining.

5. Administer laxatives, stool softeners, or propantheline bromide (Pro-Banthine), as ordered.

6. Prevent exposure to infection. If urinary tract infection is present, treat it vigorously.

7. Teach the patient a bowel and bladder program for elimination management at home, suggesting the following guidelines:
• Establish regular voiding times.
• Use Credé's maneuver.
• Restrict fluids at night or before trips.
• Observe for signs of infection.
• Use suppositories, as ordered.
• Maintain adequate fluid and fiber intake.
• Monitor times and consistency of bowel movements.

8. Additional individualized intervention: _____

Rationales

1. MS may cause elimination problems from decreased peristalsis. Evaluating the patient's status helps identify elimination problems; for example, is the elimination problem constipation or retention?

2. A regulated diet high in fiber and bulk promotes normal peristalsis to move bowel contents through the alimentary canal. Foods low in saturated fat are thought to interrupt demyelinization.

3. Increased fluid intake facilitates absorption and promotes peristalsis.

4. Mechanical or manual assistance may be necessary to overcome the effects of demyelinization on elimination. Protocols vary among institutions.

5. Medication may be required to adjust bowel absorption of metabolites and to reduce bowel spasticity problems.

6. The patient with MS is at increased risk for recurring infection, especially if urine retention is evident. (Urinary stasis is a precursor to urinary tract infection.)

7. In many cases, the patient can manage an effective elimination regimen at home; when possible, this reestablishes a sense of independence and control.

8. Rationales: _____

NEUROLOGIC DISORDERS

Target outcome criteria
Within 5 days of admission, the patient will:
• comply with dietary recommendations
• have satisfactory bowel and bladder elimination restored

• list measures to maintain effective elimination.

Nursing diagnosis: *High risk for sexual dysfunction related to fatigue, decreased sensation, muscle spasm, or urinary incontinence*

NURSING PRIORITIES: (a) Promote healthy sexual identity and (b) teach ways to minimize the effects of disease on sexual functioning.

Interventions

1. Assess the effects of MS on the patient's sexual function. During the admission interview, ask the patient how the disease has affected sexual performance.

2. Encourage the patient and spouse or partner to share sexual concerns. Offer to be available as a resource, or refer the couple to another health professional.

3. Offer specific suggestions for identified problems, such as teaching the patient to:
• initiate sexual activity when energy levels are highest.
• try different positions (for example, side-lying) if muscle spasm makes leg abduction difficult or if weakness limits activity.
• empty the bladder before sexual activity and pad the bedding, as necessary, to protect against wetness.
• try oral or manual stimulation if intercourse is difficult or unsatisfying.

4. Encourage expressions of affection between the patient and partner. If ongoing dysfunction has created anxiety about sexual encounters, suggest affectionate "play" sessions without intercourse as the goal.

5. Emphasize the importance of discussing birth control and family planning with a doctor.

6. Additional individualized interventions: _____

Rationales

1. MS is extremely variable in its course and effects. The patient may be hesitant to broach the subject of sexuality. Gentle, matter-of-fact questioning during routine assessment provides the patient an opportunity to voice concerns.

2. Even couples who have no difficulty communicating in most areas may find it hard to verbalize feelings related to sexuality. Health professionals who are comfortable discussing sexual issues may be able to facilitate dialogue in a nonthreatening way.

3. The patient needs concrete information on specific problems.
• Fatigue contributes to decreased libido.
• Muscle spasms commonly affect hip abductor and adductor muscles. Some positions require less energy expenditure.
• Urinary incontinence is more common during intercourse or masturbation.
• The MS patient may find intercourse less satisfying than before because decreased sensation makes orgasm more difficult to achieve.

4. Sexuality involves more than the act of coitus. Emphasis on playful, affectionate exchanges between partners helps reduce anxiety, promotes trust and improves the patient's body image and self-esteem.

5. An intrauterine device may be contraindicated because decreased sensation may cause complications to go undetected. Birth control pills may exacerbate MS symptoms. The familial tendency to develop MS and lack of prenatal screening for the disease may be significant factors for the patient considering having a child because women of childbearing age are the primary victims of the disease.

6. Rationales: _____

Target outcome criteria

During the admission interview, the patient will identify sexual concerns.

Throughout the hospital stay, the patient will initiate affection, especially with partner.

By the time of discharge, the patient will list three measures to minimize sexual dysfunction.

Nursing diagnosis: *Self-esteem disturbance related to progressive, debilitating effects of disease*

NURSING PRIORITY: Promote a healthy self-image and a realistic acceptance of limitations.

Interventions

1. Encourage the patient to participate in all decisions related to care planning. Discourage overdependent behavior patterns. Help the patient set goals and work toward them.

2. Facilitate the expression of feelings related to losses. Avoid overly cheerful responses while maintaining a positive outlook. See the "Grieving" plan, page 31, and the "Ineffective Individual Coping" plan, page 51.

3. Work with the family to promote maximum patient participation in familiar family roles and rituals or to identify new roles of value for the patient, such as humorist, correspondent, or arbitrator.

4. During care activities, encourage the patient to touch affected body parts, perform self-lifting activities as much as possible, and participate in grooming and wardrobe selection.

5. Provide recognition for goals achieved. Acknowledge evidence of inner strengths and growth as well as external achievements; for example, notice difficult emotional issues the patient has dealt with positively as well as activity goals achieved.

6. Additional individualized interventions: _____

_____

Rationales

1. Active participation fosters a sense of control and increases self-esteem. The patient with MS experiences loss of control in many areas; encouraging responsibility for self-care helps maintain dignity and independence. Goal setting aids in maintaining hope.

2. The patient suffering from a chronic debilitating disease may see each hospital stay as a further step in disease progression and loss of control. Healthy grieving is a realistic response to multiple losses and a normal part of acceptance. Overly cheerful responses indicate a lack of understanding of the profound changes MS entails for the patient. Empathy and realistic optimism, in contrast, show respect for the patient. The general plans of care noted suggest other interventions that may be helpful for the patient with MS.

3. Disease progression and an increasing sense of helplessness are compounded by the inability to fulfill familiar family roles. Encouraging family recognition and support of these roles minimizes distress. Physical disability may nevertheless allow the patient to assume new roles within the family, thus helping the patient maintain a sense of self-worth.

4. Acceptance of altered body image and function is essential to a healthy self-concept. Touching one's body and becoming familiar with its limitations is the first step toward acceptance. Grooming promotes a positive self-concept.

5. Chronic progressive disease may narrow a patient's world view severely. Recognizing struggles and achievements decreases the sense of isolation and aloneness. The patient can teach nurses much that may help them care for other patients. Acknowledgment of this gift may help provide a sense of meaning in difficult times and extend the patient's outlook toward others.

6. Rationales: _____

_____

NEUROLOGIC DISORDERS

Target outcome criteria
Throughout the hospital stay, the patient will:
• participate actively in care planning
• verbalize feelings related to losses
• participate in family activities to the extent possible
• show interest in appearance and grooming
• initiate independent activities
• show an interest in others.

Nursing diagnosis: *High risk for ineffective family coping related to progressive, debilitating effects of disease on family members and resultant alteration in role-related behavior patterns*

NURSING PRIORITY: Maintain family integrity while facilitating a healthy adjustment to necessary role changes.

Interventions

1. Assess the family system by observing family members' interaction with the patient, encouraging family participation in care activities, and talking with family members individually or as a group about changes brought about by the disease. See the "Ineffective Family Coping" plan, page 47.

2. Encourage family members to take turns in the caregiving role, as necessary.

3. Help the family understand and accept mental changes, if present.

4. Promote healthy habits for family members: urge adequate rest, proper dietary intake, exercise, and relaxation.

5. Help the family plan changes in the home environment to facilitate care: structural changes (ramps, rails); rearrangement of furnishings and supplies to allow easy access for the patient; transportation and care arrangements through a social services referral; and the availability of special supplies for incontinence.

6. Additional individualized interventions: _____

Rationales

1. Chronic diseases can have a devastating effect on families as well as affected individuals. As the primary support system for most patients, families must be supported and considered in care planning. Open discussion among family members facilitates mutual supportiveness and understanding. The plan noted provides interventions especially helpful for families in or at risk for crisis.

2. As the disease progresses, the patient becomes more dependent on others for care. Sharing care responsibilities helps prevent burnout, provides variety in care routines, and facilitates mutual understanding.

3. From 40% to 60% of MS patients exhibit alterations in mental function, ranging from inattention and euphoria (early in the disease) to irritability, depression, disorientation, and loss of memory (later in the disease). Understanding that these symptoms are part of the disease and not intentional helps minimize distress for both the patient and family.

4. Adequate sleep, proper food, exercise, and relaxation are essential if family members are to remain strong, supportive, and capable of caring for the patient and each other. Guilt feelings may preclude meeting personal needs unless health care providers offer encouragement.

5. Gradual progression of the disease may overwhelm the family with new demands unless careful planning is initiated. Social services may be able to offer numerous resources for patient and family support at home through volunteer, charitable, church, or public institutions.

6. Rationales: _____

Target outcome criteria
By the time of the patient's discharge, family members will:
• appear healthy and well rested
• participate actively in the patient's care
• participate in home care planning.

Discharge planning
NURSING DISCHARGE CRITERIA
Upon the patient's discharge, documentation shows evidence of:
• stable vital signs
• absence of fever
• absence of pulmonary or cardiovascular complications
• ability to manage bowel and bladder functioning independently or with minimal assistance
• absence of signs and symptoms of urinary tract infection
• ability to transfer and ambulate at prehospitalization levels or with minimal assistance, using appropriate assistive devices as ordered
• ability to tolerate adequate nutritional intake
• control of muscle spasms and pain with oral medications
• adequate home support system or referral to home care or a nursing home if indicated by inadequate home support system or inability to perform self-care.

PATIENT-FAMILY TEACHING CHECKLIST
Document evidence that the patient and family demonstrate an understanding of:
__ course and nature of MS
__ physical therapy program
__ all discharge medications' purpose, dosage, administration schedule, and adverse effects requiring medical attention (usual discharge medications include corticosteroids, antispasmodics, and stool softeners)
__ mobility aids
__ safety instructions for protection from injury related to sensory deficits
__ information regarding problems associated with immobility
__ stress reduction techniques
__ community resources
__ recommended therapeutic diet, including selection of foods low in saturated fat
__ bowel and bladder program
__ avoidance of exposure to infection.
__ date, time, and location of follow-up appointment
__ how to contact the doctor.

DOCUMENTATION CHECKLIST
Using outcome criteria as a guide, document:
__ clinical status on admission
__ significant changes in clinical status
__ pertinent laboratory data and diagnostic findings
__ physical therapy program and activity tolerance
__ medication administration
__ nutritional intake
__ fluid intake and output
__ bowel and bladder function
__ patient-family teaching
__ discharge planning.

ASSOCIATED PLANS OF CARE
Grieving
Ineffective Family Coping
Ineffective Individual Coping

References
Wilson, J.D. *Harrison's Principles of Internal Medicine,* 2039-2043, 12th ed. New York: McGraw-Hill, 1990.

NEUROLOGIC DISORDERS

Myasthenia Gravis

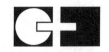

DRG information
DRG 012 Degenerative Nervous System Disorders.
    Mean LOS = 6.9 days

Introduction
DEFINITION AND TIME FOCUS
Myasthenia gravis (MG) is a chronic debilitating disease resulting from defective transmission of nerve impulses at the neuromuscular junction. Characterized by remissions and exacerbations of progressive muscle weakness, MG is estimated to occur in 1 out of 10,000 to 50,000 persons and affects more women than men. Peak incidence occurs during the 20s and 30s. When full-blown, MG causes complete dependence.

MG usually is treated pharmacologically. If symptoms persist despite medication, plasmapheresis may be used to remove autoantibodies. Thymectomy may be performed in patients with thymomas or thymic hyperplasia because these abnormal cells may trigger an autoimmune reaction; thymus gland removal decreases the response to new antigens. This clinical plan focuses on the patient admitted for initial diagnosis and pharmacologic treatment of MG.

ETIOLOGY AND PRECIPITATING FACTORS
- an autoimmune syndrome
- antibodies to acetylcholine receptors, reducing number of functional receptors on muscle cells
- smoking
- alcohol consumption
- cold weather
- prolonged exposure to sun
- stress
- menstruation
- pregnancy
- influenza

Focused assessment guidelines
NURSING HISTORY (Functional health pattern findings)

Health perception — health management pattern
- may report vague symptoms in the absence of objective findings
- may report or exhibit weak muscles, especially those involved in chewing, swallowing, and speaking
- may report or exhibit weakness of facial and extraocular muscles (may also complain of diplopia)
- may report breathlessness (related to respiratory muscle weakness)
- may report fatigue, with partial improvement of muscle strength with rest
- may report or exhibit weakness that is restricted to specific muscle groups or generalized; may be symmetric or asymmetric
- may report increased weakness with repetitive use of the muscle group

Nutritional-metabolic pattern
- may report difficulty in swallowing that worsens toward the end of meals
- may report weight loss related to decreased nutritional intake

Elimination pattern
- may report constipation

Activity-exercise pattern
- may report increasing fatigue with delayed muscle strength recovery
- may report sedentary life-style since onset of symptoms

Self-perception — self-concept pattern
- may present as helpless and unable to complete physical tasks
- may present as tired or depressed

Sexuality-reproductive pattern
- may describe impotence

Coping — stress tolerance pattern
- may report coping with symptoms by resting
- may display manifestations of ineffective coping, such as frustration, denial, and anger
- may report that stress worsens symptoms

Value-belief pattern
- may have delayed seeking medical attention because of vague and transient symptoms
- may have another autoimmune disease, such as lupus erythematosus, rheumatoid arthritis, or thyrotoxicosis, and may believe that MG symptoms are manifestations of the other disease

PHYSICAL FINDINGS
General appearance
- expressionless
- fatigued

Pulmonary
- dyspnea
- limited chest excursion
- possibly decreased tidal volume, vital capacity, and inspiratory force

Gastrointestinal
- hypoactive bowel sounds (less common)
- constipation (less common)

Neurologic
- ptosis (worsened with upward gaze), squinting, and nystagmus
- attempts to smile look snarl-like
- high-pitched, nasal voice
- progressive weakening of voice during conversation
- poorly articulated speech
- normal sensory findings

Musculoskeletal
- difficulty sitting upright, holding head up, and reaching above head
- facial drooping
- mouth hangs open
- dysphasia
- dysphagia

DIAGNOSTIC STUDIES
- acetylcholine receptor antibody titer — positive
- arterial blood gas (ABG) levels — may reveal hypoxemia or hypercapnia related to ineffective ventilation
- white blood cell count — may reveal leukocytosis related to pulmonary infection
- triiodothyronine and thyroxine — normal levels rule out thyroid disorder as cause of muscle weakness; however, abnormally high or low levels do not exclude MG because a small percentage of MG patients also have thyroid abnormalities
- magnesium — may be low because of protein-calorie malnutrition
- edrophonium test — when 2 to 10 mg of edrophonium chloride (Tensilon) is administered I.V., marked improvement in muscle strength within 60 seconds confirms MG
- electromyogram — shows rapid decreases in evoked muscle action potentials
- computed tomography scan or chest X-ray — may reveal thymoma or thymic hyperplasia

POTENTIAL COMPLICATIONS
- airway obstruction
- respiratory arrest
- aspiration
- myasthenic crisis
- cholinergic crisis
- corneal abrasion or ulceration

Collaborative problem: *Muscle weakness related to reduced number of acetylcholine receptors*

NURSING PRIORITY: Promote optimal muscle strength.

Interventions

1. Administer anticholinesterase medication orally three or four times per day, 30 to 60 minutes before meals, as ordered. Give with milk. Observe for:
- therapeutic effect — increased muscle strength
- underdosage — continuation or worsening of myasthenic symptoms (such as weakness, ptosis, dyspnea, and dysphagia)
- overdosage — cholinergic symptoms (myasthenic symptoms plus increased salivation, vomiting, diarrhea, fasciculation, and increased pulmonary secretions).

2. Keep emergency airway, suctioning, and ventilation equipment nearby. Monitor ABG measurements, as ordered.

Rationales

1. Anticholinesterases slow the breakdown of acetylcholine at the neuromuscular junction, promoting better impulse transmission to muscles and facilitating chewing and swallowing during meals. Milk prevents gastric irritation. The margin between therapeutic effects, underdosage, and overdosage varies. Anticholinesterase need may fluctuate, depending on stresses (such as emotions or infection) and the effects of other therapies.

   Underdosage may induce myasthenic crisis, an abrupt exacerbation of motor weakness caused by inadequate impulse transmission at the neuromuscular junction. Overdosage may induce cholinergic crisis, an abrupt exacerbation of motor weakness caused by prolonged action of acetylcholine at the neuromuscular junction.

   Differentiating between underdosage and overdosage can be difficult because of their similar signs and symptoms. Parasympathetic effects help to identify overdosage but are not conclusive. The edrophonium test definitively distinguishes between underdosage and overdosage.

2. Anticholinesterase overdosage or underdosage leads to respiratory muscle weakness that might require artificial ventilation. ABG measurements provide objective evidence of the adequacy of ventilation.

NEUROLOGIC DISORDERS

3. Keep atropine sulfate nearby.

4. Periodically assess muscle strength by having the patient maintain a steady upward gaze and by having the patient drink through a straw.

5. Keep a daily log of periods of fatigue and times of increased and decreased muscle strength.

6. Contact the doctor if the patient says that more or less medication is needed.

7. Administer such medications as succinylcholine (Anectine) and pancuronium (Pavulon) with caution, as ordered.

8. Observe for muscle weakness after the administration of aminoglycoside antibiotics or antiarrhythmic medications, especially quinidine (Duraquin) and procainamide (Pronestyl).

9. Additional individualized interventions: _____

_____

3. Atropine sulfate is the antidote to anticholinesterase overdosage (cholinergic crisis).

4. MG commonly affects eye muscles the most dramatically. After 1 minute of upward gazing, the patient may exhibit progressive eyelid drooping. Drinking through a straw requires repetitive use of the facial and swallowing muscles.

5. This information helps the doctor adjust the medication dosage and schedule it for optimal patient benefit.

6. The MG patient on long-term medication therapy typically can detect over- or under-dosage before clinical signs appear.

7. The MG patient is sensitive to the effects of curariform drugs.

8. The MG patient is sensitive to the neuromuscular blocking effects of the aminoglycosides and Class Ia antiarrhythmics.

9. Rationales: _____

_____

Target outcome criteria
Within 12 hours of admission, the patient will show muscle strength adequate to support ventilation, manifested by pH greater than 7.35 and $PaCO_2$ less than 45 mm Hg.

Within 2 days of admission, the patient will show improved muscle strength and the ability to turn in bed and assist with transfer to a chair.

Collaborative problem: *High risk for aspiration related to impaired swallowing*

NURSING PRIORITY: Prevent aspiration.

Interventions

1. Plan mealtimes to coincide with peak anticholinesterase effects.

2. Ask the patient for a self-evaluation of swallowing ability, and order foods of appropriate consistency: liquid, pureed, soft, or regular. Give the patient nothing by mouth if swallowing is severely impaired.

3. Provide rest periods during meals.

4. Have suctioning equipment at the patient's bedside. Stay with the patient during meals.

5. Teach the patient and family what steps to take if choking or aspiration occurs, such as back blows, abdominal thrusts, and nasotracheal suction.

Rationales

1. Oral anticholinesterase medications achieve full effect within 60 minutes of administration, with the duration of action ranging from 2 to 8 hours. The potential for aspiration increases when anticholinesterase levels are low.

2. Subjective evaluation of swallowing is usually accurate. This also allows the patient to participate in decision making, thus keeping a sense of control.

3. Chewing and swallowing make repetitive use of the same muscle groups.

4. Significant numbers of patients die from respiratory complications secondary to aspiration.

5. Back blows and abdominal thrusts can loosen food obstructing the airway. Suctioning stimulates coughing and removes sputum and debris.

6. Additional individualized interventions: _____

6. Rationales: _____

_____

_____

Target outcome criteria

Throughout the hospital stay, the patient will not aspirate.

By the time of the patient's discharge, the family will demonstrate airway clearance procedures.

Nursing diagnosis: *Activity intolerance related to muscle fatigue*

NURSING PRIORITY: Minimize fatigue and promote a tolerable level of activity.

Interventions

1. Identify sources of excess energy consumption, such as frequent telephone conversations, reading, watching television, or chewing hard or tough food.

2. Space bathing, grooming, and other activities throughout the day to avoid fatigue.

3. Rearrange the environment to keep frequently used items close by.

4. Plan a rest period before each meal. Keep meals small.

5. Additional individualized interventions: _____

_____

Rationales

1. Minimizing unnecessary actions helps conserve strength.

2. Muscles weaken rapidly when used repetitively. Several short rest periods may be more effective in restoring muscle strength than one longer rest period.

3. Keeping frequently used items within easy reach minimizes unnecessary muscle use.

4. The muscles used in chewing and swallowing weaken quickly.

5. Rationales: _____

_____

Target outcome criteria

Within 2 days of admission, the patient will show little or no fatigue.

Within 5 days of admission, the patient will be able to perform activities of daily living without assistance.

Nursing diagnosis: *Ineffective airway clearance related to decreased inspiratory force and increased secretion production*

NURSING PRIORITY: Maintain a patent airway.

Interventions

1. Demonstrate the cascade cough by having the patient take a deep breath, cough three or four times after the same inhalation, and repeat several times until the cough is productive.

2. Encourage the patient not to suppress coughs.

3. Perform chest physiotherapy (CPT) and suction every 2 to 4 hours, as needed. Evaluate lung sounds to judge efficacy.

4. Additional individualized interventions: _____

_____

Rationales

1. A deep breath followed by a single long, harsh cough is ineffective in airway clearance because it commonly causes bronchospasm. The cascade cough mimics the normal cough pattern, which moves sputum farther up the bronchial tree with each successive cough.

2. Because of pain or unpleasant sensations, the patient may try to stop the cough response to airway irritation.

3. CPT mechanically loosens secretions; suctioning helps remove them. Effective CPT clears secretions.

4. Rationales: _____

_____

NEUROLOGIC DISORDERS

Target outcome criteria
Within 12 hours of admission, the patient will have an arterial PO_2 greater than 50 mm Hg.

Within 5 days of admission, the patient will:
• show clearing or absence of gurgles
• expectorate any sputum produced
• have a temperature under 101.3° F (38.5° C).

Nursing diagnosis: *Ineffective breathing pattern related to muscle fatigue*

NURSING PRIORITY: Promote adequate ventilation.

Interventions

1. Monitor and document the respiratory rate and depth every 2 hours. Observe for changes.

2. Measure vital capacity, tidal volume, and inspiratory force before and 1 hour after administration of anticholinesterase medications. Alert the doctor if the patient's vital capacity falls below 10 ml/kg, if tidal volume falls below 5 ml/kg, or if inspiratory force falls below −20 cm H_2O or a pattern of decreasing values occurs.

3. Additional individualized interventions: _____

_____

Rationales

1. Changes in rate and depth are clues to impending respiratory muscle failure.

2. A therapeutic dose of anticholinesterase medication results in increased vital capacity, tidal volume, and inspiratory force. Both underdosage and overdosage result in muscle weakness, which is reflected as decreased vital capacity, tidal volume, and inspiratory force. Values that do not improve with I.V. administration of an anticholinesterase indicate the need for intubation and mechanical ventilation.

3. Rationales: _____

_____

Target outcome criteria
Within 12 hours of admission, the patient will have:
• no dyspnea
• an arterial PCO_2 less than 50 mm Hg
• an arterial PO_2 greater than 50 mm Hg
• a respiratory rate less than 30 breaths/minute.

Within 24 hours of admission, the patient will have:
• a regular breathing pattern
• a vital capacity greater than 15 ml/kg
• a tidal volume greater than 5 ml/kg
• an inspiratory force greater than −20 cm H_2O.

Nursing diagnosis: *Impaired verbal communication related to fatigue of facial and respiratory muscles*

NURSING PRIORITY: Establish effective communication.

Interventions

1. Avoid frequent or long conversations with the patient.

2. Provide alternative methods of communication, such as paper and pencil or a word board.

3. Additional individualized interventions: _____

_____

Rationales

1. Facial and respiratory muscles are easily fatigued.

2. Alternative methods allow communication without using facial and respiratory muscles.

3. Rationales: _____

_____

Target outcome criterion
Within 24 hours of admission, the patient will communicate needs.

Nursing diagnosis: *Nutritional deficit related to decreased oral intake*

NURSING PRIORITY: Maintain adequate oral nutrition.

Interventions

1. Collaborate with the dietitian or nutritional support service to obtain a nutritional assessment on admission, including:
• height and weight
• midarm circumference measurement
• triceps skin-fold measurement
• arm muscle circumference calculation
• creatinine height index.

2. Provide a diet with the proper balance of protein, fat, carbohydrate, and calories.

3. Serve the main meal in the morning.

4. Provide liquids in a cup.

5. Have the patient sit erect during meals.

6. Record all food and nutritional supplements consumed. Evaluate protein, calorie, vitamin, and mineral intake.

7. Consult with a dietitian about nutritional supplements, tube feedings, and total parenteral nutrition, if indicated.

8. Additional individualized interventions: _____

_____

Rationales

1. These parameters indicate nutritional status, which affects muscle performance. Colleagues with special nutritional expertise are best equipped to evaluate the patient's nutritional status.

2. A balanced diet meets nutritional needs while keeping the respiratory quotient at a normal level (0.8). (The respiratory quotient [RQ] — the ratio of carbon dioxide [CO_2] produced to oxygen consumed during metabolism — indicates the patient's ability to increase ventilation to remove excess CO_2 produced by a large carbohydrate intake. If RQ is abnormal, the work load caused by increased CO_2 production may lead to respiratory failure.)

3. The muscles used for chewing are strongest in the morning.

4. Weak facial muscles make drinking with a straw difficult.

5. Sitting erect facilitates the swallowing reflex.

6. This record of consumption provides the basis for dietary assessment; its evaluation forms the basis for further planning.

7. The dietitian's expertise helps meet the MG patient's special nutritional needs.

8. Rationales: _____

_____

Target outcome criteria
Within 2 days of admission, the patient will have arterial PCO_2 levels within normal limits.

Within 5 days of admission, the patient will have no unplanned weight loss greater than 10% of baseline body weight.

Nursing diagnosis: *Knowledge deficit related to required life-style adjustments and new medications*

NURSING PRIORITY: Provide the knowledge needed for self-care.

Interventions

1. Teach the patient and family about the disease and its implications. Find out what the doctor has stated, and reinforce that explanation. Clarify misconceptions. Stress the fluctuating nature of MG and the value of informed self-care.

Rationales

1. Because of its chronicity, MG requires a well-informed, motivated patient and family for best management. The doctor's initial explanation may have been blocked out or misinterpreted by the patient and family because of anxiety. Congruent explanations from the doctor and nurse increase confidence in caregivers.

NEUROLOGIC
DISORDERS

2. Instruct about factors that may worsen the condition — stress, infection, smoking, alcohol, exposure to cold or heat, pregnancy, and medication overdosage or underdosage.

3. Teach the patient and family signs and symptoms of crises that may require notifying the doctor or nurse, including nausea, vomiting, diarrhea, abnormal sweating, increased salivation, irregular or slow heartbeat, muscle weakness, or severe abdominal pain.

4. Teach the patient about medications, particularly:
• the importance of following the schedule exactly if the patient is to be discharged on a fixed anticholinesterase schedule
• the parameters within which the patient may adjust the dosage if following an on-demand anticholinesterase schedule
• signs of overdosage and underdosage
• the significance of alterations in GI function (such as nausea, cramping, diarrhea, or constipation)
• the need to check with the doctor before taking any additional medications, including over-the-counter ones.

5. Demonstrate how to keep a medication-response log.

6. Provide information about how to obtain a medical alert bracelet or pendant.

7. Teach ways to cope with decreased activity tolerance, including the following:
• conserving energy (for example, by using clothing that is easy to put on)
• spacing activities
• instituting safety precautions (such as hand rails in the tub or by the commode).

8. Provide the following address: The Myasthenia Gravis Foundation, 53 West Jackson Boulevard, Suite 1352, Chicago, IL 60604.

9. Additional individualized interventions: _____

_____

2. The patient and family must be aware of risk factors in order to avoid them. Involving the patient in self-management may help restore a sense of control and provide reassurance that MG does not affect intellectual capability.

3. The signs and symptoms of myasthenic and cholinergic crises are similar. Both underdosage and overdosage of anticholinesterases can cause life-threatening respiratory insufficiency.

4. A knowledgeable, confident patient and family are crucial to successful management of MG. GI dysfunction may result from long-term anticholinesterase therapy or may represent anticholinesterase toxicity. If a doctor rules out the latter, the patient may be helped by small meals, altered fluid intake, antiemetics, or other interventions. Many medications, such as narcotics, sedatives, quinidine, and aminoglycoside antibiotics, interfere with neuromuscular transmission.

5. The medication-response log helps the doctor adjust medication dosages if needed.

6. In an emergency, those providing care must know the patient's name, diagnosis, current medication dosages, and the doctor's name and number.

7. Learning methods to cope with this chronic disease may reduce frustration, decrease exacerbations, and restore self-esteem.

8. The Myasthenia Gravis Foundation provides direct services to patients and families.

9. Rationales: _____

_____

Target outcome criteria
Within 5 days of admission, the patient will:
• list signs and symptoms that should be reported to the doctor or nurse promptly
• know how to order a medical alert bracelet or pendant
• begin maintaining a medication-response log.

By time of discharge, the patient will:
• list four factors that may lead to a crisis
• verbalize intent to follow the medication schedule exactly as prescribed
• verbalize ways to cope with decreased activity tolerance.

Discharge planning

NURSING DISCHARGE CRITERIA

Upon the patient's discharge, documentation shows evidence of:
- ABG levels within normal limits
- absence of fever
- absence of airway-compromising dysphagia for at least 48 hours
- ability to tolerate adequate nutritional intake
- absence of cardiovascular and pulmonary complications
- ability to tolerate at least a minimum activity level
- ability to perform activities of daily living independently or with minimal assistance
- ability to understand and maintain a medication-response log
- adequate home support
- referral to home care or nursing home if indicated by progression of the disease, lack of home support, and potential for needing emergency care.

Additional discharge planning information: Because of the age-group and sex that MG usually strikes and the chronicity of the illness, the health care provider must assess the patient's home situation, including problems associated with child care, finances, and ability to cope with an altered life-style. In mid- and end-stage MG, patients typically need nursing home placement or around-the-clock home care assistance if they can afford it. Anticipate a social service referral for every MG patient.

PATIENT-FAMILY TEACHING CHECKLIST

Document evidence that the patient and family demonstrate an understanding of:
- ___ nature of the disease and its implications
- ___ signs and symptoms of myasthenic and cholinergic crises
- ___ activity recommendations and limitations
- ___ airway clearance procedures
- ___ all discharge medications' purpose, dosage, administration schedule, and adverse effects requiring medical attention (usual discharge medications include anticholinesterases)
- ___ community resource and support groups
- ___ how and where to obtain an emergency identification card or bracelet
- ___ when and how to contact the emergency medical system
- ___ date, time, and location of follow-up appointments
- ___ how to contact the doctor.

DOCUMENTATION CHECKLIST

Using outcome criteria as a guide, document:
- ___ clinical status on admission
- ___ significant changes in status
- ___ responses to medications
- ___ periods of fatigue or increased weakness
- ___ swallowing ability
- ___ respiratory parameters before and after medication administration
- ___ activity tolerance
- ___ patient-family teaching
- ___ discharge planning.

ASSOCIATED PLANS OF CARE

Grieving
Ineffective Family Coping
Ineffective Individual Coping
Knowledge Deficit
Total Parenteral Nutrition

References

Blazey, M.E., et al. "Nutritional Assessment of Protein Status," *Dimensions of Critical Care Nursing.* 5(6):328-32, November-December 1986.

Hickey, J.V. *The Clinical Practice of Neurological and Neurosurgical Nursing,* 3rd ed. Philadelphia: J.B. Lippincott Co., 1992.

Marshall, S.B., et al. *Neuroscience Critical Care: Pathophysiology and Patient Management.* Philadelphia: W.B. Saunders Co., 1990.

Mitchell, P.H., et al. *AANN's Neuroscience Nursing.* Norwalk, CT: Appleton and Lange, 1988.

Noroian, E.L. "Myasthenia Gravis: A Nursing Perspective," *Journal of Neuroscience Nursing* 18(2):74-80, April 1986.

Rowland, L.P. "Diseases of Chemical Transmission at the Nerve-Muscle Synapse: Myasthenia Gravis and Related Syndromes," in *Principles of Neural Science,* 2nd ed. Edited by Kandel, E.R., and Schwartz, J.H., New York: Elsevier, 1985.

Traver, G.A. "Ineffective Airway Clearance: Physiology and Clinical Application," *Dimensions of Critical Care Nursing* 4(4):198-208, July-August 1985.

NEUROLOGIC DISORDERS

Seizures

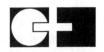

DRG information

DRG 024 Seizure and Headache. Age 17 +.
    With Complication or Comorbidity (CC).
    Mean LOS = 5.3 days
    Principal diagnoses include:
    • cerebral arteritis
    • convulsions or epilepsy (seizures)
    • benign intracranial hypertension (increased intracranial pressure)
    • reaction to spinal or lumbar puncture
    • postconcussion syndrome.
DRG 025 Seizure and Headache. Age 17 +.
    Without CC.
    Mean LOS = 3.5 days
    Principal diagnoses include selected principal diagnoses listed under DRG 024.
DRG 026 Seizure and Headache. Age 0 to 17.
    Mean LOS = 4.0 days
    Principal diagnoses include selected principal diagnoses listed under DRG 024.

Introduction
DEFINITION AND TIME FOCUS
A seizure represents uncontrolled, paroxysmal, abnormal electrical discharge in the central nervous system (CNS). The precise mechanism involved is not known, but a decreased neuronal firing threshold or excessive irritability is suspected.

Seizures are described as primary or secondary, depending on whether the cause can be identified. Primary (idiopathic) seizures appear without any identifiable cause, commonly arise in childhood, and may result from a congenital tendency. Secondary seizures are triggered by specific metabolic, structural, chemical, or physical abnormalities. Diagnostically, seizures are classified into two broad groups: partial and generalized. Partial seizures involve localized areas of brain irritability and are characterized by physical activity that corresponds to the affected area of the brain. Loss of consciousness may not occur. Generalized seizures involve both brain hemispheres and, usually, major bilateral muscle activity and loss of consciousness.

Seizures are commonly a sign of underlying abnormality, and any seizure, even in a patient with a preexisting seizure history, must be evaluated within the context of the patient's overall condition. In some patients, a single, brief seizure episode may be of minimal concern; in others, it may represent grave deterioration in the patient's neurologic status. Persistent or recurrent generalized seizures warrant immediate pharmacologic control and prompt identification and treatment of the underlying cause. Because seizures present such a wide range of physical manifestations, this plan focuses on the patient exhibiting generalized tonic-clonic seizures; you should, however, be knowledgeable about and alert for more subtle types of seizures as well.

ETIOLOGY AND PRECIPITATING FACTORS
• metabolic conditions – hyperpyrexia, hypoxia, hypoglycemia, hyperglycemia, electrolyte imbalances, uremia, fluid overload
• chemical or pharmacologic conditions – inadequate serum anticonvulsant levels, alcohol or drug overdose or toxicity, alcohol or drug withdrawal
• infections – meningitis and encephalitis
• structural or physical conditions – increased intracranial pressure (ICP), cerebral edema, cerebral or subdural hematoma, cerebral hemorrhage, eclampsia, malignant hypertension, tumor, congenital malformations
• degenerative conditions – Alzheimer's disease, multiple sclerosis, systemic lupus erythematosus
• reduced cardiac output – Stokes-Adams syncope, other arrhythmias
• idiopathic origin

Focused assessment guidelines
Note: The patient exhibiting generalized seizures cannot always provide relevant historical information, so the nursing history (functional health patterns) section of this plan has been omitted. Instead, guidelines for observing and documenting seizures are presented as an essential aid to accurate diagnosis and effective intervention. Attempt to describe findings with precision and accuracy, as follows:

Preictal phase
• Did an aura or warning precede seizure onset? What was the patient doing when the seizure began (or when the aura was noted)?

Tonic-clonic phases
• Did the patient give a shrill cry?
• Did the patient fall?
• What kind of movement was noted first?
• Where did it begin?
• Were other areas progressively involved? If so, in what pattern?
• If a tonic (rigid) phase occurred, how long did it last?
• If a clonic (jerking) phase occurred, how long did it last?
• How long did the entire seizure last?
• Was the patient incontinent?
• During the phases of the seizure, did the pupils react? Deviate?
• Did the patient lose consciousness? If so, when?

Postictal phase
- What was the patient's level of consciousness after the seizure?
- Did the patient exhibit amnesia, confusion, disorientation, or agitation when he regained consciousness?
- Did the patient have any motor, sensory, or perceptual deficits after the seizure?
- How long did the postictal phase last?

PHYSICAL FINDINGS
Note: Physical findings vary widely, depending on the type of seizure activity, the area of brain tissue involved, and the phase of the seizure (see *Physical findings in seizures*). Keep in mind that the range of physical manifestations is almost limitless.

DIAGNOSTIC STUDIES
Because a seizure represents a clinical sign, not a diagnosis, testing is usually done to determine the seizure's cause. The following tests are a partial list of possible studies that may be ordered for this purpose.
- serum glucose tests — may be ordered to rule out hypoglycemia or hyperglycemia as a cause of seizure
- serum phenytoin or serum phenobarbital levels — may be obtained to evaluate adequacy of anticonvulsant dosage in the patient with a known seizure history

- blood urea nitrogen, creatinine studies — may be obtained to evaluate renal function because uremia may induce seizures
- serum electrolytes — may be ordered because electrolyte imbalances, particularly calcium deficit, may induce seizures
- arterial blood gas values — may be obtained because hypoxia may induce seizures or result from prolonged seizures or associated respiratory depression
- toxicology screens — may be ordered if drug ingestion is suspected as a cause
- blood cultures — may be obtained to rule out sepsis as a cause of seizures
- computerized tomography (CT) scan — may identify cerebral abnormality, such as tumor, arteriovenous malformation, hemorrhage, or edema
- lumbar puncture — may identify infection, indicated by bacteria, increased white blood cell count, and decreased glucose level in cerebrospinal fluid. Increased pressure may indicate a space-occupying lesion, or bleeding may indicate hemorrhage
- electroencephalography — may identify the lesion area. Increased electrical activity and spikes are characteristic of generalized motor seizures. Repeated studies may be necessary to record actual seizure activity

PHYSICAL FINDINGS IN SEIZURES

Body system	Tonic phase	Clonic phase	Postictal phase
Neurologic	• Shrill cry, then loss of consciousness • Pupils dilated and nonreactive	• Loss of consciousness • Pupils may or may not remain dilated and nonreactive • Excessive salivation	• Deep sleep, then confusion, disorientation, amnesia • Reactive pupils
Musculoskeletal	• Opisthotonos • Rigidity • Jaw clenching • Extension of extremities • Clenched fists	• Violent, bilateral rhythmic jerking • Facial grimacing	• Flaccidity
Pulmonary	• Apnea	• Stertorous, irregular respirations	• Deep, regular respirations
Renal/Gastrointestinal		• Fecal incontinence • Urinary incontinence	
Integumentary	• Cyanosis	• Profuse diaphoresis • Flushing	
Cardiovascular	• Bradycardia	• Bradycardia or tachycardia • Hypertension	

• magnetic resonance imaging (MRI) — may reveal intracerebral abnormality
• skull X-rays — may indicate fractures or areas of calcification
• cerebral angiography — evaluates cerebral circulatory status and identifies vascular abnormalities
• ICP monitoring — may be instituted to monitor for possible increased ICP as cause of seizure

POTENTIAL COMPLICATIONS
• status epilepticus
• airway obstruction
• respiratory arrest
• aspiration pneumonia
• hyperthermia
• hypoglycemia
• renal failure
• cerebral ischemia

Nursing diagnosis: *Ineffective airway clearance related to loss of consciousness, apnea, excessive secretions, jaw clenching, or airway occlusion by tongue or foreign body*

NURSING PRIORITIES: (a) Maintain patent airway and (b) promote adequate oxygenation.

Interventions

1. If an aura or warning phase occurs, clear the patient's mouth of any foreign bodies and insert a soft cloth or gauze pad at the corner of the mouth. Never try to force the jaw open or insert an oral airway during the seizure. Turn the patient to the side and use the chin lift or jaw thrust maneuver as needed to maintain an open airway.

2. Suction the oropharynx, as needed. Provide supplemental oxygen via nasal cannula.

3. If seizures are persistent (unresponsive to drug therapy) or frequently recur, notify the doctor immediately and anticipate the need for endotracheal intubation and mechanical ventilation. See the "Mechanical Ventilation" plan, page 227.

4. After the seizure, insert a nasogastric (NG) tube and connect it to low suction, as ordered. Do not attempt to insert an NG tube during active seizure.

Rationales

1. Insertion of a soft airway protector may help keep the tongue from occluding the airway and reduce the risk of trauma to the tongue and teeth. Attempts to force the jaw open or insert objects during seizures may cause damage to the teeth or injury to the caregiver. Turning the patient to the side promotes drainage of saliva from the mouth and reduces the risk of aspiration. An apneic period of up to 60 seconds is usually followed by resumption of spontaneous respiration. If the airway becomes occluded during the tonic phase, significant hypoxia may ensue, so maintenance of an open airway is essential.

2. During the clonic and postictal phases, the obtunded patient is at risk for aspirating saliva that has accumulated during the tonic phase. Vomiting may also occur. Supplemental oxygen is indicated because seizures cause increased oxygen demands. Also, some degree of respiratory depression commonly follows generalized seizures. A cannula is preferred because a mask may hamper airway clearance if vomiting occurs.

3. Status epilepticus, in which seizure activity persists or recurs without the patient regaining consciousness, is a medical emergency. Irreversible brain damage may result from the prolonged apnea that occurs. Mechanical ventilation may be necessary to ensure adequate oxygenation while attempting to stop the seizures. The "Mechanical Ventilation" plan contains detailed interventions for the care of the patient on a ventilator.

4. Emptying the stomach of gastric contents prevents accidental aspiration should vomiting occur. Do not attempt to insert an NG tube during active seizure.

5. Additional individualized interventions: _____

5. Rationales: _____

Target outcome criterion
Throughout the seizure, the patient will maintain a clear airway.

Collaborative problem: *High risk for status epilepticus related to inadequate pharmacologic control or misidentification of underlying cause*

NURSING PRIORITIES: (a) Stop seizures and (b) treat underlying cause.

Interventions

1. Administer I.V. antiseizure medication, as ordered. Commonly ordered medications for acute seizures include the following:

• diazepam (Valium), 5 to 10 mg, I.V. push. Observe the patient closely for respiratory depression. Monitor for undesirable drug interactions, especially if the patient is also taking phenothiazines, barbiturates, narcotics, or monoamine oxidase inhibitors.

• phenobarbital (Luminal) and other barbiturate anticonvulsants. The usual dose of phenobarbital ranges from 60 to 400 mg/day. Observe the patient closely for respiratory depression, especially if the patient also received diazepam. Monitor carefully for undesirable drug interactions, especially if the patient is taking phenothiazines, warfarin (Coumadin), digoxin (Lanoxin), or disulfiram (Antabuse).

• phenytoin (Dilantin). Usual loading dose is 10 to 15 mg/kg, followed by 100 mg every 6 to 8 hours. Administer phenytoin slowly in normal saline solution, giving no more than 50 mg/minute. Observe the patient's electrocardiogram (ECG) during phenytoin administration. Monitor closely for adverse reactions or indications of possible toxicity, such as anemia, elevated serum glucose levels, GI upset, and diplopia with nystagmus.

— Monitor therapeutic blood levels, as ordered.

— Monitor carefully for possible drug interactions. Drugs that may increase serum phenytoin levels include chloramphenicol (Chloromycetin)), isoniazid (Laniazid), salicylates, sulfonamides, cimetidine (Tagamet), warfarin, and benzodiazepines; acute alcohol ingestion also may increase serum phenytoin levels. Phenytoin may increase metabolism of warfarin and digitoxin (Cristodigin). Digitoxin, reserpine (Serpasil), prednisone (Deltasone), phenobarbital, and chronic alcoholism may decrease phenytoin levels.

Rationales

1. Prolonged seizures may result in respiratory depression or arrest, cardiovascular insufficiency, or cerebral edema. Antiseizure medications suppress the ectopic focus.

• Diazepam is the initial drug of choice for generalized motor status epilepticus, although it is neither recommended nor sufficient for ongoing seizure control. It appears to act on the limbic system, thalamus, and hypothalamus to stop seizures. Respiratory depression is a common adverse reaction. The medications listed may potentiate the actions of diazepam and increase the risk of respiratory compromise.

• Like diazepam, phenobarbital depresses the central nervous system. Its precise action is unclear, but it appears to reduce cerebral oxygen consumption and may help decrease ICP. It also potentiates phenothiazines. Phenobarbital may decrease warfarin absorption and digoxin metabolism. Disulfiram may increase the likelihood of toxicity.

• Phenytoin appears to act on the motor cortex to stabilize the threshold against neuronal hyperexcitability, possibly by aiding the efflux of sodium from neurons. Phenytoin must be administered in saline solution because it precipitates in glucose-containing solutions. ECG monitoring is essential; giving phenytoin too rapidly may cause arrhythmias or cardiac arrest.

— Assessing serum phenytoin levels is essential to achieve the optimum dosage and minimize the risk of toxicity.

— Phenytoin reacts with many other medications. Achieving seizure control may involve careful balancing of several pharmacologic parameters. Be aware of the possibility of untoward reactions to avert possible toxicity or inadequate therapeutic effect.

NEUROLOGIC DISORDERS

2. Consider possible underlying causes. Assist with identification and treatment.

• head trauma

• electrolyte imbalance

• hypoxia

• hypoglycemia or hyperglycemia

• brain tumors

• infections

• cerebral hemorrhage

• toxins

3. If seizures are refractory to drug therapy, anticipate possible preparation for neuromuscular blockade or general anesthesia, with mechanical ventilation.

4. Additional individualized interventions: _____

_____

2. In a patient without a history of seizures, treating the underlying cause is paramount to seizure control.

• Secondary seizures are caused most commonly by head trauma. If the patient was admitted after an acute traumatic event, this link may be obvious. However, seizures may occur months or even years after head injury, as scar tissue creates a focus for abnormal neuronal activity, so careful history-taking is indicated.

• Electrolyte imbalances may induce seizures by altering cell membrane permeability, thus interfering with normal neuronal electrical conduction.

• Sufficient oxygen is essential for maintaining the normal neuronal ionic gradient. Any condition that lowers the level of oxygen delivered to sensitive brain tissue may contribute to seizure activity.

• Cerebral neurons are exquisitely sensitive to decreased glucose levels because glucose is their primary substrate. A sudden drop in blood glucose appears more likely to cause neurologic problems than a gradual decline. Hyperglycemia may contribute to a hyperosmolar crenation of brain cells, with resultant irritability and altered conduction pathways. Also, seizure activity increases cerebral metabolic needs and depletes stores of glucose and energy.

• Seizures are the major initial sign in as many as 18% of patients with undetected brain tumors. Tissue compression from tumor growth is usually the cause.

• Infections may contribute to seizures for several possible reasons: scarring in response to inflammatory changes, cerebral edema in acute infections, hyperpyrexia, abscesses, or autoimmune demyelinization, as in encephalomyelitis.

• Localized ischemic damage to brain tissue may cause seizures.

• Toxins may cause seizures by interfering with the cell's metabolic processes, altering cell membrane function and integrity. Some hydrocarbons, lead, mercury, and arsenic may cause seizures in high concentrations. Hypersensitive persons may develop seizures in response to certain medications, such as phenothiazines. Withdrawal from alcohol or barbiturates is a common cause of seizures because abrupt withdrawal from the CNS-depressant effects of either appears to increase neuronal irritability.

3. Status epilepticus has a mortality of about 10% and causes one-third of all seizure-related deaths. As seizures persist, cerebral vasodilation occurs, perfusion pressure drops, and irreversible cell damage follows from nutritional depletion and neuronal exhaustion. Neuromuscular blockade stops motor activity but does not directly interrupt brain electrical activity. General anesthesia causes global depression of cerebral function, interrupting the cycle of hyperexcitability at its source.

4. Rationales: _____

_____

Target outcome criteria
Following onset of seizures, the patient will:
• be recognized as being at risk for status epilepticus
• receive appropriate anticonvulsants promptly
• have underlying causes identified and treated.

Throughout the hospital stay, the patient will:
• maintain therapeutic drug levels
• receive appropriate therapy for underlying cause of seizures.

Nursing diagnosis: *High risk for injury: trauma or myoglobinuria related to excessive uncontrolled muscle activity*

NURSING PRIORITY: Prevent injury.

Interventions

1. At the seizure's onset, ensure safe patient positioning. Place pillows or padding around the patient and raise and pad the bed side rails. Do not restrain arms and legs. Maintain bed in low position.

2. During the seizure, stay with the patient. Provide privacy, as possible.

3. After motor activity stops, perform a neurologic evaluation, noting pupil size and reactivity, level of consciousness, responsiveness to stimuli, and respiratory status. Repeat the evaluation every 15 to 30 minutes until condition stabilizes. Inspect the oropharynx, tongue, and teeth for seizure-related injury.

4. Avoid excessive environmental stimulation during the postictal period.

5. If seizure was prolonged, monitor urine for possible myoglobinuria, indicated by a red or cola color. Send urine sample for myoglobin testing. Report findings to the doctor promptly.

6. Additional individualized interventions: _____

_____

Rationales

1. Violent muscle contractions may cause injury unless protective measures are instituted. Padded side rails help prevent injury if the patient strikes the rails during the seizure. Restraining arms and legs may result in fractures during the clonic phase.

2. The seizing patient is extremely vulnerable to injury because of uncontrollable muscle activity. After the seizure, the patient is commonly embarrassed and ashamed of the loss of control. Providing privacy helps protect the patient's dignity.

3. Careful monitoring of status during the postictal period is essential because respiratory depression is common. Violent seizure activity may result in mouth injury. Blood in the oropharynx and loose teeth may be aspirated.

4. Environmental stimulation, such as bright lights; loud, sudden noises; or abrupt movement may reactivate neuronal irritability and stimulate further seizures.

5. Repeated, vigorous muscle contraction releases excess amounts of myoglobin into the bloodstream from muscle cell breakdown. If the quantity is sufficient, the accumulated myoglobin may occlude the kidneys and cause renal failure. Treatment involves flushing the renal system, using fluids and diuretics.

6. Rationales: _____

_____

Target outcome criterion
During and after the seizure episode, the patient will experience no injury from muscle contractions.

NEUROLOGIC DISORDERS

Nursing diagnosis: *Knowledge deficit related to seizure management*

NURSING PRIORITY: Instruct the patient and family on seizure management.

Interventions

1. Assess the patient's and family's current level of understanding.

2. Instruct the patient and family about the disorder and the need to adhere to a medical regimen.

3. Instruct the patient and family about medications and causes of seizures.

4. Additional individualized interventions:_____

_____

Rationales

1. Determining the patient's and family's level of understanding allows the nurse to individualize learning to meet patient needs.

2. Understanding the disorder helps to increase compliance.

3. Teaching improves compliance. Failure to take medications is a common cause of recurrent seizures. Excessive stress, fatigue and environmental factors may cause seizures in susceptible individuals.

4. Rationales:_____

_____

Target outcome criteria
By the time of discharge, the patient and family will demonstrate and verbalize understanding of seizure management.

Discharge planning
NURSING DISCHARGE CRITERIA
Upon the patient's discharge, documentation shows evidence of:
• cause of seizures identified and treated
• seizures controlled
• respiratory status stable
• neurologic status stable.

PATIENT-FAMILY TEACHING CHECKLIST
Document evidence that the patient and family demonstrate an understanding of:
___ cause and implications of seizures
___ treatment modalities instituted
___ signs of possible recurrence
___ safety precautions.

DOCUMENTATION CHECKLIST
Using outcome criteria as a guide, document:
___ clinical status on admission
___ significant changes in status
___ pertinent diagnostic test findings
___ seizure episodes
___ safety precautions instituted
___ pharmacologic interventions
___ patient-family teaching
___ discharge planning.

ASSOCIATED PLANS OF CARE
Craniotomy
Drug Overdose
Hypoglycemia
Increased Intracranial Pressure
Mechanical Ventilation
Multiple Trauma
Sensory-Perceptual Alteration

References
Holloway, N. *Nursing the Critically Ill Adult,* 4th ed. Menlo Park: Addison-Wesley Co., in press.
Tucker, S., Canobbio, M., Paquette, E., and Wells, M. *Patient Care Standards: Nursing Process, Diagnosis and Outcome,* 5th ed. St. Louis: Mosby-Year Book, 1992.

EYE DISORDERS
Glaucoma

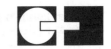

DRG information
DRG 038 Primary Iris Procedure.
　　　Mean LOS = 2.2 days
DRG 045 Neurological Eye Disorders [low tension glaucoma].
　　　Mean LOS = 3.4 days
DRG 046 Other Disorders of the Eye. Age 17+ with Complication or Comorbidity (CC) [associated with disorders of the lens or borderline glaucoma].
　　　Mean LOS = 4.2 days
Additional DRG information: Patients with DRGs 038, 045, and 046 are rarely admitted to acute-care facilities. DRG 038 patients are most commonly admitted to same-day surgery units or are treated as outpatients. This may be of concern because it reduces the amount of time available for teaching and evaluation of the patient's ability to follow discharge instructions. Documentation must contain evidence of adequate home support to assist the patient after discharge. A referral to home care should always be considered. DRGs 045 and 046 are treated in the acute-care setting if a CC necessitates admission.

Introduction
DEFINITION AND TIME FOCUS
Glaucoma is the progressive loss of visual fields resulting from increased intraocular pressure, which damages the optic nerve. The increased intraocular pressure results from an imbalance between the formation and absorption of aqueous humor. Simple chronic glaucoma is characterized by a gradual loss of peripheral vision, eventually leading to total vision loss, whereas the less common acute angle-closure glaucoma is usually characterized by a severe vision loss within a few hours of onset. This plan focuses on the patient admitted for definitive diagnosis and management of either type of glaucoma. Simple chronic glaucoma is sometimes referred to as open-angle or primary open-angle glaucoma. Other terms for acute angle-closure glaucoma include acute (congestive) glaucoma, narrow-angle glaucoma, and angleclosure or primary angle-closure glaucoma.

ETIOLOGY AND PRECIPITATING FACTORS
• simple chronic glaucoma — severe myopia; degenerative changes in the eye; swollen cataracts; ocular trauma, infection, tumor, inflammation, or hemorrhage; other factors that can narrow the trabecular meshwork openings, thus increasing resistance to aqueous humor drainage and raising intraocular pressure; and genetic predisposition
• acute angle-closure glaucoma — darkness; excitement, mydriatic medications, and other factors that can di-late the pupils and push the iris against the trabecular meshwork, thus blocking the drainage of aqueous humor through the anterior-chamber angle and increasing intraocular pressure

Focused assessment guidelines
NURSING HISTORY (Functional health pattern findings)

Health perception — health management pattern
• simple chronic glaucoma — slow onset, initially without symptoms, but then developing early symptoms, such as gradual loss of peripheral vision (tunnel vision), slightly blurred vision, persistent dull eye pain or tired feeling in the eye, or failure to detect color changes (particularly blue-green); later symptoms include blurred vision, haloes around lights, morning headaches that disappear shortly after arising, or pain behind eyeball
• acute angle-closure glaucoma — may report sudden onset of severe eye pain radiating to head, sudden blurred vision progressing to severe loss of vision within a few hours, decreased light perception, or colored haloes around lights; nausea, vomiting, and abdominal discomfort; affected eye inflamed with watery appearance, may have fixed and dilated pupil
• may have a history of frequent changes in eyeglass prescription after age 40 or of severe myopia
• if over age 40, female, black, diabetic, or with a family history, at increased risk

Nutritional-metabolic pattern
• acute angle-closure glaucoma — may report nausea, vomiting, or abdominal pain

Activity-exercise pattern
• may report a history of decreased ability to cope with ADLs
• may report fatigue in performing activities of daily living (ADLs)
• may report decreased time spent in leisure activities
• may report self-care deficit, such as inadequate grooming
• may report alterations in mobility, such as bumping into people or objects and hesitancy in walking in unfamiliar environments

Sleep-rest pattern
• may report difficulty adjusting to darkness
• may report eye pain at night or in the early morning

Self-perception — self-concept pattern
• may present self as most concerned about ability to be independent

Role-relationship pattern
• may report a decreased ability to maintain social, job, and family roles
• may report increased isolation from other people

Value-belief pattern
• may have delayed seeking medical attention because of gradual development of symptoms
• when stable, may find it difficult to comprehend or believe that lifelong treatment will be required (denial)

PHYSICAL FINDINGS
Gastrointestinal
With acute angle-closure glaucoma:
• vomiting
• abdominal pain

Neurologic
• increased intraocular pressure
• cupping of optic disk
• visual field losses with scotomas (blind spots)
• optic disk degeneration
• whiteness of optic nerve disk
• white or gray appearance of cornea
• shallow anterior chamber
• in addition (with acute angle-closure glaucoma), fixed and dilated pupil, corneal edema, hazy appearance of cornea, headache, and reddened eye

Musculoskeletal
• pained or anxious facial expression
• fatigue
• hesitancy in walking

DIAGNOSTIC STUDIES
• ophthalmoscopy—shows a white optic disk with cupping and displaced and depressed large retinal vessels
• tonometry—shows corneal indentation consistent with elevated intraocular pressure; values above 22 mm Hg indicate glaucoma, although individual norms vary
• gonioscopy—shows characteristic changes over time, small defects progressing to larger visual field defects (may have 20/20 central vision); optic disk becomes wider, deeper, and paler; impending angle closure may appear before rise in intraocular pressure
• tonography—shows characteristic changes: a flat graphic tracing with increased intraocular pressure
• visual field determination—shows characteristic loss of visual field; also shows location, size, and density of scotomas

POTENTIAL COMPLICATIONS
• total blindness
• trauma or self-injury
• nutritional deficits
• failure to thrive
• social isolation

Collaborative problem: *High risk for further vision loss related to noncompliance with the medication regimen, use of medication causing increased intraocular pressure, no response to medication therapy, or the effect of environmental variables*

NURSING PRIORITY: Prevent or minimize increases in intraocular pressure.

Interventions

1. Assess for the presence of, or any increase in, eye pain, pain around orbit, blurred vision, reddened eye, abdominal pain, nausea, vomiting, and neurologic changes, on admission and as needed.

2. Evaluate the visual fields on admission and as needed.

Rationales

1. A change from baseline assessment data may indicate increasing intraocular pressure affecting optic nerve function. With acute angle-closure glaucoma, this may indicate an emergency situation.

2. Progressive visual field losses indicate increasing intraocular pressure. Detection of subtle changes may require special equipment.

3. Assess the patient's use of medications before hospitalization by obtaining a comprehensive list of all current and past medications. Validate with the doctor the need to continue medications during the hospital stay.

3. Certain medications can cause an acute episode; many preparations can produce increased intraocular pressure, including:
• steroids (all types)
• oral and nasal inhalants
• amphetamines
• nasal decongestants (oral or spray)
• nonprescription diet capsules or tablets
• anticholinergics
• antihistamines
• antidiarrheal agents
• some antidepressant drugs
• nonsteroidal anti-inflammatory drugs.

4. Administer and document ocular medications, as ordered.

4. Consistent and timely use of medications will decrease intraocular pressure. Common medications used singly or in combination include:
• cholinergics (parasympathomimetics), such as pilocarpine hydrochloride (Pilocar) and carbachol (Carbacel), to facilitate aqueous outflow
• adrenergics (sympathomimetics), such as epinephrine (Epitrate), to decrease aqueous humor production and increase aqueous outflow
• carbonic anhydrase inhibitors, such as oral acetazolamide (Diamox), and beta-adrenergic blockers, such as timolol maleate (Timoptic), to reduce secretion of aqueous humor
• hyperosmotics, such as mannitol, used preoperatively to reduce intraocular pressure by reducing the volume of intraocular fluid.

5. Evaluate medications' effectiveness and observe for the presence of major side effects, including:
• cholinergics—headache, excessive salivation, diaphoresis, nausea, and vomiting
• adrenergics—headache, tachycardia, and tremors
• carbonic anhydrase inhibitors—paresthesias, anorexia, nausea, fatigue, and impotence
• beta-adrenergic blockers—bradycardia, hypotension, fatigue, and depression
• hyperosmotics—dehydration.

5. If symptoms persist or increase, intraocular pressure is probably increasing, and the doctor needs to be notified. Undesirable side effects may compromise other body systems.

6. Assess for signs and symptoms of increased tolerance to ocular medications related to prolonged medical therapy: increased blurring of vision, increased headache, nausea, fixed and dilated pupil, increased blood pressure, allergic reaction, and asthmatic attack.

6. An increase in signs and symptoms may indicate that the prescribed medication is no longer effective and intraocular pressure is rising. The doctor needs to be notified immediately.

7. Minimize stressful events.

7. Stress—worry, fear, excitement, or anger—increases intraocular pressure. Anticipating and preventing stress reactions helps maintain intraocular pressure at a safe level.

8. Use noninvasive techniques to reduce intraocular pressure.

8. Meditation, rest, a quiet environment, and a decrease in stimuli help decrease stress and, thus, intraocular pressure.

9. Prepare the patient for diagnostic testing.

9. Some diagnostic tests, such as tonometry, involve application of direct pressure to the eyeball. These may be done repeatedly, at different times of the day, to assess intraocular pressure. Thorough explanations of tests may decrease the patient's anxiety and ensure compliance during the procedures.

EYE DISORDERS

10. Additional individualized interventions: _____

10. Rationales: _____

Target outcome criteria
By the time of discharge, the patient will:
• show no signs or symptoms of increased intraocular pressure
• show no further decrease in vision

• list three signs of increased intraocular pressure
• list three techniques to minimize an intraocular pressure increase.

Nursing diagnosis: *Eye pain related to progressive pressure on the optic nerve*

NURSING PRIORITY: Minimize or relieve eye pain.

Interventions

1. On admission, assess the patient for presence and degree of eye pain.

2. Monitor the patient every 2 hours while awake for the occurrence of, or an increase in, eye pain.

3. On admission, teach the patient to report any eye pain or change in symptoms.

4. Assess for associated signs and symptoms, such as blurred vision, nausea, vomiting, abdominal pain, or neurologic changes.

5. Administer eye medications, as ordered. Document administration.

6. Administer analgesics judiciously, as ordered, and document their use. Assess pain relief 30 minutes after administering medication.

7. Use noninvasive pain-relief measures as well as medications. See the "Pain" plan, page 69, for details.

8. Help the patient identify and modify causes of stress.

9. Explain unfamiliar procedures and new events.

10. Additional individualized interventions: _____

Rationales

1. Eye pain in the glaucoma patient indicates increased intraocular pressure.

2. Increased eye pain, or the occurrence of eye pain not present previously, may indicate increasing intraocular pressure.

3. Early intervention is essential in preventing further damage to the optic disk.

4. The patient may not report pain, but observation of associated signs or symptoms may facilitate early intervention. Without early intervention, eye pain will eventually occur. Listed signs and symptoms may indicate increasing intraocular pressure or an episode of acute angle-closure glaucoma. Even if the patient does not report an increase in symptoms, be alert for hesitancy in walking, bumping into people or walls, or new bruises from hitting objects.

5. Eye medications are administered to permit better drainage of aqueous humor and to decrease the amount of humor produced. Consistent, accurate medication administration will reduce intraocular pressure and may prevent eye pain.

6. Continued pain can cause increased anxiety and stress, leading to increased intraocular pressure.

7. Alternative measures such as cold eye compresses may decrease painful eye spasms. Relaxation techniques and meditation, as well as a quiet room with decreased stimuli, may reduce the perception of pain.

8. Stress may increase intraocular pressure. Knowledge and modification of individual stressors, such as worry, fear, anxiety, and anger, may decrease intraocular pressure and pain.

9. The patient who is well prepared for new procedures and events experiences less stress.

10. Rationales: _____

Target outcome criteria

Within 30 minutes of the occurrence of intraocular pain, the patient will verbalize the absence or relief of pain.

By the time of discharge, the patient will:
• practice selected noninvasive pain relief measures
• identify stressors that may increase pain.

Nursing diagnosis: *High risk for injury related to decreased visual fields, medically induced blurred vision, use of eye patches, and hesitancy in walking*

NURSING PRIORITY: Prevent patient injury.

Interventions

1. Assess the patient's vision. Document blurred vision, the amount of peripheral vision, blindness, or patched eyes.

2. Assess for and document signs of decreasing vision each shift.

3. Orient the patient to the environment.

4. Ensure that items are placed within the patient's maximum field of vision.

5. Illuminate the room adequately, and provide a night light.

6. Place the bed in a low position with the wheels locked.

7. Teach the patient the side effects of medications.

8. Encourage the patient to ask for assistance, as needed. Instruct the patient to avoid activities that may increase intraocular pressure, such as coughing, vomiting, bending at the waist, squeezing the eyes, and straining at stool.

9. Additional individualized interventions: _____

_____

Rationales

1. Unable to see all or part of the environment as a result of tunnel or blurred vision, the patient may knock over, bump into, or fall over objects. Awareness of the patient's limitations helps determine what to teach about environmental hazards and if objects should be rearranged.

2. As the patient's visual acuity decreases, the potential for injury increases.

3. A thorough knowledge of surroundings, including the call system and available nurse assistance, decreases the possibility of falls or injury.

4. Placing objects within the patient's reach and sight will decrease the potential for self-injury and feelings of dependence on the health team. Thereafter, the environment should never be rearranged without first notifying the patient. Move unneeded objects out of the room so that the patient will not fall over them or bump into them.

5. When a patient has blurred or decreased vision, it is even more difficult to see in a dimly lit room. Appropriate lighting facilitates safety and decreases the patient's risk of self-injury.

6. The patient's potential for injury is reduced if the bed is at an appropriate level at all times.

7. Knowledge that vision may be further impaired after medication administration will alert the patient to the need for increased safety measures.

8. Calling for assistance may prevent falls and injuries, and instruction may keep the patient from engaging in activities that will increase intraocular pressure.

9. Rationales: _____

_____

Target outcome criteria

By the time of discharge, the patient will:
• have experienced no falls or injuries
• list safety measures necessary to prevent injury

• adjust to limitations on movement and activity.

Nursing diagnosis: *Fear related to previous vision loss, possible surgery, and possible total blindness*

NURSING PRIORITY: Comfort and support the patient.

Interventions

1. Encourage expression of feelings.

2. Provide a quiet environment.

3. Explain the need for frequent administration of ocular medications, tonometry readings, and physical assessments.

4. Support preferred coping styles.

5. Explore the patient's strengths, and introduce resources to help the patient cope with the fear of blindness.

6. Observe for excessive stress levels resulting from fear.

7. Observe for evidence of a positive response to therapy.

8. Additional individualized interventions: _____

_____

Rationales

1. Expressing fear, along with associated feelings of anger and helplessness, may assist the patient in coping. Listening attentively, providing consistency in caregivers, reassuring the patient that support is available, and communicating sensitivity to the patient's problem encourages expression of feelings. Reinforcing that the patient's response is appropriate helps to develop the trust necessary for sharing of feelings.

2. The sudden onset of symptoms and the presence of pain, as in acute angle-closure glaucoma, may be very frightening. A quiet and distraction-free environment may reduce the patient's stress while facilitating the effect of prescribed medications. As intraocular pressure and symptoms subside, fear may decrease.

3. Explaining each step of the therapy may reduce the patient's fear of the unknown and promote adjustment to the new routines.

4. Ascertaining how the patient normally copes with fear and encouraging the use of those coping strategies, while offering comfort and support, may help reduce the fear. Offering feedback about expressed feelings and supporting realistic perceptions may help the patient cope with the fear of blindness.

5. Focusing on strengths and capabilities may help the patient recognize the ability to cope with fear of the future regardless of outcome. Introducing the patient to a person coping successfully with glaucoma may also be helpful.

6. The patient may be stressed to the point of incapacitation. Early intervention is needed to prevent this reaction because treatment requires the participation of a calm, relaxed patient.

7. Reduced fear and increased comfort indicate the patient is responding in a positive manner and is coping effectively with fear.

8. Rationales: _____

_____

Target outcome criteria
Within 2 days of admission, the patient will:
• verbalize fears
• exhibit calm, relaxed facial expression, body movements, and behavior.

Nursing diagnosis: *Knowledge deficit related to the disease and surgery*

NURSING PRIORITY: Increase the patient's knowledge about the surgery.

Interventions

1. Provide preoperative teaching for the patient who will have eye surgery. (See the "Surgical Intervention" plan, page 81, for details.) Assess the patient's level of knowledge regarding the disease, and incorporate relevant pathophysiology into the teaching, as needed, to correct any misconceptions.

2. Explain noninvasive procedures, such as laser iridotomy or laser trabeculoplasty, if appropriate.

3. Explain surgical peripheral iridectomy or trabeculectomy, as appropriate.

4. Explain diathermy, cryothermy, or ultrasound therapy, as appropriate.

5. Provide instruction about the postoperative routine, precautions, and signs of complications. Explain the increased risk for injury related to the eye patch, possible poor vision in the other eye, and frustration from dependence on others and activity restrictions.

6. Administer medication as needed and encourage the patient to dim room lights and wear dark glasses.

7. Prevent infection by washing hands before administering eye drops or changing a patch, keeping the tip of the eyedropper sterile, and checking regularly for drainage.

8. Additional individualized interventions:_____

Rationales

1. The patient is awake during eye surgery and must be cooperative. Information about the procedure and correction of misconceptions allays anxieties and helps ensure cooperation. Procedures include classic surgical (cutting) techniques, such as iridectomy and trabeculectomy, and laser techniques (iridotomy and trabeculoplasty). Surgery is usually necessary with acute angle-closure glaucoma.

2. These procedures involve less risk than surgery, are more cost-effective, and can be done in an outpatient setting. Intraocular pressure is checked after 2 hours and then in 24 hours. Discomfort is usually limited to headaches and blurred vision. Glaucoma medications are continued at least until the first checkup.

3. Iridectomy is used for acute angle-closure glaucoma; trabeculectomy or iridectomy is used for simple chronic glaucoma.

4. These techniques partially destroy cells of the ciliary body to reduce aqueous production. The patient is observed for several hours before discharge.

5. The patient's understanding of the postoperative routine will help avoid complications. Intraocular hemorrhage may be related to improper positioning or increased intraocular pressure. Intraocular pressure can be increased by sneezing, coughing, bending, vomiting, straining with bowel movement, or lifting heavy objects.

6. The eye will be sensitive to light after the eye patch is removed.

7. Eye infection may cause vision loss and negate the effects of surgery.

8. Rationales: _____

Target outcome criteria
By the day of surgery, the patient will:
• verbalize understanding of preoperative instructions
• verbalize understanding of surgery and postoperative routines
• identify signs of postoperative complications and list ways to prevent them.

By the time of discharge, the patient will have demonstrated the proper technique for administration of eye drops.

EYE DISORDERS

Discharge planning

NURSING DISCHARGE CRITERIA

Upon discharge, documentation shows evidence of:
• stable intraocular pressure within acceptable limits, controlled by ocular medications or surgery
• healthy coping behaviors regarding vision loss and possibility of total blindness
• an understanding of glaucoma, glaucoma management, and signs and symptoms of increasing intraocular pressure
• an understanding of the pharmacologic regimen and the reasons for lifelong treatment.

PATIENT-FAMILY TEACHING CHECKLIST

Document evidence that the patient and family demonstrate an understanding of:
___ all discharge medications' purpose, dosage, which eye to medicate, administration schedule and technique, and adverse effects requiring medical attention (usual discharge medications include adrenergics, cholinergics, carbonic anhydrase inhibitors, and beta-adrenergic blockers)
___ infection prevention
___ need to avoid nonprescription medications
___ need to avoid medications that dilate the pupils
___ signs and symptoms indicating increasing intraocular pressure, such as aching around the eye or any changes in vision
___ date, time, and location of follow-up appointments and importance of lifelong medical supervision
___ when and how to report any reappearance of symptoms or stressful events to the ophthalmologist
___ safety precautions in taking eye medications, such as carrying medications when away from home, having a reserve bottle of eye drops at home, and knowing which local pharmacies are open late in case of emergency
___ factors that increase risk of injury
___ need to assess safety of home environment
___ safety measures to use or the need for assistance when performing tasks that require clear vision
___ circumstances that may increase intraocular pressure, such as emotional upsets, fatigue, constrictive clothing, heavy exertion, and sexual activity
___ recommended activities and precautions, such as exercise in moderation, moderate reading and television watching, maintenance of regular bowel habits, and no driving for 2 hours after administration of ocular drugs
___ transportation alternatives
___ ways to mobilize support systems
___ ways to adjust to social situations in view of vision loss and need to follow medication routine
___ need for potassium supplement or high-potassium foods if acetazolamide is prescribed
___ need to alert health care providers about diagnosis and continued need for prescribed eye drops
___ importance of wearing a medical alert tag indicating glaucoma diagnosis.

DOCUMENTATION CHECKLIST

Using outcome criteria as a guide, document:
___ clinical status on admission
___ significant changes in status, especially regarding vision, headaches, and eye pain
___ results of ophthalmoscopy, tonometry, gonioscopy, tonography, and visual field determination
___ episodes of eye pain or headache
___ episodes of nausea, vomiting, or abdominal pain
___ pain relief measures
___ serial tonometry results
___ surgery or ocular medication management
___ nutrition intake
___ patient-family teaching
___ discharge planning.

ASSOCIATED PLANS OF CARE

Grieving
Ineffective Individual Coping
Knowledge Deficit
Pain
Surgical Intervention

References

Hamrick, S. and Meredith, L.L. "Therapeutic Ultrasound, A Precise Noninvasive Therapy for Glaucoma," *AORN Journal* 47(4):950-60, April 1988.

Ignatavicius, D.D., and Bayne, M.V. *Medical-Surgical Nursing, A Nursing Process Approach*. Philadelphia: W.B. Saunders Co., 1991.

Langseth, F.G. "Transscleral Cyclophotocoagulation: A Laser Treatment for Glaucoma," *AORN Journal* 48(6):1122-27, December 1988.

Lehne, R.A., et al. *Pharmacology for Nursing Care*. Philadelphia: W.B. Saunders Co., 1990.

Thompson, J.M., et al. *Mosby's Manual of Clinical Nursing*, 2nd ed. St. Louis: Mosby-Year Book, 1989.

EYE DISORDERS
Retinal Detachment

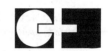

DRG information
DRG 036 Retinal Procedures.
    Mean LOS = 2.3 days
DRG 046 Other Disorders of the Eye. Age 17+ with
    Complication or Comorbidity (CC).
    Mean LOS = 4.2 days
DRG 047 Other Disorders of the Eye. Age 17+ with-
    out CC.
    Mean LOS = 2.6 days
DRG 048 Other Disorders of the Eye. Age 0 to 17.
    Mean LOS = 2.9 days

Additional DRG information: If retinal detachment cannot or should not be repaired surgically, DRG 046,
047, or 048 would be used. If surgery is attempted,
DRG 036 would be used. Although the mean LOS for
each DRG is between 2.5 and 3.8 days, it would not be
unusual for a patient with a retinal detachment to be
discharged the day of or the day after the surgical
procedure. Therefore, the patient's home support system should be carefully analyzed and a referral to
home care should *always* be considered.

Introduction
DEFINITION AND TIME FOCUS
Retinal detachment (RD) is the separation of the
neural retinal layer (rods and cones) from the pigment
epithelium layer of the retina. RD most commonly results from the entry of vitreous humor (a liquid)
through a hole or tear into the potential space between
the layers. Blindness can occur unless the separation
is treated surgically. This clinical plan focuses on the
patient admitted for surgical treatment of RD.

ETIOLOGY AND PRECIPITATING FACTORS
• myopic eye, causing thinness of the retina and vitreous degeneration
• aphakic eye (absent lens), causing distortion of the
eye
• degenerative systemic or eye disease (hypertension,
diabetic retinopathy, or tumors) that causes separation
or traction on the retina from holes, hemorrhage, or
anatomic distortion
• trauma to the head or eye that causes tearing (rip-
ping) of the retina
• strenuous physical exertion that causes separation
from increased pressure within the eye

Focused assessment guidelines
NURSING HISTORY (Functional health pattern findings)

Health perception—health management pattern
• may report vision loss: unilateral and blurred, like a
veil or like a blind being drawn over the eye
• may report flashing lights, usually lasting seconds
• may report floating spots (floaters), typically red
blood cells (RBCs)
• may be under treatment for diabetes mellitus, hypertension, or an eye condition
• may have a black eye or a history of head trauma
• if over age 40, may be at higher risk

Activity-exercise pattern
• may report an incident of heavy straining coinciding
with onset of vision changes

Cognitive-perceptual pattern
• may not recall or relate present condition to previous
occurrence of blow to head or eye
• usually does not report pain

Self-perception—self-concept pattern
• may express fears about the effects of vision loss on
mobility and work

Role-relationship pattern
• may express concern about ability to take care of
family

Value-belief pattern
• may express disbelief over suddenness of vision loss

PHYSICAL FINDINGS
Cardiovascular
• hypertension

Neurologic
• usually a sudden decrease in central and peripheral
vision

Integumentary
• if RD was caused by trauma, may have bruising
around eyes

EYE DISORDERS

Musculoskeletal
• hesitancy, awkwardness during ambulation

DIAGNOSTIC STUDIES
• laboratory data — usually reflect no significant abnormalities
• direct and indirect ophthalmoscopic measurements — show a bulging and hanging retina, curved reddish tear, and floating RBCs
• visual field and acuity examinations — show unilateral vision loss opposite the area of detachment
• biomicroscopy — may indicate proliferation of cells along retinal and vitreous surfaces (proliferative vitreoretinopathy)
• ultrasonography — identifies areas of detachment

POTENTIAL COMPLICATIONS
• permanent loss of vision
• extension of RD
• RD in other eye
• retinal hemorrhage
• infection (scleral, choroidal, or retinal)
• intolerance to scleral circling or buckling devices (bands or implants that serve to indent the eye inward)
• referred pain to face and head on affected side
• exposure of sutures or implanted devices
• endophthalmitis (inflammation of the inner eye)
• vitreal fibroblastic growth
• sympathetic ophthalmia in the other eye

Collaborative problem: *High risk for further loss of vision related to extension of detachment while awaiting surgical intervention*

NURSING PRIORITY: Prevent or minimize further vision loss during the preoperative period.

Interventions

1. Evaluate and document visual acuity and visual fields on admission, every 2 hours, and as needed.

2. Restrict movement. Place the patient on continuous bed rest. Position the head with the affected area lowermost.

3. Pad one or both eyes, as ordered, either continuously or intermittently.

4. Additional individualized interventions: _____

Rationales

1. Changes in visual acuity and visual fields may indicate worsening detachment. Sudden loss of central vision, such as inability to read, may indicate detachment in the macular area. Increased blurring or number of floaters may indicate hemorrhage.

2. Rest decreases the risk of further detachment. A dependent position helps reattachment by gravity.

3. Eye pads rest the eyes and prevent rapid eye movements, which may increase fluid accumulation between the retinal layers.

4. Rationales: _____

Target outcome criteria
Throughout the preoperative period, the patient will:
• show no further vision loss
• maintain activity and position limitations.

Collaborative problem: *High risk for loss of vision related to postoperative extension of tear or nonapproximation of retinal layers; retinal hemorrhage; or eye infection*

NURSING PRIORITY: Prevent complications that could cause further vision loss after surgery.

Interventions

1. Verify specific postoperative positioning restrictions with the doctor. Inform the patient about the restrictions. Place the patient on bed rest or limited activity for 1 to 2 days. Position the head with detached area lowermost, unless an air bubble has been injected. Position the patient who has an air bubble (injected into the eye cavity) so that the air bubble will rise against the detachment and remain there (usually this requires a face-down position with the head turned to the side just enough for the patient to breathe); maintain the face-down position for several days while the patient is in bed, eating, using the commode, or ambulating.

2. Teach the patient to avoid quick, jerking head movements, such as hair combing, face washing, teeth brushing, head turning, shampooing, and coughing; rapid eye movements, such as those involved in reading or doing crafts; vomiting; and Valsalva's maneuver.

3. After eye pads are changed (within 1 to 2 days), instruct the patient to report any vision changes or other physical symptoms immediately.

4. Give antiemetics, as needed, for nausea.

5. Give antibiotics, as ordered, to prevent infection.

6. Monitor continually for such complications as retinal hemorrhage, evidenced by vision changes and the appearance of floaters.

7. Incorporate relevant teaching into all interventions.

8. Additional individualized interventions: _____

_____

Rationales

1. Rest decreases the risk of detachment while the area is healing. Maintaining the affected area in a dependent position aids approximation of the layers and development of adhesion scars. The air bubble provides traction against the area and promotes adherence of the layers. The air bubble is absorbed into the surrounding tissue in 5 to 10 days.

2. Jerking head movements, rapid eye movements, vomiting, Valsalva's maneuver, and other quickly executed activities increase intraocular pressure—and the risk of detachment.

3. Changes in visual fields or vision acuity may indicate detachment.

4. Vomiting increases intraocular pressure and can cause detachment.

5. Infection increases the risk of vision loss.

6. Complications such as hemorrhage can increase the risk of nonapproximation of retinal layers.

7. A knowledgeable patient is more likely to comply with recommendations and to recognize complications.

8. Rationales: _____

_____

Target outcome criteria
Within the immediate postoperative period, the patient will:
• show no further vision loss
• have no nausea or vomiting
• maintain position and activity limitations
• remain free from complications, such as hemorrhage or infection.

Within 3 days of surgery, the patient will be able to describe signs and symptoms of recurrent retinal detachment.

EYE DISORDERS

Nursing diagnosis: *Eye pain related to postoperative inflammation*

NURSING PRIORITY: Relieve eye pain.

Interventions

1. Assess the patient for pain immediately after surgery and every 2 hours thereafter.

2. Administer analgesics, as ordered and needed. Document pain episodes and medication. Apply moist compresses, as ordered.

3. Keep the room dark and quiet immediately after surgery and as needed.

4. Avoid direct pressure to the eyeball.

5. Additional individualized interventions: _____

Rationales

1. Mild pain is expected after surgery; however, a sudden change in pain may indicate complications.

2. Pain increases intraocular pressure and the risk of detachment. Moist compresses reduce swelling and relieve pain.

3. Reduced light and noise may diminish the effects of photophobia caused by mydriatics and swelling.

4. External pressure may increase intraocular pressure, pain, and risk of detachment.

5. Rationales:_____

Target outcome criteria
Within 1 day after surgery, the patient will:
• verbalize the absence or relief of pain
• have no swelling
• show a relaxed posture and facial expression.

Nursing diagnosis: *Impaired physical mobility related to position and activity limitations*

NURSING PRIORITY: Prevent complications related to immobility.

Interventions

1. See the "Surgical Intervention" plan, page 81.

2. Encourage isometric, deep breathing, and range-of-motion exercises hourly while the patient is awake. Caution the patient to avoid coughing and Valsalva's maneuver.

3. Consult the doctor regarding activity progression. Maintain the head in the desired dependent position while the patient is ambulating, as ordered.

4. Instruct the patient about post-discharge activity:
• moderate, unhurried activities for the first few weeks, avoiding jerking the head or straining (such as by reading, bending the head below the waist, or driving)
• light activities by 3 weeks (such as light secretarial work)
• by 6 weeks, heavy work, sex, and exercise.

5. Additional individualized interventions: _____

Rationales

1. The "Surgical Intervention" plan contains general interventions related to postoperative immobility.

2. These activities will prevent venous stasis, skin breakdown, and atelectasis. Coughing and Valsalva's maneuver increase intraocular pressure.

3. Most patients are ambulatory by the second day after surgery. Maintaining a dependent head position will aid in scar formation and adherence of retinal layers.

4. Abrupt or vigorous changes in position associated with activity increase the risk of detachment. Lowering the head below the waist or leaning over a bowl to shampoo hair increases intraocular pressure and jeopardizes reattachment. Gradual resumption allows activity increase to parallel healing.

5. Rationales: _____

Target outcome criteria
Within 3 days after surgery, the patient will:
• have no skin breakdown
• exhibit clear lungs
• show no further vision loss.

Nursing diagnosis: *High risk for injury related to vision loss or eye pads*

NURSING PRIORITY: Prevent injuries.

Interventions	**Rationales**
1. Before surgery, after surgery, and as needed, provide orientation to the room, including the bathroom, call light, telephone, bed controls, and position of furniture.	1. Knowledge of the location of furniture and equipment needed for activities of daily living (ADLs) will help prevent patient falls and injuries.
2. Explain procedures as they are done.	2. Concurrent explanations relieve the patient's anxiety and help the patient anticipate the nurse's touch.
3. Document vision limitations on the Kardex.	3. A Kardex record will be available to other personnel to aid in providing continuity of care.
4. Additional individualized interventions: _____	4. Rationales: _____

Target outcome criteria

Within 2 hours after surgery, the patient will be reoriented to the environment.

During the hospital stay, the patient will:
• be free from injury
• be able to perform ADLs with minimal assistance.

Nursing diagnosis: *Anxiety related to fear of blindness*

NURSING PRIORITIES: (a) Reduce anxiety to a tolerable level, and (b) provide realistic reassurance.

Interventions	**Rationales**
1. During the provision of care, elicit and accept the patient's expressions of fear and anxiety. Help the patient identify and prioritize problems.	1. Identifying the most significant components of the threat of blindness helps the patient regain control and initiate contingency planning.
2. Offer realistic reassurance.	2. A large majority of retinal reattachments restore vision.
3. If the eye or eyes are patched, check the patient frequently, anticipate needs, speak when approaching the bedside, and use touch to offer reassurance.	3. Inability to see increases the sense of helplessness, further contributing to anxiety. Speaking on approach alerts the patient. Because the patient cannot perceive the usual visual cues, touch may be especially meaningful.
4. Additional individualized interventions: _____	4. Rationales: _____

Target outcome criteria

Within 3 days after surgery, the patient will:
• have a relaxed facial expression
• identify specific fears related to potential blindness

• verbalize a realistic perception of the prognosis.

EYE DISORDERS

Nursing diagnosis: *Diversional activity deficit related to postoperative activity limitation*

NURSING PRIORITY: Promote allowable activities.

Interventions

1. Provide diversional activities that do not cause rapid eye movement or head jerking, such as radio, television, conversation, books, and visitors.

2. Additional individualized interventions: _____

_____

Rationales

1. Such activities will help heal the retinal tear while relieving boredom and reducing isolation.

2. Rationales: _____

_____

Target outcome criteria
Throughout the hospital stay, the patient will:
• accept activity restriction
• have no further vision loss or other complications

• spend time daily visiting with friends and family.

Discharge planning
NURSING DISCHARGE CRITERIA
Upon discharge, documentation shows evidence of:
• absence of infection and pain
• ability to manage ADLs with minimal limitations
• ability to ambulate with minimal assistance
• stable vital signs and absence of pulmonary or cardiovascular complications
• expected amount of restored vision or ability to accept vision deficit
• ability to follow activity restrictions
• adequate home support system
• referral to home care if support system is inadequate or if further teaching is warranted
• knowledge of how to contact community resources that offer support to visually impaired persons.

PATIENT-FAMILY TEACHING CHECKLIST
Document evidence that the patient and family demonstrate an understanding of:
__ extent of vision loss (if any) and expected time period needed for further return of vision
__ all discharge medications' purpose, which eye to medicate, dosage, administration schedule, and adverse effects requiring medical attention (usual discharge medications include mydriatics)
__ activity limitations
__ signs and symptoms indicating detachment, such as changes in vision or seeing flashes of light
__ date, time, and location of follow-up appointments
__ community resources for the visually impaired.

DOCUMENTATION CHECKLIST
Using outcome criteria as a guide, document:
__ clinical status on admission
__ significant changes in status
__ pertinent laboratory and diagnostic test findings
__ vision changes
__ pain relief measures
__ activity and position restrictions
__ nutritional intake
__ other therapies
__ patient-family teaching
__ discharge planning.

ASSOCIATED PLANS OF CARE
Grieving
Ineffective Individual Coping
Knowledge Deficit
Pain
Surgical Intervention

References
Beare, P.G., and Myers, J.L., eds. *Principles and Practice of Adult Health Nursing.* St. Louis: Mosby-Year Book, 1990.
Mrochuk, J. "Introduction to Diagnostic Ophthalmologic Ultrasound for Nurses in Ophthalmology," *Journal of Ophthalmologic Nursing and Technology.* 9(6):234-39, 1990.
"Retinal Detachment," *Lippincott Manual of Nursing Practice,* 5th ed. Philadelphia: J.B. Lippincott, 1991.

Adult Respiratory Distress Syndrome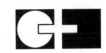

DRG information

DRG 099 Respiratory Signs and Symptoms. With Complication or Cormorbidity (CC).
Mean LOS = 4.4 days
Principal diagnoses include:
• adult respiratory distress syndrome (ARDS)
• dyspnea and other respiratory abnormalities
• hemoptysis
• cough.

DRG 100 Respiratory Signs and Symptoms. Without CC.
Mean LOS = 2.7 days
Principal diagnoses include selected principal diagnoses listed under DRG 099. The distinction is that DRG 100 excludes CC.

DRG 087 Pulmonary Edema and Respiratory Failure.
Mean LOS = 6.0 days
Principal diagnoses include:
• ARDS caused by trauma or after surgery
• respiratory failure
• pulmonary edema.

DRG 475 Respiratory System Diagnosis With Ventilator Support.
Mean LOS = 9.7 days
Principal diagnoses include:
• respiratory failure
• chronic obstructive pulmonary disease
• acute or chronic bronchitis
• pneumonia from various causes
• ARDS.

Additional DRG information: ARDS is rarely a principal diagnosis. It is usually a CC to other diseases, trauma, or surgery. Used as a secondary diagnosis, it can increase a particular DRG's weight because it qualifies as a CC. The above DRGs, however, are calculated with ARDS as a principal diagnosis.

Introduction
DEFINITION AND TIME FOCUS

ARDS is a complex, poorly understood syndrome of diffuse damage to the alveolar-capillary membrane. The most common cause of respiratory failure in the critical care setting, ARDS may represent the ultimate manifestation of several unrelated physiologic insults that produce direct or indirect pulmonary injury. Key clinical features necessary for its diagnosis include a history consistent with ARDS, moderate to severe hypoxemia, bilateral diffuse infiltrates on chest X-ray, and exclusion of other causes of pulmonary congestion, specifically left-sided heart failure.

Known by many other names (such as noncardiogenic pulmonary edema, shock lung, and postpump lung), ARDS is characterized by interstitial and alveolar pulmonary edema resulting from increased permeability of the pulmonary microvasculature. Other key pathophysiologic features include a massive pulmonary shunt, decreased lung compliance, and increased alveolar dead space. On autopsy, lungs are heavy and wet, demonstrating congestive atelectasis, and marked by hyaline membrane formation and pulmonary fibrosis.

The chemical mediators involved in ARDS are complex and poorly understood. One theory is that in sepsis, bacteria stimulate granulocytes lodged in the lung. The resulting oxidative burst releases toxic metabolites (such as free radicals) and proteolytic enzymes, both of which can cause severe pulmonary injury. Other chemical mediators include histamine, serotonin, and prostaglandins. This plan focuses on the critically ill patient with a recent diagnosis of ARDS.

ETIOLOGY AND PRECIPITATING FACTORS
• gram-negative sepsis, *Pneumocystis carinii* pneumonia, bacterial or viral pneumonia, or other infections
• aspiration of gastric contents, fresh or salt water (near drowning), or other liquids
• pulmonary contusion, nonthoracic trauma, burns, or other types of trauma
• inhalation of smoke, toxic levels of oxygen, corrosive chemicals, or other toxins
• shock
• fat embolism, cardiopulmonary bypass, massive transfusions, disseminated intravascular coagulation, transfusion reaction, or other hematologic causes
• drug overdose, particularly heroin, methadone (Dolophine), and propoxyphene (Darvon)

Focused assessment guidelines
NURSING HISTORY (Functional health pattern findings)

Health perception—health management pattern
• history of catastrophic pulmonary insult followed by a lag time of several hours to several days and then progressive dyspnea

PHYSICAL FINDINGS
General appearance
• restlessness

Pulmonary
• tachypnea
• hyperventilation
• progressive dyspnea
• fine, diffuse crackles
• increased peak inspiratory pressure (if on ventilator)

Neurologic
• deteriorating level of consciousness

Integumentary
• cyanosis

DIAGNOSTIC STUDIES

Note: No single diagnostic test exists for ARDS.
• arterial blood gas (ABG) values—reveal moderate to severe hypoxemia (partial pressure of arterial oxygen [PaO$_2$] less than 50 mm Hg), even when the inspired oxygen concentration is greater than 60%, and hypercapnia (partial pressure of arterial carbon dioxide [PaCO$_2$] greater than 50 mm Hg)
• alveolar-arterial gradient—reveals increased gradient (greater than 15 mm Hg on room air or greater than 50 mm Hg on 100% oxygen)
• shunt calculation—reveals pulmonary shunt in excess of 5%, typically 20% to 30%
• bronchial fluid protein to serum protein ratio— greater than 0.5, indicating unusually high protein concentration in the bronchial fluid (implying that a damaged alveolar-capillary membrane is allowing proteins to leak through capillary walls)

• chest X-ray—reveals bilaterally diffuse infiltrates
• lung compliance—reduced below 50 ml/cm H$_2$O, typically 20 to 30 ml/cm H$_2$O
• pulmonary capillary wedge pressure—normal or only slightly elevated (less than 15 mm Hg), indicating that left-sided heart failure is not causing pulmonary congestion
• functional residual capacity—reduced

POTENTIAL COMPLICATIONS
• respiratory arrest
• respiratory failure
• pulmonary fibrosis
• disseminated intravascular coagulation
• persistent pulmonary function abnormalities after recovery (such as mild restrictive disease, impaired gas transfer, or expiratory small airway obstruction)

Collaborative problem: *Hypoxemia related to pulmonary shunt, interstitial edema, and alveolar edema*

NURSING PRIORITIES: (a) Prevent further deterioration of lung function, (b) support the lung during healing, and (c) maintain oxygenation.

Interventions

1. Monitor for clinical signs and symptoms:

• initial insult period—persistent unexplained mild tachypnea, breathlessness, air hunger, and normal breath sounds

• latent period—persistent moderate tachypnea; increasing dyspnea; neck, chest, or abdominal muscle use; fatigue; restlessness; confusion; and crackles

• progressive pulmonary insufficiency—severe tachypnea and hyperventilation, progressive dyspnea, gurgles, and deteriorating level of consciousness

• terminal stage—depressed level of consciousness, arrhythmias, and profound shock leading to asystole.

Rationales

1. Clinical signs and symptoms, when correlated with ABG values and chest X-ray results, indicate the syndrome's progression.

• The catastrophic insult is followed by a variable lag period before signs and symptoms appear. About 60% of ARDS patients develop clinical indicators within 24 hours, 30% within 24 to 72 hours, and 10% after 72 hours. During the initial insult, signs and symptoms are mild and nonspecific. Tachypnea despite a normal PaO$_2$, the most characteristic finding, probably results from stimulation of juxtacapillary receptors in the alveolar interstitium.

• Signs and symptoms during the latent phase reflect borderline hypoxemia and interstitial edema.

• As the syndrome worsens, respiratory distress becomes marked. Increased dead space creates a need for high minute volumes while decreasing compliance creates a need for high inspiratory pressures. The continuing capillary leak produces frank alveolar edema, and the massive pulmonary shunt produces hypoxemia.

• In the terminal stage, hypoxemia refractory to therapy produces profound brain and heart dysfunction, terminating in cardiopulmonary arrest.

2. Obtain chest X-ray daily, as ordered, and monitor serial findings. Be alert for reports indicating patchy infiltrates or "white out." Also note any other abnormal findings.

3. Obtain ABG values at least every 4 hours, as ordered. Note degree of hypoxemia and any acid-base imbalance, typically:
• normal PaO_2, mild hypocapnia, and respiratory alkalosis during the insult period

• borderline hypoxemia during the latent period

• progressive hypoxemia, increasing hypercapnia, and worsening respiratory and metabolic acidosis as pulmonary insufficiency becomes more pronounced

• refractory hypoxemia, hypercapnia, and severe respiratory and metabolic acidosis during the terminal stage.

4. Continuously monitor gas exchange status, as ordered, by monitoring arterial hemoglobin saturation (SaO_2) with a pulse oximeter or monitoring mixed venous oxygen saturation ($S\bar{v}O_2$) with an $S\bar{v}O_2$ catheter. Monitoring the end tidal carbon dioxide ($EtCO_2$) level can also be helpful.

5. Prepare for endotracheal intubation if the respiratory rate exceeds 30 breaths/minute and the patient is:
• elderly, chronically ill, or suffering from preexisting pulmonary disease
• fatigued
• exhibiting an increasing $PaCO_2$.

6. Implement mechanical ventilation, as ordered. See the "Mechanical Ventilation" plan, page 227.

2. Chest X-rays are used to monitor the degree of edema and the development of complications. During the initial insult, the X-ray typically is normal. Patchy infiltrates appear during the latent period, worsen during pulmonary insufficiency, and culminate in a complete "white out" in the terminal stage.

3. ABG values provide a way to assess and document gas exchange abnormalities.

• During the insult period, tachypnea maintains a normal PaO_2, but the accompanying carbon dioxide blow-off produces hypocapnia and respiratory alkalosis.
• Borderline hypoxemia reflects early impairment of gas diffusion.
• Hypercapnia develops later because carbon dioxide is much more diffusible than oxygen. Carbon dioxide retention produces respiratory acidosis. The worsening oxygen deprivation causes cells to switch from aerobic to anaerobic metabolism, resulting in lactic acidosis.
• Refractory hypoxemia results from a massive pulmonary shunt. Interstitial edema compresses alveoli, while alveolar edema fills them with fluid. In either case, the alveoli cannot oxygenate capillary blood flowing past them. The resulting perfusion without ventilation converts the alveolar-capillary units to shunt units. Without open alveoli, supplemental oxygen cannot physically reach capillary blood.

4. Conventional ABG sampling provides only an intermittent indicator of gas exchange, and there is a delay before the results are available. Continuous monitoring provides constant, real-time data useful in detecting impending deterioration, monitoring the effects of nursing interventions, and titrating the effects of multiple interventions that may have opposing effects on oxygenation and cardiac output, such as administering dopamine (Intropin) and nitroprusside (Nipride) to a patient on positive-pressure ventilation and positive end-expiratory pressure (PEEP). Pulse oximetry monitors oxygen supplied to tissues, whereas $S\bar{v}O_2$ monitoring indicates tissue oxygen consumption. $EtCO_2$ evaluates ventilation.

5. Endotracheal intubation is usually necessary to protect the airway and allow for delivery of high levels of oxygen and PEEP. Advanced age, chronic illness, or preexisting pulmonary disease increase the likelihood the patient will be unable to tolerate the rapid respiratory rate. Fatigue and increasing $PaCO_2$ are ominous signs indicating inadequate spontaneous ventilation.

6. The widespread pulmonary congestion impairs alveolar expansion. Surfactant production decreases, making alveoli even more difficult to expand. The high inspiratory pressures required to expand alveoli and the high minute volume needed to compensate for increased physiologic dead space increase the work of breathing so markedly that patient cannot maintain spontaneous ventilation. In addition, hypoxemia makes the patient prone to respiratory arrest. Mechanical ventilation conserves the patient's energy, prevents respiratory arrest, and allows time for the lung injury to heal.

7. Implement PEEP, as ordered, typically if an inspired oxygen concentration greater than 50% is needed for more than 24 hours or if PaO_2 falls below 50 mm Hg even though oxygen concentration exceeds 60%.

7. PEEP, a mainstay in the treatment of ARDS, is believed to increase alveolar size and restore alveolar ventilation. It thus increases functional residual capacity, decreases shunting, improves ventilation-perfusion matching, and improves compliance.

8. Monitor compliance, as described in the "Mechanical Ventilation" plan, page 227.

8. Compliance objectively measures the ease of lung expansion. Decreasing compliance, implying increasing lung stiffness, indicates that ARDS is worsening. Interpreting compliance values is covered in the "Mechanical Ventilation" plan.

9. Administer medications, as ordered. Document effectiveness and observe for adverse reactions.
• corticosteroids, typically methylprednisolone (Solu-Medrol)

9. Medications have limited effectiveness in ARDS but may be prescribed empirically.
• Corticosteroid administration in ARDS is controversial. Although anecdotal reports and limited clinical and animal studies suggest possible effectiveness in certain types of ARDS, such as radiation pneumonitis, no randomized, controlled study in humans has demonstrated their effectiveness.

• antibiotics

• Antibiotics are usually prescribed for suspected or documented infection. Although many doctors prescribe them prophylactically in ARDS, such use has not been proven effective.

10. Additional individualized interventions: _____

10. Rationales: _____

_____

_____

Target outcome criteria
Within 5 days of the initial insult and continuously thereafter, the patient will:
• display eupnea
• have a respiratory rate of 12 to 20 breaths/minute
• have clear lung sounds
• display a level of consciousness equal to or better than that on admission
• have normal chest X-rays
• manifest ABG values returning to normal limits
• record an SaO_2 of 95% or better and an $S\bar{v}O_2$ of 60% to 80%, if oximetry is used.

Nursing diagnosis: *High risk for injury: complications related to single or multiple organ failure*

NURSING PRIORITY: Minimize the effects of related organ failure.

Interventions

1. Maintain adequate cardiac output. Assist with pulmonary artery (PA) catheter insertion, if indicated. Monitor PA pressures, vital signs, electrocardiogram, and urine output according to Appendix A, "Monitoring Standards."

2. Administer packed red blood cells, as ordered, to maintain the hemoglobin level at 12 to 15 g/dl.

Rationales

1. Arterial oxygen transport (the amount delivered to the tissues) depends on cardiac output and oxygen content. Close monitoring of hemodynamics is essential: Enough fluid must be given to maintain cardiac output, yet too much fluid worsens the pulmonary capillary leak. A PA catheter is also helpful in differentiating cardiac from noncardiac pulmonary edema.

2. Oxygen content depends on the hemoglobin level, hemoglobin saturation, and PaO_2. This hemoglobin level maintains normal oxygen transport.

3. Administer crystalloid or colloid I.V. fluids, as ordered. Monitor fluid administration meticulously.

4. If the patient has gastric distention, a decreased level of consciousness, or impaired airway protection reflexes, obtain an order to institute gastric drainage.

5. Provide nutritional support, as ordered. See the "Nutritional Deficit" plan, page 63.

6. Maintain strict asepsis. Monitor for signs and symptoms of infection, and document and report them promptly to the doctor. Institute aggressive treatment measures, as ordered.

7. Observe for signs of single or multiple organ failure, especially central nervous system failure, renal failure, and GI dysfunction.

8. Implement general supportive nursing measures to prevent the complications of immobility. See the "Impaired Physical Mobility" plan, page 36.

9. Additional individualized interventions: _____

_____

3. The choice of appropriate fluid in ARDS remains controversial. Crystalloids readily cross from the vascular to the interstitial space, potentially worsening edema. Colloids also cross the leaky capillary membrane, move into the interstitial space, and draw water to them via osmosis, which also worsens edema. Meticulous monitoring helps minimize development of two risk factors for ARDS: shock and fluid overload.

4. Aspiration of gastric contents is a risk factor for ARDS. Gastric drainage can prevent such aspiration.

5. The protracted period of mechanical ventilation necessary for most ARDS patients requires total parenteral nutrition to maintain pulmonary muscle strength and immunologic defense mechanisms.

6. Because sepsis is a common precursor to ARDS, monitoring for signs and symptoms of infection can prove instrumental. A major infection in an ARDS patient is an ominous sign. If the source cannot be identified, the patient is very likely to die. Identification of the source and prompt, aggressive therapy are essential.

7. Failure or dysfunction of additional organ systems appears to be associated with increased mortality in ARDS.

8. The patient on prolonged bed rest is at risk for many complications that worsen lung function, such as pneumonia, atelectasis, and pulmonary embolism. The "Impaired Physical Mobility" plan contains detailed interventions for these and other potential complications.

9. Rationales: _____

_____

Target outcome criteria
Within 24 hours of the initial insult and then continuously, the patient will:
• have a heart rate, blood pressure, and pulmonary artery and wedge pressures within normal limits
• display normal sinus rhythm
• produce an hourly urine output greater than 30 ml
• show no signs of infection.

Nursing diagnosis: *High risk for ineffective individual and family coping related to abrupt onset of life-threatening illness*

NURSING PRIORITY: Maximize the patient's and family's coping skills.

Interventions

1. Implement the measures outlined in the "Ineffective Family Coping" plan, page 47, and the "Ineffective Individual Coping" plan, page 51.

Rationales

1. Whether ARDS occurs after a catastrophic incident, such as trauma, or complicates an already critical illness, its onset can be a cruel blow to the patient and family. The stress of the disease is exacerbated by its treatment, particularly mechanical ventilation, which precludes oral communication at the time when the patient and family most need it. Using the measures detailed in the "Ineffective Family Coping" and "Ineffective Individual Coping" plans not only makes the ordeal more bearable, but also lessens anxiety-induced oxygen requirements.

2. Allow the family to interact with the patient.

2. Interaction with loved ones decreases the patient's sense of isolation and encourages a positive attitude toward treatment.

3. Encourage the patient and family to verbalize feelings about treatments, especially mechanical ventilation.

3. Becoming aware of feelings and expressing them clearly and appropriately are healthy coping behaviors.

4. Provide an alternative means of communication for the patient, such as eye blinks or paper and pencil.

4. Intubation prevents the patient from speaking. Providing an alternative means of communication increases the patient's sense of security and promotes safety.

5. Additional individualized interventions: _____

5. Rationales: _____

Target outcome criteria
See the "Ineffective Family Coping" and "Ineffective Individual Coping" plans.

Discharge planning
NURSING DISCHARGE CRITERIA
Upon the patient's discharge, documentation shows evidence of:
• stable vital signs within normal limits for the patient
• spontaneous respiratory rate of 12 to 24 breaths/minute
• patent airway without endotracheal intubation
• discontinuation of PA catheter.

PATIENT-FAMILY TEACHING CHECKLIST
Document evidence that the patient and family demonstrate an understanding of:
___ definition and pathophysiology of ARDS
___ probable cause
___ prognosis
___ rationale for mechanical ventilation, PEEP, and other therapies.

DOCUMENTATION CHECKLIST
Using outcome criteria as a guide, document:
___ clinical status on admission
___ significant changes in status
___ pertinent diagnostic test findings
___ airway care
___ tolerance of ventilator and PEEP
___ response to medications
___ fluid therapy
___ nutritional support
___ nursing care to combat effects of immobility
___ psychological coping
___ patient-family teaching
___ discharge planning.

ASSOCIATED PLANS OF CARE
Disseminated Intravascular Coagulation
Grieving
Impaired Physical Mobility
Ineffective Family Coping
Ineffective Individual Coping
Mechanical Ventilation
Multiple Trauma
Nutritional Deficit
Sensory-Perceptual Alteration

References
Bernard, G.R., and Bradley, R.B. "Adult Respiratory Distress Syndrome: Diagnosis and Management," *Heart & Lung* 15(3):250-55, May 1986.

Brandstetter, R.D. "The Adult Respiratory Distress Syndrome—1986," *Heart & Lung* 15(2):155-65, March 1986.

Celentano-Norton, L. "Mechanical Ventilation Strategies in Adult Respiratory Distress Syndrome," *Critical Care Nurse* 6(4):71-74, July-August 1986.

Elliott, C.G., et al. "Prediction of Pulmonary Function Abnormalities after Adult Respiratory Distress Syndrome (ARDS)," *American Review of Respiratory Disorders* 135(3):634-38, March 1987.

Hudson, L.D. "The Prediction and Prevention of ARDS," *Respiratory Care* 35(2):161-73, February 1990.

Karnes, N. "Don't Let ARDS Catch You Off Guard," *Nursing87* 17(5):34-38, May 1987.

Asthma

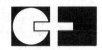

DRG information

DRG 096 Bronchitis and Asthma. Age 17 +. With
      Complication or Comorbidity (CC).
      Mean LOS = 6.0 days
      Principal diagnoses include:
      • bronchitis (acute and chronic)
      • asthma.
DRG 097 Bronchitis and Asthma. Age 17 + to 69.
      Without CC.
      Mean LOS = 4.6 days
DRG 098 Bronchitis and Asthma.
      Age 0 to 17.
      Mean LOS = 4.6 days

Additional DRG information: These DRGs, as well as many others involving respiratory disease, are very difficult to code accurately because of numerous coding nuances. The coders depend entirely on the medical record to determine the correct DRG. The DRGs listed above have very low relative weights and reimbursement rates. However, a patient presenting with these disorders and arterial blood gas (ABG) levels within certain abnormal parameters may be legitimately coded as having respiratory failure, which has a much higher weight and reimbursement rate. Pneumonia would also have a higher weight and reimbursement rate.

Introduction
DEFINITION AND TIME FOCUS

Asthma is characterized by increased responsiveness and hyperreactivity of the tracheal and bronchial smooth muscle to various stimuli, resulting in widespread narrowing of the airways (bronchoconstriction), increased mucus production, mucosal inflammation and edema, and airflow obstruction. These changes are reversible, either spontaneously or as a result of therapy. Between asthma attacks, the individual may remain symptom-free. Attacks vary in severity, from mild obstruction to profound respiratory failure. Status asthmaticus is a nonspecific term used when usual medical treatment fails to relieve severe obstruction.

Asthma is divided into two types:
• extrinsic asthma—childhood onset, usually disappears in the adult; positive family history; usually seasonal; multiple well-defined allergies; positive response to allergy skin testing (indicates an antigen-antibody response)
• intrinsic asthma—seen in adults after age 30; may be more severe in nature and continuous; associated with a history of recurrent respiratory tract infections; multiple nonspecific conditions can provoke an attack; negative response to allergy skin testing.

The adult patient admitted to the acute care setting usually has intrinsic asthma and is in acute respiratory distress. This plan focuses on the patient admitted after self-management or outpatient intervention has failed to terminate an asthma attack.

ETIOLOGY AND PRECIPITATING FACTORS

• acute episode may have numerous causes:
   —infection (viral or bacterial)
   —environmental exposure to a nonspecific allergen (such as secondhand smoke, dust, or cleaning compounds)
   —chronic sinusitis
   —weather changes (such as heat, cold, fog, or wind)
   —exercise
   —regurgitation
   —psychogenic factors
   —ingestion of aspirin (aspirin-sensitive individuals may also be sensitive to indomethacin [Indocin]; mefenamic acid [Ponstel] or tartrazine [yellow dye found in many medications])
• airway response to the causative agent may be immediate or delayed

Focused assessment guidelines
NURSING HISTORY (Functional health pattern findings)

Health perception—health management pattern
• may report increasing shortness of breath, stated as "can't catch breath," "can't inhale," or "hyperventilating"
• may report chest tightness
• describes a panicky, suffocating feeling (typically resists oxygen mask)
• may report increased coughing, often dry and nonproductive, that leaves the patient short of breath
• may report inability to move sputum out of lungs
• attack may have been in progress for some time before admission to the acute-care setting; patient may report increasing fatigue and inability to handle the attack with usual measures
• may no longer be complying with prescribed treatments
• reports using inhalers (either prescription or nonprescription type) continually, without benefit
• may identify certain events or environmental factors as major contributors to the attack's development

Sleep-rest pattern
• may state that cough disturbs sleep

Nutritional-metabolic pattern
• may report dehydration (from shortness of breath, mouth breathing, or reluctance to drink water)
• typically has not eaten since the attack's onset because of preoccupation and shortness of breath; may complain of nausea, which may be related to medication use or abuse
• if a long-term corticosteroid user, may report weight gain

Activity-exercise pattern
• may report ongoing exercise limitations because exercise can cause wheezing and shortness of breath
• if exercise is limited, may report difficulty maintaining desired level of physical conditioning

Cognitive-perceptual pattern
• may be able to describe complex strategies for self-management during an acute attack, but may report inability to put them into effect during an actual attack, when panic may overwhelm problem-solving skills and hypoxemia may impair thinking

Role-relationship pattern
• may avoid public events and activities because of embarrassment from severe dyspnea and cough; may also report that laughing can cause an attack
• may report that spouse or partner as well as family and social groups cause attacks through such environmental irritants as cigarette smoke

Self-perception — self-concept pattern
• if on maintenance corticosteroid therapy, may report changes in body image related to medication's cushingoid effects; may be very discouraged with appearance and inability to prevent or alter physiologic changes

Coping — stress tolerance pattern
• may describe fluctuations in emotions, such as:
  — denial of problem (may ignore potential irritants by refusing to give away a pet, to stop smoking, or to remove offending furniture; may refuse to learn medication routines and self-management strategies)
  — anger (may blame others for causing attack; may describe asthma as a "kid's disease"; may not feel past health habits justify disease's extent)

PHYSICAL FINDINGS
Physical parameters, which vary with the attack's severity, are good indicators of treatment outcomes.

General appearance
• anxious; maintains upright position
• fever, if infection is present

Neurologic
• initially hyperalert, awake, and oriented; may be progressively less alert, although awake and oriented, as fatigue progresses
• restlessness (from hypoxemia)
• lethargy (from increased carbon dioxide levels)

Integumentary
• color initially good; may be flushed; cyanosis a late, unreliable sign
• diaphoresis
• mucous membranes dry from rapid oral breathing and dehydration

Cardiovascular
• sinus tachycardia (related to bronchodilating medications and stress response)
• mild to moderate hypertension (related to medications and anxiety)
• paradoxical pulse becoming more pronounced (greater than 15 mm Hg) as air trapping increases
• potential arrhythmias

Respiratory
• use of accessory neck muscles during breathing, becoming more pronounced as obstruction worsens
• respiratory rate less than 30 breaths/minute, increasing as attack worsens but possibly lessening with fatigue
• prolonged exhalations
• wheezing noted; may be audible from a distance (timing varies with severity: initially expiratory, then inspiratory-expiratory, finally no wheezing — "silent" chest indicates critical airflow limitation)
• cough, possibly decreased sputum production (increased production a positive sign; can be yellow, thick, or crusted)
• speech becomes monosyllabic as airflow limitation worsens

DIAGNOSTIC STUDIES
• ABG measurements — may be obtained only in severe or prolonged attack; hypoxemia always present; carbon dioxide level used to stage attack's progress:
  — stage 1: decreased partial pressure of oxygen (PO_2) and partial pressure of carbon dioxide (PCO_2) levels (hyperventilation)
  — stage 2: decreased PO_2 level, normal PCO_2 level (increased fatigue)
  — stage 3: decreased PO_2 level (less than 50 mm Hg), increased PCO_2 level (critical hypoventilation and fatigue)
• sputum specimens — Gram stain used to detect treatable organisms; eosinophil smear done if allergens are suspected as primary cause; culture and sensitivity testing difficult to obtain because mucus is initially thick, tenacious, and difficult to mobilize; casts and plugs are present when sputum is mobilized
• complete blood count and differential — white blood cell (WBC) count increased with infection; eosinophil count increased with allergy
• serum electrolyte levels — potassium level invariably decreased
• theophylline level — may be necessary in acute phase if the patient treated self extensively with nonprescription and prescription remedies; normal level 10 to 20 mcg/ml; an elevated level may indicate medication misuse; a decreased level may indicate noncompliance

• chest X-ray—shows hyperinflation; air trapping decreases as airflow obstruction improves; between attacks, hyperinflation resolves; infiltrates are present if infection is a major cause

• pulmonary function testing (PFT)—not usually performed during an acute attack; measures of airflow rate, peak expiratory flow rate (PEFR), and forced expiratory flow rate in 1 second (FEV_1) are less than 25% of predicted value in severe obstruction; full PFT demonstrates dramatic response to bronchodilators; methacholine or histamine challenge provokes increased airway resistance

• allergen skin test—negative; positive skin test does not necessarily indicate that exposure will trigger a respiratory response

POTENTIAL COMPLICATIONS

• cardiopulmonary arrest
• cardiac arrhythmias
• rib fractures (from violent coughing)
• pneumothorax
• atelectasis
• pneumonia
• drug overdose related to noncompliance or knowledge deficit about medication use during an acute attack

---

Collaborative problem: *High risk for status asthmaticus or pulmonary arrest related to airway obstruction, hypoxemia, and progressive fatigue*

NURSING PRIORITIES: (a) Maintain effective airway clearance, and (b) promote an efficient breathing pattern.

Interventions

1. Administer oxygen via nasal cannula, 2 to 3 liters/minute or more, as ordered.

2. Administer fluid therapy orally or intravenously, as ordered. The usual fluid goal, 8 to 12 8-oz glasses (2,000 to 3,000 ml) every 24 hours, may vary with the patient's age and general status.

3. Monitor patient status continually until it stabilizes. Parameters to monitor include level of consciousness, skin color and moisture, speech pattern, use of accessory muscles for breathing, breath sounds, sputum production, respiratory rate, pulse, blood pressure, and paradoxical pulse. Obtain ABG measurements, as ordered, and expiratory flow rates. Once baselines are established, use a pulse oximeter to monitor oxygenation. Thoroughly document findings. Report changes that indicate deteriorating status.

4. Be especially alert for signs of a potentially fatal attack, and promptly report them to the doctor. Such signs include:
• previous severe asthma attacks
• FEV_1 less than 500 cc or PEFR less than 100 liters/minute
• little or no response to bronchodilator therapy in 1 hour, as evidenced in flow rate measurements
• altered level of consciousness
• cyanosis
• PO_2 less than 50 mm Hg
• PCO_2 greater than 45 mm Hg
• pulsus paradoxus
• electrocardiogram abnormality
• pneumothorax.

Rationales

1. Hypoxemia is always present in an acute asthma attack because of ventilation-perfusion imbalance. Supplemental oxygen decreases the work of breathing and reduces the potential for cardiac dysfunction.

2. The patient is usually dehydrated on admission. Hydration promotes expectoration of thickened sputum and minimizes development of impacted mucus.

3. Parameters vary with the attack's severity, the patient's response to treatment, and patient fatigue. Because of physiologic instability, parameters may change rapidly.

4. One or more of the items cited may forewarn of a fatal attack. Prompt, aggressive therapy is necessary to forestall pulmonary arrest.

5. Administer pharmacologic agents, as ordered. The medication regimen varies but typically includes:

• bronchodilators, such as beta-adrenergics and theophylline (Slo-phyllin). Beta-adrenergic agents (epinephrine [Adrenalin], terbutaline [Brethaire], isoproterenol [Isuprel], and metaproterenol [Alupent]) are given subcutaneously, inhaled from a pressurized canister or nebulizer, or taken orally; observe for such side effects as nervousness or hypertension. Theophylline (xanthine) preparations, such as aminophylline (Phyllocontin), are initially given I.V. and then orally; observe for and report any arrhythmias, tachycardia, hypotension, vomiting, or other side effects.

• corticosteroids. These are initially given I.V., then orally, with tapering as soon as possible. Aerosolized corticosteroids, with or without oral agents, may be used in some patients.

6. Initiate measures to alleviate panic, ensure safety, and promote relaxation. Place the patient in an upright position with adequate support; promote exhalation of trapped air by instructing the patient to prolong exhalation and to exhale without force; maintain a calm, reassuring attitude; reduce environmental stimulation, if possible.

7. Monitor therapeutic medication levels, and assess for associated electrolyte and glucose imbalances daily, as ordered. Report abnormal findings.

8. Initiate measures to mobilize sputum, such as postural drainage and percussion, suctioning if necessary, and controlled cough. Caution: Each of these measures can intensify hypoxemia. Use supplemental oxygen, temporarily increasing the liter flow if any respiratory distress is observed.

9. Monitor fluid balance, noting intake and output, weight, skin turgor, condition of mucous membranes, characteristics of sputum, presence or absence of edema, and urine specific gravity and hematocrit. Document and report abnormalities.

10. Do not administer narcotics or sedatives.

11. Observe for indicators for intubation, such as fatigue, further reduction in thoracic expansion, decreasing level of consciousness, PCO_2 level increased more than 10 mm Hg above the resting level, severe hypoxemia, and decreasing breath sounds. Alert the doctor immediately should any of these appear.

12. Additional individualized interventions: _____

5. Although some patients can control symptoms using relaxation techniques, pharmacologic intervention is usually necessary and is more effective when used before the attack becomes severe or prolonged.

• Cyclic adenosine monophosphate (c-AMP) is a chemical mediator that controls bronchodilation. Beta-adrenergics and xanthines stimulate production, or prevent destruction, of c-AMP and thus produce bronchodilation. Effectiveness varies with blood level.

• Corticosteroids (I.V. or oral) are believed to reduce inflammation, thereby reducing edema in bronchial mucosa. Aerosolized corticosteroids may provide beneficial effects while minimizing side effects, because they are delivered directly to the affected tissues.

6. The acutely asthmatic patient experiences extreme anxiety and panic, and may attempt to alleviate discomfort with counterproductive posturing and breathing patterns and with restless activity. Characteristically, the harder the patient attempts to breathe, the less productive the effort and the greater the amount of air trapped. Prolonged exhalation facilitates a relaxed expiratory effort and reduces air trapping.

7. Establishing a therapeutic medication regimen requires ongoing monitoring of drug levels and electrolyte status as the patient is rehydrated and stabilized. Theophylline clearance may be impaired, or electrolyte or glucose levels may be altered, or both—especially in the patient with cardiac disease, hypertension, or liver disease, or who uses other medications.

8. Once hydration is initiated, the patient must mobilize the thick, crusty mucus rapidly to prevent bronchial plugging. The fatigued patient may need assistance.

9. During an asthma attack, profuse diaphoresis and tachypnea cause fluid loss. Because the patient is usually too dyspneic and panicked to take oral fluids, significant dehydration may rapidly ensue. I.V. fluid replacement must be individualized and monitored carefully; otherwise, aggressive hydration may lead to fluid overload in the patient with compromised cardiovascular status.

10. The patient may be anxious but this is related to hypoxemia. Sedation depresses the respiratory drive and promotes hypoventilation.

11. When the work of breathing becomes overwhelming, exhaustion results. If intubation and mechanical ventilation are not initiated promptly, pulmonary arrest can ensue.

12. Rationales: _____

Target outcome criteria
Within 1 hour of beginning therapy, the patient will:
• show an improved flow rate (FEV_1 and PEFR)
• mobilize sputum
• exhibit reduced anxiety while maintaining a normal level of consciousness
• have reduced hypoxemia, with PCO_2 level at or below normal.

Once stabilized, the patient will:
• have improved breath sounds
• decrease use of accessory muscles for breathing
• exhibit stable vital signs within normal limits
• have improved ABG measurements.

Nursing diagnosis: *High risk for social isolation related to activity-induced shortness of breath, irritants, and change in body image*

NURSING PRIORITY: Improve the patient's ability to prevent or cope with breathing difficulties.

Interventions

1. After the acute episode resolves, discuss and demonstrate (through role playing) assertive strategies to be used when the patient must confront an environmental irritant (such as secondhand smoke). Have the patient return the demonstration.

2. Demonstrate strategies to be used during a coughing episode (for example, controlled cough technique or "huff" coughing) and for acute shortness of breath during an activity (for example, upright and forward posturing, with shoulder relaxation and prolonged exhalation). Coach the patient in using these strategies.

3. Teach the patient how to use a metered-dose inhaler. Discuss with the patient medication adverse reactions, such as anxiety and tremor from bronchodilators or moon face, loss of muscle tissue, and a tendency to bruise from corticosteroids. Encourage expression of frustration about the side effects' impact on socialization.

4. Help the patient identify factors that may cause attacks or contribute to them. Observing dietary intake, medications, emotional state, and environmental factors before an attack may provide clues about the patient's triggering mechanisms. Also teach the patient how to monitor peak flow rate (PFR) at home.

5. Emphasize the importance of adequate daily fluid intake.

6. Additional individualized interventions: _____

Rationales

1. The patient will be more likely to implement an assertive, nonaggressive strategy for dealing with potentially hazardous situations if several alternative responses are provided. The patient may not be aware of the right to request environmental changes or may not know how to make such requests.

2. Breathing strategies reduce forceful exhalation, which occurs during coughing or acute shortness of breath and results in increased airway obstruction.

3. Metered-dose inhalers may be used to deliver asthma medications and require instruction for proper use. Although nothing can be done to eliminate these adverse reactions, compliance with the prescribed regimen may be improved if the patient expresses feelings about such reactions to an understanding professional.

4. Once specific trigger factors have been pinpointed, the patient can take steps to minimize or eliminate exposure to them. When at increased risk for attacks, the patient can monitor PFR in the morning and at night. If the valves are abnormal, the patient may be instructed to change medication dosages, within guidelines, or to see a doctor promptly, thus preventing a major attack.

5. Dry mucous membranes may cause an attack. Dehydration worsens airway obstruction related to tenacious sputum.

6. Rationales: _____

Target outcome criteria
By the time of discharge, the patient will:
• demonstrate appropriate breathing techniques during activity-induced shortness of breath or coughing episodes
• describe assertive strategies for dealing with environmental irritants

• realistically describe body-image changes related to medication adverse effects, while continuing to comply with the medication regimen
• identify factors that may trigger attacks.

Discharge planning

NURSING DISCHARGE CRITERIA

Upon the patient's discharge, documentation shows evidence of:
• WBC count within normal parameters
• oxygen and I.V. therapy discontinued for at least 24 hours
• stable vital signs
• ABG measurements within expected parameters
• absence of cardiovascular and pulmonary complications (such as arrhythmias or atelectasis)
• tolerance of and response to oral medication regimen
• absence of dehydration signs and symptoms
• ability to tolerate adequate nutritional intake
• absence of acute shortness of breath on exertion
• ability to ambulate and perform activities of daily living at prehospitalization level
• adequate home support or referral to home care, if indicated by inadequate home support system or patient's inability to perform self-care.

PATIENT-FAMILY TEACHING CHECKLIST

Document evidence that the patient and family demonstrate an understanding of:
___ factors that trigger an asthma attack (specific to the patient, if possible)
___ home and work environment assessment and modifications to counter potential irritants
___ preventive measures for use when irritant exposure is unavoidable
___ clinical manifestations of an impending attack
___ relaxation and breathing exercises to improve control during an attack
___ all discharge medications' purpose, dose, administration schedule, and adverse effects requiring medical attention (usual discharge medications include bronchodilators and corticosteroids)
___ purpose and use of over-the-counter medications (bronchodilators, expectorants, cough suppressants, cold remedies, or sleep remedies) as well as precautions to take when using them
___ bronchial hygiene measures, including indications, schedule, and use
___ use and cleaning of respiratory therapy equipment
___ self-management plan, including decision-making strategies for beginning or mild attacks and an emergency plan for severe or progressing attacks
___ hydration requirements
___ controlled cough technique
___ exercise recommendations and limitations, if any
___ measures to control shortness of breath when performing activities
___ need for flu and pneumococcus vaccine
___ date, time, and location of follow-up appointment
___ how to contact the doctor.

DOCUMENTATION CHECKLIST

Using outcome criteria as a guide, document:
___ clinical status on admission
___ significant changes in status
___ pertinent laboratory and diagnostic test findings
___ treatments, including patient response
___ respiratory status (each shift)
___ oxygen therapy
___ medications
___ hydration status, fluid intake and output
___ patient-family teaching
___ discharge planning.

ASSOCIATED PLANS OF CARE

Ineffective Individual Coping
Knowledge Deficit

References

Cross, D., and Nelson, S. "The Role of The Peak Flow Meter in the Diagnosis and Management of Asthma," *Journal of Allergy and Clinical Immunology* 87(1 pt. 1):120-28, January 1991.

Janson-Bjerklie, S. "Status Asthmaticus," *American Journal of Nursing* 90(9):52-55, September 1990.

Petty, T. "Drug Strategies for Airflow Obstruction," *American Journal of Nursing* 87(2):180-84, February 1987.

Reed, C. "Basic Mechanisms of Asthma: Role of Inflammation," *Chest* 94(1):175-77, July 1988.

Chronic Obstructive Pulmonary Disease

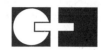

DRG information

DRG 088 Chronic Obstructive Pulmonary Disease.
  Mean LOS = 5.9 days
  Principal diagnoses include:
  • congenital bronchiectasis
  • obstructive chronic bronchitis
  • emphysema
  • chronic respiratory conditions resulting from fumes or vapors.

This DRG is seen frequently in acute care. Also, COPD patients commonly are readmitted within 15 days of previous hospitalization.

DRG 089 Simple Pneumonia and Pleurisy. Age 17 + .
  With Complication or Comorbidity (CC).
  Mean LOS = 7.2 days
  Principal diagnoses include:
  • bronchopneumonia
  • influenza with pneumonia
  • bacterial pneumonia
  • pneumonia with organism unspecified.

DRG 096 Bronchitis and Asthma. Age 17 + . With CC.
  Mean LOS = 6.0 days

DRG 097 Bronchitis and Asthma. Age 17 + . Without CC.
  Mean LOS = 4.6 days

Introduction

DEFINITION AND TIME FOCUS

Chronic obstructive pulmonary disease (COPD) is a diagnostic category applied to patients whose primary respiratory difficulty involves exhalation. This plan focuses on two diseases, emphysema and chronic bronchitis. (Asthma, another disorder sometimes included in COPD, is covered in a separate plan.)

Emphysema is permanent, nonreversible destruction of alveoli, resulting in dyspnea inappropriate for age and level of exertion. Chronic bronchitis (inflammation of the bronchi) is characterized by a chronic productive cough resulting from hyperplasia of mucus-producing cells and increased mucus production. Few patients have a "pure" disease process; most experience a combination of symptoms.

Common features of the stable state include:
• difficulty exhaling because of airway collapse, especially with increased effort (the harder the patient tries to exhale, the more difficult it becomes)
• air trapping with hyperinflation
• dyspnea
• history of smoking
• airway hypersensitivity to various stimuli
• difficulty handling secretions.

Common features of an exacerbation include ventilation-perfusion imbalance resulting in:
• increased work of breathing
• increased myocardial work
• hypoxemia
• carbon dioxide retention.

This plan focuses on the COPD patient who is admitted to the acute-care setting with an exacerbation of the disease and failure of prescribed therapies to control the symptoms.

ETIOLOGY AND PRECIPITATING FACTORS

• exacerbation caused most commonly by a viral or bacterial infection; other common causes include exposure to environmental pollutants (secondhand smoke, dust, or cleaning compounds), exercise, and weather changes (heat, cold, fog, or wind)

Focused assessment guidelines

NURSING HISTORY (Functional health pattern findings)

Health perception—health management pattern

• complains of greater than normal shortness of breath, with inability to control symptoms with prescribed or nonprescribed therapies
• may report increased fatigue and feel unable to cope with crisis
• may report increasing anxiety and panic
• may report increasing difficulty expectorating sputum

Nutritional-metabolic pattern

• may report anorexia
• may report inability to eat and digest without shortness of breath
• may report nausea, possibly associated with medications
• may report bloating, especially after eating foods known to cause flatulence
• may report difficulty maintaining adequate fluid intake (at least 8 8-oz glasses [2,000 ml] per day)
• may report symptoms of fluid and electrolyte disturbance, such as weakness, lethargy, confusion, weight changes, and muscle cramping

Activity-exercise pattern

• complains of shortness of breath with even minimal exertion or when performing activities of daily living
• may know how to control shortness of breath and panic with breathing maneuvers but may report forgetting this ability in a crisis

Sleep-rest pattern
- reports sleep pattern disturbance
- may report sleeping upright (usually in a reclining chair)
- may report shortness of breath during the night, relieved by bronchial hygiene and expectoration of secretions
- may report nervousness and trouble falling asleep
- may report chronic fatigue and sleepiness during the day
- may report nocturia (may be related to medications)
- may report morning headache

Cognitive-perceptual pattern
- may report fluctuating compliance with therapeutic regimen (may perceive regimen as complex and difficult to understand and follow)

Role-relationship pattern
- may report multiple role changes, resulting in depression, isolation, and increased dependence
- may report difficulty verbalizing feelings because emotions intensify shortness of breath

Sexuality-reproductive pattern
- may report complex interpersonal role changes with spouse or partner, with decreased desire for and frequency of sexual activity because of actual or potential shortness of breath

Coping—stress tolerance pattern
- may have difficulty expressing either positive or negative emotions because of shortness of breath
- may report fluctuating behavior, alternately passive, angry, abusive, or manipulative

Value-belief pattern
- may report ambivalence about resuscitative measures that may be necessary during hospital stay but may not ultimately improve the quality of life

PHYSICAL FINDINGS
General appearance
- apprehensive and anxious; maintains upright, tense posture
- panics easily if activity is requested
- cachectic (emphysema); plethoric (chronic bronchitis)

Cardiovascular
- typically, rapid pulse because of medications; expected upper limit for medication-induced tachycardia is 120 beats/minute
- atrial fibrillation or multifocal atrial tachycardia (common arrhythmias of COPD)
- signs of cor pulmonale and right-sided heart failure (edema, jugular venous distention, or crackles)

Pulmonary
- accentuated accessory neck muscles
- barrel chest from hyperinflation
- decreased breath sounds bilaterally
- prolonged expiratory phase
- productive cough: tapioca-like plugs (hallmark of emphysema) or copious amounts of sputum (hallmark of chronic bronchitis)
- gurgles if secretions are copious; crackles if heart failure or pneumonia is present (crackles are not a common or expected finding in COPD)
- chronic sinus drainage with accompanying sinus pain (may cause recurring infections)

Neurologic
- anxious
- if hypoxemic, restless
- if partial pressure of carbon dioxide (PCO_2) levels are increased, lethargic and sleepy

Integumentary
- skin discolors (mottling and cyanosis) easily during coughing spells, strenuous activity, or episodes of acute shortness of breath

DIAGNOSTIC STUDIES
- arterial blood gas (ABG) measurements—derangements vary with disease
  —hypoxemia: most common; more pronounced with exercise; in stable state, partial pressure of oxygen (PO_2) level should be between 55 and 65 mm Hg, because the patient may have a reduced respiratory drive when PO_2 level is greater than 65 mm Hg; in acute exacerbation, PO_2 level commonly falls below 55 mm Hg
  —increased carbon dioxide level: in stable state, PCO_2 level should be maintained at 50 mm Hg or less; during exacerbation, PCO_2 level above 50 mm Hg is very common
  —acid-base imbalance: in stable state, body compensates for respiratory acidosis; during exacerbation, both respiratory and metabolic acidosis may be present
- sputum specimens—if infection is suspected, Gram stain and culture and sensitivity tests are done to determine appropriate antibiotic
- theophylline level—normal is 10 to 15 mcg/ml (normal may be 5 to 12 mcg/ml if the patient is using other drugs); may be elevated if the patient has adjusted theophylline dose
- alpha$_1$-antitrypsin assay—uncommon; performed to determine alpha$_1$-antitrypsin deficiency in young patients with suspected emphysema
- other tests—white blood cell count, hematocrit, and serum electrolyte levels, according to suspected cause

• chest X-ray—shows hyperinflation, with flattening of the diaphragm caused by air trapping in the chest, that may worsen during exacerbation; may also show infiltrates, depending on exacerbation's cause

• pulmonary function test—usually not performed in acute exacerbation; common findings in stable state include:

  —reduced expiratory flow rates, especially with effort; airway obstruction is more pronounced as the patient tries harder to exhale

  —some response to bronchodilators in patients with chronic bronchitis; no response in patients with emphysema

  —decreased diffusion capacity in patients with emphysema predominating

POTENTIAL COMPLICATIONS

• acute respiratory failure
• cardiac arrhythmias
• depressed brain function; permanent brain injury
• other organ injury (such as kidney)
• pneumonia
• pneumothorax
• cor pulmonale

Collaborative problem: *Respiratory failure (PO$_2$ level less than 50 mm Hg, with or without PCO$_2$ level greater than 50 mm Hg) related to ventilation-perfusion imbalance*

NURSING PRIORITIES: (a) Maintain adequate airway clearance, (b) reverse hypoxemia and carbon dioxide retention, (c) maintain optimum environment for adequate function of the patient's limited respiratory reserves, and (d) resolve causative factors.

Interventions

1. Obtain and report ABG measurements as needed to determine the patient's baseline, to monitor the appropriateness of therapy, and to determine the effect of an acute episode (if the patient becomes somnolent or increasingly restless or has a sudden personality change).

2. Administer oxygen as ordered, generally 2 liters/minute during the day and 3 liters/minute at night or during activity.

3. Administer pharmacologic agents and monitor therapeutic levels, as ordered.

• bronchodilators

• antibiotics
• corticosteroids

• expectorants

4. Perform bronchial hygiene measures, as ordered. Assess lung sounds before and after all treatments and at least every 4 hours when the patient is awake. Report and document the effectiveness of any or all of the following treatments: aerosols, intermittent positive-pressure breathing, postural drainage and percussion, and suctioning (if the coughing mechanism is inadequate).

Rationales

1. ABG evaluations are the only reliable way of assessing the patient's oxygenation and carbon dioxide status. No formula exists for determining the precise percentage of oxygen a patient needs because the appropriateness of the oxygen dosage can be evaluated only by serial ABG determinations.

2. The COPD patient may have an altered respiration regulating mechanism. Instead of responding to an elevated carbon dioxide level (normal response), the COPD patient may respond only to a need for oxygen. Low percentages of oxygen are less likely to decrease the respiratory drive. Oxygen supply decreases at night (nocturnal desaturation) because of decreased intercostal muscle tone during sleep. Oxygen demand increases with activity.

3. Pharmacologic agents are ordered according to the respiratory failure's cause.

• Cyclic adenosine monophosphate (c-AMP) is a chemical mediator that controls bronchodilation. Bronchodilators (sympathomimetics and xanthines) stimulate production or prevent destruction of c-AMP, thereby producing bronchodilation. Effectiveness varies with blood level.

• Antibiotics are ordered for the specific organism.

• Corticosteroids (I.V. or oral) are believed to reduce inflammation.

• Expectorants may be used as an adjunct to fluid therapy.

4. Ventilation-perfusion abnormalities are the major reason for respiratory failure in the COPD patient. Bronchial hygiene measures open obstructed airways for more effective ventilation while conserving oxygen reserves.

5. Maintain fluid intake at 8 to 12 8-oz glasses (2,000 to 3,000 ml) of water per day.

6. Monitor, document, and report signs of infection or further deterioration in respiratory status, such as an increase or decrease of sputum, changes in the sputum's color or consistency, fever, increased shortness of breath, and changes in breath sounds.

7. If possible, reduce or eliminate environmental irritants: encourage smoking cessation, and do not use (or allow roommates or visitors to use) hair, deodorant, or room-freshening sprays or strong fragrances near the patient.

8. Additional individualized interventions:_____

_____

5. Sputum viscosity is related to the patient's hydration status. Water is the most physiologically compatible expectorant.

6. Routine monitoring and accurate documentation allows early detection of subtle changes in the patient's condition that might signal illness progression.

7. Numerous environmental substances and sprays can cause airway irritation in the COPD patient (especially when the airways are already compromised) and exacerbate the condition.

8. Rationales:_____

_____

Target outcome criteria
Within 48 hours of admission, the patient will:
• exhibit a PO_2 level greater than 50 mm Hg, with or without supplemental oxygen
• exhibit a PCO_2 level within the patient's normal range, typically less than 50 mm Hg
• exhibit fewer and shorter periods of acute shortness of breath.

By the time of discharge, the patient will:
• exhibit reduced evidence of infection or environmental irritation
• easily expectorate clear or white, thin sputum
• have lungs clear to auscultation, without gurgles or crackles.

Nursing diagnosis: *Ineffective breathing pattern related to emotional stimulation, fatigue, or blunting of respiratory drive*

NURSING PRIORITY: Maintain an effective breathing pattern.

Interventions

1. Reduce the work of breathing and lessen depletion of oxygen reserves through teaching and by promoting relaxation as follows:
• Position the patient for comfort (upright may be best, with a pillow under the elbows and the patient leaning on the overbed table).
• Remind the patient to relax the shoulders and neck muscles.
• Instruct the patient to prolong exhalation.
• Sit with the patient and encourage rhythmic breathing.
• Use a calm, unhurried manner.

2. Teach and help the patient to perform breathing exercises and coordinate breathing with activity.

3. Pace all activities according to periods of maximum bronchodilation and peak energy. Encourage energy conservation.

4. Instruct the patient in breathing techniques to use when expressing feelings that create shortness of breath (controlled cough technique or bronchial hygiene measures for public use).

5. Avoid the use of sedatives or narcotics.

Rationales

1. Inhalation normally requires muscle work and energy expenditure. Exhalation is ordinarily passive, not requiring extra energy and oxygen, but because the COPD patient in distress uses oxygen for both inhalation and exhalation, a large amount of oxygen from each inhalation is used to take and expel the next breath. Also, because shortness of breath causes anxiety, the patient tends to tighten muscle groups, thus using even more oxygen. Relaxation and easy, prolonged exhalation maximize lung expansion while minimizing energy and oxygen expenditures. Despite the value of breathing techniques, the COPD patient may forget them in a crisis and need the nurse's assistance to regain control.

2. Breath-holding during exertion dramatically increases shortness of breath.

3. Pacing allows activity while conserving energy reserves.

4. Any expression of emotion, such as happiness, anger, or sadness, affects respiratory patterns and may increase shortness of breath.

5. These agents further depress the respiratory centers and may provoke respiratory arrest.

6. Additional individualized interventions: _____

_____

6. Rationales: _____

_____

Target outcome criteria

Immediately upon admission, after coaching by the nurse, the patient will resume continuous use of breathing techniques.

Within 24 hours, the patient will pace activities to coincide with periods of maximum bronchodilation and peak energy.

Nursing diagnosis: *Nutritional deficit related to shortness of breath during and after meals and adverse reactions to medication*

NURSING PRIORITIES: (a) Maintain adequate caloric and nutritional intake, (b) reduce deterrents to eating, and (c) optimize environmental conditions to increase appetite.

Interventions

1. Use supplemental oxygen during mealtimes, as ordered.

2. Perform bronchial hygiene measures before meals. Provide mouth care, and remove secretions from the eating area.

3. Provide frequent, small meals.

4. Monitor the patient's weight and nutritional intake daily.

5. Obtain a dietary consultation as soon as the patient can take foods or fluids, with special attention to needs for:
• high-protein, low-carbohydrate, high-fat supplements

• elimination of gas-producing foods from diet

• consideration of the patient's food preferences and conformation to any dietary restrictions, such as limiting salt.

6. Additional individualized interventions: _____

_____

Rationales

1. The act of eating requires oxygen. Supplemental oxygen during meals bolsters oxygen reserves.

2. Performing hygiene measures before meals ensures maximum bronchodilation and reduces activity-related ventilation-perfusion imbalances that may cause hypoxemia. The presence of sputum may decrease appetite.

3. Small meals require less oxygen for eating and digestion than large ones.

4. During periods of exacerbation, metabolic demands may increase, creating an increased demand for calories to maintain weight. Daily assessment detects the need for dietary supplements to prevent further depletion.

5. Early dietary consultation can prevent future complications from further debilitation.

• the COPD patient has an increased respiratory rate and increased work of breathing, resulting in greater metabolic demands. A diet with a low calorie-to-nitrogen ratio will meet metabolic demands without increasing carbon dioxide production (as occurs with a high-calorie diet).

• Abdominal distention can cause diaphragmatic compression, increasing the sensation of shortness of breath.

• The patient is more likely to follow a nutritional plan that includes favorite, familiar foods. Necessary restrictions must be observed to promote an optimal state of health

6. Rationales: _____

_____

Target outcome criteria

Within 48 hours of admission, the patient will take meals without episodes of acute shortness of breath.

By the time of discharge, the patient will have a stable weight.

Nursing diagnosis: *Activity intolerance related to shortness of breath, avoidance of physical activity with resultant muscle weakness, deconditioning, depression, and (possibly) exercise-related hypoxemia*

NURSING PRIORITY: Promote a gradual return to an optimal level of activity, with absent or controlled episodes of acute shortness of breath. (Note: Progress on this priority will depend on resolving the exacerbation and its causative factors.)

Interventions

1. Instruct the patient in breathing techniques to use when performing activities of daily living (ADLs): slow and relaxed exhalation, avoidance of breath-holding, and relaxation of accessory muscles. (For more information and pictures of these techniques for use during instruction, contact the local American Lung Association chapter.)

2. Administer oxygen during activity, as ordered.

3. Before recommending an activity level, assess for stable ABG measurements and level of fitness (the pulmonary function or respiratory therapy department can assist in determining an appropriate exercise level).
   Also assess for other factors contributing to inactivity, such as family relationships, concomitant diseases (such as arthritis), or environmental conditions.

4. Develop and implement a daily walking schedule, increasing time and distance as tolerated. Before beginning, teach the patient how to control shortness of breath. This includes telling the patient to stop, lean back, position hips against a sturdy object or wall, and stand with the feet apart.

5. Before, during, and after walking, monitor the patient's response to exercise. Document these parameters along with the time and distance walked: blood pressure (before and after), pulse rate and rhythm, color, respiratory rate, and degree of shortness of breath.

6. Additional individualized interventions: _____

Rationales

1. Breathing techniques facilitate full exhalation, thereby promoting removal of stale air, increasing ventilatory efficiency, and permitting a wider range of physical activity.

2. Increased activity requires supplemental oxygen.

3. If undertaken prematurely, increased activity may worsen the exacerbation. The patient is unlikely to adhere to an activity prescription that is inappropriate in terms of ABG measurements or level of fitness or that ignores other deterrents to activity.

4. Implementing a walking schedule should start in the hospital, if possible, so that the patient can be observed and coached in appropriate breathing techniques. Gaining control over shortness of breath improves the patient's confidence in walking independently.

5. If a patient is experiencing desaturation or acidosis during the walk, these events will be reflected in vital sign changes. More sophisticated exercise testing may be needed to determine the extent of disability and the appropriate therapy.

6. Rationales: _____

Target outcome criteria
Throughout the hospital stay, the patient will increase the ability to ambulate over longer times and distances without shortness of breath, pulse changes (rate or rhythm), blood pressure drop, or a color change.

By the time of discharge, the patient will demonstrate the method for controlling activity-related shortness of breath.

Nursing diagnosis: *Sleep pattern disturbance related to bronchodilators' stimulant effect, shortness of breath, depression, and anxiety*

NURSING PRIORITY: Minimize sleep disruption.

Interventions

1. Identify the patient's normal sleep pattern as well as the abnormal pattern.

Rationales

1. The patient may have misconceptions about normal and abnormal sleep patterns. Discussion may clarify factors contributing to sleep disturbance.

2. Consult with the doctor about adjusting medications to optimize bronchodilation yet minimize stimulant effects.

2. Bronchodilators vary in their stimulant properties. Stimulants may cause myocardial irritability, nervousness, and anxiety and may increase oxygen demand.

3. Instruct the patient in performing bronchial hygiene before retiring and as needed for nocturnal dyspnea.

3. Nocturnal shortness of breath may be unavoidable; the best alternative is to teach the patient how to deal with such an episode effectively.

4. Administer oxygen therapy during the night, as ordered.

4. PaO_2 levels normally decrease at night. Although most people can tolerate the decrease, the already hypoxemic COPD patient cannot because hypoxemia-induced pulmonary vasoconstriction can cause or exacerbate cor pulmonale.

5. Monitor periods of sleeplessness, including degree of shortness of breath, pulse rate and rhythm, respiratory rate, and breath sounds. Observe which treatments seem to provide the most benefit.

5. Observing a sleeplessness episode and its resolution may provide clues for further prevention and help the patient learn to deal with future episodes.

6. Instruct the patient in relaxation techniques to be used at bedtime. (A COPD patient should not use sleeping medications unless the pulmonologist specifically prescribes them.)

6. Relaxation techniques can promote sleep and minimize oxygen demands. Sleeping medications may depress respirations in the already compromised patient.

7. Additional individualized interventions: _____

7. Rationales: _____

_____

_____

Target outcome criteria
By the time of discharge, the patient will:
• report less frequent episodes of nocturnal shortness of breath
• sleep throughout the night, without early-morning headache or excessive drowsiness during the day

• fall asleep easily at night
• report an improved sleep pattern or more easily controlled episodes of nocturnal shortness of breath, or both.

Nursing diagnosis: *High risk for injury related to failure to recognize signs and symptoms indicating impending exacerbation*

NURSING PRIORITY: Teach the patient to recognize an impending exacerbation and to seek appropriate treatment.

Interventions

1. Teach the patient the signs and symptoms of an impending exacerbation, including:
• increased or decreased sputum production
• change in the color or character of sputum over a 24-hour period
• fever (based on baseline normal temperature)
• restlessness or inability to sleep lasting more than one night
• increased fatigue or sleepiness.

Rationales

1. Early detection and intervention increase the likelihood of successful reversal or control of the episode.

2. Emphasize the need to notify the doctor promptly if these symptoms occur, rather than altering the medication regimen without the doctor's knowledge.

2. Appropriate intervention requires medical judgment.

3. Caution the patient to avoid overmedication with prescription drugs or over-the-counter remedies.

3. Overuse of some medications, such as bronchodilators, may actually increase oxygen demands. Over-the-counter remedies may contain substances, such as ephedrine, that potentiate or counteract the therapeutic effects of prescribed medication.

4. Additional individualized interventions: _____

4. Rationales: _____

_____

_____

Target outcome criteria
By the time of discharge, the patient will:
• list four indicators of an impending exacerbation
• correctly identify the rationale for notifying the doctor before adjusting the medication regimen.

Nursing diagnosis: *Altered sexuality patterns related to shortness of breath, change in body image, deconditioning, change in relationship with spouse or partner, and adverse reactions to medications*

NURSING PRIORITY: Help the patient and spouse (or partner) to discuss feelings and determine realistic expectations.

Interventions

1. Establish rapport with the patient and spouse (or partner). Discuss their feelings concerning changes in sexual functioning.

2. Help the patient learn or arrange therapies (including medication schedule, oxygen level, bronchial hygiene, and energy conservation) to optimize sexual function, as desired.

3. Additional individualized interventions: _____

_____

Rationales

1. A sense of rapport makes discussion of this sensitive topic more comfortable. Discussion will help clarify the issues involved and the expectations held by the patient and spouse (or partner).

2. As with other activities, the patient must learn to optimize therapies to accomplish desired goals.

3. Rationales: _____

_____

Target outcome criterion
By the time of discharge, the patient will describe ways to use therapies for maximum benefit in order to engage in sexual activity.

Discharge planning

NURSING DISCHARGE CRITERIA

Upon the patient's discharge, documentation shows evidence of:
• absence of fever and other signs of infection
• ABG levels within acceptable parameters
• absence of cardiovascular or pulmonary complications
• minimal shortness of breath
• lung sounds clear or as usual for patient when not in exacerbation state
• ability to tolerate ambulation with minimal limitations, same as before exacerbation and hospitalization
• ability to perform ADLs independently (or with minimal assistance) at preexacerbation level
• ability to tolerate diet with minimal shortness of breath
• stabilized weight (within 5 lb [2.5 kg] of normal weight)
• adequate home support system or referral to home care if indicated by inadequate home support, inability to perform ADLs at preexacerbation level, or need for continued assistance with bronchial hygiene measures.

Note: It is important to be aware that the patient with COPD will not be "normal" when discharged. Therefore, discharge evaluation should relate to the patient's condition before the exacerbation. The most important thing to document is the absence of acute infection, but also be alert to ABG levels on discharge. ABG levels must be within acceptable parameters, because abnormal levels on discharge commonly cause readmission within a short time.

PATIENT-FAMILY TEACHING CHECKLIST

Document evidence that the patient and family demonstrate an understanding of:
— practical energy conservation and breathing techniques
— signs and symptoms of infection or exacerbation
— all discharge medications' purpose, dose, administration schedule, and adverse reactions requiring medical attention (usual discharge medications include bronchodilators, corticosteroids, antibiotics, and expectorants)
— bronchial hygiene measures
— use, care, and cleaning of respiratory equipment
— need for drinking 8 to 12 8-oz glasses of water per day
— dietary restrictions
— daily weight monitoring
— avoiding exposure to infections and need for flu vaccination
— avoiding lung irritants, such as cold air, second-hand smoke, sprays, and dust
— exercise prescription
— referral to community agencies, as appropriate (such as Meals on Wheels, American Lung Association, Better Breathers Club, respiratory equipment company and name of representative, emergency response service, home care agency, and smoking cessation group)
— date, time, and location of next appointment
— how to contact the doctor.

DOCUMENTATION CHECKLIST

Using outcome criteria as a guide, document:
— clinical status on admission
— significant changes in status
— pertinent laboratory and diagnostic tests, such as ABG levels
— episodes of shortness of breath, including physical assessment parameters during each episode, treatment administered, and treatment outcome
— respiratory status per shift, including breath sounds; character of cough; and character, color, and amount of sputum
— administration and outcome of therapies given
— nutritional intake
— fluid intake
— exercise ability and activity level
— patient-family teaching
— discharge planning.

ASSOCIATED PLANS OF CARE

Dying
Grieving
Ineffective Individual Coping
Knowledge Deficit
Pneumonia

References

Cherniak, N. *Chronic Obstructive Pulmonary Disease.* Philadelphia: W.B. Saunders Co., 1991.

Gift, A.G., et al. "Psychologic and Physiologic Factors Related to Dyspnea in Subjects with Chronic Obstruction Pulmonary Disease," *Heart & Lung* 15(6):595-601, November 1986.

Shapiro, B.A., et al. *Clinical Application of Respiratory Care,* 4th ed. Chicago: Mosby-Year Book, 1991.

Woldum, K.M., et al. *Patient Education: Tools for Practice.* Rockville, Md.: Aspen Publishing, 1985.

Lung Cancer

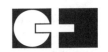

DRG information
DRG 075 Major Chest Procedures
  Mean LOS = 11.7 days
DRG 076 Other Respiratory System O.R. Procedure.
  With Complication or Comorbidity.
  Mean LOS = 0.5 days
DRG 082 Respiratory Neoplasms.
  Mean LOS = 6.7 days
DRG 410 Chemotherapy.
  Principal diagnosis: maintenance chemotherapy.
  Mean LOS = 2.7 days
DRG 409 Radiotherapy.
  Mean LOS = 6.7 days
DRG 412 History of Malignancy with Endoscopy.
  Mean LOS = 2.2 days

Introduction
DEFINITION AND TIME FOCUS
Lung cancer is a condition of aberrant cellular growth causing morphologic tissue changes within the lung. It causes 22% of all cancer in men and 35% of all cancer-related deaths in men. It is responsible for 9% of all cancer in women and 17% of all cancer-related deaths in women.

Tumors may be primary (original) or secondary (from distant metastasis). The most common types of primary lung cancer are squamous cell carcinoma (40% to 50% of cases), adenocarcinoma (25% of cases), small-cell anaplastic carcinoma (20% to 25% of cases), and large-cell anaplastic carcinoma (less than 15%).

Surgical resection, lobectomy, or pneumonectomy may be performed alone or with radiation therapy, chemotherapy, or both to treat lung cancer. However, the 5-year survival rate for persons with this disease is below 13% regardless of the treatment used. This clinical plan focuses on the patient with primary lung cancer who is admitted to an acute-care center for chemotherapy as an initial treatment.

ETIOLOGY AND PRECIPITATING FACTORS
• cigarette smoking
• exposure to carcinogens, such as asbestos, pollution, pitchblende, metals, or chemicals
• genetic predisposition

Focused assessment guidelines
NURSING HISTORY (Functional health pattern findings)

Health perception—health management pattern
• likely to report history of heavy smoking
• may report dyspnea associated with activity or anxiety; degree of dyspnea may be disproportionate to overall clinical picture
• may complain of chest pain aggravated by deep breathing (if pleura involved), cough (may be nocturnal), rust-streaked or purulent sputum, or hemoptysis
• if older than age 45 and male, at increased risk
• may complain of shoulder or arm pain if brachial plexus involved
• hoarseness common with laryngeal involvement
• may report easy bleeding from minor trauma, and slowed clot formation (cancer inhibits factor VIII [antihemophilic factor] activity)
• probably did not seek medical assistance until cough, dyspnea, weakness, and weight loss caused the patient to sense that "something was wrong"

Nutrition-metabolic pattern
• may report significant weight loss, anorexia, early satiety, changes in taste sensation, or reduced sensitivity to sweets

Elimination pattern
• may report constipation accompanied by abdominal discomfort or diarrhea

Activity-exercise pattern
• may report general fatigue and weakness

Sleep-rest pattern
• may report sleep disturbed by cough

Self-perception—self-concept pattern
• inability to carry out routine activities may cause questioning of self-worth and a feeling of powerlessness
• may express fear related to diagnosis, physical disabilities, and possible death

Role-relationship pattern
• may describe inability to assume family tasks, occupational role, and so forth
• may report feelings of loss related to changing roles and possible death
• may report loss of a significant relationship before diagnosis

Sexuality-reproductive pattern
• may report inability to be sexually active without experiencing dyspnea

Coping—stress tolerance pattern
• usually reports feeling depressed or despondent

Value-belief pattern
• may express feeling of personal control over circumstances (common in the patient with an above-average chance for successful remission)
• may equate cancer with death (common in the patient with a below-average chance for successful remission)

PHYSICAL FINDINGS
Cardiovascular
- rapid pulse rate if anemia is present
- arrhythmias if heart is involved
- edema of face or neck or distended neck veins if superior vena cava syndrome is present

Pulmonary
- cough (may be nocturnal)
- rust-streaked or purulent sputum
- crackles, wheezes, and friction rub in affected lung
- hoarseness if vocal cords are involved
- finger clubbing

Neurologic
- headache, mental confusion, and unsteady gait if central nervous system (CNS) is involved
- diminished deep tendon reflexes
- decreased mental alertness if anemia and hypoxemia are present

Musculoskeletal
- pathologic fractures with metastasis

DIAGNOSTIC STUDIES
- carcinoembryonic antigen (CEA) titer—high levels may be useful to monitor treatment responses; 50% of patients may have false-negative titers
- arterial blood gas (ABG) measurements—may reveal hypoxemia
- hemoglobin values—may be low from anemia
- hematocrit—may be low from anemia
- platelet count—may be low from bone marrow suppression
- white blood cell (WBC) count—may be low from bone marrow suppression
- sputum collection for cytology—may be useful to determine cell type (according to continuum of classes from normal to malignant)
- serum albumin level—hypoalbuminemia may indicate malnutrition
- serum creatinine level—indicates altered renal function related to chemotherapy
- 24-hour urine creatinine test—nutritional index, indicates changes in lean body weight when compared with individual's height; also indicates altered renal function related to chemotherapy

- chest X-ray—may reveal tumor position; usually does not show early tumor involvement
- computed tomography scan—outlines tumor's size, shape, and position
- bronchoscopy—useful in diagnosing centrally located lesions
- mediastinoscopy—needle biopsy of nodes useful in diagnosis and tumor staging
- radioisotopic scans—performed to assess for metastasis
- scalene node biopsy—determines lymphatic involvement

POTENTIAL COMPLICATIONS
From lung cancer:
- pleural effusion
- pneumonitis
- cardiac failure or arrhythmias
- brachial plexus involvement
- Cushing's syndrome
- hypercalcemia
- syndrome of inappropriate antidiuretic hormone secretion (SIADH)
- peripheral neuritis
- CNS degeneration
- dermatomyositis
- superior vena cava syndrome
- paralysis of diaphragm
- pathologic fractures
- disseminated intravascular coagulation

From chemotherapy:
- bone marrow suppression
- immunosuppression
- renal tubular necrosis
- liver toxicity
- cardiotoxicity
- pulmonary toxicity
- neurotoxicity
- sterility

Collaborative problem: *Hypoxemia related to aberrant cellular growth of lung tissue, bronchial obstruction, increased mucus production, or pleurisy*

NURSING PRIORITY: Optimize oxygen availability to cells.

Interventions

1. Initiate ABG measurements on admission, and monitor for changes in the partial pressure of oxygen (PO_2) daily or as the patient's clinical condition changes, as ordered.

Rationales

1. The PO_2 indicates the amount of pressure oxygen exerts against an artery. A decreased PO_2 reflects increased hypoxemia.

2. Administer humidified oxygen continuously, via mask, as ordered and according to nursing judgment.

2. Oxygen administered at higher-than-room-air concentrations increases the oxyhemoglobin saturation of available red blood cells. An increase in hemoglobin saturation increases the amount of oxygen available for cellular metabolism if circulation is not impaired. The patient with lung cancer frequently needs high concentrations of oxygen that can be provided only by mask or mechanical ventilation. An oxygen humidifier decreases the drying effect of oxygen administration on the respiratory mucosa.

3. Elevate the head of the bed during dyspneic episodes.

3. Elevating the head of the bed aids respiratory movement by allowing gravity to displace abdominal organs downward, thus decreasing pressure on the diaphragm.

4. Evaluate and document breath sounds, respiratory rate, and chest movements every 8 hours or more frequently, based on the patient's condition. Observe for dyspnea: complaints of difficulty breathing, shortness of breath, flaring nostrils, and intercostal retractions on inspiration or bulging on expiration.

4. Dyspnea is a subjective finding that indicates hypoxemia. Abnormal findings common in the patient with a lung tumor include crackles, bronchial breath sounds, pleural friction rubs, and decreased breath sounds.

5. During dyspneic episodes, stay with the patient, explain all procedures, and support the patient and family. Control the impulse to increase the oxygen rate or concentration over the prescribed level; counsel the patient and family accordingly.

5. Dyspnea is often associated with anxiety and fear of impending death. Anxiety may be decreased if the patient feels in control and has confidence in caregivers. Increasing oxygen levels may remove the hypoxic stimulus for respiration in the patient with chronic obstructive pulmonary disease, cause carbon dioxide narcosis if a face mask is used, or cause oxygen toxicity.

6. Encourage the patient to stop or decrease smoking.

6. Smoking increases mucus production, irritates respiratory mucosa, and decreases oxyhemoglobin saturation.

7. Teach pursed-lip breathing and relaxation techniques.

7. Pursed-lip breathing increases end-expiratory pressure and helps prevent alveolar collapse. Controlled breathing and relaxation decrease the anxiety associated with dyspnea.

8. Teach huff cough or cascade cough.

8. Huff cough is accomplished as the patient takes a deep breath and, with mouth open, "huffs" several times. After repeating several times, the patient coughs. The cascade cough involves taking a deep breath and then coughing until the patient feels that no air is left in the lungs. These maneuvers maximize the coughing effort and assist with removal of secretions while conserving energy.

9. Additional individualized interventions: _____

9. Rationales: _____

_____

_____

Target outcome criteria
Within 1 week of admission, the patient will:
• exhibit less dyspnea while at rest
• use pursed-lip breathing and relaxation techniques
• decrease smoking by at least one-half compared to preadmission rate

• demonstrate huff cough and cascade cough techniques on request.

Collaborative problem: *High risk for hemorrhage related to depression of platelet production by chemotherapy*

NURSING PRIORITY: Prevent or minimize hemorrhage.

Interventions

1. Caution the patient to report any bleeding immediately, including petechiae, ecchymoses, and oozing wounds.

2. Initiate and monitor serum platelet counts before, during, and after chemotherapy, as ordered.

3. Caution the patient to use a soft or sponge toothbrush for oral hygiene and to avoid spicy foods.

4. Teach the patient to monitor urine and stools for signs of bleeding and to immediately report any that occur.

5. Instruct the patient to use an electric razor for shaving or, if male, to grow a beard (unless alopecia is present).

6. Administer medications to suppress menses, as ordered.

7. Teach the patient to report any headaches, dizziness, or light-headedness immediately.

8. Avoid I.M. injections. If they are unavoidable, apply pressure for at least 5 minutes after the injection.

9. Avoid administering aspirin and aspirin-containing medications.

10. Apply ice packs to bleeding areas.

11. Administer stool softeners, as ordered.

12. Additional individualized interventions: _____

_____

Rationales

1. Hemorrhage may occur rapidly. The patient may be able to assume some responsibility for observing for signs of bleeding. Petechiae, ecchymoses, and oozing wounds indicate clotting problems.

2. Chemotherapeutic agents suppress bone marrow and affect platelet production. A patient with a platelet count lower than 20,000/mm^3 is at high risk for hemorrhage.

3. The oral mucosa may bleed if irritated from flossing or use of a hard toothbrush or a toothpick. Spicy foods also may irritate the oral mucosa.

4. Tea- or cola-colored urine or black, tarry, or blood-streaked stools indicate bleeding.

5. Nonelectric razors increase the risk of lacerating the skin while shaving.

6. Prolonged menstrual bleeding may cause severe blood loss.

7. CNS bleeding may cause headaches, dizziness, or light-headedness. Dizziness and light-headedness also may indicate hypovolemia.

8. Decreased platelet counts prolong clotting time. Direct pressure for 5 minutes stops active bleeding in most patients.

9. Aspirin decreases platelet aggregation and increases clotting time.

10. Ice causes peripheral vasoconstriction, decreasing blood flow to the area and the risk of significant hemorrhage.

11. Stool softeners promote formation of soft stools, which decrease the risk of tearing the rectal mucosa. Soft stools also help minimize straining on defecation, which increases intracranial pressure and may lead to intracranial bleeding.

12. Rationales: _____

_____

Target outcome criteria
Within 1 week of admission, the patient will:
• exhibit vital signs within normal limits
• have no evident bleeding

• employ safety measures to prevent bleeding.

Nursing diagnosis: *Pain associated with involvement of peripheral lung structures, metastasis, or chemotherapy*

NURSING PRIORITY: Relieve pain and promote comfort.

Interventions

1. Instruct the patient to report pain or discomfort immediately.

2. Monitor the patient continually for signs of pain or discomfort, such as facial grimaces, splinting of the chest (painful area), diaphoresis, or restlessness.

3. Involve the patient in pain-control strategies by using imagery and relaxation techniques. See the "Pain" plan, page 69, for details.

4. Administer pain medication, as needed, according to a set schedule or medical protocol and nursing judgment. Teach the patient or a family member how to administer pain medication after discharge.

5. Additional individualized interventions: _____

Rationales

1. Early intervention provides more effective pain relief than measures employed after the pain has peaked.

2. The patient may not report pain or discomfort. Careful observation may detect nonverbal indications that the patient is in pain.

3. Cognitive measures may decrease pain perception. The "Pain" plan contains general interventions for pain.

4. Pain medication ordered for a terminally ill patient may be given more frequently and in larger doses than routinely recommended (the patient receiving pain medication over a prolonged period may develop an increased tolerance). A set schedule may improve ongoing pain control because analgesics are more effective if given before pain becomes severe. Self- (or family) administration of medication enables the patient to control pain at home.

5. Rationales: _____

Target outcome criteria

Within 1 day of admission, the patient will:
• verbalize pain relief
• show a relaxed facial expression
• assume a relaxed posture.

By the time of discharge, the patient will:
• request pain-relief medication before pain peaks
• express an increased sense of control over pain
• demonstrate the correct procedure for administering pain medication.

Nursing diagnosis: *High risk for infection related to immunosuppression from chemotherapy and malnutrition*

NURSING PRIORITY: Prevent infection.

Interventions

1. Observe strict medical and surgical asepsis during wound care, venipuncture, or any invasive procedures.

2. Monitor and record temperature every 8 hours. Report even slight temperature elevations.

3. Instruct the patient to avoid crowds and persons with infections. Do not place the patient in reverse isolation unless laminar airflow (or other method) is available.

4. Monitor WBC counts before, during, and after chemotherapy, as ordered.

Rationales

1. The immunosuppressed patient easily contracts infections because of diminished host defenses. Maintaining strict medical and surgical asepsis decreases the risk of exposing the patient to pathogenic organisms.

2. Elevated temperature is a sign of infection. The immunosuppressed patient may show slight or no temperature elevation even when extensive infection is present.

3. The risk of infection is increased when a patient is exposed to individuals with contagious diseases. Reverse isolation is usually not effective, unless laminar airflow is used, because airborne organisms can still enter the patient's room.

4. Chemotherapy causes bone marrow depression, which may decrease the WBC count. Granulocyte counts below 1,000/mm^3 increase the patient's risk of infection.

5. Initiate routine cultures of stool, urine, sputum, naso-pharynx, oropharynx, and skin, as ordered.

5. Cultures provide information about bacterial colony growth that may produce infection. Early information about possible causes of infection guides the doctor in prescribing appropriate antibiotic therapy.

6. Instruct the female patient to use sanitary napkins instead of tampons.

6. Tampons may traumatize the vaginal mucosa and provide a favorable environment for pathogen growth.

7. Avoid using indwelling urinary catheters.

7. Indwelling catheters may introduce pathogens into the bladder and increase the risk of urinary tract infections.

8. Additional individualized interventions: _____

8. Rationales: _____

Target outcome criteria
Within 1 day of admission, the patient will isolate self from infected family members or friends.

Within 1 week of admission, the patient will:
• present no signs of infection
• have normal temperature
• present no growth from cultures.

Nursing diagnosis: *High risk for sensory-perceptual alteration related to peripheral neuropathies caused by chemotherapy*

NURSING PRIORITY: Minimize sensory-perceptual deficits caused by chemotherapy.

Interventions

1. Assess for, document, and report deficits in neurologic functioning, including paresthesias, abnormal deep tendon reflexes, or foot drop.

2. Discontinue or decrease the chemotherapy dosage, depending on the neuropathies' severity, as ordered.

3. Explain that changes in sensation are related to chemotherapy, and allow the patient to express fears related to this situation.

4. Protect the area of decreased sensory perception from injury: use a bath thermometer; assess the skin every 8 hours for signs of trauma; apply dressings to injured areas; use a night light; and avoid clutter in areas of activity to prevent abrasions, contusions, or falls.

5. Additional individualized interventions: _____

Rationales

1. Chemotherapeutic agents such as vincristine (Oncovin) may cause peripheral neuropathies.

2. Discontinuation or dosage reduction of medications, such as vinca alkaloids, may reverse adverse neurologic effects and will prevent further neuropathies.

3. Fear may be reduced when the patient confronts the situation.

4. Decreased perception at sensory nerve endings may reduce the patient's ability to judge temperature and pressure and may also reduce pain sensation. Taking preventive measures reduces the potential for injury.

5. Rationales: _____

Target outcome criteria
Within 1 week of admission, the patient will:
• have no complaints of paresthesias
• exhibit no evidence of foot drop

• have normal deep tendon reflexes.

Nursing diagnosis: *Nutritional deficit related to cachexia associated with tumor growth, anorexia, changes in taste sensation, or stomatitis*

NURSING PRIORITIES: (a) Minimize weight loss, and (b) promote return to optimum achievable body weight.

Interventions

1. Within 24 hours of admission, estimate required protein needs based on ideal body weight and serum total protein level.

2. With the patient and dietitian, develop diet plans based on calculated dietary needs and the patient's food preferences.

3. Increase dietary protein levels by adding powdered milk to gravies, puddings, and milk products.

4. Provide small, frequent feedings.

5. Document weight weekly.

6. Provide antiemetics, as ordered, before administering chemotherapeutic agents. To reduce nausea, provide diversional activities during chemotherapy and encourage the patient to lick salt or a lemon slice or sip sweetened ice water.

7. Assess the oral mucosa for stomatitis daily and document findings.

8. Provide a mild mouthwash with viscous lidocaine (Xylocaine) before meals.

9. After meals, clean the patient's mouth with ½ tsp of sodium bicarbonate and ½ tsp salt mixed with 8 oz tap water. Follow with a 1:5 solution of hydrogen peroxide and water. Rinse with the sodium bicarbonate and salt solution. Do not use the hydrogen peroxide solution if bleeding occurs in the mouth.

10. Lubricate the patient's lips with petrolatum.

11. Assess oral mucosa daily for signs of lesions from opportunistic infections, such as *Candida*.

12. Instruct the patient to swish and swallow with yogurt or buttermilk three times a day.

13. Administer oral nystatin (Mycostatin), as ordered.

Rationales

1. Caloric needs are altered by cancer-related cachexia. Serum total protein level reflects the status of visceral protein stores. Protein needs for a patient with cancer are calculated as 1 g/kg of ideal body weight (1 gram of protein = 30 kcal).

2. Patient participation allows some feeling of control. Nutritional intake should increase if the patient's likes and dislikes are considered in planning meals.

3. Powdered milk increases protein content without increasing bulk.

4. Small, frequent feedings increase total intake for the patient who experiences the early satiety common in cancer.

5. An accurate record of weight allows accurate assessment of changing nutritional needs. A patient with cancer commonly experiences significant weight loss.

6. The effects of chemotherapy on the CNS and gastric mucosa may induce vomiting. Prochlorperazine (Compazine), droperidol (Inapsine), and haloperidol (Haldol) are effective antiemetics. Marijuana and tetrahydrocannabinol are being studied for control of nausea and vomiting. Nausea associated with chemotherapy may be psychogenic (it sometimes occurs before chemotherapy is administered); diversional activities may distract the patient's attention and reduce nausea. The taste of lemon, salt, or sugar relieves nausea in some patients.

7. Chemotherapeutic agents, such as methotrexate (Folex) and fluorouracil (Adrucil), affect cells that undergo rapid replication, such as those in the GI system. Stomatitis interferes with the ability to eat.

8. The local anesthetic action of lidocaine decreases oral discomfort during meals.

9. Rinsing and cleaning with a sodium bicarbonate and salt solution and water and hydrogen peroxide reduces the bacterial count in the mouth and decreases the risk of infection. Using hydrogen peroxide in the presence of bleeding may disrupt clot formation.

10. Lubrication with petrolatum reduces lip drying and cracking.

11. *Candida* is an opportunistic organism that may cause infection in an immunosuppressed patient.

12. Yogurt and buttermilk restore to the GI tract the natural flora destroyed by chemotherapeutic agents. Growth of opportunistic organisms is decreased if normal flora are maintained.

13. Oral nystatin is effective against candidal infections.

14. Additional individualized interventions: _____

14. Rationales: _____

_____

_____

Target outcome criteria
Within 1 week of admission, the patient will:
• gain approximately 2 lb (1 kg)
• plan meals appropriately, with or without family assistance

• have no nausea or vomiting
• exhibit pink oral mucosa, with no lesions.

Nursing diagnosis: *Constipation or diarrhea related to chemotherapy*

NURSING PRIORITY: Promote normal bowel elimination.

Interventions

1. Assess and document bowel elimination pattern on admission. Determine usual bowel elimination pattern before chemotherapy.

2. Administer antidiarrheal medication, such as diphenoxylate hydrochloride (Lomotil), as ordered.

3. Assess for signs of paralytic ileus (such as diminished or absent bowel sounds and abdominal discomfort) every 8 hours. If present, report them to the doctor immediately.

4. Prevent constipation by increasing dietary fiber, providing warm fluids, and promoting the optimum amount of exercise. Do not check for fecal impaction if thrombocytopenia is present.

5. Administer stool softeners, as ordered.

6. Additional individualized interventions: _____

_____

Rationales

1. Chemotherapeutic agents may cause constipation or diarrhea. Information about previous bowel elimination pattern provides a baseline for evaluating bowel elimination during the hospital stay.

2. Diphenoxylate is an effective antidiarrheal because of its anticholinergic activity, which slows gastric motility.

3. Paralytic ileus, a medical emergency, may be caused by chemotherapeutic agents.

4. Bran, raw vegetables, fruits, and whole grain breads provide dietary fiber and promote bowel elimination. Liquids increase peristalsis. Exercise causes abdominal muscle contraction and promotes bowel elimination. Checking for fecal impaction may cause the thrombocytopenic patient to bleed.

5. Stool softeners promote bowel elimination by increasing the water content of stools and easing their passage.

6. Rationales: _____

_____

Target outcome criteria
Within 1 week of admission, the patient will:
• maintain regular bowel elimination
• have soft stools.

Nursing diagnosis: *High risk for altered urinary elimination related to possible development of renal toxicity or hemorrhagic cystitis from chemotherapy*

NURSING PRIORITY: Maintain normal urinary elimination pattern.

Interventions

1. Assess and document urinary elimination pattern on admission.

Rationales

1. Accurate assessment directs appropriate care planning.

2. Force fluids and administer allopurinol (Lopurin) before administering chemotherapeutic agents, as ordered.

2. Cyclophosphamide (Cytoxan) may cause hemorrhagic cystitis. Methotrexate may cause renal toxicity. Increasing fluid intake increases the glomerular filtration rate and reduces the risk of potentially toxic renal effects from chemotherapy. Allopurinol decreases uric acid calculi formation from chemotherapy by inhibiting uric acid synthesis.

3. Alkalinize the patient's urine before and during chemotherapy to prevent uric acid calculi formation.

3. Chemotherapy may cause uric acid calculi formation because uric acid excretion is increased in acidic urine. Fruits (such as oranges, tomatoes, and grapefruit), vegetables, and milk increase urine alkalinity and decrease uric acid calculi formation.

4. Monitor serum creatinine and 24-hour urine creatinine, as ordered, before chemotherapy.

4. Serum creatinine and 24-hour urine creatinine studies provide information about renal function. Normally functioning kidneys should clear creatinine.

5. Additional individualized interventions: _____

5. Rationales: _____

Target outcome criteria
Within 1 week of admission, the patient will:
• have urine output within normal limits
• have amber-colored urine

• have no pain on urination.

Nursing diagnosis: *Activity intolerance related to weakness from cachexia, altered protein metabolism, muscle wasting, or hypoxia*

NURSING PRIORITY: Optimize activity level without inducing dyspnea.

Interventions

1. Immediately on admission, determine what activities the patient can tolerate without dyspnea.

2. Instruct the patient to organize activities so that tasks are spaced in manageable units.

3. Teach proper body mechanics to decrease the energy expenditure associated with activities of daily living (ADLs): explain the need to slide objects rather than carry them, work close to the body, sit when possible, use gravity, and avoid unnecessary bending or reaching.

4. Additional individualized interventions: _____

Rationales

1. Dyspnea occurs as energy requirements exceed oxygen availability. Information about dyspnea-free activities guides activity recommendations.

2. Activities performed without fatigue promote comfort and decrease dyspnea.

3. The use of proper body mechanics reduces energy expenditure.

4. Rationales: _____

Target outcome criteria
Within 1 week of admission, the patient will:
• manage activities with less dyspnea
• perform ADLs with minimal assistance.

Nursing diagnosis: *Sleep pattern disturbance related to nocturnal cough*

NURSING PRIORITY: Optimize sleep patterns.

Interventions

1. Assess and document sleep patterns on admission. Discuss sleep patterns before the diagnosis was made.

2. Provide quick, efficient assistance with respiratory hygiene when coughing disrupts sleep.

3. Instruct the patient to sleep with the head elevated.

4. Exercise caution in administering sedatives and hypnotics.

5. Additional individualized interventions: _____

Rationales

1. Sleep pattern goals should be based on the patient's perception of normal sleep patterns. Sleep disruption, commonly caused by the psychological distress of diagnosis, robs the patient of energy needed to cope with the illness.

2. Sleep disturbance is minimized if care is provided quickly and efficiently.

3. Head elevation while sleeping eases the work of breathing by decreasing pressure on the diaphragm.

4. Sedatives and hypnotics may blunt respiratory drive and worsen hypoxia.

5. Rationales: _____

Target outcome criterion
Within 3 days of admission, the patient will report 8 to 10 hours of sleep in 24 hours, including 4 hours of uninterrupted sleep.

Nursing diagnosis: *Self-esteem disturbance related to weight loss, cough, sputum production, hair loss, or role changes*

NURSING PRIORITY: Promote a positive self-concept.

Interventions

1. Approach the patient with an accepting attitude.

2. Assess and document attitudes and responses related to the patient's self-concept and role changes.

3. Encourage the patient and family to share feelings.

4. Discuss methods to accentuate the patient's positive features and minimize weight loss through changes in hairstyle and clothing.

5. Encourage the use of a portable disposal unit for discarding tissues and sputum.

6. Encourage frequent contact, in person or by telephone, with loved ones.

Rationales

1. An individual needs to experience acceptance from others to develop a positive self-concept.

2. Accurate assessment of the patient's self-concept facilitates appropriate care planning.

3. Expression of feelings promotes honest, open relationships.

4. Clothing that fits well without accentuating weight loss improves general feelings of well-being. A well-groomed appearance improves self-concept.

5. Knowing how to dispose of unsightly tissues and sputum improves the patient's feelings of control and increases self-esteem.

6. Contact with others minimizes isolation and improves self-concept.

7. Discuss probable hair loss before chemotherapy starts (keep in mind that hair loss may affect all parts of the body, not just the scalp). With the patient's permission, cut hair before loss occurs. Natural hair may be used to fashion a wig, or the patient can be fitted for a wig before hair loss. The patient may want to wear a hat or scarf instead of a wig.

7. Knowledge about hair loss will decrease the anxiety associated with it. Hair loss is more manageable when hair is short. A wig, hat, or scarf helps minimize the impact of hair loss on body image and self-esteem.

8. Remind the patient that hair loss is not permanent and that hair regrows after the last dose of chemotherapeutic agent. Be sure to mention that new hair may be different in color and texture.

8. Hair regrowth usually begins within a few days to a few weeks after the last dose of chemotherapeutic agent.

9. Explain to the patient about scalp tourniquets and scalp hypothermia treatments that may diminish hair loss. Inform the patient that these procedures are time-consuming and may be unsuccessful.

9. Scalp tourniquets and scalp hypothermia treatments diminish the contact of chemotherapeutic agents with hair follicles and may decrease hair loss. The patient should be allowed to make an informed choice.

10. Additional individualized interventions: _____

10. Rationales: _____

Target outcome criteria
Within 1 week of admission, the patient will:
• wear well-fitting clothes
• express the desire to purchase a wig or wear a hat or scarf

• initiate interaction with friends, family, and health care providers.

Nursing diagnosis: *Altered sexuality patterns related to dyspnea and possible sterility*

NURSING PRIORITIES: (a) Promote acceptance of optimal expressions of sexuality, and (b) promote long-range plans for childbearing, if desired.

Interventions

1. During initial assessment, discuss any changes in patterns of sexual expression that have resulted from the diagnosis and treatments.

2. Help the patient and spouse (or partner) discuss their desires for sexual expression and intimacy. Help them differentiate between the two needs and stress the importance of love and affection in maintaining a sense of closeness with each other.

3. Discuss options for sexual expression within the patient's physical limitations. For example, if intercourse is fatiguing or impossible for physical reasons, and if the couple is receptive, suggest alternative forms of sexual and sensual expression that appeal to all senses, such as massage with scented oils, listening to music, sharing foods with various tastes and textures, and reading romantic literature.

4. Encourage the use of supplemental oxygen during intercourse.

Rationales

1. Open discussion helps the patient to develop realistic goals and expectations related to sexual expression.

2. Honest, caring communication between partners about their sexual needs promotes adjustment to cancer's impact on sexuality. Differentiating the desire for sexual activity from the desire for emotional closeness may allow the couple to focus on the strengths in their relationship rather than on a loss of a specific sexual activity.

3. Sexual expression is closely tied to self-esteem, and the patient and spouse (or partner) may find that their self-esteem suffers when they can no longer participate in intercourse. Knowledge of alternative methods of sexual and sensual gratification can restore sexual intimacy and increase self-esteem when intercourse is no longer an option.

4. Exercise increases oxygen demands.

5. Provide privacy for the patient and spouse (or partner) to maintain intimacy through such activities as private discussions and affectionate cuddling, if desired.

5. Intimacy is encouraged when individuals can share uninterrupted time.

6. Explain that reduced sexual responsiveness may be associated with fatigue or chemotherapy.

6. Knowing the reasons for reduced sexual responsiveness decreases anxiety about sexuality.

7. Explain that chemotherapy may cause sterility. If appropriate, discuss sperm banking before chemotherapy. Inform the patient that childbearing plans should be postponed for at least 18 months after the last dose of chemotherapeutic agent.

7. Chemotherapy may affect gonadal function and diminish sperm and ovum production. Sperm may be saved in sperm banks for future fertilization. Drug-induced changes in sperm and ova should be reversed by 18 months after the end of chemotherapy. Although the prognosis for these patients may be poor, discussion of future plans may help maintain hope.

8. Additional individualized interventions: _____

8. Rationales: _____

Target outcome criteria
Within 1 week of admission, the patient and spouse (or partner) will:
• discuss the desire for sexual expression and intimacy
• request time for privacy.

Discharge planning
NURSING DISCHARGE CRITERIA
Upon the patient's discharge, documentation shows evidence of:
• absence of fever and pulmonary or cardiovascular complications
• stable vital signs
• absence of infection
• nausea or vomiting and diarrhea controlled by oral medications
• adequate hydration
• normal renal function
• adequate nutritional and fluid intake
• ability to control pain using oral and subcutaneous medication
• absence of bowel complications
• coughing controlled by medication
• minimal use of oxygen to assist breathing
• ability to demonstrate or verbalize proper oxygen administration technique, including how to acquire oxygen for home use
• ability to tolerate ADLs and ambulation with minimal difficulty
• adequate home support system or, if appropriate, referral to hospice, home care, or both
• knowledge of community support programs.

PATIENT-FAMILY DISCHARGE TEACHING CHECKLIST
Document evidence that the patient and family demonstrate an understanding of:
___ diagnosis
___ effects of chemotherapy
___ prevention, detection, and management of bleeding
___ use of supplemental oxygen
___ smoking cessation
___ breathing exercises
___ all discharge medications' purpose, dose, administration schedule, and adverse effects requiring medical attention; usual discharge medications include analgesics, antiemetics, and stool softeners or antidiarrheals, as appropriate
___ pain relief measures
___ signs of and methods to prevent infection
___ signs of neurologic changes
___ dietary modifications
___ measures to control nausea and vomiting
___ measures to promote normal renal function
___ measures to decrease dyspnea
___ measures to minimize effects of changing body image
___ plans for sexual expression
___ date, time, and location of follow-up appointments
___ how to contact the doctor
___ when and how to seek emergency medical care
___ community resources.

DOCUMENTATION CHECKLIST

Using outcome criteria as a guide, document:
__ clinical status on admission
__ significant changes in status
__ pertinent laboratory and diagnostic test findings
__ response to chemotherapy
__ episodes of dyspnea
__ oxygen therapy
__ bleeding episodes
__ nutritional status
__ bowel elimination
__ urinary elimination
__ activity tolerance
__ sleep patterns
__ patient-family teaching
__ discharge planning.

ASSOCIATED PLANS OF CARE

Dying
Grieving
Ineffective Family Coping
Ineffective Individual Coping
Knowledge Deficit
Pain

References

Beare, P., and Myers, J., eds. *Principles and Practice of Adult Health Nursing.* St. Louis: Mosby-Year Book, 1990.

Campbell, C. *Nursing Diagnosis and Intervention in Nursing Practice,* 2nd ed. New York: John Wiley & Sons, 1984.

Carnevali, D., and Reiner, A. *The Cancer Experience: Nursing Diagnosis and Management.* Philadelphia: J.B. Lippincott Co., 1990.

Gordon, M. *Nursing Diagnosis: Process and Application.* 2nd ed. New York: McGraw-Hill Book Co., 1987.

Haber, J., et al. *Comprehensive Psychiatric Nursing,* 4th ed. New York: McGraw-Hill Book Co., 1992.

Lewis, C.M. *Nutrition and Nutrition Therapy in Nursing.* East Norwalk, Conn.: Appleton-Century-Crofts, 1986.

Maxwell, M.B. "Dyspnea in Advanced Cancer," *American Journal of Nursing* 85(6):672-77, June 1985.

Phipps, W., et al., eds. *Medical-Surgical Nursing: Concepts and Clinical Practice.* 4th ed. St. Louis: Mosby-Year Book, Inc., 1991.

Mechanical Ventilation

DRG information

DRG 475 Respiratory System Diagnosis With Ventila-
    tor Support.
    Mean LOS = 9.7 days
    Principal diagnoses include:
    • respiratory failure
    • chronic obstructive pulmonary disease
    (COPD)
    • acute or chronic bronchitis
    • pneumonia from various causes
    • adult respiratory distress syndrome
    (ARDS)
    • mechanical respiratory assistance.
Additional DRG information: To use DRG 475, one of
the above diagnoses must appear as the principal diagnosis. A patient with Guillain-Barré syndrome complicated by respiratory failure will not be assigned DRG
475 because the respiratory failure is a secondary diagnosis. Besides the respiratory principal diagnosis,
both mechanical ventilator assistance and endotracheal
tube insertion must be coded.

Introduction
DEFINITION AND TIME FOCUS
Mechanical ventilation (providing gas volumes sufficient to maintain alveolar ventilation) commonly is required for patients with significant breathing
abnormalities that may lead to apnea or respiratory
failure. This plan focuses on the patient receiving positive-pressure ventilation, the most common type of
mechanical ventilation in critical care.

ETIOLOGY AND PRECIPITATING FACTORS
• central respiratory depression, such as from drug
overdose, head trauma, cerebrovascular accident, anesthesia, or cardiac arrest
• airway diseases, such as asthma and bronchitis
• parenchymal diseases, such as ARDS, pulmonary
edema, pneumonia, and emphysema
• neuromuscular disorders, such as myasthenia gravis
and Guillain-Barré syndrome
• chest wall injury, such as pneumothorax, flail chest,
and major thoracic surgery

Focused assessment guidelines
NURSING HISTORY (Functional health pattern findings)

Health perception—health management pattern
• manifests sudden or progressive onset of abnormal
ventilatory patterns or airway obstruction
• if able to speak, reports severe dyspnea or air hunger
• may have history of motor vehicle accident, assault,
or other head, chest, or orthopedic trauma

• may be under treatment for long-standing chronic respiratory disease
• may have had recent major surgical procedure involving the thorax or upper abdomen
• may have history of drug or alcohol abuse
• may have history of cardiac disease

PHYSICAL FINDINGS
Pulmonary
• labored breathing
• shallow breathing
• agonal breathing or other abnormal breathing pattern
• tachypnea
• intercostal retractions
• nasal flaring
• accessory muscle use
• decreased or absent breath sounds
• crackles, gurgles, or wheezes
• increased secretions

Neurologic
• restlessness
• confusion
• agitation
• somnolence
• unconsciousness

Cardiovascular
• tachycardia (early), bradycardia (late)
• arrhythmias
• hypertension or hypotension

Integumentary
• diaphoresis
• cyanosis (central or peripheral)

DIAGNOSTIC STUDIES
• arterial blood gas (ABG) levels—reveal hypercapnia
(increased partial pressure of arterial carbon dioxide
[$PaCO_2$] greater than 50 mm Hg) in a patient who previously had normal levels (or greater than 10 mm Hg
increase above usual value in a COPD patient). ABGs
also reveal hypoxemia with a partial pressure of arterial oxygen (PaO_2) less than 50 mm Hg on supplemental oxygen
• alveolar-arterial (A-a) gradient—may be greater than
300 mm Hg on 100% oxygen
• shunt—may be greater than 30%
• minute ventilation (spontaneous)—may be less than
5 liters/minute, indicating insufficient ventilation to
remove carbon dioxide adequately, or greater than 10
liters/minute, indicating excessive work of breathing
• vital capacity (VC)—may be less than 15 ml/kg
body weight, indicating poor ventilatory reserve

• maximum inspiratory force (MIF) — may be less than 20 cm H_2O, indicating weak respiratory drive or respiratory musculature

• dead space: tidal volume (V_D:V_T) ratio — may be greater than 0.6, indicating excessive wasted ventilation

POTENTIAL COMPLICATIONS
• tension pneumothorax
• GI hemorrhage
• shock
• pneumonia
• ventilator malfunction
• airway obstruction
• long-term ventilator dependency

Collaborative problem: *Ineffective alveolar ventilation related to failure to maintain prescribed ventilator settings*

NURSING PRIORITY: Maintain settings as ordered.

Interventions

1. Confirm orders for mechanical ventilation, particularly:

• ventilator type

• inspiratory mode

— control

— assist-control

Rationales

1. Mechanical ventilation may be achieved with many combinations of modes and settings.

• Choosing the right ventilator begins with choosing the type, which is determined by how the machine controls inspiration. In the acute care setting, ventilators that can deliver a prescribed volume are indicated; these are volume-cycled ventilators. Other types include time-cycled and pressure-cycled ventilators, both of which can have variable tidal volumes and are used only for special situations.

Advances in technology and an increased need for equipment have resulted in a proliferation of different ventilators. The ventilator selected depends on the patient s ventilation requirements, type of monitoring desired, and weaning options.

• Inspiratory modes determine the type and degree of control over inspiration.

— The control mode provides complete ventilatory support by delivering a set number of breaths per minute, regardless of the patient's inspiratory efforts. The least-used mode, it is appropriate only for an apneic or paralyzed patient (such as with central nervous system dysfunction or drug-induced paralysis), or in chest trauma where negative inspiratory pressure would be detrimental (such as with flail chest). It should be emphasized that this modes prevents the patient from taking *any* additional breaths.

— Assist-control, the most common mode, is suitable for almost all initial ventilator setups. This mode ensures delivery of a preset minimum number of breaths per minute but allows the patient to initiate the breath and to breathe more rapidly if desired. If the patient initiates a breath, the machine delivers the desired volume; if the patient does not breathe, the machine supplies the breath. Because the ventilator delivers a preset volume even on patient-initiated breaths, it lessens the work of breathing while improving alveolar ventilation.

—synchronized intermittent mandatory ventilation (SIMV)

—SIMV, once used only for the difficult-to-wean patient, is now considered a standard ventilatory mode for full or partial ventilatory support. The machine delivers a preset number of mandatory breaths. In between, the patient can breathe spontaneously through the ventilator circuit. The ventilator senses each breath and synchronizes the mandatory breaths in such a way as to not "stack" breaths on top of each other. Because these spontaneous breaths depend on the negative pressure the patient can generate, their V_T may vary significantly from the ventilator V_T. Advantages of SIMV include lower mean airway pressures (reducing the risk of barotrauma—lung damage from excessive pressure—and depression of cardiac output), less risk of hyperventilation, maintenance of respiratory muscle strength, and more even ventilation throughout the lung.

—pressure support.

—Pressure support uses small amounts of pressure at the end of inspiration to increase V_T in a spontaneously breathing patient. Similar to intermittent positive-pressure breathing (IPPB) machines, pressure support can be used in combination with SIMV or as a weaning mode for a patient with inadequate spontaneous volumes.

• expiratory maneuvers

• Expiratory maneuvers determine the degree of resistance to expiration.

—positive end-expiratory pressure (PEEP)

—PEEP is used commonly with positive-pressure ventilation of the patient with alveolar collapse (from loss of surfactant, early small airway closure, or atelectasis) or alveolar filling (as with pulmonary edema). In such a patient, nonfunctioning alveoli, unable to oxygenate blood flowing through pulmonary capillaries, produce an abnormal pulmonary shunt and hypoxemia refractory to oxygen therapy. PEEP is thought to help keep alveoli from collapsing and to recruit nonfunctioning alveoli. It also increases functional residual capacity (FRC) and allows continuous gas diffusion to take place. Because PEEP improves ventilation-perfusion matching, oxygenation improves. PEEP permits lowering of inspired oxygen concentration, a valuable consideration in preventing lung damage from excessive oxygen exposure.

—continuous positive airway pressure (CPAP).

—CPAP is similar to PEEP but is used for a spontaneously breathing patient. It maintains positive airway pressure throughout the respiratory cycle. Benefits are similar to PEEP. It can be applied through a ventilator (for non-SIMV breaths), through various devices for the intubated patient not using a ventilator, or via special devices for a nonintubated patient.

2. Collaborate with the respiratory therapist to monitor prescribed settings when settings are changed, when arterial blood is drawn for ABG measurements, or when pulse oximetry or capnography is used.

2. Depending on the unit protocol, either the nurse or the respiratory therapist may be responsible for performing the ventilator checks. If the respiratory therapist performs the checks, the nurse should confirm that ventilator settings are as ordered when first assuming responsibility for the patient. Close collaboration between the nurse and the respiratory therapist is essential for optimal patient care. Checks at the times indicated ensure accuracy of the prescribed settings.

• respiratory rate: Count the machine rate and the patient's rate for one minute each and compare. Check controls for proper settings.

• With all ventilatory modes, the ventilator may not actually deliver the number of breaths set. In addition, with assist-control or SIMV, the patient can breathe above the set rate. With most volume ventilators, the rate is set with a knob.

• tidal volume: Compare delivered V_T with desired V_T, typically 10 to 15 ml/kg. On newer models, read inspired V_T from the digital readout. On models lacking a readout, measure exhaled V_T with a Wright respirometer.

• minute ventilation (MV): If the patient is on assist-control or SIMV, compare actual and desired MV. If the patient is on SIMV, also compare total and non-SIMV MV.

• inspiratory flow rate

• inspiratory-expiratory (I/E) ratio (typically 1:2 or greater)

• airway pressure (normally 20 to 40 cm H_2O and relatively constant): Monitor both peak inspiratory pressure and inspiratory plateau pressure, noting sudden changes in airway pressures or a trend of increasing pressures.

• pressure limit

• sensitivity (typically −2 cm H_2O below zero or PEEP level)

• sigh

• alarms and monitors

• V_T is the amount of air inspired or expired. V_T is set with a dial on volume ventilators. Measuring exhaled V_T indicates the amount actually received. Decreasing V_T may signify a machine, cuff, or patient leak.

• MV, the product of the respiratory rate and the V_T, determines alveolar ventilation. MV is related inversely to $PaCO_2$: as MV increases, $PaCO_2$ decreases, and vice versa. Decreased MV is associated with carbon dioxide retention and respiratory acidosis, while increased MV is associated with carbon dioxide blow-off and respiratory alkalosis.

Comparing actual and desired MVs indicates how well the machine meets the patient's ventilatory needs. Comparing total and non-SIMV MVs indicates what amount the patient's spontaneous breaths are contributing to total MV; monitoring this amount can help the doctor or respiratory therapist evaluate the patient's readiness for weaning.

• This rate is the speed of airflow per unit of time. In the volume-cycled ventilator, it is set with a knob. Slower flow rates are preferred because they cause better gas flow characteristics: less turbulence, lower mean airway pressure, and better gas distribution within the lungs. When a faster flow is needed, the patient can become quite uncomfortable. In that case, it may be necessary to increase the flow rate so that the patient has time to exhale before the next breath is triggered. Newer models contain demand valves so the patient can receive the flow needed.

• Expiration must be longer than inspiration to avoid air trapping.

• Peak inspiratory pressure is the pressure at peak inspiration. It reflects the maximum pressure necessary to overcome resistance to flow and to lung and chest wall expansion. Increased peak inspiratory pressure implies increased airway resistance, such as from secretions or bronchospasm. Plateau pressure is the pressure at end-inspiration. It reflects the pressure necessary to hold the airways open and deliver the volume of gas. Increased plateau pressure implies stiffness of lung tissue.

• This setting limits the amount of pressure that the machine can exert when delivering volume in order to prevent barotrauma. Once this level is reached, inspiration is ended even if the desired V_T has not been delivered. The pressure limit may be reached occasionally if the patient is coughing, has excessive airway secretions, or the ventilator tubing is kinked. Consistently reaching the pressure limit suggests decreased compliance or a pneumothorax.

• The sensitivity knob controls the amount of negative inspiratory pressure the patient must generate in order to trigger an inspiration.

• A sigh is a periodic deep breath delivered by the ventilator. Thought to prevent atelectasis, sighing is not commonly used. Instead, the patient is ventilated with large V_Ts to prevent atelectasis.

• Alarms need to be set for high airway pressure (usually the same as the pressure limit), low airway pressure (disconnect alarm), high and low volumes, and high and low fraction of inspired oxygen (FIO_2). Many other parameters can be monitored and alarms can be set. Newer ventilators employ microprocessors that can simultaneously and continuously monitor almost all parameters related to the ventilator.

3. In collaboration with the respiratory therapist, monitor compliance every 8 hours:

• Monitor static compliance (V_T divided by end-inspiratory [plateau] pressure) or dynamic compliance (V_T divided by peak inspiratory pressure). If PEEP is used, subtract PEEP value from pressure before dividing.

• Compare the patient's values to normal values (static: 100 ml/cm H_2O; dynamic: 50 ml/cm H_2O). Monitor compliance curves or note trend of values.

4. Evaluate pulmonary status at least every 2 hours. Note particularly the symmetry of chest excursion, bilateral breath sounds, and any adventitious sounds.

5. Additional individualized interventions: _____

_____

3. Compliance measures the resistance to expansion. It is determined by the amount of change in volume that results from a given change in pressure (volume in milliliters divided by pressure in centimeters of water pressure equals compliance [in ml/cm H_2O]). Decreased lung compliance signifies that the lungs require more pressure to ventilate; they are stiffer than usual, as in ARDS. Increased compliance, rarely a clinical problem, indicates the lungs are easier to ventilate than usual. For example, in emphysema, where elasticity is lost, lung compliance increases, though airway obstruction still may render the patient difficult to ventilate.

• Static compliance indicates compliance when the lungs are at rest, while dynamic compliance indicates compliance when airflow is occurring. Static compliance values reflect lung compliance; dynamic compliance reflects airway resistance as well.

• Comparing static and dynamic values can help identify the source of difficulty in ventilating a patient. For example, a near-normal static compliance with a low dynamic compliance suggests the problem is increased airway resistance, while low static and low dynamic compliances suggest the problem is the lung itself, such as occurs with ARDS. Compliance curves — serial plotting of pressure changes compared to volume changes — indicate trends graphically and may help to determine the best combination of pressure and volume for a patient.

4. These factors provide data about adequacy of airflow throughout the pulmonary tree and about secretions or obstructions to flow.

5. Rationales: _____

_____

Target outcome criteria
Upon institution of mechanical ventilation and continuously thereafter, the patient will:
• have bilaterally equal chest excursion and breath sounds
• manifest compliance values within usual limits for the underlying disorder

• have ABG levels within expected limits for the underlying disorder.

Collaborative problem: *High risk for hypoxemia related to insufficient oxygen delivery or inadequate PEEP level*

NURSING PRIORITY: Maintain optimal oxygenation.

Interventions

1. Compare delivered oxygen percentage to that desired, typically 100% initially and thereafter adjusted according to PaO_2. With newer models, read delivered oxygen percentage from the digital display of the built-in oxygen analyzer. With older models, use a hand-held oxygen analyzer. Initially, use pulse oximetry, if desired, to titrate the FIO_2. Confirm the pulse oximetry readings with ABG oxygenation values.

Rationales

1. The machine may or may not deliver the set oxygen percentage. The oxygen analyzer evaluates the accuracy of oxygen delivery. Too low a percentage promotes hypoxemia, whereas too high a percentage promotes oxygen toxicity (see the "High risk for injury" collaborative problem below).

2. Be aware if the FIO_2 is greater than 50%.

• With the doctor, consider the risk of oxygen toxicity in relation to the need for oxygen therapy. If possible, implement ways to reduce the oxygen dose, as ordered.

• If it is not possible to reduce the oxygen dosage, observe the patient for sharp, pleuritic chest pain (typically after about 6 hours on 100% oxygen), decreased VC and decreased compliance (typically after 18 hours), or signs and symptoms of ARDS (typically after 24 to 48 hours). Document your observations and promptly notify the doctor if any of these signs or symptoms occur.

3. Note PEEP, typically ordered if the patient cannot maintain a PaO_2 greater than 60 mm Hg on less than 50% oxygen.

• Visually monitor the PEEP level (usually 5 to 15 cm H_2O) on the PEEP gauge or inspiratory pressure gauge (instead of dropping to zero at the end of expiration, the needle drops to the PEEP level).

• Assist the respiratory therapist with titration of PEEP by correlating PEEP level with inspired oxygen percentage, the resulting PaO_2 level, and hemodynamic values. Apply PEEP in increments of 3 to 5 cm H_2O to reach a maintenance level of 5 to 15 cm H_2O, as ordered.

4. Additional individualized interventions: _____

_____

2. Prolonged exposure to high alveolar oxygen tension promotes oxygen toxicity. Although an FIO_2 greater than 60% does not cause clinically significant parenchymal abnormalities in normal lungs, an FIO_2 greater than 50% may cause serious lung dysfunction in previously damaged or susceptible lung tissue.

• Lowering the oxygen dose, as may be achieved through PEEP, helps decrease the risk of toxicity. However, the need to treat hypoxemia takes precedence over the potential danger of oxygen toxicity.

• Signs and symptoms of oxygen toxicity reflect the progression from the initial phase of tracheobronchitis through the exudative phase of alveolar-capillary membrane damage. If unchecked, the syndrome progresses to a proliferative stage resulting in pulmonary fibrosis. To assess for chest pain in an intubated patient, observe for indications of pain, such as grimacing, and analyze pain characteristics by asking the patient questions that can be answered with a "yes" or "no" signal.

3. By increasing FRC and recruiting shunt units, PEEP improves oxygen transport and allows use of a lower inspired oxygen concentration.

• Visual monitoring confirms that the prescribed PEEP level is being maintained.

• The optimal PEEP level for a given patient is a judgment based on numerous factors, including shunt reduction, lung compliance, and cardiac output. The desired goal is maintenance of an adequate PaO_2 level on less than 60% oxygen. PEEP levels above 15 cm H_2O are associated with increased barotrauma and depressed cardiac output.

4. Rationales: _____

_____

Target outcome criteria
Within 24 hours of onset of mechanical ventilation and then continuously, the patient will:
• maintain a PaO_2 level greater than 50 mm Hg
• display no signs or symptoms of oxygen toxicity.

Nursing diagnosis: *Ineffective airway clearance related to presence of endotracheal tube, increased secretions, and the underlying disease*

NURSING PRIORITY: Maintain airway patency.

Interventions

1. Provide artificial airway care according to unit protocol or as ordered, including the following:

• Support the ventilator tubing so it does not press on the edge of the patient's nose or mouth.

• Measure cuff pressures at least every 8 hours. Optimally, maintain cuff pressure at less than 20 mm Hg with a minimal leak.

Rationales

1. Meticulous airway care can prevent numerous potential complications associated with endotracheal intubation.

• Maintaining proper alignment prevents accidental extubation, tube advancement, or nasotracheal or orotracheal erosion.

• Monitoring cuff pressures permits early detection of pressures high enough to cause tracheal ischemia and necrosis.

2. Monitor endotracheal tube position. When oral or nasal endotracheal tube position is confirmed after intubation, mark the tube. Check tube placement frequently by noting the relationship between the mark and the patient's lip or nostril. Also assess breath sounds every 1 to 2 hours.

2. An endotracheal tube can migrate downward to rest against the carina, obstructing airflow and causing the patient to cough and fight the ventilator, or to enter one of the bronchi (usually the right main stem), preventing ventilation of the opposite lung. It also can migrate upward, increasing the risk of unintended extubation. Monitoring tube position and breath sounds provides adequate warning of tube movement to take corrective action.

3. Keep a manual self-inflating bag and mask connected to 100% oxygen at the bedside. If accidental extubation occurs, open the airway and ventilate with the bag and mask. Summon medical assistance.

3. Using the bag and mask provides emergency ventilation in the event of accidental extubation. Reintubation must be performed by someone skilled in the technique.

4. Change the patient's position every 1 to 2 hours. Provide chest physiotherapy as indicated.

4. Position changes help drain secretions and promote ventilation of all lung areas. Chest physiotherapy promotes secretion drainage.

5. Suction when needed, as indicated by dyspnea, coughing, gurgles, secretions visible in the tube, or a high-pressure alarm. Observe these guidelines for suctioning:

5. Intubation prevents an effective cough reflex and subsequent airway clearance. Frequent suctioning is inadvisable because of the risks of suction-induced hypoxemia, arrhythmias, bronchospasm, and loss of PEEP.

• Hyperoxygenate the patient with 100% oxygen and a self-inflating bag before, during, and after suctioning. For suctioning, use a catheter with a diameter less than 50% of endotracheal tube diameter. Suction for no more than 15 seconds. Always reset the oxygen to its previous level after hyperoxygenation. Alternatively, use an in-line suction catheter to suction the trachea without disconnecting the patient from the ventilator. Hyperoxygenate the patient before, during, and after suctioning, and make sure the ventilator is returned to its previous setting.

• Suctioning causes arterial oxygen desaturation, the degree of which depends on the presuctioning PaO_2 level, catheter size in relation to endotracheal tube size, duration of suctioning, and other factors. Following the recommended guidelines helps minimize hypoxemia. Resetting the oxygen level minimizes the risk of oxygen toxicity.

• If the patient is on PEEP, use a manual self-inflating bag with a PEEP valve or a closed suctioning system when suctioning.

• A bag with a PEEP valve minimizes loss of PEEP support. A closed suctioning system maintains the ventilator connection, including PEEP, and may minimize hypoxemia. However, if suction flow is greater than the volume delivered by the ventilator, alveolar collapse may occur, producing arterial desaturation.

• Apply suction only while withdrawing the catheter.

• This technique minimizes trauma to the endothelium.

• Monitor blood pressure, heart rate, and electrocardiogram (ECG) pattern during suctioning. If adverse reactions such as bradycardia, hypotension, or arrhythmias occur, immediately remove the suctioning catheter and ventilate the patient with 100% oxygen.

• Bradycardia, hypotension, and arrhythmias may result from stimulation of vagal fibers at the carina, hyperinflation, or hypoxemia.

• While suctioning, observe for paroxysmal coughing without deep breaths; remove the catheter if it occurs.

• Paroxysmal coughing is analogous to a sustained Valsalva's maneuver at pressures high enough to cause bradycardia and hypotension. Removing the catheter reduces airway obstruction.

• If the patient reacts adversely to traditional suctioning, consult with the doctor about administering an anticholinergic agent, such as atropine, or an anesthetic, such as lidocaine (Xylocaine), before suctioning.

• Adverse reactions should be forestalled when possible. An anticholinergic agent will prevent bradycardia caused by vagal stimulation. Lidocaine decreases coughing and, in patients with increased intracranial pressure (ICP), helps prevent further pressure increases.

6. Additional individualized interventions: _____

6. Rationales: _____

_____

_____

Target outcome criteria
Continuously during mechanical ventilation, the patient
will:
• have a patent airway
• have clear breath sounds bilaterally, as underlying
condition allows.

Collaborative problem: *High risk for injury: complications related to patient deterioration, mechanical breakdown, increased intrathoracic pressure, or bypassed defense mechanisms*

NURSING PRIORITIES: (a) Prevent complications when possible and (b) respond appropriately if complications occur.

Interventions	Rationales
ABRUPT RESPIRATORY DISTRESS	
1. Keep ventilator alarms turned on at all times.	1. The patient's life depends on this therapy, and alarms can warn of potentially fatal problems. Turning the alarms off places the patient at risk for unobserved disconnection, cardiac arrest, or other catastrophe.
2. Be familiar with troubleshooting techniques before they are needed.	2. Troubleshooting techniques are complex and vary among ventilators. Learning troubleshooting techniques in advance reduces anxiety and improves the likelihood of prompt, successful resolution of a problem.
3. Continually observe whether the patient is breathing in synchrony with the ventilator. If the patient develops sudden respiratory distress or the ventilator fails abruptly, take the following steps: • Immediately disconnect the ventilator, open the airway if necessary, and ventilate the patient using a manual self-inflating bag and 100% oxygen.	3. Breathing out of synchrony (sometimes called "fighting the ventilator" or "breathing out of phase with the ventilator") markedly increases intrathoracic pressure; failure of mechanical ventilation places the patient's life in jeopardy. • Determining whether the cause of the respiratory distress is patient- or ventilator-related is crucial. Patient-related problems (such as airway obstruction or tension pneumothorax) require immediate intervention, while distress from ventilator malfunction can be relieved by ventilating the patient manually until the exact cause can be evaluated. Manual ventilation provides a quick way to distinguish between the two categories, supplies adequate emergency ventilation, and allows rapid detection of increased airway resistance or decreased compliance.
• Once ventilation is established, reevaluate the patient. If the distress has cleared, check the ventilator settings. Obtain ABG levels immediately or evaluate oximetry readings.	• If the respiratory distress has cleared, the ventilator is at fault. ABG levels or oximetry readings may reveal hypoxemia or hypercapnia, possible indicators of inadequate mechanical ventilation. The ventilator may need to be replaced or adjusted to meet the patient's needs.
• If the distress continues, perform a rapid cardiopulmonary assessment, suction the airway if indicated, or obtain medical assistance.	• This examination may reveal the cause of the distress, such as airway obstruction or tension pneumothorax.
• Evaluate for signs of tension pneumothorax, such as a sudden unexplained increase in inspiratory pressure, shock, decreased or absent breath sounds on the affected side, tracheal deviation away from the affected side, air hunger, or intense anxiety. If any of these signs are present, anticipate immediate chest X-ray, needle thoracentesis, or chest tube insertion.	• Positive pressure ventilation increases the risk of barotrauma. Tension pneumothorax, a life-threatening emergency, may result from such factors as rupture of lung blebs, friable tissue, suture disruption, or central line insertion. Immediate chest decompression is necessary to prevent cardiopulmonary arrest from mediastinal shift.

• If the problem's source cannot be identified and patient panic is suspected, hand-ventilate at a rate faster than the patient's, gradually slow down to the ventilator rate, and then reconnect the ventilator, coaching the patient in a calm, reassuring tone to breathe with the ventilator.

• If the problem persists, implement changes in ventilator settings, sedate the patient (usually with morphine sulfate), or paralyze the patient (for example, with pancuronium bromide [Pavulon]), as ordered. If paralysis is prescribed, be sure that sedation with an amnesic agent, such as diazepam (Valium) or midazolam (Versed) also is prescribed.

4. Monitor the patient on PEEP closely for barotrauma, decreased cardiac output, water retention, and, if the patient has an ICP monitor, increased ICP.

5. Additional individualized interventions: _____

_____

• The patient may panic about the need for mechanical ventilation or the sensations associated with it. Hyperventilation may worsen the panic. Adjusting the ventilatory rate as described helps the patient gain control over hyperventilation. Conveying calmness while coaching the patient in specific maneuvers helps build a sense of trust and provides reassurance that the situation is under control.

• Persistent struggling may indicate the need for ventilator adjustments or pharmacologic support. Morphine reduces anxiety and respiratory drive. Pancuronium bromide induces apnea, eliminating the problem of "fighting" the ventilator, but does not blunt consciousness. Because paralysis can be terrifying for the fully conscious patient, sedation with an amnesic agent is indicated.

4. Because PEEP is superimposed on intrathoracic pressure already increased from mechanical ventilation, it further increases the risks of barotrauma and cardiovascular deterioration. The mechanism by which PEEP alters fluid imbalance is unclear, but it may be mediated by antidiuretic hormone (ADH), baroreceptors, renin production, or stimulation of the sympathetic nervous system. PEEP may increase pressure in the superior vena cava, thereby impeding cerebral venous drainage and raising ICP.

5. Rationales: _____

_____

DECREASED CARDIAC OUTPUT

1. Monitor the patient for signs and symptoms of decreased cardiac output, such as hypotension, tachycardia, deteriorating mental status, and arrhythmias. Report findings promptly to the doctor. Administer I.V. fluid or vasopressors, as ordered.

2. Read pulmonary artery (PA) and wedge pressures at the end of expiration.

3. If the patient is on PEEP, consult the doctor about the specific technique for reading wedge pressures. In general, leave the patient on the ventilator, and do not make any adjustments in response to the readings; instead, watch for trends over time.

4. Additional individualized interventions: _____

_____

1. The increased intrathoracic pressure associated with mechanical ventilation diminishes venous return and may cause a right-to-left shift of the interventricular septum, impinging on left ventricular filling. Also, reducing the work required for breathing and administering oxygen, sedatives, or other therapies, such as vasodilators, can cause abrupt, significant decreases in the level of sympathetic tone supporting blood pressure. Most patients placed on mechanical ventilation develop hypotension, but it usually responds well to fluid and vasopressor support.

2. PA waveforms reflect fluctuations in intrathoracic pressure. Positive pressure ventilation causes the waveforms to rise during inspiration and drop during expiration. Reading pressures at the end of expiration minimizes the effects of respiratory variation.

3. Controversy exists over the extent to which PEEP affects wedge pressures. Usually, wedge pressures obtained on the ventilator are similar to those obtained with the ventilator disconnected (probably because poorly compliant lungs do not transmit airway pressures well to the heart and pulmonary capillary bed), so the benefit of maintaining PEEP argues in favor of reading pressures on the ventilator. If there is a discrepancy, the doctor may wish to confirm by X-ray that the catheter tip lies in the basal third of the lung, where pulmonary vascular pressures are believed to be least affected by alveolar pressure.

4. Rationales: _____

_____

PULMONARY INFECTION

1. Monitor the humidifier's water level and temperature, usually set at body temperature.

1. Artificial airways bypass the upper-airway mechanisms for warming, humidifying, and purifying inspired air. Humidification is added to the ventilator to prevent mucosal dehydration and thickened secretions. The temperature is controlled to prevent loss of body heat or tracheal burns.

2. Drain condensed fluid in the ventilator tubing into a basin rather than into the humidifier.

2. This condensation, from humidified air passed through the ventilator, is contaminated and must be discarded because it increases expiratory pressure and resistance in the ventilatory circuit. It also could be aspirated.

3. Observe for signs and symptoms of pulmonary infection, such as fever, purulent secretions, or elevated white blood cell count.

3. Artificial airways provide a direct access by which contaminants may enter the lungs.

4. If signs and symptoms of infection are present, consult with the doctor.

4. Pulmonary infections are a major contributor to mortality from mechanical ventilation. Because they usually occur in debilitated patients and are caused by virulent pathogens, pulmonary infections require prompt, aggressive therapy.

5. Additional individualized interventions: _____

5. Rationales: _____

GASTROINTESTINAL BLEEDING

1. Insert a nasogastric tube, as ordered.

1. Nasogastric intubation helps prevent gastric dilatation and reduces the risk of aspiration.

2. Administer antacids, ranitidine (Zantac), or cimetidine (Tagamet), as ordered, spacing doses. Implement additional measures from the "Gastrointestinal Hemorrhage" plan, page 394, as appropriate.

2. GI hemorrhage may result from the development of a stress ulcer, a complication of prolonged mechanical ventilation. Although their exact cause is not well understood, stress ulcers are thought to result from excess gastric acid secretion and decreased gastric mucosal resistance. Antacids neutralize gastric acid; cimetidine and ranitidine decrease gastric acid secretion. Antacids should not be given concurrently with cimetidine because they may impair its absorption. The "Gastrointestinal Hemorrhage" plan contains detailed interventions for ulcer-related bleeding.

3. Additional individualized interventions: _____

3. Rationales: _____

FLUID RETENTION

1. Monitor for signs and symptoms of fluid retention. If present, consult with the doctor about treatment.

1. Fluid retention may result from the humidifier's interference with insensible water loss via the lungs, decreased lymphatic flow, or altered secretion of ADH.

2. Additional individualized interventions: _____

2. Rationales: _____

Target outcome criteria
Throughout the period of mechanical ventilation, the patient will:
• have vital signs within acceptable limits
• maintain a cardiac index of 2.5 to 4.0 liters/minute/m²
• remain free from pulmonary infection
• display no signs of GI bleeding.

Nursing diagnosis: *Fear related to inability to speak and dependence on a machine for life support*

NURSING PRIORITY: Promote acceptance of mechanical ventilation.

Interventions

1. Implement the general measures in the "Ineffective Individual Coping" plan, page 51, as appropriate.

2. Establish a communication method, such as eye blinks, magic slate, or paper and pencil. Be sure the call light is always within reach.

3. Reduce the patient's need for communication by anticipating needs, providing consistency in staffing and routines, using frequent eye contact, and reassuring the patient that monitoring is constant. Emphasize that a nurse is available immediately if needed.

4. Explain the reason for mechanical ventilation. Briefly orient the patient and family to the ventilator's features, if appropriate, stressing features (such as alarms) that may be important to them. Encourage questions. Stress the temporary nature of ventilation, if applicable.

5. Additional individualized interventions: _____

Rationales

1. Mechanical ventilation is an extremely stressful experience for most patients. The "Ineffective Individual Coping" plan contains comprehensive information on ways to decrease the stress of critical illness and facilitate positive coping.

2. Intubation prevents use of the vocal cords. Needing to communicate and being unable to do so is extremely stressful. Providing alternative methods increases security and promotes patient safety.

3. Although alternative communication methods do work, they are cumbersome and fatiguing. Reducing the need for communication helps reduce the patient's fatigue and frustration, while reassurance helps reduce fear.

4. Mechanical ventilation commonly is instituted under crisis conditions, when explanation and emotional preparation may not have been possible. Even if the patient and family were prepared, stress may have caused blocking or selective filtering of information. Briefly reviewing the procedure and encouraging questions may relieve unstated anxiety about the device.

5. Rationales: _____

Target outcome criteria
Within 2 hours of being placed on mechanical ventilation and then continuously, the patient will:
• be able to communicate needs, if conscious
• appear relaxed.

Collaborative problem: *High risk for ineffective weaning related to lack of physiologic or psychological readiness*

NURSING PRIORITY: Promote a smooth transition to spontaneous ventilation.

Interventions

1. Anticipate weaning when the patient meets these criteria: improvement in respiratory status (as manifested by an A-a gradient less than 300 mm Hg on 100% oxygen, shunt less than 20%, V_D:V_T less than 0.6, respiratory rate less than 24 breaths/minute, MV 5 to 10 liters), stable hemodynamic status, and adequate muscle strength (as manifested by VC greater than 10 to 15 ml/kg and MIF greater than -20 cm H_2O).

Rationales

1. Many factors affect the success of weaning attempts. Premature attempts to wean impose unnecessary physiologic stress on the patient, jeopardizing recovery. Meeting the listed criteria increases the likelihood that weaning will be accomplished with few or no setbacks.

2. Ascertain that the patient is rested, well nourished, oriented, able to follow commands, and not receiving any respiratory depressants.

2. Reestablishing spontaneous ventilation is physically demanding, and the patient must have adequate energy reserves to succeed. The ability to take a deep breath and cough on command helps prevent atelectasis and airway obstruction. A strong respiratory drive is essential to resume spontaneous breathing.

3. Explain weaning to the patient and family. Mention that the patient may feel short of breath initially. Stress that the patient will be attended closely during the trial of spontaneous breathing and that if it is not successful, it will be tried again later.

3. Weaning is stressful psychologically. Thorough emotional preparation promotes a sense of security. Preparing the patient for the possibility of "trying again later" may reduce the sense of failure if the weaning attempt is unsuccessful.

4. Obtain baseline vital signs, ABG levels, and pulmonary function measurements. Suction the airway.

4. These measurements provide a basis for comparison to evaluate the appropriateness of weaning. Suctioning the airway reduces the risk of aspiration because secretions may have accumulated above the cuff.

5. Implement the weaning method ordered: CPAP, SIMV, T-piece, or pressure support.

5. CPAP may facilitate weaning for the patient on PEEP by maintaining some positive pressure during the trial of spontaneous breathing. SIMV supplies periodic mandatory deep breaths; the rate can be decreased by two breaths at a time until the patient's breathing is completely spontaneous. A T-piece provides supplemental oxygen during weaning. Pressure support can increase V_T in a patient too weak to wean on a T-piece alone.

6. Monitor the blood pressure, heart rate, pulse oximeter arterial oxygen saturation (SaO_2) reading, ECG rhythm, respiratory rate, ease of breathing, level of consciousness, and level of fatigue constantly for the first 20 to 30 minutes and every 5 minutes thereafter until weaning is complete.

6. Frequent monitoring of the indicated parameters provides ongoing indications of the success or failure of the weaning attempt.

7. In collaboration with the doctor, terminate weaning if adverse reactions occur, such as a heart rate increase greater than 20 beats/minute, systolic blood pressure increase greater than 20 mm Hg, SaO_2 less than 90%, respiratory rate less than 8 or greater than 24 breaths/minute, ventricular arrhythmias, labored or erratic breathing, fatigue, or panic.

7. Attempts to persist in weaning an unstable patient may cause cardiorespiratory arrest from hypoxia or arrhythmias.

8. If weaning continues, measure the V_T, MV, and ABG values in 20 to 30 minutes. Compare to desired values for this patient, determined in collaboration with the doctor, typically V_T 300 to 700 ml, MV 5 to 10 liters, pH 7.35 to 7.45, PaO_2 greater than 70 mm Hg, and $PaCO_2$ 35 to 45 mm Hg.

8. Values at this point help determine the appropriateness of weaning.

9. If physiologic parameters indicate weaning is feasible, but the patient resists, consider the possibility of psychological dependence on the ventilator. Consult with the doctor, pulmonary nurse specialist, or psychiatric nurse clinician, as appropriate.

9. Psychological dependence is a common problem after prolonged mechanical ventilation. Possible causes for dependency include fear of dying, depression from chronic illness, and secondary gains from the illness role. Consultation with other professionals may help to uncover causes and formulate appropriate intervention to resolve underlying fears or conflicts.

10. Assist with extubation, when ordered. Confirm that someone qualified to reintubate is present.

10. The same criteria used to evaluate readiness for weaning are used to determine readiness for extubation. A patient ventilated for short periods (24 to 48 hours) usually is ready for extubation after a 30-minute trial of spontaneous breathing, while those ventilated for longer periods may require days to weeks of gradual weaning. Availability of immediate reintubation is critical because postextubation airway obstruction can be sudden and fatal.

11. Additional individualized interventions: _____

11. Rationales: _____

Target outcome criteria
During weaning and continuously thereafter, the patient will:
• maintain a clear airway
• maintain a spontaneous respiratory rate of 12 to 24 breaths/minute
• manifest ABG levels within normal limits
• display pulmonary function measurements within normal limits

• display normal sinus rhythm with no ectopic beats, or a benign variant such as sinus arrhythmia or a normal sinus rhythm with fewer than 4 premature ventricular contractions per minute
• remain alert and oriented.

Discharge planning
NURSING DISCHARGE CRITERIA
Upon the patient's discharge, documentation shows evidence of:
• respiratory status (after extubation) stable for more than 12 hours
• absence of significant arrhythmias (without I.V. antiarrhythmic drugs) for more than 12 hours
• level of consciousness stable for more than 12 hours
• vital signs within normal limits.

PATIENT-FAMILY TEACHING CHECKLIST
Document evidence that the patient and family demonstrate an understanding of:
___ reason for mechanical ventilation
___ communication measures
___ alarms
___ weaning.

DOCUMENTATION CHECKLIST
Using outcome criteria as a guide, document:
___ clinical status on admission
___ significant changes in status
___ pertinent diagnostic test findings
___ ventilator and patient checks
___ ventilator alarm status
___ airway care
___ measures to prevent or detect and treat complications
___ communication measures
___ emotional support
___ sedative or paralyzing pharmacologic agents, if used
___ weaning
___ patient-family teaching
___ discharge planning.

ASSOCIATED PLANS OF CARE
Adult Respiratory Distress Syndrome
Impaired Physical Mobility
Ineffective Individual Coping
Nutritional Deficit
Sensory-Perceptual Alteration

References
East, T. "The Ventilator of the 1990's," *Respiratory Care* 35(3):232-240, March 1990.

Holloway, N., and Jacobs, S. "Aeration Treatment Disorders," in *Nursing the Critically Ill Adult*, 4th ed. Edited by Holloway, N. Menlo Park, Calif.: Addison-Wesley Publishing Co., 1993.

Schuster, D. "A Physiologic Approach to Initiating, Maintaining, and Withdrawing Mechanical Ventilatory Support during Acute Respiratory Failure," *American Journal of Medicine* 88(3):268-78, March 1990.

Pneumonia

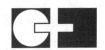

DRG information

DRG 079 Respiratory Infections and Inflammations.
Age 17+ with Complication or Comorbidity
(CC).
Mean LOS = 9.3 days
DRG 080 Respiratory Infections and Inflammations.
Age 17+ without CC.
Mean LOS = 6.8 days
DRG 081 Respiratory Infections and Inflammations.
Age 0 to 17.
Mean LOS = 6.1 days
DRG 089 Simple Pneumonia. Age 17+ with CC.
Mean LOS = 7.2 days
DRG 090 Simple Pneumonia. Age 17+ without CC.
Mean LOS = 5.6 days
DRG 091 Simple Pneumonia. Age 0 to 17.
Mean LOS = 5.2 days
Additional DRG information: Identifying the pneumonia's cause can increase the potential DRG (for example, Staphylococcal Pneumonia or Aspiration Pneumonia would place a patient into DRGs 079 to 081 rather than 089 to 091).

Introduction
DEFINITION AND TIME FOCUS
Respiratory infections account for a significant number of hospitalizations each year, particularly among the very old and the very young—the two groups most susceptible to serious respiratory illness. Respiratory infections include bacterial pneumonias (most commonly caused by pneumococci), viral pneumonias (most commonly caused by influenza and other viral diseases), tuberculosis, lung abscesses, fungal infections, bronchitis from various causes, and pulmonary empyema resulting from another disorder. Since the advent of antibiotic therapy, patients are hospitalized for treatment less commonly today than in the past. Four factors are significant in determining the need for inpatient care: the patient's age, the presence of underlying disease, the nature and severity of the patient's signs and symptoms, and the presence of immunosuppression.

This plan focuses on the patient with pneumonia who is admitted to the medical-surgical setting for diagnosis and treatment. Similar nursing interventions are applicable to most patients with respiratory infections of other types.

ETIOLOGY AND PRECIPITATING FACTORS
• for community-acquired disease:
—in otherwise healthy people, a particularly virulent organism or a high level of exposure
—in the older patient, chronic obstructive pulmonary disease, alcoholism, influenza, pulmonary neoplasms, congestive heart failure, altered consciousness, or swallowing disorders
—usual organisms include viruses, pneumococci, or *Mycoplasma pneumoniae*
• for nosocomial disease:
—compromised pulmonary defense mechanism resulting from immunosuppression, ongoing poor nutritional status, structural defects in the respiratory mucosa, depressed cough reflex, or use of an endotracheal or tracheostomy tube
—usual organisms include staphylococci, *Klebsiella pneumoniae*, and *Pseudomonas aeruginosa*
—most common mode of transmission is via hands of caregivers; incidence can be reduced by proper handwashing

Focused assessment guidelines
The manifestations of respiratory infections vary considerably, depending on the degree of inflammation, the disease stage, and the pathogenic organism involved.

NURSING HISTORY (Functional health pattern findings)

Health perception—health management pattern
• complains of fatigue, malaise, and respiratory symptoms, such as cough, pleurisy (chest pain with inspiration), and sputum production
• if disease is community-acquired, may report a recent upper respiratory infection or sinus disease; self-treatment common—may have used outdated antibiotics (prescribed for a previous illness), over-the-counter medications, or both
• may report history of smoking, alcohol abuse, or multiple stressors contributing to overall fatigue
• if disease is of nosocomial origin, may not have been admitted for a primary respiratory disorder but may have multiple risk factors, such as activity restriction, depressed inspiratory effort, depressed cough reflex, and use of respiratory equipment or an artificial airway

Nutritional-metabolic pattern
• reports anorexia during illness; may report poor nutrition before onset of respiratory illness

Activity-exercise pattern
• may report limited activity because of fatigue and shortness of breath

Sleep-rest pattern
• may report fatigue with inability to "catch up" on needed rest
• if cough is present, may disturb sleep

Cognitive-perceptual pattern
• in community-acquired disease, may wonder why the illness occurred despite good physical condition; does not relate subtle increase in stress to present illness (stresses may include excessive exercise); may have delayed seeking medical attention because the illness seemed like "just a little cold"
• in nosocomial disease, the patient and family may not understand connection between the primary reason for hospitalization and the present illness

PHYSICAL FINDINGS
General appearance
• fever—low grade or with shaking chills, depending on pathogenic organism (check the patient's normal temperature because low-grade fever may actually represent a significant elevation, such as in an older patient)

Pulmonary
• crackles
• decreased breath sounds over area of infection
• increased respiratory rate
• shallow, labored breathing (may not report shortness of breath)
• possible abnormal bronchial breath sounds heard on auscultation over area of consolidation
• fremitus—normal or increased
• possible cough
• possible sputum production and rhinorrhea—character, color, and odor of secretions depend on pathogenic organism (generally, viral organisms produce clear secretions, while bacterial organisms produce discolored and purulent secretions)

Gastrointestinal
• possible vomiting

Integumentary
• warm, moist skin
• possible cyanosis, pallor, or flushing

Lymphoreticular system
• possible cervical lymphadenopathy or tenderness in salivary glands

Musculoskeletal
• weakness

DIAGNOSTIC STUDIES
• arterial blood gas (ABG) measurements—may show hypoxemia; possible hypocapnia related to increased minute volume in response to hypoxemia
• sputum specimen (Gram stain, culture and sensitivity testing, or both)—performed to identify causative organisms; may be difficult to differentiate between colonization by an organism that is not the primary cause of infection and the pathogenic organism; even isolation of a specific pathogen does not necessarily prove pneumonia's cause
• transtracheal aspiration—may be performed in an attempt to obtain a sputum specimen free from saliva or mouth flora; an increased number of polymorphonuclear cells with few squamous cells indicates an acceptable specimen
• blood culture—may match organism in sputum, increasing likelihood that organism is causative pathogen
• bronchoscopy—may be performed to obtain a sputum specimen, identify the problem, or clear the airways
• chest X-ray—shows pulmonary infiltrates in affected areas from the inflammatory process (occasionally clear); may show pleural effusion
• thoracentesis—done to identify organism if significant pleural fluid is present on chest X-ray and sputum specimen is unobtainable
• pulmonary function tests—forced vital capacity decreased
• white blood cell (WBC) count—may be elevated but does not contribute directly to diagnosis

POTENTIAL COMPLICATIONS
• severe hypoxemia
• adult respiratory distress syndrome (ARDS)
• empyema
• sepsis
• lung abscess
• pulmonary embolism
• pneumothorax
• pericarditis
• meningitis

Collaborative problem: *High risk for hypoxemia related to inflammatory response to pathogen and inadequate airway and alveolar clearance*

NURSING PRIORITY: Optimize oxygenation and airway and alveolar clearance.

Interventions

1. Administer oxygen therapy, as ordered. Document therapy on initiation and once per shift.

2. Maintain oxygen therapy during activity, such as ambulation to the bathroom. Note activity tolerance, observing for increased fatigue, tachypnea, cyanosis, tachycardia, and other signs of impaired oxygenation.

3. Administer and document antibiotic therapy, as ordered. Monitor the results of indicated blood level studies. Monitor and document the antibiotic's adverse effects (see the "Osteomyelitis" plan, page 489).

4. Evaluate patient progress and document the following parameters once per shift and as needed: level of consciousness, sputum character and color, presence or absence of cough, temperature, pulse, respiratory rate, skin color, breath sounds, and activity tolerance.

5. Collect sputum specimens in the recommended manner. Maintain a sterile collection cup. Upon expectoration of lower respiratory tract secretions, send the specimen to the laboratory immediately to prevent overgrowth of normal oral flora. If necessary, ask the respiratory therapy department to perform a sputum induction to collect an adequate specimen.

6. Perform noninvasive measures to promote airway clearance:
• The patient who is able to cooperate should deep-breathe and cough each hour and use an incentive spirometer, as ordered.
• If the patient is unable to cooperate, perform artificial sighing and coughing each hour, using a manual resuscitation bag.
• Perform postural drainage and percussion with vibration every 4 hours or as ordered.

7. Perform nasotracheal suctioning if the patient cannot cough effectively. Suction as needed, as indicated by gurgles heard over the major airways. Follow universal precautions, including wearing eye protection and gloves.

8. Use increased levels of supplemental oxygen before and during airway clearance procedures.

Rationales

1. Until airway and alveolar clearance is achieved, supplemental oxygen is necessary to reduce the system's need to maintain high minute volumes. Although high minute volumes help compensate for hypoxemia, they may contribute to respiratory fatigue and, ultimately, respiratory failure. Usual administration is 1 to 6 liters/minute by nasal cannula.

2. Increased activity levels increase oxygen demands and further tax the already compromised system.

3. The antibiotic of choice depends on the pathogen identified. Optimum antibiotic blood levels, necessary to achieve desired results, vary among individuals. The "Osteomyelitis" plan contains a detailed discussion of selected antibiotics' adverse effects. Some adverse effects require alterations in medication levels or therapy to prevent immediate or long-term complications.

4. Changes in level of consciousness, such as increased restlessness or lethargy, can indicate deterioration and impending respiratory failure. Other parameters should improve if antibiotic and airway clearance therapy is effective.

5. Appropriate antibiotic therapy depends on accurate pathogen identification.

6. Noninvasive clearance measures move purulent, infectious secretions from the alveoli up toward the major airways, where they can be expectorated or suctioned.

7. Nasotracheal suctioning is effective only if secretions are within reach of the suction catheter, typically above the carina (at the level of Louis's angle). Because nasotracheal suctioning can damage the tracheal mucosa, it should be performed only if secretions are within reach. Following universal precautions reduces exposure to infectious organisms.

8. Measures used to clear the airways may intensify hypoxemia while they are being performed, especially if the patient has concomitant cardiovascular disease. Supplemental oxygen can be maintained via nasal prongs during nasotracheal suctioning.

9. Encourage the patient to increase fluid intake to at least 8 8-oz glasses (2,000 ml) per day.

9. Sputum's viscosity is related to the patient's overall hydration status. Fever contributes to dehydration. Adequate fluid intake promotes thinner secretions that can be expectorated more easily, decreasing the risk of hypoxemia related to sputum plugs in airway.

10. Encourage small, frequent, high-protein, high-calorie meals. If the patient cannot eat, begin total parenteral nutrition, as ordered.

10. Protein and calorie malnutrition may contribute to impaired humoral and cell-mediated host defenses. Malnutrition also weakens the patient, contributing to a less vigorous respiratory effort.

11. Monitor ABG levels, as ordered and as needed, if dyspnea increases or respiratory effort is inadequate. Report abnormalities immediately, and prepare the patient for possible ventilatory support.

11. Indications of severe hypoxemia and developing ARDS include a dropping partial pressure of oxygen (PO_2) level despite a stable or increasing level of supplemental oxygen.

12. Additional individualized interventions: _____

12. Rationales: _____

Target outcome criteria
Within 2 days of admission, the patient will:
• easily expectorate less purulent sputum
• exhibit decreased crackles
• perform pulmonary hygiene measures hourly while awake

• exhibit increased vigor and ability to perform self-care measures
• have no fever
• take oral fluids to recommended level
• have adequate dietary intake.

Nursing diagnosis: *Pain related to fever and pleuritic irritation*

NURSING PRIORITY: Minimize discomfort while promoting adequate oxygenation.

Interventions

1. See the "Pain" plan, page 69.

2. Administer antipyretics, analgesics, or both, as ordered and as needed. Use caution in administering sedatives or narcotics, if ordered. Document response.

3. Teach the patient to splint the chest wall with hands or pillows, as needed, while coughing, deep-breathing, or performing other pulmonary hygiene measures.

4. Apply a heating pad or hot packs to areas of chest wall discomfort, as ordered.

5. Additional individualized interventions: _____

Rationales

1. The "Pain" plan contains general interventions for the care of the patient in pain. This plan contains additional measures specific to pneumonia.

2. Pleuritic pain and discomfort from fever may be so severe that the patient inhibits thoracic expansion to minimize pain, increasing the likelihood of atelectasis, hypoventilation, inadequate airway clearance, and hypoxemia. Sedatives or narcotics may cause respiratory depression.

3. Splinting may help reduce unnecessary chest wall movement, which contributes to pain. Supporting painful areas helps promote fuller chest expansion.

4. Heat reduces inflammation and promotes muscle relaxation.

5. Rationales: _____

Target outcome criteria
Within 24 hours of admission, the patient will:
• demonstrate splinting technique while performing pulmonary hygiene measures (if stable)
• verbalize pain relief

• demonstrate adequate chest expansion during inspiration

Nursing diagnosis: *Knowledge deficit related to home care and preventive measures*

NURSING PRIORITY: Teach home care and preventive measures.

Interventions

1. Emphasize the importance of an ongoing pulmonary hygiene regimen. Teach the patient and family techniques for home use, based on the patient's condition and capabilities at discharge.

2. Teach the importance of rest during convalescence at home.

3. Review prophylactic measures, including the following:
• avoidance of respiratory irritants (smoke, dust, and chemical sprays)
• avoidance of crowds and persons with known infections, whenever possible
• awareness of mode of transmission (usually airborne), and that saliva and sputum contain increased concentrations of pathogens
• need for influenza vaccination, once the patient is stable, if the doctor recommends it.

4. Teach the patient and family the importance of promptly reporting symptoms that may indicate recurrence: headache, fever, dyspnea, chest pain, or other symptoms of a cold or the flu.

5. Additional individualized interventions: _____

Rationales

1. Deep-breathing exercises should be continued at home for at least 4 to 6 weeks to help reduce atelectasis and promote healing. Ongoing pulmonary hygiene measures may be indicated for the patient with a coexisting condition, such as emphysema, that is associated with a higher incidence of recurrence.

2. Respiratory infections place significant stresses on the body. Overexertion may further tax compromised defenses. Rest promotes healing.

3. Persons recovering from respiratory infections tend to be susceptible to other infections and are also at increased risk for recurrence after healing. Preventive measures may help the patient avoid further illness.

4. Early and appropriate treatment of respiratory infections results in shorter periods of illness. In older patients and other high-risk groups, a delay in reporting symptoms is associated with higher mortality rate.

5. Rationales: _____

Target outcome criteria
By the time of discharge, the patient will:
• demonstrate effective pulmonary hygiene measures for home use
• list three preventive measures

• list three symptoms indicating possible recurrence.

Discharge planning

NURSING DISCHARGE CRITERIA

Upon the patient's discharge, documentation shows evidence of:
• absence of pulmonary or cardiovascular complications (dullness on auscultation may still be present)
• ABG levels and WBC count within normal parameters
• absence of fever for at least 24 hours
• clearing pleural effusion on chest X-ray
• decreasing sputum production

• no need for supplemental oxygen for at least 48 hours
• I.V. antibiotics discontinued for at least 24 hours
• ability to tolerate adequate dietary and fluid intake
• ability to control pain using oral medications
• ability to ambulate and perform activities of daily living same as before hospitalization
• adequate home support system or referral to home care or a nursing home if indicated by an inadequate home support system or the patient's inability to care for self.

RESPIRATORY DISORDERS

PATIENT-FAMILY TEACHING CHECKLIST

Document evidence that the patient and family demonstrate an understanding of:

___ all discharge medications' purpose, dose, administration schedule, and adverse effects requiring medical intervention (usual discharge medications include antibiotics; the patient may be discharged with a bronchodilator if infectious agent has been very irritating to mucous membranes)

___ recommended dietary plan and need for ongoing fluid intake

___ realistic plan for rest and activity

___ care and use of oxygen equipment, if required for home use

___ pulmonary hygiene measures

___ preventive measures to avoid recurrence

___ symptoms requiring medical intervention

___ date, time, and location of follow-up appointments

___ how to contact the doctor.

DOCUMENTATION CHECKLIST

Using outcome criteria as a guide, document:

___ clinical status on admission

___ significant changes in status

___ pertinent diagnostic findings

___ ABG test results

___ pain relief measures

___ nutrition and fluid intake

___ oxygen therapy

___ airway clearance measures and results

___ patient-family teaching

___ discharge planning.

ASSOCIATED PLANS OF CARE

Acquired Immunodeficiency Syndrome
Chronic Obstructive Pulmonary Disease
Geriatric Considerations
Ineffective Individual Coping
Knowledge Deficit
Pain

References

Belshe, R. "Viral Respiratory Disease in the Intensive Care Unit," *Heart & Lung* 15(3):222-226, May 1986.

Caruthers, D. "Infectious Pneumonia in the Elderly," *American Journal of Nursing* 90(2):56-60, February 1990.

Craven, D., and Regan, A. "Nosocomial Pneumonia in the ICU Patient," *Critical Care Nursing Quarterly* 11(4):28-44, March 1989.

Gleckman, R.A. "Community-Acquired Pneumonia in the Geriatric Patient," *Hospital Practice* 20(3):57-60, 63, 65+, March 30, 1985.

Luckmann, J., and Sorensen, K.R. *Medical-Surgical Nursing: A Psychophysiologic Approach,* 3rd ed. Philadelphia: W.B. Saunders Co., 1987.

Stratton, C.W. "Bacterial Pneumonias—An Overview with Emphasis on Pathogenesis, Diagnosis, and Treatment," *Heart & Lung* 15(3):226-244, May 1986.

Pulmonary Embolism

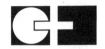

DRG information

DRG 078 Pulmonary Embolism.
  Mean LOS = 8.8 days
  Principal diagnoses include:
  • pulmonary embolism or infarction
  • air or fat embolism.

Introduction
DEFINITION AND TIME FOCUS

A pulmonary embolus (PE) is an undissolved mass deposited in a branch of the pulmonary artery that obstructs blood flow partially or completely. The severity of the associated signs and symptoms depends on the amount of lung involved and embolus size. The embolus may be massive or submassive.

In submassive embolism, numerous small emboli may occur. They usually lodge in the periphery of the pulmonary arterial bed and may or may not cause cardiopulmonary decompensation. A massive pulmonary embolus, on the other hand, obstructs more than 50% of the pulmonary arterial circulation and leads to severe, commonly life-threatening cardiopulmonary conditions. Venous thromboemboli are the most common cause of obstruction, accounting for approximately 95% of all cases; the vast majority of these arise from deep venous thrombosis in the legs. Bone fragments, air emboli, amniotic fluid, fat emboli, and septic emboli also may occur. This plan focuses on the immediate care of the symptomatic, critically ill patient with newly diagnosed thromboembolism.

ETIOLOGY AND PRECIPITATING FACTORS

• venous stasis, such as with deep venous thrombosis, immobility, burns, varicose veins, congestive heart failure, atrial fibrillation, or right ventricular infarction, or as in older adults and postpartal women
• injury of the vascular endothelium, such as with venipuncture of the legs, surgery (especially of the abdomen, pelvis, or hip), I.V. drug abuse, or trauma (particularly long-bone fractures or myocardial injury)
• hypercoagulability, such as with dehydration, oral contraceptive use, blood dyscrasias, or pregnancy.

Focused assessment guidelines
NURSING HISTORY (Functional health pattern findings)

Health perception – health management pattern
• reports sudden shortness of breath (most common symptom)

Cognitive-perceptual pattern
• complains of chest pain, similar to angina but worsened by inspiration
• may report apprehension or a sense of impending doom
• may report headache

Coping – stress tolerance pattern
• may report anxiety or fear

PHYSICAL FINDINGS
General appearance
• acute distress

Cardiovascular
• tachycardia (in 60% to 75% of patients)
• accentuated P_2 (in massive PE)
• neck vein distention (in massive PE)
• syncope
• murmur
• hypotension
• S_3 gallop (rare)

Pulmonary
• tachypnea
• crackles
• wheezes
• decreased breath sounds
• pleural friction rub
• cough (usually seen with concurrent pulmonary infarction)
• hemoptysis (usually seen with concurrent pulmonary infarction)

Neurologic
• decreased level of consciousness
• confusion
• restlessness
• hallucinations
• euphoria (rare)

Integumentary
• pallor
• cyanosis
• diaphoresis

Musculoskeletal
More than half of all patients with deep venous thrombosis in the leg have no signs or symptoms of phlebitis. If present, they include:
• swelling
• pain
• warmth
• redness

Renal
• oliguria

DIAGNOSTIC STUDIES

No diagnostic laboratory test exists for PE; laboratory data are used to rule out other conditions or provide general confirming evidence.

• arterial blood gas (ABG) levels — may reveal partial pressure of arterial oxygen (PaO_2) less than 80 mm Hg and partial pressure of arterial carbon dioxide ($PaCO_2$) less than 35 mm Hg, indicating respiratory alkalosis and increased risk for PE
• sedimentation rate — increased (a nonspecific response)
• serum bilirubin — increased if right-sided heart failure is present
• lactic dehydrogenase (LDH) — elevated
• pulmonary angiogram — considered the diagnostic standard for detecting and confirming pulmonary emboli; it reveals constant intraluminal filling defect on multiple films and sharp cutoff in vessels greater than 2.5 mm in diameter
• 12-lead electrocardiogram (ECG) — used to rule out myocardial infarction; it commonly reveals various arrhythmias, especially paroxysmal atrial tachycardia (PAT) and, in massive PE, right bundle branch block; if right-sided heart failure is present, it may reveal typical changes such as predominantly negative QRS complexes in leads 1 to 3 and inverted T waves in V_1 and V_2

• chest X-ray — may be normal, or it may reveal:
  — infiltration
  — pleural effusion
  — atelectasis
  — elevated diaphragm on affected side
  — enlarged pulmonary arteries
  — sudden cutoff of a pulmonary shadow
  — cardiac enlargement with prominent right atrial border, right ventricular dilatation, and dilated superior vena cava
  — a hump-shaped shadow on the affected side, if infarction is present
• impedance plethysmography — performed commonly because approximately 85% of pulmonary emboli arise from deep leg veins; it reveals increased pressure in veins distal to obstruction
• ventilation-perfusion lung scan — may reveal area of normal ventilation with decreased or absent perfusion

POTENTIAL COMPLICATIONS

• recurrent embolism
• atelectasis
• right ventricular failure
• shock
• cardiopulmonary arrest
• arrhythmias
• pulmonary hemorrhage (rare)
• pulmonary infarction (rare)

Collaborative problem: *Hypoxemia related to ventilation-perfusion mismatch*

NURSING PRIORITY: Maintain adequate ventilation.

Interventions

1. Assess pulmonary status at least every 2 hours. Note the presence of:
• tachypnea and dyspnea

• wheezing

• decreased or absent breath sounds

Rationales

1. Serial assessments indicate the disorder's severity and the effectiveness of interventions.

• Tachypnea, a cardinal sign, is a compensatory measure to increase oxygenation, and is attributed to stimulation of intrapulmonary receptors in the alveolar-capillary wall. Dyspnea results from apprehension or the sudden increase in alveolar dead space from alveoli that are ventilated but not perfused. Ventilation without perfusion impairs gas exchange.

• Wheezing results from pneumoconstriction following hypocapnia and platelet degranulation. Local hypocapnia constricts bronchial smooth muscle, increasing airway resistance and redirecting ventilation to better perfused areas; the resulting reduction in wasted ventilation is a protective mechanism. The thromboembolus consists of fibrin, red blood cells, and platelets; platelet degranulation releases substances that provoke bronchoconstriction and vasoconstriction.

• Normally, surfactant reduces surface tension as alveoli deflate, preventing alveolar collapse and lessening the work necessary to reinflate alveoli. Decreased surfactant production leads to atelectasis.

• crackles and gurgles

• mentation changes.

2. Monitor ABG and pulse oximeter readings levels, pulse oximeter readings, or both, as ordered.

3. Administer supplemental oxygen, as ordered.

4. Elevate the head of the bed 30 to 45 degrees. Use pillows to support the patient in a comfortable position.

5. Maintain strict bed rest. Assist with bathing, eating, and other activities that increase dyspnea.

6. Implement a program of vigorous pulmonary hygiene, including deep-breathing exercises, coughing, incentive spirometry, and frequent repositioning. Suction as necessary.

7. Assist with intubation and mechanical ventilation with positive end-expiratory pressure (PEEP), as needed. Refer to the "Mechanical Ventilation" plan, page 227, for guidelines.

8. Additional individualized interventions: _____

• Normally, surfactant also minimizes leakage of capillary fluid into alveoli by controlling alveolar surface tension. Decreased surfactant increases surface tension and allows fluid leakage, resulting in interstitial edema.

• Mentation changes reflect cerebral hypoxia.

2. ABG levels and pulse oximeter readings provide objective evidence of the degree of hypoxemia, which is useful in evaluating the PE's severity and the effectiveness of interventions.

3. Supplemental oxygen prevents the immediate consequences of hypoxemia, which may include arrhythmias, cerebral ischemia, and myocardial infarction.

4. This position promotes respiratory excursion and reduces the cardiopulmonary work load.

5. Rest conserves energy needed for breathing.

6. Adequate alveolar ventilation can reduce elevated $PaCO_2$ levels. Restoring effective aeration may prevent the onset of pneumonia from retention of secretions in the atelectatic area.

7. If the above measures fail to control hypoxemia, intubation and mechanical ventilation with PEEP may reopen collapsed alveoli. The "Mechanical Ventilation" plan details the care involved in this therapy.

8. Rationales: _____

Target outcome criteria
Within 48 hours of onset, the patient will:
• have ABG levels returning to normal limits
• have clear breath sounds bilaterally
• display no dyspnea.

Collaborative problem: *High risk for cardiogenic shock related to pulmonary arterial hypertension and right-sided heart failure*

NURSING PRIORITY: Support adequate cardiac output.

Interventions

1. Institute constant ECG monitoring, if not already present. Observe for arrhythmias, particularly PAT or right bundle branch block.

2. Maintain I.V. line patency and administer fluids, as ordered.

3. Assist with pulmonary artery (PA) catheter insertion, as ordered. Monitor pulmonary artery pressure (PAP) and pulmonary capillary wedge pressure (PCWP), as ordered, typically every hour until stable and then every 2 hours.

Rationales

1. The right ventricle may decompensate in response to the sudden elevation in pulmonary pressure. PAT or other atrial arrhythmias reflect atrial stretching from volume overload, while bundle branch block probably reflects right ventricular strain. Other arrhythmias may result from cardiac ischemia or hypoxemia; cardiopulmonary arrest may occur in massive embolism.

2. Although the PE patient is not volume depleted, I.V. access is critical for medication administration.

3. A PA catheter provides objective data useful in assessing hemodynamic function of the left and right sides of the heart.

4. Monitor for signs and symptoms of right-sided heart failure, such as neck vein distention and elevated central venous pressure readings. If any are present, notify the doctor.

5. Monitor for signs and symptoms of cardiogenic shock, such as severe hypotension and elevated PCWP. If present, notify the doctor and implement measures in the "Cardiogenic Shock" plan, page 310, as appropriate.

6. If above measures are ineffective or the PE is life threatening, prepare the patient for emergency surgery, if ordered.

7. Additional individualized interventions: _____

_____

4. Mechanical obstruction from the embolus and release of vasoconstrictors, described above, elevate pulmonary vascular resistance. The increased resistance to right ventricular ejection may cause right-sided heart failure.

5. Major obstruction to ventricular ejection produces cardiogenic shock. The "Cardiogenic Shock" plan presents detailed assessment and interventions for this complication.

6. Pulmonary embolectomy may be a life-saving operation.

7. Rationales: _____

_____

Target outcome criteria
Within 48 hours of symptom onset, the patient will have:
• blood pressure within normal limits
• cardiac rhythm within normal limits
• PAP and PCWP within normal limits
• warm and dry skin
• urine output greater than 60 ml/hour.

Collaborative problem: *High risk for complications related to recurrent emboli, anticoagulant therapy, or thrombolytic therapy*

NURSING PRIORITY: Prevent or minimize complications.

Interventions

1. Provide standard nursing care to prevent thromboemboli, such as applying antiembolism stockings; performing active or passive leg exercises; ensuring adequate fluid intake; and avoiding high Fowler's position, knee gatching, and leg massage.

2. Administer heparin, as ordered, typically by continuous low dose infusion. Monitor the partial thromboplastin time daily and maintain within prescribed therapeutic range, typically twice the control value. For excessive anticoagulation, administer protamine sulfate, as ordered.

3. Administer streptokinase (Streptase) or urokinase (Abbokinase), according to unit protocol, as ordered. Protocols vary but generally include:
• contraindications, such as recent surgery or cerebrovascular accident, active bleeding, and severe hypertension
• administration via a PA catheter or systemic infusion
• a loading dose followed by constant infusion for several hours
• maintaining thrombin time at two to five times normal
• monitoring for bleeding episodes.

4. Minimize the risk of bleeding by avoiding intramuscular injections when possible and collaborating with the doctor or clinical pharmacist to limit interactions between anticoagulants, thrombolytic agents, and other medications. Monitor for both apparent and occult bleeding, such as by observing for hematomas and by guaiac-testing gastric contents and stool.

Rationales

1. These measures help maintain peripheral venous blood flow by preventing stasis, hypercoagulability, and clot dislodgment. They also minimize clot formation.

2. Heparin is a potent anticoagulant that inactivates thrombin and blocks further clot formation. It also inhibits platelet degranulation around the thrombus and limits the release of vasoconstrictors. Subtherapeutic values place the patient at continued risk for recurrent emboli; values beyond the therapeutic range place the patient at risk for bleeding episodes. Protamine sulfate counteracts the effects of heparin.

3. Streptokinase or urokinase therapy may be ordered for the unstable patient with massive embolism. These thrombolytic agents dissolve already formed clots, decreasing symptoms. Streptokinase, the enzyme from beta-hemolytic streptococci, converts plasminogen to plasmin, producing fibrinolysis, and resulting in decreased blood viscosity, improved microcirculation, and improved oxygen delivery. Urokinase also converts plasminogen to plasmin, degrading fibrin clots, fibrinogen, and other plasma proteins. Unit protocols vary regarding details of administration.

4. Anticoagulation and thrombolytic therapy increase the risk of bleeding. Early detection permits dosage adjustment before massive hemorrhage occurs.

5. If emboli recur despite above measures, prepare the patient for surgery, as ordered.

5. Vena cava ligation or insertion of a vena cava umbrella can trap recurrent emboli, which fibrinolysis can then dissolve.

6. Additional individualized interventions: _____

6. Rationales: _____

Target outcome criteria
Throughout the hospital stay, the patient will:
• experience minor bleeding only
• display no signs of recurrent emboli.

Nursing diagnosis: *Ineffective individual and family coping related to potentially life-threatening situation*

NURSING PRIORITY: Provide emotional support to the patient and family.

Interventions

1. Implement measures in the "Ineffective Individual Coping" plan, page 51, and "Ineffective Family Coping" plan, page 47, as appropriate. If death is imminent, implement measures in the "Dying" plan, page 11, as appropriate.

Rationales

1. Pulmonary embolism is a major psychological threat, evidenced by the classic finding of a sense of impending doom. The "Ineffective Individual Coping" and "Ineffective Family Coping" plans contain measures to help the patient and family deal with the emotional aftermath of a PE. If therapeutic measures are ineffective and the patient's condition continues to deteriorate, measures in the "Dying" plan may help the patient and family cope with approaching death.

2. Additional individualized interventions: _____

2. Rationales: _____

Target outcome criteria
By the time of discharge, the patient and family will meet the outcome criteria identified in the "Ineffective Individual Coping" and "Ineffective Family Coping" plans.

Should the patient die, the family will meet the outcome criteria identified in the "Dying" plan.

Discharge planning

NURSING DISCHARGE CRITERIA

Upon the patient's discharge, documentation shows evidence of:
• stable blood pressure, pulse, and respiratory rate
• removal of PA catheter.

PATIENT-FAMILY TEACHING CHECKLIST

Document evidence that the patient and family demonstrate an understanding of:
___ underlying reasons for clot development
___ rationale for therapy
___ measures to prevent recurrence.

DOCUMENTATION CHECKLIST

Using outcome criteria as a guide, document:
___ clinical status on admission
___ significant changes in status
___ pertinent diagnostic test findings

___ oxygen therapy
___ heparin therapy
___ thrombolytic therapy
___ patient-family teaching
___ discharge planning
___ potential discharge needs.

ASSOCIATED PLANS OF CARE

Cardiogenic Shock
Dying
Ineffective Individual Coping
Ineffective Family Coping
Pain

References

Handerhan, B. "Recognizing Pulmonary Embolism," *Nursing91* February 21(2):107-10, 1991.

Williams, S. *Decision Making in Critical Care Nursing*. Philadelphia: Mosby-Decker, 1990.

Thoracotomy

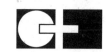

DRG information

DRG 075 Major Chest Procedures.

Mean LOS = 11.7 days

Principal procedures include:

- exploratory thoracotomy
- biopsy of diaphragm, pericardium, thymus, bronchus, or lung
- surgical collapse of lung
- incision of lung, bronchus, or thoracic vessels
- reopening of recent thoracotomy site
- pleurectomy or repair of pleura
- repair of diaphragmatic hernia, abdominal or thoracic approach.

Additional DRG information: Thoracotomy as an operative approach for other procedures may or may not be classified under DRG 075, depending on the definitive procedure accomplished.

Introduction

DEFINITION AND TIME FOCUS

A thoracotomy is an incision into the chest wall (thorax), whose location depends on the surgery's purpose. A posterolateral or anterolateral approach (through the ribs) is common with general thoracic surgery, while a median sternotomy (through the sternum) is used commonly for cardiothoracic surgery. The ribs or sternal halves are spread to gain access to the pleural cavities or the mediastinum. Common thoracotomy procedures on the lungs include exploratory thoracotomy, pneumonectomy (removal of a lung), lobectomy (removal of a lobe), segmental resection (removal of one or several lung segments), wedge resection (removal of part of a lung segment), decortication (removal of scarred, fibrous tissue over the pleura), or thoracoplasty (removal of ribs). Thoracotomies are also used to perform esophageal, diaphragmatic, aortic, or open heart procedures. A thoracotomy is a major surgical procedure that requires careful preoperative and postoperative patient management and may require mechanical ventilation and closed chest drainage. This plan focuses on preoperative care, postoperative stabilization, and initial recovery of the thoracotomy patient.

ETIOLOGY AND PRECIPITATING FACTORS

- pulmonary conditions, such as cancer, benign tumors, tuberculosis, abscesses or infection, bronchiectasis, blebs or bullae caused by emphysema, or empyema
- cardiac conditions, such as arteriosclerotic coronary arteries, valvular disease, mural wall defects, aortic aneurysm, cardiomyopathy, or congenital heart disease
- hiatal hernias or esophageal problems
- chest trauma involving one or more of the vital chest structures (lungs, heart, aorta, trachea, esophagus, or superior or inferior vena cava)

Focused assessment guidelines
NURSING HISTORY (Functional health pattern findings)

Health perception—health management pattern
- may report shortness of breath or labored breathing on exertion
- may report bloody or excessive sputum
- may report feeling more tired and having less exercise tolerance than usual
- may report swelling of feet and ankles
- may report family history of heart disease or lung conditions, such as asthma
- may report high-risk cardiac and respiratory health patterns, such as sedentary life-style, overeating, lack of exercise, stress, smoking, or exposure to respiratory toxins
- may have experienced a major traumatic accident with a blow to the chest

Nutritional-metabolic pattern
- may report loss of appetite (respiratory or cardiac problem)
- may report weight gain (cardiac problem)
- may report weight loss (respiratory problem)

Activity-exercise pattern
- may report difficulty in breathing at rest and during exercise
- may report weakness and fatigue

Cognitive-perceptual pattern
- may express fear about serious nature of illness and impending major surgery
- may report periods of dizziness

Self-perception—self-concept pattern
- may report fear of disfigurement and scarring

Role-relationship pattern
- may report fear of inability to return to work after surgical procedure
- may have a high-risk job with excessive stress or exposure to respiratory toxins

Sexuality-reproductive pattern
- may report fatigue and inability to sustain sexual activity

PHYSICAL FINDINGS
Physical findings may vary depending on the nature of the condition requiring the thoracotomy.

General appearance

• cardiac condition: may present with typical signs and symptoms of angina, acute myocardial infarction, or heart failure. See the "Acute Myocardial Infarction" plans, pages 268 and 280, for the general appearance of a patient with these problems.
• pulmonary condition: may present with respiratory distress or general debilitation depending on whether the condition is rapidly progressing or more chronic in nature
• chest trauma: may present with respiratory and cardiac distress and obvious crushing or penetrating injuries to the chest

Cardiovascular

• arrhythmias
• classic angina (substernal pain radiating to the left shoulder and arm that is relieved by nitroglycerin or rest)
• unstable angina (substernal and radiating pain that is not relieved by nitroglycerin or rest and that is more serious, prolonged, and unpredictable)
• noncardiac chest pain
• hypotension
• tachycardia

Pulmonary

• dyspnea
• shortness of breath
• tachypnea
• use of accessory muscles
• gurgles, wheezes, crackles
• chest trauma: possible open sucking wound, flail chest, paradoxical asymmetric chest movements, or orthopnea

Gastrointestinal

• hiatal hernia or esophageal problem: may have regurgitation, heartburn 30 to 60 minutes after meals, substernal pain, dysphagia, or feelings of fullness
• cardiac problem: may have nausea and vomiting

Integumentary

• cyanosis
• pallor
• chest trauma: abrasions or open wounds

DIAGNOSTIC STUDIES

Because of the various conditions for which thoracotomy may be performed, no typical laboratory data exist. This section instead presents monitoring tests.
• arterial blood gas (ABG) levels — monitor oxygenation, ventilation, and acid-base status
• cardiac enzymes, creatine phosphokinase, lactic acid dehydrogenase — may reveal cardiac tissue damage
• complete blood count — monitors red blood cell count, white blood cell (WBC) count, and platelets. Altered hemoglobin level and hematocrit reflect any potential blood loss and the blood's oxygen-carrying ability. An elevated WBC count and an elevated sedimentation rate may reflect an inflammatory response.

• serum creatinine, blood urea nitrogen levels — monitor the adequacy of renal function
• serum electrolyte panel — monitors fluid, electrolyte, and acid-base status
• urinalysis — monitors renal status including renal secretion and concentration abilities
• sputum assessment — monitors for infection
• blood coagulation studies — monitor clotting
• *For all conditions:*
—chest X-ray: may reveal abnormalities of the chest structures and heart and lung tissues
—electrocardiogram: may reveal changes associated with ischemia
—fluoroscopy: may reveal mobility abnormalities of the intrathoracic structures
—magnetic resonance imaging: may reveal abnormalities of the thoracic structures and organs
• *For cardiac or pulmonary conditions:*
—computed tomography: may reveal abnormalities of the lung, such as tumors, calcium deposits, or cavities, and abnormalities of the heart, such as enlargement
—biopsy: may aid in definitive diagnosis of lung or heart problems
—gallium scan: may reveal inflammation or tumors of the heart or lungs
• *For pulmonary conditions:*
—ventilation-perfusion pulmonary scan: may reveal areas of nonventilation and nonperfusion
—pulmonary function tests: monitor static and dynamic lung volumes and capacities
—bronchoscopy: may reveal abnormalities of the pulmonary tree
—sonogram of the lung: may reveal collections of fluid and may be used postoperatively to locate the best site for thoracentesis
—thoracentesis: may reveal abnormal fluid or tissue specimens
—bronchograms: may reveal abnormal airway structures or a tumor
• *For cardiac conditions:*
—cardiac radionuclide imaging: may reveal areas of cardiac ischemia and necrosis
—echocardiography: may reveal structural and motion abnormalities of the heart
—cardiac catheterization: may reveal abnormalities of the coronary arteries (during left-sided heart catheterization) or pulmonary artery vasculature (during right-sided heart catheterization)
• *For esophageal conditions:*
—barium swallow, esophagoscopy, motility studies: may reveal esophageal abnormalities

POTENTIAL COMPLICATIONS

• cardiac arrhythmias
• atelectasis
• pleural effusion
• pericardial effusion
• tension pneumothorax
• hemothorax
• infection

- pulmonary edema
- pulmonary embolism
- hemorrhage

- cardiac arrest
- shock
- cardiac tamponade

Nursing diagnosis: *Knowledge deficit related to preoperative and postoperative care in thoracotomy*

NURSING PRIORITY: Prepare the patient and family preoperatively for surgery and postoperative care.

Interventions	Rationales
1. Refer to the "Knowledge Deficit" plan, page 56.	1. The "Knowledge Deficit" plan contains general assessments and interventions for teaching and learning. This plan provides information specific to thoracotomy.
2. Provide information about the surgery. Document teaching and the patient's and family's response. Include the following points:	2. Preoperative teaching may allay fears and anxiety about the unknown and help the patient cooperate with care and summon energy for healing.
• purpose, goal, and general procedure	• A general understanding of thoracotomy's purpose, goal, and procedure will help orient the patient to upcoming nursing and medical care.
• type of incision	• Knowing what the incision will look like beforehand helps reduce the patient's anxiety.
• usual scar	• Knowing that the incision will heal to a thin, white line helps reduce the patient's fear of major disfigurement.
• preoperative medication	• Knowing that preoperative sedation is available helps reduce the patient's anxiety.
• anesthesia	• Teaching about the methods and effects of anesthesia helps prepare the patient for adverse reactions after surgery.
• expected location for recovery in the immediate postoperative period	• Telling the patient where recovery will take place helps reduce postoperative disorientation.
• I.V. and other lines	• A postoperative thoracotomy patient may have peripheral I.V., central I.V., and monitoring lines. The necessary tubing and equipment could be frightening without preoperative preparation.
• oxygen therapy	• All thoracotomy patients require oxygen therapy after surgery because of the atelectasis and hypoxemia produced by opening the chest and by anesthesia. The specific type of oxygen therapy depends on the surgery. Preoperative preparation about the oxygen therapy to be used may increase postoperative cooperation, particularly with the patient who will be intubated and placed on mechanical ventilation.
• chest tubes and drainage system	• Explaining the need for chest tubes and a drainage system to help reexpand the lungs and hasten recovery may allay anxiety about the invasive nature of these tubes.
• nasogastric (NG) tube	• Explaining that an NG tube reduces abdominal discomfort until the GI tract resumes function may increase patient tolerance.
• indwelling urinary catheter.	• Explaining the need to closely monitor fluid intake and output, including urine, after surgery may reduce anxiety about the catheter.
3. Describe endotracheal intubation and mechanical ventilation, if appropriate. See the "Mechanical Ventilation" plan, page 227. Document teaching and patient response.	3. Explaining intubation and mechanical ventilation, including the the temporary loss of speech, may allay anxiety about this treatment. The "Mechanical Ventilation" plan includes detailed information about caring for a mechanically ventilated patient.

4. Explain thoracotomy's general effects on the lungs and describe reexpansion methods. Coach the patient on deep breathing, coughing, and using an incentive spirometer, if ordered. Describe measurement of vital capacity and maximum inspiratory pressures. Observe return demonstrations. Document teaching and patient response.

4. Explaining the effect that opening the chest wall has on the lungs and describing reexpansion methods provide an incentive for active patient involvement. The patient's postoperative efforts to reexpand the lungs, remove secretions, and participate in respiratory function measurements may be more successful if practiced preoperatively, when the patient is under less stress and is free from pain.

5. Discuss methods to relieve postoperative pain, including pain medication and splinting the incision with a pillow during deep breathing and coughing. Document teaching and patient response.

5. Most patients describe thoracotomy pain as severe. The patient may be reassured to learn that pain relief is an important part of therapy. Explanations about the timely use of pain medication and pillow splinting may increase the patient's willingness to initiate and perform coughing and deep breathing exercises.

6. Describe and document the expected level of postoperative activity, including turning from side to side, as allowed, every 2 hours on the day of surgery; sitting in a semi-Fowler's position and sitting on the side of the bed with legs dangling on the first day after surgery; getting into a chair with assistance on the first or second day after surgery; and ambulating in the room and hallway on the second or third day after surgery. Emphasize the importance of activity despite postoperative discomfort.

6. A thoracotomy patient is likely to resist activity because of pain, fatigue, and weakness. Knowledge of expected activity and its importance provides a foundation on which the nurse can build when implementing the activity schedule.

7. Explain and demonstrate the use of antiembolism stockings. Document teaching.

7. Antiembolism stockings aid venous return and help prevent thrombus formation in the lower extremities.

8. Additional individualized interventions: _____

8. Rationales: _____

Target outcome criteria
Within 2 hours after preoperative teaching, the patient, on request, will:
• explain thoracotomy's purpose, goal, and general procedure and specific points covered during teaching
• demonstrate deep breathing, coughing, spirometer use, pillow splinting, and range-of-motion (ROM) and other exercises.

Collaborative problem: *Hypoxemia related to hypoventilation from anesthesia, pain, and analgesic medications as well as arrhythmias, atelectasis, and thickened secretions*

NURSING PRIORITY: Optimize ventilation and oxygenation.

Interventions

1. After surgery, assess the following every 15 minutes until stable, every 30 minutes for 2 hours, then every 1 to 2 hours and as needed. Document and notify the doctor of abnormal findings:

• respiratory rate, depth, and pattern; pulse rate; and blood pressure
• level of consciousness

Rationales

1. The patient usually returns from surgery with a pulmonary artery catheter, arterial line, peripheral I.V. lines, and pleural or mediastinal chest tubes, or both. Frequent assessments of the cardiopulmonary system may reveal problems and permit timely interventions.

• Hypoxemia is reflected in vital sign changes.

• Decreased oxygen delivery to the brain is reflected in changes in level of consciousness and mentation.

• bilateral breath sounds and bilateral chest movements

• accessory muscle use
• tracheal position

• color of mucous membranes, circumoral skin, and earlobes.

2. Assess percussion notes and vocal fremitus as well as the amount, color, and consistency of sputum every 1 to 2 hours and as needed.

3. Palpate the chest wall every 1 to 2 hours and as needed. Note the presence of tenderness, pain, or subcutaneous emphysema.

4. Monitor cardiac rhythm constantly. Note and report to the doctor atrial fibrillation, premature ventricular contractions (PVCs), or other cardiac arrhythmias. Refer to Appendix A, "Monitoring Standards".

5. Monitor ABG levels every shift and as needed for suspected changes in respiratory status, as ordered. Notify the doctor and document results.

6. Monitor and document arterial oxygen levels using ear or pulse oximetry twice a shift and as needed, as ordered.

7. Provide humidified oxygen for the first 1 to 2 days and as needed for respiratory distress. Document its use.

8. Medicate with analgesics for pain every 1 to 4 hours and as needed, as ordered. Monitor respiratory status to prevent respiratory depression. Document findings. Refer to the "Pain" plan, page 69, for further details.

9. Show the patient how to support the incision with the hands or a small, hard pillow as needed during deep breathing and coughing efforts. Encourage deep breathing and coughing two to three times every hour while awake.

10. Promote and document incentive spirometer use, as ordered, several times an hour while awake.

11. Provide adequate hydration. Document fluid intake.

• After thoracotomy, sounds and chest movements may be diminished over the operative area. These findings usually lessen and then disappear as recovery progresses. Adventitious sounds or persistence or worsening of diminished chest sounds and movements may reflect fluid accumulation, atelectasis, or other respiratory problems.
• Use of accessory muscles may reflect dyspnea.
• Tracheal deviation from midline may indicate increased intrathoracic pressure on the side opposite the deviation or lung collapse on the same side as the deviation.
• Cyanotic mucous membranes, circumoral skin, and earlobes may indicate hypoxemia.

2. Dullness to percussion and decreased vocal fremitus are common after surgery and reflect consolidation from atelectatic areas. Resonance to percussion and normal vocal fremitus should return gradually as recovery progresses, except in pneumonectomy. Sputum characteristics may reflect hydration status, bleeding or infection, or pulmonary edema.

3. Areas of increasing tenderness or pain imply infection or another complication. Subcutaneous emphysema may occur when an air leak increases intrapleural pressure and eventually results in air spreading throughout the surrounding tissues. Subcutaneous emphysema is usually self-limiting and reabsorbs in several days, but may indicate a need for increased pleural suction pressures.

4. Cardiac arrhythmias, including atrial fibrillation and PVCs, are common after a thoracotomy, particularly after open heart surgery. "Monitoring Standards" includes specific assessments and interventions for arrhythmias.

5. ABG levels reflect general oxygenation levels. Low PaO_2 levels may indicate a need for increased oxygen therapy and more vigorous pulmonary hygiene.

6. Oximetry monitors arterial oxygen levels without needle sticks.

7. Oxygen therapy may be required until the lungs are fully reexpanded and the breathing pattern and airway clearance are more effective.

8. Pain relief promotes effective deep breathing and coughing. Respiratory depressants such as morphine sulfate must be used cautiously to prevent inadequate ventilation, which would be counterproductive to deep breathing and coughing. The "Pain" plan contains general assessments and interventions for pain.

9. Support over the incision may decrease pain during deep breathing and coughing. Regular deep breathing and coughing promotes reexpansion of the lungs, mobilizes secretions, and prevents atelectasis.

10. Spirometers encourage deep inspiratory efforts, which are more effective in reexpanding alveoli than forceful expiratory efforts.

11. Adequate hydration promotes liquid, easily removed lung secretions. Other means of humidification, such as intermittent positive-pressure breathing, may be undesirable because of the danger of a pneumothorax.

12. Provide an overhead trapeze bar or hand pulls attached to the end of the bedframe to assist the patient to the upright position for deep breathing and coughing efforts.

13. Implement and document a progressive activity program, as allowed, typically:

• turning from side to side every 2 hours on the day of surgery, and sitting in a semi-Fowler's position and sitting on the side of the bed with legs dangling on the first postoperative day

• getting into a chair with assistance on the first or second postoperative day, and ambulating in the room and hallway on the second or third postoperative day.

14. Additional individualized interventions: _____

12. An upright position promotes lung expansion by gravity. These devices provide better mobility than does pushing against the bed.

13. Progressive activity is important to restore optimal cardiopulmonary function.

• Frequent position changes reexpand the lungs and prevent atelectasis and pooling of secretions. A patient who has had a pneumonectomy can be turned slightly toward the operative side or onto the back. Turning toward the nonoperative side could collapse the remaining lung, drain secretions into that lung, or cause a dangerous mediastinal shift. Semi-Fowler's position may aid reexpansion of the lungs by gravity, while leg dangling allows the neurovascular reflexes to adjust to the upright position.

• Early chair-sitting and ambulation may prevent thrombus formation in the lower extremities and aid adjustment to the upright position.

14. Rationales: _____

Target outcome criteria
Within 4 hours after surgery, the patient will:
• perform deep breathing and coughing
• use the incentive spirometer
• request pain medication when needed.

Within 8 hours after surgery, the patient will:
• manifest normal vital signs
• display usual level of consciousness
• display minimally diminished breath sounds and chest movements
• display trachea in normal position
• have pink mucous membranes
• display minimal dullness to percussion over operative side, except for pneumonectomy
• be free from subcutaneous emphysema
• be free from PVCs or other arrhythmias
• turn every 2 hours with assistance.

Within 2 days after surgery, the patient will:
• use a spirometer 2 to 3 times an hour while awake
• display minimal or absent crackles, gurgles, or wheezes
• manifest normal ABG levels and oximetry levels
• display minimal pain
• sit up in a chair.

Within 3 days after surgery, the patient will:
• have nearly equal bilateral breath sounds, chest expansion, and resonance to percussion, as appropriate for type of surgery
• begin to ambulate.

Collaborative problem: *High risk for respiratory distress related to pneumothorax, hemothorax, or mediastinal shift secondary to malfunction or removal of chest drainage system*

NURSING PRIORITIES: (a) Maintain patency of chest drainage system, and (b) observe for complications after chest tube removal.

Interventions

1. Maintain an intact water-seal drainage system, if used. In the event of disconnection or a broken chamber, reattach the tube or submerge it in water while the patient exhales. If reattachment is not possible or water is unavailable, leave the chest tube open to air until a new system can be attached. Notify the doctor and document occurrence. Arrange for a chest X-ray.

Rationales

1. Although most thoracotomy patients have chest tubes, chest tubes are not usually used after pneumonectomy because serous fluid collection promotes the development of fibrotic tissue in the empty space. If chest tubes are present, disconnection may allow air to enter the pleural space and cause a pneumothorax. Exhalation during reattachment may force excess air from the pleural space. Leaving the tube open to air creates the potential for a small open pneumothorax, but may be less harmful than clamping the tube and possibly causing a tension pneumothorax, especially in a patient with an air leak. A chest X-ray may be necessary to assess respiratory status.

2. Inspect the chest tube insertion site every 2 hours and as needed for the presence of:
- intact occlusive dressings

- blood or drainage on the dressing

- proper position of the chest tubes within the chest and attachment to the chest wall.

3. Observe the drainage tubing and connectors every 1 to 2 hours for proper connection and taping of connectors. Coil the tubing to prevent dependent loops.

4. Milk and strip the tubing every 1 to 2 hours and as needed, as ordered, during the first postoperative day. Document these actions.

5. Assess the drainage receptacle every 1 to 2 hours and as needed for secure attachment to the drainage tubing. If bottle drainage is used, maintain the end of the tube in the water-seal chamber ¾" (2 cm) below the water level.

6. Observe for and document tidalling (fluctuation of water level during respirations) in the submerged water-seal tube every 2 hours. To do this, turn off the suction or pinch the suction tubing temporarily.

7. Observe the water-seal chamber for intermittent bubbling during respiration every 2 hours and as needed. Document the amount of bubbling and where in the respiratory cycle it occurs.

8. If continuous bubbling occurs in the water-seal chamber, briefly clamp consecutive parts of the system, beginning at the chest wall, until the bubbling stops. If the bubbling stops when the clamp is proximal to the chest wall, notify the doctor. If the bubbling stops when the clamp is distal to the chest wall, replace the system beyond that point.

9. Maintain and document the ordered amount of suction, if used. With Emerson suction, check the pressure set on the dial and the pressure registering on the gauge. With a multiple-chamber system (such as Pleur-evac), check the water level in the suction control chamber to ensure that it equals the ordered amount of negative pressure.

10. Monitor the amount, color, and consistency of chest tube drainage every 30 minutes for 2 hours, every hour for 6 hours, and then every 2 hours and as needed. Notify the doctor if large amounts of drainage occur (more than 200 ml/hour for 3 hours). Document findings.

2. Frequent inspection may reveal problems and allow for timely interventions.
- Occlusive dressings are used to prevent air from entering the pleural space around the chest tube insertion site and to prevent accidental dislodgment of the tubes.
- Blood or drainage on the dressing may indicate recent bleeding or infection.
- Dislodgment of the tubes can create a dangerous increase of air or drainage within the pleural space, which could cause the lung to collapse.

3. The closed drainage system must be sealed to prevent air from entering the pleural space. Taped connectors are less likely to disconnect or develop air leaks. Improperly looped tubing may inhibit gravity flow of drainage.

4. This procedure assists drainage by creating negative pressure and preventing clotting and plugging of the tubes.

5. Securely attaching the drainage tubing to the drainage receptacle and placing the end of the water-seal tube below the water level prevent air from entering the drainage system and the pleural space.

6. Tidalling indicates a functioning, airtight system between the pleura and the drainage receptacle. During spontaneous ventilation, inspiration creates negative pressure in the pleura and the drainage system, which pulls the water level upward in the tubing. The level moves downward on expiration. Fluctuations are the reverse for a patient on mechanical ventilation: the positive pressure applied during inspiration pushes the water level downward, while termination of the positive pressure on expiration allows the water level to move upward. Absence of tidalling may indicate a blocked chest tube or complete lung expansion.

7. Intermittent bubbling represents drainage of air from within the pleural spaces. Bubbling occurs normally during expiration with spontaneous ventilation or during inspiration with mechanical ventilation.

8. Continuous bubbling indicates an air leak within the patient or the drainage system. Clamping as described helps isolate the leak. Bubbling that stops when the clamp is proximal to the chest wall indicates an air leak within the patient, which requires medical evaluation. Bubbling that stops with distal clamping indicates a leak in the drainage system, which requires replacement of the system.

9. Negative pressure may be required to remove secretions and air from the intrapleural space. Inadequate negative pressure may prevent drainage and reexpansion of the lungs, while excessive pressure may damage pleural tissue.

10. Large amounts of drainage may indicate bleeding and require immediate intervention to prevent shock. Absence of drainage, particularly in the immediate postoperative period, may indicate a plugged chest tube which could cause a dangerous increase in intrapleural pressure. Chest tubes commonly drain up to 500 ml in the first 8 hours, decreasing to zero drainage 3 to 4 days after surgery as the pleurae realign and the lungs reexpand.

11. Assist with removal of chest tubes 3 to 4 days after surgery.

• Before removal, note absence of chest tube drainage and tidalling with respiration as well as the return of breath sounds in the affected area.

• Medicate with an analgesic before removal, as ordered.

• Place the patient in a high Fowler's position. Have the patient take a deep breath and cough vigorously. At maximum inspiration, assist in removing the tube and tightening the purse string skin suture.

• Apply a sterile occlusive dressing.

• After removal, assess for signs and symptoms of respiratory distress, including dyspnea, pain, absent breath sounds, uneven chest movement, dull percussion sounds, cardiac arrhythmias, or anxiety.

12. If necessary, assist the doctor with reinsertion of the chest tubes or thoracentesis. Document the procedure.

13. Additional individualized interventions: _____

_____

11. Chest tubes are removed when the lungs have reexpanded.

• These signs indicate lung reexpansion.

• An analgesic helps decrease pain during removal.

• A high Fowler's position, deep breathing, and vigorous coughing may prevent a pneumothorax during tube removal and suture tightening by providing maximum lung expansion and positive intrapleural pressure.

• A sterile occlusive dressing may prevent infection and air leaks into the pleural space.

• Rarely, the patient may develop such complications as pneumothorax, hemothorax, or mediastinal shift, which may compromise the respiratory and cardiac systems. Careful assessment allows early identification and intervention.

12. Rarely, the patient may accumulate fluid or air and may require reinsertion of chest tubes or thoracentesis.

13. Rationales: _____

_____

Target outcome criteria
On admission and continuously, the patient will have a properly functioning chest drainage system.

Within 3 to 4 days after surgery, the patient will:
• have fully expanded lungs
• be free from air and fluid in the pleural space
• have chest tubes removed.

Within one week after surgery, the patient will:
• display no dyspnea
• have normal respiratory status.

Nursing diagnosis: *High risk for injury: complications related to surgical procedure, such as hemorrhage, pneumothorax, pleural effusion, atelectasis, pulmonary edema, or pulmonary embolism*

NURSING PRIORITY: Monitor for and promptly report signs and symptoms of complications.

Interventions

1. See the "Surgical Intervention" plan, page 81.

2. Monitor for signs and symptoms of hemorrhage. If present, alert the doctor immediately and document. Observe for:

• tachycardia, hypotension, low hemodynamic measurements, and excessive chest drainage

• decreasing or absent breath sounds, increasing dullness to percussion, or decreased or absent fremitus

• decreased heart sounds, paradoxical pulse greater than 10 mm Hg on inspiration, or high central venous pressure.

3. Monitor for signs of pneumothorax, including tachypnea, dyspnea, decreased or absent breath sounds, absent vocal fremitus, and hyperresonance. Notify the doctor and document their occurence.

Rationales

1. The "Surgical Intervention" plan covers general postoperative problems and interventions. This plan focuses on thoracotomy.

2. Hemorrhage may result from surgical trauma, inadequate hemostasis, or other factors. It always requires immediate medical evaluation and intervention.

• These signs may indicate hemorrhage and require a return to surgery to ligate bleeding vessels.

• These signs may reflect a hemothorax. Thoracentesis or reinsertion of chest tubes may be necessary.

• These signs may indicate cardiac tamponade, which requires immediate pericardiocentesis.

3. A pneumothorax prevents reexpansion of the lungs and may require reinserting chest tubes.

4. Monitor for signs of pleural effusion, including decreased or absent breath sounds, decreased vocal fremitus, increased dullness, and tachypnea. Notify the doctor and document their occurrence.

5. Monitor for signs of increasing atelectasis, including fever, tachypnea, tachycardia, increasing dullness, increased vocal fremitus, and bronchial or bronchovesicular breath sounds in the lung periphery. Notify the doctor and document their occurrence.

6. Monitor for signs of pulmonary edema, including tachypnea; tachycardia; dyspnea; shortness of breath; cough; crackles; wheezing; pink, frothy sputum; and anxiety. Notify the doctor and document their occurrence.

7. Continuously monitor a pneumonectomy patient for the following complications:

• hemorrhage—If a patient has a sudden, large hemoptysis, place the patient in a high Fowler's position, turned toward the operative side; summon immediate medical assistance.

• bronchopleural fistula—Observe for hemoptysis, an extensive air leak, subcutaneous emphysema, or fever.

• subcutaneous emphysema—Observe for swelling, puffiness, or crepitation of the skin.

• excessive mediastinal shift—Observe for excessive deviation of trachea at sternal notch, hypotension, tachycardia, weak peripheral pulses, or other signs of decreased cardiac output.

8. Monitor for signs and symptoms of pulmonary embolism, including chest pain, dyspnea, fever, hemoptysis, changes in vital signs, and increased central venous pressure. Notify the doctor and document. Refer to the "Pulmonary Embolism" plan, page 246, for further information.

9. Additional individualized interventions: _____

_____

4. A pleural effusion may compress the lungs, causing hypoxemia. Chest tube reinsertion may be necessary to remove the fluid and reexpand the lungs. Failure to remove the fluid may result in empyema.

5. Atelectasis (collapsed alveoli), commonly caused by poor bronchial hygiene, produces hypoxemia reflected in tachypnea and tachycardia. Dullness, increased fremitus, and abnormal breath sounds all result from consolidation.

6. Pulmonary edema is a life-threatening condition that requires immediate intervention, such as diuretics, inotropic agents, rotating tourniquets, and positive-pressure breathing. A patient with other problems, particularly cardiac problems, may be at high risk for this complication.

7. A pneumonectomy, the most traumatic form of thoracotomy, has a high incidence of complications.

• Hemorrhage may result from inadequate surgical hemostasis, development of a bronchopleural fistula, or other factors. Placing the patient in a high Fowler's position toward the operative side may prevent drainage into the remaining lung.

• A bronchopleural fistula may develop after surgery, most commonly during the first week, causing bleeding, air leaks, or infection. Depending on the size and location of the fistula, it may require surgery (to close the bronchial stump) and antibiotics.

• A bronchial stump leak may cause a large amount of subcutaneous emphysema. An air leak usually resolves over 3 days to a week but may require surgery.

• After lung removal, the mediastinum is not supported on one side and may shift. The residual pleural space should fill after surgery by a combination of mediastinal shift, diaphragm elevation, coagulation of serous drainage, and development of fibrotic tissue. If mediastinal shift is excessive, decreased cardiac output may occur, requiring mediastinal stabilization by fluid or air injection or thoracentesis.

8. Pulmonary embolism, a serious complication, may result from deep vein thrombosis and cause varying signs and symptoms depending on the size of the embolus. Prompt medical treatment is required to prevent further pulmonary tissue damage. The "Pulmonary Embolism" plan covers this disorder in detail.

9. Rationales: _____

_____

Target outcome criterion
By 3 to 7 days after surgery, the patient will display no signs of complications, such as hemorrhage, cardiac arrhythmias, hemothorax, cardiac tamponade, pneumothorax, pleural effusion, atelectasis, subcutaneous emphysema, bronchopleural fistula, or mediastinal shift.

Nursing diagnosis: *High risk for infection related to surgical incision and endotracheal intubation*

NURSING PRIORITY: Prevent infection.

Interventions

1. Monitor for and document signs of pneumonia, including fever, tachypnea, bronchial or bronchovesicular breath sounds in the periphery, increased vocal fremitus, increased dullness, and dyspnea. Notify the doctor if any of these signs occur.

2. Assess for signs and symptoms of wound infection every 2 to 4 hours and as needed. When the incision can be seen directly, observe for redness and swelling. Monitor for elevated WBC count or sedimentation rate, as ordered.

3. Monitor culture and sensitivity test results for wound drainage, as ordered.

4. Reinforce or change dressings as needed, using aseptic technique.

5. Additional individualized interventions: _____

_____

Rationales

1. Invasive chest surgery and endotracheal intubation place the patient at high risk for pneumonia. Treatment may require aggressive pulmonary hygiene, antibiotics, and positive-pressure breathing treatments.

2. Regular assessments may provide early warning of infection. Occlusive dressings may remain over the incision sites for 1 to 3 days, making direct observation of the sites difficult.

3. Culture and sensitivity tests help identify the infective organism and the most effective antibiotic treatment.

4. The dressing is usually reinforced, not changed, during the first 1 to 2 days after surgery to prevent exposure to microorganisms.

5. Rationales: _____

_____

Target outcome criteria
Within 3 days after surgery, the patient will:
• have a clean, dry, and healing wound
• display a normal temperature and vital signs
• display a normal WBC count and sedimentation rate.

By the time of discharge, the patient will have clear breath sounds, normal fremitus, and normal resonance to percussion, as appropriate to type of surgery.

Discharge planning
NURSING DISCHARGE CRITERIA
Upon the patient's discharge, documentation shows evidence of:
• stable vital signs and monitoring parameters
• clear breath sounds, bilateral lung expansion, and bilateral resonance to percussion, as appropriate
• absence of major complications
• healing surgical incision.

PATIENT-FAMILY TEACHING CHECKLIST
Document evidence that the patient and family demonstrate an understanding of:
__ surgical procedure, including expected postoperative course
__ deep breathing, coughing, and spirometer use
__ comfort measures
__ ROM and other exercises
__ purpose and mechanism of chest drainage system.

DOCUMENTATION CHECKLIST
Using outcome criteria as a guide, document:
__ clinical status on admission
__ significant changes in status

__ pertinent diagnostic test findings
__ chest drainage (amount, consistency, and color)
__ functioning of chest drainage equipment
__ complications, such as subcutaneous emphysema
__ deep breathing, coughing, and spirometer efforts
__ oxygen therapy
__ pain and effects of medication
__ activity levels and ROM and other exercises
__ patient-family teaching
__ discharge planning.

ASSOCIATED PLANS OF CARE
Mechanical Ventilation
Pain
Pulmonary Embolism

References
Alspach, J., ed. *Core Curriculum for Critical Care Nursing*, 4th ed. Philadelphia: W.B. Saunders Co., 1991.
McKenry, L., and Salerno, E. *Mosby's Pharmacology in Nursing*, 18th ed. St. Louis: Mosby-Year Book, 1992.

Abdominal Aortic Aneurysm Repair

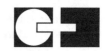

DRG information

DRG 110 Major Cardiovascular Procedures. With Complication or Comorbidity (CC).
Mean LOS = 10.5 days

DRG 111 Major Cardiovascular Procedures. Without CC.
Mean LOS = 8.1 days
Principal diagnoses include abdominal aortic aneurysm (ruptured, nonruptured, or dissecting).

Introduction
DEFINITION AND TIME FOCUS

The arterial wall consists of three tissue layers: the intima, the media, and the adventitia. In abdominal aneurysm, degeneration of the media causes the aorta to dilate, usually distal to the renal arteries. The vessel wall progressively weakens, increasing the risk of life-threatening rupture. In abdominal aortic aneurysm repair, the diseased portion of the artery (aneurysm) is surgically replaced with a synthetic polyester (Dacron) graft. The graft may be tubular or bifurcated (split into two branches), depending on the segment involved. The graft is placed in the lumen of the aneurysm so that the outer layers of the arterial wall will close over and protect the graft.

The patient undergoing abdominal aortic aneurysm repair is usually elderly, has associated cardiovascular disease, and experiences major stress from surgery. This plan focuses on preoperative care as well as the management of potential multisystem postoperative complications during the initial recovery period in the intensive care unit and the medical-surgical unit.

ETIOLOGY AND PRECIPITATING FACTORS

The most common cause of aneurysm is atherosclerosis. Risk factors for atherosclerosis include:
• cigarette smoking
• hypercholesterolemia
• hypertension
• diabetes mellitus
• obesity
• hypertriglyceridemia
• sedentary life-style
• stress
• family history of cardiovascular disease.
Other causes of aneurysm include:
• congenital disorders, such as Marfan's disease
• bacterial or fungal infections that invade the vessel wall (mycotic aneurysm)
• syphilitic aortitis
• blunt or sharp trauma
• chronic aortitis, related to Takayasu's arteritis or rheumatic spondylitis.

Focused assessment guidelines
NURSING HISTORY (Functional health pattern findings)

Health perception — health management pattern
• may report abdominal or back discomfort
• may report feeling heart beat in the abdomen
• may report a history of exercise intolerance
• may report a family history of atherosclerosis
• may report cardiac and respiratory risk factors, such as cigarette smoking; high-fat, high-cholesterol diet; or sedentary life-style

Activity-exercise pattern
• may report intermittent claudication or pain at rest
• may report shortness of breath if a heavy smoker

Sexuality-reproductive pattern
• may report impotence

Cognitive-perceptual pattern
• may express fear about impending surgery

PHYSICAL FINDINGS
Note: Physical findings may vary, depending on the aneurysm's cause and size. Aneurysms are usually asymptomatic and found by accident.

Cardiovascular
• hypertension
• arrhythmias
• diminished peripheral pulses, claudication or pain at rest, trophic changes (if associated with atherosclerosis)
• palpable abdominal mass above or at the umbilicus, extending toward the epigastrium
• carotid, femoral, or abdominal aortic bruits

Integumentary
(Integumentary changes are associated with atherosclerotic changes or distal embolization.)
• cyanosis of lower extremities
• dependent rubor, pallor on elevation
• thickened toenails
• decreased hair growth on lower extremities
• coolness of lower extremities

DIAGNOSTIC STUDIES
• arterial blood gas levels — monitor oxygenation, ventilation, and acid-base status
• complete blood count — monitors red blood cell, white blood cell (WBC) and platelets. Altered hemoglobin and hematocrit levels reflect any blood loss and the oxygen carrying ability of the blood. An elevated WBC count reflects an inflammatory response.

• serum electrolyte panel — monitors fluid, electrolyte, and acid-base status
• serum creatinine and blood urea nitrogen (BUN) — monitor renal function
• blood coagulation studies — monitors clotting
• urinalysis — monitors renal status, including secretion and concentration
• blood typing and cross-matching — necessary for blood replacement
• electrocardiography (ECG) — may reveal cardiac changes associated with ischemia
• chest X-ray — may reveal abnormalities of the chest, heart, and lungs
• abdominal X-ray — may detect calcium in the aneurysm wall
• abdominal ultrasound — may reveal the aneurysm's size
• abdominal computed tomography scan — may reveal a leaking aneurysm
• aortic arteriogram — may show aberrant renal arteries, mesenteric artery patency, and iliac artery involvement

POTENTIAL COMPLICATIONS
• myocardial infarction
• hemorrhage
• respiratory failure
• lower limb ischemia
• renal failure
• bowel ischemia
• spinal cord ischemia
• infection
• impotence

Nursing diagnosis: *Knowledge deficit regarding preoperative and postoperative care related to aortic surgery*

NURSING PRIORITY: Prepare the patient and family for the impending surgery.

Interventions

1. See the "Knowledge Deficit" plan, page 56.

2. See the "Surgical Intervention" plan, page 81.

3. Describe endotracheal intubation and mechanical ventilation. Refer to the "Mechanical Ventilation" plan, page 227.

4. Explain to the patient and family the need for close monitoring after surgery and the expected length of stay in the intensive care unit (ICU), usually 48 to 72 hours.

5. Explain the need for frequent vascular checks to assess graft patency and peripheral vascular status.

6. Explain activities that may prevent graft kinking or compression and postoperative edema in the lower extremities: reclining while sitting in a chair, avoiding leg-crossing or dangling the legs over the bedside, and elevating the foot of the bed.

Rationales

1. The "Knowledge Deficit" plan provides general patient teaching information. This plan focuses specifically on abdominal aortic aneurysm repair.

2. The "Surgical Intervention" care plan describes what to teach the patient about perioperative routines.

3. The patient undergoing abdominal aortic aneurysm repair usually requires intubation and mechanical ventilation for the first 24 hours after surgery. Explaining mechanical ventilation and weaning may allay the patient's anxiety. The "Mechanical Ventilation" plan provides detailed information about teaching a mechanically ventilated patient.

4. Explaining the expected postoperative course may minimize the patient's and family's anxiety. The length of time spent in the ICU varies among institutions.

5. Peripheral pulses are checked hourly for the first 24 hours. A Doppler ultrasound stethoscope may also be used. Knowing that frequent assessment is normal may allay the patient's fears that the surgery failed.

6. Reclining in a chair may prevent kinking of an aorta-bifemoral graft in the groin. Preventing leg-crossing or dangling the legs over the bedside and elevating the foot of the bed may prevent or decrease lower extremity edema.

7. Additional individualized interventions:_____

7. Rationales:_____

_____

_____

Target outcome criteria
Within 2 hours after preoperative teaching the patient, on request, will:
• verbalize understanding of perioperative routines
• demonstrate the ability to cough, deep breathe, and use the incentive spirometer, if applicable, and to splint the incision.

Collaborative problem: *High risk for cardiac decompensation related to changes in intravascular volume, third space fluid shift, and increased systemic vascular resistance*

NURSING PRIORITY: Promptly detect changes in cardiac status.

Interventions

1. After surgery, monitor the patient's vital signs according to unit protocol and nursing judgment (typically every 15 minutes until stable, then every hour for the first 24 hours, then every 2 hours until discharge to the medical-surgical unit, then every 4 hours until discharge from the hospital).

2. Monitor hemodynamic parameters (central venous pressure [CVP], pulmonary capillary wedge pressure [PCWP], cardiac output, and cardiac index) according to ICU protocol or doctor's orders until the pulmonary artery catheter is removed.

3. Continuously monitor heart rate and ECG for arrhythmias, particularly atrial fibrillation, until the patient is discharged to the medical-surgical unit. Document and report abnormalities to the doctor.

4. Monitor effectiveness of antihypertensive or vasopressor medications, if prescribed.

5. Monitor for fluid and electrolyte imbalances. See Appendix C, "Fluid and Electrolyte Imbalances."

6. Additional individualized interventions: _____

Rationales

1. Cardiac decompensation is the major complication that leads to morbidity following aortic surgery.

2. The patient usually returns from surgery with a pulmonary artery catheter, arterial line, peripheral I.V. lines, and an indwelling urinary catheter. Hemodynamic monitoring provides an accurate evaluation of myocardial sensitivity and guides drug and fluid therapy to prevent cardiac complications.

3. Frequent cardiopulmonary assessments may reveal problems and allow for timely interventions. (Thromboembolism from atrial fibrillation may interfere with vital arterial blood flow.)

4. Hypertension and hypotension affect graft patency.

5. The "Fluid and Electrolyte Imbalances" appendix addresses assessment parameters and interventions.

6. Rationales: _____

Target outcome criteria
Within the first 24 hours after surgery, the patient will:
• be hemodynamically stable
• be free from cardiac complications.

Collaborative problem: *High risk for hypercapnia, hypoxemia, or both related to endotracheal intubation, physiologic changes associated with aging, effects of general anesthesia, and presence of an abdominal incision*

NURSING PRIORITY: Optimize ventilation and oxygenation.

Interventions

1. Assess the patient's vital signs on admission to the ICU and every hour for 24 hours, then every 2 hours until the patient is returned to the medical-surgical unit, then every 4 hours. Note respiratory effort and the amount and character of sputum. Provide routine suctioning according to unit protocol while the patient is intubated. Document and report abnormalities.

2. See the "Mechanical Ventilation" plan, page 227.

3. Once the patient is extubated, provide supplemental oxygen, as ordered. Have the patient turn, cough, and deep breathe with an incentive spirometer every 2 hours. Monitor oxygen saturation through pulse oximetry, as ordered. See the "Mechanical Ventilation" plan for details on pulse oximetry.

4. Administer analgesics for pain, as ordered. Monitor for signs and symptoms of respiratory depression.

5. Additional individualized interventions: _____

_____

Rationales

1. Most patients undergoing abdominal aortic aneurysm repair are intubated overnight after surgery. Elevated temperature may indicate atelectasis. Respiratory effort may be minimal immediately after surgery. Suctioning promotes airway clearance.

2. The "Mechanical Ventilation" plan provides specific information on assessments and interventions for the intubated patient.

3. Supplemental oxygen may be ordered to promote adequate tissue oxygenation. Position changes and deep breathing and coughing exercises clear the airway and prevent atelectasis.

4. Pain medications may be necessary to increase the force of coughing. However, some narcotic analgesics exacerbate respiratory depression, particularly in the older patient.

5. Rationales: _____

_____

Target outcome criteria

Within 4 hours of admission, the patient will:
• exhibit bilaterally clear breath sounds
• have minimal endotracheal secretions.

Within 4 hours after extubation, the patient will:
• perform incentive spirometry without difficulty
• have bilaterally clear anterior and posterior breath sounds

---

Collaborative problem: *High risk for bleeding related to extensive retroperitoneal dissection and vascular anastomosis*

NURSING PRIORITY: Promptly detect signs and symptoms of bleeding.

Interventions

1. Monitor and document inake and output and vital signs every hour for 24 hours; monitor and document CVP, PCWP, and laboratory values according to protocol or doctor's orders. Be alert for decreased urine output, tachycardia, hypotension, decreased CVP or PCWP, and decreased hematocrit. Document and report abnormalities.

2. Assess the dressings on admission to the unit and every hour for 4 hours, then every 4 hours. Be alert for an expanding pulsatile groin mass.

Rationales

1. These signs may indicate intra-abdominal bleeding.

2. Frequent assessment allows for prompt detection of hemorrhage. An expanding pulsatile groin mass may indicate hemorrhage at the distal anastomosis of a bifurcated graft.

3. Monitor and document the amount and character of nasogastric tube drainage every 2 hours for 24 hours, then every 4 hours.

3. Bloody nasogastric drainage may indicate intra-abdominal bleeding.

4. Assess abdominal girth if retroperitoneal bleeding is suspected.

4. An increase in abdominal girth, with an accompanying increase in back pain, may suggest retroperitoneal bleeding.

5. Additional individualize interventions: _____

5. Rationales: _____

Target outcome criteria
Within 24 hours after surgery, the patient will:
• be free from signs and symptoms of hemorrhage
• have a dry, intact dressing
• have stable vital signs.

Nursing diagnosis: *High risk for injury: complications related to surgical procedure and atherosclerosis*

NURSING PRIORITY: Promptly detect complications.

Interventions

1. Monitor for decreased peripheral tissue perfusion: check peripheral pulses (both upper and lower extremities) immediately upon admission and every hour for the first 24 hours, then every 4 hours until discharge.
  Document the location and character of the pulse using this scale:
  0 = absent
  1 = detectable by Doppler ultrasound stethoscope only
  2 = weakly palpable
  3 = strong
Document evidence of capillary refill and signs of cyanosis and mottling. Notify the doctor of any changes.

2. Monitor for acute renal failure. Record hourly urine output until the indwelling urinary catheter is removed. Monitor BUN and creatinine levels, as ordered. Be alert for a urine output of less than 30 ml/hour for 2 consecutive hours and elevated BUN and creatinine levels, and notify the doctor if they occur.

3. Monitor for signs and symptoms of bowel ischemia, including diarrhea (may be positive for occult bleeding), abdominal tenderness, fever, prolonged ileus, sepsis, shock, leukocytosis, and metabolic acidosis.

4. Monitor for signs and symptoms of spinal cord ischemia. Monitor sensory and motor function of the lower extremities, as well as temperature, color, and pulses, every hour for the first 24 hours.

5. Monitor for intra-abdominal graft infection by noting temperature elevations, leukocytosis, or prolonged ileus.

Rationales

1. A decrease in peripheral tissue perfusion in the legs may result from graft thrombosis or distal embolization of atherosclerotic plaque. An arterial line may cause distal embolization, as well as arterial dissection, arteriovenous fistula, false aneurysm, and hematoma formation. Accurate assessment of perfusion is essential in the early postoperative period to detect early thrombosis formation and prevent limb loss.

2. Renal failure may result from atheromatous embolization to the renal arteries. A low urine output associated with elevated serum creatinine and BUN levels may indicate renal failure. (Creatinine clearance may be a better indicator of renal failure in the older patient.)

3. Approximately 2% of patients undergoing abdominal aortic aneurysm repair develop mesenteric artery ischemia, with a 50% mortality rate. This complication is related to low flow states, thrombosis, embolization, and fibrillatory cardiac disease. Symptoms are most likely to occur in the first 48 hours after surgery.

4. The incidence of spinal cord ischemia after abdominal aortic aneurysm repair is quite low but warrants monitoring. Interruption of the arterial supply to the spinal cord may result from hypotension or embolus to the artery, causing lower extremity paraplegia.

5. Unexplained fevers, leukocytosis, or prolonged ileus may indicate graft infection (a late complication).

6. Monitor for local wound infection by inspecting incision lines for erythema, edema, odor, and the amount and color of any drainage every 4 hours and as needed until discharge. Document and notify doctor of any changes.

6. Regular assessment may provide early warning of local wound infection.

7. Additional individualized interventions: _____

7. Rationales: _____

Target outcome criteria
Within 24 to 48 hours after surgery, the patient will:
• have adequate perfusion to the upper and lower extremities, kidneys, bowel, and spinal cord
• have any complications immediately detected, reported, and treated, as appropriate.

Before discharge, the patient will:
• have clean, dry, and intact incision lines
• be afebrile, with a WBC count within normal limits.

Nursing diagnosis: *Pain related to surgical tissue trauma or ischemia*

NURSING PRIORITY: Relieve pain.

Interventions

1. Assess patency and stability of the epidural catheter, if used. Monitor effectiveness of epidural analgesia as well as for adverse reactions.

2. See the "Pain" plan, page 69.

3. Additional individualized interventions: _____

Rationales

1. Epidural analgesia may be used to manage pain after abdominal aortic aneurysm repair.

2. The "Pain" plan specifically addresses pain assessment and management.

3. Rationales: _____

Target outcome criteria
Within 1 hour of complaint of pain, the patient will:
• verbalize adequacy of pain relief, if asked
• appear relaxed.

Discharge planning

NURSING DISCHARGE CRITERIA
Upon the patient's discharge, documentation shows evidence of:
• stable vital signs
• normal body temperature
• absence of pulmonary and cardiovascular complications
• ability to tolerate oral intake
• ability to void and defecate same as before surgery
• healing wound free from signs of infection
• ability to ambulate according to progressive activity plan
• pain controlled with oral medication
• knowledge of activity and position restrictions
• adequate home support, or referral to home health care or skilled care facility, if indicated by lack of home support or by self-care limitations.

PATIENT-FAMILY TEACHING CHECKLIST
Document evidence that the patient and family demonstrate an understanding of:
___ progressive activity and ambulation plan
___ incision care
___ signs and symptoms of wound infection or graft thrombosis
___ discharge medications' purpose, dosage, administration, and adverse effects
___ risk factors for atherosclerosis and their reduction
___ available community resources
___ date, time, and location of follow-up appointments.

DOCUMENTATION CHECKLIST

Using outcome criteria as a guide, document:
___ clinical status on admission
___ significant changes in status
___ pertinent diagnostic test findings
___ presence or absence of peripheral pulses
___ pain relief measures
___ wound site appearance and amount, color, and consistency of any drainage
___ level of activity and the patient's response to progressive ambulation
___ patient-family teaching
___ discharge planning.

ASSOCIATED PLANS OF CARE

Knowledge Deficit
Mechanical Ventilation
Pain
Surgical Intervention

References

Bensen, J., and McClellan, W. "Retroperitoneal Approach to Abdominal Aortic Aneurysm." *AORN Journal* 53(1):42, 44-6, 48 1991.

Burggraff, V., and Stanley, M. *Nursing the Elderly: A Care Plan Approach.* Philadelphia: J.B. Lippincott Co., 1988.

Cohen, J.R. "Atherosclerosis," in *Vascular Surgery for the House Officer.* Edited by Cohen, J.R. Baltimore: Williams & Wilkins, 1986.

Collins, B., and Kripp, M. "Postoperative Monitoring," in *Vascular Nursing.* Edited by Fahey, V.A. Philadelphia: W.B. Saunders Co., 1988.

Dalsing, M., Dilley, R., and McCarthy, M. "Surgery of the Aorta," *Critical Care Quarterly* 8(2):25-38, September 1985.

Hubner, C. "Preparation for Surgery," in *Vascular Nursing.* Edited by Fahey, V.A. Philadelphia: W.B. Saunders Co., 1988.

Moore, K., and Moore, S. "Abdominal Aortic Aneurysm," *Topics in Emergency Medicine* 12(2):61-65, July 1990.

Rebenson-Piano, M. "The Physiologic Changes that Occur with Aging," *Critical Care Nursing Quarterly* 12(1):1-14, June 1989.

CARDIOVASCULAR DISORDERS

CARDIOVASCULAR DISORDERS

Acute Myocardial Infarction — Critical Care Unit Phase

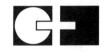

DRG information

DRG 121 Circulatory Disorders with Acute Myocardial Infarction (AMI) and Cardiovascular Complications, Discharged Alive.
Mean LOS = 8.2 days

DRG 122 Circulatory Disorders with AMI, without Cardiovascular Complications, Discharged Alive.
Mean LOS = 5.9 days

DRG 123 Circulatory Disorders, with AMI, Expired.
Mean LOS = 3.0 days

Additional DRG information: In order for any of these three DRGs to apply:
• principal diagnosis must be a Circulatory Disorder (including AMI)
• the AMI must be being treated during the initial episode of care.

DRG 121 is established when the AMI and cardiovascular complications are present. These cardiovascular complications include:
• heart aneurysm
• cardiac arrest
• atrioventricular or bundle branch blocks
• heart failure
• pulmonary embolism or infarction
• acute renal failure
• cardiogenic shock
• atrial or ventricular fibrillation or flutter
• paroxysmal atrial tachycardia
• ventricular tachycardia
• unstable angina.

DRG 123 is established when the patient expires, regardless of cardiovascular complications.

Introduction
DEFINITION AND TIME FOCUS

Acute myocardial infarction (AMI) is the death of myocardial tissue, usually resulting from coronary artery occlusion or spasm. It may present as subendocardial infarction, involving the inner myocardial layer, or transmural infarction, involving the full thickness of the myocardium. Mortality depends on the extent and location of the infarct, the patient's preexisting health status, and the speed and effectiveness of therapy.

This plan focuses on the critically ill patient admitted for diagnosis and management during an attack of severe crushing chest pain, the classic presentation in AMI.

ETIOLOGY AND PRECIPITATING FACTORS

• coronary artery disease, coronary artery spasm, hypotension, hypoxemia, severe bradycardia or tachycardia (especially with poor cardiac reserve), or other factors decreasing myocardial oxygen supply
• exercise, emotional stress, exposure to extreme heat or cold, eating, tachycardia, or other factors increasing myocardial oxygen demand

Focused assessment guidelines
NURSING HISTORY (Functional health pattern findings)

Health perception — health management pattern
• may experience sudden onset of severe chest pain — heavy, tight, crushing, or constricting quality; usually retrosternal; usually radiates to the left arm, but may radiate to the right arm, back, epigastrium, jaw, or neck; lasts longer than 30 minutes; unrelieved by rest or nitroglycerin. In some instances, AMI is painless.
• may be under treatment for angina, atherosclerosis, hyperlipidemia, hypertension, congestive heart failure (CHF), arrhythmias, cerebrovascular accident, peripheral vascular disease, or diabetes mellitus
• may have history of previous AMI, cardiac surgery, or oral contraceptive use
• may have coronary artery disease risk factors, such as obesity or cigarette smoking
• may fall into other high-risk categories — male over age 40 or postmenopausal female

Nutritional-metabolic pattern
• may report indigestion, nausea, or vomiting
• may report a diet high in calories, fat, and salt (common)

Elimination pattern
• may report feeling of fullness or bowel movement coinciding with onset of chest pain

Activity-exercise pattern
• may experience shortness of breath
• may report sporadic exercise or sedentary life-style (common)

Sleep-rest pattern
• may report sleep disturbances

Cognitive-perceptual pattern
• may report history of recurrent chest pain

Self-perception—self-concept pattern
• may express great concern about ability to return to work as soon as possible

Role-relationship pattern
• may describe self as someone on whom others depend
• may report family history of death from AMI (especially before age 50)

Coping—stress tolerance pattern
• usually anxious, tense, type A personality (aggressive, competitive, impatient)
• may report fear of death or of the unknown

Value-belief pattern
• may have delayed seeking medical attention or express disbelief over condition (denial)

PHYSICAL FINDINGS
Cardiovascular
• hypotension or hypertension
• tachycardia or, uncommonly, bradycardia
• other arrhythmias
• S_3 or S_4 heart sounds
• slowed capillary refill time (in shock)

Pulmonary
• crackles (if heart failure present)

Gastrointestinal
• vomiting
• abdominal distention

Neurologic
• restlessness
• irritability
• confusion

Integumentary
• diaphoresis
• cool, clammy skin
• variable skin color (may be normal, pale, ashen, or cyanotic)

Musculoskeletal
• pained or anxious facial expression
• tense posture

DIAGNOSTIC STUDIES
Initial laboratory data may reflect no significant abnormalities; subsequent tests may reveal the following:
• cardiac isoenzymes—show characteristic trends, particularly elevated creatine phosphokinase MB (CPK_2) and "flipped" lactic dehydrogenase (LDH) pattern (LDH_1 greater than LDH_2)
• arterial blood gas (ABG) levels—may reveal hypoxemia and acid-base abnormalities
• electrolyte panel—used to rule out disturbances affecting cardiac conduction and contractility (such as hypokalemia, hyperkalemia, hypocalcemia, hypercalcemia, or hypomagnesemia)
• white blood cell count and sedimentation rate—usually rise on second day because of inflammatory response
• blood urea nitrogen levels and creatinine clearance—may rise, indicating diminished renal perfusion
• serum cholesterol and triglyceride levels—may be elevated, indicating increased risk of atherosclerosis
• serum drug levels—may indicate subtherapeutic or toxic levels of antiarrhythmic agents, such as digitalis
• 12-lead electrocardiography (ECG)—with transmural infarction, elevated ST segment and upright T waves in hyperacute phase, progressing to deeply inverted T waves and pathologic Q waves in leads overlooking the infarcted area; with subendocardial infarction, depressed ST segment and inverted T waves
• chest X-ray—may show cardiac enlargement produced by CHF
• myocardial imaging (radionuclide) studies—demonstrate areas of poor or absent perfusion, wall motion abnormalities, and reduced ejection fraction
• echocardiography—may illustrate structural or functional cardiac abnormalities

POTENTIAL COMPLICATIONS
• arrhythmias
• sudden death
• cardiogenic shock
• CHF
• pulmonary edema
• papillary muscle dysfunction or rupture
• ventricular rupture
• pericarditis
• pulmonary embolism
• ventricular aneurysm
• cardiac tamponade

CARDIOVASCULAR DISORDERS

Collaborative problem: *High risk for cardiogenic shock related to arrhythmias, impaired contractility, or thrombosis*

NURSING PRIORITY: Optimize cardiac output and cellular perfusion.

Interventions

1. Institute and document continuous ECG monitoring on admission, with alarms on at all times. Preferably, monitor lead MCL_1 or MCL_6. See the "High risk for injury" nursing diagnosis in this plan for details about specific arrhythmias.

Rationales

1. Arrhythmias are the primary cause of death in the first 24 hours after infarction. MCL_1 and MCL_6 best differentiate supraventricular aberration from ventricular ectopy.

2. Record and analyze rhythm strips routinely every 4 hours and as needed for significant variations. Mount strips in chart.

2. Systematic analysis may warn of impending problems with impulse initiation or conduction.

3. Obtain serial 12-lead ECGs on admission, daily for 3 days, and as needed for chest pain.

3. The ECG obtained on admission provides a baseline for infarct localization. Serial ECGs monitor changes.

4. Evaluate and document hourly or as needed: level of consciousness, pulse, blood pressure, heart sounds, breath sounds, urine output, skin color and temperature, and capillary refill time.

4. Level of consciousness is a sensitive indicator of cerebral ischemia. Pulse rate may indicate fluid deficit, pulse rhythm may indicate ectopic beats, and pulse volume may indicate fluid deficit or overload. A systolic blood pressure reading more than 20 mm Hg below the patient's normal value or a systolic blood pressure of 80 mm Hg or less indicates shock. Abnormal heart sounds indicate various problems: S_3 or S_4, CHF; murmurs, incompetent or stenotic valves; and pericardial friction rub, pericarditis. Abnormal breath sounds (particularly crackles that do not clear with coughing) suggest CHF. A urine output less than 60 ml/hour suggests decreased renal perfusion. Pale, cyanotic, mottled, or cool skin indicates decreased peripheral perfusion, as does a capillary refill time greater than 3 seconds.

5. Establish and maintain a patent I.V. line on admission. Document cumulative fluid intake and output hourly.

5. An I.V. line is necessary for emergency fluid and drug administration. The usual order is for dextrose 5% in water at a keep-vein-open rate. If the patient does not need fluid, a heparin lock may be ordered instead. Intake and output records provide clues to developing fluid imbalances.

6. Administer heparin, warfarin sodium (Coumadin), or both, as ordered.

6. Heparin commonly is ordered prophylactically to minimize the risk of thromboembolism from arrhythmias or immobility. It also may be used to limit extension of a thrombus that produced an AMI. Warfarin achieves long-term anticoagulation.

7. Prepare the patient for aggressive treatment measures, as ordered, which may include:

7. Infarctions that are impending, in progress, or complicated may require immediate aggressive interventions.

• thrombolytic therapy: streptokinase (Kabikinase), alteplase (Activase), anistreplase (Eminase), or urokinase (Abbokinase)

• Thrombolytic therapy may be administered to lyse fresh clots, thus relieving the occlusion and reestablishing perfusion to the damaged area.

• emergency coronary arteriography

• Coronary arteriography normally is not performed during AMI because of the risk of furthering the infarct. It is necessary before angioplasty or emergency bypass surgery, however, to locate the site of occlusion precisely.

• percutaneous transluminal coronary angioplasty (PTCA)

• PTCA may increase coronary artery blood flow by compressing occluding lesions and dilating the vessel lumen. The resulting increase in luminal cross-sectional area improves blood flow to ischemic tissue.

• coronary artery bypass surgery.

• Emergency surgery may be necessary to bypass life-threatening lesions.

8. Additional individualized interventions: _____

8. Rationales: _____

Target outcome criteria
Within 24 hours of admission, the patient will:
• display vital signs within normal limits
• show normal skin color
• have a capillary refill time less than 3 seconds.

Within 3 days of admission, the patient will experience no life-threatening arrhythmias.

Collaborative problem: *Hypoxemia related to ventilation-perfusion imbalance*

NURSING PRIORITIES: (a) Optimize myocardial oxygen demand-supply ratio and (b) minimize the risk of further infarction.

Interventions

1. Observe for signs of hypoxemia, such as tachycardia, restlessness, irritability, or tachypnea. Monitor arterial oxygen saturation by pulse oximetry and ABG values, as ordered.

2. Administer and document oxygen therapy on admission, according to medical protocol and nursing judgment, typically 3 to 5 liters/minute by nasal cannula for the first 24 to 48 hours.

3. If blood pressure is stable within normal limits, place the patient in semi-Fowler's position.

4. During the period of acute instability, place the patient on bed rest or chair rest. Once stabilized, increase activity as tolerated. See the "Activity intolerance" nursing diagnosis, page 317, in the "Cardiogenic Shock" plan.

5. Provide adequate rest periods. Set priorities for care and group procedures. Refer to the "Sensory-Perceptual Alteration" plan, page 75, for further suggestions.

6. Additional individualized interventions: _____

Rationales

1. Cellular hypoxia commonly results from impaired coronary artery perfusion, decreased systemic perfusion, and respiratory depressant effects of analgesics and sedatives. Pulse oximetry and ABG values provide objective evidence of the degree of hypoxemia. Prompt treatment minimizes ischemic damage.

2. Supplemental oxygen will elevate arterial oxygen content and may relieve myocardial ischemia.

3. The semi-upright position facilitates breathing.

4. Rest reduces myocardial oxygen demands. Controlling oxygen demands helps limit infarct extension. Gradual resumption of activity helps promote a sense of well-being. The "Activity intolerance" nursing diagnosis contains detailed information on assessing activity tolerance and promoting safe resumption of physical activity.

5. Sleep deprivation, common in the critical care setting, can lead to increased irritability, confusion, increased sensitivity to pain, and other problems. The "Sensory-Perceptual Alteration" plan provides detailed interventions and rationales related to sleep deprivation.

6. Rationales: _____

Target outcome criteria
Within 24 hours of admission, the patient will:
• show no dyspnea
• manifest partial pressure of arterial oxygen (PaO_2) greater than 80 mm Hg
• display normal sinus rhythm or controlled arrhythmias
• have normal skin color
• rest comfortably.

Collaborative problem: *Chest pain related to myocardial ischemia*

NURSING PRIORITY: Relieve chest pain.

Interventions

1. On admission, teach the patient to report any chest pain, tightness, heaviness, or burning immediately.

2. Monitor continually for chest pain: verbalization or complaints of discomfort, sternal rubbing, tense posture, emotional withdrawal, facial grimacing, shortness of breath, diaphoresis, or restlessness.

Rationales

1. Symptoms other than obvious pain may indicate ischemia. Awareness of more subtle symptoms suggesting ischemia facilitates early intervention.

2. The patient may not report pain, but astute observation may detect associated signs and symptoms and facilitate early intervention. Shortness of breath and diaphoresis may result from sympathetic stimulation, while restlessness may reflect cerebral ischemia.

CARDIOVASCULAR DISORDERS

3. Document pain episodes: analyze pain characteristics, record a monitor rhythm strip, and obtain a 12-lead ECG.

3. Careful analysis of characteristics aids differential diagnosis of pain. The rhythm strip can document new arrhythmias, while the 12-lead ECG can document infarct extension.

4. Administer medication and document its use promptly at the onset of pain, according to medical protocol or orders. Evaluate and document blood pressure, pulse, and respirations before and after administration. Assess pain relief after 30 minutes.

4. Pain medication is more effective when given before severe pain develops. Pain may stimulate the sympathetic nervous system and increase myocardial work load. Vital sign measurements before medication administration provide objective indicators of the degree of physiologic stress imposed by pain, while those taken afterward indicate relief of such stress.

5. During the initial period of cardiovascular instability, titrate I.V. morphine, typically in 2- to 5-mg doses (if ordered), according to the level of pain and vital signs. Withhold morphine and contact the doctor if the respiratory rate is less than 12 breaths/minute or the systolic blood pressure is less than 90 mm Hg (for a previously normotensive patient), or more than 20 mm Hg below the baseline value (for a previously hypertensive patient).

5. Administering narcotics intravenously relieves pain more rapidly and reliably than by the intramuscular route because poorly perfused muscles absorb medication erratically. I.M. injections also elevate CPK levels, obscuring their diagnostic value. Morphine is the drug of choice for pain associated with AMI because it is a potent analgesic, causes peripheral vasodilation (lessening venous return and myocardial work load), and causes euphoria. The vital sign parameters listed indicate respiratory depression and excessive vasodilation, both possible adverse reactions to morphine.

6. Remain with the patient until pain is relieved.

6. The presence of a competent, confident caregiver may reassure the patient, relieving anxiety and thus lessening sympathetic stimulation.

7. Position the patient comfortably. Use noninvasive pain-relief measures and medications, as appropriate. See the "Pain" plan, page 69, for details.

7. Comfortable positioning and noninvasive pain-relief measures such as rhythmic breathing, distraction, and relaxation may reduce the perception of pain and promote endorphin release. The "Pain" plan discusses numerous alternative pain-relief strategies.

8. Additional individualized interventions: _____

8. Rationales: _____

Target outcome criteria
Within 1 to 2 hours of admission, the patient will:
• verbalize pain relief
• display no associated signs and symptoms of pain

• assume a relaxed posture
• have a relaxed facial expression.

Nursing diagnosis: *High risk for ineffective individual coping related to fear of death, anxiety, denial, or depression*

NURSING PRIORITY: Promote healthy coping.

Interventions

1. Implement measures in the "Ineffective Individual Coping" plan, page 51, as appropriate.

2. Administer tranquilizers, as ordered, typically a benzodiazepine such as diazepam (Valium), lorazepam (Ativan), or alprazolam (Xanax).

3. Additional individualized interventions: _____

Rationales

1. AMI is a major threat to psychological equilibrium and may provoke various protective responses. The "Ineffective Individual Coping" plan contains comprehensive information on evaluating and promoting healthy responses.

2. Minor tranquilizers may be used to keep anxiety at a tolerable level and avoid the deleterious physiologic effects of anxiety-triggered catecholamine release.

3. Rationales: _____

Target outcome criteria
Within 24 hours, the patient will:
• display feelings appropriate to initial stage of coping
• display the first signs of effective coping.

Nursing diagnosis: *Constipation related to diet, bed rest, immobility, or medications*

NURSING PRIORITY: Prevent or minimize constipation.

Interventions

1. Encourage intake of the prescribed diet, which is usually low in calories, salt, and fat. Limit intake of caffeine. Document intake, likes, and dislikes.

2. Supply a bedside commode when the patient's condition allows.

3. Administer stool softeners and laxatives judiciously, as ordered, and document their use. Use alternatives and supplements to stool softeners and laxatives, such as increased dietary fiber and prune juice. Encourage increased fluid intake, if appropriate to medical status.

4. Provide privacy, a room deodorizer, and television or radio noise while the patient is defecating.

5. Additional individualized interventions: _____

Rationales

1. Dietary prescriptions vary with the patient's needs. Caffeine is avoided because it is a cardiac stimulant. The patient is more likely to adhere to a diet plan that respects personal food preferences.

2. A bedside commode requires less energy to use than a bedpan so constipation can be relieved with less myocardial oxygen demand.

3. Straining to defecate produces Valsalva's maneuver, which can cause bradycardia and decrease cardiac output. Rebound tachycardia and myocardial ischemia may follow. Dependence on laxatives diminishes the urge for spontaneous defecation.

4. Without such measures, the patient may resist the urge to defecate because of embarrassment over expulsive sounds and odors.

5. Rationales: _____

CARDIOVASCULAR DISORDERS

Target outcome criteria
Within 3 days, the patient will:
• resume a regular bowel elimination pattern
• experience no straining during defecation
• have soft stool.

Nursing diagnosis: *High risk for injury: complications related to myocardial ischemia, injury, necrosis, inflammation, or arrhythmias*

NURSING PRIORITY: Prevent or minimize complications.

Interventions

1. Monitor constantly for general complications of AMI:

Rationales

1. Numerous complications can impair recovery from AMI. Many occur with any type of infarct and are associated less with its location than with the extent of myocardial damage and degree of the underlying coronary artery disease. Others have a pathophysiologic correlation with a specific type of infarct.

ARRHYTHMIAS

• Observe constantly for ventricular arrhythmias: ventricular premature beats, accelerated ventricular rhythm, ventricular tachycardia, and ventricular fibrillation.

• Observe constantly for supraventricular arrhythmias: premature atrial or junctional beats; atrial tachycardia, flutter, or fibrillation; or supraventricular tachycardia.

• Administer and document antiarrhythmic agents, as ordered. Monitor effectiveness and adverse effects. Typical agents are:

— Class IA agents, such as procainamide (Pronestyl), quinidine (Duraquin), and disopyramide (Norpace)

— Class IB agents, such as lidocaine (Xylocaine), ordered prophylactically or as needed for warning ventricular premature beats (more than 6 per minute, sequential, multifocal, or close to the preceding T wave), ventricular tachycardia, or ventricular fibrillation

— Class II agents, such as propranolol (Inderal), metoprolol (Lopressor), and atenolol (Tenormin)

— Class III agents, such as bretylium tosylate (Bretylol) and amiodarone (Cordarone)

— Class IV agents, such as verapamil (Calan), nifedipine (Procardia), and diltiazem (Cardizem)

• Implement and document emergency measures as needed, based on medical protocol and nursing judgment.

CONGESTIVE HEART FAILURE AND CARDIOGENIC SHOCK

• Implement measures in the "Cardiogenic Shock" and "Congestive Heart Failure" plans, pages 310 and 329, respectively.

INFARCT EXTENSION

• Monitor for new, increased, or persistent chest pain. Obtain a 12-lead ECG reading and administer pain medication, as ordered. Notify the doctor about the pain and any new indicators of infarction on the ECG reading.

• Ventricular arrhythmias are the most common complication of AMI. In the first few hours after infarction, they probably result from an ischemia-induced reentry mechanism, while later arrhythmias probably result from increased automaticity.

• Supraventricular arrhythmias may result from ischemia, heart failure, catecholamine stimulation, and other factors. Though less serious than ventricular arrhythmias, they may contribute to an unstable physiologic status or to thromboembolism. Tachycardias increase myocardial oxygen demand, reduce left ventricular filling time, and reduce coronary artery perfusion time. The loss of atrial "kick" (normally coordinated atrial contraction) also may reduce cardiac output.

• Arrhythmias may impair cardiac output or progress to cardiac arrest. Antiarrhythmic agents are classified according to their electrophysiologic properties.

— Used for both atrial and ventricular arrhythmias, particularly reentrant ones, Class IA drugs decrease automaticity, conduction, and repolarization.

— Class IB agents, used to prevent and treat ventricular arrhythmias, inhibit ventricular automaticity. Lidocaine also increases the threshold for fibrillation. Prophylactic lidocaine may be ordered because of AMI's high incidence of ventricular fibrillation, which commonly occurs without warning.

— Class II agents, beta-adrenergic blockers, are used to control supraventricular arrhythmias. Their complex mechanisms include suppressing sinus node automaticity and decreasing atrioventricular (AV) conduction.

— Bretylium suppresses reentrant ventricular arrhythmias and elevates the threshold for ventricular fibrillation. Amiodarone increases the refractory period and is useful in life-threatening ventricular tachyarrhythmias.

— Class IV drugs, calcium channel blockers, inhibit sinoatrial (SA) and AV automaticity and prolong AV conduction. They are particularly useful in treating supraventricular tachycardias.

• Protocols usually allow for emergency treatment of warning and lethal arrhythmias (ventricular premature beats, tachycardia, fibrillation, asystole; symptomatic sinus bradycardia; and Mobitz II second-degree and third-degree AV blocks).

• Varying degrees of myocardial failure, such as CHF or cardiogenic shock, are common during the first week after the infarction. Numerous factors place the AMI patient at risk for myocardial failure, including myocardial ischemia, hypoxemia, acidosis, hypotension, and paradoxical movement of the injured myocardial wall.

• Infarct extension may result from progressive ischemia of the myocardium secondary to swelling of damaged cells and inflammatory responses that compress surrounding tissue. Other factors that may be implicated include hypoxemia and microemboli.

PERICARDITIS

• Observe for pericardial chest pain, typically stabbing localized pain that worsens on deep inspiration and with movement. Also observe for fever, tachycardia, and pericardial friction rub.

• If signs or symptoms are present, notify the doctor. Administer anti-inflammatory agents, as ordered, typically aspirin, corticosteroids, or nonsteroidal anti-inflammatory agents.

• Monitor for indicators of pericardial effusion: weak peripheral pulses, pulsus paradoxus greater than 10 mm Hg, or a decreased level of consciousness. If present, notify the doctor promptly.

• Monitor for indicators of cardiac tamponade: Beck's triad (elevated central venous pressure [CVP], profound hypotension, and distant heart sounds), neck vein distention, tachycardia, decreased pulse pressure, paradoxical pulse, and pericardial friction rub. Summon immediate medical assistance and prepare for emergency pericardial aspiration.

VENTRICULAR ANEURYSM

• Observe for signs and symptoms of a possible ventricular aneurysm: signs and symptoms of CHF, thromboembolism, or persistent ectopy. Alert the doctor and prepare the patient for surgery, as ordered.

RUPTURE

• Monitor for signs and symptoms of papillary muscle rupture: sudden shock, a loud holosystolic murmur radiating from the apex to the left axilla, and signs of severe left ventricular failure. Obtain immediate medical assistance. Assist with treatment of cardiogenic shock or prepare the patient for surgery, as ordered.

• Observe for signs and symptoms of potential septal rupture: severe chest pain, severe heart failure, a loud holosystolic murmur at the apex and lower left sternal border, or sudden cardiac death. Initiate cardiopulmonary resuscitation (CPR), if necessary, and obtain immediate medical assistance. Implement measures to treat cardiogenic shock or prepare the patient for surgery, as ordered.

• Be alert for signs and symptoms of a possible impending myocardial rupture, especially in a patient with a transmural infarction who is on anticoagulant therapy: persistent chest pain without ECG changes, persistent hypertension postinfarct, M-shaped QRS complexes, or pericardial blood or fluid detected by an echocardiogram. Notify the doctor immediately. Assist with emergency pericardiocentesis and treatment of cardiogenic shock, as ordered.

2. Monitor constantly for complications of particular types of AMI:

• Pericardial sac inflammation is a relatively benign complication. Focal pericarditis usually develops within 5 days, while generalized pericarditis (Dressler's syndrome) typically develops within 14 days.

• Administering anti-inflammatory agents reduces the inflammation, relieving the signs and symptoms and reducing the risk of pericardial effusion.

• A pericardial effusion represents leakage of fluid across the walls of inflamed cells. The degree may vary from mild to major. Left untreated, an effusion may produce a cardiac tamponade large enough to induce cardiac arrest.

• A cardiac tamponade is a medical emergency. Because it impinges on ventricular expansion, it severely limits ventricular filling and therefore cardiac output. Immediate removal of the pericardial fluid is necessary to permit ventricular filling and prevent cardiac arrest.

• Ventricular aneurysm is thought to occur in about 10% of AMI patients. Dilation most commonly occurs in the anterolateral area, although it may also occur in the posterior or septal walls or the apical area. The systolic outward bulging of the area weakened by the infarction lessens stroke volume. In addition, clots may occur in the dilated area and embolize to other organs. Aneurysmectomy removes the bulging, weakened area and prevents potentially fatal myocardial rupture.

• Papillary muscle rupture results from necrosis of the muscles that anchor the chordae tendineae of the mitral valve. It occurs most commonly with inferior infarction involving the posterior papillary muscle, although the anterior papillary muscle may be damaged with an anteroseptal infarct. The resulting acute mitral insufficiency may severely limit cardiac output. Definitive treatment is mitral valve replacement.

• Septal rupture, a rare but life-threatening emergency, results from necrosis of the interventricular septum. It may occur in inferior or anteroseptal infarcts and is most likely if significant disease is present in both the right and left anterior descending coronary arteries. CPR and measures to combat cardiogenic shock may keep the patient alive until the ventricular septal defect can be repaired surgically.

• Rupture of the free ventricular wall, a devastating complication, occurs most commonly in the anterior or lateral walls. It may occur anywhere from 3 days to 3 weeks after the infarction, during the healing stage when leukocytic removal of myocardial debris thins the myocardial wall. Hypertension, anticoagulation, and full-thickness infarction increase the risk of rupture. The resulting massive cardiac tamponade leads to death. The invariable mortality from rupture emphasizes the urgency of action when any signs and symptoms of impending rupture are detected.

2. Certain complications correlate with a particular type of infarct, because they stem from a common pathophysiologic cause.

ANTERIOR, ANTEROSEPTAL, OR ANTEROLATERAL INFARCT

• Monitor for signs or symptoms of potential bundle branch block. Constantly monitor QRS complex width and the pattern of deflections in V_1 and V_6 (or MCL_1 and MCL_6). On serial ECGs, note axis deviation.

• Document and alert the doctor to the presence of any of the following:

   —Right bundle branch block (RBBB): QRS greater than 0.12 seconds, RSR' pattern in V_1

   —Left bundle branch block (LBBB): QRS greater than 0.12 seconds, absent Q wave, and large monophasic R wave in V_6

   —Left anterior hemiblock or left posterior hemiblock

• Observe closely for development of Mobitz II second-degree AV block or complete heart block, particularly if RBBB with left anterior hemiblock or left posterior hemiblock is present. Prepare for prophylactic pacemaker insertion, as ordered.

• Because the left anterior descending coronary artery nourishes the ventricular septum, where the bundle branches are located, an anterior infarct may produce septal ischemia or necrosis with resulting bundle branch block. Bundle branch block widens the QRS complex beyond the normal limit because it disrupts the usual sequence or speed of depolarization. Because V_1 (MCL_1) is oriented to the right ventricle and V_6 (MCL_6) to the left, the pattern of deflections in these leads best indicates the timing and sequence of bundle branch conduction.

• Untreated, bundle branch block increases risk of mortality from AMI.

   —RBBB produces delayed right ventricular stimulation, prolonging the QRS duration. It also alters the usual sequence of deflections, in which septal depolarization is followed by simultaneous depolarization of both ventricles. Instead, RBBB produces a small positive wave of septal depolarization, a large negative wave of left ventricular depolarization, and a large positive wave of right ventricular depolarization.

   —LBBB disrupts the depolarization pattern to a greater extent than RBBB. It causes loss of the normal septal Q waves in leads oriented to the left ventricle and allows the right ventricle to depolarize before the left ventricle.

   —Hemiblocks are blocks of one fascicle of the left bundle branch. Left anterior hemiblock is more common than left posterior hemiblock because the anterior fascicle is thinner and has a more vulnerable blood supply. Left anterior hemiblock is considered relatively benign, while left posterior hemiblock is more serious because it implies extensive infarction.

• Progression to a more advanced blockage is possible at any time. RBBB with hemiblock represents blockage of two of the three fascicles responsible for ventricular conduction, leaving the patient dependent on a single fascicle. Mobitz II block is an ominous sign because it represents intermittent blockage of all three fascicles, implies extensive myocardial necrosis, and commonly heralds complete heart block. Prophylactic pacemaker insertion prevents ventricular asystole if complete heart block occurs.

INFERIOR INFARCT

• Monitor for sinus bradycardia and AV block, particularly first-degree AV block and Mobitz I second-degree AV block.

   —Correlate rhythm with clinical status, noting the presence of hypotension, altered level of consciousness, chest pain, or increased ventricular premature beats.

   —If the patient is symptomatic, administer atropine, as ordered and according to unit protocol. Notify the doctor and document the episode.

• Although these rhythms may occur with any type of infarct from excess vagal stimulation, they are most common in inferior infarction. An inferior infarct typically results from occlusion of the right coronary artery, which nourishes the SA node in about 90% of the population and the AV node in about 55%. Ischemia of the SA node produces sinus arrhythmias, while AV nodal ischemia above the bundle of His produces progressive slowing of impulse conduction through the AV node. Such ischemia usually is transient and responds promptly to administration of atropine.

   —The clinical signs listed indicate the arrhythmia is decreasing cardiac output.

   —Atropine blocks vagal stimulation, thereby increasing SA node impulse formation and AV node conduction.

• Observe for indicators of right ventricular infarction, such as:

- neck vein distention, positive hepatojugular reflux, positive Kussmaul's sign (increased neck vein distention on inspiration), or elevated CVP or right atrial pressure with normal or mildly elevated pulmonary capillary wedge pressure.
- widely split S_2, right ventricular S_3 or S_4 heart sounds (audible at the third to fourth intercostal space at the left sternal border), or tricuspid insufficiency murmur

- bradycardia, AV blocks, and hypotension.

• If the patient is dehydrated on admission, be especially alert for the above signs after I.V. hydration.

• When recording 12-lead ECGs on a patient with suspected inferior or posterior infarction, routinely record right ventricular leads, such as V_{4R}.

• If indicators of right ventricular infarction are present, alert the doctor. Obtain a chest X-ray and other noninvasive diagnostic studies, as ordered.

• If right ventricular infarction is confirmed, collaborate with the doctor to modify therapy.

- Avoid diuretics. Administer fluid boluses, as ordered, typically to maintain right atrial pressure at 20 to 25 mm Hg and pulmonary capillary wedge pressure at 15 to 18 mm Hg.

- Administer inotropes and vasodilators judiciously, as ordered.

• Monitor hemodynamic parameters and clinical indicators of the effectiveness of therapy closely.

• Right ventricular infarction may occur with inferior or posterior left ventricular infarction because all these areas are perfused by the right coronary artery. Right ventricular infarction occurs in about 30% of inferior AMIs.

- These signs reflect the increased venous pressure that results from impaired right ventricular compliance and inability to pump blood effectively.

- The wide S_2 split reflects delayed pulmonary valve closure, the result of prolonged right ventricular ejection caused by the increased right ventricular volume and pressure. The S_3 or S_4 sound indicates decreased right ventricular compliance, while the tricuspid insufficiency murmur reflects a functional valvular insufficiency secondary to right ventricular dilatation.
- Bradycardia probably reflects SA nodal ischemia, blocks indicate AV nodal ischemia, and hypotension results from impaired right ventricular stroke volume.

• Because the AMI patient may be dehydrated from nausea, vomiting, and diaphoresis, signs of right ventricular infarction may appear only after rehydration.

• The routine 12-lead ECG is not helpful in detecting right ventricular infarction, although it will reveal signs of concomitant inferior or posterior infarction. Right ventricular leads typically reveal Q waves, ST segment elevation, and T wave inversion with acute right ventricular infarction.

• A chest X-ray and other diagnostic studies provide objective evidence of right ventricular infarction. With right ventricular infarction alone, the chest X-ray typically is clear. An echocardiogram helps differentiate right ventricular infarction from cardiac tamponade, while radionuclide studies identify areas of infarction or decreased right ventricular ejection fraction. Diagnostic studies also help differentiate hypotension resulting primarily from right ventricular dysfunction from that resulting from left ventricular dysfunction—an important distinction because the therapy for each is quite different.

• Although the treatment of right ventricular infarction differs from that for left ventricular infarction, the goal is the same: to improve left ventricular filling pressure and thereby optimize cardiac output.

- Because strong right ventricular contraction is absent with right ventricular infarction, blood flow from the right to the left side of the heart becomes passive and dependent on preload. Diuretics lower preload. Fluid is administered, rather than limited as in left ventricular infarction, to improve preload-dependent right ventricular systolic ejection, thereby increasing left ventricular filling pressure and cardiac output.
- Inotropes may increase right ventricular contractility. Vasodilators may be used to decrease pulmonary vascular resistance; the resulting right ventricular afterload reduction may improve left ventricular filling, while the simultaneous left ventricular afterload reduction may improve left ventricular systolic emptying.

• The association of right ventricular infarction with left ventricular infarction can be confusing to interpret and a challenge to manage. The treatment of right ventricular infarction described above must take into consideration the therapy for left ventricular infarction. Continual surveillance is necessary to make sure that therapies are modified as necessary to achieve optimal cardiac output.

CARDIOVASCULAR DISORDERS

3. Additional individualized interventions: _____

3. Rationales: _____

Target outcome criteria
Within 24 hours of admission, the patient will:
• display normal sinus rhythm or a controlled arrhythmia with a ventricular rate of 60 to 100 beats/minute
• manifest strong, bilaterally equal peripheral pulses.

Within 3 days of admission, the patient will:
• have hemodynamic values within expected limits
• have clear breath sounds
• have clear heart sounds with decreasing or no S$_3$ or S$_4$, rub, or new murmurs
• experience no further chest pain
• show decreasing or no neck vein distention.

Nursing diagnosis: *Knowledge deficit related to diagnostic procedures, therapeutic interventions, and long-range implications for life-style changes*

NURSING PRIORITY: Educate the patient and loved ones about health status, as appropriate.

Interventions

1. Implement measures in the "Knowledge Deficit" plan, page 56, as appropriate.

2. Defer a formal rehabilitation and education program until the period of physiologic instability has passed. In the meantime:

• Establish rapport. Use eye contact, reflective listening, and nonverbal communication. Emphasize and display consistency as much as possible.

• Assess immediate learning needs, encourage questions, and provide brief explanations, correcting any misconceptions; repeat as necessary.

• As appropriate, provide brief information about the pathophysiology of AMI, risk factor reduction, medications, dietary recommendations, activity restrictions, rehabilitation programs, community agencies, and support groups. Consult the "Acute Myocardial Infarction: Stepdown Unit Phase" plan, page 280.

• Note and document long-range learning needs. Upon discharge to the general medical-surgical unit, communicate them to the new unit's staff.

3. Additional individualized interventions: _____

Rationales

1. The "Knowledge Deficit" plan contains detailed information helpful in assessing and meeting learning needs for all patients. This plan focuses on information specific to AMI.

2. Implementing a major teaching program during this period is inappropriate because physiologic recovery is a higher priority. Nevertheless, capitalizing on unexpected teaching opportunities provides a way to assess learning needs and meet immediate concerns.

• Excessive anxiety interferes with learning. Establishing rapport through consistent, caring contact helps promote trust and relaxation, which are conducive to retention of new information.

• AMI usually raises major questions for the patient and family related to health and life-style. Responding to expressed needs displays sensitivity to the patient and family. Brief, repeated explanations may be necessary because high anxiety levels or medication effects may cause the patient to unconsciously screen out information.

• Judicious selection of initial teaching content helps prevent information overload. The "Acute Myocardial Infarction: Stepdown Unit Phase" plan contains comprehensive information on long-range learning needs and rehabilitation programs, usually addressed after the patient has become physiologically stable.

• Documentation and communication of long-range learning needs allows continuity of care and personalization of ongoing educational efforts.

3. Rationales: _____

Target outcome criteria
Within 48 hours of admission, the patient and family will:
• provide feedback indicating an adequate knowledge base for immediate needs (for example, by asking appropriate questions and by respecting dietary restrictions)
• begin to identify long-range learning needs.

Discharge planning
NURSING DISCHARGE CRITERIA
Upon the patient's discharge, documentation shows evidence of:
• stable blood pressure within normal limits without I.V. inotrope or vasodilator support
• stable cardiac rhythm with arrhythmias (if any) controlled by oral, sublingual, or transdermal medications or by permanent pacemaker
• spontaneous ventilation.

PATIENT-FAMILY TEACHING CHECKLIST
Document evidence that the patient and family demonstrate an understanding of:
___ extent of infarction
___ activity restrictions
___ recommended dietary modifications
___ smoking-cessation program as needed
___ common emotional changes
___ community resources for life-style modification support and cardiac rehabilitation.

DOCUMENTATION CHECKLIST
Using outcome criteria as a guide, document:
___ clinical status on admission
___ significant changes in status
___ pertinent diagnostic test findings
___ chest pain
___ pain relief measures
___ rhythm strip analyses
___ use of emergency protocols
___ hemodynamic trends and other data
___ I.V. line patency
___ oxygen therapy
___ other therapies
___ nutritional intake
___ patient-family teaching
___ discharge planning.

ASSOCIATED PLANS OF CARE
Cardiogenic Shock
Congestive Heart Failure
Grieving
Impaired Physical Mobility
Ineffective Family Coping
Ineffective Individual Coping
Knowledge Deficit
Pain

References
Holloway, N., ed. *Nursing the Critically Ill Adult,* 4th ed. Menlo Park, Calif.: Addison-Wesley Publishing Co., 1993.

Kline, E. "Clinical Controversies Surrounding Thrombolytic Therapy in Acute Myocardial Infarction," *Heart & Lung* 19(6): 595-601, November 1990.

McMillan, J., and Little-Longeway, C. "Right Ventricular Infarction," *Focus on Critical Care* 18(2):158-63, April 1991.

Miracle, V. "Understanding the Different Types of MI," *Nursing88* (18):53-63, January 1988.

Rodgers, M. "Pericarditis: A Different Kind of Heart Disease," *Nursing90* 20(2):52-58, February 1990.

Topol, E., and Wilson, V. "Pivotal Role of Early and Sustained Infarct Vessel Patency in Patients with Acute Myocardial Infarction," *Heart & Lung* 19(6): 583-593, November 1990.

Walter, L. "Alternative Therapy in Atherosclerotic Heart Disease," *Heart & Lung* 18(3):316-20, May 1989.

CARDIOVASCULAR DISORDERS

CARDIOVASCULAR DISORDERS

Acute Myocardial Infarction – Stepdown Unit Phase

DRG information
(see "Acute Myocardial Infarction – Critical Care Unit Phase," page 268)
DRG 121 Circulatory Disorders. With AMI and Cardio-
vascular Complication. Discharged Alive.
Mean LOS = 8.2 days
DRG 122 Circulatory Disorders. With AMI. Without
Cardiovascular Complication. Discharged
Alive.
Mean LOS = 5.9 days

Introduction
DEFINITION AND TIME FOCUS
Acute myocardial infarction (AMI) is necrosis (death)
of the myocardium resulting from an interrupted or diminished supply of oxygenated blood from the coronary arteries. This plan focuses on the patient who
has passed through the critical stage of AMI and is
ready to begin recovery. For information about problems seen in the critical care phase, see the "Acute
Myocardial Infarction – Critical Care Unit Phase" plan.

ETIOLOGY AND PRECIPITATING FACTORS
The underlying disease is usually atherosclerosis that
results in coronary occlusion or thrombosis, although
severe coronary spasm may also be a cause. Contributing factors include:
• increased myocardial oxygen demand, such as from
physical exertion, emotional stress, heavy meals,
tachycardia, hyperthyroidism, hypertension, valvular
insufficiency, and pregnancy
• decreased myocardial oxygen supply, such as from vasoconstriction, smoking, air pollution, anemia, bradycardia, hypotension, and sleep.

Focused assessment guidelines
NURSING HISTORY (Functional health pattern findings)

Health perception – health management pattern
• may have history of chest pain or previous infarction
• may be under treatment for hypertension, diabetes
mellitus, congestive heart failure, arrhythmias, hyperthyroidism, or anemia
• may have cardiac risk factors, such as smoking, obesity, hyperlipidemia, high-stress occupation, sedentary
life-style, or positive family history
• if white male over age 40, is at increased risk
• if postmenopausal female, is at increased risk
• may not comply with treatment program (diet, exercise, and medication)

Nutritional-metabolic pattern
• usually describes diet high in calories, fat, and salt

Elimination pattern
• may report constipation

Activity-exercise pattern
• may report lack of energy for personal care and
activities
• commonly describes sedentary life-style, lack of regular exercise, and lack of leisure activities

Sleep-rest pattern
• may report difficulty sleeping because of unfamiliar
surroundings, noise, or anxiety
• may report need for frequent rest periods

Cognitive-perceptual pattern
• may report recurring chest pain

Self-perception – self-concept pattern
• may express realization of vulnerability and mortality

Role-relationship pattern
• may express concern over inability to continue in
usual family roles
• may express concern for family's ability to manage
• may express concern about ability to return to work
• may express financial concerns

Sexuality-reproductive pattern
• may express concern about decreased libido and resumption of sexual activities

Coping – stress tolerance pattern
• usually type A personality (aggressive, ambitious,
competitive, work-oriented, time-driven, impatient, and
hostile)
• usually anxious, expressing fear of sudden death,
loss of employment, and loss of independence
• may be depressed over losses
• may deny seriousness of illness

Value-belief pattern
• may express need for spiritual counseling

PHYSICAL FINDINGS
Cardiovascular
• normal sinus rhythm or controlled arrhythmias
• S_3 or S_4 (less common)
• hypotension (related to medications)

Pulmonary
- shortness of breath
- crackles (less common)
- tachypnea secondary to pain or anxiety

Musculoskeletal
- weakness
- fatigability

DIAGNOSTIC STUDIES
- cardiac enzymes—after an infarct, creatine phosphokinase levels should return to normal within 3 to 4 days, lactic dehydrogenase levels within 7 to 10 days; sustained or regained elevations indicate further cell death (expanding or recurrent infarction)
- electrolyte levels—should be within normal limits; however, hypokalemia is not uncommon because of diuretic therapy
- cholesterol and triglyceride levels—may be elevated
- blood urea nitrogen and creatinine levels—should be within normal ranges; however, may be elevated if blood supply to kidneys is diminished
- serum drug levels—should be within therapeutic range
- white blood cell count—should be returning to normal 5 to 7 days after infarct
- erythrocyte sedimentation rate—may remain elevated for several weeks
- chest X-ray—may show cardiomegaly; if congestive heart failure is present, may show lung congestion, pleural effusion, and pulmonary edema
- telemetry—may show arrhythmias

- 12-lead ECG—abnormal ST segment elevation, signifying ischemia, and depressed or inverted T wave, indicating injury (may be present for days to weeks or longer); abnormal Q waves, signifying necrosis (may remain indefinitely)
- echocardiography—may show valvular dysfunction, mural thrombi, dilated chambers, abnormal wall motion, and decreased cardiac output
- exercise stress test—submaximal tests, used to measure exercise capacity and to help set activity and exercise guidelines, may show intolerance, as evidenced by arrhythmias, chest pain, shortness of breath, claudication, ST segment changes, and blood pressure changes
- thallium scan—used to detect location and extent of infarction and scarring; when performed during exercise, can reveal ischemic areas that are adequately perfused at rest

POTENTIAL COMPLICATIONS
- pulmonary edema ✓
- thromboembolism
- ventricular aneurysm
- extension of the infarction ✓
- recurrent myocardial infarction
- arrhythmias
- angina ✓
- congestive heart failure ✓
- valvular dysfunction ✓
- pericarditis, Dressler's syndrome
- shoulder-hand syndrome

CARDIOVASCULAR DISORDERS

Nursing diagnosis: *Activity intolerance related to myocardial ischemia, decreased contractility, or arrhythmias*

NURSING PRIORITIES: (a) Minimize the risk of further infarction, and (b) implement safe measures to increase activity or exercise tolerance.

Interventions

1. Using telemetry, continuously monitor heart rate, rhythm, and conduction, as ordered. Document every 4 hours.

2. Promote physical comfort and rest.

3. Prohibit smoking and intake of stimulants, such as coffee, tea, and other beverages that contain caffeine.

Rationales

1. A myocardial infarction may produce arrhythmias by promoting reentry and increased automaticity. Early detection allows for prompt treatment and prevention of life-threatening arrhythmias. Activity or exercise may cause new arrhythmias, or a change in preexisting arrhythmias, which can result in decreased cardiac output.

2. Rest reduces myocardial oxygen needs and allows the heart to heal. Physical comfort reduces anxiety as well as oxygen demand. Controlling the extent of myocardial ischemia limits the infarction's size.

3. Stimulants increase the heart rate, thus increasing oxygen demands. Smoking decreases oxygen availability because hemoglobin molecules have a greater affinity for carbon monoxide (present in smoke) than for oxygen.

4. Encourage the patient to perform activities of daily living (ADLs) and diversional activities, as permitted and tolerated. Allow the patient to make as many decisions as possible.

4. Participation in ADLs and diversional activities increases the patient's sense of well-being and decreases anxiety. Making decisions about care activities and their timing, when possible, increases the patient's sense of control.

5. Implement the prescribed activity or exercise program according to unit protocol, starting with low-energy activities, such as range-of-motion (ROM) exercises, and progressing to full self-care. Encourage regular rest periods.

5. Progressive activity increases the heart's strength and collateral circulation. Starting with low-energy activities avoids creating an oxygen demand that exceeds supply. Alternating activity or exercise with rest periods prevents fatigue. Early ROM exercises decrease the risk of thromboembolism and other deleterious effects of bed rest.

6. Assess and document intolerance to activity or exercise, as evidenced by:
• a pulse rate greater than 110 beats/minute or increased more than 20 beats/minute over baseline
• a pulse rate that does not return to baseline within 5 minutes
• new arrhythmias or a change in preexisting arrhythmias
• a blood pressure decrease during activity
• chest pain, diaphoresis, or dyspnea
• dizziness, increased weakness or fatigue, or syncope
• ST segment elevation (if monitored).
   Monitor vital signs before and after activity or exercise and every 5 to 15 minutes during each session, depending on the patient's tolerance.

6. Exercise places increased demands on the heart that it may not be able to meet. AMI decreases contractility. Cardiac output may be reduced, resulting in decreased blood pressure and tissue perfusion. The heart rate may increase as a compensatory mechanism to maintain cardiac output. The absence or presence of symptoms helps determine when the activity or exercise program should be increased or stopped.

7. Stress the importance of avoiding Valsalva's maneuver and isometric exercises.

7. Valsalva's maneuver may lead to bradycardia and a corresponding decrease in cardiac output and tissue perfusion. Isometric exercises cause a greater increase in blood pressure and heart rate than isotonic exercises do because sustained muscle tension impedes blood flow. The resultant increase in afterload increases myocardial work and myocardial oxygen demand.

8. Provide supplemental oxygen as ordered, using nursing judgment.

8. The healing myocardium requires a constant supply of oxygen. Supplemental oxygen increases arterial oxygen tension and may increase activity tolerance.

9. Administer vasodilators, as ordered, and monitor the patient's response. Also monitor for side effects, particularly hypotension.

9. Vasodilators dilate coronary arteries and peripheral blood vessels, thus increasing myocardial oxygen supply while decreasing demand.

10. Teach the patient to monitor pulse rate before and after activity or exercise.

10. Pulse rate best reflects the cardiac work load during activity or exercise.

11. Stress the importance of complying with the activity or exercise program and with rest requirements.

11. Regular periods of activity improve myocardial healing. Fatigue is to be avoided because fatigued muscles require increased oxygen.

12. Encourage family members to support the patient's activity or exercise program.

12. Support from family members, as well as health care professionals, can motivate the patient to increase activity and exercise in accordance with the therapeutic plan and individual tolerance.

13. Additional individualized interventions: _____

13. Rationales: _____

Target outcome criteria
By the time of discharge, the patient will:
• present vital signs within normal limits
• perform self-care activities independently
• ambulate independently
• comply with the recommended activity and exercise program.

Nursing diagnosis: *High risk for ineffective individual coping related to anxiety, denial, or depression*

NURSING PRIORITY: Encourage healthy coping.

Interventions

1. Encourage verbalization of feelings.

2. Anticipate feelings of denial, shock, anger, anxiety, and depression.

3. Explain the grieving process to the patient and family.

4. Evaluate the meaning of the patient's altered body image and role responsibilities.

5. Assess daily for indicators of anxiety, such as apprehensive expression, tense posture, continuous talking, difficulty remembering explanations, sweaty palms, tachycardia, shaky voice, tremulousness, disturbed sleep, and indecision.
• Introduce yourself and other caregivers to the patient and family.

• Assign a primary care nurse, and limit the number of other nurses caring for the patient.
• Care for the patient calmly and confidently.

• Explain the purpose and routine nature of frequent assessments.
• Repeat explanations as necessary.

• Orient the patient to the unit.

• Administer minor tranquilizers, as ordered, using nursing judgment. Document their use.

• Help the patient explore ways to resolve unfinished business.

Rationales

1. The patient may perceive reactions as bizarre or otherwise inappropriate and may need "permission" to express them.

2. These are normal responses to loss. They may become exaggerated in the face of overwhelming, life-threatening experiences and intense psychological threats.

3. The patient and family may be bewildered and alarmed about their emotional responses.

4. Response varies because of the unique meaning of loss to the individual.

5. Systematic assessment and comparison with previous findings increases the likelihood that coping problems will be detected early. Anxiety may result from fear of the unknown, unfamiliar surroundings, unfinished business, or other causes.
• Introductions reduce the depersonalizing effects of the hospital environment and lay the foundation for establishing rapport and trust.
• Continuity of caregivers promotes trust.

• Calm, confident behavior provides nonverbal reassurance of the caregiver's competence.
• Explaining that frequent assessment is normal dispels fears that the patient's condition is deteriorating.
• Anxiety interferes with memory; repetition enhances learning.
• Orientation increases the predictability of experiences, reducing the need for vigilance (wary watchfulness) and defining the patient's role in care.
• Minor tranquilizers may help calm the patient during periods of physiologic instability but can interfere with psychological adjustment by creating an air of unreality and by disturbing rapid-eye-movement (REM) sleep. A benzodiazepine such as diazepam (Valium), lorazepam (Ativan), or alprazolam (Xanax) is usually given.
• The patient may feel compelled to keep appointments, conduct business, and so forth, and may need assistance in determining realistic ways to handle such situations. The patient may also need such reassurances as "It's okay to let go" and "People will understand that your health needs come first now."

CARDIOVASCULAR DISORDERS

6. Assess daily for indicators of denial, such as refusal to discuss the AMI, minimal acceptance of its significance, apparent lack of concern about status, verbal acknowledgment that the AMI has occurred while ignoring diet and activity restrictions, and ongoing attempts to continue usual activities.

6. Early detection allows prompt resolution of denial. Denial may be associated with the patient's current grieving process or previous coping pattern.

• Evaluate the impact of denial on the patient's health.

• Some denial is normal and may be a healthy initial response to an overwhelming situation. Denial that promotes self-destructive behavior, however, requires intervention.

• If the patient verbalizes denial, listen nonjudgmentally.

• Confronting denial and forcing the patient to "face facts" prematurely may cause distraught behavior.

• If denial is demonstrated through acting-out behavior, document it, express concern, and promote greater patient control over the environment. Involve the patient in solving the problem, compromising and modifying restrictive aspects of care, and allow choices where appropriate.

• These interventions promote a greater sense of control for the patient and are more likely to promote behavioral changes than are confrontation and threats.

• Be alert for topics the patient consistently fails to raise or refuses to discuss when prompted.

• The patient may avoid topics that are especially anxiety producing.

• Encourage the patient to focus on remaining abilities.

• The patient may be preoccupied with or panicked about perceived losses and may need encouragement to focus on strengths.

• Encourage the resumption of full self-care, as physical abilities allow.

• Enforced dependence contributes to low self-esteem.

• Consult psychiatric resources for further assistance, if needed.

• A psychiatric clinical specialist, psychiatrist, or social worker can provide additional insight and guidelines for further intervention.

7. Assess daily for indicators of depression, such as excessive concern about heart; focus on past physical accomplishments; negative feelings about the body; feelings of sadness, helplessness, or hopelessness; lack of appetite; insomnia or excessive sleeping; psychosomatic complaints (such as headache, neckache, backache, or stomachache); apathy; frequent crying episodes (or desire to cry); and poor personal hygiene.

7. Accurate interpretation of cues helps the nurse intervene appropriately. Depression is most likely to result from body-image changes and altered role performance.

• Assess for and document specific psychological, spiritual, and pathophysiologic causes of depression as well as the depressive effects of medications.

• Treatment of depression is most effective when it focuses on specific causes and patient concerns.

• Assess and document the patient's sleep pattern. Promote restful sleep by grouping procedures, minimizing external stimuli, and providing relaxation measures at bedtime.

• Depression may contribute to sleep disturbances (especially feeling less than fully rested on awakening). Depression also can result from lack of REM sleep.

• Encourage verbalization of feelings and crying.

• Sharing feelings can help the patient identify causes of depression. Because crying is discouraged in American society, the patient may need permission and active encouragement to release pent-up tears.

• Assist with realistic problem solving.

• The patient who has mental "tunnel vision" may need help identifying and evaluating options.

• When pessimism is expressed, point out hopeful aspects of the situation.

• Depression may be self-perpetuating. Focusing on hopeful, positive factors may encourage the patient to break the cycle of depressive thoughts.

• Encourage physical activity, as appropriate, and document responses.

• Depression is immobilizing, and lack of activity reinforces depression. Physical activity usually elevates mood.

• Help the patient identify and implement enjoyable diversions.

• Boredom may encourage an unhealthy preoccupation with illness. Pleasurable diversions include reading, doing crossword puzzles, listening to music, participating in arts and crafts (which involve the patient directly), and watching television (a passive activity).

• Share information on the patient's status, as appropriate. Emphasize even small signs of progress.

• A depressed person tends to focus on negative thoughts. Emphasizing even small gains may help the patient recognize signs of recovery.

8. Additional individualized interventions: _____

8. Rationales: _____

Target outcome criteria
Within 3 days of admission to the intermediate care unit, the patient will:
• appear less anxious by exhibiting a calm expression, relaxed posture, dry palms, steady voice and hands, no tremors, and a normal heart rate. The patient will also sleep easily, have no morning insomnia, be comfortable with silences, and be able to recall explanations and make reasonable decisions.
• confront denial (if present), and express concern about the AMI by discussing problems, gradually showing other signs of grief (such as crying, anxiety, or anger), taking responsibility for cooperating with the health plan, and allowing others to take over business affairs

• exhibit less depression (if present), participate in self-care, show a return of appetite, sleep restfully, discuss problems openly, talk about feelings without uncontrollable crying, express interest in learning about life-style modifications, make appropriate decisions, and express an intention to use available resources.

Nursing diagnosis: *Altered sexuality pattern related to physical limitations secondary to cardiac ischemia and medications*

NURSING PRIORITY: Provide information to the patient and spouse (or partner) regarding resumption of sexual activity.

Interventions

1. Obtain a sexual history, including incidence of chest pain during or after foreplay and intercourse.

2. Encourage the patient and spouse (or partner) to verbalize fears and anxieties. Provide time for joint and individual discussion.

3. Be aware of personal feelings about sexuality and if unable to counsel the couple effectively, make an appropriate referral.

4. Provide printed material about AMI and resumption of sexual activities.

5. Inform the patient that some medications can cause impotence or decrease libido. Encourage discussion with the doctor if such problems occur.

6. Discuss ways to decrease the effects of sexual activity on the cardiovascular system, such as through medications and positioning.

Rationales

1. The history provides baseline information and identifies previous sexual problems.

2. Verbalizing fears and anxieties may help identify important issues and allow an opportunity to correct misconceptions.

3. Unawareness of personal feelings may inhibit sensitivity to sexual concerns. The caregiver's discomfort may keep the couple from expressing their concerns.

4. Accurate information may allay fears and anxieties and dispel misconceptions. Providing printed material will avoid misinterpretation and may increase the likelihood of resumption of sexual activity.

5. Awareness of possible pharmacologic causes of sexual dysfunction helps decrease the patient's anxiety. Some commonly used medications with these adverse effects are antihypertensives (such as methyldopa [Aldomet], reserpine [Serpasil], guanethidine [Ismelin], and clonidine [Catapres]); diuretics (such as spironolactone [Aldactone] and hydrochlorothiazide [Esidrix]); and beta blockers (such as propranolol [Inderal] and nadolol [Corgard]).

6. Nitroglycerin or another vasodilator may be prescribed before intercourse to reduce the heart's work load. Some positions place less demand on the myocardium than others.

7. Emphasize that sexual activity should be avoided after large meals or alcohol intake, in extreme temperatures, and under conditions of fatigue or increased stress.

7. Digestion of a large meal requires increased visceral blood flow and increases cardiac work load. In low doses, alcohol increases heart rate and cardiac output; in higher doses, alcohol causes myocardial depression and corresponding decreases in heart rate and cardiac output. Stress causes catecholamine release, increasing cardiac work load and oxygen demand.

8. As ordered, evaluate activity tolerance by means of low-level treadmill exercise testing or two-flight stair climbing, followed by a resting ECG.

8. These tests provide specific information that can be used in counseling and as a guide for resuming sexual activity. The myocardial oxygen requirement for two-flight stair climbing is similar to that required for sexual activity. Walking on a treadmill at 3 to 4 miles/hour without ECG changes or excessive increases in blood pressure and heart rate indicates that the patient is more than able to meet the cardiac work requirements of sexual activity.

9. Teach symptoms that should be reported to the doctor if they occur during foreplay or intercourse, particularly increased heart rate and respirations persisting 10 minutes after activity, extreme fatigue the day after sexual activity, and chest pain during intercourse.

9. These symptoms indicate that the activity is too strenuous and that the increased myocardial oxygen demand is not being met.

10. Additional individualized interventions: _____

10. Rationales: _____

Target outcome criteria
Within 1 week of admission, the patient will:
• verbalize understanding of sexual activity's effects on cardiovascular function
• list three recommendations for minimizing myocardial stress during sexual activity.

Nursing diagnosis: *Knowledge deficit related to newly diagnosed, complex disease and to unfamiliar therapy*

NURSING PRIORITY: Assist in identifying cardiac risk factors and ways to modify life-style.

Interventions

1. To increase understanding of the disease:

• Describe the basic anatomy and physiology of the heart, how atherosclerosis develops, and the pathophysiology of chest pain and AMI.

• Discuss angina's symptoms and what to do if it occurs. Instruct the patient to call the doctor if chest pain is unrelieved by nitroglycerin (see *Medication therapy after myocardial infarction* for guidelines).

• Instruct the patient about medication therapy (see *Medication therapy after myocardial infarction*).

2. To increase compliance with necessary dietary modifications:
• Explain the rationale for a diet low in calories (if the patient is obese), saturated fats, and salt.

Rationales

1. The patient who understands the disease is more likely to implement therapeutic recommendations.
• Comprehension of AMI's pathophysiology provides a basis for understanding therapy.

• The prepared patient is more likely to react appropriately when angina occurs.

• Accurate information dispels misconceptions, reduces anxiety, and increases patient compliance.

2. Obesity, hypertension, and hyperlipidemia greatly increase the risk of coronary heart disease (CHD).
• Reducing weight and salt intake helps decrease blood pressure. Reducing saturated fat intake decreases blood lipid levels and increases the level of high-density lipoproteins (HDLs), which protect against atherosclerosis. Explanations improve patient compliance.

MEDICATION THERAPY AFTER MYOCARDIAL INFARCTION

Drug	Action	Administration	Patient teaching	Possible adverse reactions
Vasodilator (such as nitroglycerin or long-acting nitrates)	Primarily dilates peripheral blood vessels, reducing myocardial work load	Can be given by mouth before meals. Sublingual: 1 tablet every 5 minutes for a maximum of three tablets; if no relief, call doctor. Dermal: patch or cream	Take prophylactically before activities, as prescribed, or at onset of chest pain. Take sitting or lying down to prevent postural hypotension. If no relief after three tablets, do not drive self to hospital: call an ambulance. Record number of tablets taken. Check expiration date. Carry nitroglycerin at all times. Wear medical alert bracelet. Avoid alcohol, which has added vasodilating effect. Replace tablets at 4 months. If ointment or patch is prescribed, follow guidelines for correct application, skin care, site rotation, and frequency of change.	Transient headache, flushing, faintness, dizziness, or hypotension
Beta blocker (such as propranolol [Inderal], metoprolol [Lopressor], or atenolol [Tenormin])	Blocks beta adrenergic receptors to decrease blood pressure, heart rate, and contractility; also decreases automaticity to slow sinus rate, suppress ectopic beats, and improve myocardial oxygenation	Initially given I.V., then by mouth	Monitor pulse rate and blood pressure; report pulse rate under 60 beats/minute, irregular, or changed. Do not stop abruptly—may cause chest pain or myocardial infarction.	Bradycardia, hypotension, dizziness, nausea, vomiting, diarrhea, or bronchoconstriction
Calcium channel blocker (such as verapamil [Calan], nifedipine [Procardia], diltiazem [Cardizem])	Blocks transport of calcium across cell membrane, resulting in vasodilation and decreased contractility; verapamil also increases refractory period of atrioventricular node and decreases sinoatrial node rate	By mouth, 1 hour before meals or 2 hours after meals	Monitor pulse rate and blood pressure; report pulse rate under 50 beats/minute.	Postural hypotension, bradycardia, headache, dizziness, syncope, nausea, edema, or constipation
Aspirin	Antiplatelet action; decreases aggregation	By mouth daily, or every other day, usually with food	Report ongoing gastrointestinal upset or burning, dark tar-like stool, or easy bruising or bleeding	Gastrointestinal upset and irritation; gastrointestinal bleeding; increased bruising

• Take a dietary history, and help the patient identify eating patterns.

• Have the dietitian help the patient plan a diet low in calories, fat, and salt that fits the patient's life-style, culture, and socioeconomic status.

• Discuss the role of exercise in reducing weight, blood pressure, and serum lipid levels.

• Stress the need for the entire family to follow the modified diet.

• The dietary history provides baseline information and identifies patterns that need to be changed.

• The patient is more apt to adhere to a prescribed diet if it is acceptable and affordable.

• Exercise decreases blood pressure, weight, triglyceride levels, and anxiety. It also increases HDL levels.

• Obesity, hypertension, and hyperlipidemia have familial tendencies. Compliance is more likely if the patient can share family meals.

• Give information about antilipemic medications (if prescribed), including action, dosage, scheduling, and side effects.

• Provide a list of weight-reduction programs, if appropriate.

• Give printed diet information for home use.

3. To stress the importance of hypertension management:

• Explain the risks of high blood pressure.

• Discuss medication therapy, including action, dosage, scheduling, and adverse effects, such as electrolyte imbalances, sexual dysfunction, orthostatic hypotension, lethargy, headache, flushing, nausea, vomiting, and palpitations.

• Describe ways to reduce salt intake, based on the diet history.

• Emphasize the need for follow-up visits.

• Provide printed information about antihypertensive medications.

• Stress the importance of contacting the doctor if any of these symptoms occur: chest pain, dizziness, headache, blurred vision, edema, nausea, vomiting, nose bleeds, or shortness of breath.

4. To stress the importance of smoking cessation:

• Explain the rationale for quitting.

• Discuss the benefits of not smoking.

• Help the patient identify needs currently met by smoking, then explore substitutes.

• Discuss with the patient's spouse, partner, or family the need to assist and support the patient's efforts to stop smoking.

• Provide a list of community smoking cessation programs.

• Antilipemics inhibit lipid synthesis. Information about medications will help the patient assume responsibility for self-care.

• Programs can provide motivation and increase compliance.

• Giving the patient printed material will avoid misinterpretation and increase compliance.

3. Hypertension is a significant predictor of CHD: the risk of heart disease increases in direct proportion to increases in systolic and diastolic blood pressure.

• Hypertension increases afterload and makes the heart increase its rate and force of contraction over a period of time. Left ventricular hypertrophy occurs, resulting in an increase in cardiac work load and oxygen demand. Also, a structural change in the coronary arteries accelerates atherosclerosis.

• Noncompliance is a common problem with antihypertensive medication therapy. Lack of symptoms makes it difficult to convince patients they have a serious health problem requiring lifelong treatment and follow-up care; adverse effects may further increase noncompliance. The patient should know that the doctor can change medications or dosage if adverse effects occur.

• Reduced salt intake decreases fluid volume and myocardial work load. Although the relationship between salt intake and hypertension is not well understood, a reduced intake in susceptible people is known to decrease blood pressure. Excessive salt intake causes fluid retention, which increases blood volume and peripheral vascular resistance and can lead to elevated blood pressure. Reducing salt intake also enhances the effectiveness of most antihypertensives.

• Follow-up visits provide opportunities to monitor blood pressure, response to medication and other forms of treatment, and early development of complications.

• Giving the patient printed material helps prevent misinterpretation and increase compliance.

• These symptoms, which indicate increased hypertension, cardiac failure, or both, require therapeutic intervention.

4. Smoking increases the risk of premature heart disease three to six times; smoking cessation markedly decreases that risk.

• Smoking causes vasoconstriction, alters coagulation, and increases carbon monoxide levels and platelet aggregation. Also, nicotine (a stimulant) increases heart rate and the occurrence of arrhythmias.

• Knowledge of these benefits makes smoking cessation during the hospital stay a growth-promoting experience. The many benefits include improved senses of smell and taste, improved lung function, increased longevity, monetary savings, and gratitude from nonsmokers.

• Smoking satisfies complex needs. For a smoking cessation program to be successful, it must address those needs, ideally with less harmful substitutes.

• Support from others provides motivation and encouragement to stop smoking.

• These programs offer support, motivation, and methods.

5. To promote stress reduction:

• Discuss stress and its effect on the cardiovascular system.

• Help the patient identify stressors and learn health-promoting behaviors.

• Identify the characteristics of type A behavior, and review their relationship to AMI.

• Teach stress reduction techniques, such as progressive relaxation, guided imagery, and aerobic exercise within recommended guidelines. Provide referral to an outpatient stress reduction program, as needed, and to a cardiac rehabilitation program, where available.

6. Additional individualized interventions: _____

_____

5. Stress is an important risk factor for AMI recurrence.

• Tension and psychological stress cause sympathetic stimulation, increasing blood pressure, pulse rate, and cardiac work load.

• Behavior modification is necessary for stress reduction and promotion of optimal health. The program should include specific and regular times for recreation and relaxation.

• Correlations exist between type A behavior patterns and the prevalence of CHD.

• Decreasing stress reduces myocardial oxygen demands and increases the patient's feeling of well-being.

6. Rationales: _____

_____

Target outcome criteria
By the time of discharge, the patient will:
• verbalize knowledge of preventive health measures
• verbalize a willingness to adhere to prescribed therapy
• list personal risk factors
• explain the rationale for dietary modifications
• identify specific ways to reduce salt and fat intake

• have begun a smoking cessation program, if appropriate
• identify two personal stressors and ways to cope with them
• verbalize understanding of the medication regimen.

Discharge planning
NURSING DISCHARGE CRITERIA
Upon the patient's discharge, documentation shows evidence of:
• absence of chest pain
• tolerance of activity without signs of orthostatic hypotension, dyspnea, pain, or shortness of breath
• angina controlled by medication
• oxygen therapy discontinued for at least 48 hours before discharge
• ECG within expected parameters
• arrhythmias (if present) controlled by oral medication
• I.V. lines discontinued for at least 48 hours before discharge
• ability to tolerate ambulation and perform activities of daily living
• vital signs within expected parameters for at least 48 hours before discharge
• absence of fever and of pulmonary or cardiovascular complications
• blood chemistries and laboratory values within expected parameters
• ability to tolerate diet and any diet restrictions
• normal elimination pattern
• referral to an outpatient cardiac rehabilitation program (if applicable).

PATIENT-FAMILY TEACHING CHECKLIST
Document evidence that the patient and family demonstrate an understanding of:
__ the disease and its implications
__ measuring radial pulse rate accurately
__ all discharge medications' purpose, dosage, administration schedule, and adverse effects requiring medical attention (usual discharge medications include nitrates, beta blockers, antiarrhythmics, calcium antagonists, antihypertensives, and inotropes)
__ need for risk factor modification
__ prescribed diet
__ prescribed activity or exercise program
__ need for regularly scheduled rest periods
__ signs and symptoms to report to health care providers
__ need for follow-up care
__ when to resume sexual activity
__ availability of community resources
__ how to contact the doctor.

DOCUMENTATION CHECKLIST
Using outcome criteria as a guide, document:
— status on admission
— significant changes in status
— pertinent laboratory and diagnostic test findings
— telemetry monitoring
— chest pain
— interventions for pain relief
— dietary intake
— medical therapies, including medications
— emotional status
— activity tolerance
— patient-family teaching
— discharge planning.

ASSOCIATED PLANS OF CARE
Dying
Geriatric Considerations
Grieving
Ineffective Family Coping
Ineffective Individual Coping
Knowledge Deficit
Pain

References

Gleeson, B. "Teaching Your Patient About His Antian-ginal Drugs," *Nursing91* 21(2):65-72, February 1991.

Gleeson, B. "Loosening the Grip of Anginal Pain," *Nursing91* 21(1):33-40, January 1991.

McCann, M.: "Sexual Healing After Heart Attack," *American Journal of Nursing* 89(9):1132-40, September 1989.

Schell, M. "Cholesterol, Lipoproteins, Lipid Profiles: A Challenge in Patient Education," *Focus on Critical Care.* 17(3):203-11, June 1990.

Angina Pectoris

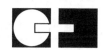

DRG information
DRG 140 Angina Pectoris.
  Mean LOS = 3.8 days
  Principal diagnoses include:
  • angina pectoris
  • intermediate coronary syndrome
  • acute heart ischemia without acute myo-
    cardial infarction (AMI).

Introduction
DEFINITION AND TIME FOCUS
Angina pectoris is transient insufficient coronary blood flow caused by obstruction, constriction, or spasm of the coronary arteries. Angina is characterized by brief episodes of substernal or retrosternal chest pain, commonly felt beneath the middle and upper third of the sternum. Angina pain commonly radiates to the left shoulder, left arm, neck, jaw, or upper abdomen. The cells within the heart muscle do not die in angina as they do in AMI because the hypoxia is transient.

Angina may be classified as stable or unstable (also known as preinfarction or crescendo) angina. The patient also may experience nocturnal angina, which occurs while sleeping, or angina decubitus, which occurs only when the patient is supine, disappearing when the patient stands. Variant (Prinzmetal's) angina occurs at rest, usually during the same time each day, and may be caused by coronary artery spasm. These categories differ according to cause, precipitating factors, descriptions of pain, and electrocardiography (ECG) findings. This plan focuses on the patient admitted for diagnosis and medical management during an initial acute attack.

ETIOLOGY AND PRECIPITATING FACTORS
Classic angina:
• any condition that decreases oxygen delivery by the coronary arteries, increases the cardiac work load, or increases myocardial need for oxygen, such as atherosclerosis, severe aortic stenosis, mitral stenosis or regurgitation, hypotension, hyperthyroidism, marked anemia, ventricular arrhythmias and early menopause, oral contraceptive use, or hypertension
• classic coronary artery disease risk factors, such as physical or emotional stress, physical inactivity, obesity, smoking, increased serum cholesterol level (above 200 mg/dl), and diabetes mellitus
• genetic factors, such as hypertension and type II familial hyperlipoproteinemia

Prinzmetal's angina:
• coronary artery spasm

Focused assessment guidelines
NURSING HISTORY (Functional health pattern findings)

Health perception—health management pattern
• reports sudden onset of substernal chest pain, pressure, or both; not sharply localized—may radiate to arms, shoulders, neck, jaw, upper abdomen; untreated, usually lasts 2 to 5 minutes, not more than 30 minutes
• typically describes pain as "pressure," "tightness," "aching," or "squeezing;" rest or nitroglycerin provides relief
• typically reports recent emotional stress, heavy exercise, a large meal, or exposure to cold (classic angina)
• typically reports cyclical pain in absence of precipitating factors (Prinzmetal's angina)
• may be under treatment for hypertension, hyperlipidemia, or diabetes mellitus
• may have left ventricular hypertrophy
• may be obese or smoke cigarettes
• may have history of chronic stress, type A behavior, or sedentary life-style
• if white male over age 40, white female over age 50, or black male or female under age 45 with hypertension, at increased risk

Nutritional-metabolic pattern
• may report nausea or indigestion
• may report feeling of fullness
• when stable, likely to report diet high in calories, cholesterol, saturated fat, and caffeine
• may report pain episode after large, heavy meal

Activity-exercise pattern
• typically describes shortness of breath during chest pain episode
• when stable, commonly reports sedentary life-style with only sporadic exercise
• may report transient chest pain episodes during increased activity, alleviated by rest

Sleep-rest pattern
• when stable, may report sleep disturbance such as chest pain during dreams or when lying flat

Cognitive-perceptual pattern
• may report feeling of impending doom during chest pain

Self-perception—self-concept pattern
• may have difficulty believing something is physically wrong during pain-free intervals

Role-relationship pattern
• may report family history of coronary artery disease
• may report perception of responsibility for others
• may be involved in multiple high-stress roles, such as business executive, president of community group, and parent of teenager
• commonly concerned that hospitalization will prevent resumption of occupation and life-style

Sexuality-reproductive pattern
• may have history of oral contraceptive use
• may report previous chest pain episodes during sexual activity
• may verbalize concern over resuming normal sexual relations

Coping—stress tolerance pattern
• typically shows type A personality traits, such as overreaction to stress, exaggerated sense of urgency, excessive aggressiveness, and competitiveness
• may be in high-stress occupation
• typically has delayed securing medical attention because chest pain subsided with rest (denial)

Value-belief pattern
• may display compulsive striving for achievement

PHYSICAL FINDINGS
Cardiovascular
• increased heart rate
• elevated blood pressure at onset of pain
• arrhythmias
• S_3 and S_4 gallop
• transient jugular venous pressure elevations

Pulmonary
• shortness of breath during chest pain episode
• abnormal breath sounds, particularly crackles

Neurologic
• anxiety
• restlessness

Integumentary
• cool, clammy skin
• diaphoresis

Musculoskeletal
• pained facial expression
• clenched fists
• tense, rigid posture

DIAGNOSTIC STUDIES
• cardiac enzyme and isoenzyme levels—no elevations, or minor elevations without pattern characteristic of AMI
• complete blood count—may show decreased hemoglobin level, hematocrit, and red blood cell level, suggesting anemia-induced angina
• serum cholesterol, lipid profile—may be elevated, indicating increased risk for coronary artery disease
• serum electrolyte levels—used to determine imbalances, particularly in potassium levels, that can cause arrhythmias
• serum drug levels—may indicate toxic or subtherapeutic levels of cardiotonics or antiarrhythmics
• 12-lead ECG—resting ECG usually normal in angina, with ischemic changes during chest pain: classic angina, inversion of T waves and ST segment depression; Prinzmetal's angina, ST segment elevation
• treadmill or exercise test—may reveal chest pain and ECG signs of ischemia on exertion, especially ST segment and T wave changes; ventricular arrhythmias; and downsloping or horizontal ST segment depression
• myocardial perfusion studies—may show ischemic areas of the myocardium (imaged with thallium 201) as cold spots
• echocardiogram—may illustrate structural problems, such as valvular disease or stenoses
• cardiac catheterization and angiography—used to visualize blockage and to demonstrate coronary artery patency and ability to adequately perfuse myocardium

POTENTIAL COMPLICATIONS
• sudden death
• AMI
• intractable, unstable, or crescendo angina
• arrhythmias, especially ventricular arrhythmias
• decreased ventricular function

Nursing diagnosis: *Chest pain related to myocardial ischemia*

NURSING PRIORITY: Identify and relieve chest pain.

Interventions

1. Assess and document chest pain episodes according to the following criteria: location, duration, quality (on a scale of 1 to 10), causative factors, aggravating factors, alleviating factors, and associated signs and symptoms.

Rationales

1. Many conditions can produce chest pain. The nurse must carefully assess the chest pain in order to differentiate angina from pain related to other causes, such as pleuritic, gastric, or musculoskeletal disorders

2. Assess the patient for nonverbal signs of chest pain: restlessness; clenched fists; rubbing of the chest, arms, or neck; chest clutching; and facial flushing or grimacing.

2. Patients differ in the ways they express pain and in the meaning pain has for them. Denial of cardiac symptoms is common initially. An increase or change in the degree or intensity of pain may indicate increasing myocardial ischemia.

3. Obtain a 12-lead ECG immediately during acute chest pain.

3. Resting ECGs are usually normal in myocardial ischemia. Ischemic changes may be noted only during periods of actual chest pain.

4. Administer sublingual nitroglycerin promptly at the onset of pain, as ordered. (The typical protocol is one 0.15 to 0.6 mg tablet every 5 minutes to a maximum of three tablets.) Assess pain relief after 15 to 20 minutes. Evaluate and document blood pressure, pulse rate, respirations, and pain before and after medication administration. If the pain is unrelieved after 15 to 20 minutes (or after three tablets), notify the doctor immediately.

4. Nitrates decrease myocardial oxygen demands by causing vasodilation, which reduces preload and afterload and thus decreases cardiac work load and oxygen consumption. Pain unrelieved by nitroglycerin suggests extended ischemia or myocardial cell death.

5. Implement measures to improve myocardial oxygenation: institute oxygen therapy, place the patient on bed rest in semi- to high-Fowler's position, and minimize environmental noise and distractions.

5. These measures reduce the heart's oxygen demand and help alleviate chest pain and ensuing anxiety. Chest and head elevation eases lung ventilation. Sitting with the shoulders pulled slightly back allows unrestricted movement of the diaphragm. Decreasing anxiety reduces circulating catecholamine levels, thus decreasing blood pressure and myocardial oxygen consumption.

6. Stay with the patient during chest pain episodes.

6. The presence of a competent caregiver may decrease anxiety and promote patient comfort. It also allows for immediate intervention if problems occur.

7. Monitor and document the therapeutic effects of beta blockers (such as propranolol [Inderal], metoprolol [Lopressor], and nadolol [Corgard]), calcium channel blockers (such as verapamil [Calan] and nifedipine [Procardia]), and vasodilators (such as hydralazine [Apresoline] and prazosin [Minipress]). Monitor for bradycardia, hypotension, arrhythmias, signs and symptoms of congestive heart failure, constipation, and exacerbation of ischemic symptoms from medication therapies.

7. Beta blockers block the myocardial response to sympathetic stimulation, thus decreasing oxygen demand and preventing or relieving anginal pain. Beta blockers also decrease heart rate, blood pressure, and myocardial contractility. Calcium channel blockers dilate the coronary arteries, thus decreasing coronary artery spasm and improving myocardial perfusion. Vasodilators that act on the arterial system may lessen the hypertensive response to exertion, which may prevent anginal attacks.

8. Establish and maintain I.V. access.

8. I.V. access is necessary for possible emergency medication administration or until the differential diagnosis is completed. The usual order is for a heparin lock or dextrose 5% in water to keep the vein open.

9. Additional individualized interventions: _____

9. Rationales: _____

Target outcome criteria
Within 30 minutes of chest pain onset, the patient will:
• verbalize absence or relief of pain
• display relaxed facial expression and body posture
• display normal depth and rate of respirations
• show no restlessness, grimacing, or other signs and symptoms of pain.

Within 1 hour of chest pain onset, the patient will:
• display vital signs within normal limits
• increase participation in appropriate activities
• show no life-threatening arrhythmias.

CARDIOVASCULAR DISORDERS

Collaborative problem: *High risk for arrhythmias or AMI related to myocardial hypoxia and ischemia*

NURSING PRIORITIES: (a) Optimize cardiac oxygenation and perfusion, and (b) decrease myocardial oxygen demands.

Interventions

1. Monitor, report, and document signs and symptoms of arrhythmias, such as irregular apical pulse, pulse deficit, pulse rate below 60 or above 100 beats/minute, syncope, dizziness, palpitations, chest "fluttering," or abnormal configurations on rhythm strips or 12-lead ECGs.

2. Administer antiarrhythmic medications, as ordered, noting and documenting their effectiveness and adverse effects.

3. Decrease myocardial oxygen demands by restricting activity (based on the arrhythmia's severity), maintaining oxygen therapy, and providing a calm, supportive environment.

4. Monitor, report, and document signs and symptoms of inadequate tissue perfusion, such as decreasing blood pressure; cool, clammy skin; cyanosis; diminished peripheral pulses; decreased urine output; increased restlessness and agitation; or respiratory distress.

5. Monitor and report signs and symptoms of developing MI, such as chest pain lasting longer than 30 minutes and unrelieved by administration of a short-acting nitrate, elevation of creatine phosphokinase isoenzymes, ST segment elevation, or pathological Q wave on a 12-lead ECG.

6. Additional individualized interventions: _____

Rationales

1. Ventricular irritability secondary to myocardial ischemia can lead to life-threatening ventricular arrhythmias. Prompt arrhythmia identification is essential for stabilizing the patient's cardiovascular condition.

2. Common antiarrhythmic medications include lidocaine (Xylocaine), procainamide (Pronestyl), quinidine (Cardioquin), bretylium (Bretylol), and atropine. Lidocaine is the medication of choice for dangerous premature ventricular contractions (more than 6 per minute, sequential, multifocal, or early diastolic), which are common with myocardial hypoxia and ischemia.

3. Activities that increase myocardial oxygen demands may potentiate arrhythmia development by promoting increased automaticity and impeding electrical conduction through the myocardium.

4. Arrhythmias may lead to decreased cardiac output, resulting in inadequate tissue perfusion. Prompt recognition is essential to minimize damage and complications.

5. When myocardial ischemia is severe or prolonged, irreversible injury (tissue necrosis) occurs. Chest pain that does not respond to nitroglycerin within 30 minutes strongly suggests AMI.

6. Rationales:_____

Target outcome criteria

Within 30 minutes of chest pain onset, the patient will have stable vital signs.

Within 24 hours of admission, the patient will:
• display an apical or radial pulse rate of 60 to 100 beats/minute
• show normal sinus rhythm on ECG or arrhythmias controlled with drugs
• have no syncope, palpitations, or skipped beats
• have no pulse deficit.

Within 3 days of admission, the patient will:
• have no elevation of cardiac enzymes
• have a resting ECG negative for ST segment elevation and Q waves
• have normal blood pressure, pulse, and respirations
• display clear lungs
• maintain normal urine output.

Nursing diagnosis: *Activity intolerance related to development of chest pain on exertion*

NURSING PRIORITY: Promote gradual activity restoration, balancing myocardial oxygen supply and demand.

Interventions

1. Instruct the patient to stop immediately any activity that causes chest pain. If chest pain occurs, maintain the patient in Fowler's position, and administer oxygen therapy, as ordered.

2. Instruct the patient to avoid Valsalva's maneuver, such as by not straining at bowel movements or avoiding heavy lifting.

3. Document activity tolerance, and instruct the patient to increase activity gradually; monitor pulse rate before and after activity; use chest pain, fatigue, or marked tachycardia as an indication to stop; and pace activities to avoid sudden demands on the heart.

4. Promote physical rest and emotional comfort.

5. Additional individualized interventions: _____

_____

Rationales

1. Pain may be relieved by stopping the physical activity that preceded its onset. Changing from a supine to a sitting position decreases central blood volume because blood pools in the extremities, reducing the heart's oxygen demand. Fowler's position allows maximum lung expansion; oxygen therapy decreases the heart's work load.

2. Valsalva's maneuver induces parasympathetic stimulation, which can cause bradycardia and decrease cardiac output, leading to increased ischemia.

3. Physical activity increases myocardial oxygen demand and can cause chest pain. An activity prescription is determined for each patient to maintain cardiovascular stability and prevent fatigue.

4. Fear and anxiety increase sympathetic nervous system responses, increasing myocardial oxygen demand. Relaxation increases the patient's ability to cooperate and participate in therapeutic activities.

5. Rationales: _____

_____

Target outcome criteria
Within 24 hours of admission, the patient will tolerate bed rest without chest pain.

Within 72 hours of admission, the patient will:
• ambulate to the bathroom and chair without chest pain
• have normal bowel elimination without straining.

Nursing diagnosis: *Altered health maintenance related to cardiovascular risk factors*

NURSING PRIORITY: Minimize the development of complications from modifiable risk factors.

Interventions

1. Teach the patient about factors that may cause anginal attacks after discharge, such as strenuous exercise, changes in sexual habits or partners, exposure to extreme cold, strong emotions, stress, or smoking. Teach ways to decrease the risk of chest pain, such as using sublingual nitroglycerin prophylactically; monitoring pulse rate before and after activity; and stopping activity if chest pain, dyspnea, or palpitations ensue. Use the patient's experience as a basis for teaching. Document the patient's response to teaching.

2. Instruct the patient to maintain a diet low in saturated fat and cholesterol and to achieve ideal body weight. Document current height and weight.

Rationales

1. Teaching the patient ways to avoid anginal attacks will decrease anxiety and may increase participation in self-care. Controlling risk factors may minimize the disease's progress and lessen its impact on the patient's life-style. Relating teaching to the patient's experience capitalizes on the principle that adults learn better when material is relevant to their needs and integrated with prior experience.

2. Exacerbation of coronary artery disease may be related to increased dietary intake of cholesterol, which contributes to increased plaque formation and narrowing of coronary arteries. Obesity elevates blood pressure and places a greater demand on the heart.

CARDIOVASCULAR DISORDERS

3. Provide six light meals per day rather than three heavy ones.

3. Although subject to debate, large meals are believed to require an increased blood supply to the GI tract for digestion, increasing myocardial work. An anginal attack may be caused by a large, heavy meal. Small meals prevent epigastric fullness or indigestion that might be mistaken for anginal pain. In addition, small meals place less demand on myocardial oxygen consumption during digestion, reducing the risk of angina.

4. Encourage avoidance of foods and beverages high in caffeine.

4. Coffee, tea, chocolate, and colas contain varying amounts of caffeine, which is a myocardial stimulant that increases myocardial oxygen consumption.

5. Discourage cigarette smoking.

5. Nicotine causes vasoconstriction, is a cardiac stimulant, and reduces oxygen availability.

6. Instruct the patient in stress-reduction techniques.

6. Unresolved anxiety and a stressful life-style increase myocardial oxygen demands, so they are risk factors for cardiovascular disease. Decreasing stress levels may decrease circulating catecholamine levels, thus decreasing blood pressure and overall myocardial oxygen consumption.

7. Start the patient on a cardiovascular fitness regimen when approved by the doctor.

7. Supervised exercise enhances cardiovascular fitness while minimizing the chance of another cardiac event.

8. Additional individualized interventions: _____

8. Rationales: _____

Target outcome criteria
Within 3 days of admission, the patient will:
• verbalize knowledge of diet, life-style, and health habit modifications
• eliminate smoking

• indicate specific plans made for appropriate life-style modifications.

Nursing diagnosis: *Knowledge deficit related to unfamiliarity with diagnostic or therapeutic procedures*

NURSING PRIORITY: Teach the patient about upcoming procedures.

Interventions

1. See the "Knowledge Deficit" plan, page 56.

Rationales

1. The "Knowledge Deficit" plan provides helpful interventions for patient teaching. This plan contains additional specific information for the patient undergoing an invasive diagnostic or corrective procedure.

2. Explain hospital protocol for cardiac catheterization to the patient and family. Include procedural steps, risks and benefits, pre- and post-procedure care, possible complications, and post-procedure activity restrictions.

2. Currently, the most accurate way to determine the extent of coronary artery disease is through cardiac catheterization. A special catheter is inserted through a distal vein or artery (usually the femoral) and advanced into the right or left chambers of the heart. During angiography, radiopaque contrast dye is injected through the catheter to trace coronary artery bloodflow. Teaching the patient about the procedure will decrease anxiety and enhance cooperation.

3. Based on the results of cardiac catheterization, the patient may require percutaneous transluminal coronary angioplasty (PTCA) or coronary artery bypass graft surgery (CABG). Assess the patient's level of anxiety, fear, and understanding of the planned procedure. Begin patient teaching as soon as appropriate and clarify any misconceptions.

3. When the coronary arteries are significantly blocked, when the patient develops intractable angina, or when medical management no longer controls anginal attacks, the doctor usually recommends further interventions. PTCA is an invasive, nonsurgical procedure in which a balloon-equipped catheter is passed under fluroscopy into a partially blocked coronary artery. When the balloon is inflated, it stretches the artery, opening the lumen and relieving the blockage. CABG is indicated for the patient who either does not respond to PTCA or has more significant blockage. CABG uses a saphenous or mammary vein graft to bypass one or more blocked coronary arteries. The patient will be more receptive to teaching about the procedure if anxieties and fears are addressed first. Adequate preparation helps ensure cooperation.

4. For the patient undergoing CABG, see the "Cardiac Surgery" plan, page 299.

4. This plan specifies nursing care for the patient undergoing cardiac surgery.

5. Additional individualized interventions:_____

5. Rationales:_____

CARDIOVASCULAR DISORDERS

Target outcome criterion
Prior to invasive procedures, the patient will, on request, verbalize knowledge of the procedure, risks and benefits, pre- and post-procedure care, possible complications, and post-procedure activity restrictions.

Discharge planning

NURSING DISCHARGE CRITERIA
Upon the patient's discharge, documentation shows evidence of:
• absence of chest pain, or angina controlled by oral or sublingual medications
• stable vital signs for at least 48 hours
• absence of fever and pulmonary or cardiovascular complications
• ability to perform activities of daily living and ambulate without chest pain
• blood chemistry studies within expected parameters
• normal sinus rhythm or arrhythmias controlled with drugs
• ability to tolerate activity at prescribed levels
• ability to tolerate diet and dietary restrictions
• normal voiding and bowel movements
• ability to list activities that may cause angina
• referral to outpatient cardiac programs (if applicable).

PATIENT-FAMILY TEACHING CHECKLIST
Document evidence that the patient and family demonstrate an understanding of:
__ angina's pathophysiology and implications
__ recommended modifications of risk factors (smoking, stress, obesity, lack of exercise, diet high in fat and cholesterol)
__ prescribed dietary modifications
__ resumption of daily activities

__ all discharge medications' purpose, dose, administration schedule, adverse effects, and toxic effects (usual discharge medications include nitrates, beta blockers, calcium channel blockers, or antilipemic drugs)
__ common emotional adjustments
__ community resources for life-style and risk factor modification, such as stress- and weight-reduction groups, cardiac exercise programs, and smoking cessation programs
__ signs and symptoms indicating need for medical attention, such as chest pain unrelieved by three nitroglycerin tablets within 20 minutes, new pattern of anginal attacks, palpitations or skipped beats, syncope, dyspnea, or diaphoresis
__ date, time, and location of follow-up appointments
__ how to contact the doctor.

DOCUMENTATION CHECKLIST
Using outcome criteria as a guide, document:
__ clinical status on admission
__ significant changes in status
__ chest pain episodes—precipitating, aggravating, and alleviating factors
__ pertinent laboratory and diagnostic test results
__ pain relief measures
__ oxygen therapy
__ I.V. therapy
__ use of protocols
__ nutritional intake

___ response to medications
___ emotional response to illness; coping skills
___ activity tolerance
___ patient-family teaching
___ discharge planning.

ASSOCIATED PLANS OF CARE
Acute Myocardial Infarction—Stepdown Unit Phase
Ineffective Individual Coping
Knowledge Deficit
Pain

References

Andreoli, K., et. al. *Comprehensive Cardiac Care*, 6th ed. St. Louis: Mosby-Year Book, 1987.

Canobbio, M. *Cardiovascular Disorders*. St. Louis: Mosby-Year Book, 1990.

Cardiac Problems. Nurse Review Series. Springhouse, Pa.: Springhouse Corp., 1986.

Cardiovascular Care Handbook. Springhouse, Pa.: Springhouse Corp., 1986.

Carpenito, L. *Handbook of Nursing Diagnosis*, 4th ed. Philadelphia: J.B. Lippincott Co., 1991.

Gordon, M. *Manual of Nursing Diagnosis 1991-1992*. St. Louis: Mosby-Year Book, 1991.

Huang, S.L., et al. *Coronary Care Nursing*, 2nd ed. Philadelphia: W.B. Saunders Co., 1989.

Luckman, J., and Sorensen, K. *Medical-Surgical Nursing: A Psychophysiological Approach*, 3rd ed. Philadelphia: W.B. Saunders Co., 1987.

Underhill, S., et al. *Cardiac Nursing*, 2nd ed. Philadelphia: J.B. Lippincott Co., 1989.

Zorb, L., et al. *Cardiac Diagnostic Testing*. Gaithersburg, Md.: Aspen Publishing, 1991.

CARDIOVASCULAR DISORDERS
Cardiac Surgery

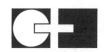

DRG information

Cardiac surgery may be classified under several DRGs, depending on the principal operating room procedure and whether cardiac catheterization was performed.

DRG 104 Cardiac Valve Procedure With Pump and With Cardiac Catheterization.
Mean LOS = 18.3 days
Principal operating room procedures include:
• open-heart mitral, aortic, pulmonary, or tricuspid valvuloplasty without replacement
• replacement of mitral, aortic, pulmonary, or tricuspid valve with biological or mechanical prosthesis
• implantation or replacement of automatic cardioverter defibrillator, total system.

DRG 105 Cardiac Valve Procedure With Pump and Without Cardiac Catheterization.
Mean LOS = 13.0 days

DRG 106 Coronary Bypass With Cardiac Catheterization.
Mean LOS = 13.9 days
Principal operating room procedures include aorto-coronary bypass of 1, 2, 3, 4, or more coronary arteries.

DRG 107 Coronary Bypass Without Cardiac Catheterization.
Mean LOS = 11.2 days

DRG 108 Other Cardiothoracic or Vascular Procedures With Pump.
Mean LOS = 12.9 days
Principal operating room procedures include:
• open chest coronary angioplasty to remove artery obstruction, with pump
• biopsy of pericardium
• cardiotomy
• excision of aneurysm or other heart lesion
• open chest cardiac massage
• procedures on structures adjacent to heart valves
• pericardiotomy
• pericardiectomy
• repair of atrial or ventricular septa with tissue graft or prosthetic device
• total repair of certain congenital cardiac anomalies
• closed cardiac valvotomy.

Additional DRG information: Hundreds of additional vascular operating room procedures also are classified under DRG 108. The above list details only coronary procedures. Other cardiac surgical procedures not addressed in the following plan (such as permanent pacemaker insertion) have still other DRG numbers.

Introduction
DEFINITION AND TIME FOCUS

Cardiac surgery can correct numerous structural and physiologic problems. During surgery, the surgical team stops the heart and collapses the lungs; cardiopulmonary bypass (CPB) maintains systemic perfusion and gas exchange during this time. CPB causes some predictable physiologic and hemodynamic changes during the early postoperative period. Nursing care during this period focuses on assessing for anticipated changes, maintaining organ function, preventing complications, and providing emotional support to the patient and family. This clinical plan focuses on the patient in the critical care unit during the first 1 to 3 days after coronary artery bypass graft (CABG) or valve repair or replacement. It assumes that a cardiovascular nurse specialist or a similarly qualified person provided preoperative teaching and that a formal postoperative teaching and rehabilitation program has been planned. (For teaching guidelines on cardiovascular health promotion, risk factor modification, and rehabilitation, see Underhill et al., 1989.)

ETIOLOGY AND PRECIPITATING FACTORS

• severe coronary artery disease of one or more vessels, particularly the left anterior descending coronary artery
• acute myocardial infarction (AMI), especially if complicated by cardiogenic shock, infarct extension, uncontrollable failure, papillary muscle rupture, or septal rupture
• unstable or crescendo angina pectoris
• previous bypass grafting with recurrent angina or angiographic evidence of graft closure
• ventricular aneurysm
• valvular stenosis or insufficiency with hemodynamic compromise

Focused assessment guidelines
NURSING HISTORY (Functional health pattern findings)

Health perception—health management pattern
• may have history of acute or chronic coronary artery disease or valvular dysfunction
• may have a condition refractory to less invasive therapies, such as medication. Note: Remaining health pattern findings are those of the underlying disease; refer to "Acute Myocardial Infarction—Critical Care Unit Phase," page 268, "Acute Myocardial Infarction—Stepdown Unit Phase," page 280, "Congestive Heart Failure," page 329, and "Cardiogenic Shock," page 310, for examples.

PHYSICAL FINDINGS
Because the preoperative physical findings are those of the underlying disorder, they are not repeated here; instead, this section presents typical postoperative findings.

General appearance
• increase of 2 to 18 lb (1 to 8 kg) above preoperative weight

Cardiovascular
• blood pressure variable
• arrhythmias
• heart sounds variable; may have early flow murmur or audible clicking after valve replacement
• chest tube drainage variable
• peripheral pulses usually equal bilaterally
• slow capillary refill

Pulmonary
• variable rate and depth, depending on ventilator settings
• breath sounds usually diminished in left base
• crackles or gurgles

Neurologic
• level of consciousness variable (patient usually can be awakened)
• confusion
• disorientation

Integumentary
• cool skin
• dry skin
• pallor
• generalized edema
• serosanguinous oozing from incisions

Gastrointestinal
• absent bowel sounds
• nasogastric tube drainage variable
• pain may be increased or paralytic ileus prolonged with use of abdominal arterial bypass conduits (gastroepiploic or inferior epigastric arteries)

Renal
• polyuria

DIAGNOSTIC STUDIES
The following tests are performed before surgery for baseline data. This section details common early postoperative findings.
• hemoglobin level and hematocrit — decreased because of hemodilution; hematocrit is usually about 25% or lower
• coagulation panel — reveals prolonged prothrombin time (PT) and partial thromboplastin time (PTT), reflecting intraoperative heparinization, and decreased platelet level, reflecting history of antiplatelet medication (aspirin, dipyridamole [Persantine]), and platelet destruction by CPB equipment, especially roller and filtration unit
• serum glucose level — elevated from stress-induced glycogenolysis and decreased insulin production
• serum electrolyte values — vary, depending on preoperative status, replacement during surgery, fluid shifts, and other factors
• cardiac isoenzymes — may be elevated if AMI is present (slight elevation normal after surgery)
• 12-lead electrocardiography (ECG), resting and stress — findings vary, depending on preexisting disorders (such as AMI), acid-base status, electrolyte status, or medications
• chest X-ray — reveals cardiac size, mediastinal position, and pulmonary status; postoperatively, it confirms endotracheal tube, chest tube, central venous pressure line, and pulmonary artery catheter placement
• preoperative cardiac catheterization and coronary arteriography — reveal critical coronary artery occlusion, poor left ventricular function, or hemodynamically significant valve stenosis or insufficiency (manifested by elevated left ventricular end-diastolic and pulmonary pressures, cardiac index (CI) less than 2.5 liter/minute/m^2, ejection fraction less than 0.30, tight valve areas, increased valvular gradients, occlusive lesions, or shunts)
• echocardiography — compares preoperative and postoperative function (especially for valve repairs)

POTENTIAL COMPLICATIONS
• cardiogenic shock
• hypovolemic shock
• AMI
• heart failure
• endocarditis
• graft occlusion
• thromboembolism
• atelectasis
• cerebrovascular accident
• hemorrhage

Collaborative problem: *High risk for low cardiac output syndrome related to hypothermia, excessive vasoconstriction, myocardial depression, arrhythmias, cardiac tamponade, or graft occlusion*

NURSING PRIORITY: Maintain optimal cardiac output.

Interventions

1. Monitor blood pressure continuously with an arterial catheter. Maintain mean arterial pressure (MAP) within desired limits; determine limits in consultation with the surgeon. In general, report a systolic blood pressure less than 80 mm Hg or greater than 150 mm Hg, a diastolic blood pressure greater than 100 mm Hg, or a MAP less than 60 mm Hg or greater than 90 mm Hg. Report any value abnormal for the patient.

2. Measure cardiac output (CO), as ordered, typically every hour until normal and then every 2 hours. If not using a computerized monitoring system, calculate CI by dividing CO by body surface area (obtain body surface area value from a chart or nomogram); calculate SVR by subtracting right atrial pressure (RAP) from MAP and dividing the result by CO. Follow the trend of CI and SVR values, comparing them with normal ranges and previous values.

3. Monitor pulmonary artery diastolic pressure (PADP) continuously until stable. Monitor RAP, pulmonary artery systolic pressure (PASP), and pulmonary capillary wedge pressure (PCWP), as ordered, typically every hour until stable. Compare with preoperative values and desired limits; determine limits in consultation with the surgeon.

4. Provide constant ECG monitoring. Observe for indicators of possible myocardial damage (such as ST-segment deviation, T-wave inversion, or pathologic Q waves) and for preexisting arrhythmias, new ventricular arrhythmias, and arrhythmias associated with the specific surgical procedure (see *Arrhythmias associated with cardiac surgery,* page 302). If present, assess for underlying causes, treat according to standing orders (usually with medications or temporary pacing), and document their occurrence.

Rationales

1. Low cardiac output syndrome, a common postoperative problem, may result from preexisting abnormalities or the stress of surgery. Arterial monitoring provides the most direct and accurate blood pressure measurements. Because perfusion is directly related to blood pressure, maintaining optimal MAP ensures adequate organ perfusion. Hypothermia, used during surgery to lower metabolic demand and protect organs from ischemia, induces vasoconstriction, which increases systemic vascular resistance (SVR) and the risk of hypertension. Stress triggers the release of catecholamines, antidiuretic hormone (ADH), and aldosterone, which also may produce hypertension. Persistent hypertension can cause leaking or rupture of suture lines. The causes of hypotension are discussed later in this plan.

2. CO may drop in the postoperative period because of decreased preload from a fluid volume deficit (discussed below), increased afterload from elevated SVR, or impaired contractility (discussed below). Any of these factors may cause the already stressed heart to fail. CO measurements and CI calculations provide objective data on the adequacy of output, while SVR values show the degree of resistance to ventricular ejection. Increased afterload and hypertension both increase myocardial work load. SVR values typically are elevated in the early postoperative period. SVR and blood pressure values should return to normal gradually as rewarming occurs.

3. PADP is a useful indirect indicator of left ventricular performance. RAP reflects central venous pressure; PASP, the force of right ventricular ejection; and PCWP, left ventricular function. These values provide objective data for assessing the patient's fluid volume, cardiovascular function, and pulmonary status.

4. Constant monitoring provides early warning of possible myocardial damage or arrhythmias. Underlying causes may include pain, anxiety, hypokalemia, preexisting conditions (such as chronic atrial fibrillation), hypoxemia, and volume depletion. Arrhythmias usually respond to standard protocols, such as lidocaine (Xylocaine) administration for premature ventricular beats. In many patients, pacing wires are inserted during surgery and brought out through the chest wall. If necessary, they can be connected to a pacemaker to provide a stable rhythm until cardiac irritability or the underlying cause resolves.

ARRHYTHMIAS ASSOCIATED WITH CARDIAC SURGERY

Certain cardiac procedures place the patient at risk for arrhythmias related to the underlying pathophysiology of the disorder or to the procedure itself.

Surgery	Likely ECG changes	Significance
Coronary artery bypass grafting	• ST segment (ischemic) changes • Ventricular ectopy • New Q waves	• Related to myocardial ischemia, residual air in the coronary arteries, or an occluded graft • Related to surgical manipulation, ischemia, or hypoxemia • Indicate perioperative myocardial infarction
Aortic valve replacement	• ST segment (ischemic) changes • Left bundle branch block	• Related to embolization of valve debris (such as calcium or tissue) • Related to left ventricular hypertrophy
Mitral valve repair or replacement	• Atrial fibrillation • ST segment (ischemic) changes • Heart block	• Related to preoperative left atrial enlargement • Related to embolization of valve debris • Usually associated with valve disease
Tricuspid valve repair or replacement	• Heart block	• Related to surgical manipulation of the bundle of His

5. Monitor for indicators of myocardial ischemia caused by graft occlusion: ECG changes, angina pectoris (must be differentiated from sternal incisional pain), or cardiac enzymes (creatine phosphokinase-MB [CPK-MB]) elevated above expected postoperative level (consult surgeon for acceptable level). Expect slight elevations 4 to 7 hours after CABG, and higher elevations after valve replacement or repair than after CABG. Immediately report an elevation greater than 50 U/liter or any other significant changes.

6. Monitor level of consciousness; apical pulse rate; skin color, warmth, and temperature; peripheral pulse rates; and urine output every 15 minutes to 1 hour until normal and stable. Report any abnormalities to the surgeon promptly.

7. Monitor core body temperature continuously (via bladder or rectal probe or pulmonary artery catheter) or every hour (with a rectal thermometer) until normal and then every 4 hours.

8. If body temperature is low, cover the patient with warmed blankets until it returns to normal. As the temperature rises, monitor for signs of fluid volume deficit. If the temperature rises above 101° F (38.3° C), assess for underlying causes; administer antipyretics, such as acetaminophen (Tylenol), as ordered; and use a hypothermia blanket, as ordered, for high fever.

9. Administer vasodilators, such as sodium nitroprusside (Nipride), as ordered. Refer to the "Congestive Heart Failure" plan, page 329, for details regarding administration. Correlate vasodilator administration with body temperature and rewarming.

5. Early graft occlusion results from thrombus formation caused by poor run-off, graft injury, or faulty anastomosis. Late graft closure is related to subintimal thickening of the graft.

The normal stress of surgery causes a slight CPK-MB elevation a few hours after CABG. An elevation greater than 50 U/liter after 18 to 30 hours may indicate a perioperative AMI. Higher CK-MB levels are normal after valve surgery because of greater tissue trauma.

6. These parameters indicate the adequacy of central and peripheral perfusion. Abnormalities may signal the development of numerous complications and warrant medical evaluation.

7. The patient's body temperature is usually low after surgery from induced hypothermia and heat loss from the open chest. The temperature then typically rises somewhat above normal (because of the inflammatory response after surgery) and gradually returns to normal in approximately 3 days.

8. Gradual rewarming gives the heart time to adjust to the expanded vascular bed as vasoconstriction lessens. As body temperature rises, vasodilation may unmask a previously hidden fluid volume deficit. Temperatures above 101° F suggest a cause other than the normal inflammatory response, such as dehydration or sepsis. Fever increases cardiac work load, therefore reducing body temperature reduces stress on the heart. Aspirin usually is avoided because it decreases platelet aggregation and may contribute to bleeding.

9. Vasodilators achieve controlled dilation of the vascular bed and reduce hypertension. Because afterload reduction lessens resistance to ventricular ejection, it also lessens myocardial work load. The "Congestive Heart Failure" plan covers vasodilator administration. Because vasodilators, fever, and rewarming all cause vasodilation, their effects must be correlated to avoid excessive vascular bed expansion.

10. Administer positive inotropic agents, as ordered, typically dopamine (Intropin) or dobutamine (Dobutrex). Refer to the "Congestive Heart Failure" plan, page 329, for details on administration.

10. Mild, transient depression of contractility is common because of hypothermia and myocardial edema. Dopamine improves contractility through its beta,-adrenergic effects but may cause tachycardia and arrhythmias. Dobutamine also increases contractility but is less likely to cause tachycardia and arrhythmias. An inotrope may be used for the first 12 to 24 hours in an uncomplicated recovery; in cases of preoperative myocardial depression or intraoperative infarction, it may be used for a longer period. The "Congestive Heart Failure" plan presents administration of inotropic agents.

11. Monitor for indicators of cardiac tamponade, even when mediastinal chest tubes are draining freely. Observe for rapid hypotension, marked central venous pressure elevation, neck vein distention, muffled heart sounds, paradoxical pulse, or decreased QRS voltage on ECG; also observe for a sudden decrease in chest tube drainage.

11. Cardiac tamponade results when blood or fluid accumulates in the pericardium. Clotted chest tubes can produce tamponade; however, patent tubes do not necessarily reduce the risk of tamponade because fluid can accumulate in areas not drained by the tubes. Tamponade can rapidly interfere with ventricular filling and cardiac output.

12. If tamponade with cardiac decompensation occurs, immediately notify the doctor. Assemble supplies and equipment for open chest massage and maintain fluid replacement.

12. Cardiac decompensation is a medical emergency. Opening the chest allows evacuation of blood or fluid while cardiac massage perfuses the brain and other vital organs.

13. Additional individualized interventions: _____

13. Rationales: _____

Target outcome criteria
Within 24 hours after surgery, the patient will:
• have a MAP of 70 to 90 mm Hg
• have a regular supraventricular rhythm with a ventricular rate of 60 to 100 beats/minute (normal sinus rhythm is ideal)
• have peripheral pulses bilaterally equal and full

• have warm, dry arms and legs
• have a temperature of 98.6° to 101° F (37° to 38.3° C)
• display no signs of cardiac tamponade
• have RAP, PADP, PASP, and PCWP within desired limits.

Collaborative problem: *High risk for endocarditis or other infection related to perioperative contamination*

NURSING PRIORITIES: (a) Promote wound healing and (b) prevent nosocomial infection.

Interventions

1. Identify conditions that place the patient at high risk for endocarditis or another infection: previous endocarditis; valvular heart disease; rheumatic heart disease; Marfan's syndrome; congenital heart disease; presence of foreign bodies, such as a pacemaker or prosthetic valves or grafts; or presence of invasive lines or a urinary catheter.

2. Administer prophylactic antibiotics, as ordered.

3. Use strict aseptic technique during wound care and dressing changes.

4. Assess for signs and symptoms of endocarditis or other infection: elevated temperature; elevated white blood cell count; incision red, tender, or draining; changes in urine color, odor, clarity, or amount; malaise, weakness, diaphoresis, and easy fatigability; new murmur after valve surgery; or positive wound, blood, or urine cultures.

Rationales

1. These conditions increase the risk of endocarditis and other infections.

2. Antibiotics are routinely administered for 24 to 48 hours after surgery (until invasive lines are removed).

3. Aseptic technique prevents cross-contamination and transmission of bacteria to incision sites.

4. These are common findings for endocarditis or other infection.

CARDIOVASCULAR DISORDERS

5. If signs and symptoms of endocarditis or other infection develop, notify the doctor promptly. Obtain wound cultures and administer antibiotics as ordered. See the "Surgical Intervention" plan, page 81, for further details.

5. Because of the high mortality rate associated with post-operative endocarditis or other infection, prompt, aggressive treatment is indicated. Cultures help to identify specific sites of infection, while antibiotics fight the organism involved. The "Surgical Intervention" plan contains general information on infection control.

6. Additional individualized interventions: _____

6. Rationales: _____

Target outcome criteria
After surgery, the patient will display no signs or symptoms of endocarditis.

Within 48 hours after surgery (or after invasive lines are removed), the patient will require no additional antibiotics.

Collaborative problem: *Interstitial edema related to hemodilution, excessive fluid replacement, and stress adaptation syndrome*

NURSING PRIORITY: Restore normal fluid volume.

Interventions

1. Expect signs and symptoms of interstitial fluid overload; monitor degree of overload and speed of resolution:

• Monitor generalized edema and tissue turgor.

• Monitor daily weights. Compare with preoperative and previous day's values.

• Monitor for neck vein distention or S_3 heart sound, and, if present, notify the doctor.

2. Administer I.V. solutions, as ordered. Unless the patient is hypovolemic, limit fluid intake from all sources to 100 ml/hour or less.

3. Monitor intake and output measurements, usually hourly on the first postoperative day and then every 8 hours.

4. Administer I.V. diuretics, such as furosemide (Lasix), if ordered.

Rationales

1. During CPB, hemodilution is achieved with I.V. crystalloid solution. Because hemodilution decreases blood viscosity and peripheral vascular resistance, it minimizes microcirculatory sludging, thus protecting organs from ischemia during surgery.

• Hemodilution lowers plasma oncotic pressure, which allows fluid to shift from the vascular to interstitial spaces, producing generalized edema.

• Weight gain from hemodilution may approach 18 lb (8 kg). Daily weight comparisons provide objective evidence of the degree of fluid retention and the speed with which fluid is mobilized and excreted after surgery.

• Although most of the excess fluid is in the interstitial space, central blood volume may increase. These findings may reflect such an increase or may result from cardiac dysfunction (described below), and require medical evaluation.

2. Early hypovolemia is common, and I.V. fluids may be needed initially to compensate for interstitial fluid shifts, to increase plasma volume, and to optimize preload. Hemodilution during bypass pushes fluids to the interstitial space; however, this fluid shifts back into the vascular space between the second and fifth postoperative day. This fact, in addition to the large number of I.V. lines, can cause fluid overload unless total intake is monitored.

3. The stress reaction triggered by surgery causes the release of ADH, the secretion of aldosterone, and sympathetic stimulation of the kidneys, all of which result in fluid retention. Monitoring intake and output records provides objective data on which to gauge fluid retention and base therapeutic decisions.

4. Aggressive diuresis may be used to eliminate excess interstitial fluid.

5. Monitor for signs and symptoms of electrolyte imbalance, particularly hypokalemia. See Appendix C, "Fluid and Electrolyte Imbalances," for details. If hypokalemia is present:
• observe for arrhythmias
• add potassium to I.V. fluids, as ordered
• monitor serum levels closely, typically every 4 hours in the first 24 hours
• monitor for hyperkalemia.

6. Additional individualized interventions: _____

5. Hypokalemia is very common after surgery. It may result from preoperative diuretic administration, hemodilution, or postoperative diuresis. Supplemental I.V. potassium usually is necessary. Close monitoring of serum potassium level is essential to guide replacement and to avoid hyperkalemia from potassium administration and potassium release from hemolyzed blood cells.

6. Rationales: _____

Target outcome criteria
Within 24 hours after surgery, the patient will have a 24-hour fluid output greater than intake.

Within 3 days after surgery, the patient will:
• return to preoperative weight
• have normal serum electrolyte levels.

Collaborative problem: *Hypovolemia related to bleeding or diuresis*

NURSING PRIORITY: Maintain normal fluid volume.

Interventions

1. Monitor PT, PTT, and platelet counts, as ordered. Consult the surgeon about reportable values, particularly prolonged PT, prolonged PTT, low platelet level, or other coagulation deficiencies.

2. Monitor hemoglobin levels and hematocrit. Consult the surgeon about reportable values, particularly declining ones. Have blood and blood products available.

3. Measure and document chest tube drainage. If drainage is constant or increasing, bright red, or exceeds 200 ml/hour, notify the surgeon.

4. Maintain autotransfusion system, if used.

5. Observe for other signs of bleeding, such as excessive oozing from incisions, petechiae, and ecchymoses. If hemoglobin levels, hematocrit, or coagulation values are abnormal, test urine, feces, and vomitus for occult blood.

6. Monitor vital signs for tachycardia or hypotension.

Rationales

1. Blood loss has multiple causes during and after surgery. During surgery, some blood loss is inevitable, and heparin is used to prevent clotting in the extracorporeal circuit. This anticoagulation is reversed with protamine sulfate, but inadequate reversal may result in bleeding. Heparin rebound also may occur from the release of heparin stored in the tissues. The CPB equipment, especially the roller pump and filtration unit, damages platelets. Finally, the patient may have a history of antiplatelet medication use. All of these factors may alter normal coagulation, so values below normal are expected after surgery. Reportable values vary among surgeons.

2. Hemoglobin and hematocrit values are low after surgery as a result of hemodilution. As postoperative diuresis occurs, the values should return to normal. Failure to do so implies continued bleeding. Usually, the patient will be transfused when the hematocrit drops below 25%.

3. Postoperative bleeding includes oozing of incisions and suture disruption. Excessive or bloody drainage warrants surgical exploration.

4. Conserving the patient's blood avoids allergic reactions and the risks associated with bank blood.

5. Although laboratory tests provide valuable objective data of bleeding tendencies, they are no substitute for astute clinical assessment. Signs of frank or occult bleeding may be the first indication of abnormal coagulation.

6. Vital sign changes are usually nonspecific, relatively late indicators of bleeding; however, tachycardia is a compensatory response to hypovolemia, while hypotension can reflect significant blood loss or cardiac depression.

CARDIOVASCULAR DISORDERS

7. Administer protamine sulfate, platelet concentrate, fresh frozen plasma, or red blood cells, as ordered.

7. Protamine sulfate treats anticoagulation from inadequate heparin reversal. Platelet concentrate restores missing platelets, while fresh frozen plasma replaces platelets, clotting factors, and volume. Red blood cells provide hemoglobin.

8. Monitor for urine output greater than 1 liter/hour for the first 4 hours, or increasing output thereafter. Also observe for urine output less than 0.5 ml/kg/hour. Monitor specific gravity every 2 hours for the first 24 hours. Report abnormal urine output and specific gravity values. Monitor serum glucose levels, as ordered. Correlate glucose values with urine output.

8. Mannitol, usually administered during surgery to maintain cardiac output, produces osmotic diuresis. In addition, diuretics may be administered after surgery to eliminate retained fluid. Urine output may be as much as 1 liter/hour for the first 4 hours. Oliguria with high specific gravity may indicate hypovolemia, while oliguria with low specific gravity may indicate renal damage. Hyperglycemia results from stress-induced glycogenolysis and decreased insulin production, producing osmotic diuresis. Correlating glucose levels with urine output may identify hyperglycemia as the cause of excessive diuresis.

9. Additional individualized interventions: _____

9. Rationales: _____

Target outcome criteria
Within 3 hours after surgery, the patient will manifest chest tube drainage less than 200 ml/hour and declining.

Within 4 hours after surgery, the patient will have a urine output greater than 0.5 ml/kg/hour.

Within 24 hours after surgery, the patient will:
• display minimal drainage from incisions
• have vital signs within normal limits
• show hemoglobin levels, hematocrit, PT, PTT, and platelet levels returning to normal
• experience no signs or symptoms of excessive bleeding.

Collaborative problem: *High risk for hypoxemia related to alveolar collapse, increased pulmonary shunt, increased secretions, capillary leak, or pain*

NURSING PRIORITY: Maintain oxygenation and ventilation.

Interventions

1. Monitor pulmonary status and provide conscientious postoperative care to prevent pulmonary complications. Refer to the "Surgical Intervention" plan, page 81.

Rationales

1. Many factors place the patient undergoing cardiac surgery at risk for impaired gas exchange. Lung collapse during CPB results in atelectasis, and reduced surfactant production makes the lungs more difficult to expand after surgery. Hemodilution promotes interstitial fluid accumulation. CPB also activates complement and kinin systems, creating a capillary leak syndrome. Microcirculatory clotting increases pulmonary shunt. Anesthesia irritates the airways, increasing production of secretions, and depressed ciliary action impairs secretion removal. After surgery, lingering anesthetic effects and narcotics cause respiratory depression, while pain and splinting reduce lung expansion. As a result, close observation of pulmonary status and aggressive pulmonary hygiene are important after surgery. The "Surgical Intervention" plan details the nursing measures used to achieve these goals.

2. Monitor $S\bar{v}O_2$ through a pulmonary artery catheter to assess oxygen supply-demand balance.

2. Fiber-optic oximetry allows continuous monitoring of oxygen balance.

3. Monitor arterial oxygen saturation with pulse oximetry.

3. Monitoring arterial oxygen saturation alerts the clinician to potential hypoxemia.

4. Provide care according to the "Mechanical Ventilation" plan, page 227.

4. The patient undergoing cardiac surgery usually is mechanically ventilated for several hours after surgery to reexpand collapsed alveoli and lessen cardiopulmonary work load. The "Mechanical Ventilation" plan details appropriate nursing care.

5. Additional individualized interventions: _____

5. Rationales: _____

_____

_____

Target outcome criteria
Within 24 hours after surgery, the patient will:
• have a spontaneous respiratory rate of 12 to 24 breaths/minute
• maintain arterial blood gas levels within normal limits.

Nursing diagnosis: *High risk for sensory-perceptual alteration related to sensory overload or deprivation from unit environment, anesthesia, cerebral ischemia or infarction, or prolonged CPB*

NURSING PRIORITY: Optimize sensory-perceptual processing.

Interventions

1. Implement measures in the "Sensory-Perceptual Alteration" plan, page 75, as appropriate.

2. For the first 5 postoperative days, assess for indicators of sensory-perceptual alteration every 4 hours while the patient is awake or more frequently if the patient is disoriented. If present, reassure the patient and family that these alterations are usually transient, continue implementing the measures in the "Sensory-Perceptual Alteration" plan, and arrange for early transfer to a telemetry unit, if the patient's condition allows.

3. Assess for indicators of cerebral ischemia or infarction: change in mental status or level of consciousness (compare with preoperative status), motor weakness, hemiparesis, change in pupil size, or slurred speech.

4. Additional individualized interventions: _____

_____

Rationales

1. The "Sensory-Perceptual Alteration" plan describes interventions to reduce or eliminate sensory-perceptual dysfunction in any acutely ill patient.

2. Sensory-perceptual alteration may result from many factors in the critical care setting, including anxiety, sensory deprivation and overload, and sleep disruption; personality also plays a role. In addition, prolonged CPB, decreased cardiac output, hypotension, and vasoactive medications can contribute to disorientation. It usually resolves by the time the patient is transferred from the unit. Measures in the "Sensory-Perceptual Alteration" plan are helpful, as is early transfer to a less hectic environment.

3. Cerebrovascular accident is one of the most serious complications of open heart surgery. It is more common in older patients, who are more likely to have atherosclerotic disease of the aorta or carotid and vertebral arteries. Possible causes include carotid disease and emboli from the heart (thrombi, calcium fragments from diseased valves, or air remaining in the cardiac chambers).

4. Rationales: _____

_____

Target outcome criterion
By the end of the first postoperative week, the patient will return to a normal level of mentation.

Nursing diagnosis: *Knowledge deficit related to postoperative care*

NURSING PRIORITY: Educate the patient and family about the early postoperative period, as needed.

Interventions

1. Refer to the "Knowledge Deficit" plan, page 56.

2. Ascertain whether preoperative teaching was provided. If the patient and family did receive preoperative teaching, reinforce explanations, as necessary. If emergency surgery was performed, provide explanations as the opportunity arises.

3. Encourage questions.

4. Begin discharge planning. Evaluate needs for discharge teaching. Explain to the family that detailed discharge education will be done after discharge to the telemetry unit. Document and communicate needs to staff members on the new unit when the patient is transferred.

5. Tailor education to the nature of the patient's surgery. For CABG, teach about risk factors; life-style modifications related to diet, exercise, and stress; antiplatelet medication regimen (aspirin and dipyridamole). For valve repair or replacement, teach about signs and symptoms of infection, antibiotic prophylaxis before invasive procedures, anticoagulation medication (in patients with mechanical valves or history of chronic atrial fibrillation), signs and symptoms of valve failure, and signs and symptoms of thromboembolism

6. Additional individualized interventions: _____

Rationales

1. The "Knowledge Deficit" plan contains general information on assessing and meeting learning needs.

2. Before elective cardiac surgery, the patient and family usually receive extensive teaching. However, anxiety may limit retention of information, and for the patient, pain and medications affecting consciousness further limit recall. In emergency cardiac surgery, preoperative preparation is minimal, so teaching should be done as the opportunity arises.

3. Questions provide an opportunity for dealing with initial concerns, clarifying misconceptions, and eliminating knowledge gaps.

4. Discharge planning is most effective when awareness of its importance pervades all phases of the hospital stay. Detailed discharge education is most appropriate after the patient is physiologically stable. Early identification of needs sets the stage for later teaching, while documentation and communication enhance continuity of care.

5. An adult is more likely to learn information specific to personal needs. Coronary artery disease is progressive; knowledge of risk factors and potential life-style changes may retard disease progression. Antiplatelet medications decrease risk of thrombus formation and may maintain graft patency. The success of valve repair or replacement depends on both patient-related and prosthetic valve-related factors.

6. Rationales: _____

Target outcome criterion
Throughout the unit stay, the patient (after extubation) and family will verbalize questions and concerns.

Discharge planning

NURSING DISCHARGE CRITERIA

Upon the patient's discharge, documentation shows evidence of:
• blood pressure within normal limits for 12 hours without I.V. drugs
• normal sinus rhythm or acceptable variant for 12 hours without I.V. antiarrhythmic drugs

• CI, SVR, and other hemodynamic values within desired limits
• removal of pulmonary artery catheter, arterial line, chest tubes, and indwelling urinary catheter
• spontaneous ventilation within normal limits for at least 12 hours
• arterial blood gases, hemoglobin, hematocrit, electrolytes, and coagulation panel within normal limits.

PATIENT-FAMILY TEACHING CHECKLIST

Document evidence that the patient and family demonstrate an understanding of:
___ signs and symptoms of prosthetic valve malfunction
___ need for follow-up laboratory studies (PT if taking anticoagulants)
___ signs and symptoms of endocarditis
___ surgical procedure
___ anticipated postoperative course
___ rationale for interventions
___ common emotional reactions
___ medications (warfarin [Coumadin], antiplatelet therapy)
___ discharge planning.

DOCUMENTATION CHECKLIST

Using outcome criteria as a guide, document:
___ clinical status on admission
___ significant changes in status
___ pertinent diagnostic test findings
___ CI, SVR, and other hemodynamic parameters
___ diuretic, inotropic, or vasodilator administration
___ routine postoperative care
___ emotional response
___ fluid and electrolyte status
___ pulmonary care
___ complications, if any, and related interventions
___ patient-family teaching
___ discharge planning.

ASSOCIATED PLANS OF CARE

Cardiogenic Shock
Congestive Heart Failure
Grieving
Hypovolemic Shock
Impaired Physical Mobility
Ineffective Coping
Knowledge Deficit
Mechanical Ventilation
Pain
Sensory-Perceptual Alteration
Surgical Intervention

References

Berne, R., and Levy, M. *Cardiovascular Physiology,* 6th ed. St. Louis: Mosby-Year Book, 1991.

Guzzetta, C., and Dossey, B. *Cardiovascular Nursing: Holistic Practice.* St. Louis: Mosby-Year Book, 1992.

Hudak, C., et al. *Critical Care Nursing: A Holistic Approach,* 5th ed. Philadelphia: J.B. Lippincott Co., 1990.

Kinney, M., et al. *Comprehensive Cardiac Care,* 7th ed. St Louis: Mosby-Year Book, 1991.

Sabiston, D., and Spencer, F. *Surgery of the Chest,* 5th ed. Vols. I and II. Philadelphia: W.B. Saunders, 1990.

Seifert, P. "Cardiac Surgery," in *Alexander's Care of the Patient in Surgery,* 9th ed. Edited by Meeker, M., and Rothrock, J. St. Louis: Mosby-Year Book, 1991.

Seifert, P. "Surgery for Acquired Valvular Heart Disease," *Journal of Cardiovascular Nursing* 1(3):26-40, May 1987.

Shinn, J. "Cardiopulmonary Bypass," in *Nursing the Critically Ill Adult,* 3rd ed. Edited by Holloway, N. Menlo Park, CA: Addison-Wesley Publishing Co., 1988.

Thelan, L., et al. *Textbook of Critical Care Nursing: Diagnosis and Management.* St. Louis: Mosby-Year Book, 1990.

Underhill, S., et al. *Cardiac Nursing,* 2nd ed. Philadelphia: J.B. Lippincott Co., 1989.

Cardiogenic Shock

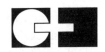

DRG information

DRG 121 Circulatory Disorders with Acute Myocardial Infarction and Cardiovascular Complication. Discharged Alive.
Mean LOS = 8.2 days

When an acute myocardial infarction (AMI) causes cardiogenic shock, or an AMI occurs later in the same admission, the AMI takes precedence in DRG grouping, with cardiogenic shock as the cardiovascular complication.

DRG 123 Circulatory Disorders with Acute Myocardial Infarction. Expired.
Mean LOS = 3.0 days

This DRG is used if the person with AMI dies.

DRG 127 Heart Failure and Shock.
Mean LOS = 6.2 days
Principal diagnoses include:
• heart failure
• shock without trauma.

Introduction
DEFINITION AND TIME FOCUS

Cardiogenic shock occurs when the heart fails to produce a cardiac output (CO) sufficient to meet metabolic demands, producing hypotension, vasoconstriction, and peripheral hypoperfusion. A major problem in critical care, cardiogenic shock usually results from a loss of 40% or more of functional myocardium, although it may result from heart failure from any cause. Signs and symptoms result from the backup of fluid behind the failing ventricle (backward failure) or from decreased stroke volume (forward failure). When CO is significantly decreased and physiologic compensatory mechanisms are ineffective, cardiogenic shock results. Because cardiogenic shock is associated with an 80% mortality rate, this plan focuses on the patient with acute heart failure and the interventions necessary to prevent or decrease the complications of cardiogenic shock.

ETIOLOGY AND PRECIPITATING FACTORS
• increased preload, such as in severe valvular stenosis or insufficiency, ruptured interventricular septum, papillary muscle rupture, or rupture of chordae tendineae
• decreased myocardial contractility, such as in massive AMI, cardiomyopathy, ventricular aneurysm, myocarditis, or cardiac tamponade
• increased afterload, such as in systemic hypertension, pulmonary hypertension, or massive pulmonary embolism
• severely abnormal heart rate, such as in severe tachycardia, bradycardia, or conduction disturbances

Focused assessment guidelines
NURSING HISTORY (Functional health pattern findings)

Health perception—health management pattern
• may report fatigue, weakness, or shortness of breath
• if under treatment for chronic congestive heart failure, may report failure to comply with low-salt diet or medication regimen

Nutritional-metabolic pattern
• may report anorexia, nausea, or vomiting

Activity-exercise pattern
• may report dyspnea on exertion or at rest
• may report palpitations
• may report dizziness or fainting (syncope)

Sleep-rest pattern
• may complain of insomnia, paroxysmal nocturnal dyspnea, or nocturia
• may report using several pillows to elevate head (orthopnea)

Coping—stress tolerance pattern
• may report marked anxiety, apprehension, or sense of impending doom

PHYSICAL FINDINGS
Cardiovascular
• hypotension
• tachycardia or other arrhythmias
• S_3 or S_4 heart sounds or both
• weak or irregular pulses
• decreased pulse pressure

Pulmonary
• crackles, usually bibasilar
• air hunger
• hyperventilation

Gastrointestinal
• decreased bowel sounds

Integumentary
• cyanosis
• diaphoresis
• pallor

Renal
• oliguria

DIAGNOSTIC STUDIES

• arterial blood gas (ABG) analysis—may reveal respiratory alkalosis (early stage) or hypoxemia and respiratory acidosis (late stage)
• serum digitalis level—may reveal subtherapeutic range
• 12-lead electrocardiography (ECG)—reveals sinus tachycardia, frequent premature ventricular contractions, atrial fibrillation, or other arrhythmias
• pulmonary artery pressures—reveal elevated pulmonary artery diastolic pressure and pulmonary capillary wedge pressure (PCWP)

• chest X-ray—reveals pulmonary infiltrates or cardiac enlargement
• complete blood count—may reveal dilutional changes
• gated blood pool imaging—may reveal reduced ejection fraction
• echocardiography—may reveal chamber enlargement, ventricular dyskinesia, or valvular abnormalities

POTENTIAL COMPLICATIONS

• cardiac arrest
• pulmonary edema
• fluid and electrolyte imbalance

Collaborative problem: *High risk for hypoxemia related to pulmonary congestion, decreased systemic perfusion, or both*

NURSING PRIORITY: Maintain optimal gas exchange.

Interventions

1. Monitor pulmonary status as needed, typically every 15 minutes until stable and then every 2 hours. Observe for:

• crackles, gurgles, wheezes, dyspnea, orthopnea, shallow respirations, accessory muscle use, cough, or S_3 or S_4 heart sounds

• tachypnea, cyanosis, restlessness, irritability, confusion, somnolence, or slow or irregular respirations

• elevated PCWP.

2. Monitor ABG values as ordered, typically every 4 hours until stable or as needed. Obtain chest X-rays, as ordered.

Rationales

1. Baseline and ongoing monitoring of pulmonary status provides data to guide priorities and interventions.

• Left ventricular end-diastolic pressure (LVEDP) most directly determines the strength of left ventricular contraction and the resulting adequacy of stroke volume. As the heart fails, decreased ventricular compliance raises LVEDP beyond the optimal stretch of myocardial fibers and, according to the Frank-Starling mechanism, optimal contractility. The elevated LVEDP is transferred to the pulmonary capillary bed and increases hydrostatic pressure in pulmonary capillaries, producing pulmonary congestion (backward failure). Elevated pulmonary capillary hydrostatic pressure causes fluid to shift across capillary walls into the interstitium and eventually into the alveoli. Crackles may result when pulmonary interstitial fluids compress the alveoli or when fluid accumulates in them. Gurgles and wheezes indicate fluid accumulation in the large airways. Interstitial edema produces dyspnea, shallow respirations, and accessory muscle use, while alveolar edema produces orthopnea, and cough. S_3 and S_4 heart sounds reflect decreased ventricular compliance or volume overload.

• Fluid-filled alveoli cannot oxygenate the capillary blood flowing past them, producing a pulmonary shunt and hypoxemia. Tachypnea is an early compensatory mechanism for hypoxemia, while cyanosis is a late sign. Decreased CO (forward failure) produces cerebral ischemia, resulting in an altered level of consciousness. Ischemia of medullary and pontine respiratory centers causes altered breathing patterns.

• PCWP correlates with the degree of pulmonary congestion. Usually, a PCWP of 18 to 20 mm Hg correlates with the onset of congestion, 20 to 25 mm Hg with moderate congestion, 25 to 30 mm Hg with severe congestion, and more than 30 mm Hg with pulmonary edema.

2. ABG values provide evidence of hypoxemia and accompanying respiratory and metabolic acidosis, while chest X-rays provide evidence of pulmonary fluid infiltration.

3. If pulmonary congestion is present, place the patient in semi- or high-Fowler's position.

3. Elevating the head of the bed improves diaphragmatic excursion, facilitating ventilation.

4. Administer supplemental oxygen, as ordered, typically by nasal cannula at 6 liters/minute. If the patient has chronic obstructive pulmonary disease (COPD), administer at 2 liters/minute.

4. Supplemental oxygen helps saturate hemoglobin, raising arterial oxygen content and improving oxygen transport. A cannula is less likely to produce the feelings of suffocation that an air-hungry patient experiences with a mask. A high oxygen flow rate can suppress the hypoxic drive to breathe in a COPD patient and induce respiratory arrest.

5. Monitor peripheral oxygen saturation (SPO_2) continuously by pulse oximetry.

5. Continuous pulse oximetry is a safe, noninvasive method for early detection of hypoxemia. SPO_2 reflects arterial oxygen saturation (SaO_2). SPO_2 trends provide important information about the effects of therapy on SaO_2.

6. Suction as needed.

6. In heart failure, the lungs may produce sputum so rapidly that the patient cannot clear it spontaneously. Prompt suctioning not only improves gas exchange but also lessens the patient's anxiety.

7. Assist with insertion of a pulmonary artery (PA) catheter, as ordered. A fiberoptic PA catheter for continuous venous oxygen saturation ($S\bar{v}O_2$) monitoring may be indicated.

7. The multiple therapies used in cardiogenic shock can affect the determinants of CO. Interpreting these effects based on clinical signs alone can be confusing. A PA catheter allows objective CO measurement and PCWP monitoring. PCWP monitoring is particularly important because it provides the most direct bedside indication of left ventricular function. In mitral valve or pulmonary disease, however, PCWP does not necessarily reflect left ventricular performance. $S\bar{v}O_2$ monitoring continuously reflects CO and helps determine if the body's oxygen supply can meet tissue oxygen demand. Evaluation of tissue oxygenation provides early identification of hemodynamic changes and immediate evaluation of therapeutic interventions.

8. Monitor PA pressure every hour, PCWP every 2 hours, and cardiac index (CI) every 4 hours, or as ordered. (CI equals CO divided by body surface area, determined from a DuBois nomogram). Note both individual values and trends.

8. Objective measurements of PCWP and PA diastolic pressure provide a means of evaluating left ventricular filling pressure, while CI indicates adequacy of CO. CI takes the patient's size into consideration, so it provides a more precise indication of the adequacy of CO than does CO alone. Isolated values provide immediate data, while trends indicate whether cardiogenic shock is resolving or worsening over time.

9. Determine the presence and severity of heart failure according to PCWP and CI. (See *Classification of heart failure by hemodynamic subsets*.)

9. Classification by hemodynamic status is used to distinguish disease patterns and plan therapy.

10. Anticipate medical therapy. Administer therapy as ordered.

10. Anticipation of therapy allows systematic planning and adequate patient preparation. Goals and therapeutic measures follow logically from the characteristics of each subset.

• For patients with no signs of failure (Subset I), observe for its development.

• Patients in Subset I have acceptable PCWP and CI. However, because critically ill patients decompensate rapidly, continuing observation is warranted.

• For patients with pulmonary congestion only (Subset II), administer medication, as ordered.

• Patients in Subset II have an elevated PCWP and good CI. Drug therapy is designed to decrease circulating blood volume, thereby relieving pulmonary congestion.

• If blood pressure is normal, administer diuretics, typically furosemide (Lasix) or bumetanide (Bumex). Document effectiveness and monitor for side effects, especially excessive diuresis or electrolyte imbalances (particularly hypokalemia).

• Diuretics reduce preload rapidly and effectively, improving ventricular compliance. Because diuretics block renal fluid reabsorption and increase renal tubular flow, potassium excretion increases. Excessive diuresis and hypokalemia are exaggerations of diuretics' therapeutic effects.

CLASSIFICATION OF HEART FAILURE BY HEMODYNAMIC SUBSETS

Subset	Classification
• Subset I: pulmonary capillary wedge pressure (PCWP) 18 mm Hg and cardiac index (CI) 2.2 liters/minute/m² (no failure)	• A PCWP of 18 mm Hg is the level above which signs of pulmonary congestion appear and a CI of 2.2 liters/minute/m² is the level below which signs of peripheral hypoperfusion appear. Increased PCWP and depressed CI are the "final common pathways" for almost all signs of heart failure. In Subset I, a relatively normal PCWP and CI indicate the absence of heart failure.
• Subset II: PCWP greater than18 mm Hg and CI greater than 2.2 liters/minute/m² (pulmonary congestion)	• In Subset II, PCWP is elevated, but CI is relatively normal. Clinically, the patient shows signs of pulmonary congestion.
• Subset III: PCWP less than 18 mm Hg and CI less than 2.2 liters/minute/m² (peripheral hypoperfusion)	• In Subset III, PCWP is relatively normal, but CI is depressed. Clinically, the patient shows signs of peripheral hypoperfusion.
• Subset IV: PCWP greater than 18 mm Hg and CI less than 2.2 liters/minute/m² (pulmonary congestion and peripheral hypoperfusion)	• In Subset IV, PCWP is elevated and CI is depressed. Clinically, the patient presents with both pulmonary congestion and peripheral hypoperfusion.

From: Forrester, J., et al. "Medical Therapy of Acute MI by Application of Hemodynamic Subsets," *New England Journal of Medicine* 295(23): 1356-62, December 1976. Used with permission.

CARDIOVASCULAR DISORDERS

• If blood pressure is elevated, administer vasodilators, typically:

—venodilators, such as nitroglycerin or morphine. Observe for and report side effects, especially hypotension and, with morphine, respiratory depression.

—arteriolar dilators, such as sodium nitroprusside (Nipride). Monitor for and report side effects, especially hypotension, signs of hypoxemia, and thiocyanate and cyanide toxicity.

• When blood pressure is high enough to cause pulmonary congestion and reduce oxygenation, the patient's condition is too serious to wait for the action of diuretics. By expanding the vascular bed, vasodilators allow the vessels to accommodate the same amount of fluid in a larger area, thus lowering pressure. Vasodilation also lowers preload, which improves left ventricular performance.

—Nitroglycerin produces significant venodilation and relatively little arteriolar dilation. Used primarily for its venodilating properties, nitroglycerin decreases preload and pulmonary congestion. It also redistributes myocardial blood flow, causing greater dilation of large vessels than of small ones, thus increasing flow to ischemic areas. As myocardial perfusion improves, more efficient contraction increases CO. Morphine, the drug of choice in pulmonary edema, also induces vasodilation. The resulting reductions in preload, afterload, and myocardial work all improve CO. Morphine also induces euphoria, particularly helpful in lessening the severe anxiety present with pulmonary edema.

—Although sodium nitroprusside dilates both arteriolar and venous beds, it is used primarily for its arteriolar effects. Because sodium nitroprusside reduces afterload, systolic emptying is improved and myocardial work decreases. As a result, it produces a greater increase in CO than nitroglycerin. Hypotension results from excessive dosage. Hypoxemia may result from reversal of pulmonary vasoconstriction, a compensatory mechanism that shunts blood to better-aerated alveoli. Thiocyanate and cyanide toxicity may develop from accumulation of toxic metabolites with long-term use, high dosage, or impaired liver or renal perfusion.

11. If administering morphine sulfate, observe for and report hypotension, nausea, and vomiting. Titrate doses to achieve desired effects without causing respiratory depression.

11. Morphine decreases pain, anxiety, catecholamine stimulation, and tachypnea, lessening the work of breathing. In a patient with respiratory center depression, however, they cause further depression and may trigger respiratory arrest. Titrating doses minimizes the risk of side effects. Morphine sulfate decreases the brain's oxygen requirement by nearly 50%, thereby decreasing the arterial blood flow required to oxygenate the brain. Antiemetics may be administered with morphine sulfate to control nausea and vomiting.

12. Alert the doctor immediately if the patient develops severe dyspnea, pink frothy sputum, marked neck-vein distention, or describes a sense of impending doom.

12. These findings indicate pulmonary edema, a life-threatening condition. Immediate medical intervention is crucial.

13. Additional individualized interventions: _____

13. Rationales: _____

Target outcome criteria
Within 3 days, the patient will:
- show no signs or symptoms of hypoxemia
- have ABG levels within normal limits
- display a level of consciousness similar to or better than that before admission
- be free from restlessness, irritability, confusion, or somnolence

- have a PCWP within normal limits
- have lungs clear to auscultation
- have a normal chest X-ray.

Collaborative problem: *Inadequate CO related to heart rate abnormalities or diminished contractility*

NURSING PRIORITY: Maintain adequate CO.

Interventions

1. Observe for signs and symptoms of decreased CO, such as:

- arterial hypotension, tachycardia, narrowed pulse pressure, weak peripheral pulses

- restlessness, irritability, confusion, somnolence

- weakness and fatigue

- cool, mottled, or cyanotic skin

- decreased urine output.

Rationales

1. Cardiogenic shock is considered a form of heart failure because of several interrelated mechanisms. Decreased contractility makes the heart unable to move blood efficiently. The resulting distention causes ventricular fibers to exceed optimal stretch according to the Frank-Starling curve, so the ejection fraction falls and systemic perfusion suffers. Failure of the left ventricle affects all body systems.

- Systemic vascular resistance (SVR) increases initially in an attempt to maintain mean arterial pressure. Pulse pressure narrows because the decreased CO lowers systolic pressure, while the increased SVR elevates diastolic pressure. Tachycardia, although a compensatory response to decreased CO, may actually impair it further by limiting ventricular filling time.

- Changes in level of consciousness or mentation reflect cerebral hypoxemia or ischemia.

- Weakness and fatigue result from diminished skeletal muscle perfusion, excessive work of breathing, and sleep disturbances.

- Skin changes reflect shunting away from skeletal muscles as the body attempts to preserve perfusion of core organs.

- Decreased urine output reflects diminished renal perfusion resulting from decreased circulating blood volume and intense sympathetic vasoconstriction of afferent arterioles.

2. Monitor the ECG continuously. Document and report significant findings (see Appendix A, "Monitoring Standards," for details).

3. For patients with hypoperfusion only (Subset III):

• If heart rate is elevated, administer fluids. Document effectiveness and observe for side effects, especially fluid overload.

• If heart rate is depressed, assist with pacemaker insertion. Document effectiveness and observe for pacemaker malfunction.

4. For patients with pulmonary congestion and peripheral hypoperfusion (Subset IV), administer medications, as ordered.

• If blood pressure is depressed, administer positive inotropes, typically:

— digitalis preparations. Observe for and report signs of toxicity, including gastrointestinal distress, bradycardia, atrioventricular block, premature beats, and atrial tachycardia with block.

— dopamine hydrochloride (Intropin). Observe for and report hypotension, tachyarrhythmias, ectopic beats, vasoconstriction with high doses, and I.V. fluid infiltration.

— dobutamine hydrochloride (Dobutrex). Monitor for and report side effects, especially tachycardia and arrhythmias.

— combined inotrope and vasodilator therapy, such as dopamine and sodium nitroprusside or amrinone (Inocor). With dopamine and sodium nitroprusside, monitor for and report adverse reactions, especially chest pain or increased ventricular arrhythmias. With amrinone, observe for and report adverse reactions, including arrhythmias, hypotension, and GI distress.

• If blood pressure is normal, administer vasodilators. See the "High risk for hypoxemia" collaborative problem above for details.

2. Because CO depends on the heart rate and stroke volume, arrhythmias can affect CO significantly; a dramatic drop in CO can cause cardiac arrest. Continuous monitoring allows for prompt treatment of arrhythmias.

3. Measures for patients in Subset III are designed to increase CO, thereby increasing peripheral perfusion.

• Tachycardia is a primary compensatory response to hypovolemia. Administering fluid increases preload and thus increases CO. The resulting increase in circulating blood volume restores peripheral perfusion and relieves tachycardia because as stroke volume increases, heart rate returns to normal.

• Because heart rate is a primary determinant of CO, bradycardia with hypoperfusion indicates a need to restore the normal heart rate. Pacemaker insertion provides an immediate way to increase the heart rate while the underlying problem, such as heart block, is identified and resolved.

4. Patients in Subset IV have an elevated PCWP and depressed CI, so the treatment goals are to lower PCWP and improve CI.

• Elevated PCWP, depressed CI, and depressed blood pressure strongly suggest depressed myocardial contractility. Positive inotropic agents increase myocardial contractility, thus improving CI and lowering PCWP as fluid is moved more efficiently through the heart.

— Digitalis improves contractility, but it also slows heart rate and cardiac conduction. It also may provoke various arrhythmias by increasing automaticity.

— Dopamine has complex dose-related pharmacologic actions. In heart failure, midrange doses of dopamine (2 to 10 mcg/kg/minute) increase renal perfusion via dopaminergic effects, and increase heart rate and contractility via beta$_1$-adrenergic stimulating effects.

— Dobutamine, primarily a direct beta$_1$ stimulator, is a potent inotropic agent with less effect on heart rate than dopamine. As such, it significantly improves contractility with less tendency to cause arrhythmias than dopamine.

— Two synergistic drugs improve CO better and more safely than either agent used alone. For example, dopamine and sodium nitroprusside in combination reduce preload, augment contractility, and reduce afterload better than if used singly. However, both agents may decrease myocardial oxygen supply. Amrinone has both inotropic and vasodilating properties that lessen pulmonary congestion and improve CO. It is used commonly for short-term management of heart failure patients unresponsive to other therapies.

• Patients with congestion, hypoperfusion, and normal blood pressure may benefit from afterload reduction achieved through vasodilation.

5. For patients in Subsets III and IV who do not respond to fluid and drug therapy, assist with intra-aortic balloon pump (IABP) counter pulsation. Monitor augmentation as necessary, every 15 minutes until stable and then every hour. Document the effectiveness of counterpulsation, and observe for complications and IABP malfunction.

5. IABP counterpulsation increases coronary artery perfusion, contractility, and vital organ perfusion and reduces afterload and myocardial oxygen demand. Balloon inflation during diastole displaces blood from the aorta, augmenting coronary artery and peripheral perfusion by increasing the diastolic pressure. Balloon deflation at the end of diastole decreases pressure in the ascending aorta, thus reducing LVEDP and work load.

6. Additional individualized interventions: _____

6. Rationales: _____

Target outcome criteria
Within 3 days, the patient will have:
• blood pressure within normal limits
• heart rate within normal limits, ideally 60 to 80 beats/ minute

• CI greater than 2.2 liters/minute/m^2 and PCWP less than 18 mm Hg
• strong, bilaterally equal peripheral pulses.

Nursing diagnosis: *Activity intolerance related to hypoxemia, weakness, or diminished cardiovascular reserve*

NURSING PRIORITY: Promote rest.

Interventions

1. Assess for signs and symptoms of activity intolerance, such as heart rate increase greater than 25%, blood pressure increase greater than 25%, any heart rate or blood pressure decrease, chest pain, arrhythmias, decreased level of consciousness, or complaints of weakness or fatigue.

2. Place the patient on complete bed rest. Assist with activity, as needed. Implement measures in the "Impaired Physical Mobility" plan, page 36, as appropriate.

3. Pace nursing care to promote rest. If possible, allow at least 90 minutes of uninterrupted sleep at a time.

4. When the patient's condition stabilizes, increase activity gradually, as ordered.

• Maintain supplemental oxygen.

• Monitor the patient's response to increased activity. Slow or discontinue activity progression if the patient shows any signs of intolerance.

5. Additional individualized interventions: _____

Rationales

1. A dysfunctional myocardium may be unable to adjust stroke volume and oxygen during exertion. The unmet oxygen needs may cause tachycardia and myocardial or cerebral ischemia. Anaerobic metabolism resulting from impaired skeletal muscle perfusion results in weakness or fatigue.

2. Bed rest decreases myocardial work load. Assisting with activity conserves cardiovascular and energy reserves. The "Impaired Physical Mobility" plan contains measures to counteract the complications of immobility.

3. The numerous medical and nursing measures necessary to treat heart failure and cardiogenic shock may interrupt rest and exhaust the patient. The average sleep cycle lasts 90 minutes. Providing at least this much uninterrupted rest at a time allows the patient to progress through both rapid eye movement (REM) sleep, which helps restore psychological equilibrium, and non-REM sleep, which helps restore physiologic well-being.

4. A gradual activity increase allows neurovascular compensatory mechanisms to adjust to increased demands.

• Supplemental oxygen helps meet increased tissue oxygen demands during exercise.

• Close monitoring allows the nurse to match exercise level with energy resources.

5. Rationales: _____

> **Target outcome criterion**
> By time of discharge, the patient will show no signs or symptoms of activity intolerance during self-care activities.

Discharge planning

NURSING DISCHARGE CRITERIA

Upon the patient's discharge, documentation shows evidence of:
• blood pressure within 30 mm Hg of normal value for at least 12 hours without I.V. vasodilators
• no significant arrhythmias for at least 12 hours without I.V. antiarrhythmic agents
• stable hemodynamic status for at least 12 hours without IABP counterpulsation
• absence of arterial and PA line
• stable respiratory status for at least 12 hours without mechanical ventilation.

PATIENT-FAMILY TEACHING CHECKLIST

Document evidence that the patient and family demonstrate understanding of:
___ cause and implications of cardiogenic shock
___ purpose of medications
___ rationales for other therapeutic interventions
___ need for continued treatment of underlying cause, including life-style modifications if appropriate.

DOCUMENTATION CHECKLIST

Using outcome criteria as a guide, document:
___ clinical status on admission
___ significant changes in status
___ pertinent laboratory and diagnostic test findings
___ hemodynamic measurements
___ oxygen therapy
___ response to cardiac assist devices, such as a pacemaker or IABP
___ fluid therapy or restrictions
___ response to inotropes, vasodilators, or other drugs
___ dietary modifications
___ activity restrictions
___ patient-family teaching
___ discharge planning.

ASSOCIATED PLANS OF CARE

Acute Myocardial Infarction—Critical Care Unit Phase
Hypovolemic Shock
Impaired Physical Mobility
Knowledge Deficit

References

Forrester, J., et al. "Medical Therapy of Acute MI by Application of Hemodynamic Subsets," *New England Journal of Medicine* 295(23):1356-62, December 1976.

Hardy, G. "Assessment Techniques: SvO$_2$ Continuous Monitoring Techniques," *DCCN: Dimensions in Critical Care Nursing* 7(1):8-17, January-February, 1988.

Holloway, N., and Kern, L. "Cardiovascular Disorders," in *Nursing the Critically Ill Adult,* 3rd ed. Edited by Holloway, N. Menlo Park, Calif.: Addison-Wesley Publishing Co., 1988.

Joseph, D., and Bastes, S. "Intra-Aortic Balloon Pumping: How to Stay on Course," *American Journal of Nursing* 90(9):42-47, September, 1990.

Kenner, C., Guzzetta, C., and Dossey, B. *Critical Care Nursing: Body-Mind-Spirit*, 2nd ed. Boston, MA: Little, Brown and Co., 1985.

Roberts, S. "Cardiogenic Shock: Decreased Coronary Artery Tissue Perfusion," *DCCN: Dimensions in Critical Care Nursing* 7(4):196-207, July-August, 1988.

Szaflarski, N., and Cohen, N. "Use of Pulse Oximetry in Critically Ill Adults," *Heart & Lung* 18(5):444-53, September 1989.

CARDIOVASCULAR DISORDERS

Carotid Endarterectomy

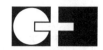

DRG information
DRG 005 Extracranial Vascular Procedures.
> Mean LOS = 5.8 days
> Includes Carotid Endarterectomy with synthetic or tissue patch graft.

Introduction
DEFINITION AND TIME FOCUS
Carotid endarterectomy is the surgical removal of atherosclerotic plaque from the inner lining of the carotid artery to widen the vessel lumen. Endarterectomy increases cerebral blood flow and reduces the risk of cerbrovascular accident (CVA).

The surgical incision is made along the anterior sternocleidomastoid muscle to expose the carotid bifurcation, the most common site of plaque formation. The diseased artery is dissected away from surrounding tissue and nerves and clamped above and below the obstruction. Once the plaque is removed, the artery is sutured or closed with a vein or synthetic polyester (Dacron) patch graft.

Carotid endarterectomy is generally viewed as preventive surgery and is best performed before the patient shows significant neurologic loss. The patient may have had transient ischemic attacks (TIAs) or a CVA with minimal residual neurologic deficits. Symptoms usually occur when the artery is 70% occluded.

This plan focuses on the immediate postoperative care of a patient undergoing elective carotid endarterectomy for an atherosclerotic lesion of an internal carotid artery.

ETIOLOGY AND PRECIPITATING FACTORS
Atherosclerosis is the underlying cause in 90% of extracranial carotid disease, resulting in partial or complete occlusion. Indicators for surgery include:
• TIAs or reversible ischemic neurologic deficits (RINDS) with arteriographic evidence of an atherosclerotic carotid lesion. TIAs and RINDs usually affect the face and extremities on the side opposite the involved cerebral hemisphere as a result of temporarily insufficient blood supply to focal brain areas. TIAs resolve in 24 hours or less with no residual deficits, while RINDs last from 24 hours to a week.
• CVA from a carotid lesion with severe stenosis of the internal carotid artery and a good recovery (mild or no residual neurologic deficits) at least five weeks after the CVA. A CVA is characterized by hemiplegia and sensory loss on the side of the body opposite the involved hemisphere and visual field defects on the same side as the involved hemisphere.

• asymptomatic carotid bruits with severe stenosis of one internal carotid artery and total occlusion of the opposite carotid artery, bilateral stenosis, a markedly ulcerated plaque, or stenosis in the artery to the dominant hemisphere
• recurrence of stenosis after endarterectomy

Focused assessment guidelines
NURSING HISTORY (Functional health pattern findings)

Health perception—health management pattern
• may have history of TIAs, RINDs, or completed CVA
• may be under treatment for hypertension or diabetes mellitus
• may have history of atherosclerosis elsewhere, such as coronary artery disease (angina) or peripheral arterial occlusive disease (intermittent claudication)
• may have history of acute myocardial infarction (AMI)
• may have risk factors such as smoking, obesity, and sedentary life-style; high stress levels; high serum cholesterol, lipoprotein, and triglyceride levels; vasospasms of cerebral arteries; clotting abnormalities; polycythemia; or substance abuse
• if a black male, at increased risk
• if over age 45, at increased risk; if over age 65, risk increases further
• may not comply with antihypertensive regimen or may not have sought medical attention for many years

Nutritional-metabolic pattern
• may describe diet high in calories, fat, cholesterol, and salt
• may report transient or ongoing difficulty swallowing

Elimination pattern
• may report transient or ongoing bowel or bladder incontinence

Activity-exercise pattern
• with history of TIAs, RINDs, or CVA, may describe sedentary life-style and lack of regular exercise because of transient visual deficits (blurred vision, diplopia, blindness in one eye, or tunnel vision), motor deficits (contralateral weakness or paralysis in arm, hand, or leg), or vertigo (less common); may have minimal residual deficits that interfere with activity and exercise
• may be afraid of falling because of previous TIAs, RINDs, or CVA

Cognitive-perceptual pattern
• may report dizziness
• may report slowed mentation or clumsiness associated with prior TIAs or CVA

Sleep-rest pattern
• with history of TIAs or CVA as a result of thrombosis, symptoms may have developed during sleep or shortly after awakening

Self-perception — self-concept pattern
• may report altered self-concept, particularly if residual neurologic deficits are present

Role-relationship pattern
• may report fear of inability to perform usual roles because of residual neurologic deficits or fear that TIA or CVA will occur during role performance

PHYSICAL FINDINGS
Clinical manifestations will vary depending on the extent of the disease at the bifurcation and the adequacy of collateral blood supply to the affected area. The patient may remain asymptomatic if there is sufficient collateral blood supply.

General appearance
• may have some residual facial drooping from CVA

Neurologic
• transient motor and sensory deficits, such as numbness, weakness, or paralysis of the face, hand, arm, or leg on the side opposite the lesion (contralateral); less commonly, gait disturbance (ataxia)
• visual deficits, such as transient scotoma (area of poor vision surrounded by normal vision), tunnel vision, diplopia, blurred vision, or amaurosis fugax (transient blindness in one eye, lasting 10 minutes or less) on same side as affected carotid artery
• speech difficulties, such as transient motor or expressive aphasia if the dominant hemisphere is involved

Cardiovascular
• hypertension
• carotid bruit localized to site of carotid bifurcation: characteristically loud, harsh, high-pitched systolic murmur that extends into diastole, associated with a decreased carotid pulse (no bruit is heard in about 20% of patients with significant obstruction of internal carotid artery)
• decreased facial and superficial temporal pulses on side of lesion

Musculoskeletal
• minimal residual weakness on side opposite lesion

DIAGNOSTIC STUDIES
Screening tests are recommended prior to arteriography. Commonly used noninvasive tests include:

• oculoplethysmography — reveals significant disruption of blood flow to the ophthalmic artery, an important branch of the internal carotid artery, when carotid stenosis is present
• B-mode ultrasonography — reveals restricted blood flow when carotid stenosis is present
• carotid Doppler ultrasound — differentiates thrombotic from ulcerative plaques in the stenosed carotid artery
• Doppler imaging — detects abnormal carotid blood flow and ulcerative plaques within carotid arteries; highly accurate
• carotid phonoangiography — identifies origin of bruits and estimates severity of stenosis
• computed tomography scan — reveals ischemia and hemorrhage and identifies other causes of symptoms (such as tumors, hematomas, or cerebral aneurysms); discovery of a cerebral infarction may alter timing of surgery and indicate need for an intraluminal shunt during surgery; serves as baseline in event of perioperative neurologic deficit

Commonly used invasive tests include:
• digital subtraction angiography (DSA) — provides anatomic detail of the aortic arch, subclavian and vertebral arteries, and extracranial carotid arteries; identifies moderate to severe carotid artery stenosis; may be used in place of standard angiography for the asymptomatic patient in whom noninvasive tests demonstrate a significant stenosis; if DSA appears normal in symptomatic patients, standard angiography should be performed because minor stenoses and small ulcerations may be overlooked
• cerebral arteriography — identifies exact location and extent of atherosclerotic lesions; indicated if noninvasive screening reveals severe obstruction with harsh, bilateral bruits or progressive atherosclerosis elsewhere (recommended for all patients being considered for surgery)
• blood urea nitrogen and creatinine levels — monitor renal function before and after angiography or DSA, because dyes used in these tests may affect renal function
• hemoglobin level and hematocrit — provide baseline for comparison with postoperative values to detect bleeding
• coagulation panel — may be increased if the patient takes antiplatelet medications, such as aspirin, before surgery provides a baseline for comparison with postoperative values to detect clotting abnormalities
• electrolyte panel — provides a baseline for comparison with postoperative values because electrolyte imbalances may occur after surgery (existing electrolyte imbalances are corrected before surgery)
• arterial blood gases (ABGs) — provide a baseline for comparison because hypoxemia is a major concern after surgery
• electrocardiography (ECG), treadmill exercise test, myocardial perfusion scans, and coronary angiography — screen for cardiac disease (AMI is the leading cause of death after carotid endarterectomy)

POTENTIAL COMPLICATIONS
• blood pressure lability (hypertension most common, hypotension less common)
• AMI
• cerebral ischemia or CVA
• cranial nerve injury
• airway obstruction secondary to hemorrhage and hematoma formation
• acute respiratory insufficiency

• hyperperfusion syndromes (rare), such as ipsilateral vascular type headaches, seizures, or intracerebral hemorrhage
• increased intracranial pressure secondary to cerebral hemorrhage
• rarely, vocal cord paralysis
• infection

Collaborative problem: *Blood pressure lability related to carotid sinus dysfunction, hypovolemia secondary to intraoperative or postoperative bleeding or fluid imbalance, acute myocardial infarction (AMI), or hypoxia*

NURSING PRIORITY: Maintain blood pressure within prescribed limits.

Interventions

1. Assess blood pressure every 15 minutes for the first hour, then every hour or as needed for the first 24 hours after surgery. Ideally, use an arterial line for the first 24 hours or until the blood pressure stabilizes. If medication is needed to control blood pressure, assess blood pressure every 15 to 30 minutes, and as needed.

2. Implement measures to control hypertension:
• Administer antihypertensive medications, such as sodium nitroprusside (Nipride), to maintain a systolic blood pressure at 120 to 150 mm Hg, diastolic blood pressure at 70 to 90 mm Hg, or mean arterial pressure (MAP) at 86 to 110 mm Hg, or as ordered. Notify the doctor immediately if the medication cannot maintain blood pressure within this range.
• Administer pain medication as ordered.
• Provide a quiet, restful environment.
• Maintain activity restrictions as ordered, usually bedrest for the first 24 hours.
• Maintain fluid restrictions as ordered.

3. Implement measures to control hypotension:

• Assess fluid intake and output every hour or as needed for the first 24 hours. If a pulmonary artery catheter is in place, assess cardiac output, wedge pressure, and central venous pressure every hour or as needed for the first 24 hours.

• If hypotension results from fluid loss, replace fluids as ordered.

• Assess for evidence of AMI (ECG changes, elevated creatine phosphokinase (CPK) and positive CPK-MB isoenzyme levels, and chest pain); if hypotension is caused by AMI, see the "Acute Myocardial Infarction—Critical Care Unit Phase" plan, page 268, for further interventions.

Rationales

1. Baroreceptors at the carotid bifurcation normally control blood pressure. Surgical manipulation of these baroreceptors may impair carotid sinus reflexes, causing blood pressure instability. Additionally, hypovolemia and hypoxia contribute to fluctuating blood pressure. If uncontrolled, extreme hypertension or hypotension can cause a CVA. Blood pressure is most accurately measured with an arterial line.

2. Surgical trauma may render the carotid sinus insensitive to increasing blood pressure, resulting in hypertension. Because surgery increases blood supply to the cerebrum, capillaries are more prone to rupture when hypertension occurs, causing intracerebral bleeding and cerebral infarction. As blood pressure exceeds the limits of cerebral autoregulation (MAP of 60 to 120 mm Hg), increased pressure forces more blood into the cerebrum, leading to increased intracranial pressure and cerebral ischemia (see the "Increased Intracranial Pressure" plan, page 134). Research shows that stimuli (particularly noxious stimuli), hypervolemia, pain, and stress increase blood pressure. Hypertension may also cause the graft site to rupture.

3. Hypotension is less common after surgery than hypertension. The carotid sinus may be hypersensitive after surgery if the removed plaque had been dampening pressure signals. Frequent checks of the indicated parameters alert the nurse to hypotension and help differentiate between two common causes, hypovolemia and AMI.

• Frequent assessment provides early warning of developing problems.

• Fluid volume replacement increases cardiac output, thus increasing blood pressure and cerebral perfusion.

• Hypotension may result from fluid deficit or myocardial dysfunction.

• Administer vasopressors, such as dopamine (Intropin) or dobutamine (Dobutrex), to maintain blood pressure within the limits specified above, as ordered.

• Administer pain medications judiciously.

• Monitor the incision and drainage system for bleeding and drainage.

4. Maintain oxygenation as ordered, usually 2 to 5 liters by nasal cannula after extubation.

5. Additional individualized interventions: _____

_____

• Hypotension, whether caused by hypovolemia or decreased contractility with an AMI, results in decreased cerebral perfusion, decreased oxygenation, and cerebral ischemia and possible infarction. Short-acting drugs such as dopamine or dobutamine increase cardiac contractility, thus increasing cardiac output and blood pressure.

• Pain medications keep the patient comfortable while maintaining blood pressure within desired limits.

• Excessive bleeding or drainage indicates the need for prompt intervention to prevent hypovolemia.

4. Hypoxemia contributes to blood pressure fluctuations because the heart rate increases to supply additional oxygen to vital organs, thus increasing cardiac output and blood pressure. Conversely, if the carotid body has been damaged, there may be a loss of the normal circulatory response to hypoxia. Because hypoxia causes the cerebral arteries to dilate, blood flow to the cerebrum increases, potentially increasing intracranial pressure and causing ischemia.

5. Rationales: _____

_____

Target outcome criteria
Within 24 hours after surgery, the patient will:
• maintain systolic or diastolic blood pressure or MAP within desired limits without antihypertensive or vasopressor drugs
• exhibit fluid balance, as evidenced by approximately equal intake and output, blood pressure within desired limits, and pulmonary artery pressures within normal limits

• have ABGs within normal limits
• exhibit little or no bleeding from the surgical site.

Collaborative problem: *High risk for cerebral ischemia related to carotid artery clamping during surgery or vasospasm from clamping and manipulating cerebral vessels, hypovolemia secondary to blood loss, cerebral vessel compression from hematoma or edema, cerebral embolization from manipulation of the arteries, marked fluctuations in blood pressure, or thrombosis at the endarterectomy site*

NURSING PRIORITY: Prevent or minimize cerebral ischemia.

Interventions

1. Assess level of consciousness, orientation, pupillary reaction, and motor and sensory function hourly or as needed for the first 24 hours. Document and report immediately decreased level of consciousness; change in orientation; pupillary changes, such as unequal pupils, a sluggish or absent pupillary reaction to light, or pupil deviated from midline position; motor and sensory deficits such as paresthesias, motor weakness, or contralateral hemiparesis; and slurred speech or seizures. When the patient is fully recovered from anesthesia, report any visual disturbances (such as blurred or dimmed vision, diplopia, or ipsilateral change in visual field) or headache.

Rationales

1. Cerebral ischemia or infarction is a major concern after endarterectomy. Depending on the extent of ischemia, symptoms vary from mild ischemia to CVA. Assessing frequently for signs of decreased cerebral perfusion reduces the risk of permanent damage, as appropriate action can be taken immediately.

2. Assess blood pressure, pulse, and respiratory rate hourly or as needed for the first 24 hours after surgery. Report increased or decreased pulse rate, marked fluctuations in blood pressure, and changes in respiratory rate and pattern (refer to the "High risk for hypoxemia" and "Blood pressure lability" problems in this plan).

3. Assess for patency of the internal carotid artery by lightly palpating the superficial temporal and facial arteries hourly, or by monitoring vital signs. Document and report any change from the baseline assessment.

4. Assess for signs of bleeding: increased neck circumference, bright red blood on the dressing, deviated trachea and respiratory distress (see the "High risk for hypoxemia" problem in this plan), or increased drainage in the collection system, if used. Monitor vital signs. Document and immediately report any changes from baseline. Assess hemoglobin and hematocrit values and bleeding times, as ordered, and report changes that indicate bleeding, such as decreasing hemoglobin and hematocrit and increasing bleeding times.

5. If bleeding is present, prepare the patient for corrective procedures, such as noninvasive or invasive testing, surgery to correct a suture line bleed, or arteriotomy and thrombectomy to remove a thrombus. Consult the "Surgical Intervention" plan, page 81, for details.

6. Implement measures to promote adequate cerebral blood flow, as ordered:
• Detect and treat hypovolemia.
• Maintain drain patency by keeping tubing free from kinks and emptying the collection device as necessary.
• Change or reinforce the dressing as necessary.
• Apply an ice pack at the incision line, as ordered.
• Support the patient's head and neck during position changes and maintain body alignment.
• Administer corticosteroids, if ordered, and monitor for therapeutic and nontherapeutic effects.
• Control hypertension with antihypertensive medications, such as sodium nitroprusside.
• Control hypotension with fluid replacement or vasopressors, such as dopamine or dobutamine.
• Maintain activity restrictions.

7. Implement measures to minimize injury, if signs and symptoms of cerebral ischemia occur:

• Continue the measures above to promote cerebral blood flow.

• Assess and report progression of sign and symptoms.

• Maintain the patient on bedrest with head of bed flat, unless contraindicated.

• Initiate seizure precautions.

• Provide emotional support to the patient and family.

2. Changes such as increased pulse and respiratory rates and decreased blood pressure may indicate hypovolemia caused by fluid deficit or bleeding. Hypovolemia leading to decreased cardiac output, hypertension, and hypoxia increases the risk of cerebral ischemia. Bradycardia contributes to decreased cardiac output and may be caused by vagal nerve stimulation.

3. Strong palpable pulses indicate good flow through the carotid artery and are a useful adjunct to other assessments.

4. The patient undergoing carotid endarterectomy usually receives aspirin before surgery, sometimes up until the time of surgery, as well as heparin during surgery. Immediate detection of increased bleeding is therefore a high priority because decreased circulating blood volume increases the potential for cerebral ischemia. In addition to compromising cerebral blood flow, hematomas may cause tracheal compression, obstructing the airway. The patient may require further surgery to detect the cause of bleeding.

5. Prompt detection and correction of cerebral ischemia's cause may minimize damage. Adequate patient preparation for testing or surgery helps allay anxieties. The "Surgical Intervention" plan provides detailed information for this problem.

6. These measures promote cerebral circulation, help prevent hematoma formation, or reduce edema and stress at the suture line, reducing the risk of bleeding.

7. Minimizing injury reduces the risk of permanent neurologic damage.

• Promoting cerebral blood flow reduces the risk of further injury.

• The progression of signs and symptoms alerts the nurse to the need for more aggressive intervention. Continued deterioration, bleeding, hematoma formation, or increased intracranial pressure may require further surgery.

• The supine position improves blood flow to the brain.

• Cerebral ischemia may trigger seizures.

• Keeping the family informed about what is happening may help to reduce anxiety and secure their cooperation in the patient's care.

8. Additional individualized interventions: _____   8. Rationales: _____

_____   _____

Target outcome criteria
Within 24 hours after surgery, the patient will:
• exhibit signs of adequate cerebral blood flow as evidenced by alertness and orientation, intact motor and sensory function, and normal pupil reactions
• maintain blood pressure within normal limits

• have hemoglobin and hematocrit values and bleeding times within prescribed limits
• exhibit little or no bleeding.

Collaborative problem: *Cranial nerve injury (particularly cranial nerves III, VII, IX, X, XII) related to surgical trauma or blood accumulation and edema in the surgical area*

NURSING PRIORITY: Detect and minimize neurologic impairment.

Interventions

1. Assess cranial nerve function hourly for the first 24 hours after surgery or as needed. Check for the following:

• full extraocular movements (EOMs)

• ability to smile and clench teeth symmetrically; general facial symmetry present

• swallows easily, uvula in the midline position, gag reflex intact, speaks clearly with normal tones, symmetrical movements of vocal chords and soft palate

• shoulders symmetrical, able to rotate head to side and shrug shoulders against resistance

• tongue midline, able to protrude tongue in the midline position and move it laterally with normal movements; able to speak, eat, and swallow without difficulty

• facial sensation, particularly in the earlobe and over the mastoid process.

2. Compare cranial nerve assessment to preoperative or recovery room baseline. Immediately report the following: incomplete EOMs, ipsilateral facial drooping (loss of nasolabial fold, drooping of corner of mouth or lower eyelid), difficulty swallowing, absent or diminished gag reflex, hoarse speech, early voice fatigue, unilateral shoulder sag, difficulty raising arm on affected side to horizontal position or raising shoulder against resistance, ipsilateral tongue deviation, dysphagia, tongue biting while eating, or loss of facial sensation.

Rationales

1. The cranial nerves lie close to the endarterectomy site. Clamping of or trauma to the nerves during surgery can impair their normal function. Nerves also may be severed accidentally during dissection to access the carotid artery.

• Normal EOMs indicate that the oculomotor nerve (cranial nerve III) is intact.

• These findings demonstrate normal facial nerve (cranial nerve VII) function.

• These findings demonstrate normal glossopharyngeal (cranial nerve IX) and vagus nerve (cranial nerve X) function (these two nerves are tested together).

• These movements indicate normal spinal accessory nerve (cranial nerve XI) function.

• These capacities demonstrate hypoglossal nerve (cranial nerve XII) function.

• These sensations show normal greater auricular nerve function.

2. An awareness of preexisting deficits facilitates prompt detection of cranial nerve damage. Dysfunction may be caused by stretching of the nerves during retraction, pressure from blood accumulation, or edema in the surrounding tissues. Prompt detection of cranial nerve damage facilitates appropriate interventions to minimize complications and injury to the patient.

CARDIOVASCULAR DISORDERS

3. Implement measures to reduce edema or accumulation of fluid in the surgical area:
• Elevate the head of the bed as prescribed.
• Maintain patency of surgical drains, if present.
• Keep the head and neck in the midline position when the patient is supine. Support the patient's head and neck when turning.
• Keep the head and neck in correct alignment with pillows or rolls when the patient is turned to the side.
• Apply an ice pack at the incision line, as ordered.
• Monitor for therapeutic and nontherapeutic effects of corticosteroids, if administered.

3. Reducing edema and fluid accumulation in the surgical area minimizes pressure on the cranial nerves, reducing the potential for dysfunction. Corticosteroids are used to reduce edema.

4. If nerve damage occurs, particularly to the facial, hypoglossal, vagus, or glossopharyngeal nerves, implement measures to prevent injury to the patient:

• Keep suctioning equipment at the bedside and perform oral, pharyngeal, or tracheal suctioning as needed.

4. Compensating for nerve deficits reduces the risk of injury.

• Suctioning excess secretions reduces the risk of aspiration and subsequent aspiration pneumonia. This is particularly important for the endarterectomy patient, who should avoid hypoxemia (see the "High risk for hypoxemia" problem in this plan).

• Withhold oral fluids and food until the gag reflex returns.

• Withholding fluids and food when the gag reflex is absent prevents aspiration.

• Assess the patient's ability to chew and swallow before offering fluids or food.

• Assessing ability to chew and swallow helps the nurse gauge the risk of aspiration.

• Place the patient in high Fowler's position, unless contraindicated, during and after oral intake.

• Placing the patient in this position facilitates swallowing and decreases the risk of aspiration.

• Instill isotonic eyedrops or tape the eyelids shut if the patient's blink reflex is decreased or absent.

• Artificial tears and taping help prevent corneal irritation and permanent eye damage.

5. If the vagus or glossopharyngeal nerve is damaged (as shown by hoarseness, difficulty speaking clearly, or asymmetrical movement of vocal cords), implement measures to facilitate communication: Maintain a quiet environment. Establish a means of communication with the eyes (blinking for yes and no). Provide pencil and paper, magic slate, flash cards, or pictures. Pay close attention when the patient communicates.

5. The inability to communicate effectively can be very stressful, if not terrifying. Providing the patient with a means of communication or signaling helps reduce anxiety.

6. If nerve damage occurs, provide emotional support to the patient and family by listening and providing information as appropriate.

6. The effects of cranial nerve damage can be frightening for both the patient and family. Providing the opportunity to express concerns and giving appropriate information can relieve anxiety and stress

7. Initiate appropriate referrals for follow-up care when cranial nerve damage persists.

7. Nerve damage is usually not permanent, but the symptoms may take months to resolve. Working with such health care team members as the speech pathologist, physical therapist, or dietitian facilitates recovery and should begin as soon as the deficits are discovered.

8. Additional individualized interventions: _____

8. Rationales: _____

Target outcome criteria
Within 24 hours after surgery, the patient will manifest no signs and symptoms of cranial nerve damage.

If damage has occurred, within 72 hours after surgery the patient will:
• experience beginning resolution of cranial nerve damage as evidenced by a gradual improvement in facial muscle tone, movements and sensation, ability to chew and swallow, speech, and shoulder movements
• begin therapy for more severe cranial nerve damage, such as speech therapy or physical therapy.

Collaborative problem: *High risk for AMI related to atherosclerosis and trauma of surgery*

NURSING PRIORITY: Promptly detect and treat AMI.

Interventions

1. Assess for chest pain (see the "Acute Myocardial Infarction – Critical Care Unit Phase" plan, page 268). Also evaluate laboratory and diagnostic tests specific to cardiac function: 12-lead ECG, arrhythmia monitoring, CPK, and CPK isoenzymes. Document and report immediately ECG changes consistent with AMI, CPK elevations and positive CPK-MB isoenzymes, elevated ST segment, and premature ventricular contractions during continuous monitoring. Compare to baseline values.

2. Assess blood pressure, pulse rate, and respiratory rate, central venous pressure, and urine output hourly, or as ordered. If a PA catheter is used, assess wedge pressure every 2 hours and cardiac output or index every 4 hours, or as ordered. Correlate abnormal findings with laboratory and diagnostic test results.

3. Administer nitroglycerin, as ordered, until preoperative cardiac medications can be resumed.

4. Implement the measures in the "Acute Myocardial Infarction – Critical Care Unit Phase" plan for the patient with AMI.

5. Additional individualized interventions: _____

Rationales

1. Because generalized atherosclerosis is common in patients undergoing endarterectomy, coronary artery disease is usually present. AMI is the leading cause of death after endarterectomy. Continuous cardiac monitoring after surgery may detect ischemia and arrhythmias. Early detection of ischemia or an AMI facilitates prompt treatment and may help prevent cardiovascular complications.

2. Decreased blood pressure, cardiac output, and cardiac index, along with increased pulse and respiratory rates, wedge pressure, and central venous pressure help to differentiate an MI from other postoperative complications. Laboratory and diagnostic test results also help rule out other complications. Urine output is one of the best indicators of cardiac output, particularly if a pulmonary artery catheter is not in place.

3. Nitroglycerin may be ordered for the patient with known coronary artery disease to increase blood flow and decrease cardiac work load by vasodilation.

4. The "Acute Myocardial Infarction – Critical Care Unit Phase" plan provides detailed information about the care of the patient with an AMI.

5. Rationales: _____

Target outcome criterion
Within 24 hours after surgery, the patient will exhibit stable cardiac status as evidenced by vital signs within normal limits and a stable ECG with no evidence of further infarction.

CARDIOVASCULAR DISORDERS

Collaborative problem: *High risk for hypoxemia related to airway obstruction from tracheal compression or aspiration*

NURSING PRIORITIES: (a) Minimize or prevent airway obstruction and aspiration, and (b) maintain oxygenation.

Interventions

1. Assess airway patency every 15 minutes for the first hour after surgery and then hourly, as needed, for 24 hours. Assess respiratory rate and effort, respiratory pattern, chest excursion, position of trachea, breath sounds, level of consciousness, and color. Document and report immediately increased respiratory rate, accessory muscle use, unequal chest excursion, altered level of consciousness (such as lethargy, restlessness, or confusion), pale to cyanotic color, shortness of breath, tracheal deviation, stridor, wheezing, or labored respirations.

2. Assess oxygenation levels by continuous pulse oximetry or ABG levels, as needed. Also monitor ABG levels to ensure that pH and partial pressure of arterial carbon dioxide also stay within normal limits. Document and report oxygen saturation below 95%, or as ordered, and ABG values outside the prescribed limits.

3. If airway obstruction occurs, prepare to assist with endotracheal intubation or drainage of an incisional hematoma. Anticipate intubation even if signs of hypoxemia have not yet developed.

4. Assess for bleeding and hematoma formation:

• Assess neck size closely every 15 minutes for the first hour, then hourly, as needed, for the first 24 hours after surgery. To maintain accuracy, mark the point at which the circumference is measured on the dressing. Observe for blood on the dressing. Document and immediately report excessive bleeding or a sudden increase in the neck's circumference.

• Check for bleeding behind the neck of the supine patient. If a bulky neck dressing makes inspection difficult, use the quality of respirations and ability to swallow as guidelines.

• Monitor hemoglobin and hematocrit values, as ordered, and report any decreases.

• If a drain is present, maintain patency, and note the amount of drainage. Document and report excessive drainage.

5. Evaluate the patient's ability to swallow.

6. Assess for an intact gag reflex, ability to swallow and speak clearly with normal tones, and symmetrical movements of the vocal cords and soft palate.

Rationales

1. Maintaining a patent airway is essential. The most common cause of acute postoperative airway obstruction is compression of the trachea by a hematoma or edema at the surgical site. Tracheal deviation and signs of hypoxemia, including altered level of consciousness, labored respirations, and wheezing or stridor, are key assessment findings for the obstructed airway.

2. Pulse oximetry provides ongoing noninvasive monitoring of arterial oxygen saturation. ABG values provide objective documentation of acid-base status and are a helpful adjunct to observations of respiratory status. Acidosis or hypercapnia may increase cerebral edema.

3. Although usually done in the operating room, emergency drainage of a life-threatening hematoma in the neck may be performed at the patient's bedside. Drainage may be necessary before an endotracheal tube can be inserted. The postoperative carotid endarterectomy patient must avoid hypoxemia because sufficient damage to the carotid body impairs ventilatory and circulatory responses to hypoxia. Therefore, the patient may be intubated before hypoxemia develops.

4. Bleeding can lead to hypovolemia, while hematoma formation may compress the airway.

• Neck size increases with a developing hematoma. Closely observing neck size, ensuring consistency in measurements, and monitoring for bleeding promotes early detection of hypoxia.

• Blood may pool, promoting hematoma formation posterior to the incision.

• Decreasing hemoglobin and hematocrit values may indicate slow bleeding.

• Excessive bleeding through a drain may lead to hypovolemia and hypotension.

5. Edema that exerts pressure on the trachea and esophagus makes swallowing difficult and increases the risk of airway obstruction.

6. Damage to the laryngeal branches of the vagus nerve prevents closure of the glottis, which can lead to aspiration and subsequent aspiration pneumonia. Pneumonia may cause hypoxia, a potentially dangerous condition after carotid endarterectomy.

7. Keep suctioning equipment at the bedside for oral, pharyngeal, or endotracheal suctioning as needed.

7. Prompt suctioning can prevent aspiration.

8. Implement measures to increase gas exchange and prevent hypoxemia:

8. Facilitating gas exchange helps prevent hypoxemia and the complications associated with it.

• Elevate the head of the bed as ordered, as soon as vital signs are stable.

• An upright position facilitates diaphragmatic excursion.

• Encourage deep breathing every two hours. Remind the patient to yawn and sigh periodically. Provide frequent position changes after vital signs have stabilized, minimizing stress on the operative site by supporting the head and maintaining proper alignment when turning and positioning the patient. Suction secretions as necessary.

• These measures lessen postoperative atelectasis.

• Discourage the patient from coughing during the first 24 hours after surgery.

• Coughing during the first 24 hours can cause excessive pressure on the incision and may cause it to rupture.

• Evaluate respiratory rate and effort before administering analgesics or sedation.

• Analgesics and sedatives can depress the respiratory center, promoting hypoxemia.

• Maintain supplemental oxygen as ordered.

• Supplemental oxygen increases blood oxygen content.

9. Additional individualized interventions: _____

9. Rationales: _____

Target outcome criteria
Within 24 hours after surgery, the patient will:
• have a patent airway as evidenced by normal respiratory rate and effort, normal breath sounds, and appropriate level of consciousness
• have ABG values within normal limits

• produce minimal drainage from the incision
• display trachea in the midline position.

Discharge planning

NURSING DISCHARGE CRITERIA
Upon the patient's discharge, documentation shows evidence of:
• patent airway
• stable blood pressure within normal limits without I.V. inotrope or vasodilator support
• ABG measurements within normal limits
• no bleeding from incision
• stable neurologic function
• absence of cardiovascular, respiratory, or neurologic complications
• normal fluid and electrolyte balance
• absence of infection
• absence or control of seizures
• absence of headaches.

PATIENT-FAMILY TEACHING CHECKLIST
Document evidence that the patient and family demonstrate an understanding of:
__ extent of surgery
__ extent of neurologic deficits, if any
__ rehabilitation, if needed
__ risk factors for atherosclerosis
__ need for life-style modifications
__ recommended dietary modifications

__ life-style modification programs, such as stress management, cardiovascular fitness, weight loss, smoking-cessation and alcohol rehabilitation programs, as needed
__ community resources for life-style modification support
__ all discharge medications' purpose, dosage, schedule, and adverse effects
__ signs and symptoms to report to health care provider.

DOCUMENTATION CHECKLIST
Using outcome criteria as a guide, document:
__ clinical status on admission
__ significant changes in status, especially regarding motor, sensory, or visual deficits, or episodes of hypertension or hypotension
__ wound condition
__ pertinent laboratory and diagnostic test findings
__ episodes of headaches or seizures
__ respiratory support measures
__ pain relief measures
__ nutritional status
__ preoperative teaching
__ patient-family teaching
__ rehabilitation needs
__ discharge planning.

ASSOCIATED PLANS OF CARE
Acute Myocardial Infarction — Critical Care Unit Phase
Cerebrovascular Accident
Increased Intracranial Pressure
Ineffective Individual Coping
Knowledge Deficit
Pain
Surgical Intervention

References

Dossey, B., et al., *Essentials of Critical Care Nursing, Body, Mind, and Spirit*. Philadelphia: J.B. Lippincott Co., 1990.

Fahey, V., ed. *Vascular Nursing*. Philadelphia: W.B. Saunders Co., 1988.

Fode, N. "Carotid Endarterectomy: Nursing Care and Controversies," *Journal of Neuroscience Nursing* 22(1):25-31, February 1990.

Hudak, C., et al. *Critical Care Nursing*, 5th ed. Philadelphia: J.B. Lippincott Co., 1990.

"Tightening the Reins on Carotid Endarterectomy," *Emergency Medicine* 22(5):62-73, March 15, 1990.

Congestive Heart Failure

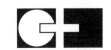

DRG information

DRG 127 Heart Failure and Shock.
            Mean LOS = 6.1 days
Additional DRG information: DRG 127 is the most
prevalent DRG in the United States (4.9% of all prospective payment system discharges); however, heart
failure commonly accompanies other diagnoses, especially other cardiac diagnoses. In these cases, DRG
127 is not likely to be the principal DRG.

Introduction
DEFINITION AND TIME FOCUS
Congestive heart failure (CHF) is the end result of several disease states in which cardiac output fails to
meet the body's metabolic demands, resulting in pulmonary and systemic congestion. Inadequate cardiac
output stimulates the sympathetic nervous system, resulting in increased heart rate, myocardial contractility, vasoconstriction, and salt and water retention.
Cardiac and peripheral oxygen demands also increase.
If the underlying problem cannot be corrected, these
compensatory mechanisms lead to progressive fluid retention and further deterioration of cardiac efficiency.
This plan focuses on the care of the patient admitted
for treatment of an acute exacerbation of chronic CHF
or treatment of CHF resulting from an acute event
(such as acute myocardial infarction [AMI]).

ETIOLOGY AND PRECIPITATING FACTORS
• conditions that reduce myocardial contractility, such
as cardiomyopathies, ischemic cardiac disease, ventricular aneurysms, or constrictive pericarditis
• conditions that increase fluid volume and lead to circulatory overload (increased preload), such as too-
rapid infusion of I.V. fluids, increased sodium intake, or
inadequate diuretic therapy
• conditions that alter cardiac rhythm, such as severe
bradycardia in the presence of decreased contractility,
or tachycardia severe enough to decrease cardiac filling time and diminish cardiac output
• conditions that increase resistance to blood flow out
of the heart (increased afterload), such as arteriosclerotic heart disease, hypertensive heart disease, or pulmonary hypertension
• conditions that interfere with blood flow through the
heart, such as valvular insufficiency or stenosis
• conditions that increase oxygen demands beyond the
heart's capabilities, such as hyperthyroidism, fever,
pregnancy, or anemia

Focused assessment guidelines
NURSING HISTORY (Functional health pattern findings)

Health perception—health management pattern
• may be under long-term treatment for heart failure or
a precipitating disease, such as hypertensive heart
disease
• may have no experience with signs and symptoms if
episode occurs in response to an acute event, such as
an AMI
• may report noncompliance with prescribed diet, medications, or activity restrictions
• may complain of peripheral edema or fatigue (common)

Nutritional-metabolic pattern
• may complain of anorexia (common); occasionally, reports nausea or vomiting from congested peripheral
circulation or from medication adverse effects
• may exhibit weight loss and cachexia from decreased
caloric intake and poor nutrient absorption

Elimination pattern
• may report altered urinary patterns (from diuretic
treatment or decreased renal blood flow)
• may report constipation (from edema of the GI tract)

Activity-exercise pattern
• may report inability to participate in exercise or leisure activities (common)
• may report difficulty participating in everyday activities because of fatigue or shortness of breath

Sleep-rest pattern
• may report disturbed sleep patterns from dyspnea
and nocturia (common)
• may sleep on 2 or 3 pillows because of orthopnea
(common)
• may report paroxysmal nocturnal dyspnea

Cognitive-perceptual pattern
• may demonstrate failure to understand problem and
treatment protocols (if heart failure is an acute event)
• may report headaches, confusion, or memory impairment

Self-perception—self-concept pattern
• may describe body-image disturbances related to
edema and decreased activity level

Role-relationship pattern
• may describe difficulty fulfilling role responsibilities because of fatigue, weakness, or decreased activity tolerance (common)

Sexuality-reproductive pattern
• may report decreased libido and impotence or orgasmic dysfunction related to fatigue or medications

Coping—stress tolerance pattern
• may report anxiety related to shortness of breath
• may complain of anxiety related to chronic illness
• may grieve for loss of former level of health and loss of former roles and function
• may anticipate premature death

PHYSICAL FINDINGS
Cardiovascular
• tachycardia
• S_3 heart sound
• S_4 heart sound with summation gallop (with tachycardia)
• atrial and ventricular arrhythmias
• jugular vein distention
• systolic murmur (in advanced CHF)
• decreased peripheral pulses

Pulmonary
• dyspnea
• crackles
• nonproductive cough
• progressive bilateral diminishing of breath sounds, beginning at bases

Neurologic
• increased irritability
• impaired memory
• confusion (rare)

Gastrointestinal
• abdominal distention
• vomiting
• tenderness over liver
• liver enlargement

Renal
• decreased urine output

Integumentary
• dependent edema, such as in feet and sacrum
• cyanosis
• clubbing of fingers (in chronic failure)

Musculoskeletal
• weakness and easy fatigability
• muscle wasting (rare)

DIAGNOSTIC STUDIES
• serum electrolyte levels—electrolyte imbalances may occur from fluid shifts, diuretic therapy, or response of organ systems to decreased oxygen and increased congestion
  —hyponatremia: volume overload causes dilutional hyponatremia; sodium restriction and diuretics may also lead to low serum sodium level
  —hypokalemia: most common diuretics cause potassium loss
  —hyperkalemia: can occur with oliguria or anuria
• arterial blood gas (ABG) measurements
  —lowered PO_2 related to pulmonary congestion
  —elevated PCO_2 (respiratory acidosis) may be from pulmonary edema or hypoventilation
• prothrombin time (PT), partial thromboplastin time (PTT)—obtained to determine baseline before beginning anticoagulant therapy or to evaluate clotting status during anticoagulant therapy
• blood urea nitrogen (BUN) and creatinine levels—elevated, reflecting decreased renal function
• bilirubin, aspartate aminotransferase, lactic dehydrogenase levels—elevated, indicating decreased liver function
• urinalysis—reveals proteinuria and elevated specific gravity
• chest X-ray—may reveal enlarged cardiac silhouette (common), distended pulmonary veins from redistribution of pulmonary blood flow, and interstitial and alveolar edema (common)
• electrocardiogram—nonspecific diagnostically, but useful in identifying rhythm disturbances, conduction defects, axis deviations, and hypertrophy
• echocardiography—can identify valvular abnormalities, chamber enlargement, abnormal wall motion, hypertrophy, pericardial effusions, and mural thrombi
• MUGA scan (multigated blood pool imaging)—demonstrates decreased ejection fraction and abnormal wall motion

POTENTIAL COMPLICATIONS
• cardiogenic shock
• pulmonary edema
• AMI
• arrhythmias
• thrombolytic complications
• renal failure
• liver failure

Collaborative problem: *Decreased cardiac output related to decreased contractility, altered heart rhythm, fluid volume overload, or increased afterload*

NURSING PRIORITY: Maintain optimum cardiac output.

Interventions

1. Monitor and document heart rate and rhythm, heart sounds, blood pressure, pulse pressure, and the presence or absence of peripheral pulses. Compare to the baseline assessment. Report abnormalities to the doctor, particularly tachycardia, a new S_3 heart sound or systolic murmur, hypotension, decreased pulse pressure or pulse loss, or increased arrhythmias.

2. Administer cardiac medications, as ordered, and document the patient's response. Observe for therapeutic and side effects:

• inotropic agents (digitalis derivatives) — monitor for anorexia, pulse rate below 60 beats/minute or above 100 beats/minute, irregular heart rate, nausea, vomiting, and visual disturbances. Withhold the dose and contact the doctor if any of these signs occur.

• diuretics such as hydrochlorothiazide (Esidrix) and furosemide (Lasix) — monitor for hypovolemia and hypokalemia. (See Appendix C, "Fluid and Electrolyte Imbalances," for details.)

• nitrates such as isosorbide dinitrate (Isordil) — monitor for signs of hypovolemia.

• afterload reducers (vasodilators) such as hydralazine (Apresoline) — monitor for hypotension.

3. Observe for signs and symptoms of hypoxemia, such as confusion, restlessness, dyspnea, arrhythmias, tachycardia, and cyanosis. Ensure adequate oxygenation with proper positioning (semi-Fowler's or upright) and supplemental oxygen, as ordered.

4. Ensure adequate rest by monitoring the noise level, limiting visitors, grouping diagnostic tests (such as by ordering multiple blood tests on one blood sample, when possible), and spacing therapeutic interventions.

Rationales

1. One of the earliest signs of worsening heart failure is increased heart rate. A new S_3 heart sound or a systolic murmur may reflect increased fluid volume, leading to increased cardiac congestion and failure. Hypotension can reflect decreased cardiac output from impaired myocardial contractility or overdiuresis. Diminished pulse pressure or peripheral pulse loss can indicate a decrease in cardiac output. Increased arrhythmias can reflect an increased number of premature atrial or ventricular contractions — signs of increasing failure or medication toxicity.

2. Pharmacotherapeutic agents may relieve CHF by altering preload, contractility, or afterload — major determinants of cardiac output. However, many of these agents have narrow therapeutic ranges or side effects that can worsen the underlying disease.

• Inotropic agents increase contractility but also can increase myocardial oxygen consumption and cardiac work, increasing CHF. Digitalis, one of the most common medications used, has a narrow therapeutic range. Early toxic side effects include anorexia; later, severe bradyarrhythmias, tachyarrhythmias, and irregular cardiac rhythms can compromise cardiac output. Signs of digitalis toxicity are more common in patients with decreased renal function.

• Diuretics decrease preload but can cause true hypovolemia, from excessive fluid loss, or hypokalemia, from potassium loss.

• Nitrates cause venodilation, reducing preload but also increasing the risk for relative hypovolemia from redistribution of blood volume to the periphery.

• Afterload reducers lower resistance to ventricular ejection but may lower blood pressure enough to compromise organ perfusion.

3. Prompt detection of hypoxemia allows timely intervention. The semi-Fowler's position prevents abdominal organs from pressing on the diaphragm and interfering with its movement. An upright position permits a severely dyspneic patient to use accessory muscles for breathing; it also redistributes blood to dependent areas, decreasing blood return to the heart and reducing preload in a patient with volume overload. A patient who has difficulty maintaining an arterial oxygen level (PaO_2) above 60 mm Hg may benefit from supplemental oxygen.

4. Rest reduces myocardial oxygen consumption.

5. Monitor fluid status:

• Obtain accurate daily weights.

• Maintain an accurate intake and output record.

• Assess the lungs for crackles, decreased sounds, and a change from vesicular to bronchial breath sounds.

• Assess for dependent edema and increasing dyspnea.

• Assess for signs of dehydration.

6. Assess for increasing confusion.

7. Decrease the patient's fear and anxiety by providing information and by eliciting concerns and responding to them. See the "Ineffective Individual Coping" plan, page 51, for details.

8. Additional individualized interventions: _____

_____

5. Fluid volume may be increased from the heart's inability to maintain adequate flow and pressure through the kidneys.

• Rapid weight gain (1 to 2 lb [2 to 4 kg] a day) indicates fluid retention and the need for increased diuresis.

• Accurate intake and output records can warn of early fluid excess.

• Crackles, decreased sounds, and bronchial breath sounds indicate fluid in the lungs and signal increasing left-sided heart failure.

• Dependent edema and dyspnea are signs of increasing right-sided and left-sided heart failure respectively.

• Fluid volume may be decreased from excessive diuresis.

6. When cardiac output is decreased, cerebral perfusion suffers, producing confusion.

7. Fear and anxiety activate the sympathetic nervous system and increase heart rate, myocardial contractility, and vasoconstriction. All these factors increase myocardial oxygen consumption. The "Ineffective Individual Coping" plan contains general interventions to reduce anxiety.

8. Rationales: _____

_____

Target outcome criteria
By the time of discharge, the patient will:
• exhibit heart rate under 100 beats/minute
• have warm, dry skin
• exhibit optimal systolic blood pressure, as manifested by capillary refill time of less than 3 seconds, and minimal or absent peripheral edema
• have no S_3 heart sound

• have stable cardiac rhythm with any life-threatening arrhythmias under control
• have lungs clear to auscultation
• perform activities of daily living (ADLs) without incapacitating dyspnea
• have mental status within normal limits.

Nursing diagnosis: *Fluid volume excess related to decreased myocardial contractility, decreased renal perfusion, and increased sodium and water retention*

NURSING PRIORITY: Optimize and monitor volume status and electrolyte balance.

Interventions

1. See Appendix C, "Fluid and Electrolyte Imbalances."

2. Monitor hourly fluid intake and output and 24-hour fluid balance. Weigh the patient daily.

3. Administer I.V. solutions, as ordered. Avoid saline solutions.

Rationales

1. The "Fluid and Electrolyte Imbalances" appendix describes the causes, signs and symptoms, laboratory findings, and treatments of these disorders.

2. Intake and output monitoring provides an objective method of tracking fluid gains or losses, while 24-hour summaries indicate net fluid balance. Daily weight measurements are a rough measure of fluid status; a weight change of 2.2 lb (1 kg) corresponds with a 1-liter change in fluid balance.

3. The type and amount of I.V. fluid ordered depends upon the patient's current condition and the cause of heart failure. Saline solutions can cause water retention.

4. If the patient is placed on fluid restriction:

• explain the rationale to the patient and family

• establish a fluid intake schedule, teach the patient how to record oral fluids, and use microdrip tubing or an infusion pump to control I.V. intake.

5. Monitor creatinine and BUN levels and report increasing values.

6. Monitor sodium and potassium levels. Report abnormal values and signs of imbalances.

7. Additional individualized interventions: _____

_____

4. Fluid restriction helps limit excessive preload.

• The patient and family are more likely to comply with fluid restriction if they understand the reasons behind it. Thirst is a powerful need and restricting fluids may cause the patient to feel deprived or punished. Explaining the rationale may help the patient view the situation positively.

• Regular fluid intake, consistent measurements, and use of microdrip tubing or infusion devices help ensure maintenance of fluid restrictions.

5. Creatinine and BUN levels reflect decreased renal perfusion from worsening heart failure. The BUN level rises disproportionately; the BUN-creatinine level ratio can increase from the normal of 10:1 to as high as 40:1.

6. Hyponatremia can cause decreased blood pressure, confusion, headache, and seizures; hypokalemia, weakness, fatigue, ileus, and ventricular fibrillation; and hyperkalemia, bradycardia and ventricular asystole.

7. Rationales: _____

_____

Target outcome criteria
By the time of discharge, the patient will:
• have fluid intake and output in approximate balance
• exhibit sodium, potassium, creatinine, and BUN levels within expected parameters.

Nursing diagnosis: *Activity intolerance related to bed rest and decreased cardiac output*

NURSING PRIORITIES: (a) Prevent complications of bed rest, and (b) increase activity level without exceeding cardiac energy reserves.

Interventions

1. Determine cardiac stability by evaluating blood pressure, heart rhythm and rate, and indicators of oxygenation, such as level of consciousness and skin color.

2. When the patient is stable, institute a graduated activity program according to unit protocol. Begin with regular position changes and range-of-motion (ROM) exercises during bed rest. Then, as tolerated, progress to active ROM exercises, chair sitting, and ambulation.

Rationales

1. Activity increases myocardial contractility, heart rate, blood pressure, and myocardial oxygen consumption. If cardiac output is already compromised (as in tachycardia or severe arrhythmias), activity will reduce it further.

2. Bed rest has many detrimental effects, including cardiac deconditioning, increased risk of atelectasis and pneumonia, and skin breakdown. It also promotes venous stasis, further increasing the risk of thromboembolism from depressed myocardial contractility and atrial fibrillation—an arrhythmia common in CHF because of atrial distention. Position changes and exercises that involve a change in muscle length (such as active or passive limb flexion) improve peripheral circulation and reduce the risks associated with immobility.

CARDIOVASCULAR DISORDERS

3. Evaluate patient tolerance to new activities. Monitor blood pressure and pulse; respiratory rate, pattern, and depth; level of consciousness and coordination; and patient reports of energy and strength. Discontinue activity, and resume it later at a slower pace, if any of the following occur:
• pulse rate greater than 30 beats/minute above resting level (or greater than 15 beats/minute if taking beta blockers)
• systolic blood pressure 15 mm Hg or more below resting level
• diastolic blood pressure 10 mm Hg or more above resting level
• new or increased pulse irregularity
• dyspnea, slowed respiratory rate, or shallow respirations
• decreased level of consciousness or loss of coordination
• chest or leg pain
• fatigue disproportionate to activity level
• profound weakness.

3. A too-rapid activity increase can exacerbate heart failure, myocardial ischemia, or peripheral vascular insufficiency. It also may cause hypotension, syncope, or cardiovascular collapse. At the very least, activity goals that exceed the patient's capabilities may cause a psychological setback.

4. Alternate activity with rest periods.

4. Bed rest and inactivity cause cardiac and muscle deconditioning. Initially, even short periods of activity can induce symptoms of cardiac compromise. Regular rest prevents depletion of cardiac reserves.

5. Administer anticoagulants, as ordered. Monitor appropriate coagulation studies and report results that exceed set limits.

5. Heparin inactivates thrombin, preventing fibrin clot formation. Warfarin sodium (Coumadin) interferes with vitamin K production, decreasing synthesis of several clotting factors. The therapeutic PTT should be 2 to 2½ times normal; the therapeutic PT, 1½ to 2½ times normal.

6. Teach the patient how to avoid Valsalva's maneuver (forced expiration against a closed glottis), such as by exhaling when changing position and increasing fiber intake to promote bowel elimination.

6. Valsalva's maneuver increases intrathoracic pressure and decreases blood return to the heart. When the breath is released, venous return increases by reflex. Valsalva's maneuver has been associated with syncope and premature ventricular contractions.

7. Additional individualized interventions: _____

7. Rationales: _____

Target outcome criteria
By the time of discharge, the patient will:
• exhibit no evidence of thrombophlebitis or pulmonary embolism
• maintain a normal bowel pattern
• perform ADLs (feeding, bathing, and dressing) independently, with no significant change in heart rate or blood pressure

• walk in hall with no significant change in heart rate and blood pressure and no complaints of chest pain or profound fatigue.

Nursing diagnosis: *Nutritional deficit related to decreased appetite and unpalatability of low-sodium diet*

NURSING PRIORITY: Ensure adequate intake of nutrients needed for healing and increased energy requirements.

Interventions

1. Keep a daily record to monitor calorie intake. Consult with the dietitian to identify the patient's calorie needs.

Rationales

1. Calorie needs vary with the patient's illness stage, activity level, and weight.

2. Assess the patient's food preferences, and plan meals to meet treatment requirements and patient needs.

2. A low-sodium diet reduces cardiac preload by decreasing water retention. Unfortunately, low-sodium diets may be unpalatable to the patient accustomed to seasoned foods. The patient may be more compliant if food preferences are considered whenever possible.

3. Additional individualized interventions: _____

_____

3. Rationales: _____

_____

Target outcome criterion
By the time of discharge, the patient will meet daily calorie requirements.

Nursing diagnosis: *Knowledge deficit related to complex disease process and treatment*

NURSING PRIORITY: Prepare the patient to implement necessary life-style modifications to prevent recurrent episodes of CHF, if possible.

Interventions

1. Once the patient is stable, institute a structured teaching plan only as the condition allows. See the "Knowledge Deficit" plan, page 56, for details.

2. Briefly explain the pathophysiology of heart failure. Relate the explanation to the patient's signs and symptoms.

3. Emphasize the patient's role in controlling the disease and the importance of medical follow-up.

4. With the dietitian, instruct the patient and family about the prescribed diet, usually one low in sodium, fat, cholesterol, and (if the patient is overweight) calories. Explain the rationale for such dietary restrictions as reducing sodium intake. Provide a list of high-sodium foods and suggest alternatives to salt, such as lemon juice and herbs. Recommend low-sodium cookbooks. Stress the importance of family support in making the necessary life-style changes.

5. Explain the rationale for activity restrictions. Provide specific information about recommended activities. Teach the patient to monitor activity tolerance by measuring pulse rate before and after activity and by watching for symptoms of over exertion. (See the "Activity intolerance" nursing diagnosis in this plan for details.)

Rationales

1. The acutely ill patient usually is unable to tolerate sustained teaching. Planned teaching is more efficient and effective than haphazard instruction. The "Knowledge Deficit" plan describes assessing readiness to learn and selecting teaching methods.

2. Although extensive teaching should be deferred until the patient is stable, a brief explanation may help the patient understand the rationales for therapy. An adult learns best when the information relates directly to personal experience. Relevant information is helpful, but excessive detail can overwhelm and confuse.

3. Heart failure commonly becomes chronic or recurrent. The patient's active participation in implementing and monitoring treatment can be instrumental in limiting the disease's progression.

4. Many of the therapies for chronic or recurrent heart failure involve life-style modifications, such as a low-sodium diet, that may affect other family members. Other changes may involve habits the patient finds pleasurable, such as smoking. In either case, family support can smooth the transition to a more healthful life-style. Successful management of CHF requires lifelong life-style modifications; changing eating habits is one of the most difficult. Understanding the reason for restrictions may help motivate the patient to establish and maintain the prescribed diet.

5. Vague instructions to "take it easy" leave the patient confused and may impair adjustment to an altered lifestyle, thus creating a "cardiac cripple." Providing information specific to the patient's condition lessens uncertainty and facilitates adjustment to recommended activity levels.

6. Teach about discharge medications—typically inotropes, diuretics, vasodilators, or anticoagulants. Provide information sheets, and review the medications' purpose, dosage, schedule, adverse effects, and toxic effects. Stress the importance of taking doses on time. Suggest labeling a pillbox with days and times for doses.

6. Successful CHF management typically involves a long-term, complex drug regimen. Information about those medications better equips the patient and family to manage therapy at home. Understanding the drugs' purpose may increase the patient's motivation to take them; understanding dosage may increase accuracy. A properly labeled pillbox may decrease confusion and improve compliance.

7. Emphasize the importance of self-monitoring for signs and symptoms of increasing heart failure, such as ankle or leg swelling, breathlessness, tachycardia, and new or increased pulse irregularity.

7. An alert, informed patient and family are the first line of defense against recurrence or aggravation of heart failure. Knowing what to observe for and what measures to take increases the likelihood that the patient will receive prompt treatment. Early detection of increasing heart failure allows prompt adjustment of the therapeutic regimen. The patient is best able to identify subtle physiologic changes.

8. Discuss with the patient and family an emergency plan, if needed, including:
• a medical alert bracelet
• circumstances that warrant emergency medical care, such as severe chest pain, marked difficulty breathing, and cessation of breathing
• access to emergency care
• cardiopulmonary resuscitation classes for the family.

8. The patient with heart failure is at increased risk for other cardiovascular complications, such as AMI or cardiac arrest. Planning increases the likelihood of prompt, appropriate action in an emergency.

9. Review the plan for follow-up care—the doctor's name and telephone number and the date, time, and location of the next appointment.

9. Management of CHF requires consistent follow-up care.

10. Additional individualized interventions: _____

10. Rationales: _____

Target outcome criteria
By the time of discharge, the patient will:
• state intent to follow dietary recommendations
• demonstrate correct method for measuring pulse rate
• list five signs or symptoms of activity intolerance, on request
• give name, purpose, dosage, schedule, and possible adverse effects for all discharge medications

• verbalize understanding of when to seek emergency medical care
• have made first appointment for follow-up care.

Nursing diagnosis: *High risk for noncompliance related to complicated treatment regimen, health beliefs, or negative relationship with caregivers**

NURSING PRIORITY: Maximize compliance.

Interventions

1. Observe for indicators of noncompliance, such as exacerbation of signs and symptoms, development of complications, failure to keep follow-up appointments, reports of behavior contrary to health recommendations, failure to seek health care when indicated, despairing remarks about health status, or belligerent exchanges with caregivers.

Rationales

1. Noncompliance can have serious repercussions. Early identification of a problem increases the likelihood of its successful resolution.

---

*Note: NANDA defines noncompliance as the informed decision to refuse a prescribed treatment. As such, it is more than just a deviation from therapeutic recommendations. The diagnosis is controversial; many nurses believe it is value-laden and thus inappropriate. The intent here is to use the term neutrally, not to label a patient negatively. To respect the patient's right to self-determination is to recognize the right to refuse therapy. This section's goal is to help the nurse identify and eliminate factors that may be confused with noncompliance so that the diagnosis is not applied prematurely, the patient's rights are protected, and the potential for compliance remains intact.

2. Evaluate the extent and result of noncompliance.

3. Differentiate noncompliance from other problems, such as knowledge deficit, lack of family support, memory deficits, adverse effects of treatment, transportation difficulties, denial, poor self-esteem, or self-destructive behavior. Consult the "Ineffective Individual Coping" plan, page 51, and the "Knowledge Deficit" plan, page 56, for possible interventions. Take appropriate steps, such as providing information or making necessary referrals, as indicated.

4. Initiate discussion of the situation with the patient and family, involving a psychiatric clinician or other health care team members as needed.

5. Express concern for the patient as a person.

6. Emphasize the seriousness of CHF and the importance of self-care. Use the patient's situation to explain how noncompliance affects health, and emphasize the positive effects of compliance.

7. Discuss the following with the patient:
• life priorities
• perception of prognosis
• feelings about the illness's length
• complexity of treatment
• degree of confidence in caregivers
• health care beliefs.

8. Consider the patient's cultural and spiritual heritage.

9. Ask the patient about satisfaction with caregivers. Also, examine caregivers' attitudes: if nontherapeutic, either help establish more positive attitudes or assign other caregivers to the patient.

10. Validate conclusions about reasons for behavior with the patient and loved ones.

11. Collaborate with other caregivers to reevaluate the goals and implementation of care. Consider possible modifications.

12. Search for alternative solutions. Ask what the patient wants or is willing to do to bring about agreement to the plan of care.

13. Use creative negotiation strategies to set goals with the patient. Consider changing the agreement's scope, shortening its length, or making trade-offs.

2. If noncompliance is limited to areas of minor consequence in the overall plan of care, no further action may be necessary.

3. Numerous problems may masquerade as noncompliance. Identifying problems accurately increases the likelihood of appropriate intervention and resolution.

4. Open discussion can help reveal the reasons for noncompliance. The patient, family, and health care team members all can contribute insights and observations helpful in reevaluating the plan of care.

5. Expression of human caring and warmth may help break the cycle of negativity, if present, and free emotional energy for improved self-care. Nurturing behavior also may help establish rapport and trust.

6. Failure to accept an illness's seriousness can be linked to noncompliance. Discussion that incorporates the patient's experiences is most effective in making points "come alive."

7. Apparent deliberate noncompliance may actually reflect preoccupation with more pressing needs, such as food and shelter. The patient's perception of expected outcomes may be overly pessimistic. Prolonged illness, complex treatment, lack of confidence in caregivers, and health care beliefs that differ from caregivers' beliefs increase the likelihood of noncompliance.

8. The patient is less likely to accept treatment that clashes with cultural or spiritual beliefs.

9. The patient's level of dissatisfaction with caregivers influences noncompliance. A caregiver's negative attitude that results from frustration may be changed through expression and peer support. A negative attitude that results from burnout or personality clashes, however, may be best handled by removing the caregiver from the situation.

10. Labeling a patient noncompliant may stigmatize the patient and affect future caregivers' behavior. Obtaining feedback about the accuracy of conclusions helps avoid erroneous assumptions and inappropriate interventions.

11. Insisting on a plan to which the patient objects may create a power struggle between patient and caregivers. Flexibility and adaptability are more likely to achieve the desired ends.

12. Focusing on what the patient wants or is willing to do interrupts negativism and recasts the situation in a positive light. Such refocusing may free energy for creative problem solving and increase the patient's sense of control.

13. If full agreement is not possible, partial or temporary agreement may be. The patient may be willing to trade compliance in one area (such as medications) for greater freedom in another (such as food intake).

14. If the patient makes an informed choice not to follow the recommendations, and if negotiation is not possible:

• avoid punitive responses, and accept the decision

• keep open the option for treatment

• respect the patient's readiness to die.

15. Additional individualized interventions: _____

_____

14. Patients have the right of self-determination.

• Exhibiting rejecting or other punitive behavior is disrespectful and may provoke the patient to terminate contact with health care resources.

• As the patient's condition changes, resistance may soften.

• Every person has the right to die with dignity. The patient's decision to refuse care may be a rational choice to live out the remaining period of life in a meaningful way.

15. Rationales: _____

_____

Target outcome criteria
Within 2 days of admission, the patient will:
• identify areas of potential noncompliance
• identify reasons for potential noncompliance

• verbalize willingness and ability to follow modified therapeutic plan, when possible.

Discharge planning
NURSING DISCHARGE CRITERIA
Upon the patient's discharge, documentation shows evidence of:
• stable vital signs
• absence of fever and pulmonary or cardiovascular complications
• ability to tolerate adequate nutritional intake
• stable cardiac rhythm with arrhythmias controlled
• shortness of breath no worse than usual
• peripheral edema within acceptable limits or no worse than usual
• ABG measurements within acceptable parameters
• clear lung fields shown on chest X-ray within 48 hours of discharge
• absence of supplemental oxygen for at least 48 hours before discharge
• absence of signs and symptoms of dehydration
• mental status within normal limits
• laboratory values within expected parameters
• absence of urinary or bowel dysfunction
• ability to perform ADLs and ambulate same as before admission
• adequate home support system, or referral to home care if indicated by inadequate home support or inability to perform ADLs
• referral to community heart failure support group.

PATIENT-FAMILY TEACHING CHECKLIST
Document evidence that the patient and family demonstrate an understanding of:
___ cause and implications of CHF
___ signs and symptoms of increasing CHF
___ all discharge medications' purpose, dosage, administration schedule, and adverse effects requiring medical attention (usual discharge medications include inotropes, diuretics, vasodilators, or anticoagulants)
___ need for life-style modifications
___ dietary restrictions
___ activity restrictions
___ plan for follow-up care
___ plan for emergency care
___ how to contact the doctor.

DOCUMENTATION CHECKLIST
Using outcome criteria as a guide, document:
___ clinical status on admission
___ significant changes in clinical status
___ pertinent laboratory and diagnostic findings
___ intake and output
___ nutritional intake
___ response to activity progression
___ response to illness and hospitalization
___ family's response to illness
___ patient-family teaching
___ discharge planning.

ASSOCIATED PLANS OF CARE
Acute Myocardial Infarction—Critical Care Unit Phase
Acute Myocardial Infarction—Stepdown Unit Phase
Chronic Renal Failure
Dying
Grieving
Ineffective Individual Coping
Knowledge Deficit

References

Clark, S. "Quality of Life for Clients with Progressing Cardiac Disability," in *Nursing in Cardiac Rehabilitation: Issues and Intervention Strategies.* Edited by Jillings, C. Frederick, MD: Aspen Press, 1988.

Doyle, B. "Nursing Challenge: The Patient with End-Stage Heart Failure," in *Cardiac Critical Care Nursing.* Edited by Kern, L. Rockville, MD: Aspen Press, 1988.

Fukada, N. "Outcome Standards for the Client with Chronic Congestive Heart Failure," *Journal of Cardiovascular Nursing* 4(3):59-70, May 1990.

Laurent-Bopp, D. "Heart Failure," in *Cardiac Nursing,* 2nd ed. Edited by Underhill, S., et al. Philadelphia: J.B. Lippincott, 1989.

Schactman, M., and Crawford, M. "Dobutamine Rescue for Intractable Congestive Heart Failure," *American Journal of Nursing* 88(12):1642-43, December 1988.

Stanley, R. "Drug Therapy of Heart Failure," *Journal of Cardiovascular Nursing* 4(3):17-34, May 1990.

VanParys, E. "Assessing the Failing State of the Heart," *Nursing 87* 17(2):42-50, February 1987.

Watson, J. "Fluid and Electrolyte Disorders in Cardiovascular Patients," *Nursing Clinics of North America* 22(4):797-803, December 1987.

CARDIOVASCULAR DISORDERS

Femoral Popliteal Bypass

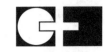

DRG information
DRG 110 Major Cardiovascular Procedures. With Complications or Comorbidities (CC).
 Mean LOS = 10.5 days
DRG 111 Major Cardiovascular Procedures.
 Without CC.
 Mean LOS = 8.1 days

Introduction
DEFINITION AND TIME FOCUS
Femoral popliteal bypass is one of several surgical revascularization techniques used to relieve symptoms of acute or chronic ischemia of the lower extremities. Femoral popliteal bypass involves using an autologous graft (usually the saphenous vein) or synthetic graft (polytetra florethylene or Dacron) to route arterial blood from the femoral artery around a blocked popliteal artery, thus reestablishing blood flow in the tibial arteries. If revascularization fails, amputation is the treatment of last resort.

Femoral popliteal bypass may be the primary treatment or an adjunct to other revascularization techniques, such as pulsed laser with angioplasty, rotablator catheter angioplasty (atherectomy), or intravascular stent placement. These newer, less invasive approaches to revascularization are associated with problems characteristic of any evolving technology, such as unsuitable design, insufficient technical guidance, and operator inexperience. These new techniques also carry a higher reported incidence of rapid thrombus formation, vessel perforation, vessel dissection, and rapid reocclusion of the manipulated vessel.

This plan focuses on postoperative care for the patient undergoing femoral popliteal bypass surgery.

ETIOLOGY AND PRECIPITATING FACTORS
Acute occlusion (Note: Acute occlusion is usually treated with anticoagulants, antiplatelet agents, vasodilators, embolectomy, or plasty repairs. Femoral popliteal bypass may be used when these approaches fail or the vessel is destroyed.)
• traumatic transection or occlusion
• disorders associated with embolus formation, such as endocarditis, aneurysms of the left ventricle or aorta, and atrial fibrillation
• collagen diseases and vasospastic disorders, such as throbangities obliterans (Buerger's disease)
• diagnostic procedures, such as angiography

Chronic occlusion (Note: Chronic occlusion may present with signs and symptoms of long-term ischemia or with evidence of acute limb-threating ischemia. A stenosis of 60% or greater will produce significant symptoms. The typical blockage ranges in length from 1½" to 9½" [4 cm to 24 cm].)

• atherosclerosis, especially in a person over age 60 with a coexisting vascular disorder
• aneurysm of the popliteal artery
• chronic infection
• restenosis of previous grafts

Focused assessment guidelines
NURSING HISTORY (Functional health pattern guidelines)

Nutritional-metabolic pattern
• may be obese
• may have type I or type II diabetes mellitus
• may be following a low-salt, low-cholesterol diet to control cardiovascular disease
• may present with a severe nutritional deficit related to multisystem vascular insufficiency or advanced age

Elimination pattern
• may report sudden onset of severe abdominal distress if ischemia is associated with multiple emboli and infarction of mesenteric vessels
• may report symptoms of acute renal failure if ischemia is associated with multiple emboli and infarction of the renal or arcuate arteries
• may report symptoms of chronic renal failure associated with hypertension and diabetes
• may report neurosensory impairment of bowel function (constipation or diarrhea) associated with long-term diabetes
• may report constipation associated with decreased physical activity
• may be unable to perform activities of daily living

Activity-exercise pattern
• typically reports sedentary life-style before onset of symptoms
• typically reports limited mobility related to the onset of ischemic muscle pain with physical activity
• may experience leg muscle weakness associated with ischemic changes
• may report a sports- or work-related injury (dislocation of the knee)
• may report fractures resulting from muscle weakness and sensory loss
• may be unable to perform activities of daily living

Sleep-rest pattern
• may report sleep disturbance related to ischemic pain occurring at rest

Cognitive-perceptual pattern
• may report low self-esteem as a result of inability to exercise or perform usual activities
• may report depression
• may have a history of cerebrovascular accident (CVA) with residual neurologic damage

Role-relationship pattern
• may report diminished social interaction related to inability to maintain usual activities
• may report history of chronic alcohol abuse
• may have diminished cognitive abilities associated with previous CVA

Sexuality-reproductive pattern
• if diabetic, may report decreased libido
• if diabetic male, may report impotence
• if female, may report developing symptoms after menopause
• if age 60 or older, may exhibit atrophy of secondary sex characteristics
• may report oral contraceptive use or the recent birth of a child (uncommon)

Coping—stress tolerance pattern
• may have history of cigarette smoking
• may have history of chronic alcohol abuse

PHYSICAL FINDINGS
Cardiovascular
• hypertension
• decreased or absent peripheral pulses
• bruits over abdominal aorta, femoral artery, or popliteal artery
• decreased capillary filling
• dependent rubor or cyanosis
• atrial fibrillation
• ventricular, aortic, or popliteal aneurysm

Renal
• chronic renal failure
• acute renal failure

Pulmonary
• symptoms of congestive heart failure or chronic obstructive pulmonary disease

Gastrointestinal
• diarrhea or constipation
• paralytic ileus

Neurologic
• decreased sensory perception (heat, cold, pressure, and pain) in affected extremities
• decreased proprioception in affected extremities
• altered cognitive function

Integumentary
• thinning
• hair loss
• paresthesia
• ulcerations that fail to heal
• skin cool or cold to touch
• gangrene

Musculoskeletal
• weakness
• atrophy

DIAGNOSTIC STUDIES
• multiplane (retrograde femoral or translumbar) arteriography—visualizes abdominal aorta and vessels in the lower extremities
• ultrasound Doppler and Duplex waveform analyses—demonstrate direction and velocity of arterial flow
• 99mTc-hexametazime-labeled leukocyte imaging—radioactive scan, localizes infection in grafts from previous bypass procedures
• ankle-brachial index (ABI)—noninvasive hemodynamic study, estimates the degree of arterial occlusion (a normal ABI is 1.0; single vessel occlusion, 0.5 to 1.0; multiple vessel occlusion, below 0.5)
• toe-ankle index (TAI)—noninvasive hemodynamic study, estimates degree of occlusion (normal TAI is above 0.65)
• stress tests—estimate the degree of disease based on development of claudication
• serum cholesterol—may be elevated if arterial occlusion is related to systemic vascular disease
• serum triglycerides—may be elevated if symptoms are related to systemic vascular disease
• blood glucose—may be elevated because diabetes mellitus is commonly associated with peripheral vascular disease
• blood urea nitrogen—may be elevated if hypertension has affected renal function
• liver function tests—may be altered in the patient with a history of alcohol abuse

POTENTIAL COMPLICATIONS
• hematoma formation
• infection
• emboli or thrombi
• gangrene
• skin ulcers

Collaborative problem: *Arterial insufficiency related to arterial graft occlusion, reperfusion injury, or coexisting microangiopathy associated with diabetes or microemboli*

NURSING PRIORITY: Maintain arterial flow.

Interventions

1. Assess and document appearance of surgical site. Include type of dressing, extent of drainage, and any drainage devices (such as a Hemovac).

2. Note the contours of the surgical site and compare with the opposite side. Observe for masses, ecchymoses, and skin changes. Monitor hemoglobin and hematocrit values.

3. Measure calf circumference hourly for the first 24 hours, then as condition warrants. Observe for decreased capillary refill; diminished or absent pulses; mild pain beginning in the feet and lateral to the tibia, progressing to pain unrelieved by narcotics; decreased range of motion and ABI; or cold, cyanotic skin. Document findings.

4. Position the leg to avoid hyperextension and undue pressure on the graft site.

5. Observe for symptoms of fluid volume deficit or hypotension. Document findings.

6. Administer ordered drugs and monitor for adverse reactions. If the antiplatelet medication will be continued after discharge, teach the patient about administration and possible side effects.

7. Observe for signs and symptoms of reperfusion injury (same as for severe hypoxia—cyanosis, coldness, and pain—with pulses still present). Maintain adequate hydration. If cyanosis, coldness, or pain occur, check for presence of peripheral pulses. Notify physician of findings promptly and administer treatment as ordered, typically mannitol.

8. Additional individualized interventions: _____

Rationales

1. Baseline assessment permits later comparison of data. A surgical drain may be in place to remove lymph or blood. Drainage should be minimal and bright red initially, becoming serous within 24 hours.

2. Disruption of graft anastomosis, hemorrhage of soft tissues, or drainage from severed lymph vessels can produce enough fluid to occlude the graft. Fluid collection causes the skin at the site to become taut with a dimpled appearance. A mass will be palpable. Surgical fluid removal is necessary if graft occlusion is imminent. Ecchymoses indicate arterial bleeding and possible disruption of the anastamosis. Decreased hemoglobin and hematocrit values may indicate bleeding also.

3. These symptoms suggest anterior compartment syndrome caused by tissue edema and hemorrhage. Emergency fasciotomy may be necessary to relieve symptoms.

4. Hyperextension of the knee or pressure from body weight can retard venous flow, increasing tissue edema. Pressure also can diminish arterial flow through the graft. The resulting thrombosis calls for an emergency embolectomy.

5. The patient is at greatest risk for shunt occlusion immediately after surgery. Factors which decrease blood pressure could cause shunt collapse.

6. Antiplatelet drugs, such as dipyridamole (Persantine) and aspirin, and anticoagulant drugs, such as heparin and warfarin (Coumadin), usually are ordered. Urokinase (Abbokinase) or streptokinase (Kabikinase) may be used to reverse shunt occlusion. The patient is usually continued on antiplatelet therapy after discharge.

7. In reperfusion injury, reperfused tissues typically demonstrate initial improvement, only to undergo severe hypoxic changes within 2 hours after surgery. Reperfused cells produce high levels of free oxygen radicals, which injure cells. Adequate hydration lessens the risk of reperfusion injury. The presence of peripheral pulses differentiates arterial reocclusion (in which pulses are absent) from reperfusion injury. Mannitol helps control reperfusion injury by acting as a free-radical scavenger.

8. Rationales: _____

Target outcome criteria
Within 24 hours after surgery and then continuously,
the patient will have:
• no ischemic pain
• measurable peripheral pulses.

Nursing diagnosis: *Impaired skin integrity related to surgical incision and possible preexisting stasis ulcers*

NURSING PRIORITIES: (a) Promote wound healing and (b) prevent infection.

Interventions	**Rationales**
1. Maintain strict aseptic technique in caring for the surgical wound, drains, and stasis ulcers of the feet and legs.	1. The arterial graft lies close to the skin surface. As a result, infection at the surgical site can extend quickly to the shunt. In addition, lymph channels are severed during surgery, so debris from infected stasis ulcers drains into the surgical site, fostering infection at the graft.
2. Do not administer injections on the affected side.	2. Edema, tissue swelling, and the severing of lymph channels all slow circulation on the affected side, resulting in unpredictable drug absorption.
3. Assess for signs of infection: fever, chills, malaise, increased pain at the surgical site, signs of arterial insufficiency distal to the site, incisional edema, drainage, and redness. Instruct the patient to observe for signs of infection daily for 90 days after surgery.	3. Tissue hypoxia before surgery increases the risk of infection. Infection with shunt occlusion can occur as late as 90 days after surgery.
4. Administer antibiotics and observe for adverse reactions.	4. Antibiotics are prescribed routinely because the risk of infection with subsequent shunt loss is high.
5. Reposition the patient and perform skin care every 2 hours. Consider using a specialty bed or mattress for the patient with a chronic mobility problem, such as a multisystem disorder, obesity, or advanced age. Document your actions.	5. The skin, particularly on bony prominences, is prone to breakdown. Ulcers may already be present.
6. Monitor and document fluid and food intake.	6. Adequate hydration and nutrition are necessary for wound healing and prevention of skin breakdown.
7. Additional individualized interventions: _____	7. Rationales: _____

Target outcome criteria
By the time of discharge, the patient will:
• demonstrate evidence of wound healing
• display no symptoms of infection.

Nursing diagnosis: *Impaired physical mobility related to surgery and preexisting disability*

NURSING PRIORITY: Help the patient return to highest level of self-care and mobility possible.

Interventions

1. Before surgery, instruct the patient about positioning the affected extremity: avoiding hyperextension of the knee, leg-crossing, any position that puts pressure on the popliteal space, sitting for more than 20 minutes, or wearing clothing that restricts arterial flow.

2. After surgery, maintain the patient on bedrest as ordered, usually for 24 to 48 hours. Position the affected joint as ordered.

3. Encourage active range-of-motion (ROM) exercises of all unaffected joints 3 to 4 times daily or, if the patient is unable, perform passive ROM exercises.

4. Collaborate with the health care team to design an appropriate rehabilitation program. Instruct the patient accordingly.

5. Additional individualized interventions: _____

Rationales

1. Preoperative teaching helps the patient avoid positions that could cause shunt occlusion.

2. Bedrest is usually maintained until shunt patency is ensured. Positioning depends on the type of surgery.

3. Exercise maintains joint flexibility and prevents postoperative complications associated with bedrest.

4. Extensive reconditioning may be necessary for the patient with long-term hypoxic injury to muscles and nerves or a history of myocardial infarction or CVA. Patient compliance with the rehabilitation regimen depends on an understanding of the prescribed treatment.

5. Rationales: _____

Target outcome criteria
Upon discharge, the patient will:
• demonstrate no complications associated with immobility
• demonstrate improved mobility

• verbalize an understanding of the prescribed treatment regimen.

Nursing diagnosis: *Pain associated with the surgical incision*

NURSING PRIORITY: Control pain.

Interventions

1. See the "Pain" plan, page 69.

2. Identify and document the source and degree of pain, using an analog scale. Instruct the patient to report unrelieved pain.

3. Elevate the affected extremity.

4. Administer pain medication, as necessary, and observe for adverse reactions.

5. Additional individualized interventions: _____

Rationales

1. General interventions for pain control are detailed in the "Pain" plan.

2. Prolonged or increasing pain could indicate hematoma or seroma formation at surgical site. Unrelieved pain distal to the surgical site indicates anterior compartment syndrome, described under the "Arterial insufficiency" collaborative problem above, or shunt occlusion.

3. Moderate elevation, so as to not impair arterial flow, helps decrease tissue edema and swelling associated with surgical trauma.

4. Narcotic analgesics are used judiciously in the early postoperative period.

5. Rationales: _____

Target outcome criterion
Upon discharge, the patient will report pain controlled with oral medication.

Discharge planning

NURSING DISCHARGE CRITERIA
Upon the patient's discharge, documentation shows evidence of:
• wound healing
• vital signs within limits for age and coexisting disorders
• absence of infection
• shunt patency
• absence of or minimal reports of pain
• restored arterial flow.

PATIENT-FAMILY TEACHING CHECKLIST
Document evidence that the patient and family demonstrate an understanding of:
__ medication regimen
__ proper positioning
__ desirable life-style changes, such as smoking cessation
__ rehabilitation regimen
__ dates and times of follow-up care
__ symptoms of infection
__ symptoms of arterial insufficiency
__ symptoms requiring medical intervention.

DOCUMENTATION CHECKLIST
Using outcome criteria as a guide, document:
__ clinical status on admission
__ significant changes in the preoperative state
__ completion of preoperative checklist
__ preoperative teaching
__ clinical status on admission from postanesthesia unit
__ amount and character of drainage from wounds or drains
__ tube patency
__ pain relief measures
__ activity tolerance
__ nutritional intake
__ elimination status
__ pertinent laboratory finding
__ patient-family teaching
__ discharge planning
__ clinical status upon discharge.

ASSOCIATED PLANS OF CARE
Amputation
Pain
Surgical Intervention

References

Agrifoglio, G., et al. "Thrombectomy for Late Graft Limb Occlusion," *Journal of Cardiovascular Surgery* (Torino) 31:617-20, September-October 1990.

Ala-Kulju, K., et al. "Effect of Antiplatelet and Anticoagulant Therapy on Patency of Femorotibial Bypass Grafts," *Journal of Cardiovascular Surgery* (Torino) 31:651-55, September-October 1990.

Ameli, F. "Predictors of Surgical Outcome in Patients Undergoing Aortobifemoral Bypass Reconstruction," *Journal of Cardiovascular Surgery* (Torino) 31:333-39, May-June 1990.

Guyton, A. *A Textbook of Medical Physiology*, 8th edition. Philadelphia: W.B. Saunders Co., 1991.

Insall, R., et al. "New Isotopic Technique for Detecting Prosthetic Arterial Graft Infection," *British Journal of Surgery* 77(11):1295-98, November 1990.

Lancashire, M., et al. "Popliteal Aneurysms Identified by Intra-arterial Streptokinase: A Changing Pattern of Presentation," *British Journal of Surgery* 77(12):1388-90, December 1990.

Luckman, J., and Sorenson, K. *Medical-Surgical Nursing: A Psychophysiological Approach* Philadelphia: W.B. Saunders Co., 1987.

Rosenthal, D. "Prosthetic Above-knee Femoropopliteal Bypass for Intermittent Claudication," *Journal of Cardiovascular Surgery* 31:462-68, 1990.

Valentine, D., et al. "Intermittent Claudication Caused by Atherosclerosis in Patients Aged Forty Years and Younger," *Surgery, Gynecology and Obstetrics* 172(1):7-8, 1991.

Wesorick, B. *Standards of Nursing Care. A Model For Clinical Nursing Practice.* Philadelphia: J.B. Lippincott Co., 1990.

CARDIOVASCULAR DISORDERS

CARDIOVASCULAR DISORDERS

Hypovolemic Shock

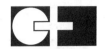

DRG information

DRG 127 Heart Failure and Shock.
        Mean LOS = 6.1 days
Note: Hypovolemic shock is more likely to be coded by its cause than by DRG 127 because the principal diagnosis or procedure determines the DRG. For example, hypovolemic shock caused by gastrointestinal hemorrhage would be coded as DRG 174, Gastrointestinal Hemorrhage with Complication or Comorbidity.

Introduction
DEFINITION AND TIME FOCUS

Hypovolemic shock is a complex, life-threatening process of microcirculatory dysfunction and altered cellular metabolism resulting from decreased blood volume. Sympathetic stimulation mediates hypovolemic shock's systemic effects, which include constriction of precapillary sphincters and venules. The resulting low capillary pressure promotes an interstitial-to-intravascular fluid shift that temporarily compensates for diminished circulating blood volume and maintains capillary flow. As shock progresses, however, this powerful compensatory mechanism fails. Decompensation results in capillary hypoxemia and acidosis, which promote sphincter relaxation, allowing capillary pressure to rise. Increased capillary permeability permits fluid to leak into the tissues, and the resulting decreased circulating blood volume increases hypoxemia and acidosis, creating a vicious circle that ultimately causes irreparable damage.

On a cellular level, shock disrupts vital processes. Delicate sodium-potassium transport mechanisms are paralyzed, allowing sodium to accumulate inside the cell and produce swelling. Mitochondrial depression impairs energy production; oxygen deprivation causes cells to switch from aerobic to an aerobic metabolism. Anaerobic metabolism, an inefficient energy-generating process, also depletes glucose stores and produces lactic acid, creating metabolic acidosis. As cells die, lysosomal destruction releases proteases and other enzymes. These enzymes wreak havoc on surrounding cells' integrity and trigger release of vasoactive substances, including myocardial depressant factor, that cause myocardial depression and severe vasodilation, further accelerating the vicious circle. This plan focuses on the critically ill patient with hypovolemic shock.

ETIOLOGY AND PRECIPITATING FACTORS
• hemorrhage
• severe dehydration
• excessive diuresis
• burns
• surgical or accidental trauma
• diabetes mellitus or diabetes insipidus

Focused assessment guidelines
NURSING HISTORY (Functional health, pattern findings)

Health perception–health management pattern
• may have a history of a history of diabetes mellitus, pancreatitis, hypertension, hemorrhage (internal or external), or other factors affecting fluid balance
• may have undergone a recent invasive procedure, especially abdominal or genitourinary surgery
• may have a history of recent trauma (particularly to the chest, abdomen, or spinal cord) or burns

Nutritional-metabolic pattern
• may describe intense thirst

Elimination pattern
• may describe increased urination or severe diarrhea (early) or oliguria (late)

Activity-exercise pattern
• typically complains of weakness and fatigue

Cognitive-perceptual pattern
• commonly shows reduced alertness or restlessness or anxiety

PHYSICAL FINDINGS
Cardiovascular
• orthostatic hypotension (early)
• supine hypotension (late)
• tachycardia
• arrhythmias
• decreased or thready peripheral pulses
• capillary filling time greater than 3 seconds

Pulmonary
• tachypnea

Neurologic
• altered level of consciousness, ranging from confusion, irritability, or restlessness (early) to coma (late)

Integumentary
• altered skin temperature, ranging from coolness (early) to coldness (late)
• pallor
• mottling
• cyanosis

Gastrointestinal
• pale or cyanotic oral mucous membranes

Renal
• oliguria or anuria

DIAGNOSTIC STUDIES

- complete blood count (CBC) — may vary, depending on shock stage; typically, decreased hemoglobin level and red blood cell count, variable hematocrit
- blood glucose level — elevated, reflecting stress-induced sympathetic stimulation
- blood urea nitrogen (BUN) and creatinine levels — elevated, reflecting decreased renal perfusion
- serum electrolyte levels — may vary, depending on the underlying problem and shock stage. Commonly, hypernatremia reflects increased renal sodium retention in response to volume losses; hypokalemia reflects urinary potassium losses in exchange for sodium; and hyperkalemia reflects acidosis, decreased glomerular filtration, and cell necrosis
- arterial blood gas (ABG) levels — reveal increased pH level and decreased $PaCO_2$ in early shock, reflecting respiratory alkalosis caused by hyperventilation, or decreased pH level, increased $PaCO_2$, and decreased bicarbonate level in late shock, reflecting respiratory acidosis caused by hypoventilation and metabolic acidosis caused by anaerobic metabolism
- clotting profile — may reveal coagulopathy, shown by decreased platelet level, decreased fibrinogen level, and increased fibrin split products
- serum osmolality — may increase, reflecting fluid loss
- urine osmolality or specific gravity — increase, reflecting water retention
- 12-lead electrocardiogram (ECG) — may reveal arrhythmias or changes reflecting myocardial ischemia, acute myocardial infarction (AMI), or electrolyte imbalances
- chest X-ray — may reveal pneumothorax or hemothorax

POTENTIAL COMPLICATIONS

- renal failure
- adult respiratory distress syndrome
- disseminated intravascular coagulation (DIC)
- liver failure
- irreversible brain damage

Collaborative problem: *Hypovolemic shock related to blood loss, diuresis, dehydration, or third-space fluid shift*

NURSING PRIORITY: Restore fluid volume.

Interventions

1. If the patient has active external bleeding (for example, from an arm laceration), apply direct, continuous pressure and elevate the area, if possible.

2. Observe for signs and symptoms of fluid loss:

- minimal volume loss: Slight tachycardia; normal supine blood pressure; positive postural vital signs (systolic blood pressure decrease greater than 10 mm Hg or pulse increase greater than 20 beats/minute); capillary refill time greater than 3 seconds; urine output greater than 30 ml/hour; cool, pale extremities; and anxiety

- moderate volume loss: Rapid, thready pulse; supine hypotension; cool truncal skin; urine output 10 to 30 ml/hour; severe thirst; and restlessness, confusion, or irritability

Rationales

1. Direct pressure to bleeding sites mechanically controls hemorrhage and aids clot formation by obstructing flow.

2. Signs and symptoms correlate with the approximate percentage of volume loss.

- Powerful compensatory mechanisms produce these signs, which correlate with blood volume loss between 10% and 15%. Medullary vasomotor center stimulation via the baroreceptor reflex causes tachycardia and vasoconstriction. Also, antidiuretic hormone and aldosterone release causes renal retention of sodium and water. All of these mechanisms help to maintain blood volume and normal supine blood pressure. However, postural vital signs are positive because homeostatic mechanisms cannot compensate for the added stress of a position change. Prolonged capillary refill time and slight oliguria reflect decreased circulating volume. Cool, pale skin with normal mental status reflects shunting of blood away from the periphery to preserve function of the brain and heart.

- These signs correlate with a volume loss of approximately 25%. As circulating blood volume drops to this level, compensatory mechanisms are no longer sufficient and decompensation occurs. Oliguria reflects decreased renal perfusion, while mental changes indicate decreased cerebral perfusion.

• severe volume loss: Marked tachycardia and hypotension; weak or absent peripheral pulses; cold, mottled, or cyanotic skin; urine output less than 10 ml/hour; and unconsciousness.

3. Elevate the patient's legs above heart level, unless there is active bleeding from the head and neck or suspected increased intracranial pressure or cardiogenic shock.

4. Obtain initial and serial diagnostic tests, including CBC, blood typing and cross-matching, serum electrolyte levels, ABG levels, urinalysis, 12-lead ECG, and chest X-ray.

5. Insert and maintain the following, as ordered:

• two or more large-bore I.V. lines

• indwelling urinary catheter.

6. Assist with insertion of a central venous pressure (CVP) catheter or pulmonary artery (PA) catheter, if ordered. Monitor urine output and CVP or pulmonary capillary wedge pressure (PCWP) every 15 minutes to 1 hour. Determine the frequency of measurement according to the depth of shock and rapidity of its progression.

7. Administer a fluid challenge, if ordered. See *Fluid challenge algorithm* for details.

8. Administer blood products and crystalloid or colloid I.V. solutions, as ordered.

9. Assist with insertion of an arterial line, if ordered. Monitor blood pressure continuously and measure mean arterial pressure (MAP) electronically.

• If an arterial line is not in place, measure cuff blood pressure every 5 to 15 minutes until stable, then every hour. Monitor MAP electronically or calculate it by adding one-third of pulse pressure to diastolic pressure, or by using this formula:

$$\frac{SP + (DP \times 2)}{3}$$

where SP equals systolic pressure and DP equals diastolic pressure.

• Maintain MAP within the desired range—usually at least 70 mm Hg. Consult with the doctor about the appropriate range for the patient.

• These signs reflect a volume loss of at least 40% and severely decreased vital organ perfusion.

3. Elevation promotes venous drainage from the legs and increases circulating blood volume as much as 800 ml. This measure will exacerbate the conditions indicated, however.

4. Serial data provide objective evidence of the disorder's severity and the effectiveness of interventions.

5. These invasive measures will combat shock.

• Large-bore I.V. lines allow rapid infusion of large fluid volumes.

• An indwelling catheter facilitates monitoring of urine output, the most easily assessed indicator of renal perfusion.

6. CVP measurements can be used to guide fluid volume replacement and may be ordered for patients with lesser degrees of shock. For patients with severe shock, a pulmonary artery catheter is preferred because it allows measurement of PCWP, which reflects left ventricular filling pressures more accurately than CVP does. Frequent measurements help determine the degree of shock and evaluate the effectiveness of interventions.

7. A fluid challenge involves administration of a fluid bolus over a limited period. It allows assessment of hemodynamic response to rapid volume administration, which helps identify hypovolemic shock.

8. Various I.V. solutions may be used; their advantages and drawbacks remain controversial. Colloids—solutions containing protein—help expand intravascular volume through osmosis; however, proteins may leak into the interstitial space, causing such complications as pulmonary edema. Crystalloid solutions—solutions containing salt, sugar, or both—do not cause protein leakage but require relatively large volumes because they leave the vascular space quickly.

9. Direct blood pressure measurement is preferred because it provides more accurate data than cuff measurements. MAP reflects the average pressure at which organs are perfused.

• Cuff blood pressure measurements and arithmetic MAP calculation, though less desirable than intra-arterial measurement, provide valuable data. MAP is closer to diastolic blood pressure than to systolic blood pressure because diastole is about twice as long as systole in the cardiac cycle.

• Maintaining MAP within the desired range provides for adequate organ perfusion. In most cases, MAP must be maintained above 70 mm Hg in a previously normotensive patient. A higher MAP is appropriate for the patient with chronic hypertension. An MAP that is too low promotes ischemia; an MAP that is too high contributes to such complications as cerebral and pulmonary edema.

FLUID CHALLENGE ALGORITHM

Measure central venous pressure (CVP) or pulmonary capillary wedge pressure (PCWP); administer 10-minute fluid challenge

If CVP or PCWP <12	If CVP or PCWP 12 to 18	If CVP or PCWP >18
Infuse at 20 ml/min	Infuse at 10 ml/min	Infuse at 5 ml/min

Measure CVP or PCWP again and compare to baseline

If CVP increases ≤2 or PCWP increases ≤3	If CVP increases 3 to 4 or PCWP increases 4 to 6	If CVP increases >5 or PCWP increases >7 (at any time)
Repeat challenge	Discontinue infusion and observe for 10 minutes	Discontinue challenge

Has CVP fallen to within 2 or PCWP fallen to within 3 of initial value?

Yes → Repeat challenge

No → Discontinue challenge

Data reprinted from M.H. Weil and E.C. Rackow, "A Guide to Volume Repletion," *Emergency Medicine* 16(8):101-110, ©1984 by Cahners Publishing Company. CVP values are in cm H$_2$O; PCWP values are in mm Hg.

CARDIOVASCULAR DISORDERS

10. During all fluid administration, monitor the trend of hemodynamic measurements and urine output. Observe for signs of fluid overload, such as crackles, neck vein distention, or a third heart sound (S$_3$).

10. Because the shock patient is hemodynamically unstable and has compromised compensatory mechanisms, volume administration may cause rapid progression from fluid depletion to fluid overload. If not detected promptly, fluid overload may cause pulmonary edema, congestive heart failure, or cerebral edema.

11. Additional individualized interventions: _____

11. Rationales: _____

_____

_____

Target outcome criteria
Within 48 hours, the patient will:
• maintain arterial pressure within normal limits
• maintain strong peripheral pulses
• maintain capillary refill time less than 3 seconds
• maintain CVP or PCWP within normal limits

• show no signs of fluid overload
• have warm, dry skin
• return to previous level of consciousness – ideally, alert and oriented.

Collaborative problem: *Hypoxemia related to ventilation-perfusion imbalance and diffusion defect*

NURSING PRIORITY: Maintain ventilation and oxygenation.

Interventions

1. Provide standard nursing care related to impaired gas exchange: maintain airway patency; monitor respiratory status; suction as necessary; provide supplemental oxygen, as ordered; and assist with intubation and mechanical ventilation, if indicated.

2. Monitor oxygen saturation through continuous pulse oximetry. Monitor ABG levels, as ordered – typically at least every 4 hours.

3. Additional individualized interventions: _____

_____

Rationales

1. Numerous factors may cause ventilation-perfusion imbalance in shock, including atelectasis, microemboli, pulmonary congestion, and impaired capillary perfusion. The general measures listed apply to the care of any critically ill patient.

2. Pulse oximetry determines oxygen saturation rapidly and continuously. ABG results indicate oxygenation status and degree of acid-base imbalance. Hyperventilation, a compensatory response to hypoxemia, is common in early hypovolemic shock and can lead to respiratory alkalosis. Combined metabolic acidosis (from lactic acid production in anaerobic metabolism) and respiratory acidosis (from decreased capillary perfusion) characterize late hypovolemic shock.

3. Rationales: _____

_____

Target outcome criteria
Within 48 hours, the patient will:
• maintain a patent airway
• have clearing breath sounds bilaterally

• show ABG levels within expected limits.

Nursing diagnosis: *High risk for injury: complications related to ischemia*

NURSING PRIORITY: Prevent or minimize complications.

Interventions

1. Prevent paralytic ileus and stress ulcers. Withhold food and fluids; insert a nasogastric tube connected to suction, as ordered. Administer cimetidine (Tagamet), ranitidine (Zantac), sucralfate (Carafate), or antacids, as ordered. Monitor bowel sounds.

Rationales

1. Paralytic ileus may result from mesenteric ischemia. The resulting gastric distention provokes vomiting, which can lead to chemical pneumonitis if aspiration occurs. Withholding food and fluids reduces stress on the stomach. Nasogastric drainage decompresses the stomach. The medications listed reduce the risk of stress ulcers by decreasing hydrochloric acid secretion or coating the gastric mucosa.

2. Observe for signs and symptoms of adult respiratory distress syndrome (ARDS), such as tachypnea, progressive dyspnea, increased inspiratory pressure (if the patient is on a ventilator), deteriorating ABG or pulse oximetry values, or lung compliance less than 50 ml/cm H_2O. If you detect these problems, document them and alert the doctor. Implement measures described in the "Adult Respiratory Distress Syndrome" plan, page 193, as appropriate.

2. Shock ranks as a major risk factor for ARDS because of such factors as decreased perfusion, hypoxemia, increased capillary permeability, and high oxygen levels used in treatment. The plan for ARDS describes this ominous complication and related care.

3. Observe for signs and symptoms of AMI, such as severe chest pain, shortness of breath, hypotension, diaphoresis, pained facial expression, elevated cardiac isoenzymes, or ECG showing ST-segment displacement, T-wave inversion, or pathologic Q waves. See the "Acute Myocardial Infarction—Critical Care Unit Phase" plan, page 268, for more details.

3. Decreased perfusion, catecholamine stimulation, hypoxemia, and increased afterload all may cause AMI. The AMI plan gives details on this complication.

4. Observe for signs and symptoms of DIC, such as blood oozing from multiple sites, repeated bleeding episodes, acral cyanosis, petechiae, ecchymoses, hematomas, prolonged prothrombin time, prolonged partial thromboplastin time, decreased fibrinogen level, decreased platelet count, or elevated fibrin split products level. See the "Disseminated Intravascular Coagulation" plan, page 625, for details.

4. Shock is a major risk factor for DIC because of such factors as capillary sludging; acidosis; and sepsis, trauma, or other underlying causes. The "Disseminated Intravascular Coagulation" plan describes this devastating development in depth.

5. Observe for signs and symptoms of acute renal failure, such as oliguria or anuria, weight gain, neck vein distention, crackles, dependent edema, or elevated BUN and serum creatinine levels. As appropriate, implement measures described in the "Acute Renal Failure" plan, page 548.

5. Constriction of renal blood vessels is an early compensatory mechanism in shock. Although this constriction limits glomerular filtration, thus conserving fluid volume, it impairs renal perfusion, which may result in acute renal failure. The "Acute Renal Failure" plan describes this complication in detail.

6. Observe for signs and symptoms of liver failure, such as drowsiness, intellectual deterioration, personality changes, septicemia, fever, hyperkinetic circulation, jaundice, hepatomegaly, ascites, easy bruising, increased prothrombin time, elevated serum aspartate aminotransferase level, or increased bilirubin level. See the "Liver Failure" plan, page 430.

6. Although shock may damage the liver's parenchymal cells, prompt correction of shock may allow these cells to regenerate. Early detection of liver failure may prevent severe damage to this critical organ. The "Liver Failure" plan presents the pathophysiology of this disorder and related care.

7. Additional individualized interventions: _____

7. Rationales: _____

_____

_____

Target outcome criterion
By the time of discharge, the patient will show no signs of the complications described above.

Nursing diagnosis: *High risk for ineffective individual coping, ineffective family coping, or both related to threat to life*

NURSING PRIORITY: Provide emotional support to the patient and family.

Interventions

1. Implement measures described in the "Ineffective Individual Coping" plan, page 51, and the "Ineffective Family Coping" plan, page 47, as appropriate.

Rationales

1. Families (and alert patients) are aware that shock is life threatening, and they react to the possibility of death in various ways. Measures to help them cope with their realistic fear and other emotional responses are described in these plans.

2. Additional individualized interventions: _____

2. Rationales: _____

_____

Target outcome criteria
By the time of discharge, the patient will meet outcome criteria identified in the "Ineffective Individual Coping" plan.

Discharge planning

NURSING DISCHARGE CRITERIA
Upon the patient's discharge, documentation shows evidence of:
• blood pressure within normal limits without I.V. inotrope or vasopressor support
• pulse and respirations within normal limits
• ABG levels within expected limits for recovery stage
• urine output within normal limits
• no evidence of major complications.

PATIENT-FAMILY TEACHING CHECKLIST
Document evidence that the patient and family demonstrate an understanding of:
___ cause and significance of shock
___ expectations for recovery
___ purpose of monitoring devices
___ rationales for therapeutic interventions.

DOCUMENTATION CHECKLIST
Using outcome criteria as a guide, document:
___ clinical status on admission
___ significant changes in status
___ pertinent diagnostic test findings
___ care for invasive monitoring lines
___ fluid administration
___ use of inotropes, vasopressors, or other pharmacologic agents
___ measures to support ventilation and oxygenation
___ emotional support
___ patient-family teaching
___ discharge planning.

ASSOCIATED PLANS OF CARE
Adult Respiratory Distress Syndrome
Disseminated Intravascular Coagulation
Impaired Physical Mobility
Ineffective Family Coping
Ineffective Individual Coping
Liver Failure
Major Burns
Mechanical Ventilation
Multiple Trauma
Pulmonary Embolism

References
Bumann, R., and Speltz, M. "Decreased Cardiac Output: A Nursing Diagnosis," *DCCN: Dimensions of Critical Care Nursing* 8(1):6-15, January-February 1989.

Futrell, A. "Decreased Cardiac Output: Case for a Collaborative Diagnosis,"*DCCN: Dimensions of Critical Care Nursing* 9(4):202-09, July-August 1990.

Jones, D. "Fluid Therapy in the PACU," *Critical Care Nursing Clinics of North America* 3(1):109-20, March 1991.

Kuhn, M. "CCRN Challenge: Colloids vs. Crystalloids," *Critical Care Nurse* 11(5):37-51, May 1991.

Rice, V. "Shock, a Clinical Syndrome: An Update. Part 1. An Overview of Shock," *Critical Care Nurse* 11(4):20-27, April 1991.

Rice, V. "Shock, a Clinical Syndrome: An Update. Part 2. The Stages of Shock," *Critical Care Nurse* 11(5):74-89, May 1991.

Rice, V. "Shock, a Clinical Syndrome: An Update. Part 3. Therapeutic Management," *Critical Care Nurse* 11(6):34-39, June 1991.

Rice, V. "Shock, a Clinical Syndrome: An Update. Part 4. Nursing Care of the Shock Patient," *Critical Care Nurse* 11(7):28-43, July-August 1991.

Sommers, M. "Fluid Resuscitation Following Multiple Trauma," *Crtical Care Nurse* 10(10):74-83, November-December 1990.

Weil, M., and Rackow, E. "A Guide to Volume Repletion," *Emergency Medicine* 16(8):100-5, 108-10, April 30, 1984.

Permanent Pacemaker Insertion

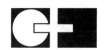

DRG information

DRG 115 Permanent Cardiac Pacemaker Implant.
With Acute Myocardial Infarction (AMI),
Heart Failure, or Shock.
Mean LOS = 12.1 days

DRG 116 Permanent Cardiac Pacemaker Implant.
Without AMI, Heart Failure, or Shock.
Mean LOS = 5.8 days

Introduction
DEFINITION AND TIME FOCUS

Permanent pacemaker insertion may be required when the patient experiences symptoms of decreased cardiac output secondary to irreversible or uncontrolled arrhythmias. Irreversible bradycardia results from atrioventricular (AV) heart block (typically Mobitz Type II second- or third-degree), sinus bradycardia, sinus arrest, or sinoatrial (SA) block. Tachyarrhythmias unresponsive to other treatments also may benefit from a permanent pacemaker, as may sick sinus (tachycardia-bradycardia) syndrome. This plan focuses on managing the patient who has had a permanent pacemaker inserted transvenously. The lead is inserted through a vein — commonly the cephalic, jugular, or subclavian — and positioned with fluoroscopy in the right ventricle. Lead attachment to the endocardium is either passive, with fibrosis occurring at the contact point, or active, with the lead screwed into the muscle. A subcutaneous pocket is made in the upper chest or abdominal region, and the pulse generator box is placed in it. The distal end of the lead is connected under the skin to the generator box. The procedure is commonly done under local anesthesia.

ETIOLOGY AND PRECIPITATING FACTORS

• idiopathic sclerotic degeneration of the SA node
• coronary artery disease, especially with significant disease or infarction involving the artery to the SA node (right coronary artery in 55% of the population, circumflex in 45%) or the AV node (right coronary artery in 90%, circumflex in 10%)
• rheumatic heart disease
• cardiomyopathy
• congenital heart disease, such as ventricular septal defect or transposition of the great vessels
• surgical trauma or edema affecting the cardiac conduction system
• myocarditis
• hypersensitive carotid sinus syndrome

Focused assessment guidelines
NURSING HISTORY (Functional health pattern findings)

Note: Findings vary, depending on the underlying condition.

Health perception — health management pattern
• may report syncope, dizziness, and light-headedness (Adams-Stokes disease)
• may be under treatment for arrhythmias
• may also be under treatment for angina, atherosclerosis, hypertension, or congestive heart failure
• may report a history of myocardial infarction (MI), congenital heart disease, or cardiac surgery
• typically an older male

Nutritional-metabolic pattern
• may report swelling of extremities and weight gain

Activity-exercise pattern
• may report shortness of breath, fatigue, and activity intolerance

Cognitive-perceptual pattern
• may report chest pain
• may report palpitations

Self-perception — self-concept pattern
• may express concern over anticipated changes in body image and functioning
• may express concern over follow-up care and restrictions

PHYSICAL FINDINGS
(before pacemaker insertion)

Cardiovascular
• arrhythmias — bradycardia, irregular rhythms, or (uncommonly) tachycardia
• hypotension
• venous engorgement or jugular vein distention
• S_3 or S_4 heart sounds
• decreased peripheral pulses
• slow capillary refill

Pulmonary
• crackles
• shortness of breath
• paroxysmal nocturnal dyspnea
• orthopnea

Neurologic
- dizziness
- syncope
- seizures
- transient ischemic attacks

Integumentary
- cool, clammy skin
- edema

Renal
- weight gain (from fluid retention)

Gastrointestinal
- liver enlargement
- positive hepatojugular reflux

DIAGNOSTIC STUDIES
- electrolyte panel—used to rule out disturbances affecting cardiac conduction and contractility (hypokalemia or hyperkalemia, and hypocalcemia or hypercalcemia)
- serum drug levels—may reveal subtherapeutic or toxic medication levels that may affect heart rate and rhythm (medications that may affect heart rate or rhythm include digoxin [Lanoxin], quinidine, amiodarone (Cordarone), beta blockers, calcium channel blockers, narcotics, and some psychotropics and antihypertensives)

- blood urea nitrogen and creatinine levels—may reflect low renal perfusion from low cardiac output
- triiodothyronine (T_3) and thyroxine (T_4) levels—may be low, indicating that hypothyroidism may be depressing cardiac impulse formation or conduction
- 12-lead electrocardiogram (ECG)—may reveal electrical activity not obvious in a single-lead rhythm strip and may help identify the arrhythmia
- Holter monitor—may be used to confirm sick sinus syndrome or other transient arrhythmias
- chest X-ray—may show cardiac enlargement
- electrophysiology studies—may allow induction and identification of symptom-causing arrhythmias

POTENTIAL COMPLICATIONS
- arrhythmias
- infection
- thrombosis or embolism
- tamponade or perforation of myocardium
- hematoma or hemorrhage
- lead fracture
- pneumothorax
- hiccups (diaphragmatic pacing)
- tricuspid insufficiency
- painful subcutaneous pocket or pocket erosion
- pacemaker syndrome

Collaborative problem: *High risk for arrhythmias related to pacemaker malfunction or catheter displacement*

NURSING PRIORITY: Maintain optimal cardiac rhythm.

Interventions

1. Initiate constant ECG monitoring for 48 to 72 hours after pacemaker insertion or as ordered. Keep alarms on at all times. Set the low limit at 3 beats less per minute than the pacer setting. Set the high limit 10 beats/minute above the anticipated maximum cardiac rate. Place monitoring electrodes 2″ (5 cm) away from the generator box. Change the monitoring electrode sites if the pacer appears to be malfunctioning.

2. Document in the plan of care the patient's intrinsic rate and rhythm. Also indicate the pacemaker type (refer to *Generic pacemaker code*) and rate.

3. Record and document rhythm strips every shift and mount them in the patient's chart. Analyze the strips: Appropriately paced beats will show a pacer spike artifact followed by a depolarization wave that differs from the intrinsic waveform. Notify the doctor promptly if problems occur with impulse initiation or conduction:

Rationales

1. Continuous monitoring facilitates early problem detection. If the pacemaker is functioning properly, the cardiac rate should not go below the pacer setting. The risk of tachyarrhythmias cannot be ignored. Monitoring electrodes placed near the generator box or in lead locations where the ECG amplitude is small may result in failure to record intrinsic beats.

2. This information is necessary for correct ECG interpretation.

3. Systematic documentation provides an objective, organized means of analyzing pacer activity. Waveforms of paced and intrinsic beats differ because of independent conduction paths.

GENERIC PACEMAKER CODE

The North American Society of Pacing and Electrophysiology and the British Pacing and Electrophysiology Group have recommended a sequence of five letters to designate pacemaker capabilities. Note that the first three positions are used for antibradyarrhythmia function exclusively.

Chamber paced (Position I)	Chamber sensed (Position II)	Response to sensing (Position III)	Programmability, rate modulation (Position IV)	Antitachyarrhythmia function (Position V)
O = none A = atrium V = ventricle D = dual (A and V)	O = none A = atrium V = ventricle D = dual (A and V)	O = none T = triggered I = inhibited D = dual (T and I)	O = none P = simple programmable M = multiprogrammable C = communicating R = rate modulation	O = none P = pacing (antitachyarrhythmia) S = shock D = dual (P and S)

From: Bernstein, A.D., et al. "The NASPE/BPEG Generic Pacemaker Code for Antibradyarrhythmia and Adaptive Rate Pacing and Antitachyarrhythmia Devices," *PACE* 10:794-99, July-August 1987. Used with permission.

• failure to sense — pacer spikes occur despite the patient's intrinsic rate

• The sensitivity setting may be such that the pacemaker does not consistently detect intrinsic low-amplitude cardiac electrical activity. Failure to sense also may result from fibrosis at the lead tip, lead fracture, or a dislodged lead. Failure to sense may result in inappropriate, unnecessary pacing and may cause R-on-T phenomenon, in which a pacer spike falls on the downslope of the preceding T wave, triggering ventricular tachycardia or ventricular fibrillation.

• failure to capture — pacing spikes not followed by cardiac depolarization

• Failure to capture results when the voltage of the pacemaker stimulus is insufficient to trigger depolarization. It may result from fibrosis at the lead-myocardial junction, a weak battery, the effect of cardiac drugs, electrolyte imbalance, or a dislodged or malpositioned lead.

• failure to pace — absence of pacing spikes when the intrinsic rate is below the pacer setting.

• Failure to pace may result from a fractured lead wire, malfunction at the lead-generator connection, power source depletion, or oversensing — the sensing of noncardiac electrical activity, such as muscle activity near the generator box, power lines, other sources of electrical noise, or cross talk in dual chamber pacemakers.

4. Obtain 12-lead simultaneous ECG recordings daily for 3 days and as needed.

4. A 12-lead recording shows pacer function and cardiac electrical activity more accurately than a single-lead rhythm strip. Simultaneous tracings help to confirm pacing spikes and intrinsic beats that may vary in amplitude in different leads and therefore may not be obvious in one particular lead.

5. Administer cardiac medications, as ordered, and document their effectiveness and adverse effects.

5. Cardiac medications may be indicated for treatment of underlying cardiac problems, such as coronary artery or valvular disease.

6. Monitor blood pressure, apical pulse, and respirations every 4 hours or as ordered.

6. Deviation from postoperative baseline vital signs may indicate pacemaker failure or other complications.

7. Maintain and document I.V. line patency, as ordered.

7. The I.V. line may be needed to administer emergency medications.

8. Maintain the patient on bed rest with turning limitations and with the head of the bed elevated 30 to 45 degrees for 48 to 72 hours, or as ordered.

8. With passive lead placement, activity and positioning limitations are needed temporarily to maintain lead placement until fibrosis develops around the electrode tip and anchors it in place. Limitations may be less restrictive with active lead attachment.

9. If use of the affected arm is restricted, perform limited passive range-of-motion (ROM) exercises with the arm every hour during the first 24 hours after surgery.

10. Assess chest X-ray daily for 3 days.

11. Additional individualized interventions: _____

_____

9. Movement restrictions may be ordered to reduce the chance of lead displacement. Passive ROM exercises may prevent frozen shoulder.

10. Chest X-rays may be used to confirm lead placement.

11. Rationales: _____

_____

Target outcome criteria

Immediately after surgery and throughout the hospital stay, the patient will:
• display a cardiac rate no less than pacemaker setting
• display ECG evidence of appropriate pacer sensing, firing, and capturing.

Within 3 days after surgery, the patient will:
• have decreased or no signs and symptoms of low cardiac output (if present before surgery)
• visit the pacemaker clinic for a definitive check of pacemaker functioning.

Nursing diagnosis: *High risk for infection related to surgical disruption of skin barrier*

NURSING PRIORITIES: (a) Promote incisional healing by primary intention, and (b) prevent or promptly detect infection.

Interventions

1. Check the primary dressing for drainage. Circle any drainage, and write the date and time when first discovered.

2. Reinforce the primary dressing as needed for 24 hours. Do not change the primary dressing without an order from the doctor.

3. After removing the primary dressing, check the incision for excessive redness, swelling, warmth, and drainage.

4. Perform wound care, as ordered.

5. Administer antibiotics, as ordered.

6. Monitor body temperature every 4 hours. Notify the doctor if the patient's oral temperature exceeds 100° F (37.8° C).

7. Monitor the white blood cell (WBC) count, as ordered.

8. Culture purulent drainage, if present, as ordered.

Rationales

1. This is an objective method of monitoring for bleeding and incisional drainage.

2. Reinforcement protects the incision and aids hemostasis while providing a protective barrier against microorganisms. Removing the primary dressing increases the risk of accidentally disrupting the incision and causing bleeding.

3. These signs may reflect infection.

4. The pacemaker pocket is the most common entry site for infectious organisms, which can migrate along the pacing wires to the heart. A clean, dry incision promotes healing.

5. Antibiotics may be prescribed prophylactically because pacemaker insertion is an invasive procedure that involves implanting a foreign object into the heart. Also, the disruption of the skin barrier provides a potential portal of entry for infectious organisms into the heart.

6. Commonly, elevated temperature is a systemic response to infection.

7. The WBC count increases in response to infectious organisms.

8. WBCs and cellular debris accumulate locally in response to infectious organisms. Proper treatment requires identifying the causative agent and its medication sensitivity.

9. Additional individualized interventions: _____

9. Rationales: _____

Target outcome criteria
Within 1 day after surgery and throughout the hospital stay, the patient will:
• have a dry and intact incision
• experience no fever.

By the time of discharge, the patient will:
• have a WBC count within normal limits
• show no signs of infection.

Nursing diagnosis: *Bathing, feeding, and toileting self-care deficit related to bed rest and activity limitations*

NURSING PRIORITY: Assist with bathing, feeding, and toileting while bed rest is required.

Interventions

1. Assist with bathing and oral hygiene daily, as needed.

2. Assist the patient at mealtime. Elevate the head of the bed, as ordered.

3. Supply a bedpan and urinal, as needed.

4. Administer stool softeners and laxatives judiciously, as ordered, and document their use. Encourage alternatives or supplements to stool softeners and laxatives, such as increased dietary fiber (if possible) and prune juice.

5. After arm use is no longer restricted, encourage the patient to move the arm and resume self-care.

6. Additional individualized interventions: _____

Rationales

1. Bed rest and arm movement limitations prevent the patient from sitting up and using bathing and oral hygiene supplies.

2. The patient may be unable to reach or manipulate items on the meal tray while on bed rest. Raising the head of the bed facilitates swallowing and minimizes the risk of aspiration.

3. The patient will be unable to use the bathroom.

4. Straining to defecate requires considerable energy and may produce vagal-mediated arrhythmias. Laxative dependence diminishes the urge for normal defecation.

5. The patient may be hesitant to use the arm initially for fear of dislodging the electrode.

6. Rationales: _____

Target outcome criteria
While on bed rest, the patient will:
• accept self-care assistance
• observe activity restrictions.

Within 3 days after surgery, the patient will:
• resume normal self-care activities
• perform normal bowel elimination without straining.

Nursing diagnosis: *Knowledge deficit: self-care after discharge related to unfamiliar therapeutic intervention*

NURSING PRIORITY: Teach the information and skills necessary for optimal self-care.

Interventions

1. Explain potential signs and symptoms of decreased cardiac output that should be reported to the doctor, such as shortness of breath, low or erratic pulse, light-headedness, chest pains, decreased exercise tolerance, prolonged fatigue or weakness, or recurrence of preimplant symptoms.

Rationales

1. These signs and symptoms may indicate pacemaker malfunction.

2. Discuss signs and symptoms of extraneous stimulation that should be reported, such as muscle, arm, or skin twitching near the generator box or prolonged and rapid hiccups.

2. These signs and symptoms may result from electrode or lead malposition and adjacent tissue stimulation.

3. Teach the patient to recognize and report signs and symptoms of pocket infection, such as fever or chills and incisional drainage, redness, swelling, or pain.

3. Infection may not be apparent until after discharge.

4. Teach the patient to check the radial pulse at the same time daily after resting for 5 minutes; reinforce guidelines for reporting significant changes, particularly a decrease of 3 to 5 beats/minute below the pacer setting or an erratic, persistent high rate.

4. Changes in pacemaker function may be detected by regular assessment.

5. Emphasize the importance of complying with the follow-up monitoring regimen (by in-person appointments or a telephone monitoring device).

5. Pacemaker function can be evaluated most accurately by an ECG. Periodic checks using a donut-shaped magnet help determine when a new battery is needed.

6. Emphasize the need to inform health care providers about the pacemaker. The patient should wear a medical alert bracelet and carry a wallet identification card with pacemaker specifications.

6. Certain procedures, such as electrocautery, physical therapy, and nuclear magnetic resonance imaging, may be contraindicated. A medical alert bracelet and pacemaker specifications will help ensure faster treatment if an emergency occurs.

7. Discuss potential environmental hazards, such as power plants and radar stations, electromagnetic power fields, anti-theft devices, radio and television transmitters, and running car engines.

7. Exposure to electromagnetic power sources may alter pacemaker function. Most home electric appliances, including microwave ovens, are not a problem if in proper working order.

8. As specified by the doctor, instruct the patient about resuming activity and any limitations on travel, exercise, bathing and showering, tight clothing, and sexual activity.

8. Gradual resumption of activities according to patient tolerance generally is encouraged. Activities involving abrupt, forceful arm movement (such as tennis and golf) that may cause lead fracture may be limited for several weeks. Contact sports typically are not allowed. Tight clothing over the incision may impair healing.

9. Teach the purpose, dose, administration schedule, and adverse effects of all medications.

9. Knowledge may increase compliance.

10. Provide written material for all patient-teaching topics.

10. Written material reinforces and serves as a reference for this detailed information.

11. Additional individualized interventions: _____

11. Rationales: _____

Target outcome criteria
By the time of discharge, the patient will:
• demonstrate accurate pulse rate measurement
• list significant, reportable signs and symptoms
• verbalize activity expectations and limitations and environmental hazards
• explain initial follow-up arrangements or appointments

• state the purpose, dose, administration schedule, and adverse effects of medications
• verbalize understanding of the need to inform health care providers about the pacemaker.

Nursing diagnosis: *High risk for body-image disturbance related to dependence on prosthetic device*

NURSING PRIORITY: Promote positive incorporation of the pacemaker into the patient's body image.

Interventions	**Rationales**
1. Assess the patient's adaptation to change, including perceptions and personal meaning of limitations.	1. The changes caused by pacemaker implantation may vary in significance among patients. Many patients welcome the increased activity tolerance and show signs of improved self-image. For others, however, loss of a body function may trigger the grieving process.
2. Encourage the patient to ask questions and verbalize feelings.	2. Verbalization enables the nurse to listen to, assess, and validate the patient's feelings, thus facilitating adjustment to change.
3. Encourage the patient to look at the incision and the pacemaker site.	3. Willingness to view the incision and site may reflect beginning acceptance and adjustment.
4. Assess for maladaptive coping behaviors, such as manipulating the generator box, verbalizing inability to make life-style or health-promoting changes, crying or a flat affect, lack of participation and interest in activities, or anxiety.	4. These behaviors may indicate that the patient is having difficulty adjusting to the physical change and the need for pacemaker dependence.
5. If indicated, consult the "Grieving" and "Ineffective Individual Coping" plans, pages 31 and 51 respectively.	5. These plans contain generalized interventions related to these problems.
6. Additional individualized interventions: _____	6. Rationales: _____

Target outcome criteria
By the time of discharge, the patient will:
• participate actively in self-care
• ask appropriate questions and show interest in learning about the pacemaker

• show no evidence of maladaptive coping.

Discharge planning
NURSING DISCHARGE CRITERIA
Upon the patient's discharge, documentation shows evidence of:
• normal body temperature
• absence of angina and arrhythmias
• ECG within expected parameters, indicating appropriate pacemaker settings, sensing, firing, and capturing
• vital signs within acceptable parameters
• absence of pulmonary and cardiovascular complications
• absence of redness, swelling, and drainage at incision site
• WBC count within normal parameters
• ability to transfer, ambulate, and perform activities of daily living (ADLs) same as before hospitalization
• adequate home support system or referral to home care if indicated by inadequate support system and the patient's inability to perform ADLs.

PATIENT-FAMILY TEACHING CHECKLIST
Document evidence that the patient and family demonstrate an understanding of:
___ symptoms of pacemaker failure or complications
___ symptoms of infection
___ type of pacemaker, set rate, and operating method
___ need for daily pulse rate measurement
___ how to obtain a wallet identification card and medical alert bracelet
___ need to inform other health care providers about pacemaker
___ plan for resuming activities
___ limitations and precautions
___ all discharge medications' purpose, dose, administration schedule, and adverse effects requiring medical attention (usual discharge medications may include oral analgesics and other medications based on the patient's needs and underlying disorder)
___ follow-up monitoring
___ how to contact the doctor.

CARDIOVASCULAR DISORDERS

DOCUMENTATION CHECKLIST

Using outcome criteria as a guide, document before surgery:

___ clinical status on admission

___ 12-lead ECG reading

___ chest X-ray and results

___ urinalysis results

___ SMA and complete blood counts

___ patient teaching

___ telemetry strip documentation

___ surgical skin preparation

___ I.V. line patency and site condition.

Using outcome criteria as a guide, document after surgery:

___ clinical status on return from postanesthesia recovery unit

___ significant status changes

___ telemetry strip documentation

___ 12-lead ECG reading

___ incision status and care

___ I.V. line patency and site condition

___ chest X-ray and results

___ pacemaker clinic check for correct functioning before discharge

___ patient-family teaching

___ discharge planning.

ASSOCIATED PLANS OF CARE

Acute Myocardial Infarction—Stepdown Unit Phase

Angina Pectoris

Congestive Heart Failure

Geriatric Considerations

Grieving

Ineffective Individual Coping

Pain

Surgical Intervention

Thrombophlebitis

References

Andreoli, K. *Comprehensive Cardiac Care*, 6th ed. St. Louis: Mosby-Year Book, 1987.

Carpenito, L. *Nursing Diagnosis: Application to Clinical Practice*, 4th ed. Philadelphia: J.B. Lippincott Co., 1992.

Stafford, M. "Monitoring Patients with Permanent Cardiac Pacemakers," *Nursing Clinics of North America* 22(2):503-19, June 1987.

Underhill, S., et al. *Cardiac Nursing*, 2nd ed. Philadelphia: J.B. Lippincott Co., 1989.

Welch, T. "Pacemaker Implant: Implications for Perioperative Nurses," *AORN* 49(1):257-67, January 1989.

CARDIOVASCULAR DISORDERS
Thrombophlebitis

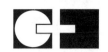

DRG information
DRG 128 Deep Vein Thrombophlebitis.
　　　　Mean LOS = 7.7 days
DRG 130 Peripheral Vascular Disorders.
　　　　With Complication or Comorbidity (CC).
　　　　Mean LOS = 6.0 days
DRG 131 Peripheral Vascular Disorders. Without CC.
　　　　Mean LOS = 4.4 days

Introduction
DEFINITION AND TIME FOCUS
Thrombophlebitis is the severe, acute inflammation of small- and medium-sized veins associated with secondary thrombus formation. It can occur in superficial or deep veins. The most common site of superficial thrombophlebitis is the saphenous vein; the most common sites of deep-vein thrombosis are the iliofemoral vein, popliteal veins, and small calf veins. This plan focuses on the patient admitted for diagnosis and management of acute lower-extremity thrombophlebitis.

ETIOLOGY AND PRECIPITATING FACTORS
• venous stasis from prolonged bed rest, sitting, or standing; varicose veins; low cardiac output; obesity; or limb paralysis
• hypercoagulability from dehydration or oral contraceptive use
• vessel wall trauma from venipunctures, leg injury, venous disease, infection, or chemical irritants, such as I.V. antibiotics or potassium chloride
• vascular narrowing or degeneration from hypertension, hypercholesterolemia, diabetes, kidney disease, cerebrovascular accident, or smoking

Focused assessment guidelines
NURSING HISTORY (Functional health pattern findings)

Health perception — health management pattern
• may report acute onset of local pain (relieved by elevation of extremity), tenderness, edema, erythema, warmth, induration, or febrile reaction
• may have known risk factors
• may have a history of recent vessel cannulation or vessel trauma

Activity-exercise pattern
• may report a sedentary life-style or occupation that requires standing for long periods
• may report recent prolonged bed rest or immobility

Role-relationship pattern
• may report a family history of cardiac risk factors

PHYSICAL FINDINGS
Cardiovascular
• local edema
• engorged vessel
• positive Homan's sign

Integumentary
• local erythema
• warmth
• local induration
• ulceration

DIAGNOSTIC STUDIES
• complete blood count — white blood cell count may reflect inflammatory response and systemic infection
• partial thromboplastin time (PTT) and prothrombin time (PT) — may indicate clotting defects or hypercoagulability
• cholesterol levels — may be elevated, suggesting increased risk for atherosclerosis
• serum glucose levels — may be elevated, reflecting stress response or diabetes
• triglyceride levels — may be elevated, indicating increased risk of atherosclerosis
• Doppler ultrasound blood flow detector test — determines venous return, may identify thrombolic occlusion
• plethysmography — may show segmental occlusion
• venography — may indicate loss of significant venous return
• ^{125}I fibrinogen leg scanning — may reflect vascular insufficiency

POTENTIAL COMPLICATIONS
• venous ulcer
• pulmonary embolus
• phlegmasia cerulea dolens (sudden, marked leg swelling and cyanosis related to iliofemoral venous thrombosis)

Collaborative problem: *Venous insufficiency related to obstruction and stasis*

NURSING PRIORITY: Promote venous blood flow.

Interventions

1. Assess calves and thighs daily for signs and symptoms of thrombophlebitis. Early signs include swelling, erythema, edema, tenderness, venous patterning, or engorgement along the vein. Later signs include pain, cording, and a positive Homan's sign (not always present). Avoid deep palpation. If swelling is suspected or present, measure and record leg circumference, placing a reference mark on the leg. Repeat the measurement daily, comparing the latest measurement with previous values.

2. Notify the doctor immediately if new signs and symptoms develop or existing ones worsen.

3. Implement activity restrictions:
• Maintain complete bed rest, usually for 3 to 7 days.
• Elevate the extremity at least 30 degrees continuously, unless contraindicated.
• Avoid using the knee gatch, pillows under the knees, and, when the patient is allowed out of bed, leg crossing and prolonged sitting.

4. Encourage the patient to perform gentle foot and leg exercises every hour. Consult the doctor about appropriate exercises, which may include isometric exercises (quadriceps setting or plantar flexion against a footboard) or isotonic exercises (active or passive foot and leg flexion and extension and ankle rotation).

5. Increase fluid intake to 8 8-oz glasses (2,000 ml) a day, unless contraindicated.

6. Consult the doctor about using antiembolism stockings.

7. Teach the patient stress-control measures, as needed, such as progressive relaxation techniques, breathing exercises, and visualization. Encourage smoking cessation and refer the patient to appropriate resources for help.

8. Administer medications, as ordered: anti-inflammatory agents, such as ibuprofen (Advil) and indomethacin (Indocin), and anticoagulants, such as heparin, warfarin sodium (Coumadin), or aspirin.

Rationales

1. Early signs and symptoms result from vessel wall inflammation; later ones, from thrombus formation. Homan's sign (pain in the calf on dorsiflexion of the foot), commonly believed to indicate deep-vein thrombosis, is an unreliable indicator. Absent in many cases of deep-vein thrombosis, Homan's sign can be produced in any painful calf condition. Deep palpation may dislodge a clot. Leg circumference monitoring provides an objective method to evaluate swelling; using a reference mark ensures consistency.

2. New or worsening signs of thrombophlebitis require prompt medical attention. Superficial thrombophlebitis, although not dangerous, is painful. Untreated deep-vein thrombophlebitis can be life-threatening if the thrombus moves to the lungs.

3. Bed rest and elevation improve venous flow by using gravity to reduce the pressure gradient between the extremity and the heart. Also, bed rest reduces oxygen requirements, limits the risk of thrombus dislodgement, and promotes fibrinolytic breakdown and clot absorption. The remaining measures avoid increased popliteal pressure, which compresses veins and impedes venous return.

4. The pumping effect of muscle action promotes venous return. Gentle exercise minimizes further thrombus formation, but overly vigorous exercise may dislodge clots. Isometric exercises, generally recommended after surgery, increase venous flow but also may increase blood pressure. Because this effect may be detrimental, particularly to the patient with cardiovascular disease, some doctors prefer isotonic exercises, which cause a more desirable cardiovascular response.

5. Increased fluid intake increases vascular volume and reduces viscosity, thus improving blood flow.

6. Superficial veins may be dilated and tortuous, particularly in the older patient. Antiembolism stockings may support venous return by compressing superficial veins and redirecting blood flow to deeper veins.

7. Stress-related catecholamine release and smoking induce vasoconstriction.

8. Anti-inflammatory agents are the primary treatment for superficial thrombophlebitis. Anticoagulants may be used if a superficial thrombus extends or threatens the deep venous system in the groin. Anticoagulants are the mainstay of treatment for deep venous thrombophlebitis. Heparin interferes with platelet aggregation, conversion of prothrombin to thrombin, and conversion of fibrinogen to fibrin, thereby minimizing further clot formation. Warfarin sodium interferes with the vitamin K activity necessary for clotting. Aspirin interferes with platelet aggregation.

9. Monitor clotting studies, as ordered: PTT if the patient is receiving heparin, PT if the patient is receiving warfarin sodium. Report values outside the desired range to the doctor before the next scheduled anticoagulant dose.

10. Observe for signs of bleeding, such as oozing at intravenous or intramuscular injection sites, epistaxis, bleeding gums, ecchymoses, hematuria, or melena.

11. Increase the patient's activity level, as ordered.

12. Observe for signs of chronic venous insufficiency: dependent ankle edema, induration, shiny skin, varicosities, and stasis ulcers. Consult the doctor if these signs are present.

13. Additional individualized interventions: _____

9. Dosages are adjusted to maintain PT and PTT within a therapeutic range. The typical ranges desired are 2 to 2½ times control values.

10. Excessive anticoagulant dosages increase the risk of bleeding.

11. Muscle movement compresses vessels, improving venous return.

12. Repeated episodes of deep-vein thrombosis can cause chronic venous insufficiency from venous valvular destruction.

13. Rationales: _____

Target outcome criteria
Within 3 days of admission, the patient will:
• show improved color and temperature of affected area
• have decreased edema
• perform leg exercises as instructed
• maintain fluid intake within desired range
• show no evidence of bleeding.

Nursing diagnosis: *Pain related to vessel obstruction, inflammation, and edema*

NURSING PRIORITY: Relieve pain.

Interventions

1. See the "Pain" plan, page 69.

2. Promote venous flow, as described in the previous problem.

3. Handle the affected extremity gently. Use a bed cradle.

4. Apply warm, moist heat to the affected area, as ordered.

5. Administer analgesics, as ordered, observing for therapeutic and adverse effects. Question the use of indomethacin or aspirin if the patient is receiving an anticoagulant.

6. Administer anti-inflammatory agents, as ordered.

7. Additional individualized interventions: _____

Rationales

1. The "Pain" plan contains multiple interventions for pain relief.

2. Eliminating the pain's cause is the most effective relief measure.

3. The thrombophlebitic extremity is extremely sensitive; even slight pressure or movement may be painful. A bed cradle keeps the weight of linens off the extremity.

4. Heat is soothing and causes vasodilation, improving blood flow.

5. The appropriate type and amount of analgesic depends on the degree of pain and the use of anticoagulants. Indomethacin and aspirin, which may be used to control pain, increase anticoagulant activity and may be inappropriate for the patient taking heparin or warfarin.

6. Reducing inflammation reduces pain.

7. Rationales: _____

CARDIOVASCULAR DISORDERS

Target outcome criterion
Within 1 hour of reporting pain, the patient will verbalize relief.

Collaborative problem: *High risk for thromboembolism related to dislodged thrombus*

NURSING PRIORITY: Prevent or promptly detect thromboembolism.

Interventions

1. Monitor for signs and symptoms of either a massive pulmonary embolism (profound shock, cyanosis, diaphoresis, and a sense of impending doom) or a lesser pulmonary embolism (tachypnea, dyspnea, pleuritic chest pain [sharp, stabbing pain that worsens on inspiration or coughing], and restlessness).

2. Alert the doctor promptly if any signs or symptoms of pulmonary embolism appear. If signs of massive pulmonary embolism occur, place the patient in the high Fowler's position, administer oxygen at 6 liters/minute by nasal prongs, monitor vital signs, and summon immediate medical assistance. Refer to the "Pulmonary Embolism" plan, page 246.

3. During acute thrombophlebitis, maintain bed rest as ordered.

4. Caution the patient against rubbing the painful area.

5. Help the patient avoid Valsalva's maneuver. Teach the patient to exhale during defecation, and provide fluid, high-fiber foods, prune juice, or other measures to promote passage of soft stool.

6. Observe for persistent or recurrent thrombophlebitis. If present, consult with doctor about further treatment.

7. Additional individualized interventions: _____

Rationales

1. Pulmonary embolism is the most common pulmonary complication in hospitalized patients. Deep venous thrombophlebitis is the primary risk factor for embolus development.

2. Pulmonary emboli can cause local areas of pulmonary dysfunction and increase the risk of massive embolism. Massive pulmonary embolism, in which 50% or more of the pulmonary vascular bed is occluded, is a medical emergency. Treatment may include full cardiopulmonary support, surgical intervention, I.V. streptokinase (Kabikinase), and heparin. The "Pulmonary Embolism" plan contains further details on this disorder.

3. Bed rest decreases the likelihood that muscle contractions will dislodge a clot.

4. Rubbing may cause the clot to break free and embolize.

5. A sudden increase in intrathoracic pressure, such as that produced by Valsalva's maneuver, may dislodge the clot.

6. Persistent or recurrent thrombophlebitis increases the risk of pulmonary embolism. Treatment may include prolonged anticoagulant therapy or insertion of an inferior vena caval umbrella to trap clots.

7. Rationales: _____

Target outcome criteria
Within 24 hours of thrombophlebitis onset, the patient will:
• maintain activity restrictions
• exhale during defecation
• show no signs of pulmonary embolism.

By the time of discharge, the patient will show no signs of persistent or recurrent thrombophlebitis.

Nursing diagnosis: *Knowledge deficit related to postdischarge care*

NURSING PRIORITY: Educate the patient and family about continuing therapy and preventing recurrence.

Interventions

1. Teach the patient and family about factors that may increase the risk of recurrence. Discuss measures that may reduce or eliminate risk factors, including weight control through diet and exercise, smoking cessation, drug therapy for hypertension, and careful diabetes control.

2. Teach the patient ways to improve venous flow: exercising feet and legs hourly while awake; increasing fluid intake to at least 8 8-oz glasses (2,000 ml) a day (unless contraindicated); elevating extremity when sitting or lying down; participating in prescribed activity program; avoiding girdles, garters, knee-high stockings, and other constricting clothing; using antiembolism stockings; avoiding leg crossing; and avoiding oral contraceptives.

3. Teach the patient and family to observe for signs and symptoms of recurrence.

4. Teach the patient how to care for extremities: maintaining clean, dry skin; carefully monitoring any skin lesions; and protecting skin from injury.

5. Teach the patient and family about oral anticoagulant therapy, if prescribed. Also teach ways to minimize the risk of bleeding, such as using an electric shaver and avoiding aspirin. (See the "Cerebrovascular Accident" plan, page 100, for further details.)

6. Emphasize the importance of following the doctor's recommendations for regular medical follow-up, including laboratory test monitoring. Also stress the value of wearing a medical alert bracelet or necklace, and tell the patient how to obtain one.

7. Additional individualized interventions: _____

_____

Rationales

1. Thrombophlebitis commonly recurs, particularly if risk factors are not eliminated. Teaching measures to eliminate or reduce risk factors may avert further problems.

2. These methods prevent the classic causes of thrombophlebitis: venous stasis, vessel trauma, and hypercoagulability.

3. Early detection promotes early treatment.

4. Impaired circulation in the extremities predisposes the patient to stasis ulcers.

5. A patient with uncomplicated deep venous thrombophlebitis usually takes warfarin for 4 to 6 weeks after discharge. Complications may warrant lifelong anticoagulant therapy. The "Cerebrovascular Accident" plan contains further details related to anticoagulant therapy.

6. Thrombophlebitis may recur or develop into chronic venous insufficiency. Conscientious medical follow-up provides the greatest protection against future life-threatening episodes or chronicity. Monitoring laboratory parameters, such as PT for the patient taking warfarin, helps the doctor maintain therapeutic dosage. A medical alert bracelet or necklace increases the likelihood of appropriate treatment should the patient be unable to communicate in a medical emergency.

7. Rationales: _____

_____

Target outcome criteria
By the time of discharge, the patient will:
• be able to list personal risk factors
• be able to list the signs and symptoms of thrombophlebitis
• be able to identify five ways to improve venous flow
• be able to correctly describe the details of anticoagulant administration, if prescribed, and how to minimize bleeding risk

• verbalize the importance of regular medical follow-up
• verbalize intent to obtain a medical alert bracelet or necklace.

Discharge planning

NURSING DISCHARGE CRITERIA

Upon the patient's discharge, documentation shows evidence of:
• absence of heat, pain, swelling, or inflammation at affected site
• PTT or PT within acceptable parameters
• absence of pulmonary or cardiovascular complications
• absence of fever
• vital signs within normal parameters
• absence of bowel or bladder dysfunction
• heparin therapy discontinued for 24 hours
• anticoagulation controlled with oral medication
• presence of bilateral pedal pulses
• absence of pain and pallor in the affected lower extremity
• ability to perform activities of daily living (ADLs), transfers, and ambulation same as before hospitalization
• adequate home support system, or referral to home care or a nursing home if indicated by lack of home support system or inability to perform ADLs, transfers, and ambulation.

PATIENT-FAMILY TEACHING CHECKLIST

Document evidence that the patient and family demonstrate an understanding of:
___ signs and symptoms of recurring thrombophlebitis
___ continued use of antiembolism stockings
___ all discharge medications' purpose, dosage, administration schedule, and adverse effects requiring medical attention (usual discharge medications include oral anticoagulants and anti-inflammatory medications)
___ allowable activity level
___ importance of wearing medical alert identification if the patient remains on anticoagulant therapy
___ need to modify risk factors
___ procedure for obtaining follow-up laboratory tests, such as PT
___ date, time, and location of follow-up appointment
___ how to contact the doctor.

DOCUMENTATION CHECKLIST

Using outcome criteria as a guide, document:
___ clinical status on admission
___ significant changes in status
___ pertinent laboratory data and diagnostic test findings
___ pain relief measures
___ effect of position changes and extremity elevation
___ application and effect of warm, moist compresses
___ anticoagulant administration
___ any change in clotting studies
___ any bleeding tendencies
___ administration of other pharmacologic agents, such as an anti-inflammatory or antibiotic

___ level of activity and the patient's response to progressive ambulation
___ patient-family teaching
___ discharge planning.

ASSOCIATED PLANS OF CARE

Cerebrovascular Accident
Ineffective Individual Coping
Knowledge Deficit
Pain
Surgical Intervention

References

Alfaro, R. *Application of Nursing Process: A Step-by-Step Guide to Care Planning.* Philadelphia: J.B. Lippincott Co., 1986.
Baum, P. "Heed the Warning Signs of Peripheral Vascular Disease (PVD)," *Nursing85* 15(3):50-57, March 1985.
Braunwald, E. *Harrison's Principles of Internal Medicine*, 12th ed. New York: McGraw-Hill Book Co., 1990.
Hurst, J., ed. *The Heart*, 7th ed. New York: McGraw-Hill Book Co., 1989.
Iyer, P., et al. *Nursing Process and Nursing Diagnosis*. Philadelphia: W.B. Saunders Co., 1986.
Kenner, C., et al. *Critical Care Nursing: Body-Mind-Spirit*, 2nd ed. Boston: Little, Brown & Co., 1985.
Kneisl, C., and Ames, S. *Adult Health Nursing: A Biopsychosocial Approach* . Menlo Park, Calif.: Addison-Wesley Publishing Co., 1986.
Patrick, M., et al. *Medical-Surgical Nursing*. Philadelphia: J.B. Lippincott Co., 1986.
Raffensperger, E., et al. *Clinical Nursing Handbook*. Philadelphia: J.B. Lippincott Co., 1986.
White, R. "Diagnosis and Therapy of Emergent Vascular Diseases," in *Textbook of Critical Care*, 2nd ed. Edited by Shoemaker, W., et al. Philadelphia: W.B. Saunders Co., 1988.

Anorexia Nervosa and Bulimia Nervosa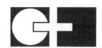

DRG information
Anorexia nervosa:
DRG 428 Disorders of Personality and Impulse Control.
     Mean LOS = 6.4 days
Bulimia nervosa:
DRG 432 Other Diagnoses of Mental Disorders.
     Mean LOS = 4.3 days

Introduction
DEFINITION AND TIME FOCUS
Anorexia nervosa and bulimia nervosa are complex psychiatric disorders characterized by abnormal eating patterns and eating-related behaviors. The defining criteria for anorexia nervosa and bulimia nervosa are in a state of evolution (Love and Seaton, 1991) — in part because many patients move between the diagnostic categories over time. As a result, a patient may not fit neatly into either category. The following information is based on current definitions and understanding of the disorders.

Anorexia nervosa involves dramatic weight loss unrelated to organic causes: intentional starvation, ritualistic or compulsive eating behaviors, and bizarre delusional disturbances in body image are part of the typical picture. Although the patient is obsessed by thoughts of food, the need for control overrides the desire to eat. Limiting food intake provides a sense of control. Bulimia nervosa is characterized by binge-purge cycles in which the patient consumes large quantities of high-calorie food, then uses laxatives or purgatives, fasts excessively, or induces vomiting to rid the body of the calories consumed. The binges usually occur at least twice weekly, during periods of stress. Anorexia nervosa involves weight loss of dangerous proportions, whereas bulimia nervosa may be characterized by normal or even above-normal weight with frequent, sometimes abrupt fluctuations. Usually, the bulimic patient displays more insight into the abnormal character of threatening behaviors, and hides them from family and friends. The anorexic patient is less able to recognize potentially harmful eating behaviors because of a severely altered body image. In either disorder, life-threatening physical complications related to the physiologic effects of malnutrition may occur.

Anorexia nervosa has been reported to have the highest death rate of any psychiatric disorder. Up to 25% of bulimics also suffer from clinical depression; a similar number attempt suicide. Many patients with eating disorders also have substance abuse problems and characteristics typical of personality disorders. Treatment recommendations also vary widely. Some clinicians advocate rigorous behavior-modification techniques; others use in-depth psychotherapy, psychoanalysis, family therapy, or a combination of approaches. Because the etiology and perpetuating factors for eating disorders vary among individuals, multiple treatment approaches are needed. When the patient with an eating disorder is admitted to an inpatient medical-surgical unit, the immediate focus is likely to be controlled nutritional replenishment, prevention of complications, restoration of physiologic equilibrium, and initiation or continuation of appropriate psychiatric treatment.

This plan focuses on the anorexic or bulimic patient admitted for diagnosis and management of severely disruptive and potentially dangerous eating patterns.

ETIOLOGY AND PRECIPITATING FACTORS
No clear-cut or consistent factors have been identified as causing these disorders. Instead, a combination of complex psychodynamic, familial, and societal factors appears to be involved.
- psychodynamic
  - developmental deficits related to issues of loss, separation, sexuality, autonomy, and power
  - sense of powerlessness or lack of control
- familial
  anorexia nervosa:
  - perfectionistic or overprotective families
  - pattern of avoiding family conflicts
  - lack of conflict-resolution skills
  bulimia nervosa:
  - perfectionistic or overprotective families, or families lacking clear interpersonal boundaries or roles
- societal
  - emphasis on being thin and exercising as a basis for peer acceptance
  - thinness as the societal image of female beauty
- cultural
  - seen in all economic, cultural, and religious groups
  - less common among blacks and southern Europeans
  - predominantly affects adolescent girls and young women

Focused assessment guidelines
NURSING HISTORY (Functional health pattern findings)

Health perception – health management pattern
Anorexia nervosa:
• onset may have followed a successful diet taken to extremes (a typical finding in adolescent girls)
• may report pleading, punitive measures, or arguments by others to eat, with no effect on eating patterns
• may report frequent pressure to seek treatment
Bulimia nervosa:
• onset may have followed actual or impending separation from home (a typical finding in young adult women age 18 to 25)
• may have begun as a quick weight-loss attempt and escalated to a compulsive need to binge, followed by vomiting
• may have had an undiagnosed anorexic episode in adolescence
• may report a history of drug or alcohol abuse

Nutritional-metabolic pattern
Anorexia nervosa:
• likely to report absence of hunger
• may report various reasons for restricting food intake, such as GI discomfort, food allergies, or dislike of certain foods
• may urge others to eat, such as brothers or sisters
• may report rituals occurring at mealtimes, with an excessive amount of time spent over each meal
• may express an interest in recipes and cooking
• likely to eat low-calorie, low-fat, low-carbohydrate, and "diet" foods
• family may report that the patient hides or hoardes food
Bulimia nervosa:
• may complain of difficulty breathing after bingeing
• likely to report planning of, or preoccupation with, bingeing and purging
• typically reports secretive binge eating but may binge with others (a group binge)
• may report a history of hiatal hernia
• may report esophageal or GI discomfort
• likely to report eating high-carbohydrate foods during a binge but eating balanced meals or "diet" food at regular meals

Elimination pattern
Anorexia nervosa:
• likely to report chronic constipation
• may report self-induced or spontaneous vomiting
Bulimia nervosa:
• may report constipation or diarrhea
• likely to report constipation if laxative abuse is discontinued

• may report permanent loss of bowel reactivity once laxatives are discontinued (rare)
• may report vomiting, most commonly self-induced and not usually accompanied by nausea
• may also report spontaneous regurgitation

Activity-exercise pattern
Anorexia nervosa:
• may report a high energy level
• may report exercising secretly after meals
• may report a history of rigidly scheduled and compulsive exercise
• may report emotional distress when exercise is not possible or is interrupted
• may report an extremely structured and active lifestyle
Bulimia nervosa:
• all of the above, plus may report lethargy after bingeing

Sleep-rest pattern
• may report sleep disturbances
• may report dreams about food or eating
• may report nocturnal binges after delaying food intake during the day

Cognitive-perceptual pattern
Anorexia nervosa:
• may exhibit dichotomous thinking – that is, an all-or-nothing attitude toward many issues and "good-bad" perception of staff members
• may report preoccupation with food, weight, and diets
• typically denies feelings of hunger, along with any other needs
• typically denies seriousness of weight loss, weight loss itself, and body-image distortion
• may report blurred vision
• may report difficulty concentrating
• may report auditory disturbances
• may report dizziness or headaches
Bulimia nervosa:
• may exhibit dichotomous thinking
• may report preoccupation with food, weight, or diets
• may acknowledge need for treatment and report distress over bingeing; less commonly, reports distress about purging behavior

Self-perception – self-concept pattern
• may report guilt over worrying others or being a burden because of disorder
• may exhibit body-image distortion: for example, may report "feeling fat" despite being at normal or below-normal weight
• may report feelings of inadequacy, hopelessness, rejection, and self-loathing

Role-relationship pattern

Anorexia nervosa:
• may describe self as compliant and introverted or shy with others; may avoid socializing with peers
• commonly reported by others as being "a good child" who had no problems before the onset of the eating disorder

Bulimia nervosa:
• same as above, or may report temper outbursts followed by guilt

Sexuality-reproductive pattern

Anorexia nervosa:
• commonly reports sexual inactivity
• commonly denies masturbating
• reports feelings of shame, guilt, or disgust regarding sexuality or sexual functioning
• denies having any sexual desires
• may report amenorrhea
• may report a history of sexual abuse by others

Bulimia nervosa:
• same as above, or reports episodes of sexual promiscuity that are impulsive or compulsive in nature

Coping – stress tolerance pattern

Anorexia nervosa:
• may exhibit a perfectionistic, obsessive, and compulsive personality
• may report a feeling of well-being from control of body size through food restriction and exercise
• may attempt to manipulate staff in an effort to gain control

Bulimia nervosa:
• same as above, or may exhibit a pattern of losing control through impulsive behaviors, then regaining control through purging, vigorous exercise, or (less commonly) self-mutilation

Value-belief pattern

Anorexia nervosa:
• may express belief that to negate needs and desires is "good" and that to "give in" to needs and desires is "bad"
• may equate being thin with being happy

Bulimia nervosa:
• same as above
• may wish to be anorexic, expressing shame over loss of control
• more commonly than the anorexic, may express distress over symptoms and behaviors

PHYSICAL FINDINGS
General appearance

Anorexia nervosa:
• 20% to 25% below normal weight for height and frame (common)
• absence of secondary sexual characteristics

Bulimia nervosa:
• low-normal to high-normal weight range (common)
• obese (less common)

Cardiovascular

Anorexia nervosa:
• hypotension
• bradycardia
• hypothermia
• dehydration
• edema, possibly generalized

Bulimia nervosa:
• arrhythmias
• finger clubbing
• dehydration
• rebound water retention (on cessation of purging)

Gastrointestinal

Anorexia nervosa:
• vomiting
• abdominal distention
• constipation or diarrhea

Bulimia nervosa:
• erosion of dental enamel
• irritation of esophagus or chronic hoarseness
• reddened throat
• swollen salivary glands, especially parotids
• steatorrhea
• constipation or diarrhea

Neurologic

Anorexia nervosa:
• hyperactivity
• poor motor control
• paresthesias
• hypersensitivity to noise and light

Bulimia nervosa:
• seizures
• weakness and lethargy

Integumentary

Anorexia nervosa:
• pallor
• hair loss
• growth of lanugo
• poor skin turgor

Bulimia nervosa:
• dry skin and hair
• pale color

Musculoskeletal

Anorexia nervosa:
• emaciated appearance
• loss of muscle mass, muscle weakness

Bulimia nervosa:
• tetany (rare)

Genitourinary

Anorexia nervosa:
• chronic or persistent vaginal and urinary tract infection

DIAGNOSTIC STUDIES*

• complete blood count (CBC) with differential — may indicate anemias or leukopenia, blood dyscrasias associated with malnutrition, or leukopenia
• urinalysis and culture and sensitivity testing — may indicate renal dysfunction, dehydration, or infection related to malnourished state
• chemistry panel — may indicate electrolyte imbalances, such as hypokalemia, hypocalcemia, hypernatremia, hypoglycemia, or hypercholesterolemia
• growth hormone level — may be high
• luteinizing hormone level — may be low because of decreased body fat
• follicle-stimulating hormone level — may be low
• thyroid function (T_3, T_4, renal uptake, and plasma T_3 levels) — may be underactive
• fasting plasma cortisol levels — may be high
• testosterone levels (in males) — may be low
• dexamethasone suppression test (if indicated) — may show nonsuppression of adrenal response
• chest X-ray — may indicate pulmonary edema or congestive heart failure
• electrocardiography — may indicate arrhythmias

POTENTIAL COMPLICATIONS

• cardiac arrest (from hypokalemia)
• arrhythmias
• starvation
• amenorrhea or irregular menses (exact cause unknown)
• dental caries or erosion (from vomiting)
• peripheral myopathy and cardiomyopathy (with ipecac syrup use)
• bone decalcification
• gastric dilation and perforation (from refeeding)
• congestive heart failure
• blood disorders (from malnutrition)
• osteoporosis (from hypocalcemia)
• insulin-dependent (type I) diabetes (relationship to eating disorders is not clearly understood)
• liver damage
• renal damage

Nursing diagnosis: *Nutritional deficit related to inadequate food intake or purging behavior*

NURSING PRIORITY: Establish and monitor safe and controlled refeeding.

Interventions

1. On admission, perform a baseline nutritional assessment, noting weight in relation to height, body protein stores, skin and hair condition, and fluid and electrolyte status. See the "Nutritional Deficit" and "Total Parenteral Nutrition" plan, pages 63 and 411 respectively, for further details.

2. With the doctor and dietitian, plan the type, amount, and route of refeeding based on the patient's nutritional needs and ability to comply with the refeeding plan. Discuss the plan in advance with the patient and consider using a written contract. Include a clear explanation of the alternatives (tube feeding or total parenteral nutrition) if the patient does not comply with the plan for oral food intake. If a nasogastric (NG) tube is used, remove it after each feeding.

3. Provide emotional support while closely monitoring intake and output of food and fluids. Avoid authoritative attitudes. Convey an attitude of warm yet firm support and consistent expectations.

Rationales

1. Baseline assessment of nutritional status is essential to developing a refeeding plan. The "Nutritional Deficit" and "Total Parenteral Nutrition" plans contain detailed information on nutritional assessment.

2. Refeeding must be carefully controlled in order to avoid too-rapid weight gain with subsequent psychological and physiologic trauma. Resistance to eating may be so strong that tube feeding or total parenteral nutrition must be instituted. A written contract and clear understanding of the alternatives to oral intake provide choices and may minimize manipulative behavior. If the patient does not eat, an NG tube may be inserted for feeding of a previously specified amount of liquid nutrients. This method is controversial. If it is used, a matter-of-fact, nonpunitive attitude is essential to minimize feelings of powerlessness. The patient may try to siphon food out of the stomach if the tube is left in place.

3. Feelings of powerlessness increase as refeeding begins. A careful tally of intake and output is essential in assessing the feeding plan's adequacy. Consistency reduces manipulative behavior.

---

*Initial laboratory data may reflect no abnormalities or may reflect signs of malnutrition or starvation.

4. Set and maintain specific limits regarding the amount of time allowed for meals or tube feedings, the amount of intake, and the privileges linked to compliance. Ensure that the patient and all personnel working with or around the patient are aware of these limits.

5. Provide one-to-one supervision during and for 1 to 2 hours after meals if the patient has a history of purging.

6. Weigh the patient before breakfast and after voiding, ensuring that the patient is wearing only a hospital gown. Reward meeting weight goals by increasing privileges.

7. Monitor vital signs at least every 8 hours.

8. Observe for signs and symptoms of hypokalemia and hypovolemia: weakness, irregular pulse, paresthesias, and hypotension. Maintain a normal fluid and electrolyte balance, including administering I.V. electrolyte replacements, as ordered by the doctor. See Appendix C, "Fluid and Electrolyte Imbalances," for details.

9. When the patient refuses to eat, avoid excessive attentiveness while carrying out alternative feeding measures.

10. Ensure that the patient is referred for psychiatric care from an eating disorders specialist.

11. Additional individualized interventions: _____

_____

4. Limit-setting conveys caring and clear expectations, minimizing manipulative behavior. If all personnel (including housekeepers and laboratory technicians) are not made aware of the limits, the patient may be able to circumvent the diet plan.

5. The patient may refuse to eat, hide or hoard food, or purge in an attempt to control weight gain. Being with the patient during times of stress is a way to provide emotional support.

6. Weight gain provides an objective measurement of nutritional status improvement. Weighing at the same time daily ensures consistency. The patient may try to hide objects in street clothes to simulate weight gain. Weight gain increases the patient's anxiety. Increasing privileges reinforces healthy behavior.

7. Hypotension and bradycardia can result from malnourishment and dehydration. Vital signs should improve as refeeding is instituted.

8. Hypokalemia-induced arrhythmias may be fatal, and severe hypovolemia can provoke cardiovascular collapse. Specific signs, symptoms, and interventions associated with hypokalemia and hypovolemia are contained in the "Fluid and Electrolyte Imbalances" appendix.

9. Providing extra attention, even if negative, when the patient refuses food may be perceived as an indirect reward for such behavior, contributing to the self-destructive cycle.

10. Treating the nutritional deficit and other life-threatening manifestations is essential, but ongoing psychiatric therapy is also necessary for definitive treatment of these complex disorders.

11. Rationales: _____

_____

GASTROINTESTINAL DISORDERS

Target outcome criteria
Throughout the hospital stay, the patient will:
• verbalize an understanding of the diet plan and feeding alternatives
• gain weight according to preestablished goals
• show improving vital signs as refeeding progresses
• show no evidence of arrhythmias.

Nursing diagnosis: *Powerlessness related to inability to identify and meet emotional, physical, sexual, and social needs and to familial and societal expectation to focus on others' needs*

NURSING PRIORITIES: (a) Help the patient identify emotional, physical, sexual, and social needs, and (b) explore ways to meet these needs.

Interventions

1. Be aware that the issue of control permeates all aspects of the patient's personal life.

Rationales

1. Fear of losing control may relate to anxiety over many issues. Controlling food intake may be the only way the patient knows how to control the self or others.

2. Encourage the patient to participate in unit activities that foster socialization and mutual sharing.

2. The patient with an eating disorder tends to be isolated because of feelings of shame or a fear of "not measuring up" to others. If these feelings are explored in a group setting, as they occur, the patient will receive and learn to seek feedback from others. This learning process increases the patient's sense of power and control.

3. Encourage self-nurturing behaviors while discouraging self-destructive behaviors. Observe for signs of depression, anxiety, or suicide potential, such as withdrawal, lack of eye contact, agitation, frequent references to death or self-destructive activities, or sudden improvement in a previously depressed patient. Ask if the patient has a plan for suicide

3. Once needs are identified and attempts are made to meet them, the patient may try to sabotage any progress. The patient with an eating disorder believes that personal needs are "bad" and that wanting needs to be fulfilled is also "bad." The patient may be so uncomfortable with these needs that suicide seems an acceptable option. Sudden improvement of mood in a previously depressed patient may indicate the patient has decided to commit suicide. Most patients are honest about their plans for self-harm.

4. Give the patient positive reinforcement for expressing and meeting personal needs in spite of fears of losing control.
• Encourage expression of anger, and help the patient learn assertive conflict-resolution skills, especially in family interactions.
• Help the patient identify non-food-related goals.
• Provide opportunities for creative expression.

4. Once needs can be identified and met without a loss of control, the patient will be able to achieve a sense of satisfaction from self-nurturing behaviors.
• The family may need guidance to react supportively to expressions of anger instead of withdrawing affection.

• Identifying goals promotes a sense of self-control.
• Creative expression may facilitate recognition of previously "unacceptable" feelings.

5. Additional individualized interventions: _____

5. Rationales: _____

Target outcome criteria
Within 1 week of admission, the patient will identify one non-food-related goal.

Several weeks to months after discharge, the patient will:*
• establish a regular pattern of socializing and sharing with others without undue anxiety
• engage spontaneously in self-nurturing behaviors without trying to sabotage any progress made
• respond to familial and societal expectations in ways that do not negate personal goals
• participate in creative activity.

Nursing diagnosis: *Self-esteem disturbance related to perfectionism, sense of inadequacy, or dysfunctional family dynamics*

NURSING PRIORITY: Promote a healthy self-image.

Interventions

1. Provide a positive role model for the patient by displaying a consistent, caring, truthful attitude and realistic self-acceptance.

2. Relate to the patient as a person with positive characteristics and interests apart from eating behaviors and food.

Rationales

1. If the family unit is dysfunctional, the patient may have had limited opportunity for role or behavior testing. A "safe" setting such as the hospital may encourage healthful identification and experimentation.

2. Emphasizing other personal aspects helps the patient to base self-esteem on factors other than physical characteristics.

---

*Because of their long-term nature, these criteria will not be met during any one hospital stay. They are included here so the nurse is aware of them and can recognize and reward steps toward meeting them.

3. Promote activities that have a high probability of success, beginning with simple tasks and gradually increasing the amount of effort required. Making the bed, cleaning the room, and helping another patient with room-cleaning are examples of related tasks that require increasing effort. Praise and recognize successes.

4. Refer the patient to an occupational or physical therapist as appropriate. Consult with other therapists to ensure consistency in the treatment plan.

5. If family dysfunction is identified, encourage family members to consider family therapy.

6. Observe the patient's interactions with others, and provide support and positive reinforcement when the patient is able to identify emotions and express them clearly, particularly "negative" feelings such as anger. Encourage assertiveness.

7. Encourage the patient to explore family and societal beliefs and attitudes about food, eating, and body image.

8. Additional individualized interventions: _____

3. Success, even in simple activities, provides a sense of satisfaction and helps decrease depression and feelings of inadequacy. Helping others involves increased effort and promotes realistic self-appraisal as the patient receives positive feedback from others.

4. Diversionary activity decreases boredom and improves the patient's general feeling of well-being. Adjunctive therapies may also provide opportunities for goal achievement.

5. The patient's behavior usually reflects the family's underlying psychopathology.

6. The patient with an eating disorder may be using eating behaviors as a means of self-assertion, even though this is self-destructive. Learning that it is acceptable to express feelings directly and forcefully may decrease attachment to eating behaviors as a coping device and promote a more positive self-image.

7. The family and society can teach unrealistic and perfectionistic attitudes. The patient needs support to question such attitudes.

8. Rationales: _____

Discharge planning

NURSING DISCHARGE CRITERIA
Upon the patient's discharge, documentation shows evidence of:
• stable vital signs
• stabilizing weight
• electrolytes and CBC within normal parameters
• I.V. lines or total parenteral nutrition, if used, discontinued for at least 48 hours
• adequate oral intake
• ability to comply with refeeding regimen
• absence of cardiovascular or pulmonary complications
• motivation to continue psychiatric treatment on an outpatient basis
• referral for ongoing psychiatric follow-up.

PATIENT-FAMILY TEACHING CHECKLIST
Document evidence that the patient and family demonstrate an understanding of:
___ physical status at time of discharge
___ warning signs of hypokalemia, dehydration, or any other physical complications of fasting, bingeing, or purging
___ all discharge medications' purpose, dosage, administration schedule, and adverse effects requiring medical attention
___ diet plan
___ community support resources
___ helpful attitudes and behaviors family members can exhibit toward the patient
___ attitudes and behaviors to avoid

___ awareness that treatment for an eating disorder is long-term and involves the family as well as the patient
___ date, time, and location of follow-up appointments
___ emergency telephone numbers to use when the patient or family is in crisis.

DOCUMENTATION CHECKLIST
Using outcome criteria as a guide, document:
___ clinical status on admission and discharge
___ significant changes in clinical status
___ completion of all diagnostic studies and laboratory tests indicated by clinical status on admission, with repeat testing of all abnormal findings
___ eating pattern before and at discharge
___ exercise pattern
___ daily weights
___ any occurrence of vomiting, prohibited exercise, or unprescribed use of laxatives or diuretics
___ daily mental status checks, including assessment for depression, suicide potential, and body-image distortion
___ sleep patterns
___ complete intake and output records, especially use of I.V., total parenteral nutrition, or tube feeding
___ patient-family teaching, including medication teaching
___ discharge planning.

GASTROINTESTINAL DISORDERS

ASSOCIATED PLANS OF CARE
Chronic Renal Failure
Ineffective Family Coping
Ineffective Individual Coping
Nutritional Deficit
Total Parenteral Nutrition

References

Burgess, A.W. *Psychiatric Nursing in the Hospital and Community,* 5th ed. Norwalk, CT: Appleton & Lange, 1990.

Deering, C.G., and Niziolek, C. "Eating Disorders: Promoting Continuity of Care," *Journal of Psychosocial Nursing* 26(11):6-8, 10-11, 15, November 1988.

Garner, D., and Garfinkel, R., eds. *Handbook of Psychotherapy for Anorexia Nervosa and Bulimia.* New York: Guilford Press, 1985.

Keller, O.L. "Bulimia: Primary Care Approach and Intervention," *Nurse Practitoner* 11(8):42-46, August 1986.

Kneisl, C.R., and Ames, S.W. *Adult Health Nursing: A Biopsychosocial Approach.* Menlo Park, Calif.: Addison-Wesley Publishing Co., 1986.

Love, C.C., and Seaton, H. "Eating Disorders: Highlights of Nursing Assessment and Therapeutics," *Nursing Clinics of North America* 26(3):677-97, 1991.

Schultz, J.M., and Dark, S.R. *Manual of Psychiatric Care Plans.* Glenview, IL: Scott Foresman, 1986.

Colostomy

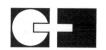

DRG information

DRG 146 Rectal Resection. With Complication
or Comorbidity (CC).
Mean LOS = 13.0 days
DRG 147 Rectal Resection. Without CC.
Mean LOS = 9.5 days
DRG 148 Major Small and Large Bowel Procedure.
With CC.
Mean LOS = 13.9 days
DRG 149 Major Small and Large Bowel Procedure.
Without CC.
Mean LOS = 9.4 days

Introduction

DEFINITION AND TIME FOCUS

A colostomy is a surgically created opening (stoma)
between the abdominal wall and the colon that permits fecal diversion. A colostomy may be created because of trauma, inflammation, or obstruction of the
distal bowel, or when the distal bowel is resected, as
in proctocolectomy (excision of colon and rectum) or
abdominoperineal (AP) resection (removal of rectum).
Colostomies may be designated according to location,
construction, or duration:

• location — Although a colostomy may be constructed
anywhere in the large bowel, the two most common locations are the transverse colon and the descending
colon.
• construction — Common surgical construction methods
(see *Types of colostomies*) include:

— end colostomy (bowel is divided; proximal bowel
is brought out as a stoma and distal bowel is either
removed — as in AP resection of the distal colon and
rectum — or "oversewn" and left in place — as in
Hartmann's procedure)
— double-barreled colostomy (bowel is divided and
both ends are brought out as stomas; the proximal
stoma drains stool and the distal stoma drains only
mucus)
— loop colostomy (entire loop of bowel is brought
out through the abdominal wall and stabilized over
a rod, bridge, or catheter until granulation to the
abdominal wall occurs; the bowel's anterior wall is
opened to provide fecal diversion; the posterior
bowel wall remains intact).
• duration — A colostomy is classified as permanent (no
potential for reversal) if the rectum and anus are removed or as temporary (potential for reversal) if the
rectum and anus remain.

This plan focuses on preoperative assessment of
teaching needs and on the postoperative phase, the
"active teaching" phase, between initial recovery or
stabilization and discharge.

ETIOLOGY AND PRECIPITATING FACTORS

• disease conditions requiring removal of the distal
bowel (for example, colorectal cancer or pelvic malig-
nancies)
• infectious or inflammatory conditions of the distal
bowel requiring fecal diversion (for example, diverticulitis or Crohn's disease)

TYPES OF COLOSTOMIES

End colostomy: Sigmoid
colon

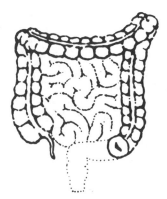

Double-barreled colostomy:
Transverse colon

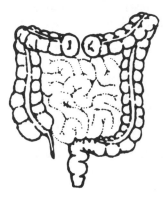

Loop colostomy: Transverse
colon

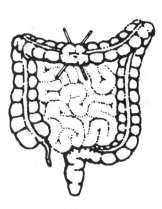

• trauma to the distal bowel requiring fecal diversion (as in a gunshot or stab wound)
• extensive surgery of the distal bowel requiring protective fecal diversion (for example, low anterior colon resection)
• obstruction of the distal bowel (as in obstructing tumor)

Focused assessment guidelines
NURSING HISTORY (Functional health pattern findings)

Note: Because a colostomy may be performed for widely varied conditions, no typical presenting picture exists; therefore, the nursing history and physical findings sections are omitted in this plan. The following are guidelines for preoperative assessment.

Health perception—health management pattern
• Determine the diagnosis or reason for colostomy. Determine the planned procedure, prognosis, and the patient's potential for independence as a basis for discharge planning and teaching.
• Explore the patient's perceptions concerning colostomy and its impact on health status and life-style. (Note: Previous contact with a person with an ostomy will affect the patient's expectations and adaptation.)
• Identify any allergies, particularly to topical agents such as tape; the patient with such allergies may react to colostomy products.

Nutritional-metabolic pattern
• Assess diet and fluid intake when planning patient teaching. Assess the home diet for adequate fiber and fluid intake and for consumption of gas-producing foods.
• Assess nutritional status (skin turgor, mucous membranes, hair condition, height and weight, and recent weight loss). Be alert to signs of nutritional deficiency that may predispose the patient to postoperative complications, such as wound infection or delayed healing.

Elimination pattern
• Determine usual bowel patterns. Assess the preoperative frequency and character of bowel movements as a basis for colostomy management and patient teaching (particularly important in selecting a management approach for a descending or sigmoid colostomy).

Activity-exercise pattern
• Assess independence and any limitations in activities of daily living. The amount of independence is significant in planning for colostomy management and patient-family teaching. The patient's manual dexterity and coordination are particularly significant in selecting appropriate equipment, such as a pouch system or clip.

Cognitive-perceptual pattern
• When planning teaching, assess the patient's understanding of the diagnosis, prognosis, surgical procedure, and management of colostomy.
• Assess for any sensory deficits, such as in visual and auditory acuity, when planning self-care instruction; most patients requiring colostomy are over age 60, so sensory loss is common.
• Base teaching strategies on the patient's learning style and sensory strengths; for example, if a patient with diminished visual acuity learns best by doing, self-care instruction should involve much practice (with a magnifying mirror) but minimal reading.

Self-perception—self-concept pattern
• Self-concept and self-esteem correlate with adaptation potential; be alert to consistent self-derogatory statements or inappropriate affect, which may indicate low self-esteem.
• Emotional response is variable. It is common for a patient to have negative feelings regarding colostomy.
• Openness in expressing feelings is affected by the patient's personality and the nurse's communication skills.

Role-relationship pattern
• Assess areas of concern about roles and relationships. Patients commonly express concern about a colostomy's effect on relationships, with major concern relating to spouse or partner reaction.
• Young and middle-aged adults commonly express concern about their ability to resume preoperative roles and responsibilities.
• Older adults commonly express concern about their ability to maintain independence and to manage the cost of ostomy supplies.
• Assess family dynamics, particularly dependence-independence issues. Older patients may desire their spouse's or a family member's involvement in care, while younger adults may value independence and privacy.

Sexuality-reproductive pattern
• Assess the patient's and partner's openness with each other and in discussing sexuality, preoperative sexual patterns, and other major concerns.
• A common concern is how the colostomy affects intimate relationships—that is, sexual attractiveness and function.

Coping—stress tolerance pattern
• The patient's and family's responses to colostomy are highly variable and reflect coping patterns.
• Assess the patient's feelings about support groups, to determine the appropriateness of referral to the United Ostomy Association.

Value-belief pattern
• Response to colostomy is affected by cultural beliefs and familial response to illness, surgery, and elimination.

DIAGNOSTIC STUDIES
Studies vary according to the patient's condition and the underlying disorder; they may include:
• complete blood count — may reveal low hemoglobin or hematocrit values that indicate continuing or unreplaced blood loss; may also reveal elevated white blood cell count indicating infection, usually intra-abdominal
• electrolyte panel — detects or rules out electrolyte abnormalities that affect fluid balance (for example, hyponatremia or hypernatremia) and GI tract function (for example, hypokalemia or hyperkalemia)
• chemistry panel — detects electrolyte imbalances and nutritional deficits that affect wound healing (for example, hypoproteinemia) and monitors liver and kidney function, which may be affected by underlying disease, such as metastatic disease, or by treatment, such as antibiotic therapy
• serum drug levels — peak and trough levels may detect toxic or subtherapeutic levels of prescribed antibiotics or other drugs
• carcinoembryonic antigen (CEA) levels — may be done before and after surgery for comparison; if elevated before surgery, effective surgical resection should result in decreased CEA level
• flat plate or upright abdominal X-ray — may be done before surgery to rule out colon perforation (in a trauma patient) or colon obstruction (in a patient with suspected malignancy); done after surgery as needed to differentiate postoperative ileus (visualized as air-filled loops of bowel) from mechanical obstruction (visualized as air-fluid levels and dilated proximal bowel)

• computed tomography scan of abdomen — may be used before or after surgery to rule out intra-abdominal abscess or to detect metastatic lesions
• stool guaiac (Hemoccult) test — preliminary study to rule out GI bleeding; positive study requires further workup to rule out malignancy, hemorrhoidal bleeding, inflammatory bowel disease, or upper tract bleeding; negative study inconclusive because of high incidence of false-negative results
• barium enema with air and contrast — rules out diverticular disease and detects filling defects that indicate colon lesions (such as polyps and tumors)
• sigmoidoscopy or colonoscopy — rules out colon lesions and allows removal of polyps or biopsy of suspicious lesions

POTENTIAL COMPLICATIONS
• prolonged ileus
• wound infection or dehiscence
• mechanical bowel obstruction
• stomal necrosis
• stomal retraction
• peritonitis or intra-abdominal abscess
• thrombophlebitis or deep vein thrombosis
• sexual dysfunction (in AP resection)
• nonhealing perineal wound (in AP resection)
• bladder dysfunction (in AP resection)

GASTROINTESTINAL DISORDERS

Collaborative problem: *High risk for stomal necrosis related to the surgical procedure, bowel wall edema, or traction on the mesentery*

NURSING PRIORITIES: (a) Optimize blood flow to the bowel wall, and (b) prevent complications related to circulatory impairment.

Interventions

1. Assess and document stoma color every 8 hours during the first 4 days after surgery (or until the stoma remains pink for 3 days).

2. If the stoma is ischemic or necrotic, check the viability of the proximal bowel by inserting a test tube into the stoma and using a flashlight to assess the mucosa for ischemia. Document your findings.

3. Document and notify the doctor promptly if necrosis extends to the end of the test tube (see above).

Rationales

1. Healthy bowel tissue is pink; a dusky blue color indicates ischemia; a brown or black color indicates necrosis. Ischemia may or may not progress to necrosis.

2. A distal stoma is most likely to necrose because it is farthest from the mesenteric blood supply. Stomal necrosis does not necessarily represent a surgical emergency (the stoma may be allowed to "slough" as long as the proximal bowel is viable).

3. Necrosis extending to the fascia represents a surgical emergency because of the threat of perforation and peritonitis.

4. Implement measures to prevent or minimize abdominal distention:
• Examine the abdomen for distention every 8 hours during the first 4 days after surgery.
• If distention is present, monitor its degree by measuring abdominal girth at the umbilicus.
• If distention is present, notify the doctor and request an order to insert an NG tube.
• If a nasogastric (NG) tube is present, irrigate as needed to maintain patency.

4. Severe abdominal distention may cause mesenteric stretching, which places blood vessels under tension; this stress may decrease blood flow to the distal bowel and stoma. Using the umbilicus as the reference point for measuring abdominal girth promotes consistency and accuracy of measurements.

5. Additional individualized interventions: _____

5. Rationales: _____

Target outcome criterion
Within the first 4 days after surgery, the patient will display a pink and viable stoma.

Collaborative problem: *High risk for stomal retraction related to mucocutaneous separation*

NURSING PRIORITIES: (a) Optimize wound healing and granulation of the stoma to the abdominal wall, and (b) prevent stomal retraction.

Interventions

1. Assess and document the integrity of the mucocutaneous suture line at each pouch change.

2. Initiate and document nutritional support measures for the patient at risk for nutritional deficiency, based on the recommendations of a nutritional resource nurse or dietitian.

3. Request vitamin A supplements for the patient receiving steroids.

4. For the patient with a loop colostomy stabilized by a rod or bridge, expect that the loop support will not be removed until the stoma granulates to the abdominal wall.

5. If mucocutaneous separation occurs, alter the pouch system to prevent fecal contamination of exposed subcutaneous tissue. Fill the separated area with absorptive powder or granules; cover with tape strips, then pectin-based paste. Apply a pouch sized to fit closely around the stoma.

6. Additional individualized interventions: _____

Rationales

1. Breakdown of the stoma or skin suture line is a major contributing factor to stomal retraction.

2. Nutritional deficiency causes negative nitrogen balance. Because wound repair depends on adequate protein stores, the suture line may break down.

3. Vitamin A partially compensates for corticosteroids' negative effects on wound healing; by supporting macrophage activity and wound repair, vitamin A helps prevent suture line breakdown.

4. Loop support removal before abdominal wall attachment may cause stomal retraction.

5. An optimal environment for healing includes protection from secondary infection, absorption of exudate, and maintenance of a clean, moist surface. The absorptive agent and tape strips prevent fecal contamination and absorb exudate. Using paste and a pouch sized for the stoma provides a secure seal.

6. Rationales: _____

Target outcome criteria
By the time of discharge, the patient will:
• display a stoma granulated to the abdominal wall
• exhibit a healed mucocutaneous suture line
• show no stomal retraction.

Nursing diagnosis: *High risk for impaired skin integrity: peristomal breakdown related to fecal contamination of skin*

NURSING PRIORITIES: (a) Maintain an intact pouch seal, and (b) prevent peristomal skin breakdown.

Interventions

1. Have an enterostomal therapy nurse mark the optimal stoma site before surgery, if possible.

2. Assess the patient's abdominal contours and select a pouch system that matches those contours: for example, try an all-flexible system for a stoma in a crease or fold.

3. Use the following principles in preparing and applying the pouch:
• Use a drainable pouch.

• Remove peristomal hair.
• Use a skin sealant (such as Skin Prep) under the tape.

• Use a pouch with a barrier ring sized to fit closely around the stoma; use barrier paste (such as Stomahesive) to fill in the gaps.
• If an adhesive-only pouch is used, size it to clear the stoma by 1/8" (3 mm). (It should be used with a barrier ring and paste.)

4. Change the pouch routinely every 5 to 7 days and as needed if leakage or complaints of peristomal burning or itching occur.

5. Inspect the skin at each pouch change, and treat any denudation by dusting the area with absorptive powder (such as karaya). Seal the area by blotting it with water or sealant.

6. Additional individualized interventions: _____

Rationales

1. For best results, the stoma should be located in an area free from creases or folds, within the patient's view, and within the rectus muscle. Site selection is best done before surgery, when the patient can be evaluated lying down, sitting, and standing.

2. Accurately matching the pouch system to abdominal contours optimizes the pouch-to-skin seal and minimizes leakage.

3. Good technique provides maximum security and skin protection.
• A drainable pouch can be emptied as needed without being removed.
• Hair removal prevents folliculitis.
• The copolymer film prevents epidermal stripping with pouch removal.
• This procedure prevents fecal material from contacting skin and causing breakdown.

• Inflexible pouch edges placed too close to the stoma can damage it during peristalsis. Exposed skin must be protected.

4. Routine changes before leaks can occur protect skin and provide the patient with a sense of control. Burning or itching may indicate fecal contamination of skin.

5. Powder provides an absorptive protective layer over the area of breakdown; sealing provides a surface for pouch adherence.

6. Rationales: _____

Target outcome criteria
Throughout the postoperative phase, the patient will display peristomal skin free from breakdown.

By the time of discharge, the patient will have had an intact pouch for 3 days.

Nursing diagnosis: *Knowledge deficit related to unfamiliarity with altered bowel functioning involved in a descending or sigmoid colostomy**

NURSING PRIORITY: Help the patient select options most appropriate for personal physical status and life-style.

Interventions

1. Assess the patient's candidacy for bowel function regulation by irrigation. Consider the following factors:
- Is the colostomy permanent?

- Do stomal complications, such as hernia or prolapse, exist?
- Is the patient mentally and physically able to learn and perform the procedure?
- What were the preoperative bowel patterns?

- Is the patient to receive radiation?

- Does the patient have adequate home facilities?

2. If the patient meets feasibility criteria, discuss management options:
- wearing a pouch continuously, emptying as needed and changing every 5 to 7 days
- daily or every-other-day irrigations to stimulate bowel movements, wearing a security pouch between irrigations.

3. Help the patient explore the options based on personal priorities, such as tolerance of the pouch versus the time required for regular irrigations.

4. Establish a teaching plan based on the patient's decision.

5. Additional individualized interventions: _____

Rationales

1. Irrigation is usually contraindicated if:

- the colostomy is temporary (because of the time factor and potential for bowel dependence)
- the patient has a peristomal hernia (potential for perforation) or prolapse (potential for worsening of prolapse)
- the patient has coordination problems or learning difficulties
- the patient has a preoperative history of diarrhea (less likely to achieve control than the patient with a preoperative history of regular stools or constipation)
- the patient is to receive radiation therapy (because diarrhea is a usual side effect)
- the patient has no running water or indoor plumbing in the home.

2. Colostomy irrigations are not necessary because peristalsis and bowel movements continue; however, regular irrigations induce evacuation and promote colonic "dependence" on their stimulating effects, providing increased control over bowel function. Thus, regulation by irrigation is a management option.

3. Exploring the pros and cons of various options and discussing the patient's concerns and priorities facilitates decision making and increases the patient's sense of self-control.

4. The patient must be able to perform colostomy care before discharge.

5. Rationales: _____

Target outcome criterion
By 2 days before discharge, the patient will describe options considered and select a preferred approach.

---

*Note: The stoma's location in the GI tract determines stool consistency and frequency and affects selection of a management approach. With a descending or sigmoid colostomy, output is soft to solid, frequency is similar to preoperative patterns, and output may be regulated by irrigation. With a transverse colostomy, output is mushy, occurs after meals and unpredictably, and cannot be regulated by irrigation.

Nursing diagnosis: *High risk for body-image disturbance related to loss of control over fecal elimination*

NURSING PRIORITIES: (a) Prevent or minimize alteration in body image, and (b) enhance the patient's sense of control over bowel functions.

Interventions

1. Teach the patient measures for odor control, such as performing regular pouch care; using an odor-proof pouch; using pouch deodorant, if desired; using a room deodorant when the pouch is emptied; altering diet to reduce fecal odor, if desired; and using over-the-counter internal deodorants, if desired, such as bismuth subgallate.

2. Teach the patient measures to reduce and control flatus, such as identifying gas-forming foods; understanding the "lag time" between ingestion and flatulence; muffling sounds of flatus; and using pouch filters that deodorize flatus.

3. Teach the patient how to conceal the pouch under clothing; wearing a knit or stretchy layer next to the skin holds the pouch close to the body and helps conceal large or bulky stomas.

4. Discuss the normal emotional response to colostomy with the patient and family. Allow the patient and family to explore their feelings about the colostomy. Assess the patient's usual coping strategies. Present helpful coping strategies, such as discussing feelings and seeking information.

5. Offer information on the United Ostomy Association; arrange for an ostomy visitor if the patient wishes.

6. Discuss colostomy management during occupational, social, and sexual activity. Help the patient to role-play difficult situations, such as telling someone about the stoma.

7. Additional individualized interventions: _____

Rationales

1. Odor control is a major concern of most patients; instruction in odor-control methods increases feelings of control and confidence and reduces feelings of embarrassment and shame. Onions, garlic, beans, and cabbage generally increase odor; orange juice, buttermilk, and yogurt may decrease odor. Bismuth reduces flatus and odor and thickens stool; it is contraindicated in the patient with renal failure or on anticoagulant therapy.

2. Inability to control flatus may lead to social embarrassment and self-deprecation. The patient can time the intake of any gas-forming foods so that flatulence occurs during "safe" periods. Filters keep the pouch flat by allowing flatus to escape and prevent odor by first deodorizing flatus.

3. The ability to dress normally and look the same as before surgery diminishes alterations in body image and enhances self-concept.

4. Discussing the normal emotional response and accepting negative feelings gives the patient and family permission to explore their feelings. Accepting feelings enhances self-concept and promotes adaptation. Discussing various coping strategies may provide the patient with new or more effective ways to handle emotions.

5. Contact with others who have ostomies reduces isolation and increases perception of the colostomy as manageable, thus enhancing the patient's sense of control.

6. Preparing for such activities increases coping skills and the likelihood that the patient will manage them successfully. Role playing helps the patient prepare for difficult situations, which increases the sense of control and enhances self-concept.

7. Rationales: _____

Target outcome criteria

By 3 days before discharge, the patient will:
• observe and perform stoma care
• discuss feelings about the stoma with loved ones.

By the time of discharge, the patient will:
• describe the colostomy as manageable
• achieve adequate self-care
• describe plans for resuming preoperative life-style.

GASTROINTESTINAL DISORDERS

Nursing diagnosis: *High risk for sexual dysfunction related to change in body image or damage to autonomic nerves**

NURSING PRIORITIES: (a) Facilitate the resumption and maintenance of intimate relationships, and (b) minimize alteration in sexual function.

Interventions

1. Discuss with the patient (and spouse or partner, if possible) the importance of openness and honesty as well as the fact that both must adapt to the ostomy.

2. Teach the patient measures for securing and concealing the pouch during sexual activity, such as using a small pouch or wearing a pouch cover, a "tube top" or cummerbund around the midriff, or crotchless panties.

3. For a female with a wide rectal resection, discuss the possible need for artificial lubrication.

4. For a male with a wide rectal resection, explain potential interference with erection and ejaculation; explain that no loss of sensation or orgasmic potential will occur; explore alternatives to intercourse as indicated; and reinforce the importance of intimacy, whether or not it involves intercourse.

5. Additional individualized interventions: _____

Rationales

1. Both the patient and spouse (or partner) may have concerns and negative feelings that can affect their sexual relationship. Openness in discussing feelings may help resolve these.

2. The stoma and pouch affect overall body image and feelings of sexual attractiveness. Securing and concealing the pouch help prevent leakage and allow the patient to focus on sexuality and sharing rather than on the pouch and stoma.

3. Wide rectal resection may damage parasympathetic nerves thought to mediate vaginal lubrication.

4. Wide rectal resection may damage parasympathetic nerves controlling erection and sympathetic nerves controlling ejaculation. Sensation and orgasm, mediated by the pudendal nerve, remain intact. Intimacy—emotional closeness—is a human need separate from the desire for sexual expression. It can be met in ways other than sexual behavior, such as sharing feelings and affectionate touching.

5. Rationales: _____

Target outcome criteria
By the time of discharge, the patient will:
• share feelings about stoma with spouse or partner
• describe any alteration in sexual function (if applicable)

• describe measures for pouch management during sexual activity (if applicable).

Discharge planning
NURSING DISCHARGE CRITERIA
Upon the patient's discharge, documentation shows evidence of:
• absence of fever
• stable vital signs
• absence of pulmonary or cardiovascular complications
• healing wound with no signs of redness, swelling, or drainage
• ability to change and empty pouch using proper technique

• ability to tolerate diet
• absence of skin problems around stoma
• absence of bladder dysfunction
• absence of abdominal distention
• restored bowel function
• ability to perform activities of daily living and ambulate same as before surgery
• ability to control pain with oral medications
• adequate home support system or referral to home care if indicated by inadequate home support system or inability to manage colostomy care at home.

---

*Nerve damage applies only to the patient with rectal resection, particularly wide resection for cancer treatment.

PATIENT-FAMILY TEACHING CHECKLIST

Document evidence that the patient and family demonstrate an understanding of:
___ reason for colostomy
___ colostomy's impact on bowel function
___ normal stoma characteristics and function
___ pouch-emptying procedure
___ pouch-changing procedure
___ peristomal skin care
___ colostomy irrigation procedure (if applicable)
___ management of mucous fistula stoma (if applicable)
___ flatus and odor control
___ management of diarrhea and constipation
___ normal adaptation process and feelings after colostomy
___ community resources available for support
___ recommendations affecting resumption of preoperative life-style
___ potential alteration in sexual function (if applicable)
___ sources of colostomy supplies and reimbursement procedures for them
___ signs and symptoms to report to the doctor
___ need for follow-up appointment with the doctor (and enterostomal therapy nurse, if available)
___ how to contact the doctor.

DOCUMENTATION CHECKLIST

Using outcome criteria as a guide, document:
___ clinical status on admission
___ significant changes in clinical status
___ GI tract function (bowel sounds, NG tube output, and colostomy output)
___ stoma color and status of mucocutaneous suture line
___ oral intake and tolerance
___ episodes of abdominal distention, nausea, and vomiting
___ incision status (any signs of infection)
___ stoma location and abdominal contours
___ management plan, including pouch system selected (and decision about irrigation for the patient with a descending or sigmoid colostomy)
___ peristomal skin status
___ emotional response to colostomy and discussion of coping strategies
___ patient-family teaching
___ discharge planning.

ASSOCIATED PLANS OF CARE

Grieving
Ineffective Family Coping
Ineffective Individual Coping
Knowledge Deficit
Pain
Surgical Intervention

References

Alfaro, R. *Application of Nursing Process: A Step-by-Step Guide.* Philadelphia: J.B. Lippincott Co., 1986.

Dobkin, K., and Broadwell, D. "Nursing Considerations for the Patient Undergoing Colostomy Surgery," *Seminars in Oncology Nursing* 2(4):249-55, November 1986.

Hampton, B., and Bryant, R., eds. *Ostomies and Continent Diversions: Nursing Management.* St. Louis: Mosby-Year Book, 1992.

Mash, N., et al. *Standards of Care: Patient with Colostomy.* Irvine, CA: International Association of Enterostomal Therapy, 1989.

GASTROINTESTINAL DISORDERS

GASTROINTESTINAL DISORDERS

Duodenal Ulcer

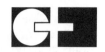

DRG information

DRG 174 GI Hemorrhage. With Complication or Comorbidity (CC).
Mean LOS = 5.5 days
Principal diagnoses include:
• acute or chronic duodenal ulcer with hemorrhage
• acute or chronic duodenal ulcer with or without obstruction.

DRG 175 GI Hemorrhage. Without CC.
Mean LOS = 3.9 days

DRG 176 Complicated Peptic Ulcer.
Mean LOS = 5.9 days
Principal diagnoses include:
• acute or chronic duodenal ulcer with or without perforation
• acute or chromic duodenal ulcer with or without obstruction or hemorrhage.

DRG 177 Uncomplicated Peptic Ulcer.
With CC.
Mean LOS = 5.2 days
Principal diagnoses include acute or chronic duodenal ulcer without hemorrhage, obstruction, or perforation.

DRG 178 Uncomplicated Peptic Ulcer. Without CC.
Mean LOS = 3.9 days

Introduction
DEFINITION AND TIME FOCUS
Duodenal ulcer results from an inflammatory and ulcerative process that affects the first portion of the duodenum within 1⅛″ (3 cm) of the gastroduodenal junction. This plan focuses on the duodenal ulcer patient admitted with signs and symptoms that have not been controlled through outpatient management. Long-term maintenance medication therapy is generally recommended instead of surgical treatment; therefore, the plan focuses on medical treatment.

ETIOLOGY AND PRECIPITATING FACTORS
Gastric acid secretion is necessary for duodenal ulcers to develop. Pathophysiologic abnormalities that influence gastric acid secretion are:
• increased parietal cell and chief cell mass (related to gastrinomal gastrin-secreting tumor or familial or genetic factors)
• increased basal secretory or postprandial secretory drive (related to gastrinoma or antral G cell hyperfunction)
• rapid gastric emptying (related to familial or genetic factors)
• *Campylobacter pylori* infection (present in majority of patients with duodenal ulcers)
• impaired mucosal defense (related to ingestion of aspirin, corticosteroids, or phenylbutazone [Butazone] and to other factors such as stress or infectious agents).

Focused assessment guidelines
NURSING HISTORY (Functional health pattern findings)

Health perception—health management pattern
• may report steady, gnawing, burning, aching, or hungerlike discomfort high in the right epigastrium; pain occurs 2 to 4 hours after meals, usually does not radiate, and is relieved by food or antacids
• at increased risk if male, age 40 to 60, with type O blood, a cigarette smoker, or with chronic emotional stress
• may report ingestion of certain drugs that contribute to duodenal ulceration, such as aspirin, corticosteroids, phenylbutazone, or indomethacin (Indocin)
• may report family history of ulcers

Nutritional-metabolic pattern
• may have history of excessive alcohol consumption
• may report nausea (vomiting not common)
• appetite usually good

Elimination pattern
• may report feeling of fullness, gaseous indigestion, or constipation

Activity-exercise pattern
• may report fatigue
• may report exacerbation of pain following unusual physical exertion

Sleep-rest pattern
• may report sleep disturbances from pain, commonly occurring between 12:00 and 3:00 a.m.

Coping—stress tolerance pattern
• may report stressful life events—such as occupational, educational, or financial problems or family illness—preceding development or exacerbation of signs and symptoms
• may deny signs and symptoms during pain-free periods (symptoms commonly disappear for weeks or months and then recur)

PHYSICAL FINDINGS
Gastrointestinal
• localized tenderness in epigastrium over ulcer site

DIAGNOSTIC STUDIES
• routine laboratory studies—add little to the workup
• more sophisticated GI studies, such as serum pepsinogen I or fasting gastrin levels—may be ordered based on the suspected cause of the duodenal ulcer; a high serum pepsinogen I level and a high fasting gastrin level provide evidence for gastrinoma or antral G cell hyperfunction
• endoscopy—reveals the ulcer's location and allows for biopsy and cytology

• screening test for *Campylobacter pylori* (available in near future)—likely to be positive
• single- or double-contrast radiography—may be ordered along with endoscopy to locate ulcer

POTENTIAL COMPLICATIONS
• duodenal obstruction
• perforation
• hemorrhage

Collaborative problem: *High risk for GI hemorrhage related to extension of duodenal ulcer into the submucosal layer of the intestinal lining*

NURSING PRIORITY: Observe for, prevent, or promptly treat hemorrhage.

Interventions

1. Observe for and report signs of GI hemorrhage. Describe any hematemesis, melena, or other signs of intestinal bleeding, including amount, consistency, and color. Test all stools and emesis with a guaiac reagent strip (Hemoccult).

2. Institute nasogastric (NG) intubation, if ordered. Keep the tube patent by instilling 30 ml of saline solution every 2 to 4 hours, then removing the same amount by mechanical suction.

3. Institute continuous saline lavage, if ordered. Instill aliquots of room-temperature fluid (500 to 1,000 ml), then remove the same amount by gentle suction and gravity drainage.

4. If the patient is bleeding actively, check vital signs hourly (more frequently if unstable). Alert the doctor immediately to any deterioration, as indicated by decreasing alertness, dropping systolic blood pressure, tachycardia, narrowing pulse pressure, or restlessness or agitation.

5. Treat hypovolemia, if present. Keep the patient warm, administer I.V. fluids and blood transfusions, as ordered, and provide oxygen at 2 to 6 liters/minute via nasal cannula.

6. Prepare the patient for surgery, if indicated.

7. Maintain the patient on bed rest after the bleeding episode. Begin the prescribed medication regimen, as ordered.

8. Additional individualized interventions: _____

Rationales

1. Hematemesis of frank red blood indicates active bleeding, while coffee-ground emesis indicates old bleeding. Guaiac testing unmasks occult bleeding.

2. NG intubation reveals the presence or absence of blood in the stomach, helps assess the rate of bleeding, and provides a route for saline lavage. If the tube is not patent, the patient may vomit stomach contents.

3. Continuous lavage indicates the rapidity of bleeding and cleans the stomach should endoscopy be necessary. Iced saline may impair coagulation. Experimental evidence suggests that room-temperature water lavage may be as effective as iced saline lavage.

4. Loss of blood volume leads rapidly to hypovolemic shock. Untreated, shock may progress to irreversible tissue ischemia; death follows quickly. Early detection of active bleeding and aggressive fluid replacement are essential to prevent shock.

5. Restoring intravascular volume and supplementing oxygen transport reduce the effects of blood loss on tissues until bleeding can be controlled.

6. Surgery may be indicated if bleeding continues longer than 48 hours, recurs, or is associated with perforation or obstruction. The preferred surgery is parietal cell vagotomy.

7. Rest aids hemostasis and decreases GI tract activity. A medication regimen (as in the following nursing diagnosis) is the usual therapy before surgery is considered.

8. Rationales: _____

GASTROINTESTINAL DISORDERS

Target outcome criteria
Within 24 hours of admission, the patient will:
• show evidence that any bleeding has ceased, such as normal NG drainage and negative guaiac testing
• have vital signs within normal limits.

Nursing diagnosis: *Pain related to increased hydrochloric acid secretion or increased spasm, intragastric pressure, and motility of upper GI tract*

NURSING PRIORITIES: (a) Promote stomach and intestinal healing, and (b) teach about risk factors and measures to prevent recurrence.

Interventions

1. Administer ulcer-healing medications and document their use, as ordered. Medications may include one or a combination of the following:
• histamine (H_2)-receptor antagonists (cimetidine [Tagamet], ranitidine [Zantac], famotidine [Pepcid], and nizatidine [Axid]), usually given with meals and at bedtime
• antacids, given after meals and at bedtime unless otherwise ordered
• anticholinergics
• sucralfate (Carafate).

2. Provide bed rest and a quiet environment, minimizing visitors and telephone calls.

3. Teach and reinforce the role of diet in ulcer healing. Help the patient identify specific foods that may increase discomfort.

4. Encourage adequate caloric intake from the basic food groups at regular intervals. Encourage frequent small meals.

5. Teach and reinforce required life-style changes to reduce physical and emotional stress. Help the patient identify specific personal stressors and recognize the relationship between increased stress and ulcer pain. As appropriate, present information on relaxation techniques, exercise, priority setting, time management and personal organization, building and nurturing relationships, the importance of "play" time, and assertiveness techniques.

6. Encourage the patient who smokes to quit.

7. Teach the patient signs and symptoms indicating ulcer recurrence and bleeding, including pain, hematemesis, dark or tarry stools, pallor, increasing weakness, dizziness, or faintness.

8. Additional individualized interventions: _____

Rationales

1. Increased hydrochloric acid secretion results in edema and inflammation of gastric mucosa. H_2-receptor antagonists inhibit gastrin release, antacids buffer hydrochloric acid, anticholinergics decrease hydrochloric acid secretion, and sucralfate binds to proteins at the base of the ulcer to form a protective barrier against acid and pepsin. Studies indicate ulcer healing occurs within 4 to 6 weeks of beginning a medication regimen.

2. Ulcer symptoms are usually reduced by rest and a quiet environment.

3. Dietary restrictions other than avoidance of excessive alcohol and caffeine are not currently recommended. Promotion of specific diets is highly controversial; none has been scientifically proven to promote healing. Identifying personal food intolerances aids diet planning.

4. Food itself acts as an antacid, neutralizing stomach acid 30 to 60 minutes after ingestion.

5. Stressful life situations, such as occupational, financial, or family problems, are reported more commonly in patients with duodenal ulcers that require longer than 6 weeks to heal. Identifying cause-and-effect relationships helps the patient make necessary life-style changes.

6. Research indicates that patients who smoke have impaired ulcer healing and a higher mortality rate when compared to nonsmokers.

7. Early identification of ulcer recurrence and bleeding may permit intervention before bleeding becomes severe.

8. Rationales: _____

Target outcome criteria
Within 2 days of admission, the patient will:
• verbalize absence or relief of pain
• identify dietary intolerances
• observe dietary recommendations in menu selection
• identify personal stressors, on request

• demonstrate interest in stress-reduction measures
• list signs and symptoms of ulcer recurrence and bleeding.

Discharge planning

NURSING DISCHARGE CRITERIA
Upon the patient's discharge, documentation shows evidence of:
• stable vital signs
• absence of signs and symptoms of GI hemorrhage
• hemoglobin within expected parameters
• absence of pain
• ability to tolerate nutritional intake as ordered
• ability to verbalize diet and medication instructions
• ability to perform activities of daily living and ambulate as before hospitalization
• adequate home support system or referral to home care if indicated by inadequate home support system or inability to perform self-care.

PATIENT-FAMILY TEACHING CHECKLIST
Document evidence that the patient and family demonstrate an understanding of:
___ nature and implications of disease
___ pain relief measures
___ all discharge medications' purpose, dose, administration schedule, and adverse effects requiring medical attention (usual discharge medications include antacids or H_2-receptor antagonists, or both)
___ recommended dietary modifications
___ need for smoking cessation program (if applicable)
___ stress reduction measures
___ signs and symptoms of ulcer recurrence and GI bleeding
___ date, time, and location of follow-up appointment
___ how to contact the doctor.

DOCUMENTATION CHECKLIST
Using outcome criteria as a guide, document:
___ clinical status on admission
___ significant changes in status
___ pain relief measures
___ nutritional intake and intolerances
___ pertinent diagnostic test findings
___ medication administration
___ patient teaching
___ discharge planning.

ASSOCIATED PLANS OF CARE
Esophagitis and Gastroenteritis
Gastrointestinal Hemorrhage
Ineffective Individual Coping
Knowledge Deficit
Pain

References

Bardhan, K. "Treatment of Duodenal Ulceration: Reflections, Recollections and Reminiscences," *Gut* 30(11):1647-55, November 1989.

Brunner, L., and Suddarth, D. *Textbook of Medical-Surgical Nursing*, 6th edition. Philadelphia: J.B. Lippincott Co., 1988.

Graham, D. "*Campylobacter pylori* and Peptic Ulcer Disease," *Gastroenterology* 96(2 Pt. 2 Suppl.):615-25, February 1989.

Lipsy, R., et al. "Clinical Review of Histamine$_2$ Receptor Antagonists," *Archives of Internal Medicine* 150(4):745-51, April 1990.

McCarthy, D. "Nonsteroidal Anti-inflammatory Drug-Induced Ulcers: Management by Traditional Therapies," *Gastroenterology* 96(2 Pt. 2 Suppl.):662-74, February 1989.

Sleisenger, M., and Fordtran, J. *Gastrointestinal Disease: Pathophysiology, Diagnosis, Management*, 4th edition. Philadelphia: W.B. Saunders Co., 1988.

GASTROINTESTINAL DISORDERS

Esophagitis and Gastroenteritis

DRG information

DRG 182 Esophagitis, Gastroenteritis, and Miscellaneous Digestive Disorders. Age 17+. With Complication or Comorbidity (CC).
Mean LOS = 4.9 days

DRG 183 Esophagitis, Gastroenteritis, and Miscellaneous Digestive Disorders. Age 0 to 17. Without CC.
Mean LOS = 3.5 days

DRG 184 Esophagitis, Gastroenteritis, and Miscellaneous Digestive Disorders.
Age 0 to 17.
Mean LOS = 3.2 days

Introduction
DEFINITION AND TIME FOCUS

Esophagitis and gastroenteritis are nonspecific inflammatory conditions of the mucosa of the esophagus and the stomach and small bowel, respectively. Esophagitis is usually related to inadequate cardiac sphincter tone, resulting in gastric reflux and subsequent irritation. Gastroenteritis is most commonly caused by bacteria or viruses that produce severe vomiting, diarrhea, and abdominal cramping. Both conditions may cause temporary discomfort (which can be treated on an outpatient basis) or serious, even life-threatening, illness if the patient is elderly, debilitated, or otherwise at increased risk. This plan focuses on the patient admitted for diagnosis and treatment of acute esophagitis or gastroenteritis.

ETIOLOGY AND PRECIPITATING FACTORS

• infectious agents—fungal (moniliasis), viral (herpes simplex), and bacterial (staphylococcus, *Helicobacter pylori*)
• drugs and chemical agents—gastric acid reflux; bile reflux; ingestion of caustic substances (such as lye); medications such as aspirin, steroids, indomethacin (Indocin), antibiotics
• trauma or physical factors—excessive ingestion of alcohol, spicy foods, or coffee; cigarette smoking; ingestion of very hot or very cold substances; nasogastric intubation; radiation therapy; severe physical stress from surgery, sepsis, burns, accidents, or heavy weight lifting; excessive emotional stress

Focused assessment guidelines
NURSING HISTORY (Functional health pattern findings)

Health perception—health management pattern
• may present with various nonspecific symptoms
• symptoms may be acute, as from infection or ingestion of a caustic substance, or gradual (reflux esophagitis)
• may have delayed seeking medical attention because of vagueness of symptoms (reflux esophagitis)
• may report tendency to self-medicate with multiple over-the-counter remedies for GI upset
• may be receiving radiation therapy for diabetes, scleroderma, or other disease that makes esophageal or gastric mucosa more susceptible to infection and inflammation
• may be receiving treatment for sepsis, trauma, burns, immunologic disorder, endocrine disorder, liver disease, pancreatitis, or pulmonary disease

Nutritional-metabolic pattern
• with esophagitis, may report heartburn, dysphagia, or odynophagia (pain on swallowing); with gastroenteritis, typically complains of epigastric or abdominal discomfort, nausea, vomiting, diarrhea, or fever
• may report hematemesis and food regurgitation
• may report eructation and epigastric fullness after meals
• may report anorexia or weight loss
• mouth may appear swollen and inflamed
• may report history of excessive alcohol consumption, aspirin ingestion, cigarette smoking, or ingestion of caustic substance
• may report habitually eating excessive amounts of spicy foods, consuming very hot or cold substances, and eating late at night

Elimination pattern
• may report cramping, abdominal distention, diarrhea, increased flatus, or melena

Activity-exercise pattern
• may report sudden or chronic fatigue

Sleep-rest pattern
• may report restlessness
• may report awakening at night because of pain or with regurgitated food on pillow

Cognitive-perceptual pattern
• pain intensity and description depend on cause of problem (for example, acute gastritis may cause epigastric discomfort and abdominal cramping, and caustic chemical ingestion may cause immediate localized pain and odynophagia)
• may report morning hoarseness (laryngitis)
• may report salty salivary secretions (water brash)
• if symptoms result from ingestion of a caustic substance, may report altered taste (from damage of salivary glands)

Coping—stress tolerance pattern
• may report high levels of stress at work or home

PHYSICAL FINDINGS
Gastrointestinal
Esophagitis
- hematemesis
- eructation
- dysphagia

Gastroenteritis
- vomiting
- diarrhea
- eructation
- hyperactive bowel sounds
- flatulence
- hematemesis
- melena

Cardiovascular
(if hypovolemia present)
- hypotension
- tachycardia

Neurologic
(if hypovolemia present)
- dizziness
- restlessness
- irritability

Integumentary
(if hypovolemia present)
- pallor
- cool, clammy skin
- poor skin turgor

Musculoskeletal
(when in pain)
- tense posture
- facial grimacing

DIAGNOSTIC STUDIES
For esophagitis and gastroenteritis:
- complete blood count (CBC) — may show decreased hemoglobin or hematocrit, possibly indicating GI blood loss; elevated white blood cell count may indicate infection or inflammation
- serum electrolyte levels — may be studied to detect signs of fluid imbalance from blood loss, vomiting, or diarrhea (hypokalemia common with significant vomiting or diarrhea)
- serum amylase and lipase levels — elevations indicate pancreatitis as cause of symptoms

For esophagitis:
- barium swallow — detects inflammation, ulceration, esophageal strictures, and gastric reflux
- esophagoscopy — allows direct visualization of the esophagus to detect inflammation, ulceration, strictures, and hiatal hernia; biopsy of mucosa or brushing for cytology may be used for tissue diagnosis
- esophageal manometry — may reveal decreased esophageal sphincter pressure, as seen with gastroesophageal reflux; may detect peristaltic abnormalities responsible for infections or inflammatory changes in the esophagus
- acid perfusion test (Bernstein test) — if the patient has pain or burning during perfusion of acid (via a tube) into esophagus, may indicate esophagitis
- pH reflux test — a pH less than 4 may indicate gastroesophageal reflux (normal esophageal pH is greater than 5)

For gastroenteritis:
- esophagogastroduodenoscopy — allows direct visualization of esophagus, stomach, and duodenum; biopsy of mucosa or brushing for cytology may be performed for tissue diagnosis; Clotest may be performed to detect the urease enzyme of *Helicobacter pylori*
- upper GI series — radiographically visualizes lining of esophagus, stomach, and duodenum; may detect inflammation, ulcerations, or strictures
- guaiac test — occult blood in stool may indicate blood loss

POTENTIAL COMPLICATIONS
For esophagitis:
- ulcerative esophagitis
- hemorrhage
- esophageal stricture
- aspiration pneumonia
- Barrett's epithelium — columnar (gastric) epithelium in the esophagus resulting from chronic gastroesophageal reflux; places the patient at great risk for adenocarcinoma of the esophagus
- carcinoma of the esophagus
- inflammatory polyps of the vocal cords
- lung abscess

For gastroenteritis:
- hemorrhage
- gastric or duodenal ulcer
- gastric outlet obstruction

Nursing diagnosis: *High risk for fluid volume deficit related to vomiting, diarrhea, or GI hemorrhage*

NURSING PRIORITY: Reestablish and maintain fluid and electrolyte balance.

Interventions

1. Monitor and record the patient's vital signs every 15 minutes if bleeding or every 4 hours if stable. Unless the patient is syncopal, frankly hypotensive, or severely tachycardic when supine, assess for orthostatic blood pressure and pulse rate changes every 8 hours: take the patient's blood pressure and pulse while supine, then have the patient sit up and measure blood pressure and pulse rate again. Document your findings.

2. Withhold oral foods and fluids until vomiting has subsided. Begin I.V. fluids, as ordered. Monitor CBC and serum electrolyte levels, as ordered, and report abnormalities. See Appendix C, "Fluid and Electrolyte Imbalances."

3. Administer antiemetics, antidiarrheals, and anticholinergics, as ordered.

4. Monitor and record the effectiveness of medications.

5. Assess the patient's skin for signs of dehydration—poor skin turgor, dry skin and mucous membranes, and pallor. Also assess for thirst.

6. Monitor and record intake and output each shift. Include all vomitus, diarrhea, tube drainage, and blood loss in output, and all blood products and I.V. fluids in input. Record hourly urine outputs in the unstable patient. Record daily weights. Test all GI output with guaiac reagent strips (Hemoccult).

7. Assess and record the patient's level of consciousness, muscle strength, and coordination at least every 8 hours. Report changes promptly.

Rationales

1. Tachycardia and hypotension may indicate hypovolemia or shock. Orthostatic changes (a blood pressure decrease of 10 mm Hg or more or a pulse rate increase of 20 beats/minute or more) may indicate hypovolemia.

2. Allowing the patient to eat and drink may cause more vomiting and lead to metabolic alkalosis, hypokalemia, or hyponatremia. The "Fluid and Electrolyte Imbalances" appendix provides details related to specific abnormalities.

3. Antiemetics, such as prochlorperazine (Compazine), promethazine (Phenergan), and chlorpromazine (Thorazine), prevent activation of the vomiting center in the brain stem. Adverse reactions include sedation, blurred vision, and restlessness.
   Antidiarrheals, such as diphenoxylate with atropine (Lomotil), loperamide (Imodium), and kaolin and pectin (Kaopectate), may be used to decrease fluid loss from diarrhea. Diphenoxylate with atropine and loperamide are synthetic opium alkaloids that decrease intestinal motility, thereby decreasing diarrhea. They are contraindicated in patients with obstruction or diarrhea caused by infectious agents.
   Because kaolin and pectin act by adsorbing liquids, bacteria, toxins, nutrients, and drugs, loss of essential nutrients may occur with prolonged use.
   Anticholinergics, such as dicyclomine hydrochloride (Bentyl) and propantheline bromide (Pro-Banthine), decrease gastric acid secretion and GI tone and motility and effectively control nausea and vomiting in acute gastritis. Adverse reactions include urine retention, dryness of mucous membranes (including dry mouth), dizziness, flushing, and headache.

4. Lack of effectiveness may indicate the need to reevaluate the pharmacologic regimen.

5. Poor skin turgor, dry skin and mucous membranes, and increased thirst may indicate hypovolemia resulting from decreased extracellular fluid volume.

6. Accurate monitoring of intake and output alerts caregivers to imbalances that may cause hypovolemic shock. Oliguria (less than 30 ml of urine per hour) indicates decreased glomerular filtration rate; this may result from decreased blood flow, as in hypovolemia. Weight loss may reflect fluid loss. Checking GI output for occult blood may provide early detection of bleeding.

7. Confusion, dizziness, or stupor may indicate hypovolemia and electrolyte imbalance. A decreased level of consciousness reflects cerebral hypoxemia caused by decreased circulating blood volume. Vomiting and diarrhea can cause electrolyte loss. Sodium loss may cause confusion and delirium; potassium loss may cause muscle weakness.

8. If the patient develops a GI hemorrhage, consult the "Gastrointestinal Hemorrhage" plan, page 394.

8. The "Gastrointestinal Hemorrhage" plan contains detailed information on this complication.

9. Additional individualized interventions: _____

9. Rationales: _____

Target outcome criteria
Within 2 hours of admission, the patient will:
• display stable vital signs
• experience no vomiting
• maintain adequate urine output (greater than 60 ml/hour).

Nursing diagnosis: *Pain related to inflammation of the esophagus, stomach, and duodenum*

NURSING PRIORITY: Relieve pain.

Interventions

1. See the "Pain" plan, page 69.

2. Assess and document the pain's characteristics: onset, location, duration, and severity; radiation to back, neck, or shoulder; relationship to activity or position changes; relationship to eating patterns and bowel movements; and relationship to ingestion of spicy foods, coffee, alcohol, hot or cold liquids, or certain medications. Notify the doctor of any findings. Assess and document pain relief measures.

3. Administer antacids (typically hourly and 1 hour after meals), histamine (H_2)-receptor antagonists (1 hour before meals and at least 30 minutes before sucralfate administration), sucralfate (Carafate), antibiotics, and antifungal medication, as ordered.

4. Monitor and record the effectiveness of medications.

5. Assist and instruct the patient to rest, physically and emotionally. Help the patient identify personal stressors and ways to minimize their effects. Limit the number of visitors. Coordinate patient care to minimize interruptions. Keep room lights low. Teach stress-relieving techniques such as deep breathing and relaxation exercises.

Rationales

1. Pain associated with esophagitis and gastroenteritis may be subtle, as in abdominal cramping or heartburn, or may be more acute, such as sharp substernal pain similar to angina. The "Pain" plan provides general interventions for pain. This plan contains additional information related to esophagitis and gastroenteritis.

2. Accurate assessment is important in determining the pain's cause and formulating a medical diagnosis. Substernal burning pain (heartburn) and odynophagia are commonly associated with esophagitis. Epigastric pain while eating and abdominal cramping and tenderness are associated with acute gastritis.

3. Antacids are most effective if given 1 hour after meals to neutralize increased gastric acid secretion stimulated by food ingestion. Antacids are effective for about 30 minutes in the fasting stomach and should be given hourly for optimum neutralization of gastric acid. In case of severe pain, antacids may be given every 30 to 60 minutes.
   H_2-receptor antagonists decrease gastric acid secretions and lower gastric pH by blocking H_2. They are poorly absorbed if given with meals, antacids, or sucralfate.
   Sucralfate provides a protective coating for the gastric lining and is not absorbed. It may be ordered crushed and mixed with water to form a slush that coats the esophagus.
   Antibiotics should be given after meals. Combination therapy (two different antibiotics and bismuth salt) is given to treat *Helicobacter pylori* infection.

4. Lack of effectiveness may indicate improper administration, inadequate dosage, the need to change medications, or new or complicating factors.

5. Stress stimulates the vagus nerve, which increases gastric mucosal blood flow, gastric acid secretion, and gastric motility. These factors may increase pain and inhibit healing.

GASTROINTESTINAL DISORDERS

6. Instruct the patient and family about pain-prevention measures. If pain causes the patient to awake at night or if the pain is worse on awakening, instruct the patient to sleep with the head of the bed elevated and to avoid eating for 2 to 3 hours before bedtime. Advise the patient to avoid bending, lifting heavy objects, and wearing constrictive clothing. Administer stool softeners, if prescribed, to avoid straining during bowel movements. Assess the patient's diet and habits to identify known causes of pain, such as spicy foods, alcohol, caffeinated products, aspirin, and smoking.

6. Eating stimulates gastric acid secretion. The patient with esophagitis should avoid eating for 3 hours before bedtime and elevate the head of the bed to prevent gastric reflux during sleep. Bending, lifting, wearing constrictive clothing, and straining decrease esophageal pressure and increase intra-abdominal pressure. Spicy foods, alcohol, caffeinated products, and aspirin irritate the gastric lining, increasing discomfort, and should be avoided. Cigarette smoking stimulates increased gastric secretion, which may contribute to further inflammation.

7. Additional individualized interventions: _____

7. Rationales: _____

Target outcome criteria
Within 2 hours of admission, the patient will:
• verbalize pain relief
• rest comfortably in a relaxing environment

• have stable vital signs.

Nursing diagnosis: *Nutritional deficit related to nausea and vomiting, dysphagia, and mouth soreness*

NURSING PRIORITY: Reestablish nutritional balance.

Interventions

1. Assess the patient's ability to retain oral food and fluids, noting any nausea, vomiting, or regurgitation; dysphagia for solids, liquids, or both; and complaints of mouth pain or soreness. Record all observations.

2. Monitor intake and output. Withhold oral foods and fluids until vomiting subsides. If total parenteral nutrition (TPN) is ordered, infuse the solution at the prescribed rate. (See the "Total Parenteral Nutrition" plan, page 411.) Administer oral nutritional and vitamin supplements as ordered. Record daily weights and calorie counts.

3. Explain the dilatation procedure, if ordered, for dysphagia, and assist when needed.

4. Assist the dietitian in teaching the patient how to plan a well-balanced, nutritious diet. Teach the patient with esophageal strictures who cannot eat solids to puree foods and drink nutritional supplements. Instruct the patient with acute gastritis to eat frequent small meals instead of three large meals a day. Tell the patient to restrict or avoid spicy foods, alcohol, and caffeinated products, if necessary. Record all patient teaching.

Rationales

1. Careful assessment of symptoms aids differential diagnosis. Mouth pain or soreness may indicate fungal infection or occur after ingestion of a caustic substance. Dysphagia may result from stricture formation from reflux esophagitis or ingestion of a caustic substance.

2. Food and fluids may cause further vomiting, increasing the risk of such complications as Mallory-Weiss tears (tearing of the esophageal mucosa, usually after forceful or prolonged vomiting). TPN may be necessary if oral intake is contraindicated for an extended period. The TPN plan contains details about this therapy. Nutritional supplements are indicated for the patient with esophageal strictures who is unable to swallow solid foods or for the patient who is unable to maintain metabolic balance because of anorexia, nausea, or mouth soreness.

3. Esophageal strictures, a common cause of dysphagia in esophagitis, can result from ingestion of a caustic substance, gastric reflux, or chronic infection (such as moniliasis). Carefully explaining the dilatation procedure helps alleviate the patient's anxiety. (Because dilatation procedures vary widely, consult institution protocol for details.)

4. Dietary instruction aims to establish a balanced diet and ultimately return the patient's weight to normal. Thorough teaching may prevent subsequent problems and complications. Careful documentation of teaching provides a record for other caregivers so that reinforcement and review may be provided, as appropriate.

5. Additional individualized interventions: _____

5. Rationales: _____

Target outcome criteria
Within 2 hours of admission, the patient will verbalize relief of nausea and vomiting.

Within 24 hours of admission, the patient will discuss nutritional needs with the dietitian.

Discharge planning
NURSING DISCHARGE CRITERIA
Upon the patient's discharge, documentation shows evidence of:
• stable vital signs
• absence of pulmonary or cardiovascular complications
• hemoglobin and hematocrit values within expected parameters
• ability to tolerate adequate nutritional intake
• adequate hydration
• absence of pain
• urine output and bowel function same as before onset of acute illness
• stabilizing weight
• ability to follow prescribed diet
• ability to ambulate and perform activities of daily living same as before hospitalization.

PATIENT-FAMILY TEACHING CHECKLIST
Document evidence that the patient and family demonstrate an understanding of:
___ disease and implications
___ all discharge medications' purpose, administration schedule, dosage, and adverse effects requiring medical attention (usual discharge medications include antacids, H_2-antagonists, anticholinergics, antibiotics, or antifungal medications)
___ recommended dietary modifications or TPN administration, if patient is being discharged on TPN
___ recommended life-style modifications, including smoking cessation and stress reduction
___ importance of medical follow-up, which may include weekly visits for dilatation
___ how to contact the doctor
___ signs and symptoms of complications
___ available community resources such as Alcoholics Anonymous, as indicated.

DOCUMENTATION CHECKLIST
Using outcome criteria as a guide, document:
___ clinical status on admission
___ significant changes in status
___ description of pain
___ pain relief measures
___ episodes of nausea and vomiting
___ description of vomitus
___ description of stools
___ bleeding episodes

___ fluid intake and output
___ stress relief measures
___ pertinent laboratory and diagnostic test findings
___ nutritional status
___ patient-family teaching
___ discharge planning.

ASSOCIATED PLANS OF CARE
Gastrointestinal Hemorrhage
Ineffective Individual Coping
Knowledge Deficit
Pain
Total Parenteral Nutrition

References
Conti-Nibali, S., Sferlazzas, C., Fera, M., Saitta, G., Tedeschi, A., and Magazzu, G. "*Helicobacter pylori* Infection: A Simplified Diagnostic Approach," *The American Journal of Gastroenterology* 85(12): 1573-75, December 1990.

Glupeznski, Y., and Burette, A. "Drug Therapy for *Helicobacter pylori* Infection: Problems and Pitfalls," *The American Journal of Gastroenterology* 85(12):1545-51, December 1990.

Graham, D. "The Whos and Whens of Therapy for *Helicobacter pylori*," *The American Journal of Gastroenterology* 85(12):1552-55, December 1990.

Hoffman, S., Marshall, B., Dye, K., and Caldwell, S. "Gastric Urease, *Campylobacter pylori* and the Interpretation of Clotest," *Gastroenterology Nursing* 11(4):217-20, Spring 1989.

Sleisenger, M., and Fordtran, J. *Gastrointestinal Disease, Pathology, Diagnosis, Management,* vol. 2, 4th ed. Philadelphia: W.B. Saunders Co., 1989.

GASTROINTESTINAL DISORDERS

Gastrointestinal Hemorrhage

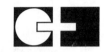

DRG information

DRG 174 Gastrointestinal Hemorrhage. With Complication or Comorbidity (CC).
   Mean LOS = 5.5 days
   Principal diagnoses include:
   • GI hemorrhage — site or etiology unspecified
   • hemorrhage of anus or rectum
   • acute ulcer (gastric, peptic, duodenal, jejunal, or a combination of sites) with hemorrhage
   • esophageal varices with hemorrhage.

DRG 175 Gastrointestinal Hemorrhage. Without CC.
   Mean LOS = 3.9 days
   Principal diagnoses include selected principal diagnoses listed under DRG 174. The distinction is that patients grouped under DRG 175 have no CC.

Introduction
DEFINITION AND TIME FOCUS

In the acute care setting, severe gastrointestinal (GI) bleeding is most commonly associated with upper GI pathology; although bleeding can occur anywhere in the GI tract, lower GI bleeding is usually less severe. Bleeding may result from an underlying condition, such as ulcers, invasive tumors, or esophageal varices. (Gastritis and gastric ulcers are estimated to account for up to 80% of all GI bleeding episodes.) Bleeding may also develop as an untoward effect of therapeutically administered medications, such as anti-inflammatory drugs or anticoagulants. Trauma, burns, sepsis, and other conditions may cause stress ulcers, which usually manifest as sudden, severe, and painless bleeding. Regardless of the cause, acute GI bleeding may be life-threatening without prompt diagnosis and treatment. Delay in diagnosis is associated with a higher mortality rate and increased complications. This plan focuses on the patient experiencing an acute episode of upper GI bleeding.

ETIOLOGY AND PRECIPITATING FACTORS

• gastric irritation or altered gastric pH, as with medication use (for example, salicylates, steroids, or other anti-inflammatory drugs), alcohol or caffeine abuse, toxic or allergic reactions, ingestion of corrosive substances, peptic or gastric ulcer, gastritis, and stress reactions
• altered gastric function or circulation, as with tumors, portal hypertension or esophageal varices, or Mallory-Weiss laceration of gastric mucosa
• altered blood coagulation, as with anticoagulant use blood dyscrasias, cancer, shock, sepsis, uremia, and disseminated intravascular coagulation (DIC)

Focused assessment guidelines
NURSING HISTORY (Functional health pattern findings)

Health perception–health management pattern
• commonly gives a history of gastric ulcer or gastritis
• may have history of heavy alcohol intake or cigarette smoking (associated with gastritis and esophageal varices)
• may give a history of long-term steroid, salicylate, or other anti-inflammatory therapy

Nutritional-metabolic pattern
• commonly complains of nausea
• may complain of a feeling of fullness in the abdomen
• may complain of thirst
• may complain of heartburn

Elimination pattern
• may describe dark or tarry stools
• may give history of "coffee-ground" emesis

Activity-exercise pattern
• commonly describes weakness and easy fatigability

Cognitive-perceptual pattern
• if bleeding is related to ulcer disease, may complain of gnawing, aching, or burning abdominal pain, which may be relieved by eating
• if bleeding is related to stress ulcer, may be painless

Coping–stress tolerance pattern
• likely to express extreme fear in reaction to sight of own blood

PHYSICAL FINDINGS
General appearance
• frightened or anxious facial expression

Cardiovascular
• tachycardia
• orthostatic hypotension
• weak, thready peripheral pulse

Gastrointestinal
• melena
• hematemesis (associated with upper GI bleeding)
• "coffee-ground" vomitus (indicates slower upper GI bleeding)
• hematochezia (bright, bloody stools — usually indicates lower GI bleeding but may occur with rapid upper GI hemorrhage)

Pulmonary
• hyperventilation

Neurologic
- restlessness
- decreased alertness (with shock)

Integumentary
- pallor
- diaphoresis

DIAGNOSTIC STUDIES
- blood urea nitrogen (BUN) levels — elevated because of digestion of blood proteins in the GI tract and accumulated blood breakdown by-products
- complete blood count (CBC) — obtained for baseline; may reflect minimal abnormalities for up to 36 hours if bleeding is slow. Eventually, reduced hemoglobin, hematocrit, and red blood cell count reflect overall blood loss; reticulocyte count may be elevated in response to bleeding
- blood typing and cross-matching — obtained in anticipation of blood replacement; in acute bleeding, type-specific, non–cross-matched blood may be administered as an emergency measure
- prothrombin time, partial thromboplastin time — obtained for baseline and for evaluation of altered coagulation status as cause of bleeding. Further clotting studies may also be obtained if coagulation defects are suspected
- gastric aspiration — provides information regarding amount and time of bleeding; results are used to guide further intervention. For example, a small aspiration of material resembling coffee grounds may indicate "old" bleeding that only warrants close observation of the patient; aspiration of fresh bright red blood is evidence of active hemorrhage and demands prompt intervention

- endoscopic examination, including flexible fiber-optic endoscopy — provides visualization of bleeding site and associated pathology; may permit direct coagulation of bleeding sites via endoscope or tissue biopsy
- abdominal angiography — allows visualization of abdominal vasculature; used to locate bleeding sites and may be used for localized treatment by infusion of vasopressin (Pitressin) or injection of clot formation material (embolization)
- computed tomography scan — may be used to detect tumors or polyps
- barium studies — may be used to identify gastric erosions or tumors as bleeding source if angiography is not available; used as a last resort in patients with active bleeding as barium obscures the field for subsequent endoscopic or angiographic assessment

POTENTIAL COMPLICATIONS
- shock
- renal failure
- DIC
- hepatic encephalopathy
- myocardial ischemia or infarction

Collaborative problem: *High risk for hypovolemic shock related to blood loss*

NURSING PRIORITIES: (a) Assess amount of blood loss, (b) restore blood and fluid volume, and (c) help identify the source or cause and provide treatment.

Interventions

1. See the "Hypovolemic Shock" plan, page 346.

2. Assess the amount of blood loss using the following procedures:
- Maintain accurate intake and output records, including precise measurement of all vomitus and stools. Unless output is visibly bloody, guaiac test it.

Rationales

1. The "Hypovolemic Shock" plan provides detailed interventions for assessment and treatment of the patient in actual or impending shock.

2. Prevention of shock depends on accurate status assessment.
- Direct measurement of bloody output is essential to guide replacement therapy. Guaiac testing provides objective assessment for the presence of occult blood. Careful monitoring of urine output is vital because a drop in hourly urine output (less than 60 ml/hour) may signal the development of shock.'

• Evaluate vital signs every 4 hours, or more frequently if indicated; include evaluation of orthostatic changes unless the patient is syncopal, frankly hypotensive, or severely tachycardic when supine. Note and report promptly to the doctor a systolic blood pressure decrease of more than 10 mm Hg or a pulse increase of more than 20 beats/minute.

• Compensatory neurovascular mechanisms may be able to maintain normal supine blood pressure when blood loss is less than 500 ml. Moving from a supine to a sitting position adds an orthostatic stress that may unmask hidden hypotension. A pulse increase of 20 to 30 beats/minute with no change in blood pressure correlates with a blood loss of 500 ml, while a pulse increase of more than 30 beats/minute and systolic blood pressure drop of more than 10 mm Hg may indicate a blood loss of 1,000 ml or more. Although many critically ill patients are too unstable to tolerate orthostatic assessment, it may provide useful data in the stable patient. However, when clear evidence of hypotension already exists, the test may accelerate shock progression.

• If the patient is in a critical care unit, evaluate hemodynamic pressures and electrocardiography (ECG) findings according to Appendix A, "Monitoring Standards," or unit protocol.

• These parameters provide additional data useful in judging the degree of shock present.

• Obtain appropriate laboratory studies, as ordered, including CBC, BUN, and creatinine for baseline and ongoing monitoring.

• Hemoglobin and hematocrit values reflect blood volume status but may show no changes initially. BUN and creatinine levels are of greater diagnostic value. An elevated BUN level in the presence of normal creatinine level indicates a likely blood loss of more than 1,000 ml.

• Assess the patient frequently for clinical signs of hypovolemia. Note constellations of signs and symptoms, such as those of mild shock (for example, anxiety, perspiration, or weakness); moderate shock (for example, hyperactive bowel sounds, tachycardia, or thirst); or severe shock (for example, pallor, cool and clammy skin, decreased level of consciousness, decreased urine output, and thready pulse).

• Clinical parameters help define stages of blood loss. Signs and symptoms of mild shock (less than 500 ml blood loss) are nonspecific. Signs of moderate shock (500 to 1,000 ml blood loss) reflect progressive activation of sympathetic nervous system compensatory mechanisms and other homeostatic mechanisms. Signs of severe shock (more than 1,000 ml blood loss) reflect ischemia of core organ systems.

• Insert and maintain a gastric tube, as ordered, and check drainage for blood.

• Gastric intubation permits removal and accurate measurement of accumulated blood from the stomach. It is also therapeutic because blood in the stomach may stimulate vomiting and excess gastric acid secretion, both of which may cause or accelerate bleeding. Finally, blood that passes into the intestines is broken down into ammonia, which may have toxic metabolic effects.

3. Replace blood loss by:

3. Replacement therapy is essential to prevent hypovolemia and hypoxemia related to reduced hemoglobin level.

• establishing and maintaining I.V. access with one or two large-bore cannulas

• A large-bore cannula is necessary for rapid infusion of blood and fluids.

• rapidly administering I.V. crystalloid solution (such as lactated Ringer's solution)

• Crystalloid solutions effectively expand plasma volume. Rapid administration averts cardiovascular collapse.

• administering and monitoring the response to transfusion of packed red blood cells, fresh frozen plasma, or other blood components as well as volume expanders, such as plasma protein fraction (Plasmanate) or albumin, as ordered. Prepare the patient for emergency surgery if blood pressure does not increase in response to 1 liter of fluid given over 10 minutes or if hemoglobin and hemtocrit values fail to increase in response to blood product administration.

• Restoration of circulating volume and replacement of blood components are essential to minimize cell death from hypoxemia. If congestive heart failure is present, packed cells may be administered with minimal additional fluid to avert fluid overload. The hematocrit should increase with each unit of packed cells administered. Persistent bleeding is present if hematocrit does not improve. For other patients, volume expanders may be indicated. Albumin, for example, provides an osmotically induced fluid expansion equal to five times its volume. Blood that has been stored for a period of time may be deficient in some clotting factors, so the administration of fresh frozen plasma or other components may be needed. Emergency surgery is indicated to identify and correct the cause of massive bleeding.

4. Initiate measures to stop bleeding, as ordered, such as:

4. As many as 90% of upper GI hemorrhages cease spontaneously, but severe bleeding constitutes a medical or surgical emergency, and prompt corrective treatment is warranted.

• maintaining activity restrictions, which usually include strict bed rest

• performing gastric lavage, usually with room temperature or iced normal saline solution, with or without addition of norepinephrine (Levophed) to the solution. If norepinephrine is used, the usual dilution is 2 ampules to 1,000 ml normal saline solution in a continuous irrigation.

• administering vasopressin I.V., unless the patient has a history of coronary artery disease or other vascular problems. The dose range is 0.02 to 0.06 mcg/minute I.V. or through an arterial catheter placed near the bleeding site. Monitor the ECG during administration.

• preparing the patient with uncontrollably bleeding esophageal varices, if a poor surgical risk, for injection sclerotherapy; after injection, observe for rebleeding, chest pain, fever, and other complications

• preparing the patient for laser therapy, if ordered

• assisting with insertion, monitoring, and maintaining the placement of a Sengstaken-Blakemore tube or other compression tubes. Elevate the head of the bed. Suction the oropharynx, nasopharynx, and upper esophagus frequently. Irrigate the tube at least every 2 hours. Maintain proper balloon pressures. Maintain proper positioning by verifying balloon placement by X-ray, as ordered, and maintaining traction on the balloon. Cut and remove the tube immediately if airway compromise occurs.

• administering vitamin K₁ (phytonadione, Aqua-MEPHYTON) I.M., as ordered

• preparing the patient for surgery if medical treatment is unsuccessful (bleeding requires more than 2 units of blood per hour to maintain blood pressure, requires more than 6 to 8 units of blood within 24 hours, exceeds more than 2,500 ml in the first 24 hours, or recurs during therapy).

• Activity may increase intra-abdominal pressure and accelerate bleeding.

• Gastric lavage removes accumulated blood and clots and clears the stomach for endoscopic examination. Iced lavage, which was traditionally ordered based on the theory that gastric cooling decreased blood flow, has become controversial as a therapeutic measure. Some studies have demonstrated prolonged clotting times in response to iced irrigation. Norepinephrine may be added for its local vasoconstrictive effects, although its value has not been proven. Systemic effects are minimized when norepinephrine is administered in this way because the drug is metabolized in the liver immediately after gastric absorption.

• Vasopressin causes vasoconstriction and contraction of smooth muscle in the GI tract. It also increases reabsorption of water in the renal tubules. However, its use may cause myocardial ischemia, infarction, or hypertension, particularly in a patient with cardiovascular disease.

• Injection sclerotherapy is a definitive treatment involving injection of a coagulating substance into a bleeding vessel. This produces intense inflammation and scarring, and stops bleeding in approximately 80% of cases. Hemorrhage may recur, requiring multiple treatments. Chest pain and fever (typically appearing within 6 hours and lasting 3 days) result from the inflammatory process.

• Laser coagulation therapy may be used when endoscopy indicates active bleeding, fresh clots, or a duodenal ulcer or gastric erosion with a visible vessel.

• Compression balloon tubes, such as the Sengstaken-Blakemore tube, may be used to control hemorrhage temporarily in patients with esophageal varices. However, the high rebleeding rate, significant discomfort, and risk of aspiration limit the tubes' usefulness. The balloon applies direct pressure against bleeding vessels, while the gastric tube permits continued decompression and aspiration. Elevating the head of the bed helps prevent esophageal reflux and associated irritation. When the tube is in place, the patient is unable to swallow salivary secretions. Also, nasal secretions may be increased because of local irritation from the tube. Irrigation ensures patency of the tube and prevents gastric distention.

Excessive pressure may result in perforation, inflammation, or ulceration of the esophagus or gastric mucosal lining, while insufficient pressure may render the tube ineffective or contribute to its displacement.

X-ray verification and maintenance of traction help ensure correct positioning. If the tube becomes displaced, it may obstruct the airway. Cutting the tube deflates the gastric and esophageal balloons and permits immediate removal.

• The patient receiving I.V. feedings or multiple antibiotics for a prolonged period may develop vitamin K deficiency because this catalyst for clotting factor production is either obtained through a normal diet or synthesized by intestinal bacteria. Replacement therapy may be necessary to restore normal clotting status.

• If bleeding does not stop, surgery is indicated to identify and correct the problem.

GASTROINTESTINAL DISORDERS

5. Administer medications to control gastric acidity, typically histamine (H_2)-blockers such as cimetidine (Tagamet) or ranitidine (Zantac) I.V. during acute bleeding episodes. Monitor gastric aspirate pH and adjust dosage, as ordered, to maintain a pH greater than 4.0. Observe for drug interactions, especially if the patient is also receiving theophylline (Slo-Phyllin), procainamide (Promine), or warfarin (Coumadin). Observe for signs of toxicity if cimetidine and lidocaine (Xylocaine) are administered concurrently.

6. Prepare the patient and family for and assist with diagnostic procedures, as ordered, such as endoscopic examination, angiography, or other studies.

7. Additional individualized interventions: _____

_____

5. Gastric hyperacidity, indicated by a low pH, is a primary contributor to ulcer development and the need for dosage increases. H_2 blockers inhibit the action of histamine, raising gastric pH. Cimetidine and ranitidine reduce theophylline clearance, increasing the risk of theophylline toxicity; impair metabolism of procainamide, possibly producing toxicity; and impair metabolism of warfarin, increasing the risk of bleeding. Cimetidine reduces liver clearance of lidocaine.

6. Identification of the site and cause of the bleeding is essential because delay in diagnosis is associated with a higher mortality rate.

7. Rationales: _____

_____

Target outcome criteria
Within 24 hours of detection of bleeding, the patient will:
- exhibit systolic blood pressure greater than 90 mm Hg
- exhibit normal heart rate
- have urine output of at least 60 ml/hour
- show no orthostatic changes in vital signs
- have warm, dry skin
- exhibit gastric pH greater than 4.0.

Nursing diagnosis: *High risk for injury: complications related to undetected bleeding, inadequate organ perfusion, accumulation of toxins, electrolyte imbalance, release of procoagulants, or ulcer perforation*

NURSING PRIORITY: Prevent or promptly detect and treat complications.

Interventions

1. Continue to perform guaiac tests on all gastric contents and stools at least daily, even after the patient's condition has stabilized.

2. Immediately report and thoroughly investigate any complaint of chest pain, particularly in a patient with preexisting cardiac disease.

3. Monitor renal and hepatic function, including hourly urine outputs, daily BUN and creatinine levels, and daily weight. Note daily serum electrolyte values, including serum calcium, particularly if the patient has received multiple blood transfusions.

4. Observe for bleeding from other sites, such as epistaxis or petechiae. See the "Disseminated Intravascular Coagulation" plan, page 625.

5. Immediately report any complaint of sudden, severe abdominal pain or rigidity, and prepare the patient for surgery if these occur.

Rationales

1. As much as 200 ml of blood may be lost daily without detectable clinical signs. Early detection allows prompt treatment.

2. Blood loss reduces the level of circulating hemoglobin, thus compromising normal delivery of oxygen to tissues. If coronary circulation is already impaired, this reduction may cause ischemic changes or myocardial infarction.

3. Hemorrhage and the resulting hypovolemia may cause renal and hepatic hypoperfusion, eventually leading to kidney or liver failure. Liver dysfunction, commonly associated with esophageal varices, contributes to elevated blood ammonia levels and can result in hepatic encephalopathy. Hypocalcemia is a common adverse effect of multiple transfusions because calcium binds with the preservative in stored blood.

4. Bleeding from other sites may signal the development of DIC, a grave complication of hemorrhage. The plan for this disorder contains detailed interventions.

5. These signs and symptoms may indicate gastric perforation, which causes peritonitis, sepsis, and shock unless promptly treated. Immediate surgical intervention is warranted to remove gastric contents from the peritoneal cavity.

6. Additional individualized interventions: _____

6. Rationales: _____

Target outcome criteria
Throughout the hospital stay, the patient will:
• exhibit decreasing BUN and normal creatinine values
• display electrolytes within normal limits
• maintain urine output greater than 60 ml/hour
• remain alert and oriented.

Nursing diagnosis: *Fear related to sight of blood and distressing physical symptoms*

NURSING PRIORITY: Reduce the patient's fear.

Interventions

1. Provide care promptly, explaining all interventions to the patient in simple terms. Avoid expressing dismay or revulsion at the sight of bleeding; assume a calm, confident, matter-of-fact manner. Acknowledge the patient's fear by saying, for example, "I know it must be pretty scary to see all this blood, but we treat this condition often. We will be replacing your blood by giving you transfusions and extra fluids."

2. Encourage verbalization of feelings by using active listening skills. See the "Ineffective Individual Coping" plan, page 51.

3. Accept expressions of anxiety related to the possibility of death. See the "Dying" plan, page 11.

4. Additional individualized interventions: _____

Rationales

1. The sight of blood is normally extremely threatening to the patient, who justifiably may fear bleeding to death. Anxiety may interfere with the patient's ability to comprehend, but simple explanations about what is happening may reassure the patient that needed care is being given. Recognizing the normalcy of the patient's fear reduces the patient's sense of isolation. Patients typically are quite concerned about bloody excreta and losing bowel control. Calm acceptance may minimize shame related to these losses of bodily control.

2. Verbalizing feelings helps the patient identify specific fears and begin to mobilize coping strategies. The "Ineffective Individual Coping" plan details interventions that may be helpful in promoting coping behaviors.

3. Issues of death are always of acute importance for the patient with a critical condition. The "Dying" plan contains specific interventions useful in caring for patients and families confronting issues of mortality.

4. Rationales: _____

Target outcome criterion
After initial stabilization, the patient will verbalize personal feelings related to the condition, if desired.

Nursing diagnosis: *Knowledge deficit related to potential recurrent bleeding*

NURSING PRIORITY: Teach assessment techniques and preventive measures.

Interventions

1. See the "Knowledge Deficit" plan, page 56.

2. Defer detailed teaching until the patient is alert and physiologically stable. Then, as indicated by condition, discuss with the patient:

• precipitating or contributing factors of bleeding episode, for example, alcohol consumption or medication use

Rationales

1. The "Knowledge Deficit" plan contains detailed interventions related to patient and family teaching.

2. The patient's condition may limit teaching, but abbreviated teaching may lay the groundwork for more detailed education before discharge.

• Awareness of contributing factors over which the patient has control may decrease the likelihood of a recurrence.

• signs and symptoms indicating possible recurrence, for example, melena, coffee-ground vomitus, weakness, or dizziness

• other causes of dark stools, for example, intake of iron, beets, berries, or greens

• dietary recommendations, as ordered, for example, avoidance of caffeine.

3. Additional individualized interventions: _____

_____

• Early medical attention if bleeding recurs may avert the need for a prolonged hospital stay.

• Knowing other causes may avert undue alarm.

• Careful dietary management may be the primary preventive therapy for some conditions.

3. Rationales: _____

_____

Target outcome criteria
Before discharge, the patient will (as condition allows):
• list any precipitating or contributing factors identified
• describe signs and symptoms of possible recurrence of bleeding

• verbalize understanding of any dietary recommendations.

Discharge planning

NURSING DISCHARGE CRITERIA
Upon the patient's discharge, documentation shows evidence of:
• stable vital signs within normal limits
• urine output of at least 60 ml/hour
• normal or decreasing BUN values
• normal serum electrolytes
• normal skin perfusion
• gastric pH of 4.0 or greater
• negative guaiac test of stools or vomitus
• level of consciousness stable for more than 12 hours
• balanced fluid intake and output.

PATIENT-FAMILY TEACHING CHECKLIST
Document evidence that the patient and family demonstrate an understanding of:
___ cause and site of bleeding
___ precipitating or contributing factors
___ signs and symptoms indicating possible recurrence of bleeding
___ dietary recommendations, if any.

DOCUMENTATION CHECKLIST
Using outcome criteria as a guide, document:
___ clinical status on admission
___ significant changes in status
___ pertinent diagnostic test findings
___ bleeding episodes
___ fluid and blood replacement measures
___ fluid intake and output
___ emotional response
___ pharmacologic interventions
___ procedures to stop bleeding
___ patient-family teaching
___ discharge planning.

ASSOCIATED PLANS OF CARE
Acute Renal Failure
Disseminated Intravascular Coagulation
Dying
Hypovolemic Shock
Impaired Physical Mobility
Ineffective Individual Coping
Knowledge Deficit
Liver Failure
Nutritional Deficit
Pancreatitis

References

DeBourgh, G. "Gastrointestinal Disorders," in *Nursing the Critically Ill Adult,* 4th ed. Edited by Holloway, N. Menlo Park, Calif.: Addison Wesley Publishing Co., 1993.

Dworken, H. "Gastrointestinal Hemorrhage," in *Textbook of Critical Care,* 2nd ed. Edited by Shoemaker, W., et al. Philadelphia: W.B. Saunders Co., 1989.

Konopad, E., and Noseworthy, T. "Stress Ulceration, A Serious Complication in Critically Ill Patients," *Heart and Lung* 17(4):339-47, July 1988.

Luckmann, J., and Sorensen, K. *Medical-Surgical Nursing: A Psychophysiologic Approach,* 3rd ed. Philadelphia: W.B. Saunders Co., 1987.

Ragan, J.A. "Lasers in Gastroenterology," *Nursing Clinics of North America* 25(3):685-96, September 1990.

Rikkers, L., ed. "Management of Variceal Hemorrhage," *Surgical Clinics of North America* 70(2): 251-486, April 1990.

Savino, J., Berman, H., and Del Guercio, L. "A Multidisciplinary Approach to Gastrointestinal Bleeding," in *Textbook of Critical Care,* 2nd ed. Edited by Shoemaker, W., et al. Philadelphia: W.B. Saunders Co., 1989.

Sleisenger, M.H., and Fordstran, H.S. *Gastrointestinal Disorders,* 4th ed. Philadelphia: W.B. Saunders Co., 1988.

Van DeVelde-Coke, S. "The Gastrointestinal System," in *Core Curriculum for Critical Care Nursing,* 3rd ed. Edited by Alspach, J., and Williams, S. Philadelphia: W.B. Saunders Co., 1985.

Inflammatory Bowel Disease

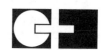

DRG information

DRG 179 Inflammatory Bowel Disease.
  Mean LOS = 7.1 days
  Principal diagnoses include:
  • proctocolitis
  • regional enteritis.
DRG 182 Esophagitis, Gastroenteritis, and Miscella-
  neous Digestive Disorders. Age 17 + . With
  Complications or Comorbidity (CC).
  Mean LOS = 4.9 days
  Principal diagnoses include:
  • diverticulitis
  • infectious diarrhea.
DRG 183 Esophagitis, Gastroenteritis, and Miscella-
  neous Digestive Disorders. Age 17 + . With-
  out CC.
  Mean LOS = 3.5 days
DRG 184 Esophagitis, Gastroenteritis, and Miscella-
  neous Digestive Disorders. Age 0 to 17.
  Mean LOS = 3.2 days

Introduction
DEFINITION AND TIME FOCUS
Inflammatory bowel disease (IBD) is a broad diagnostic category that includes ulcerative colitis, Crohn's
disease (regional enteritis), appendicitis, diverticulitis,
infectious diarrhea, functional bowel disorders, and hu-
morally mediated diarrheal syndromes. Hospitalized
IBD patients may be acutely ill and may demonstrate
similar management problems. This plan focuses on
the problems associated with acute exacerbations of
ulcerative colitis and regional enteritis.

  Ulcerative colitis and regional enteritis involve local defects characterized by excavation of the bowel
surface from sloughing of necrotic inflammatory tissue. The ulcerations in regional enteritis are transmural, involving all layers of the bowel; those of
ulcerative colitis begin in the crypts of Lieberkühn
and usually involve the mucosa and submucosa. The lesions in ulcerative colitis are usually confined to the
descending large bowel and sigmoid colon and are continuous in nature; the defects in regional enteritis occur predominantly in, but are not confined to, the
terminal ileum and tend to alternate with areas of normal bowel surface.

ETIOLOGY AND PRECIPITATING FACTORS
• exact cause unknown — infectious agents, genetic or
familial tendencies, immunologic mechanisms, and
stress-related psychological factors may be involved
• stressful event, possibly preceding an acute attack
by 4 to 6 months
• bacterial infection, possibly occurring several weeks
before an acute attack

• age — attacks are more severe, with a higher mortality rate, after age 40 in regional enteritis and after
age 60 with ulcerative colitis

Focused assessment guidelines
NURSING HISTORY (Functional health pattern findings)

Health perception — health management pattern
• may report gradual or acute onset of abdominal
cramping, anorexia, and weight loss related to fear of
intake of food and fluids that increase cramping; low-
grade fever (may be high-grade if perforation present);
change in bowel habits with increasing frequency of
stools (in ulcerative colitis, stools may exceed 15 per
day, be accompanied by urgency and tenesmus, and
contain blood, mucus, or pus)
• may report a history of acute exacerbations
• may report a drug regimen that includes corticosteroids or immunosuppressants
• may report family history of disorder
• typically in Caucasian populations, but an unexplained increase in regional enteritis among Blacks
has been observed
• may demonstrate growth retardation (seen in childhood onset of IBD)

Nutritional-metabolic pattern
• typically reports anorexia with weight loss
• may present with signs and symptoms of chronic
malnutrition
• may report intake of fatty foods or other dietary indiscretions; if disease is chronic, may report being on
a low-residue, low-fiber, bland diet

Elimination pattern
• reports increasing frequency of bowel movements
(may have been gradual or acute in onset)
• reports abdominal pain and possible audible bowel
sounds (borborygmi) before onset of discomfort
• may report bright-red rectal bleeding with fecal incontinence, particularly with ulcerative colitis
• may exhibit visible peristaltic waves over the abdomen

Activity-exercise pattern
• typically reports malaise and fatigue
• may report muscle weakness

Sleep-rest pattern
• may report sleep disturbance related to abdominal
discomfort and nocturnal defecation

Self-perception—self-concept pattern
• may have low self-esteem, compensated for by ambitious, hard-driving life-style

Role-relationship pattern
• may use dependent behavior to cope with feelings of anger, hostility, and anxiety
• may report family history of similar GI problems

Sexuality-reproductive pattern
• with chronic disease, may demonstrate altered ability to cope with human relationships
• typically demonstrates delayed development of secondary sex characteristics and sexual function if IBD begins before puberty
• may experience decreased fertility

Coping—stress tolerance pattern
• may express feelings of hopelessness and despair
• may use somatization (recurrent, multiple physical complaints with no organic cause), expressions of helplessness, crying, excessive demands on staff time, and excessive praise as mechanisms for individual coping

PHYSICAL FINDINGS
Cardiovascular
• hypotension
• tachycardia
• arrhythmias

Renal
• decreased output
• fecal material in urine (if bladder fistula present)

Gastrointestinal
• diarrhea
• weight loss
• hyperactive or hypoactive bowel sounds
• abdominal tenderness and mass
• abdominal distention and rigidity
• rectal bleeding
• liver tenderness

Neurologic
• restlessness
• irritability
• blurred vision (uncommon)
• iritis (uncommon)
• conjunctivitis (uncommon)
• uveitis (uncommon)

Integumentary
• poor skin turgor
• pallor
• pustules (uncommon)
• erythematous lesions (uncommon)
• pyoderma gangrenosum (uncommon skin infection)

• icterus (if hepatitis present)
• draining fistulas (particularly around umbilicus or surgical scars)
• ecchymoses

Musculoskeletal
• muscle weakness
• joint pain and tenderness
• rheumatoid spondylitis (uncommon)

DIAGNOSTIC STUDIES
• complete blood count—may reveal moderate elevation in white blood cell (WBC) count, unless perforation is present (which causes a major elevation above normal); hematocrit and hemoglobin values are decreased with chronic blood loss; if blood loss is sudden and dramatic, hematocrit and hemoglobin values may not immediately reflect the change in blood volume; the red blood cell (RBC) count may reflect megaloblastic anemia if the part of the ileum responsible for vitamin B absorption is affected
• electrolyte profile—sodium, potassium, and chloride may be deficient with persistent or acute loss of fluids from the GI tract with inadequate replacement
• total protein levels—decreased because a significant amount of protein is lost in inflammatory exudate in the bowel and through bleeding of damaged tissues, which can deplete albumin and other plasma proteins
• blood urea nitrogen (BUN) level—decreased because significant nutritional deficits cause the catabolism of body proteins; reflected in negative nitrogen balance
• bleeding and clotting time—prolonged because vitamin K synthesis decreases as bowel surfaces are destroyed; liver involvement may disturb clotting factor synthesis, altering clotting mechanisms
• stool studies—culture and sensitivity testing and examination for ova and parasites are usually ordered to rule out an infectious origin for the symptoms; a guaiac test is usually positive for occult blood; fat may also be found in stools (steatorrhea) if destruction of bowel surfaces impairs bile reabsorption
• liver function tests—hepatitis is a complication of IBD, consequently elevated bilirubin and liver enzyme levels may be observed
• alkaline phosphatase levels—increased if arthritic skeletal involvement or hepatitis is present
• urine studies—culture and sensitivity testing may be ordered if a fistula to the bladder is suspected; opportunistic infections may also occur in the genitourinary tract from overall immunosuppression
• tuberculin skin test—tuberculosis of the cecum may mimic symptoms of IBD
• antibody titers—anticolon antibodies are demonstrated commonly in patients with ulcerative colitis but not usually observed in other IBD patients
• carcinoembryonic antigen—may be ordered for patients with ulcerative colitis as they tend to develop colon cancer after 10 years with the disorder

• barium enema—in ulcerative colitis, demonstrates the characteristic obliteration of haustral folds, blurring of bowel margins, and narrowing and stenosis of the large bowel; in regional enteritis, changes usually found in the small bowel but may occur in the large bowel, so distinguishing between the two disorders on the basis of a barium enema is difficult; procedure may be omitted if abscess or fistula is suspected because the bowel preparation for the procedure, and the procedure itself, may aggravate the condition
• carotene and Shilling tests—reflect the intestine's absorptive capacity; estimate degree of damaged bowel surface in regional enteritis
• protoscopy or colonoscopy—demonstrates hyperemic, edematous, friable bowel mucosa; if lesion is beyond the ileocecal valve, narrowing and stenosis of the valve may be evident
• rectal biopsy—inflammation and abcesses of the crypts are evident in ulcerative colitis; biopsy usually does not contribute to regional enteritis
• computed tomography scan—reveals abdominal masses that could be fistulas or abcesses
• upper GI series—lesions in regional enteritis can occur at any point along the GI tract and tend to alternate with segments of normal tissue; upper GI series reveals the extent of involvement and indicates segments where scarring and stenosis may obstruct intestinal flow

• skeletal X-rays—used to demonstrate the presence and extent of arthritic changes and ankylosing spondylitis, which can occur with IBD

POTENTIAL COMPLICATIONS
• malnutrition
• bowel obstruction
• arrhythmias
• peritonitis
• hepatitis
• toxic megacolon
• malabsorption syndrome
• gangrenous skin lesions
• ankylosing spondylitis
• exudative retinopathy
• kidney stones
• pericarditis
• carcinoma of the colon

Collaborative problem: *High risk for cardiac arrhythmias related to electrolyte depletion*

NURSING PRIORITY: Maintain electrolyte levels within normal limits.

Interventions

1. Monitor and record fluid losses. Evaluate serum electrolyte levels daily, as ordered. Monitor apical and radial pulses, changes in tendon reflexes, and muscle strength every 4 hours or more frequently, depending on the severity of the patient's condition.

2. Administer and document electrolyte replacement therapy.

3. Notify the doctor immediately of any evidence of arrhythmias, for example, pulse irregularity, syncopal episodes, or altered level of consciousness. See Appendix C, "Fluid and Electrolyte Imbalances."

4. Additional individualized interventions: _____

Rationales

1. Diarrhea and internal fluid sequestration can cause significant electrolyte loss. Frequent observations for signs of alterations in the cellular membrane potential are necessary. Reminders to the doctor to order electrolyte determinations may also be necessary.

2. Normal saline or Ringer's lactate solution and potassium supplements usually are ordered during the acute stage, when oral replacement may be contraindicated.

3. Cardiac arrest can occur without warning in severe hypokalemia or hyperkalemia. The "Fluid and Electrolyte Imbalances" appendix provides details on specific imbalances.

4. Rationales: _____

Target outcome criteria
Within 24 hours of admission, the patient will show vital signs within normal limits.

Within 3 days of admission, the patient will:
• have serum electrolyte levels within normal limits
• display normal cardiac rate and rhythm.

Nursing diagnosis: *High risk for fluid volume deficit related to decreased fluid intake, increased fluid loss through diarrhea or internal sequestration of fluid, or hemorrhage*

NURSING PRIORITY: Maintain fluid balance or replace fluid loss to improve cellular perfusion.

Interventions

1. Measure and document hourly urine outputs with specific gravity determinations for the acutely ill patient. Report a urine output of less than 30 ml/hour. Weigh the patient daily.

2. Maintain accurate records of the type and amount of fluid lost.

3. Monitor and record skin color, turgor, and temperature; level of consciousness; body temperature; and vital signs every 1 to 4 hours, depending on the severity of the patient's condition. Note trends.

4. Auscultate and palpate the abdomen, and observe for increasing pain. Document evidence of distention and changes in bowel sounds.

5. Administer and document fluid replacement, as ordered.

6. Additional individualized interventions: _____

Rationales

1. Urine output and specific gravity determinations provide an immediate, objective indication of the need for volume replacement. Weight loss may indicate loss of fluid volume.

2. The type and amount of fluid lost will guide replacement therapy.

3. A persistent or dramatic change in the parameters listed indicates either sequestration of fluid or blood volume loss. Hypovolemia is indicated by hypotension, tachycardia, and signs of decreased peripheral perfusion.

4. Sudden, acute distention, increased pain, and loss of or diminished bowel sounds can be early indications of serious bowel injury. Increased bowel activity may also indicate early obstruction or increasing tissue damage and inflammation.

5. The preferred route for fluid replacement is by mouth. However, the IBD patient may be too ill, or oral replacement may increase distressing symptoms. I.V. fluids usually include volume expanders such as normal saline solution. Whole blood or packed RBCs may also be ordered if hypotension is related to blood loss.

6. Rationales: _____

Target outcome criteria
Within 24 hours of admission, the patient will:
• display vital signs within normal limits
• maintain urine output of at least 30 ml/hour
• show good skin turgor.

Within 3 days of admission, the patient will maintain urine output within normal limits.

Nursing diagnosis: *Nutritional deficit related to decreased nutrient intake, increased nutrient loss, and possible decreased bowel absorption*

NURSING PRIORITIES: (a) Maintain or increase body weight, and (b) improve general nutritional status.

Interventions

1. Estimate and document the extent of the nutritional deficit based on body weight; character, color, and texture of hair and skin; the presence or absence of corneal plaques, cracked and bleeding gums and mucous membranes, muscle wasting and weakness, and anemia; changes in visual acuity; and decreased BUN level.

Rationales

1. Rapidly reproducing cells, such as those of the hair, skin, mucous membranes, and retinas, tend to be the first to demonstrate the changes characteristic of nutritional deficit. Later manifestations of a severe deficit include muscle wasting, weakness, decreased BUN level, and anemia.

2. Collaborate with the patient, family, and other health team members to set goals and plan for normal nutritional maintenance.

2. The IBD patient tends to ignore dietary recommendations and may eat irritating foods. The IBD patient also learns to associate food and fluid intake with unpleasant sensations and may voluntarily decrease intake to avoid distressing symptoms. The patient must have the support of both family and caregivers for the dietary plan to succeed.

3. Administer medications, as ordered, to control peristalsis before meals.

3. The presence of food in the gut stimulates peristalsis and causes increased discomfort and diarrhea. Diphenoxylate hydrochloride with atropine sulfate (Lomotil) or camphorated opium tincture (Paregoric) are commonly used.

4. Serve small, frequent meals rather than three large meals a day. Assess patient response.

4. Small, frequent meals tend to be better tolerated and cause fewer distressing symptoms.

5. Administer I.V. nutritional supplements, such as fat emulsions (Intralipid) and vitamins, or total parenteral nutrition, as ordered. See the "Total Parenteral Nutrition" plan, page 411, for further details.

5. I.V. nutritional supplements or total parenteral nutrition may be indicated for the IBD patient who cannot take anything by mouth, to rest the gut and promote healing, and for the patient too malnourished to tolerate surgery. Vitamin B_{12} is useful in reversing anemia associated with decreased blood cell formation and for treating immunosuppression associated with chronic inflammation. The "Total Parenteral Nutrition" plan contains details about this therapy.

6. Additional individualized interventions: _____

6. Rationales: _____

Target outcome criteria
Within 2 days of admission, the patient will comply with the agreed-upon treatment plan.

By the time of discharge, the patient will:
• gain mutually agreed-upon weight
• perform activities of daily living (ADLs)
• tolerate diet without undue distress.

Nursing diagnosis: *High risk for infection related to bowel perforation, immunosuppression, and general debilitation*

NURSING PRIORITY: Prevent opportunistic infections.

Interventions

1. Monitor and record vital signs, body temperature, bowel sounds, breath sounds, urine character and odor, and the presence or absence of abdominal distention, joint pain, hepatic tenderness, icterus, increasing malaise, and exudative skin or eye lesions.

2. Administer antibiotics, as ordered.

3. Obtain specimens for culture and sensitivity testing, as ordered, before beginning antibiotic therapy.

4. Practice careful aseptic technique for all nursing procedures.

5. Question orders for extensive bowel preparation for the patient with abdominal tenderness or masses, decreased or absent bowel sounds, or abdominal distention or rigidity.

Rationales

1. The patient with IBD is susceptible to many opportunistic infections. Close observation is necessary because such infections may not produce the usual dramatic rise in body temperature and WBC count, as a result of medication-related immunosuppression and the condition's chronicity.

2. Typically, broad-spectrum antibiotics, such as sulfasalazine (Azulfidine), are ordered as a prophylactic measure.

3. Culture and sensitivity testing tend to be inaccurate when performed after initiation of antibiotic therapy.

4. The IBD patient tends to be immunosuppressed, as noted previously.

5. Enemas and purgatives are irritants that can cause or exacerbate detrimental changes in the patient with acute abdominal pathology.

GASTROINTESTINAL DISORDERS

6. Additional individualized interventions: _____

6. Rationales: _____

Target outcome criteria
By time of discharge, the patient will:
• have a normal body temperature
• show no signs of infection.

Nursing diagnosis: *Pain related to abdominal and possible skeletal pathology*

NURSING PRIORITY: Prevent or control pain.

Interventions

1. Assess and document complaints of pain. Be especially alert for sudden and severe abdominal pain, guarding, rigidity, or distention, and for vomiting, and report their occurrence to the doctor immediately.

2. Administer appropriate analgesic medication, as ordered. Teach the patient about nonpharmacologic pain control measures. See the "Pain" plan, page 69.

3. Administer anti-inflammatory medications, as ordered, and document their therapeutic and adverse effects.

4. Additional individualized interventions: _____

Rationales

1. Changes in the character and severity of abdominal pain may indicate a life-threatening condition, such as perforation of the GI tract.

2. Narcotic analgesics are administered judiciously in IBD because they tend to mask potentially life-threatening conditions. Medications that inhibit GI motility and abdominal cramping, such as diphenoxylate hydrochloride with atropine sulfate or camphorated opium tincture, may be ordered. Skeletal discomfort related to arthritis is best handled with gentle exercise, warm soaks, and frequent repositioning because many of the oral anti-inflammatory medications used to control skeletal pain are GI irritants. The "Pain" plan contains general interventions for pain control.

3. Control of IBD reduces distressing and painful symptoms. Common medications used to suppress inflammation include hydrocortisone sodium succinate (Solu-Cortef), methylprednisolone sodium succinate (Solu-Medrol), and dexamethasone (Decadron).

4. Rationales: _____

Target outcome criteria
Within 3 days of admission, the patient will verbalize pain relief.

By the time of discharge, the patient will:
• verbalize rationale for pain-control measures
• use nonpharmacologic pain-control methods, as appropriate.

Nursing diagnosis: *Sleep pattern disturbance related to uncomfortable sensations, possible anxiety related to hospitalization, nocturnal defecation, or change in usual sleep environment*

NURSING PRIORITY: Promote adequate rest and sleep.

Interventions

1. Ask the patient to describe the usual sleep environment; when possible, modify the patient's surroundings to match that environment.

2. Avoid performing prolonged or painful procedures within the hour before bedtime.

3. Group all nursing procedures that must be done while the patient sleeps.

4. Encourage the patient to express fears. Offer reassurance as appropriate.

5. Allow the patient to follow rituals that promote sleep at home.

6. Reposition the patient for comfort, and offer soothing back rubs.

7. Provide a bedside commode for night use. Administer antidiarrheal medication at bedtime.

8. Additional individualized interventions: _____

Rationales

1. An unfamiliar environment may inhibit sleep.

2. Autonomic nervous system stimulation, with increased catecholamine secretion, may interfere with sleep.

3. The sleep cycle is 90 to 120 minutes long. Grouping nursing procedures allows the patient to complete sleep cycles.

4. Some patients may equate sleep with death. They may need to be reassured that the staff will be available to meet their needs.

5. At home, most individuals follow sleep rituals, such as reading, that help them fall asleep.

6. If the patient is on bed rest, immobility can increase discomfort.

7. These measures help minimize sleep disturbance related to nocturnal defecation.

8. Rationales: _____

Target outcome criteria
Within 2 days of admission, the patient will verbalize feelings of being at ease and rested.

Throughout the hospital stay, the patient will experience adequate rest and sleep.

Nursing diagnosis: *Impaired perianal skin integrity related to frequent stools and altered nutritional status*

NURSING PRIORITY: Prevent skin breakdown.

Interventions

1. Provide and document perianal care after each bowel movement.

2. Institute and document a skin care routine, based on the patient's general condition, to be performed every 2 to 4 hours.

3. Promote and document food and fluid intake, paying special attention to protein consumption.

Rationales

1. The acid secretions and digestive enzymes from diarrhea quickly excoriate the perianal area. A protective ointment, such as lanolin and petrolatum (A&D), is commonly used because the skin is vulnerable to breakdown.

2. Anticipating and preventing skin breakdown on other body surfaces is important because tissue damage heals slowly, if at all, in the critically ill IBD patient.

3. Adequate intake of nutrients (especially protein) and fluids is necessary for tissue repair.

GASTROINTESTINAL DISORDERS

4. Additional individualized interventions: _____

4. Rationales: _____

Target outcome criterion
By the time of discharge, the patient will show no evidence of skin breakdown.

Nursing diagnosis: *Social isolation related to dependent behavior*

NURSING PRIORITIES: (a) Decrease use of dependent behavior, and (b) facilitate direct expression of feelings.

Interventions

1. Identify dependent behavior for patient, self, staff, and family.

2. Collaborate with staff and family to set limits on unacceptable behavior. Ensure that all staff members agree to maintain the limits and to share concerns with each other.

3. Avoid bargaining about or justifying limits. Enforce them without apology.

4. Discuss the patient's feelings concerning limits. Encourage expression of feelings of anxiety, hostility, and anger.

5. Investigate somatic complaints immediately and matter-of-factly.

6. If behavioral problems persist, consult a psychiatric clinical nurse specialist or other mental health professional.

7. Additional individualized interventions: _____

Rationales

1. Dependent behavior may be manifested by crying, expressions of hopelessness, endless requests for staff attention, or excessive praise of staff. Although such behavior represents an attempt to control and manage underlying feelings of anger, hostility, and anxiety, it commonly provokes social isolation, reinforcing negative feelings.

2. Limit setting and consistent enforcement allow the patient to know exactly what is expected and interrupts the cycle of dependency and isolation. The dependent patient may attempt to turn staff members against each other through manipulative behavior.

3. Engaging in dialogue concerning limits creates doubt about their enforcement.

4. The patient may have difficulty identifying feelings. A nonjudgmental atmosphere provides a way to recognize and discuss uncomfortable emotions.

5. Somatization is an attention-getting behavior used by people with inadequate coping skills. The seriousness of the illness warrants investigation of complaints; avoid prolonged discussions of physical complaints, however, and focus instead on the patient's feelings.

6. A mental health professional can offer expertise for dealing with manipulative behavior and the staff's negative response to such behavior.

7. Rationales: _____

Target outcome criteria
By the time of discharge, the patient will:
• decrease use of ineffective coping behaviors
• express anger, hostility, and anxiety appropriately.

Nursing diagnosis: *High risk for altered sexuality patterns related to diminished physical energy and persistence of uncomfortable physical symptoms*

NURSING PRIORITY: Encourage the discussion and expression of sexual desires.

Interventions

1. Initiate discussion about values, beliefs, and feelings concerning sexuality. Assess for sexual dysfunction. Include the patient's spouse or partner in discussions, if possible.

2. Allow the patient to discuss feelings, values, and beliefs concerning sexuality in a nonjudgmental atmosphere. It is important to be aware of personal feelings about sexuality. If you are too uncomfortable to counsel the patient and spouse or partner effectively, make an appropriate referral.

3. To the extent possible, allow the patient and spouse or partner uninterrupted private time together.

4. Construct a teaching plan for sexual expression. Address energy conserving positions for intercourse, timing activity to coincide with peak energy levels, alternatives to intercourse, specific patient concerns, and potential interactions between contraceptives and medications used to treat IBD.

5. Additional individualized interventions: _____

Rationales

1. Discussions concerning sexuality are difficult for many patients to initiate, although the topic may be of considerable importance. The nurse must anticipate that altered sexual function is common in patients who have chronic or debilitating illnesses and who have diminished energy and persistent, uncomfortable physical sensations. The IBD patient may also be facing surgery for fecal diversion; thus, body-image changes and altered sexual function should be anticipated.

   The patient may or may not communicate openly with the spouse or partner. Both may welcome frank discussions of sexual matters.

2. The nurse's values and beliefs concerning sexual behavior may interfere with the ability to provide professional care. If this occurs, referral to another professional may provide acceptance and counsel to benefit the patient and partner.

3. Sexuality can be expressed in many forms besides sexual intercourse, such as cuddling and fondling. The IBD patient may be hospitalized for prolonged periods and needs privacy to express intimate feelings.

4. The sexual intercourse guidelines for cardiac patients can be modified to meet the needs of the patient with chronic IBD who has diminished physical energy and uncomfortable physical sensations. Patient teaching should also cover the potential interactions between various types of contraceptives and the medications used to treat chronic IBD.

5. Rationales: _____

Target outcome criteria
By the time of discharge, the patient will:
• discuss sexual feelings openly with partner
• identify techniques for minimizing physical demands of sexual activity.

Discharge planning
NURSING DISCHARGE CRITERIA
Upon the patient's discharge, documentation shows evidence of:
• absence of fever
• absence of signs and symptoms of infection
• stable vital signs
• ability to tolerate oral nutritional intake
• I.V. lines discontinued for at least 24 hours before discharge
• stabilized weight
• ability to control pain using oral medications
• ability to perform perianal care
• controlled bowel movements
• absence of skin breakdown
• electrolyte levels within acceptable parameters
• ability to ambulate and perform activities of daily living (ADLs)
• adequate home support system, or referral to home care if indicated by inability to perform ADLs and perianal care independently, by inadequacy of the home support system, or by the need to reinforce teaching.

GASTROINTESTINAL DISORDERS

PATIENT-FAMILY TEACHING CHECKLIST

Document evidence that the patient and family demonstrate an understanding of:

___ extent of disease

___ all discharge medications' purpose, dose, administration schedule, and adverse effects requiring medical attention (usual discharge medications include steroids and immunosuppressants)

___ recommended dietary modifications (usual diet is low fiber, low residue, and bland)

___ community support groups and resources, including an ostomy club, when appropriate

___ resumption of normal role activity

___ signs and symptoms indicating exacerbation of illness

___ date, time, and location of follow-up appointments

___ how to contact the doctor.

DOCUMENTATION CHECKLIST

Using outcome criteria as a guide, document:

___ clinical status on admission

___ significant changes in status

___ pertinent laboratory and diagnostic findings

___ pain relief measures

___ I.V. line patency

___ fluid intake

___ acute abdominal pain episodes

___ use of emergency protocols

___ nutritional intake

___ other therapies

___ patient-family teaching

___ discharge planning.

ASSOCIATED PLANS OF CARE

Colostomy
Grieving
Ineffective Individual Coping
Pain
Total Parenteral Nutrition

References

Corbett, J. *Laboratory Tests and Diagnostic Tests with Nursing Diagnoses.* East Norwalk, Conn.: Appleton & Lange, 1987.

Guyton, A. *Textbook of Medical Physiology.* (8th ed.) Philadelphia: W.B. Saunders Co., 1991.

Luckman, J., and Sorenson, K. *Medical Surgical Nursing.* Philadelphia: W.B. Saunders Co., 1987.

Sodeman, W., and Sodeman, T. *Pathologic Physiology. Mechanisms of Disease.* Philadelphia: W.B. Saunders Co., 1989.

Spencer, R., Nichols, L., Lipkin, G., Sabo, H., and West, F. *Clinical Pharmacology and Nursing Management.* Philadelphia: J.B. Lippincott Co., 1989.

GASTROINTESTINAL DISORDERS
Total Parenteral Nutrition

DRG information
DRG 296 Nutritional and Miscellaneous Metabolic Disorders. Age 17 +. With Complication or Comorbidity (CC).
Mean LOS = 6.1 days
DRG 297 Nutritional and Miscellaneous Metabolic Disorders. Age 17 +. Without CC.
Mean LOS = 4.1 days
DRG 298 Nutritional and Miscellaneous Metabolic Disorders. Age 0 to 17.
Mean LOS = 3.2 days
Principal diagnoses include:
• anorexia
• dehydration
• malnutrition.

Additional DRG information: Total parenteral nutrition (TPN) is used to treat numerous disorders. The diagnosis necessitating its use determines the DRG assigned. Examples of diagnoses and DRGs that may require TPN are listed above. Several others associated with cancer could also require TPN but were omitted here for brevity.

Introduction
DEFINITION AND TIME FOCUS
TPN is the delivery of nutrients solely through the central venous infusion of glucose, amino acids, fats, vitamins, and trace elements in sufficient quantities to maintain or replete body cell mass and promote anabolism. (The term central venous alimentation also describes this method of providing nutrients.) The patient requiring TPN typically exhibits one of four problems:
• cannot eat — the patient may have an obstruction or ileus at any point along the GI tract or may be at risk for aspiration if fed orally
• will not eat — the geriatric, cancer, or anorexic patient may be unwilling to ingest food
• should not eat — the patient may have a disease or condition aggravated by oral intake, such as intestinal fistula, severe pancreatitis, small-bowel obstruction, or inflammatory bowel disease
• cannot eat enough — the patient has such a severe disease or degree of injury that sufficient nutrients cannot be provided enterally. Examples are short-bowel syndrome, multiple trauma, and major burns.
TPN is indicated when:
• the enteral route is unavailable for nutritional support.
• the patient has lost 10% to 15% of body weight.
• the patient is not permitted food or fluids for more than 7 days.
Safe delivery of TPN depends on four basic principles of care:
• aseptic technique in catheter placement
• aseptic technique in catheter care

• proper preparation and delivery of the TPN solution
• careful patient monitoring.
This plan focuses on the patient who requires TPN to maintain nutritional status during the hospital stay.

Focused assessment guidelines
NURSING HISTORY (Functional health pattern findings)

Health perception — health management pattern
• may be chronically ill or have an acute condition that increases nutritional needs

Activity-exercise pattern
• may report decreased energy level
• may report generalized weakness or weak extremities related to muscle wasting

Nutritional-metabolic pattern
• may report nausea, vomiting, diarrhea, or constipation
• may report lack of appetite
• may report recent weight loss
• may report lack of interest in food
• may have improperly fitting dentures
• may be chronically thirsty
• may prefer salty beverages

PHYSICAL FINDINGS
Note: The clinical signs of malnutrition are rarely observed and may not be recognized as clinically significant.

Musculoskeletal
• generalized muscle wasting and weakness (muscle mass and major organs are spared unless the patient has moderate to severe malnutrition)
• edematous extremities

Integumentary
• skin — subcutaneous fat loss, scaly dermatitis (primarily on legs and feet), pellagrous dermatitis, seborrheic dermatitis of face, nasolabial seborrhea (greasy and scaly skin of the nasolabial folds of the nose, from riboflavin deficiency), follicular hyperodosis (thinning of the innermost layer of the epidermis, possibly from vitamin A deficiency), dilated veins, petechiae, purpura, poor skin turgor, dry mucous membranes
• hair — increased pluckability, lack of luster, alopecia, sparsity, decreased pigmentation
• nails — brittle, lined, increased rigidity, thin, flattened or spoon-shaped

MAJOR ELEMENTS MONITORED IN T.P.N.

■ **glucose** — serum levels may be elevated above 200 mg/dl when TPN infusion is begun, decreasing to 150 to 200 mg/dl after 24 to 48 hours as body adjusts to increased glucose load. (Serum glucose levels greater than 200 mg/dl indicate glucose intolerance or hyperglycemia. Levels less than 60 mg/dl indicate hypoglycemia, the more dangerous of the two states; without glucose, the brain cannot function and death is imminent if hypoglycemia continues.)

■ **electrolytes** — sodium, potassium, and chloride levels obtained for baseline and as guide for replacement therapy. (Fluid and electrolyte management is the most important aspect of TPN, because the patient requiring nutritional repletion typically has fluid and electrolyte abnormalities. Electrolytes are provided as needed to replace loss from fistulas, nasogastric [NG] drainage, diarrhea, or excessive output or — in an appropriate ratio — to promote lean muscle mass, nutritional repletion, and positive nitrogen balance.)

■ **magnesium** — low serum levels may occur in intestinal malabsorption syndrome, bowel resection, intestinal fistula, or in patients with extended NG suction. (Magnesium requirements increase with nutritional repletion related to new tissue synthesis: 0.35 to 0.45 mEq/kg/day is sufficient to prevent magnesium depletion in patients receiving TPN. Magnesium levels need to be monitored at least every week and twice a week for patients in renal failure. The normal range of magnesium is 1.4 to 2.2 mEq/liter.)

■ **phosphorus** — low serum levels occur in patients receiving TPN because of increased use of phosphorus for glucose metabolism. (For each kilocalorie of TPN administered, 2 mEq/dl of phosphorus is required. Serum levels should be measured weekly. Serum phosphorus levels below 1 mg/dl will produce clinical signs and symptoms of hypophosphatemia. The normal range is 2.5 to 4.5 mg/dl.)

Neurologic
- lethargy
- hyporeflexia
- decreased proprioception
- disorientation
- confabulation
- paresthesias
- weakness of legs
- irritability
- seizures
- flaccid paralysis
- confusion

Gastrointestinal
- tongue — baldness, glossitis, edema
- lips — cheilosis, angular stomatitis

Glandular
- parotid enlargement
- thyroid enlargement

DIAGNOSTIC STUDIES
See *Major elements monitored in TPN.*

POTENTIAL COMPLICATIONS
- sepsis
- mechanical injury from catheter
  - pneumothorax, hemothorax
  - arterial puncture
  - air emboli
  - catheter emboli
  - catheter and venous thrombosis
- metabolic disorders
  - hypoglycemia
  - fluid and electrolyte abnormalities
  - hyperglycemia
  - essential fatty acid deficiency

Eye
- xerosis (dryness) of conjunctivae
- keratomalacia (a condition linked to vitamin A deficiency that causes softening of the cornea; early signs include xerotic spots on conjunctivae and xerotic, insensitive, and hazy cornea)
- corneal vascularization
- blepharitis (scaly inflammation of eyelid edges)
- Bitot's spots (gray, triangular conjunctival spots, linked to vitamin A deficiency)
- "spectacle eye" (inflammation of the periorbital skin associated with a vitamin B [biotin] deficiency)

Nursing diagnosis: *High risk for injury related to complications of TPN catheter insertion, displacement, use, or removal*

NURSING PRIORITY: Prevent or promptly treat complications that may result from TPN catheter.

Interventions

1. Observe for signs and symptoms of respiratory distress and shock during insertion of the central venous catheter (CVC), including tachypnea, tachycardia, dropping systolic blood pressure, dyspnea, use of accessory muscles for respiration, and decreased or absent breath sounds on side of insertion.

2. Maintain the patient in Trendelenburg's position during CVC insertion.

3. After CVC insertion, assess for bilateral breath sounds in all lung fields and ensure that a chest X-ray is obtained. Monitor the patient's respiratory status and breath sounds at least every 8 hours thereafter.

4. Do not begin administering the TPN solution until the position of the catheter tip is confirmed by chest X-ray.

5. Use locking (Luer-Lok) connections, or tape the connections securely.

6. Before opening the I.V. system to the air, instruct the patient to perform Valsalva's maneuver (hold the breath and bear down), or clamp the catheter. If the patient is unable to perform Valsalva's maneuver, change the tubing only during exhalation.

7. Observe for signs and symptoms of air emboli, such as extreme anxiousness, sharp chest pain, cyanosis, or churning precordial murmur. If air emboli are suspected, position the patient in Trendelenburg's position on the left side, administer oxygen, and notify the doctor immediately.

8. During dressing changes, observe for a suture at the insertion site of a temporary CVC, a suture at the exit site of a permanent CVC, or increased external catheter length.

9. Observe for inability to withdraw blood; complaints of chest pain or burning; leaking fluid; and swelling around the insertion site, shoulder, clavicle, and upper extremity.

Rationales

1. After using a local anesthetic, the doctor inserts the catheter into the subclavian or internal jugular vein and positions the tip in the superior vena cava. He then sutures the catheter in place and applies an occlusive dressing. The lungs or an artery may be punctured during subclavian venous cannulation. The artery may bleed to the point of compressing the trachea, causing life-threatening respiratory distress. A puncture of the lung creates a pneumothorax, causing respiratory compromise from entry of air into the pleural space and collapse of all or part of the lung on the venipuncture side.

2. Trendelenburg's position increases venous pressure in the upper half of the body. This prevents air influx into the venous system through the insertion needle or I.V. catheters when their lumens are open to air.

3. Bilateral breath sounds and symmetrical pain-free chest movement indicate fully inflated lungs. Chest X-ray confirms placement of the catheter tip in the superior vena cava and rules out hemothorax, chylothorax (from puncture of a lymph vessel), and pneumothorax.

4. The hyperosmolar TPN solution irritates veins smaller than the superior vena cava. Thrombophlebitis can result if the TPN solution is infused into the jugular, subclavian, or innominate vein.

5. Secure connections are essential to prevent accidental tubing disconnection. Accidental disconnection may cause bleeding, loss of catheter patency from clot formation, air emboli, hub contamination, and sepsis.

6. Valsalva's maneuver increases intrathoracic pressure, forcing blood through the area of least resistance (in this case, the catheter) and preventing inflow of air. Air will enter the catheter only as the patient inhales. (Negative intrathoracic pressure allows the lungs to fill with air. If the I.V. catheter is open to the air during inhalation, air can be pulled into the bloodstream as well.)

7. Small amounts of air may produce no symptoms. Large amounts, however, may cause an air lock in the heart, in which case no blood can pass through the heart. The patient may die from cardiac arrest related to blocked blood flow and resultant ischemia.
   Trendelenburg's and the left lateral recumbent positions allow air to collect at the apex of the right ventricle. Small amounts of air may pass into the pulmonary circulation and be reabsorbed. Large amounts of air in the heart may need to be aspirated through a catheter passed into the right atrium.

8. A suture at the insertion or exit site stabilizes the catheter. Increased external catheter length indicates movement and possible catheter displacement.

9. These may indicate catheter displacement and vein thrombosis.

GASTROINTESTINAL DISORDERS

10. Observe for visible collateral circulation on the chest wall.

10. Development of collateral circulation on the chest wall is a sign of vein thrombosis.

11. When the catheter is being removed, be sure that:

• the patient is supine

• the patient performs Valsalva's maneuver before the catheter is removed

• a completely sealed airtight dressing is applied over the insertion site after the CVC is removed.

11. Conscientious attention to the details of catheter removal is important for several reasons:
• The supine position allows a clear view while removing stitches and the catheter and applying a sealed dressing.
• Air can be sucked in through the CVC sinus tract if the catheter is pulled out during inhalation, causing air emboli.
• The CVC sinus tract allows air to enter the venous system with each inhalation if an airtight dressing is not applied.

12. When the catheter is removed, measure its length and observe for jagged edges.

12. To ensure that the entire catheter was removed, the catheter should be measured and inspected for breaks.

13. Additional individualized interventions: _____

13. Rationales: _____

Target outcome criteria
While the CVC is in place, the patient will:
• exhibit unrestricted, pain-free inhalation and exhalation
• exhibit symmetrical chest movement
• exhibit normal respirations

• present a normal chest X-ray
• have a patent catheter
• show no fluid infiltration
• show no evidence of catheter emboli.

Nursing diagnosis: *Nutritional deficit related to inability to ingest nutrients orally or digest them satisfactorily, or to increased metabolic need*

NURSING PRIORITY: Provide for adequate nutritional intake.

Interventions

1. Administer the ordered TPN solution.

2. Infuse TPN solution at a constant rate with an infusion pump.

• Check the volume of solution, flow rate, and patient tolerance every half hour.

• Do not interrupt the flow of TPN solution.

Rationales

1. TPN solution composition is based on the individual patient's calculated needs. Usual nutrient requirements for critically ill patients include calories, 2,000 to 3,000 kcal/day; protein, 0.8 to 2 g/kg/day; fat, 30% of nonprotein calories; trace elements (variable), supplied by trace element formula added to solution; and vitamins (variable), supplied by 10 ml/day of multivitamin preparation added to solution.

2. The infusion pump regulates the flow rate with greater accuracy than a standard I.V. set, decreasing the likelihood of accidentally infusing a bag of TPN solution too quickly.

• This prevents a hyperglycemic, hyperosmolar load. (The hyperosmolar state results in osmotic diuresis that can lead to dehydration, lethargy, and coma.)

• Turning TPN on and off at intervals creates fluctuations in the serum glucose level. The pancreas responds to high or low serum glucose by altering the secretion of glucagon and insulin. This system keeps the serum glucose level within the normal range; if changes in flow rate are made too quickly, the body cannot adjust and signs and symptoms of hypoglycemia or hyperglycemia may occur.

• Do not attempt to "catch up" if the TPN infusion is behind schedule or "slow down" if it is ahead of schedule. Set the I.V. infusion to the ordered rate.

• When discontinuing TPN, lower the rate to 50 ml/hour for 3 to 4 hours.

3. Ensure that the TPN infusion does not stop suddenly, or take appropriate corrective action:

• For a clotted catheter, hang dextrose 10% in water at another I.V. site to infuse at the ordered TPN rate.

• During cardiopulmonary arrest, stop the TPN infusion and provide one or more boluses of dextrose 50% in water, as ordered.

4. Monitor fingerstick glucose levels and laboratory serum glucose levels every 6 hours, as ordered. Maintain serum glucose level at 100 to 200 mg/dl. Monitor urine glucose and acetone levels every 6 hours.

5. Observe for signs and symptoms of the following problems:

• hypoglycemia—weakness; agitation; tremors; cold, clammy skin; serum glucose level less than 60 mg/dl; and urine tests negative for sugar and acetone

• hyperglycemia—thirst, acetone breath, diuresis, dehydration; serum glucose level above 200 mg/dl; urine positive for glucose and varying from negative to large amounts of acetone

• protein overload—elevated blood urea nitrogen and creatinine levels

• If TPN on gravity drip has fallen behind the ordered drip rate, there will be less glucose circulating in the blood and less insulin secreted to handle the glucose (insulin decreases serum glucose levels by transporting glucose into the cells to be converted to glycogen for storage). A rapid infusion of TPN solution results in a rapid rise in serum glucose to above normal levels without a corresponding increase in insulin production. (The body takes 30 to 60 minutes to sense the high serum glucose level and respond by increasing insulin production.)

The physiologic effect of high serum glucose levels is dehydration. Water is drained out of the interstitial spaces into the vascular system in an attempt to equalize serum and interstitial glucose levels. This results in dehydrated interstitial spaces, causing excessive thirst and hunger. The kidneys sense the increased vascular volume and excrete the excess fluid and glucose. Dehydration, if not treated, will lead to lethargy, confusion, and coma.

• Slowing the TPN rate to 50 ml/hour for 3 to 4 hours allows the body to sense the lower serum glucose level and adjust to it. The pancreas responds by decreasing insulin production. These mechanisms prevent development of hypoglycemia, which can occur if TPN is discontinued too rapidly.

3. If the TPN infusion stops suddenly, another source of glucose must be supplied to prevent hypoglycemia. The high levels of insulin in the bloodstream will deplete the serum glucose level to less than 60 mg/dl within an hour.

• Brain cells cannot function without glucose as an energy source. Another source of I.V. glucose prevents a rapid drop in the serum glucose level.

• This precaution prevents accidentally giving a bolus of TPN solution during an emergency. One or more boluses of dextrose prevents hypoglycemia and allows more control. In an emergency situation, a rapidly decreasing serum glucose level may otherwise go unnoticed.

4. Monitoring serum glucose levels evaluates the patient's tolerance of the glucose load being infused. Levels greater than 200 mg/dl may indicate that the body is not using glucose, and additional insulin may be necessary to increase conversion of glucose to glycogen. Levels greater than 200 mg/dl also may indicate new stressors: Medications, surgery, and sepsis all can cause hyperglycemia. To handle the stress, the body increases the amount of glucose available for energy. Blood glucose checks may be less frequent if hyperglycemia does not exist. Monitoring urine glucose indicates renal glucose spillage and production of ketones.

5. The complex nature of TPN therapy places the patient at risk for numerous complications:

• The brain cannot survive without glucose. Death may occur within an hour if glucose levels are not restored to normal.

• Monitoring for signs and symptoms of hyperglycemia promotes early identification of glucose intolerance and its cause. This may be related to a new stress such as sepsis. Unchecked, hyperglycemia leads to osmolar diuresis, causing dehydration, thirst, confusion, lethargy, seizures, and coma.

• Protein overload can cause osmotic diuresis.

• hyperosmolar overload — thirst, headache, lethargy, seizures, and urine positive for glucose and negative for acetone

• Hyperosmolar hyperglycemic nonketotic syndrome (HHNKS) may occur if the TPN solution is infused over too short a time. A serum osmolar level above 300 mOsm/kg water pulls fluid into the vascular bed to dilute the osmolar load. The excess vascular fluid results in osmotic diuresis. Also, HHNKS may occur with simultaneous infusion of TPN solution and tube feeding. To prevent this problem, decrease the TPN rate as the tube feeding rate is increased.

• electrolyte imbalances (see Appendix C, "Fluid and Electrolyte Imbalances") — hypocalcemia (numbness and tingling), hypokalemia (muscle weakness, cramps, paresthesia, lethargy, confusion, ileus, and arrhythmias), hypomagnesemia (confusion, positive Chvostek's sign, and tetany), hyponatremia (lethargy and confusion), and hypophosphatemia (weakness, signs of encephalopathy, and poor resistance to infection). Monitor serum electrolyte levels as ordered, typically daily until stable and then 2 to 3 times a week.

• The "Fluid and Electrolyte Imbalances" appendix contains general information on these disorders; this section covers information specific to TPN. Fluid and electrolyte status requires careful monitoring for several reasons: (a) Increased glucose metabolism and protein synthesis tend to deplete potassium and phosphate; if they are not replaced appropriately with TPN, a deficit may result. (b) The primary diagnosis may alter fluid and electrolyte balance. Fluid and electrolyte losses from fistulas, diarrhea, or nasogastric tubes can cause electrolyte and acid-base abnormalities. (c) To promote lean body mass repletion and positive nitrogen balance, electrolytes have to be supplied in a specific ratio: phosphorus 0.8 g, sodium 3.9 mg, potassium 3 mEq, chloride 2.5 mEq, and calcium 1.2 mEq for every gram of nitrogen infused.

• vitamin and trace mineral deficiencies (see *Signs and symptoms of vitamin and trace mineral deficiencies*).

• Vitamins and trace minerals are necessary for vital processes. Vitamins may function as hormones and as catalysts in enzyme systems. Minerals serve as co-enzyme activators and as major factors in the regulation of acid-base and fluid and electrolyte balance.

Deficiencies of vitamins and minerals result from inadequate intake, inability to digest and absorb, poor utilization of nutrients, excess losses, and increased requirements related to medication or severity of illness.

6. Infuse I.V. fat emulsion as ordered through one of three infusion methods:

6. Fat emulsions are used as an adjunct to TPN therapy to prevent essential fatty acid deficiency. Fats also can be used as a source of calories if calories from TPN alone are not sufficient. For example, if hyperglycemia is a consistent problem and insulin cannot control the serum glucose level, the glucose infusion is decreased and the lost calories are supplied as fat.

SIGNS AND SYMPTOMS OF VITAMIN AND TRACE MINERAL DEFICIENCIES

Vitamin deficiencies are avoided by adding 1 unit of a multivitamin preparation to the TPN solution every day. Trace mineral deficiencies will usually not develop until 2 to 4 weeks after oral intake has stopped.

Water-soluble vitamins	Fat-soluble vitamins	Trace mineral deficiencies
vitamin B complex blepharitis, periorbital fissures, cheilosis, glossitis, weakness, paresthesias of legs, dermatoses **vitamin C (ascorbic acid)** bleeding gums, joint and muscle aching	**vitamin A** night blindness, Bitot's spots **vitamin D** bone tenderness **vitamin E** myopathy, creatinuria **vitamin K** prolonged blood clotting	**chromium** glucose intolerance, mental confusion **copper** depigmentation of skin and hair within 2 to 4 weeks, kinky hair **iodine** enlarged thyroid, impaired memory, hoarseness, hearing loss **manganese** transient dermatitis **molybdenum** night blindness, irritability **selenium** muscle pain and tenderness **zinc** hypogeusesthesia (abnormally diminished sense of taste); moist, excoriated rash in paranasal, anal, and groin areas

• through a separate I.V.

• through a Y-connector added between the TPN catheter and the I.V. tubing

• as a 3-in-1 solution.

7. If 3-in-1 solution is used, ensure that it is mixed in a ratio of calcium, less than or equal to 15 mEq/liter; phosphorus, less than or equal to 30 mEq/liter; and magnesium, less than or equal to 10 mEq/liter.

8. Check that the infusion pump delivers the correct volume of 3-in-1 solution. Adjust the infusion rate as needed to ensure delivery of the desired volume.

9. Observe for fat separation in the 3-in-1 solution as indicated by a yellow ring around the edges of the solution. Stop the infusion if this occurs, and replace the solution bag with a fresh one.

10. Culture the 3-in-1 solution if the patient develops sepsis.

11. If a separate fat infusion is used, administer it slowly over the first 15 to 20 minutes (1 ml/minute for a 10% fat infusion or 0.5 ml/minute for a 20% fat infusion). Observe for dyspnea, pain at the I.V. site, or chest or back pain. If any of these signs or symptoms occur, stop the infusion and notify the doctor. Otherwise, increase the rate as ordered.

12. If the fat emulsion is to be infused in a second I.V., infuse it over 4 hours (for a 10% fat emulsion) or 8 hours (for a 20% fat emulsion). Do not allow fat emulsions to hang more than 12 hours unless mixed in a 3-in-1 solution.

13. Do not use I.V. filters with fat emulsion infusions. When infusing fats on a long-term basis (longer than 3 months), ensure that thiosalicylate-free tubing is used.

14. Encourage walking or mild exercise to promote nitrogen retention and nutrient use.

15. Weigh the patient at the same time, with the same amount of clothing, on the same scale every day.

• Infusing fats separately prevents breakdown of the emulsion and decreases the risk of fat emboli.

• The Y-connector allows fats to infuse with minimal mixing with the TPN solution, preventing breakdown of the fat emulsion and decreasing the risk of fat emboli. Fats appear to float on top of the TPN solution when administered through a Y-connector.

• The pharmacy can mix carbohydrates, protein, and fat in one bag to hang over a 24-hour period. This method saves nursing time, because there is no extra I.V. or Y-connector to add, and pharmacy time, because only one bag must be mixed and dispensed. These solutions are also cost-effective because they use less I.V. tubing and fewer I.V. catheters. Most important, the patient is spared the pain of venipuncture for a fat emulsion I.V.

7. The milky color of 3-in-1 solutions obscures particulate matter. The ratio listed prevents precipitate formation.

8. When fats are added to a TPN solution, the solution's increased viscosity may alter infusion pump delivery.

9. The 3-in-1 solution can separate if it is not mixed properly or if it hangs for more than 24 hours. Separation may cause fat emboli.

10. If it becomes contaminated, the 3-in-1 solution is more likely to support microbial growth than a TPN solution without fat.

11. Allergic reactions to the fat emulsion may be local or systemic. Slow administration allows time to observe for an allergic reaction before a dangerous amount of antigen is administered. Signs and symptoms listed indicate possible allergic reactions.

12. The patient with renal failure or congestive heart failure (CHF) may not tolerate an additional 500 ml of fluid 2 to 3 times per week. The slower infusion rate allows the body to assimilate the emulsion and prevents hyperlipidemia.

13. The fat emulsion particle size exceeds the filter pore size, so the solution will not infuse through the filter. Fats leach thiosalicylate from ordinary tubing; it can accumulate in the body, with unknown effects.

14. Exercise improves use of nutrients and promotes lean muscle mass development rather than the storage of fatty acids. Exercise also prevents muscle wasting, which occurs with inactivity.

15. Weighing is necessary to determine if nutritional goals are being met. Weight is also used to assess the patient's fluid status. Weight gain of more than ½ lb (1.3 kg) a day may indicate fluid retention.

GASTROINTESTINAL DISORDERS

16. When oral intake resumes, initiate a daily calorie count and measure fat intake. Observe for nausea, vomiting, or diarrhea.

16. Daily monitoring of fat intake and calories provides guidelines for therapy. When the patient is taking 10 g of fat per day orally, I.V. fat emulsions can be discontinued. When the patient can consume 1,000 calories/day or half of the estimated caloric intake without nausea, vomiting, or diarrhea, TPN can be discontinued.

17. Observe for changes in muscle strength and energy level.

17. Increased strength, energy level, and sense of well-being indicate that TPN is meeting the body's nutritional needs.

18. Additional individualized interventions: _____

18. Rationales: _____

Target outcome criteria
Within 24 hours of starting TPN and throughout TPN therapy, the patient will:
• maintain negative urine glucose level
• maintain serum glucose level of 100 to 200 mg/dl
• show no signs or symptoms of hypoglycemia, hyperglycemia, HHNKS, electrolyte imbalance, or vitamin or trace metal deficiencies.

Within 7 days of starting TPN, the patient will:
• exhibit weight gain of less than ½ lb/day
• exhibit increased muscle strength
• exhibit increased energy level
• verbalize increased sense of well-being.

Nursing diagnosis: *High risk for fluid volume excess or deficit related to fluid retention, altered oral intake, or osmotic diuresis*

NURSING PRIORITY: Maintain optimal fluid balance.

Interventions

1. See Appendix C, "Fluid and Electrolyte Imbalances."

2. Observe for edema, increased pulse rate, and increased blood pressure. If any of these signs are present, consult with the doctor about decreasing overall fluid administration.

3. Observe for thirst, dry mucous membranes, dry skin, decreased urine output, and increased urine specific gravity.

4. Assess breath sounds each shift.

5. Record fluid intake and output each shift. Maintain approximate balance.

6. Weigh the patient daily. For every liter lost or gained, weight should change approximately 2 lb (1 kg). Generally, maintain weight gain at less than ½ lb/day.

Rationales

1. The "Fluid and Electrolyte Imbalances" appendix contains further details related to fluid and electrolyte disorders.

2. Edema, increased pulse rate, and increased blood pressure may be signs of excess fluid volume. This may result from the body's inability to tolerate the increased cardiac and renal work load imposed by TPN or from the underlying disease itself (for example, CHF or renal failure). Edema in the malnourished patient is also often related to protein depletion, in which circulating serum protein levels are lower than protein levels in the interstitial spaces. This inequality causes fluids to shift into the interstitial spaces to equalize protein-to-fluid ratios.

3. These may be signs and symptoms of fluid deficit or dehydration.

4. Crackles or gurgles may indicate fluid overload.

5. An intake consistently lower than output indicates a fluid deficit and the need for additional fluid to prevent dehydration and renal failure. An intake higher than output may reflect fluid overload and result in pulmonary complications.

6. Daily weight is another way to determine whether the patient is being given too much or too little fluid. Weight gain over ½ lb/day is too rapid and reflects fluid retention.

7. Additional individualized interventions: _____

_____

7. Rationales: _____

_____

Target outcome criteria
Throughout TPN therapy, the patient will:
- maintain fluid intake that approximately equals output
- exhibit no signs or symptoms of fluid imbalance
- maintain urine output greater than 200 ml/8 hours
- exhibit weight gain less than ½ lb/day.

Nursing diagnosis: *Knowledge deficit related to lack of experience with TPN*

NURSING PRIORITY: Teach the patient and family about TPN.

Interventions

1. Briefly explain the purpose and method of TPN therapy.

- Explain that in TPN calories and nutrients infuse directly into the bloodstream until the patient can resume oral intake.
- Define the roles of the dietitian, nurse, pharmacist, doctor, and other health care team members in TPN.
- Explain that the TPN solution contains carbohydrate, protein, fat, vitamins, and electrolytes and will provide all the calories and protein the patient needs.
- Describe the route and equipment used, the length of time TPN may be infused, and the patient's responsibilities.
- Provide the patient and family with written material on TPN therapy.

2. If the patient is to receive TPN at home, take the following steps:

- Collaborate with the nutrition support service to determine appropriate teaching strategies.

- Teach the signs, symptoms, and necessary actions for managing complications, such as infection, abnormal serum glucose levels, air emboli, clotted catheter, and displaced catheter. Ask the patient to report any signs or symptoms to the nutrition support team.
- Review the information, and answer questions. Ask the patient "what if" questions.

- Provide written instructions on home TPN protocols.

3. See the "Knowledge Deficit" plan, page 56, for further details.

4. Additional individualized interventions: _____

_____

Rationales

1. A general understanding of TPN provides a framework within which to understand the specific details of therapy.
- This defines TPN in terms the patient can understand.

- Describing the roles of the health care team members ensures patient awareness of resources.
- Describing the TPN solution may reassure the patient and family.

- A thorough understanding of TPN administration, clear expectations, and acceptance of responsibility for self-monitoring promote optimum therapeutic benefit.
- Written material reinforces the nurse's explanation.

2. TPN is a complex therapy requiring substantial expertise on the patient's part for successful home management.
- The nutrition support service can provide expert advice on adapting teaching to the home setting. The patient receiving TPN at home will need to be followed by the service (or by a home care agency specializing in TPN management).
- Knowledge of how to detect and manage complications may increase the patient's confidence about managing this therapy at home. Prompt reporting facilitates timely intervention.

- Reviewing, clarifying, and using practical "what if" examples promote understanding and boost problem-solving skills.
- Written information reinforces teaching and provides a permanent reference.

3. The "Knowledge Deficit" plan contains interventions related to patient teaching.

4. Rationales: _____

_____

GASTROINTESTINAL DISORDERS

Target outcome criteria
Within 48 hours of starting TPN, the patient or family will:
• describe TPN on request
• discuss medical reasons for TPN
• discuss the role of the nutrition support service staff

• use appropriate problem-solving skills
• list signs and symptoms of complications.

Nursing diagnosis: *High risk for infection related to invasive CVC, leukopenia, or damp dressing*

NURSING PRIORITY: Prevent or detect and promptly treat infection.

Interventions

1. Follow hospital protocol for dressing changes. Use sterile technique and universal precautions. Apply a clear, completely sealed dressing.

2. Inspect the dressing every 8 hours, and change it any time it is unsealed or damp.

3. Observe the insertion site every 8 hours for signs of infection. Report any redness, swelling, pain, or purulent drainage.

4. Follow hospital protocol for tubing changes and antibacterial preparation at all connections before changing I.V. tubing.

5. Follow pharmacy or nutrition support service recommendations for I.V. filters.

6. Infuse only TPN solution through the TPN catheter. Do not use the TPN line for injecting medications or drawing blood samples.

7. Use only solutions prepared in the pharmacy under a laminar flow hood. Do not make any additions on the unit. If additions are necessary, request that they be made in the pharmacy under a laminar flow hood.

8. Return cloudy or precipitated solution to the pharmacy.

9. Allow each bag or bottle to hang no more than 24 hours.

10. Monitor for signs of infection:
• increased pulse and respiratory rates
• temperature above 101° F (38.3° C)
• white blood cell (WBC) count over 10,000/mm³
• serum glucose level over 200 mg/dl
• glycosuria
• chills, diaphoresis, or lethargy.

11. Additional individualized interventions: _____

Rationales

1. Good technique decreases the risk of infection. Dressing change frequency ranges from every day to once a week.

2. Moisture and exposure to air encourages microbial growth at the insertion site. Colonization may lead to sepsis.

3. These signs may indicate infection of the insertion site.

4. Using proper technique when changing and disconnecting tubing decreases the risk of TPN line contamination. Tubing changes usually are performed every 24 to 96 hours.

5. The use of I.V. filters is controversial. Some hospital pharmacies filter solutions rather than add filters to I.V. tubing on the unit.

6. Using the TPN catheter for other solutions provides another possible source of contamination and increases the risk of sepsis.

7. Preparing the solution in a sterile area decreases the risk of contamination. The laminar flow hood minimizes contamination from airborne microorganisms.

8. Cloudy solution indicates possible bacterial contamination. Precipitate may occlude the catheter or cause thrombus formation.

9. Infusing solutions over longer periods allows for rapid multiplication of any microorganisms inadvertently introduced during mixing of the TPN solution.

10. A change in vital signs or WBC count, hyperglycemia, glycosuria, chills, or diaphoresis may indicate developing infection.

11. Rationales: _____

Target outcome criteria
Throughout TPN therapy, the patient will:
• be afebrile
• present urine negative for glucose
• show no infection or inflammation at the catheter site

• maintain serum glucose level between 100 and 200 g/dl.

Discharge planning

NURSING DISCHARGE CRITERIA

Upon the patient's discharge, documentation shows evidence of:
• absence of fever
• stabilizing weight
• absence of pulmonary or cardiovascular complications
• electrolytes within acceptable parameters
• WBC counts within normal parameters
• absence of redness, swelling, pain, and drainage at catheter site
• absence of nausea and vomiting
• ability to perform activities of daily living (ADLs), transfer, and ambulate same as before hospitalization
• adequate home support system, or referral to home care or a nursing home if indicated by an inadequate home support system or the patient's inability to perform ADLs, transfers, and ambulation
• a plan for follow-up by nutrition support service or home care agency specializing in TPN for the patient receiving TPN at home.

PATIENT-FAMILY TEACHING CHECKLIST

If the patient is to receive TPN at home, document evidence that the patient and family demonstrate an understanding of:
___ preventing complications
___ actions to take if complications do occur
___ where and how to obtain supplies
___ catheter site care
___ procedure for TPN administration
___ community resources
___ date, time, and location of follow-up appointments
___ how to contact the doctor.

DOCUMENTATION CHECKLIST

Using outcome criteria as a guide, document:
___ nutritional status on admission
___ any significant changes in status
___ CVC insertion—difficulties or complications; length of catheter; position and any change in position; signs of infection, thrombosis, emboli, or other post-insertion complication
___ dressing and tubing changes
___ TPN solution and fat emulsion—for each bag or bottle, record date, time, name of nurse hanging solution; all ingredients; rate of infusion
___ patient-family teaching
___ discharge planning.

ASSOCIATED PLANS OF CARE
Knowledge Deficit
Nutritional Deficit

References
Alpers, D., Clouse, R., and Stenson, W. *Manual of Nutritional Therapeutics,* 2nd ed. Boston: Little, Brown & Co., 1988.

Bozzetti, F., Bonfanti, G., Regalia, E., Calligaris, L., and Cozzaglio, L. "Catheter Sepsis from Infusate Contamination," *Nutrition in Clinical Practice.* 5(4):156-159, 1990.

Bursztein, S., Elwyn, D., Askanazi, J., and Kinney, J. *Energy Metabolism, Indirect Calorimetry, and Nutrition.* Baltimore: Williams and Wilkins, 1989.

Camp-Sorrell, D. "Advanced Central Venous Access: Selection, Catheters, Devices, and Nursing Management," *Journal of Intravenous Nursing* 13(6):361-68, 1990.

Dean, R. *Training Manual for Total Parenteral Nutrition,* 2nd ed. Chicago: Precept Press, 1990.

Freund, H., and Rimon, B. "Sepsis during Total Parenteral Nutrition," *Journal of Parenteral and Enteral Nutrition* 14(1):39-41, 1990.

Grant, J., and Kennedy-Caldwell, C. *Nutritional Support in Nursing.* Philadelphia: Grune and Stratton, 1988.

Hermann-Zaidins, M., and Touger-Decker, R. *Nutritional Support in Home Health.* Rockville, Md.: Aspen, 1989.

Kennedy-Caldwell, C., and Guenter, P. *Nutritional Support Nursing,* 2nd ed. Silver Springs, Md.: American Society for Parenteral and Enteral Nutrition, 1988.

Maki, D. "Catheter Infection," presented at the 14th Clinical Congress, San Antonio: American Society for Parenteral and Enteral Nutrition, 1990.

Murphy, L., and Lipman, T. "Central Venous Catheter Care in Parenteral Nutrition: A Review," *Journal of Parenteral and Enteral Nutrition* 11(2):190-200, 1987.

Rombeau, J. *Atlas of Nutritional Support Techniques.* Boston: Little, Brown and Co., 1989.

Rombeau, J., and Caldwell, M. *Enteral and Tube Feeding,* 2nd ed. Philadelphia: W.B. Saunders Co., 1990.

Schlichtig, R., and Ayres, S. *Nutritional Support of the Critically Ill.* Chicago: Year Book Medical Publishers, 1988.

Speer, E. "Central Venous Catheterization," *Journal of Intravenous Nursing* 13(1):30-39, 1990.

GASTROINTESTINAL DISORDERS

HEPATOBILIARY AND PANCREATIC DISORDERS

Cholecystectomy

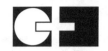

DRG information

DRG 195* Total Cholecystectomy with Common Duct
Exploration (CDE). With Complications or
Comorbidity (CC) for the following proce-
dures:
- exploration of duct to relieve obstruction
- exploration of duct to remove stone.
Mean LOS = 11.0 days
DRG 196 Total Cholecystectomy with CDE. Without
CC.
Mean LOS = 8.2 days
DRG 197* Total Cholecystectomy without CDE. With
CC.
Mean LOS = 8.6 days
DRG 198 Total Cholecystectomy. Without CDE or CC.
Mean LOS = 5.5 days
PRO alert: In many states, professional review organizations (PROs) are closely reviewing cases falling into
these DRGs because of suspicions that these procedures
often are performed unnecessarily. PROs also are focusing their postoperative reviews on pulmonary
symptoms because of the frequency of these complications. PRO review guidelines include the following:
1. Documentation in the nursing admission history
must describe preoperative pulmonary status.
2. High-risk patients, such as those with a history of
smoking, obesity, pulmonary disease, chronic cough, alcohol abuse, or insulin-dependent diabetes, must be
identified.
3. Preoperative evaluation and education of high-risk
patients must include:
- incentive spirometry and documentation of teaching
- training in proper breathing and coughing techniques
- prophylactic antibiotics as ordered by the doctor
- a chest X-ray within 30 days of surgery.
4. Postoperative documentation should include:
- ambulation within 24 hours
- heparin ordered for high-risk patients
- use of compression stockings, when indicated
- monitoring of white blood cell count
- chest X-ray.
The nurse should be particularly attentive to documenting nursing activities involved with assessing
pulmonary status, preventing postoperative complications, obtaining diagnostic tests (as ordered by the
doctor), and implementing medical treatments for pulmonary symptoms.

Introduction
DEFINITION AND TIME FOCUS
Cholecystitis (inflammation of the gallbladder) is an
extremely common disorder usually associated with
cholelithiasis (gallstone formation), although choleli-

*Most commonly occurring DRG in this category

thiasis may present without symptoms. Most gallstones
are composed of cholesterol and a matrix to which the
cholesterol adheres. The mechanism and cause of stone
formation are unknown, although infection, stasis, and
genetic causes have been suggested. Cholecystitis may
be acute or chronic. Patients who require hospitalization usually present with an acute attack of intense
pain, nausea, and vomiting; for these patients, cholecystectomy (surgical removal of the gallbladder) is the
most common treatment. This procedure is usually performed with choledochostomy (exploration of the common and hepatic bile ducts) to remove stones that may
be causing obstruction.
    Cholecystectomy is performed through various ap-
proaches:
- traditional — surgical incision and direct visualization
with surgical or laser dissection
- endoscopic — endoscopic visualization with surgical or
laser dissection.
    Laser cholecystectomy with direct visualization
(via a right subcostal incision) or endoscopic visualization (via a small puncture at the umbilicus) is usually done on an outpatient basis, with immediate
postoperative care provided at the ambulatory surgery
center, followed by home health care. Endoscopic visualization with surgical dissection is also an outpatient
procedure and may be followed by a short hospital
stay (less than 24 hours). Postoperative care is the
same as for traditional cholecystectomy patients, however, recovery is accelerated. These new techniques are
reserved for uncomplicated cases.
    This plan focuses on preoperative and postopera-
tive care for the patient with acute cholecystitis who
requires traditional cholecystectomy with surgical dissection.

ETIOLOGY AND PRECIPITATING FACTORS
- stones lodged in the gallbladder neck
- other causes unknown, but possibilities include kinking of the neck of the gallbladder, adhesions, edema,
neoplasms, extensive fasting, anesthesia, narcotics, dehydration, pancreatic enzymes refluxing into the gallbladder, and inadequate blood supply

Focused assessment guidelines
NURSING HISTORY (Functional health pattern findings)

Health perception — health management pattern
- may report pain, initially situated in midepigastrium
that becomes pronounced in the right upper quadrant
(RUQ); pain is initially mild but persistent and intensi-
fies as inflammation spreads; pain may be referred to
the right scapula or right shoulder and is exacerbated
by movement, coughing, and deep breathing

• may have history of diabetes, extensive bowel resections, or hemolytic anemia
• if over age 50, is at increased risk

Nutritional-metabolic pattern
• may report intolerance of heavy meals or fatty foods
• may report indigestion leading to anorexia
• may report nausea, possibly with vomiting

Elimination pattern
• may report flatulence
• may report change in color of urine or stool (indicates obstructed bile flow)
• may report pruritus

Activity-exercise pattern
• may report sedentary life-style; if so, is at increased risk for gallstones and therefore cholecystitis

Sleep-rest pattern
• may report pain that disturbs sleep

Sexuality-reproductive pattern
• women with more than one child are at increased risk for cholelithiasis
• women who use oral contraceptives are at increased risk for cholelithiasis

PHYSICAL FINDINGS
General
• elevated temperature
• obesity

Eyes
• icteric sclera

Mouth
• jaundiced mucous membranes

Cardiovascular
• rapid, irregular pulse
• hypertension

Pulmonary
• short and shallow respirations

Abdomen
• pain in RUQ, referred to right scapula and intensified by deep breathing or percussion above right costal margin
• localized rebound tenderness in RUQ
• distention
• light-colored stools

Urinary
• dark, frothy urine

Integumentary
• jaundice, especially on inner aspects of forearms
• bruising

DIAGNOSTIC STUDIES
• white blood cell count — typically 10,000 to 15,000/mm^3, although it may not be elevated
• serum bilirubin level (direct and indirect) — may be elevated when gallstones obstruct the bile duct
• prothrombin time (PT) — may be prolonged because bile is necessary for vitamin K absorption (prothrombin synthesis depends on vitamin K)
• alkaline phosphatase level — may be elevated because normal excretion through the biliary system may be impeded
• oral cholecystogram — may not visualize gallbladder because of biliary duct obstruction or inability of the gallbladder to concentrate the dye; repetition may be ordered to rule out inadequate preparation
• cholangiogram — may show gallstones or strictures in biliary tree
• ultrasonography — may show gallstones

POTENTIAL COMPLICATIONS
• perforation of the gallbladder
• hemorrhage
• empyema of the gallbladder
• subphrenic or hepatic abscess
• fistulas
• pancreatitis
• cholangitis
• pneumonia

Collaborative problem: *High risk for peritonitis related to possible preoperative perforation of the gallbladder*

NURSING PRIORITIES: (a) Detect perforation and (b) minimize possible complications.

Interventions

1. Monitor vital signs every 2 hours for 12 hours, then every 4 hours if stable. Document and report abnormalities, especially fever, tachycardia, or dropping blood pressure.

Rationales

1. Early detection of changes in vital signs will alert caregivers to possible perforation and the need for emergency surgery. Temperature changes indicate further inflammation or response to antibiotics.

2. Assess the abdomen during vital signs checks, particularly noting bowel sounds, distention, firmness, and presence or absence of a mass in the RUQ. Document and report any changes.

3. Note the location and character of pain during vital signs checks. Document and report any changes.

4. Maintain antibiotic therapy, as ordered.

5. Additional individualized interventions: _____

_____

2. Muscle rigidity and a palpable mass in the RUQ suggest peritonitis. In peritonitis, an initial period of hypermotility is followed by hypoactive or absent bowel sounds.

3. RUQ pain that becomes generalized may indicate perforation.

4. Antibiotics excreted through the biliary tree are given to prevent or treat infection and to decrease the risk of perforation from a friable or necrotic gallbladder wall.

5. Rationales: _____

_____

Target outcome criteria
Within 24 hours of admission, the patient will:
• display vital signs within normal limits
• verbalize reduction of pain

• show lessening of abnormal abdominal signs.

Collaborative problem: *High risk for hemorrhage related to decreased vitamin K absorption and decreased prothrombin synthesis*

NURSING PRIORITIES: (a) Prevent hemorrhage and (b) detect clotting abnormalities so that they can be corrected before surgery.

Interventions

1. Monitor the PT, as ordered. Alert the doctor to an abnormally prolonged PT.

2. Administer vitamin K, as ordered.

3. Observe for bleeding from the gums, nose, or injection sites and for blood in the urine or stool. Document and report bleeding.

4. Give injections using small-gauge needles. If an increased bleeding tendency is noted, limit the number of injections or venipunctures as much as possible, and apply direct pressure for at least 5 minutes after such procedures.

5. Apply gentle pressure to injection sites instead of massaging them.

6. Additional individualized interventions: _____

_____

Rationales

1. Prothrombin is manufactured in the liver and depends on vitamin K for synthesis. Bile is necessary for vitamin K absorption; thus, PT may be prolonged if an obstruction interferes with bile excretion.

2. Administration of vitamin K will correct any deficiency and promote prothrombin synthesis.

3. Observing for bleeding aids in detecting coagulation problems.

4. Small-gauge needles reduce the risk of bleeding at injection sites. Minimizing the number of punctures reduces the risk of significant blood loss. Direct pressure controls bleeding and allows clot formation.

5. Gentle pressure reduces the trauma at injection sites and controls bleeding.

6. Rationales: _____

_____

Target outcome criteria
Within 48 hours of admission, the patient will:
• have PT levels approaching normal
• show no evidence of bleeding.

Nursing diagnosis: *Pain related to gallbladder inflammation*

NURSING PRIORITY: Relieve RUQ pain.

Interventions

1. See the "Pain" plan, page 69.

2. Administer medications, as ordered, and document their effectiveness. Meperidine (Demerol) is the analgesic of choice; papaverine hydrochloride (Parabid), amyl nitrite, or sublingual nitroglycerin (Nitrostat) may be ordered.

3. Additional individualized interventions: _____

_____

Rationales

1. Generalized interventions regarding pain management are included in the "Pain" plan.

2. Specific medications are most appropriate for pain from cholecystitis. Meperidine is less likely than morphine to cause spasm of the biliary tree. Papaverine hydrochloride exerts a nonspecific spasmolytic effect on smooth muscle. Amyl nitrite diminishes spasm of the biliary ducts and partially counteracts the spasmogenic effects of narcotics. (Other drugs with similar action may be ordered, depending on the doctor's preference.) Nitroglycerin relieves pain and relaxes smooth muscle.

3. Rationales: _____

Target outcome criteria
Within 1 hour of admission, the patient will:
• verbalize pain relief
• display easy, deep, and regular respirations.

Collaborative problem: *High risk for postoperative infection related to obstruction or dislodgment of external biliary drainage tube*

NURSING PRIORITIES: (a) Prevent or promptly detect complications and (b) maintain patency of the drainage system.

Interventions

1. Monitor vital signs every 4 hours. Document and report abnormalities.

2. Assess the abdomen every shift, noting any abdominal pain or rigidity. Document and report any changes.

3. Assess for signs of infection at the T-tube insertion site. Document and report any redness, swelling, warmth, or purulent drainage. Teach the patient and family to recognize and report signs of infection.

4. Assess for signs of T-tube obstruction. Document and report pain in the RUQ, bile drainage around the T-tube, nausea and vomiting, clay-colored stools, jaundice, or dark yellow urine.

5. Assess for signs of tube dislodgment — decreased drainage or a change in tube position.

6. Using sterile technique, connect the T-tube to a closed gravity drainage system, and attach sufficient tubing so it does not kink or pull as the patient moves.

Rationales

1. Elevated temperature may indicate infection (either wound infection or bile peritonitis).

2. Generalized abdominal pain and rigidity, combined with an elevated temperature, may indicate bile peritonitis.

3. Early detection of infection facilitates prompt treatment.

4. These signs indicate the backup of bile into the common bile duct and liver.

5. Prompt detection and treatment of tube dislodgment reduces the risk of complications (such as peritonitis) from bile leakage.

6. After choledochostomy, a T-tube is inserted into the hepatic duct and the common bile duct to allow bile drainage and maintain patency until edema subsides. A closed biliary drainage system ensures sterility. Providing enough tubing reduces the risk of obstructing or dislodging the T-tube.

HEPATOBILIARY AND PANCREATIC DISORDERS

7. Monitor the amount and character of any drainage. Measure and record the drainage once per shift.

7. Initially, all bile output (500 to 1,000 ml/day) may flow through the T-tube. Within 7 to 10 days, however, most of the bile should flow into the duodenum. Monitoring the amount of drainage permits early detection of an obstructed or dislodged tube.

8. Monitor and record the patient's stool color.

8. Stools will be light colored initially, when most of the bile is flowing out through the T-tube. Stools should gradually become normal in color as bile passes into the duodenum. Persistence of light-colored stools for more than 7 days may indicate tube obstruction.

9. Place the patient in low Fowler's position upon return from surgery.

9. Low Fowler's position facilitates T-tube drainage.

10. If the patient will be discharged with a T-tube in place, teach the patient and family how to care for the drainage system, including the expected amount of drainage, frequency of bag emptying and dressing changes, techniques for site care and dressing changes, and signs to report to the doctor (excessive drainage, leakage, and signs of obstruction).

10. To successfully manage the T-tube at home, the patient and family need to know about routine care, as well as what to do about potential complications.

11. Additional individualized interventions: _____

11. Rationales: _____

Target outcome criteria
Throughout the period of external biliary drainage, the patient will:
• display vital signs within normal limits
• show no signs of infection or peritonitis
• show no signs of tube obstruction
• show no signs of tube dislodgment.

Nursing diagnosis: *High risk for postoperative ineffective breathing pattern related to high abdominal incision and pain*

NURSING PRIORITIES: (a) Maintain optimal air exchange and (b) prevent atelectasis.

Interventions

1. Monitor respiratory rate and character every 4 hours. Note the depth of respirations. Document and report abnormalities.

Rationales

1. After cholecystectomy, the patient may breathe shallowly to avoid pain associated with deep breathing.

2. Auscultate breath sounds once per shift. Document and report changes.

2. Breath sounds may be diminished at the bases, especially on the right side.

3. Instruct and coach the patient in diaphragmatic breathing.

3. Diaphragmatic breathing increases lung expansion by allowing the diaphragm to descend fully.

4. Assist the patient to use the incentive spirometer — 10 breaths/hour during the day and every 2 hours at night.

4. Using the incentive spirometer promotes sustained maximal inspiration, which fully inflates alveoli.

5. Turn the patient every 2 hours.

5. Position changes promote ventilation of all lung lobes and drainage of secretions.

6. Assess pain and administer pain medication, as needed, before breathing exercises and ambulation.

6. The pain-free patient is better able to take deep breaths, and therefore is more likely to cooperate with prescribed pulmonary hygiene measures and activity level.

7. Assist the patient to splint the incision with a pillow or bath blanket while coughing.

7. Splinting relieves stress and pulling on the incision.

8. Encourage the patient to increase ambulation progressively.

8. Ambulation promotes adequate ventilation by increasing the depth of respirations.

9. Additional individualized interventions: _____

9. Rationales: _____

Target outcome criteria
Throughout the postoperative period, the patient will:
• maintain a respiratory rate of 12 to 24 breaths/minute
• display nonlabored, deep respirations

• have audible, clear breath sounds in all lobes.

Nursing diagnosis: *High risk for nutritional deficit related to preoperative nausea and vomiting, postoperative NPO status, nasogastric suction, altered lipid metabolism, and increased nutritional needs during healing*

NURSING PRIORITIES: (a) Maintain optimal nutritional status and (b) teach the patient and family about postoperative dietary recommendations.

Interventions

1. Maintain I.V. fluid replacement, as ordered. See Appendix C, "Fluid and Electrolyte Imbalances."

2. Once peristalsis returns, remove the NG tube and encourage a progressive dietary intake, as ordered.

3. Clamp the T-tube during meals, as ordered.

4. Teach the patient and family about a fat-restricted diet, as ordered. Involve a dietitian in meal planning and home care teaching.

5. Suggest small, frequent meals.

6. Instruct the patient to minimize alcohol intake during recovery.

7. Prepare the patient for the possibility of persistent flatulence.

8. Additional individualized interventions: _____

Rationales

1. During the immediate postoperative period, the patient will receive nothing orally until peristalsis returns. The patient may also have a nasogastric (NG) tube in place to reduce distention and minimize the pancreatic stimulation normally triggered by gastric juices. Gastric suction and NPO status increase the risk of fluid and electrolyte disorders.

2. Patients usually are able to take clear liquids 24 to 48 hours after surgery and gradually increase to a full diet, with fat restrictions as ordered.

3. Clamping the T-tube during meals may aid fat absorption by allowing additional bile to flow into the duodenum.

4. After cholecystectomy, the liver must store and release all bile for lipid digestion; thus, fat absorption may be altered, especially if postoperative edema limits hepatic bile excretion. Fat intake usually is limited for 1½ to 6 months, depending on the doctor's preference and the patient's response to gradual increases in fat intake. A dietitian can help ensure that the patient's diet compensates for the calories normally provided by fats.

5. Large meals may contribute to distention and increase discomfort.

6. Pancreatitis is a common complication after cholecystectomy. Alcohol intake commonly triggers acute pancreatic inflammation.

7. Flatulence is common after surgery. Typically, these patients have other gastrointestinal disorders (such as hiatal hernia or ulcer) that may cause persistent symptoms, such as bloating and nausea. Dietary modifications and treatment of the underlying disorder may reduce symptoms.

8. Rationales: _____

Target outcome criteria
Throughout the hospital stay, the patient will have normal fluid and electrolyte status.

By the time of discharge, the patient will:
• list three general dietary considerations
• identify specific foods that may need to be restricted.

Nursing diagnosis: *High risk for altered oral mucous membrane related to NPO status and possible NG suction*

NURSING PRIORITY: Maintain integrity of the oral mucous membrane.

Interventions

1. Assess the oral mucous membrane once per shift for dryness, cracks, coating, or lesions.

2. Assist the patient with gentle mouth care at least twice daily or as needed. Ensure that water and oral hygiene materials are within the patient's reach.

3. Apply lubricant to the lips every 2 hours while the patient is awake or more frequently as needed.

4. Additional individualized interventions: _____

Rationales

1. Early identification of potential problems facilitates prompt treatment.

2. NPO status and NG suction (as well as any previously existing nutritional deficits) may contribute to fragility of the oral mucosa and increase the risk of infection or injury. Frequent mouth care reduces accumulation of bacteria and decreases discomfort associated with NPO status.

3. Lubricant keeps lips smooth and moist.

4. Rationales: _____

Target outcome criteria
Throughout the period of NPO status, the patient will:
• have an intact, moist oral mucous membrane
• display no evidence of inflamed oral mucosa.

Discharge planning
NURSING DISCHARGE CRITERIA
Upon the patient's discharge, documentation shows evidence of:
• absence of wound infection
• absence of fever
• stable vital signs
• absence of pulmonary and cardiovascular complications
• ability to tolerate diet as ordered
• ability to ambulate same as before surgery
• ability to perform activities of daily living (ADLs) independently
• adequate support system after discharge
• referral to home care if indicated by inadequate home support system or inability to perform ADLs.

PATIENT-FAMILY TEACHING CHECKLIST
Document evidence that the patient and family demonstrate an understanding of:
___ signs and symptoms of wound infection
___ dietary modifications (patient may be on a low-fat diet for up to 6 months; a normal diet is resumed as soon as tolerated)
___ resumption of normal activities
___ resumption of sexual activity
___ all discharge medications' purpose, dosage, administration schedule, and adverse effects (postoperative patients may be discharged with oral analgesics)
___ if discharged with a T-tube, routine care and signs to report to the doctor
___ date, time, and location of follow-up appointment
___ how to contact the doctor.

DOCUMENTATION CHECKLIST
Using outcome criteria as a guide, document:
__ clinical status on admission
__ significant changes in status
__ pertinent laboratory and diagnostic test findings
__ wound assessment
__ amount and character of T-tube drainage
__ pain relief measures
__ pulmonary hygiene measures
__ observations of oral mucous membrane
__ nutritional intake
__ gastrointestinal assessment
__ patient-family teaching
__ discharge planning.

ASSOCIATED PLANS OF CARE
Knowledge Deficit
Pain
Pancreatitis
Surgical Intervention

References

Carpenito, L.J. *Nursing Diagnosis: Application to Clinical Practice,* 3rd ed. Philadelphia: J.B. Lippincott Co., 1989.

Govoni, L.E., and Hayes, J.E. *Drugs and Nursing Implications,* 6th ed. East Norwalk, Conn.: Appleton & Lange, 1988.

Kneisl, C.R., and Ames, S.W. *Adult Health Nursing: A Biopsychosocial Approach.* Reading, Mass.: Addison-Wesley Publishing Co., 1986.

Long, B.C., and Phipps, J.J. *Essentials of Medical-Surgical Nursing: A Nursing Process Approach,* 2nd ed. St. Louis: C.V. Mosby Co., 1988.

Thompson, J.M., et al. *Mosby's Manual of Clinical Nursing,* 2nd ed. St. Louis: C.V. Mosby Co., 1989.

HEPATOBILIARY AND PANCREATIC DISORDERS

Liver Failure

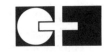

DRG information

DRG 205 Disorders of Liver Except Malignancy, Cirrhosis, or Alcoholic Hepatitis. With Complications or Comorbidity (CC).
Mean LOS = 6.7 days
Principal diagnoses include:
- acute or chronic liver failure
- various types of hepatitis
- hepatomegaly
- jaundice, unspecified etiology
- hepatic infarction
- liver abscess.

DRG 206 Disorders of Liver Except Malignancy, Cirrhosis, or Alcoholic Hepatitis. Without CC.
Mean LOS = 3.8 days
Principal diagnoses include selected principal diagnoses listed under DRG 205. The distinction is that a case assigned DRG 206 has no CC.

Introduction
DEFINITION AND TIME FOCUS

The liver is an essential organ for life, with metabolic, secretory, excretory, and vascular functions. Metabolic functions include glycogen formation, storage, and breakdown; glucose formation; fat storage, breakdown, and synthesis; amino acid deamination; ammonia conversion; and synthesis of plasma proteins, including clotting factors. Secretory functions include bile production and bilirubin conjugation. Excretory functions include detoxification of hormones and drugs. Vascular functions include blood storage and filtration.

In liver failure, which can result from almost all forms of liver disease, parenchymal cells are progressively destroyed and replaced with fibrotic tissue. Once chronically damaged, the liver will never regain normal structure. However, because liver cells retain an enormous regenerative capacity, functional compensation may be attained if precipitating factors are eliminated. This plan focuses on the critically ill patient presenting with acute symptoms of liver failure. These symptoms include hepatic encephalopathy, fluid and electrolyte imbalance from ascites, and related complications of liver failure.

ETIOLOGY AND PRECIPITATING FACTORS
- Laënnec's (alcoholic) cirrhosis with an acute episode of alcohol ingestion, hypovolemia from rapid diuresis or shock, gastrointestinal bleeding, or infection
- acute hepatic failure caused by fulminant hepatitis, hepatotoxic chemicals, or biliary obstruction

Focused assessment guidelines
NURSING HISTORY (Functional health pattern findings)

Health perception–health management pattern
- complains most commonly about weakness and fatigue
- may have been under treatment for chronic alcoholism, hepatitis, or biliary obstructive disease

Nutritional-metabolic pattern
- commonly has diet history that includes excessive alcohol consumption and fat intolerance
- usually reports anorexia and resulting weight loss
- may report ingestion of certain drugs, such as large doses of acetaminophen (Tylenol), tetracycline (Tetracyn), or antituberculosis drugs such as isoniazid (Laniazid)

Elimination pattern
- may report clay-colored stools or dark urine resulting from jaundice

Activity-exercise pattern
- may report psychomotor defects

Sleep-rest pattern
- may report increased drowsiness

Cognitive-perceptual pattern
- patient's family commonly reports intellectual deterioration and slurred speech in beginning stages of hepatic encephalopathy
- patient's family may report personality changes or altered moods

Sexuality-reproductive pattern
- male patient may be impotent because of endocrine changes
- female patient may report erratic menstruation

Role-relationship pattern
- may have job involving hepatotoxic chemicals such as vinyl chloride

PHYSICAL FINDINGS
General appearance
- fever unaffected by antibiotics; reason for fever is unknown

Cardiovascular
• hyperkinetic circulation: flushed extremities, bounding pulse, and capillary pulsations that result primarily from liver cell failure but also may occur with the opening of many normal but functionally inactive arteriovenous anastomoses

Pulmonary
• cyanosis

Neurologic
• hyperactive reflexes, positive Babinski's reflex
• various stages of encephalopathy with resultant altered level of consciousness

Gastrointestinal
• fetor hepaticus: sweetish, slightly fecal breath smell, presumably intestinal in origin
• hepatomegaly, splenomegaly
• ascites
• distant bowel sounds and muffled percussion notes

Endocrine
• male: hypogonadism, gynecomastia
• female: gonadal atrophy

Integumentary
• jaundiced skin, sclera, and mucous membranes from failure to metabolize bilirubin
• vascular spiders: consist of central arteriole with radiating small vessels; usually in vascular territory of superior vena cava (above nipple line)
• palmar erythema: hands warm, palms bright red from estrogen excess
• easy bruising from inadequate clotting factors
• "paper money skin": numerous small blood vessels which resemble silk threads in a dollar bill

DIAGNOSTIC STUDIES
• complete blood count—may reveal decreased hematocrit and hemoglobin values, which reflect the liver's inability to store hematopoietic factors (such as iron, folic acid, and vitamin B_{12}); decreased white blood cell (WBC) and thrombocyte levels, which appear with splenomegaly; and elevated WBC count, which may indicate infection
• increased prothrombin time—reflects decreased synthesis of prothrombin, impaired vitamin K absorption, or both
• enzyme tests—may show elevated serum aspartate aminotransferase (formerly glutamic-oxaloacetic transaminase [SGOT]), serum alanine aminotransferase (formerly glutamic-pyruvic transaminase [SGPT]), alkaline phosphatase, and lactic dehydrogenase values, which reflect hepatocellular or biliary tissue dysfunction and necrosis
• protein metabolite tests (serum albumin and total protein levels)—may reflect impaired protein synthesis

• lipid and carbohydrate tests—may reveal decreased serum cholesterol levels, reflecting impaired hepatic synthesis, or increased levels, reflecting obstructive pathology; elevated serum ammonia values, reflecting impaired hepatic synthesis of urea; and decreased serum glucose levels, which accompany malnutrition
• bilirubin levels (total and direct)—increased in liver disease
• urine and stool tests—may reveal increased urine urobilinogen and reduced fecal urobilinogen values, which accompany jaundice
• testosterone level—reduced
• abdominal ultrasound—may be performed if biliary obstruction is suspected
• abdominal X-rays—may reveal liver enlargement
• angiography or superior mesenteric arteriography—important for evaluation of portal hypertension
• liver scan—reveals abnormalities in hepatic structure
• liver biopsy—indicates extent of hepatic tissue changes
• electroencephalography (EEG)—may show generalized slowing of frequency, which substantiates encephalopathy
• endoscopy—helps locate gastrointestinal bleeding site

POTENTIAL COMPLICATIONS
• hepatorenal failure
• disseminated intravascular coagulation
• bleeding esophageal varices

Collaborative problem: *Deteriorating neurologic status related to hepatic encephalopathy syndrome*

NURSING PRIORITIES: (a) Monitor changes in psychomotor skills, mental status, and speech, and (b) eliminate factors that decrease hepatocellular function.

Interventions

1. Assess neurologic status hourly. Describe the changes observed, typically:
• Stage 1: confusion, altered mood or behavior, psychomotor deficits
• Stage 2: drowsiness, inappropriate behavior
• Stage 3: stupor, marked confusion, and inarticulate speech (although the patient may speak or obey simple commands)
• Stage 4: coma, but response to painful stimuli still present
• Stage 5: deep coma; no response to painful stimuli.

2. Assess for asterixis (flapping tremor of the wrist).

3. Auscultate the chest and assess respiratory rate hourly. Administer oxygen therapy via nasal prongs, as ordered. Anticipate more aggressive measures, such as intubation, if the encephalopathy progresses to coma.

4. Stop intake of dietary protein. Also stop administration of all drugs containing nitrogen, such as ammonium chloride, urea (Ureaphil), and methionine, as ordered.

5. Administer neomycin (Mycifradin) via nasogastric tube, if ordered. The usual dose is 1 g.

6. Administer lactulose (Cephulac) via nasogastric tube, if ordered. The usual dose is 10 to 30 ml. Monitor for diarrhea; if it occurs, consult with the doctor about reducing the dose.

7. Stop any diuretic therapy, as ordered.

8. Administer neutral, acid-free enema solutions, as ordered.

9. Avoid all sedatives metabolized primarily by the liver. If the patient is uncontrollable, administer half the usual dose of barbiturate, as ordered. Morphine and paraldehyde (Paral) are absolutely contraindicated.

Rationales

1. Symptoms vary; therefore, close monitoring is important. The encephalopathy syndrome results from impaired nitrogen metabolism, passage of toxic substances of intestinal origin (ammonia, active amines, and short-chain fatty acids) to the brain, and numerous other metabolic abnormalities occurring in hepatocellular failure. The toxic substances are thought to interfere with glucose metabolism and cerebral blood flow. Chronic exposure of brain cells to these substances through repeated bouts of encephalopathy results in irreversible damage.

2. This sign, caused by impaired flow of proprioceptive information to the brain stem reticular formation, indicates that the patient is in the early stages of encephalopathy.

3. The patient with long-standing liver disease will have developed decreased oxygen saturation and decreased diffusing capacity before the onset of encephalopathy. Therefore, respiratory support measures are commonly required.

4. Intake of dietary protein and drugs containing nitrogen increase the accumulation of nitrogenous substances that the liver cannot break down.

5. Neomycin decreases the intestinal bacteria that produce ammonia.

6. Although lactulose's exact mechanism of action is unclear, it may be instrumental in chelating ammonia (NH_3), acting as an osmotic agent for inducing diarrhea, changing gut pH resulting in excretion of ammonium (NH_4^+), or changing gut flora to decrease the growth of ammonia-forming bacteria. Diarrhea is a sign of excessive dosage.

7. If the patient has hepatic cirrhosis, the most common cause of hepatic encephalopathy is excessive diuresis from diuretic therapy. The resulting hypovolemia further reduces hepatic perfusion, causing the encephalopathy.

8. Purging the intestines reduces ammonium absorption and may result in improvement of clinical symptoms and EEG readings.

9. The patient in impending coma is extremely sensitive to sedatives. Drugs metabolized primarily by the liver are particularly dangerous because toxic accumulations can occur rapidly from the impaired hepatic perfusion. Some sedation may be necessary, however, if the patient becomes agitated as hepatic failure worsens and toxic metabolic substances accumulate. Long-acting, short-chain barbiturates that are excreted largely by the kidney are preferred. Morphine and paraldehyde may cause coma.

10. Teach the patient and family about necessary interventions, as appropriate. Emphasize causes of changes in neurologic status and rationales for methods to reduce encephalopathy.

10. Although patient teaching may be of limited success because of altered level of consciousness, brief and repeated explanations may help the patient feel more secure psychologically. Teaching family members may help them understand mood swings and behavior changes.

11. Additional individualized interventions: _____

11. Rationales: _____

_____

_____

Target outcome criteria
Within 24 to 48 hours of admission, the patient will:
• awaken and display improved neurologic status
• display a decreased need for respiratory support.

Collaborative problem: *High risk for fever related to liver disease or infection*

NURSING PRIORITY: Assist in determining the cause of fever.

Interventions

1. Assess temperature every 4 hours. If elevated, assess more frequently. Consult with the doctor about abnormal readings.

2. Observe for cloudy, concentrated urine and pain upon urination, if a catheter is not in place. Avoid catheterization, if possible.

3. Auscultate lung fields at least every 2 hours. Also assess respiratory rate, skin color, and level of cyanosis.

4. Auscultate bowel sounds at least every 4 hours. Observe for abdominal rigidity, increased abdominal girth, or vomiting.

5. If infection is diagnosed, assist with treatment, as ordered; for example, administer antibiotics. If the fever stems solely from liver disease, provide symptomatic care, such as frequent linen changes.

6. Additional individualized interventions: _____

Rationales

1. Continuous low-grade fever rarely exceeding 100.4° F (38° C) is seen in about one-third of patients with liver disease. This fever is unaffected by antibiotics and attributable to liver disease alone, although the reason for it is unknown. However, the patient may have fever from infection. The liver normally is bacteriologically sterile and filters bacteria from the bloodstream. Cirrhosis allows bacteria to pass into the circulation. Differentiation of possible causes of fever is necessary for effective treatment.

2. These signs indicate urinary tract infection. Avoiding catheterization reduces the risk of infection. Remember, urine may be dark amber because of jaundice.

3. Respiratory difficulties may indicate aspiration pneumonia. Pulmonary arteriovenous shunting from liver disease and the resultant decreased oxygen saturation place the patient at increased risk for pneumonia.

4. Spontaneous peritonitis is known to occur in patients with liver disease.

5. Infection requires prompt, aggressive treatment because it promotes protein accumulation from tissue catabolism. Low-grade fever may remain if fever results solely from liver disease. Frequent linen changes reduce discomfort from diaphoresis.

6. Rationales: _____

_____

Target outcome criteria
Within 24 to 48 hours of admission, the patient will:
• have the cause of fever determined
• have appropriate therapy initiated.

Collaborative problem: *Fluid and electrolyte imbalance related to ascites*

NURSING PRIORITY: Restore a more normal fluid balance.

Interventions

1. Closely monitor fluid and electrolyte status, including strict intake and output measurements, hourly determination of urine specific gravity, daily weights, and assessment of lung fields at least every 2 hours for crackles or gurgles.

2. Percuss and palpate the abdomen every 4 hours. Do not rely solely on abdominal girth measurements.

3. Maintain strict bed rest.

4. Implement therapy, as ordered:
• dietary restrictions, typically sodium intake of 0.5 g/day and fluid intake of 1 liter/day
• diuretic administration, typically furosemide (Lasix) or spironolactone (Aldactone)
• postoperative care after peritoneovenous (LeVeen) shunt insertion.

5. Teach the patient and family about necessary interventions, as appropriate.

6. Additional individualized interventions: _____

_____

Rationales

1. Close monitoring of fluid status is necessary to judge the degree of cardiovascular and pulmonary compromise imposed by ascites. In liver failure, ascites develops from lowered plasma oncotic pressure, portal venous hypertension, and sodium and water retention. The lowered plasma oncotic pressure results from the liver's failure to synthesize albumin. This lowered oncotic pressure, combined with increased hydrostatic pressure from portal hypertension, causes fluid to shift into interstitial spaces (third spacing) in the peritoneal cavity. The resulting depletion of effective intravascular volume causes the renal tubules to retain sodium and water via the aldosterone effect.

2. Percussion and palpation allow evaluation of changes in fluid shifting. Dullness on percussion in the flanks is the earliest sign of ascites and indicates approximately 2 liters of fluid. The liver and spleen may be palpated if only moderate amounts of fluid are present; with tense ascites, it is difficult to palpate abdominal viscera. A fluid thrill indicates a large amount of free fluid. It is a very late sign of fluid under tension. Abdominal girth measurements are unreliable as gaseous distention is common.

3. Recumbency increases renal perfusion and the kidneys' ability to excrete excess fluid.

4. The rate of ascitic fluid reabsorption is limited to 700 to 900 ml a day. Limiting sodium and water intake reduces ascitic fluid production, while diuretic administration increases fluid excretion. Shunt insertion controls ascites in less than 5% of patients with liver failure.

5. Understanding the effects of ascites and treatment methods improves the patient's and family's cooperation with the treatment plan, increasing the likelihood of its effectiveness.

6. Rationales: _____

_____

Target outcome criteria
Within 4 days of admission, the patient will:
• manifest urine output of at least 60 ml/hour
• display urinary sodium excretion greater than 10 mEq/day

• show lessened ascites and edema, as evidenced by decreased weight and improved respiratory status.

Collaborative problem: *High risk for gastrointestinal hemorrhage related to esophageal varices*

NURSING PRIORITY: Monitor for, prevent, or promptly treat hemorrhage.

Interventions

1. Observe for and report signs of esophageal bleeding, such as hematemesis. Anticipate drug treatment with vasopressin (Pitressin) or propranolol (Inderal), or insertion of a gastric compression tube. See the "Gastrointestinal Hemorrhage" plan, page 394, for specific nursing interventions.

2. Additional individualized interventions: _____

Rationales

1. The mechanism of esophageal varices formation is unclear; they are thought to be caused by excessive portal venous backflow into the esophageal vasculature. Hematemesis of frank red blood indicates active bleeding. Vasopressin constricts blood vessels and smooth muscle in the GI tract, while propranolol lowers blood pressure. A compression tube may control bleeding varices temporarily. The "Gastrointestinal Hemorrhage" plan contains detailed information on detecting and treating bleeding varices.

2. Rationales: _____

Target outcome criteria
Within 24 hours of detection of bleeding, the patient will:
• exhibit vital signs within normal limits
• have warm, dry skin.

Nursing diagnosis: *Nutritional deficit related to catabolism from liver disease*

NURSING PRIORITY: Restore metabolism to an anabolic state.

Interventions

1. Implement dietary prescriptions, as ordered. Maintain high caloric intake, usually 1,600 calories/day, by administering high carbohydrate I.V. infusions, as ordered. If jaundice is present, do not administer oral fat or fat infusions.

2. If encephalopathy is present, stop protein intake. Once encephalopathy has subsided, begin protein intake at 20-g/day increments. Monitor closely for recurrence of encephalopathy.

3. Emphasize to the patient and family the importance of dietary restriction.

4. Additional individualized interventions: _____

Rationales

1. Dietary control of precursors to toxic metabolites plays an important role in the control of symptoms. High-caloric intake is necessary to meet energy needs. Jaundice indicates decreased bile salt levels, which impair fat absorption.

2. Inability to metabolize protein causes the blood ammonia level to rise, producing encephalopathy. Restricting protein intake helps eliminate symptoms. Gradual reintroduction of protein allows careful determination of the amount the patient can metabolize safely. Recurrence of symptoms indicates the need for permanent protein restriction.

3. The necessary restrictions may make the diet unpalatable and difficult to accept. Understanding the rationale increases the patient's motivation to follow recommendations and the likelihood of family support.

4. Rationales: _____

Target outcome criterion
Within 96 hours of admission, the patient will tolerate protein intake.

HEPATOBILIARY AND PANCREATIC DISORDERS

Nursing diagnosis: *High risk for impaired skin integrity related to jaundice, increased bleeding tendencies, malnutrition, and ascites*

NURSING PRIORITY: Maintain or restore skin integrity.

Interventions

1. Monitor skin condition. Particularly note the presence of vascular spiders.

2. Monitor prothrombin time, as ordered.

3. Turn the patient and rub bony prominences every 2 hours. Implement additional measures in the "Impaired Physical Mobility" plan, page 36, as appropriate.

4. Provide symptomatic treatment of pruritus, as necessary; for example, bathe the skin with cool water.

5. Additional individualized interventions: _____

Rationales

1. Careful monitoring of skin status, commonly overlooked, allows early detection of skin problems to which liver failure patients are particularly susceptible. Vascular spiders can bleed profusely.

2. Liver failure impairs the synthesis of clotting factors. A prolonged prothrombin time increases the risk of skin bruising and breakdown.

3. Malnutrition and ascites predispose the patient to pressure ulcer formation. The "Impaired Physical Mobility" plan itemizes detailed information on potential skin problems.

4. Pruritus, which results from jaundice, can cause extreme discomfort. Treatment may be limited because phenothiazides and antihistamines are contraindicated if the patient has encephalopathy.

5. Rationales: _____

Target outcome criterion
Within 48 hours of admission, the patient will have no apparent skin breakdown.

Discharge planning

NURSING DISCHARGE CRITERIA
Upon the patient's discharge, documentation shows evidence of:
• improved neurologic status
• absence of respiratory complications
• adequate urine output
• reduction of ascites and weight
• normal temperature or stable low-grade fever
• resumption of I.V. or oral protein and fat intake.

PATIENT-FAMILY TEACHING CHECKLIST
Document evidence that the patient and family demonstrate an understanding of:
___ relationship between alcohol consumption and exacerbation of liver disease
___ causes of changes in neurologic status and relationship to liver disease
___ effects of ascites and methods of treatment
___ importance of diet in liver disease.

DOCUMENTATION CHECKLIST
Using outcome criteria as a guide, document:
___ clinical status on admission
___ significant changes in status
___ pertinent laboratory and diagnostic test findings
___ weight
___ fluid intake and output measurements
___ fluctuations in fever and associated symptoms
___ skin integrity
___ any signs of GI bleeding
___ patient-family teaching
___ discharge planning.

ASSOCIATED PLANS OF CARE
Gastrointestinal Hemorrhage
Impaired Physical Mobility
Nutritional Deficit
Sensory-Perceptual Alteration

References

Briones, T. "Gastrointestinal System," in *Core Curriculum for Critical Care Nursing,* 4th ed. Edited by Alspach, J. Philadelphia: W.B. Saunders Co., 1991.

Keith, J. "Hepatic Failure: Etiologies, Manifestations, and Management," *Critical Care Nurse* 5(1):60-86, January 1985.

Luckmann, J., and Sorensen, K. *Medical-Surgical Nursing: A Psychophysiologic Approach,* 3rd ed. Philadelphia: W.B. Saunders Co., 1987.

Sherlock, S. *Diseases of the Liver and Biliary System.* Boston: Blackwell Scientific Publications, 1987.

Pancreatitis

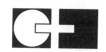

DRG information

DRG 204 Disorder of Pancreas Except Malignancy.
   Mean LOS = 6.1 days
   Principal diagnoses include:
   • pancreatitis
   • benign neoplasm of pancreas, except islets of Langerhans
   • injury to any portion of the pancreas.

Introduction
DEFINITION AND TIME FOCUS

Pancreatitis (inflammation of the pancreas) is an auto-digestive disorder in which premature activation of pancreatic proteolytic enzymes damages the organ itself. The exact physiologic mechanism is unknown, but theoretically duodenal reflux or spasm, or blockage of pancreatic ducts by gallstones or edema, may result in the backup of pancreatic secretions. Pancreatitis may be a complication of surgery for other biliary tract or gastrointestinal disease; numerous other causative factors have also been implicated.

   Depending on the nature and severity of the disorder, significant edema, tissue necrosis, and life-threatening hemorrhage may result. Pancreatitis may be either acute or chronic. Chronic pancreatitis causes progressive loss of pancreatic function and may be associated with repeated bouts of acute pancreatitis. This plan focuses on the care of the patient who is admitted for diagnosis and management of an episode of acute pancreatitis.

ETIOLOGY AND PRECIPITATING FACTORS
• alcohol abuse
• cholecystitis or cholelithiasis
• abdominal surgery
• trauma
• peptic or duodenal ulcer
• hyperparathyroidism
• viral hepatitis
• mumps
• hyperlipidemia
• anorexia nervosa
• ischemia related to shock
• metabolic disorders
• use of certain medications: thiazide diuretics, steroids, sulfonamides, oral contraceptives, tetracycline, acetaminophen (in excessive doses)

Focused assessment guidelines
NURSING HISTORY (Functional health pattern findings)

Health perception–health management pattern
• commonly complains of severe abdominal pain in epigastric or umbilical region that radiates into back or flank
• may note that pain increases when supine or when food is taken and after administration of certain narcotics
• may have history of gallbladder disease or alcoholism with recent dietary indiscretion or drinking binge

Nutritional-metabolic pattern
• commonly describes nausea or vomiting
• may complain of anorexia
• may note recent weight loss

Elimination pattern
• may note increased flatus
• may describe steatorrhea (associated with chronic disease)

Activity-exercise pattern
• may prefer hunched sitting position because of pain
• may become dizzy or faint when standing

Cognitive-perceptual pattern
• may complain of shoulder pain or frequent hiccups (if diaphragmatic irritation is present)
• may complain of pleuritic-like pain that increases with deep inspiration

Coping–stress tolerance pattern
• may habitually use unhealthy coping mechanisms (such as alcoholism)

PHYSICAL FINDINGS
General appearance
• hunched posture
• restlessness

Cardiovascular
• fever
• tachycardia
• hypotension

Pulmonary
If pleural effusion is present:
- reduced chest excursion
- crackles
- tachypnea

Gastrointestinal
- abdominal distention
- guarding
- reduced or absent bowel sounds
- ascites

Neurologic
- seizures
- stupor
- neuromuscular irritability

Integumentary
- jaundice
- pallor
- diaphoresis
- Cullen's sign (ecchymosis around umbilicus)
- Grey Turner's sign (ecchymosis in flank, retroperitoneal, and groin area)
- cool extremities
- cyanosis (if advanced shock)

Musculoskeletal
If hypocalcemia is present:
- tetany
- positive Chvostek's sign
- positive Trousseau's sign

Renal
- oliguria (if acute tubular necrosis is present)

DIAGNOSTIC STUDIES
- serum amylase level—elevated in acute pancreatitis; although not specific for pancreatitis, increased enzyme levels occur during pancreatic inflammation
- amylase-creatinine clearance ratio—indicates acute pancreatitis if greater than 5%
- urine amylase level—elevated for the first 3 to 5 days of illness; it reflects pancreatic secretion better than serum value; in acute pancreatitis, renal clearance of amylase is markedly increased
- serum calcium level—decreased, usually less than 8 mg/dl (unless hyperparathyroidism is present, in which instance value may be normal)

- complete blood count (CBC)—likely to reveal leukocytosis; hemoglobin and hematocrit values vary depending on fluid status, hemorrhage, or degree of compensation
- serum and urine glucose levels—may be elevated because of altered insulin production
- serum lipase level—elevated
- serum and urine bilirubin levels—elevated
- serum albumin value—usually less than 3.2 g/dl
- serum triglyceride levels—may be elevated
- serum electrolyte levels—may reveal hypokalemia or hyponatremia
- computed tomography (CT) scan—visualizes tumors, dilated pancreatic ducts, calcification, or pseudocyst
- abdominal ultrasound—may provide evidence of inflammation, edema, gallstones, calcified pancreatic ducts, abscess, organ enlargement, hematoma, or pseudocyst (cavities of exudate, blood, and pancreatic products that may expand and compress other organs)
- abdominal X-rays—may reveal areas of calcification or adhesions, or identify indicators of reduced bowel motility
- upper GI X-rays—may show enlarged pancreas or may reveal stomach displacement from pseudocyst formation
- chest X-ray—may reveal diaphragmatic elevation if abscess formation or peritonitis is present; may identify areas of atelectasis or effusion
- I.V. cholangiography—used to rule out acute cholecystitis as cause of symptoms
- paracentesis—may reveal elevated amylase levels or blood, both associated with acute pancreatitis

POTENTIAL COMPLICATIONS
- hypovolemic shock
- hemorrhage
- adult respiratory distress syndrome
- renal failure
- pulmonary edema
- myocardial infarction
- peritonitis or sepsis
- pleural effusion
- abscess formation
- hyperglycemia or diabetes mellitus
- paralytic ileus
- pseudocyst formation

Collaborative problem: *High risk for hypovolemic shock related to hemorrhage, fluid shifts, hyperglycemia, or vomiting*

NURSING PRIORITY: Maintain fluid volume.

Interventions

1. Monitor vital signs, fluid intake and output, hemodynamic pressures, and electrocardiography findings according to Appendix A, "Monitoring Standards," or unit protocol. Immediately report any findings indicating hypovolemia.

2. Maintain I.V. access through peripheral or central lines. Monitor I.V. fluid replacement, usually with lactated Ringer's solution, dextrans, or albumin. If hemorrhage is suspected, anticipate and monitor transfusion, as ordered.

3. Assess serum glucose or fingerstick glucose and urine ketone levels every 4 to 6 hours or more frequently if severe hyperglycemia is present. Administer regular insulin, as ordered, and monitor and document effects.

4. Monitor serum electrolytes daily, as ordered, including serum calcium. See Appendix C, "Fluid and Electrolyte Imbalances." Stay alert for characteristic signs of severe hypocalcemia: neuromuscular irritability and tetany.

5. Maintain continuous gastric drainage with low suction, as ordered, preferably with a double-lumen tube. Administer anticholinergic medications, if ordered. Test gastric drainage for blood at least every 8 hours. Withhold food and fluids.

6. Administer I.V. dopamine (Intropin) or other vasopressor, as ordered, if hypotension persists.

7. Prepare the patient for the surgery if hemodynamic parameters do not stabilize in response to therapeutic interventions.

8. Additional individualized interventions: _____

Rationales

1. The damaged pancreas releases several substances that have systemic vasoactive effects. Kinins increase vascular permeability and cause vasodilation, increasing the likelihood of shock. Elastase and chymotrypsin cause necrosis and damage blood vessels, which may cause hemorrhage. In addition, pancreatic fluid and blood entering the peritoneum may cause chemical irritation of the bowel and bowel atony, resulting in fluid shift into interstitial spaces (third spacing) as fluid leaks out of the damaged intestine. Reduced renal blood flow may lead to acute tubular necrosis.

2. Rapid I.V. infusion of large volumes of fluid or blood is the primary immediate treatment indicated for hypovolemia. Untreated, hypovolemia quickly results in circulatory collapse and tissue death.

3. Injury to the insulin-producing islet cells of the pancreas commonly decreases insulin production and causes at least transient hyperglycemia. If damage is severe, particularly if chronic pancreatitis is also present, overt diabetes mellitus may develop. Hyperglycemia may contribute further to functional hypovolemia as the body responds to the hyperosmolar state with further fluid shifts.

4. Fluid shifts associated with acute pancreatitis may result in various electrolyte imbalances, including hypokalemia and hyponatremia. Hypocalcemia is a common finding, possibly from the bonding of calcium with fatty substances. Clinically significant hypocalcemia is associated with a poorer prognosis.

5. Draining gastric secretions removes a stimulus for pancreatic secretions, thus reducing the release of vasoactive substances and allowing the damaged pancreas to rest. A double-lumen tube is preferable for continuous suction because the air vent minimizes the risk of damage to the gastric mucosa. Anticholinergic use is controversial because such medication may contribute to ileus; some practitioners believe anticholinergics effectively reduce pancreatic secretions, but this is unproven. Withholding food and fluids prevents stimulation of gastric secretions.

6. In acute pancreatitis, the release of myocardial depressant factor from the pancreas is thought to reduce cardiac output. Dopamine has a positive inotropic effect on the heart, increasing cardiac output, and a dopaminergic effect on the kidneys, improving renal blood flow.

7. Persistent shock indicates the need for surgical intervention to stop bleeding, relieve duct obstruction, drain an abscess or pseudocyst, or evaluate other possible intra-abdominal pathology.

8. Rationales: _____

Target outcome criteria
Within 24 hours of admission and then continuously, the patient will:
• have vital signs within normal limits for patient
• display serum glucose, urine glucose, and ketone levels returning to normal

• have serum electrolyte levels returning to normal.

Nursing diagnosis: *Pain related to edema, necrosis, autodigestive processes, abdominal distention, abscess formation, ileus, or peritonitis*

NURSING PRIORITIES: (a) Monitor, evaluate, and relieve pain, and (b) treat underlying cause.

Interventions

1. Assess pain, noting location, character, severity, radiation, frequency, and any accompanying symptoms. Immediately report changes in pain quality or location, particularly if abdominal rigidity, reduced or absent bowel sounds, palpable abdominal mass, or other indications of generalized peritonitis or abscess occur. See the "Pain" plan, page 69.

2. Ensure that blood samples for serum amylase and lipase levels are obtained before administering analgesics.

3. Medicate, as ordered, with narcotic analgesics, usually meperidine (Demerol). Observe for increased pain after narcotic administration and collaborate with the doctor to adjust pain control regimen, as indicated.

4. Administer antacids, as ordered, clamping the gastric tube for 30 minutes after administration. When oral intake is resumed, avoid simultaneous administration of antacids with oral cimetidine (Tagamet).

5. If the patient's condition permits, begin teaching dietary and life-style measures that reduce discomfort and help avert recurrence of acute attacks. Include family members in all teaching. Address the following considerations:
• need for lifelong avoidance of alcohol
• low-fat diet, depending upon presence of gallbladder disease
• avoidance of caffeine or other substances linked to increased gastric secretions.

6. Additional individualized interventions: _____

Rationales

1. Evaluating the nature of the patient's pain is essential for early detection of complications. Typically, the pain accompanying acute pancreatitis is severe, steady, and felt across the entire abdomen, and it commonly radiates to the back or flank. Tenderness to deep palpation may occur; however, the abdomen usually remains soft. Abdominal rigidity and reduced bowel sounds may indicate peritonitis; a mass may indicate abscess or pseudocyst. Prompt surgical intervention is warranted if these occur. The "Pain" plan contains general interventions for any patient in pain.

2. Many analgesics, including meperidine (Demerol) and morphine, may elevate serum amylase and lipase levels, limiting the usefulness of these findings in diagnosis.

3. The severity of pain associated with acute pancreatitis generally warrants narcotic analgesia. Morphine is thought to increase spasm of Oddi's sphincter and thus is usually avoided for these patients. However, other analgesics, including meperidine, may also have such effects to some degree.

4. Antacids reduce gastric acidity and associated discomfort; some products may also act to relieve flatulence and distention. Antacids may impair cimetidine absorption if given at the same time.

5. The patient's condition may limit teaching, but introductory material can lay the groundwork for more thorough discussion after the patient has stabilized. Alcohol is a common factor in the recurrence of acute pancreatitis, although the exact physiologic mechanism is not known. Gallbladder disease may indicate the need for a low-fat diet to avoid exacerbating symptoms. Caffeine causes increased gastric acid secretion and thus increases pancreatic activity.

6. Rationales: _____

Target outcome criterion
Within 2 hours of the onset of pain, the patient will verbalize pain relief.

Nursing diagnosis: *High risk for injury: complications related to pulmonary insults, hypovolemia, alcoholism, or other factors*

NURSING PRIORITY: Prevent or detect and promptly treat complications.

Interventions

1. Assess lung sounds, sputum production, skin color, and respiratory rate and effort frequently, at least every 2 hours. Report decreased breath sounds, crackles, productive cough, increased respiratory rate or effort or other signs of respiratory complications immediately. Monitor arterial blood gas levels daily or as ordered, and report abnormal results.

2. Encourage deep breathing, coughing, incentive spirometer use, and position changes at least every 2 hours.

3. Assess for indicators of paralytic ileus, perforated viscus, or peritonitis, such as reduced or absent bowel sounds, vomiting, increased abdominal distention, rigid or boardlike abdomen, and tympany.

4. Monitor for signs and symptoms of pseudocyst development, such as increasing tenderness, palpable mass, upper abdominal pain, diarrhea, and worsening of general condition despite interventions.

5. After any surgical intervention, assess for and report any indications of colonic, enteric, or pancreatic fistula. Observe for signs of a fistula opening to the skin: pinpoint openings at wound edges or within the wound, green or yellow wound drainage, and excoriated wound edges. If the fistula opens to the skin, collect drainage, provide frequent meticulous skin care, measure drainage pH, and replace fluids and electrolytes as ordered. Also observe for signs of an internal fistula: electrolyte imbalance, hypovolemia, fever, and peritonitis. If the fistula is internal, anticipate surgery.

6. Assess for and report indications of disseminated intravascular coagulation (DIC), such as bleeding or oozing from wounds, drains, or puncture sites; purpura of the chest or abdomen; petechiae; hematuria; melena; or epistaxis. Guaiac test all drainage. See the "Disseminated Intravascular Coagulation" plan, page 625, for details.

7. Assess for early indications of renal impairment, such as oliguria or anuria, increased urine osmolality, and elevated blood urea nitrogen level.

8. Be alert for indications of alcohol withdrawal syndrome, such as agitation, tremors, insomnia, hypertension, and anxiety. If alcoholism is a likely contributing factor to the patient's condition, consult with the doctor regarding measures to prevent or minimize alcohol withdrawal syndrome.

Rationales

1. The patient with acute pancreatitis is at increased risk for pulmonary complications from edema, fluid shifts, diaphragmatic irritation, and possible decreased myocardial contractility. Adult respiratory distress syndrome, pulmonary edema, pleural effusion, or pneumonia may occur. Endotracheal intubation and mechanical ventilation may be required for adequate oxygenation if respiratory impairment is a factor. Early intervention reduces the risk of significant hypoxic damage.

2. Abdominal distention, pain, and the use of narcotic medications may contribute to reduced chest expansion, predisposing the patient to pulmonary abnormalities. These measures help reexpand atelectatic areas and improve clearance of pulmonary secretions.

3. These conditions may arise as a result of chemical irritation of the bowel, necrosis, and abscess formation associated with acute pancreatitis. Without immediate surgical intervention, sepsis may develop.

4. Pseudocysts are pockets, left in the pancreas after tissue necrosis, in which blood, tissue debris, and pancreatic secretions accumulate. They may resolve spontaneously, rupture and cause chemical peritonitis, or grow so large that they compress other organs. Intervention may include drainage, with percutaneous aspiration guided by CT scan, or surgical resection.

5. Fistulas, abnormal openings from body cavities or hollow organs to other cavities or the skin surface, can result from impaired wound healing around surgical anastomosis sites or an anastamotic leak. Pancreatic fistulas are more common when necrosis of the head or midportion of the pancreas leaves a viable, juice-secreting tail behind. Because pancreatic secretions have a high enzyme content, drainage collection minimizes skin excoriation; it also helps predict fluid replacement needs. The pancreas produces bicarbonate, so an alkaline pH confirms pancreatic fistula drainage. Fluid and electrolyte loss from fistula drainage can cause dehydration, hypokalemia, and hyponatremia.

6. DIC is a major potential complication associated with acute pancreatitis, possibly from release of tissue fragments, toxins associated with shock, or other physiologic mechanisms. Early detection allows prompt treatment. The "Disseminated Intravascular Coagulation" plan contains interventions for this disorder.

7. Hypovolemia may decrease renal perfusion and lead to acute renal failure. Renal impairment may also occur in acute pancreatitis when volume status is normal; the mechanism involved is unclear, but may involve DIC.

8. Because excessive alcohol intake is a common factor in acute pancreatitis, always consider the possibility of overt or hidden alcoholism. Untreated, the withdrawal syndrome may progress rapidly to seizures, hallucinations, hyperthermia, other severe complications, or death.

HEPATOBILIARY AND PANCREATIC DISORDERS

9. Additional individualized interventions: _____

9. Rationales: _____

Target outcome criteria
Throughout the hospital stay, the patient will:
• perform pulmonary hygiene measures as instructed
• show no evidence of complications

• receive prompt treatment if complications develop.

Nursing diagnosis: *Nutritional deficit related to vomiting, pain, gastric suction, nothing by mouth (NPO) status, and impaired digestion*

NURSING PRIORITY: Maintain or restore adequate nutritional intake.

Interventions

1. Assess nutritional status. See the "Nutritional Deficit" plan, page 63, for details.

2. Administer total parenteral nutrition (TPN), as ordered, and monitor patient response, including careful monitoring of glucose levels. Consult the "Total Parenteral Nutrition" plan, page 411, for details.

3. As the patient's condition permits, institute dietary teaching, as indicated, including:
• diabetic diet
• use of pancreatic enzymes, if recommended
• avoidance of alcohol and caffeine.

4. Additional individualized interventions: _____

Rationales

1. Baseline assessment of nutritional status is essential for planning appropriate maintenance or replacement therapy. The "Nutritional Deficit" plan provides details on evaluating nutritional status.

2. Oral nutrient intake during an acute pancreatitis episode tends to exacerbate pain and increase pancreatic activity. In the patient requiring prolonged NPO status, TPN may be indicated to avert malnutrition. Increased protein and calories are necessary for healing and for maintenance of the body's immunologic defenses. In pancreatitis, glucose levels may be elevated because of damage to the insulin-producing islet cells in the pancreas; if hyperglycemia has been present, the additional glucose in the TPN solution makes insulin dosage adjustment necessary. Enteral products may be contraindicated during the initial phases of pancreatitis.

3. Careful dietary teaching may help the patient avoid recurrences. A diabetic diet may be necessary because of reduced insulin production. Oral intake of pancreatic enzymes helps correct deficiencies. Alcohol and caffeine avoidance eliminates common triggers of acute pancreatitis.

4. Rationales: _____

Target outcome criterion
Throughout the hospital stay, the patient will maintain adequate nutritional intake (see the "Nutritional Deficit" plan for specific criteria).

Discharge planning
NURSING DISCHARGE CRITERIA
Upon the patient's discharge, documentation shows evidence of:
• stable vital signs
• normal electrolyte values
• serum glucose controlled by medication, as needed
• pain controlled by medication
• absence of pulmonary or cardiovascular complications
• normal bowel sounds and elimination
• normal urine output
• adequate nutritional intake.

PATIENT-FAMILY TEACHING CHECKLIST
Document evidence that the patient and family demonstrate an understanding of:
— disease, precipitating factors, and prognosis
— dietary considerations
— diabetic teaching, as condition requires
— signs and symptoms indicating recurrence or complications
— pain relief measures.

DOCUMENTATION CHECKLIST
Using outcome criteria as a guide, document:
— clinical status on admission
— significant changes in status
— pertinent laboratory and diagnostic test findings
— fluid intake and output
— bowel function
— patient-family teaching
— discharge planning.

ASSOCIATED PLANS OF CARE
Adult Respiratory Distress Syndrome
Diabetic Ketoacidosis
Disseminated Intravascular Coagulation
Ineffective Individual Coping
Knowledge Deficit
Nutritional Deficit
Pain
Pulmonary Embolism
Total Parenteral Nutrition

References
Brozenec, S., and Patras, A. "Gastrointestinal Surgery," in *Critical Care Nursing of the Surgical Patient.* Edited by Shekleton, M., and Litwak, K. Philadelphia: W.B. Saunders Co., 1991.

Fain, J., and Amato-Vealey, E. "Acute Pancreatitis: A Gastrointestinal Emergency," *Critical Care Nurse* 8(5):47-61, July-August 1988.

Hennessy, K. "Nutritional Support and Gastrointestinal Disease," *Nursing Clinics of North America* 24(2):373-82, June 1989.

Jeffres, C. "Complications of Acute Pancreatitis," *Critical Care Nurse* 9(4):38-46, April 1989.

Luckmann, J., and Sorenson, K. *Medical-Surgical Nursing: A Psychophysiologic Approach,* 3rd ed. Philadelphia: W.B. Saunders Co., 1987.

Reber, H., ed. "The Pancreas," *Surgical Clinics of North America* 69(3):447-686, June 1989.

Sarles, H., Bernard, J., and Gullo, L. "Pathogenesis of Chronic Pancreatitis," *Gut* 31(6):629-31, June 1990.

Singh, M., and Simsek, H. "Ethanol and the Pancreas," *Gastroenterology* 98(4):1051-62, April 1990.

Stanten, R., and Frey, C. "Comprehensive Management of Acute Necrotizing Pancreatitis and Pancreatic Abscess," *Archives of Surgery* 125(10):1269-75, October 1990.

HEPATOBILIARY AND PANCREATIC DISORDERS

Amputation

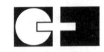

DRG information
DRG 213 Amputation for Musculoskeletal System and Connective Tissue Disorders.
Mean LOS = 9.7 days
Additional DRG Information: DRG 213 is only provided as a rough guideline. Determining the correct DRG for amputations depends on the underlying disease or type of trauma, and the site and level of amputation.

Introduction
DEFINITION AND TIME FOCUS
Amputation is the surgical removal of an irreparably damaged or diseased limb. An amputation may be immediate because of the nature of an injury (such as from a motor vehicle accident or burn), or offered together with a prosthesis to improve function. The stump is closed with sutures or staples unless massive infection was present before surgery, in which case a guillotine-like surgery is performed and the wound is left unsutured. Traction may be applied to prevent skin retraction and to allow healing.
    This plan focuses on providing care after amputation of an upper or lower extremity.

ETIOLOGY AND PRECIPITATING FACTORS
• advanced peripheral vascular disease (especially when associated with diabetes mellitus, infection, and smoking)
• trauma (such as that from crushing injuries, motor vehicle accidents, or industrial accidents)
• thermal injury (such as that from frostbite, chemical exposure, or burns)
• tumors
• congenital anomalies

Focused assessment guidelines
NURSING HISTORY (Functional health pattern findings)

Health perception — health management pattern
• may be under treatment for diabetes mellitus, atherosclerotic arterial occlusive disease, or osteomyelitis
• if a smoker with peripheral vascular disease, likelihood of amputation is significantly increased

Activity-exercise pattern
• if lower limb is involved, may experience difficulty in ambulation, leading to an altered exercise pattern
• may report severe pain associated with exercise in lower limbs if peripheral vascular disease is present

Sleep-rest pattern
• may report interrupted sleep pattern associated with discomfort

Cognitive-perceptual pattern
• may report tingling or burning sensation or paresthesia

Self-perception — self-concept pattern
• may experience difficulty accepting body-image change
• may verbalize concern about returning to work

Role-relationship pattern
• may voice concern about relationships and rejection by others
• may verbalize fear of role change

Coping — stress tolerance pattern
• may have failed to seek or follow medical treatment for problem, necessitating amputation
• may use denial to deal with current experience

PHYSICAL FINDINGS
Integumentary
(in affected extremity)
• shiny skin
• skin atrophy
• skin cool to touch
• cyanosis or rubor of extremities when in dependent position
• thickened nails
• stasis ulcer
• edema
• nonhealing wound
• palpable mass

Cardiovascular
• capillary refill time greater than 3 seconds
• severe, cramping pain with exercise, usually relieved by rest
• decreased pulse amplitude
• diminished or absent peripheral pulses

Musculoskeletal
• limited limb movement
• limited ambulation
• pain
• contractures
• protective holding of affected extremity

DIAGNOSTIC STUDIES
• wound culture and sensitivity — if infection is present, may identify causative microorganism and identify appropriate antibiotics
• complete blood count — elevated white blood cell count indicates infection
• erythrocyte sedimentation rate — elevation indicates an inflammatory response

- X-rays—may reveal skeletal trauma, anomalies, or a mass
- computed tomography scan—may reveal primary and metastatic tumors, infection, or trauma
- arteriography and Doppler flow studies—may confirm circulatory inadequacy in major arteries or veins
- biopsy—confirms presence of a malignant or benign mass
- physical and occupational therapy evaluation—extent of gross and fine motor function determines ability to use assistive devices (such as prosthesis, crutches, or walker)

POTENTIAL COMPLICATIONS
- hemorrhage
- infection
- flexion contracture
- psychopathologic adaptation to limb loss

Collaborative problem: *High risk for hemorrhage related to amputation*

NURSING PRIORITY: Maintain circulatory volume.

Interventions

1. Assess the surgical site immediately upon the patient's arrival on the unit after surgery. Document your findings, including the type of dressing and a description of any drainage and drainage devices, such as a Hemovac.

2. Observe and document signs of oozing on the dressing. Reinforce the dressing as required. Do not remove the dressing until ordered. Document the amount of supplies used and the frequency of reinforcement.

3. Maintain an I.V. line. Document its site, appearance, and patency.

4. Keep a tourniquet at the bedside. Apply it to the limb or apply direct pressure to the artery if significant bleeding occurs. Notify the doctor immediately, remain with the patient until the doctor arrives, and document the events.

5. Additional individualized interventions: _____

Rationales

1. Baseline assessment permits comparison of data, assisting in ongoing status evaluation. A drain or portable wound suction device may be in place to remove fluid or blood that might interfere with granulation. Observed drainage will be minimal and serosanguineous. Increased amounts of bright red drainage may indicate hemorrhage.

2. A small amount of oozing from the incision is normal. Documenting the supplies used and drainage characteristics helps other caregivers assess status changes. Initially, most postamputation dressings are pressure or pressure-cast dressings; premature removal may result in undesirable edema, bleeding, or both.

3. Loss of circulating blood volume results in vessel constriction, increasing the difficulty of venipuncture. An established line provides a route for rapid fluid replacement if necessary.

4. If hemorrhage occurs, immediate tourniquet application prevents significant blood loss and shock. If bleeding is severe, direct arterial pressure may be necessary. The patient may be frightened by the amount of blood lost; the nurse's presence is reassuring.

5. Rationales: _____

Target outcome criteria
Within 1 day after surgery, the patient will:
- have vital signs that are stable and within normal limits.
- have decreased drainage.

Within 3 days after surgery, the patient will have no hemorrhage.

Nursing diagnosis: *Pain related to postoperative tissue, nerve, and bone trauma*

NURSING PRIORITIES: (a) Relieve pain, (b) provide reassurance, and (c) teach about phantom limb phenomena.

Interventions

1. See the "Pain" plan, page 69.

2. Monitor for pain continually. Listen to complaints of discomfort and observe for tense posture, tightening fists, diaphoresis, and increased pulse rate.

3. Document pain episodes, noting location, characteristics, radiation, frequency, severity, and associated findings.

4. When pain occurs, administer medication promptly, as ordered. Evaluate and document the patient's response. Taper the frequency of intramuscular medication administration after the third or fourth postoperative day, as ordered; substitute oral medication, as ordered and as needed.

5. Evaluate the dressing or cast for tightness each time the patient complains of pain and every 3 to 4 hours. Document the findings. If circulation, sensation, or movement is impaired, notify the doctor and reapply the dressing more loosely.

6. Reposition the patient or the affected limb every 2 to 3 hours. Document repositionings.

7. Gently massage the stump every 4 hours after the surgeon removes the dressing. Avoid using emollients. Evaluate and document the patient's response.

8. Explain the cause of phantom limb sensation and pain. Inform the patient that this may last as long as 6 months (rarely longer), although phantom limb pain may arise again even years later.

9. Use nonpharmacologic pain relief measures between doses of pain medication and when the patient does not experience pain relief. Consider diversion, activity, backrub, relaxation techniques, imagery, or cutaneous stimulation (such as counterirritation with oil of wintergreen). Consider consulting the doctor about a transcutaneous electrical nerve stimulation device.

10. Additional individualized interventions: _____

Rationales

1. The "Pain" plan provides general guidelines and interventions for pain.

2. Pain is what the patient states it is; early detection and intervention promote patient comfort. Pain stimulates the sympathetic nervous system, resulting in physical symptoms.

3. Documentation provides a baseline to help others interpret pain-related behaviors.

4. Early administration of pain medication is more effective in controlling pain than waiting until the pain becomes severe. Pain normally begins to diminish in intensity three or four days after surgery.

5. Decreased circulation causes tissue hypoxia and increases the pain response.

6. Pain increases with external pressure or fatigue. Changing position relieves pressure and the risk of complications from immobility.

7. Massage increases circulation to the traumatized area. Emollients can cause skin maceration.

8. Phantom limb sensation is the feeling or perception of the amputated limb. Phantom limb pain, a separate phenomenon, is the awareness of pain in the amputated body part. Unfortunately, treatment methods for persistent phantom limb pain are of limited value. The cause of these relatively uncommon phenomena is unknown. Knowing that phantom limb sensation and pain are normal responses to amputation may reassure the patient.

9. These methods decrease awareness of painful stimuli.

10. Rationales: _____

Target outcome criteria
Within 4 hours after surgery, the patient will:
• verbalize pain relief
• show no associated pain behaviors.

Within 1 day after surgery, the patient will verbalize understanding of phantom limb pain and sensation.

Within 3 days after surgery, the patient will decrease requests for pain medication.

Nursing diagnosis: *High risk for infection related to interrupted skin integrity*

NURSING PRIORITY: Promote wound healing.

Interventions

1. Observe the incision line for redness, edema, or exudate during each dressing change. Document all findings. If a plaster cast is in place, check for signs of tissue necrosis: "hot" spots, drainage on the cast, unrelieved pain, or foul odor.

2. Protect the stump from contamination and trauma. If the patient is incontinent, protect the limb with a plastic covering. Always use sterile technique during dressing changes.

3. Always rewrap dressings securely but not tightly. Do not apply tape to skin.

4. Encourage the patient to follow the prescribed diet. Document the patient's likes and dislikes, and assist with menu selection. Promote intake of foods high in protein, vitamins, calories, and minerals.

5. Bathe the stump daily with mild soap and water after a dressing is no longer necessary. Dry it thoroughly and leave it exposed to air twice daily for at least 20 minutes.

6. Teach the signs and symptoms of stump breakdown. Examine the stump daily for edema, redness, and skin breaks. Teach the patient to examine the stump regularly after discharge, such as during exercise or bathing.

7. Teach stump-toughening exercises. Have the patient push the stump against a soft pillow four to six times daily. Increase resistance gradually. Document progress.

8. Additional individualized interventions: _____

_____

Rationales

1. Assessment of the incision line during the first dressing change provides baseline data for future comparison. Histamine release causes the classic signs of inflammation. Diminished tissue perfusion, resulting from decreased circulation secondary to external pressure, causes cell death. Tissue necrosis results in pain, a sensation of local heat, drainage, and odor.

2. Exposing the stump to microorganisms increases the risk of infection. Trauma causes tissue death and slows healing.

3. Tight dressings may inhibit blood flow to the healing wound, reducing the availability of oxygen and essential nutrients. Tape can cause tissue trauma during removal.

4. Preexisting diseases, such as diabetes, may require that the patient follow a specific diet. Additional amounts of protein, calories, vitamins, and minerals are needed for wound healing.

5. Hygiene is essential to maintaining healthy skin that can tolerate a prosthesis. Moist skin allows maceration to occur.

6. Early detection of stump breakdown allows prompt treatment. Undetected complications jeopardize the patient's rehabilitation program and may make further amputation necessary.

7. Fragile, delicate skin will not withstand the pressure a prosthesis will apply. Toughening the skin prepares the patient to wear a prosthesis and reduces the chance of infection related to skin breakdown.

8. Rationales: _____

_____

Target outcome criteria
By the time of discharge, the patient will:
• show no signs or symptoms of infection
• list signs of stump breakdown

• demonstrate stump-toughening exercises.

Nursing diagnosis: *High risk for loss of joint function related to impaired physical mobility*

NURSING PRIORITY: Maintain range of motion (ROM) in affected joint.

Interventions

1. Promote joint extension. Do not use pillows under a lower-extremity stump; raise the foot of the bed instead. Use slings and pillows under an upper-extremity stump.

2. Place the patient in the prone position for 30 minutes four times daily and for sleep (for lower-limb amputation), if not contraindicated.

3. Do not allow the knee to bend over the edge of the chair or bed if the patient had a below-the-knee amputation.

4. Institute ROM exercises for the affected limb two to three times daily, beginning on the first day after surgery. Gradually increase the frequency on subsequent days. Evaluate and document the patient's response.

5. Provide a trapeze bar over the patient's bed.

6. Plan activities around the time of pain medication administration. Be alert for medication effects that can decrease alertness or increase the patient's potential for injury.

7. Position personal belongings, water, the telephone, and the call light within the patient's reach at all times, particularly if an arm was amputated.

8. Instruct a patient with a lower-extremity amputation to call for assistance when getting out of bed. Keep the bed in the low position at all times.

9. Teach transfer techniques appropriate to the patient's amputation (for example, repositioning in bed, or bed-to-chair or bed-to-wheelchair transfer). Document the teaching and the patient's use of the techniques.

10. Teach muscle-strengthening exercises specific to the limb amputated. Gluteal-setting exercises for above-the-knee amputation, hamstring-setting exercises for below-the-knee amputation, and straightening the flexed proximal joint against resistance are examples of valuable exercises. Include exercises for increasing triceps strength, such as pushing against the bed with the fists and raising the buttocks off the bed. Tell the patient to exercise twice daily, gradually increasing frequency as muscle strength increases.

11. Explain that stance will be altered. Teach abdominal and gluteal muscle-tightening exercises to perform while standing. Have the patient practice balancing on the toes, and bending the knee and hopping while holding onto a chair. Remain with the patient during these exercises.

Rationales

1. Proper positioning promotes venous return and decreases edema without causing flexion contracture.

2. The prone position facilitates normal joint alignment in extension.

3. Allowing the stump to hang in a dependent position decreases venous return and increases edema. Flexion contracture may occur if the stump remains bent.

4. ROM exercises are directed toward maintaining normal joint mobility. Disuse can cause permanent shortening of the muscles, resulting in contractures.

5. A trapeze increases mobility in bed, allows the patient to be more independent, and prevents exclusive use of the heel or elbow for pushing when the patient moves (this may contribute to skin breakdown).

6. Pain prevents full participation in activities. Narcotics may cause orthostatic hypotension and fainting from vascular dilation.

7. Being able to reach needed items promotes independence and increases self-confidence in a patient with an altered self-concept.

8. Muscle weakness and impaired balance after a lower-limb amputation may result in an injury.

9. Learning transfer techniques reestablishes the patient's independence and promotes a feeling of security when moving in and out of bed.

10. Optimal muscle strength is required to maintain balance while using assistive devices, such as crutches, a walker, or a prosthesis.

11. An altered center of gravity requires increased muscle strength, balance, and coordination to compensate for the amputated extremity. Remaining with the patient during practice provides reassurance and helps prevent injury related to loss of balance.

12. Consult with the doctor concerning physical therapy or occupational therapy referrals.

12. Early intervention by physical and occupational therapy specialists increases the patient's rehabilitation potential.

13. After a lower-extremity amputation, reinforce skills of ambulation, crutch walking, or use of assistive devices learned during physical therapy. Encourage the patient to use these techniques whenever ambulating.

13. Consistent use of learned methods increases the patient's skill, self-confidence, and awareness of their importance.

14. Ensure appropriate referral for home care if self-care ability or motivation is a problem. Emphasize the importance of ongoing rehabilitative follow-up.

14. Inadequate follow-up may lead to functional limitations or further limb compromise. Ongoing follow-up allows early detection of problems.

15. Additional individualized interventions: _____

15. Rationales: _____

_____

_____

Target outcome criteria
By the time of discharge, the patient will:
• display no signs of joint contracture
• demonstrate independent use of transfer techniques
• use assistive devices independently
• demonstrate muscle-strengthening exercises
• initiate discussion of follow-up plans.

Nursing diagnosis: *Body-image disturbance related to loss of a body part*

NURSING PRIORITY: Promote acceptance of the loss of a body part.

Interventions

1. Show an accepting attitude toward the patient. Anticipate a period of mourning for the lost limb. See the "Grieving" plan, page 31.

2. Spend time with the patient each shift. Encourage verbalization of feelings about the amputation. Clarify areas of misunderstanding and reassure the patient that feelings are normal.

3. Encourage family and friends to interact with the patient. Explain the patient's response, if necessary. Refer family members to a counselor, as needed.

4. Encourage the patient to look at the stump and to help in its care during the early postoperative period. Do not force this, however, if the patient is hesitant.

5. Introduce the patient to others with similar amputations who have adapted successfully.

Rationales

1. Acceptance helps the patient feel valued as an individual. The patient may experience various manifestations of the grieving process, such as directing anger and frustration toward staff and family members. The "Grieving" plan contains detailed information on assisting with the grieving process.

2. Clarifying knowledge and encouraging expression of feelings helps the patient pass through the stages of grief.

3. The demonstration of acceptance and love by family and friends is essential to completing the grieving process.

4. Acknowledging the stump helps the patient recognize reality and promotes acceptance of an altered body image. Acceptance is a highly individualized process; forcing the patient to look at the stump may provoke undue distress.

5. Seeing someone who has adapted successfully demonstrates that the amputation does not have to interfere with a normal life-style. Peers may provide realistic encouragement and practical help in adapting to the change.

6. Provide information about an appropriate prosthesis and its use, reinforcing the teaching of the prosthetist or physical therapist.

6. Replacement of the amputated body part with a prosthesis gives the body a more normal appearance and increases the patient's participation in daily activities. Knowing that a prosthesis is available provides the patient with a goal to work toward.

A prosthesis may be applied immediately after surgery. This reduces residual limb edema, loss of muscle strength, and complications of immobility and also promotes healing through increased tissue perfusion at the operative site as a result of early ambulation. More importantly, immediate application of a prosthesis improves the patient's psychological outlook.

A prosthesis also may be applied 1 to 6 months after surgery. This occurs when wound healing is delayed because of infection, peripheral vascular disease, or the patient's debilitated status.

7. Consult a member of the clergy, psychiatric clinician, or social worker if the patient is unable to progress through the grieving process. See the "Ineffective Individual Coping" plan, page 51.

7. Special assistance may be necessary to help the patient accept the amputation. Maladaptation to amputation may result in severe depression or suicidal behavior.

8. Additional individualized interventions: _____

8. Rationales: _____

Target outcome criteria
By the time of discharge, the patient will:
• verbalize feelings regarding amputation
• participate in stump care

• express knowledge about the availability of a prosthesis (if appropriate).

Discharge planning
NURSING DISCHARGE CRITERIA
Upon the patient's discharge, documentation shows evidence of:
• stable vital signs
• absence of pulmonary or cardiovascular complications
• a healing incision with no signs of swelling, redness, inflammation, or drainage
• absence of fever
• absence of contractures
• pain controlled by oral medication
• ability to tolerate diet
• ability to perform stump care independently or with minimal assistance
• ability to perform activities of daily living (ADLs) independently or with minimal assistance
• completion of initial physical therapy program with appropriate assistive devices
• ability to transfer and ambulate independently or with minimal assistance (with a lower-extremity amputation)
• adequate home support, or referral for home care or to a rehabilitation setting if indicated by lack of home support system; inability to perform ADLs, stump care, and safe transfers; or continued need for physical therapy.

PATIENT-FAMILY TEACHING CHECKLIST
Document evidence that the patient and family demonstrate an understanding of:
__ underlying disease and implications
__ all discharge medications' purpose, dosage, administration schedule, and adverse effects requiring medical attention (discharge medications are prescribed only if the patient has an infection or a preexisting condition, such as diabetes mellitus; patient may be prescribed pain medication to be taken as needed)
__ prescribed diet
__ necessary equipment and supplies
__ care of stump and prosthesis
__ phantom limb sensation and pain
__ signs of wound inflammation and infection that require medical attention
__ prescribed exercises for the residual limb
__ need for smoking cessation program (if appropriate)
__ name and telephone number of contact person for additional information or answers to questions
__ date, time, and location of follow-up appointments
__ how to contact the doctor
__ available community resources.

DOCUMENTATION CHECKLIST
Using outcome criteria as a guide, document:
___ clinical status on return from surgery
___ significant changes in status
___ pertinent laboratory and diagnostic test findings
___ pain at surgical site
___ phantom limb pain
___ phantom limb sensation
___ pain relief measures
___ mobility and positioning
___ dressing changes
___ appearance of wound
___ drainage devices
___ I.V. line patency
___ oxygen therapy
___ nutritional intake
___ psychological status
___ physical therapy, occupational therapy, or both
___ assistive devices, such as a walker, crutches, or prosthesis
___ patient-family teaching
___ discharge planning.

ASSOCIATED PLANS OF CARE
Diabetes Mellitus
Grieving
Ineffective Individual Coping
Knowledge Deficit
Pain
Surgical Intervention

References
Guyton, A.C. *Textbook of Medical Physiology*, 8th ed. Philadelphia: W.B. Saunders Co., 1991.
Lewis, S.M., and Collier, I.C. *Medical-Surgical Nursing: Assessment and Management of Clinical Problems.* New York: McGraw-Hill Book Co., 1987.
Long, B.C., and Phipps, W.J. *Essentials of Medical-Surgical Nursing.* St. Louis: C.V. Mosby Co., 1989.

Fractured Femur

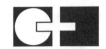

DRG information
DRG 210 Hip and Femur Procedures, Except Major Joint. Age 17 +. With Complication or Comorbidity (CC).
Mean LOS = 12.0 days

DRG 211 Hip and Femur Procedures, Except Major Joint. Age 17 + Without CC.
Mean LOS = 9.6 days

DRG 212 Hip and Femur Procedures, Except Major Joint. Age 0 to 17.
Mean LOS = 4.5 days
Principal procedures for DRGs 210, 211, and 212 include:
• fixation of bone without fracture reduction
• closed and open reduction with internal fixation
• open reduction without internal fixation.

PRO alert: DRG 210 is a frequently occurring DRG. Professional review organizations (PROs) are scrutinizing discharge planning criteria for this category because patients assigned this DRG commonly complain of premature discharge. Therefore, daily nursing documentation must describe the patient's progress with activities of daily living (ADLs), transfers, and ambulation. Upon discharge, the patient's ability to perform ADLs and transfers must be documented carefully.

Introduction
DEFINITION AND TIME FOCUS
The femur, which connects the hip joint and the knee joint, is the longest and strongest bone in the body. It follows, therefore, that most fractures of the femur are the result of traumatic accidents involving considerable force.

The two primary classifications of femur fractures are:
• proximal end fractures, involving the portion of the femur that engages with the acetabulum (These fractures may be further classified into two subtypes: intracapsular, involving the head and neck of the femur within the hip joint, and extracapsular, involving the area from the femoral neck distally to about 2″ [5 cm] below the lesser trochanter.)
• femoral shaft fractures, involving the distal portion of the femur.

This plan focuses on preoperative and postoperative care of the patient admitted to the hospital for treatment of a femur fracture. See the "Total Joint Replacement in a Lower Extremity" plan, page 516, for more information on fractures involving the hip joint.

ETIOLOGY AND PRECIPITATING FACTORS
• proximal end fractures—fall injuries most common, with osteoporosis a significant contributing factor in older patients
• femoral shaft fractures—high-impact traumatic accidents, most often in younger patients

Focused assessment guidelines
NURSING HISTORY (Functional health pattern findings)

Health perception—health management pattern
• if older, may have history of coexisting medical conditions (such as heart disease, diabetes, or hypertension) that contributed to the fall or caused it
• if younger, may be the first contact with an inpatient setting

Activity-exercise pattern
• in proximal end fractures, may be able to walk but, more typically, cannot bear weight
• in femoral shaft fractures, usually unable to bear weight
• weight bearing may begin within 24 hours with rod insertion

Cognitive-perceptual pattern
• typically complains of severe, localized pain in the affected limb
• may complain of numbness or tingling in the affected limb

Value-belief pattern
• in proximal end fractures, commonly expresses disbelief that injury is severe; an older patient may insist that only pain relief is necessary; may deny need for surgical intervention

PHYSICAL FINDINGS
Cardiovascular
• edema at injury site or distally
• tachycardia
• hypotension
• with severe vascular involvement, absent pulse, reduced pulse rate, or reduced or absent pulse amplitude in the affected limb

Pulmonary
• hyperventilation, tachypnea

Musculoskeletal
- deformity at injury site (for example, external rotation or shortening)
- severe pain with movement of affected limb
- ecchymosis
- crepitus

Integumentary
- diaphoresis
- pallor (if significant blood is lost)

DIAGNOSTIC STUDIES
(may reveal no significant abnormalities initially, unless related to coexisting condition)
- complete blood count — performed before surgery to establish baseline; may reveal extent of blood loss associated with the injury (loss of up to 1.5 liters may occur); decreased hemoglobin and hematocrit values result from dilution by crystalloid fluid replacement during resuscitation; white blood cell count may be elevated in response to injury
- blood typing and cross-matching — performed in preparation for blood replacement if significant blood loss is present or incurred during surgery
- chemistry panel — obtained before surgery to establish baseline and assess for underlying imbalances that may have contributed to the injury or that may affect intraoperative care (for example, potassium imbalances, which can cause increased cardiac irritability during anesthesia); blood urea nitrogen and creatinine levels evaluate renal function
- prothrombin time and partial thromboplastin time — performed before surgery to establish baseline; usually are normal unless an underlying bleeding disorder is present; older patients may be started on anticoagulant therapy after surgery to minimize the risk of thromboembolism

- urinalysis — performed for baseline evaluation of renal function
- serum drug levels — performed if medication overdose or noncompliance is suspected as contributing factor to injury
- femur X-ray — identifies location and type of fracture
- chest X-ray — routinely obtained before surgery to rule out associated injuries or preexisting conditions affecting surgical care (such as cardiomegaly or congestive heart failure)
- 12-lead electrocardiography (ECG) — obtained before surgery to establish baseline and to identify preexisting cardiac abnormalities, if any; may be especially significant in older patients or in those with blunt trauma to the chest (possible cardiac contusion) in addition to the leg injury

POTENTIAL COMPLICATIONS
- shock
- hemorrhage
- pulmonary embolism
- fat embolism
- thrombophlebitis
- aseptic necrosis of the femoral head
- nonunion of the affected portions
- osteomyelitis
- pneumonia
- arthritic deformities

Collaborative problem: *High risk for preoperative complications related to nature of traumatic injury*

NURSING PRIORITIES: (a) Prepare the patient to undergo surgery in optimal physical condition and (b) prevent, or identify and promptly treat, preoperative complications.

Interventions

1. Ensure adequacy of respirations. Auscultate the lungs and note any evidence of unequal chest excursion, unequal or diminished breath sounds, pain with respiration, cyanosis, restlessness, or dyspnea. Report any respiratory difficulty to the doctor immediately, and prepare to support ventilation or insert chest tubes, if indicated.

Rationales

1. High-impact accidents, such as those which cause femoral fractures, have a high incidence of multisystem injuries, including chest trauma. Pulmonary or chest abnormalities may indicate tracheal injury, pneumothorax, rib fractures, or other complications. In older patients, preexisting medical conditions may involve cardiac or central nervous system functions, affecting respiratory capability and adequacy.

2. Assess for signs of bleeding, and maintain circulatory volume. Report increasing pulse rate, decreasing blood pressure, pallor, diaphoresis, or decreasing alertness. Establish and maintain an I.V. line as ordered, usually with Ringer's lactate solution initially. If an open fracture is bleeding, apply direct, continuous pressure to the area and notify the doctor.

2. Femoral fractures are associated with significant blood loss because of the vascularity of long bones and the proximity of large vessels. The parameters noted are signs of shock and require immediate intervention. Intravenous infusions help replace fluids lost from bleeding; Ringer's lactate expands blood volume and replaces electrolyte losses. Direct pressure controls active bleeding until it can be stopped surgically.

3. Assess the limb's neurovascular status. Note weakened or absent pulses, mottling, cyanosis, paresthesias, or loss of sensation. Compare pulse rates bilaterally. Avoid moving the limb unnecessarily. Report deficits to the doctor immediately.

3. Blood vessels and nerves in the fracture area may be displaced or severed by bone fragments or by edema and deformity. Movement may cause further injury. Inadequate perfusion of the limb may result in permanent functional impairment or loss of the affected portion.

4. Control pain. Administer analgesics as ordered during the preoperative period, making sure all medications are noted on the surgical checklist. Apply cold packs to the fracture area. Maintain traction or splinting as ordered.

4. Pain contributes to increasing anxiety, stresses the cardiovascular system, and may contribute to increased muscle tension and associated displacement at the injury site. Noting medications on the checklist ensures that their effects are considered in the administration of anesthetics. Cold packs help minimize edema by causing local vasoconstriction. Traction and splints may help reduce muscle spasms and pain.

5. If an open fracture is present, ensure that tetanus and infection prophylaxis are considered before surgery. Cover the wound with a sterile dressing.

5. Tetanus immunization, if not current, should be updated because open wounds associated with trauma are considered tetanus-prone. Any break in skin integrity predisposes the patient to infection. Covering the wound minimizes further contamination from airborne bacteria.

6. Prepare the patient for surgery, if indicated. See the "Surgical Intervention" plan, page 81, for details.

6. Depending on the location and type of fracture, a femoral fracture may be treated with traction or a cast; however, surgery is usually the treatment of choice. Various surgical procedures are used to repair these fractures, including placement of a prosthesis, pins, intramedullary rods, or nails and bone grafts. Proper preoperative preparation helps minimize postoperative problems. General interventions for the surgical patient are included in the "Surgical Intervention" plan.

7. Additional individualized interventions: _____

7. Rationales:_____

Target outcome criteria
Before surgery, the patient will:
• have normal respirations or, if abnormal, respiratory problems treated
• show stable vital signs
• have no uncontrolled bleeding
• have neurovascular findings within expected limits, with the doctor aware of current status
• verbalize reduction in the pain's severity
• have had tetanus and infection prophylaxis begun, if indicated
• have had preoperative teaching and preparation.

Collaborative problem: *High risk for postoperative complications related to the initial trauma injury, surgical intervention, or immobility*

NURSING PRIORITIES: (a) Prevent, or identify and promptly treat, postoperative complications and (b) promote healing.

Interventions

1. See the "Pain" and "Surgical Intervention" plans, pages 69 and 81 respectively.

Rationales

1. General guidelines for care of the surgical patient and for pain management are included in these plans.

2. Assess vital signs according to postoperative protocol or more often if unstable. Check dressings and drains for bleeding. Report any abnormalities in vital signs; excessive bleeding, if any, from the wound, surgical sites, drains, or graft sites; increasing edema; or ecchymosis. Assess for associated injuries if a high-impact trauma was involved.

2. As noted previously, femoral fractures may cause massive bleeding. Tachycardia and hypotension may indicate inadequate fluid replacement, excessive blood loss related to injury and repair, or other undetected injuries.

3. Assess neurovascular status at least once every hour or more often if compromised. Note weakened or absent pulses, mottling, cyanosis, paresthesias, loss of sensation, or a significant increase in edema after surgery. Be especially alert for signs of compartment syndrome: progressive pain exacerbated by stretching, sensory deficits, paralysis, tense or hard swelling, or decreasing distal pulses. Notify the doctor immediately if neurovascular status becomes impaired.

3. Careful assessment ensures prompt intervention should the limb's neurovascular status be compromised after surgery. Increasing edema may put pressure on surrounding vascular structures, impairing oxygenation of tissue. Immediate intervention is needed to restore circulation. Compartment syndrome is a complication caused by muscle swelling in which increased tissue pressure causes circulatory impairment and ischemia. This condition may occur immediately after injury or may develop over several days. Immediate treatment (fasciotomy) may avert permanent damage.

4. Maintain a patent I.V. line and administer fluids as ordered, usually for at least 24 hours after surgery.

4. I.V. infusions replace fluid losses related to bleeding, restricted oral intake, preexisting dehydration, or tissue loss during surgery. Also, maintaining venous access allows administration of I.V. medication.

5. Administer antibiotics, if ordered. Observe the wound carefully and report any increase in erythema or swelling or any fever, purulent drainage, or other signs of infection.

5. I.V. antibiotics are usually ordered during the initial postoperative period, particularly for the patient with an open fracture or increased susceptibility to infection. Infected bone wounds can be particularly serious; untreated, they may lead to osteomyelitis and bone disintegration. If the patient is already on antibiotic therapy when the infection develops, a different antibiotic may be indicated because the causative organism may be resistant to current therapy.

6. Prevent complications associated with immobility.

6. Immobility predisposes the patient to serious complications.

• Encourage the patient to perform gentle range-of-motion exercises for unaffected extremities; encourage alternate flexion and extension or quadriceps-setting exercises for the affected limb, as permitted. Increase activity level as permitted and as tolerated.

• Exercise, as allowed, decreases venous stasis and helps maintain muscle tone.

• Apply antiembolism stockings or sequential compression pants, as prescribed.

• Antiembolism stockings or sequential compression pants increase venous return and may help prevent thrombus formation.

• Provide a trapeze to assist movement.

• A trapeze allows the patient to assist with repositioning.

• Encourage coughing and deep breathing hourly while the patient is awake.

• Pulmonary hygiene measures help prevent postoperative lung infections related to immobility, anesthesia, decreased respiratory effort, and accumulation of secretions.

• Urge adequate fluid intake, when allowed, forcing fluids unless contraindicated. Document intake and output.

• Forcing fluids helps maintain hydration, liquefy secretions, maintain renal function, and minimize risk of urinary infection from stasis. Documenting intake and output identifies fluid imbalances.

• Provide clean, dry bedding and a special bed or mattress as needed; reposition the patient at least every 2 hours, and provide frequent skin care, with special attention to bony prominences.

• The immobilized patient is at increased risk for skin breakdown from constant pressure. A warm, moist environment encourages bacterial growth. Special beds and careful skin care prevent pressure ulcers.

• Encourage verbalization of feelings. Provide diversionary activities.

• Prolonged immobilization contributes to depression, anxiety, and frustration. Verbalizing feelings to an accepting caregiver may help decrease stress. Diversionary activities decrease boredom and give the patient some sense of self-control.

7. Observe for signs and symptoms of embolism, as follows:

• fat embolism—tachycardia, dyspnea, pleuritic pain, pallor and cyanosis, petechiae, crackles, wheezing, nausea, syncope, weakness, altered mentation, ECG changes, or fever; in the affected limb, pallor, numbness, or coldness to touch

• pulmonary embolism—sudden chest pain, dyspnea, tachycardia, cough, hemoptysis, anxiety, syncope, ECG changes, hypotension, or fever

• thrombophlebitis—positive Homan's sign, pain in calf, swelling, or redness locally in the limb.

Report any signs to the doctor immediately, and initiate treatment, as ordered.

8. Maintain proper immobilization of the affected limb, depending on the fracture site and the type of repair. Usually, adduction, external rotation, and acute hip flexion should be avoided in a patient with a proximal end fracture; lateral pressure or overpulling with traction must be avoided in a patient with a femoral shaft fracture. Verify specific positioning orders with the doctor.

9. Observe for and report immediately any sudden, sharp pain, shortening or rotation of the affected limb, or persistent muscle spasm.

10. Encourage adequate nutritional intake, especially of protein-rich foods and foods high in vitamins and minerals.

11. Additional individualized interventions: _____

_____

7. The nature of the injury and the period of postoperative immobility predispose the patient to this complication.

• Fat embolism occurs most often with long-bone fractures, usually within the first 3 days after injury. The exact physiologic mechanism is unknown. Fat emboli may lodge in the lungs, heart, brain, or extremities, and associated lipase release may cause tissue irritation.

• Pulmonary embolism is usually a later complication, occurring 10 to 24 days after injury. Signs may be related to obstruction from a blood clot that travels to the lungs and from reflex vasoconstriction.

• Thrombophlebitis usually occurs in the lower extremities as the result of clot formation and obstruction of superficial veins, although thrombi can occlude major vessels as well.

Immediate intervention is required because these complications may be life-threatening. Treatment may include ventilatory support, corticosteroids, anticoagulants, or thrombolytic agents.

8. Movement of the fracture site may displace bone fragments and interfere with healing. Positioning of the affected limb depends on the fracture location and the surgical approach; common rules do not hold true for all patients. Verifying positioning recommendations and careful positioning avert dislocation during turning.

9. These signs and symptoms may indicate dislocation of the joint or necrosis of the femoral head in a patient with a proximal end fracture. Immediate intervention is needed to prevent permanent damage.

10. Healing requires additional calories and protein. Deficits in vitamins and minerals (particularly vitamins B and C and calcium) retard healing and can contribute to long-term bone disorders, such as osteomalacia. Careful dietary assessment and monitoring may be required for the patient with impaired renal, hepatic, or pulmonary function.

11. Rationales: _____

_____

Target outcome criteria
Within 2 hours of arrival on the unit after surgery, the patient will:
• have vital signs within normal limits
• have no signs of excessive bleeding, neurovascular impairment, or infection
• have no uncontrolled pain
• manage coughing and deep breathing well
• maintain proper positioning.

Within 24 hours after surgery, the patient will:
• perform exercises as permitted
• show no signs of skin breakdown
• show no signs of embolism
• verbalize awareness of positioning restrictions
• take adequate food and fluids orally, if permitted.

Nursing diagnosis: *Knowledge deficit related to changes in allowable activity level and ongoing care of injury after discharge*

NURSING PRIORITIES: (a) Reinforce the doctor's recommendations for home care, and (b) identify potential problems related to home care and intervene as appropriate.

Interventions	Rationales
1. See the "Knowledge Deficit" plan, page 56.	1. General interventions for patient and family teaching are included in this plan.
2. Provide patient and family teaching related to positioning, activity restrictions, cast care, crutch walking, use of a cane or walker, diet, complications, and medications. Verify recommendations with the doctor, and incorporate teaching throughout the hospital stay.	2. Home care recommendations vary widely, depending on the nature of the fracture and repair, the patient's age and condition, and any associated or preexisting conditions. The patient may be more responsive to continuous, repetitive instruction during inpatient care routines than to a large amount of information just before discharge.
3. Assess available resources for home care, and make appropriate referrals.	3. Depending on the factors mentioned above and on the family support structure, the patient may require home medical or nursing assistance or other follow-up care to ensure an uncomplicated recovery.
4. Additional individualized interventions: _____	4. Rationales: _____

Target outcome criteria
By the time of discharge, the patient and family will:
• verbalize and demonstrate understanding of positioning and activity restrictions or recommendations and care of the injury
• verbalize understanding of the recommended diet and medication regimen

• identify signs and symptoms of complications
• receive appropriate referrals for home care and follow-up.

Discharge planning
NURSING DISCHARGE CRITERIA
Upon the patient's discharge, documentation shows evidence of:
• stable vital signs
• absence of pulmonary or cardiovascular complications
• healing incision with no signs of swelling, redness, inflammation, or drainage
• ability to control pain using oral medication
• absence of fever
• hemoglobin levels within expected parameters
• ability to perform ADLs independently or with minimal assistance
• ability to transfer independently or with minimal assistance
• ability to demonstrate weight-bearing restrictions when transferring
• ability to verbalize activity restrictions
• completion of initial ambulation training with the appropriate assistive device
• ability to tolerate diet
• normal voiding and bowel movements

• referral to home care if indicated by inability to perform ADLs and safe transfer technique or by continued need for physical therapy
• adequate home support or, if home support is not adequate, ability to verbalize agreement with temporary placement in a nursing home to convalesce and continue physical therapy.

PATIENT-FAMILY TEACHING CHECKLIST
Document evidence that the patient and family demonstrate an understanding of:
___ site and nature of injury and repair
___ implications of injury
___ all discharge medications' purpose, dosage, administration schedule, and adverse effects requiring medical attention (discharge medications may include antibiotics, analgesics, anticoagulants, and antispasmodics)
___ signs and symptoms of complications
___ activity and positioning restrictions and recommendations
___ care of cast, if present
___ dietary recommendations

___ when and how to access the emergency medical
system
___ home care and follow-up referrals
___ date, time, and location of follow-up appointments,
and availability of transportation, if indicated
___ how to contact the doctor.

DOCUMENTATION CHECKLIST
Using outcome criteria as a guide, document:
___ clinical status on admission
___ preoperative assessment and treatment
___ postoperative assessment and treatment
___ significant changes in status
___ pertinent laboratory and diagnostic findings
___ pain relief measures
___ recommendations for and tolerance of activity and
positioning
___ nutritional intake
___ fluid intake and output
___ bowel status
___ patient-family teaching
___ discharge planning.

ASSOCIATED PLANS OF CARE
Geriatric Considerations
Impaired Physical Mobility
Knowledge Deficit
Pain
Pulmonary Embolism
Surgical Intervention
Thrombophlebitis
Total Joint Replacement in a Lower Extremity

References

Dolan, J. *Critical Care Nursing: Clinical Management
through the Nursing Process.* Philadelphia: F.A. Davis
Co., 1990.
Emergencies. Nurse's Reference Library. Springhouse,
Pa.: Springhouse Corp., 1985.
Holloway, N. *Nursing the Critically Ill Adult: Applying
Nursing Diagnosis,* 3rd ed. Reading, Mass.: Addison-
Wesley Publishing Co., 1988.
Hudak, C., et al. *Critical Care Nursing: A Holistic Ap-
proach.* Philadelphia: J.B. Lippincott Co., 1990.
Luckmann, J., and Sorensen, K. *Medical-Surgical
Nursing: A Psychophysiological Approach,* 3rd ed.
Philadelphia: W.B. Saunders Co., 1987.
Shoemaker, W., et al. *Textbook of Critical Care.* Phila-
delphia: W.B. Saunders Co., 1989.
Smith, L., and Glowac, B. "New Frontiers in the Man-
agement of the Multiple Injured Patient," *Critical
Care Nursing Clinics of North America* 1(1):2, 1989.
Trunkey, D., and Lewis, F. *Current Therapy of Trauma,*
3rd ed. Toronto: B.C. Decker, 1991.

Low Back Pain – Conservative Medical Management

DRG information

DRG 243 Medical Back Problems.
        Mean LOS = 5.0 days

PRO alert: Low back pain is usually treated on an outpatient basis. In fact, one of the criteria professional review organizations (PROs) look at is whether conservative outpatient management was tried before hospitalization. (This documentation would be found in the doctor's history and physical notes or in the discharge summary.) Therefore, the plan of care, once the patient is hospitalized, must include frequent monitoring of pain and pain management — for example, every 4 hours. For a back pain case to be covered in an acute-care setting, the following must be documented:
• onset of sudden, acute pain or, if chronic pain is present, failure of outpatient management
• severe, debilitating pain requiring that pain medication be administered intramuscularly
• the patient's inability to undergo outpatient radiology testing
• bed rest ordered and complied with.

In many cases, if myelography or magnetic resonance imaging (MRI) is positive, the patient will need a laminectomy, and documentation needs to address the future plans and potential timing for this surgery. If a patient with a positive myelogram or MRI test is discharged and readmitted within 15 days (soon to be 30 days), the PRO would consider this fragmented care — "care that could have or should have been performed during the first admission." In such a case, the hospital would not be paid for the second admission. Thus, documentation at the first discharge must address treatment plans if conservative management proves unsuccessful. The patient's understanding of treatment plans should also be documented, especially when a myelogram or MRI indicates a laminectomy is necessary. This is important because if the patient decides to be discharged for conservative treatment, the PRO will not consider this "fragmented care." This necessary documentation is the doctor's responsibility. Nurses should be aware of the need for this documentation, however, and document related nursing care, such as pain relief attempts and discharge teaching.

Introduction
DEFINITION AND TIME FOCUS

Low back pain requiring medical management results from localized injury such as muscle strain or sprain, from degenerative changes in the vertebral facets, or from abrupt dislocation of an intervertebral disk of the lumbar spine. Usually a disabling condition, it is one of the most common health problems reported. This plan focuses on the patient admitted for diagnosis and conservative management during an episode of acute or chronic back pain and limited mobility.

Note: This plan does not address back pain from visceral conditions, such as pancreatitis, renal calculi, gynecologic diseases, spinal cord infections, or spinal tumors.

ETIOLOGY AND PRECIPITATING FACTORS
• poor posture, scoliosis, or exaggerated lordotic curve
• congenital malformation, spondylolisthesis, or spondylosis
• degenerative changes in the vertebrae from osteoarthritis or osteoporosis
• muscle or ligament tears, or degenerative disk
• muscle deconditioning or excessive physical activity
• history of stooping, bending, improper body mechanics, heavy lifting, or sudden movement
• obesity

Focused assessment guidelines
NURSING HISTORY (Functional health pattern findings)

Health perception – health management pattern
• if outpatient management was tried, may report failure to follow medical recommendations for back pain control because of personal and family attitudes that conflict with the therapeutic regimen
• may report occupation requiring manual labor, leading to mechanical stress on the back muscles, or sedentary work, leading to deconditioning of muscles
• may describe present health status as a threat to job security
• may describe self-care activities, including use of over-the-counter medication and visits to chiropractor

Nutritional-metabolic pattern
• may report dietary intake that exceeds therapeutic recommendations

Elimination pattern
• may describe change in bowel or bladder elimination, such as difficulty urinating or constipation

Activity-exercise pattern
• commonly describes a recent change in normal activity level, including activities of daily living (ADLs), work-related activities, and leisure activities
• commonly reports emotional intolerance to confinement of bed rest

Sleep-rest pattern
• may report sleep often interrupted by low back pain or referred pain
• may report "bed-rest fatigue"

Cognitive-perceptual pattern
• generally reports disabling acute or chronic pain, or both
• usually does not understand, or is misinformed about, diagnosis and treatment
• may report decreased tactile sensation in body area distal to injury site
• may have experienced a significant decrease in sensory-perceptual stimulation because of bed rest

Self-perception — self-concept pattern
• may express concern about loss of independence
• may describe feelings of low self-esteem

Role-relationship pattern
• may report decreased ability to maintain social, occupational, and family roles, leading to a sense of isolation
• may report family resentment concerning inability to perform roles

Sexuality-reproductive pattern
• commonly describes altered sexual functioning

Coping — stress tolerance pattern
• may report concern about financial security
• may describe frustration with bed rest routine
• may express anxiety about long-term implications of condition

Value-belief pattern
• may express values or beliefs that conflict with long-term therapeutic regimen and life-style changes

PHYSICAL FINDINGS
Musculoskeletal
• sprains or strains
  — painful and limited spinal motion
  — paravertebral muscle tenderness
  — weak abdominal muscles
  — no increase in pain with dorsiflexion of foot
  — painful, limited spinal motion

• disk problems (abrupt and degenerative)
  — pain in low back region
  — increased sciatic pain with movement, activity, or straight-leg raising (associated with L2-3 or L3-4 disk herniation)
  — pain or numbness in neck, shoulders, or arms (associated with cervical disk herniation)
  — pain radiating down one or both lower extremities
• vertebral problems (degenerative conditions)
  — painful, limited spinal motion
  — pain in the low back

Neurologic
• sprains or strains
  — no abnormal findings — for example, deep tendon reflexes are present
• disk problems (abrupt and degenerative)
  — positive neurologic signs, such as absent deep tendon reflexes
  — sensory deficit noted on one or both extremities corresponding to level of lesion

DIAGNOSTIC STUDIES
Note: no specific laboratory data apply to lower back pain.
• lumbar spine X-ray — usually unrevealing
• computed tomography scan and MRI — indicate the spinal canal diameter, showing disk displacement
• myelography — may be normal or may show narrowing of the disk space
• electromyography — tests the electrical potential of skeletal muscles; helpful in localizing the site of nerve root pressure related to ruptured disk
• epidural phlebography (injection of contrast medium into anterior internal vertebral blood vessel) — may reveal altered venous flow over area of disk herniation

POTENTIAL COMPLICATIONS
• herniation of intervertebral disk
• major neurologic deficits distal to lesion
  — paralysis
  — nerve damage
  — loss of urinary bladder and bowel control
  — muscle atrophy

Nursing diagnosis: *Impaired physical mobility related to acute pain and limitations imposed by the therapeutic regimen*

NURSING PRIORITIES: (a) Promote healing, (b) prevent complications associated with immobility, and (c) prepare the patient for participation in a long-term rehabilitation program.

Interventions

1. Maintain strict and complete bed rest for 1 to 6 weeks, using a firm mattress or a bed board. Supervise bathroom privileges if ordered.

Rationales

1. Bed rest with bathroom privileges only is the essential ingredient in the conservative treatment of low back pain. Bed rest allows inflammation to subside so the affected disk shrinks back away from the spinal nerve on which it has impinged.

2. Evaluate neurologic function in the lower extremities daily, and report new or increasingly abnormal findings to the doctor. Assess the following parameters: deep tendon reflexes, sensation (presence in both extremities, sharp and dull differentiation, and position and temperature awareness), and muscle strength (bilateral symmetry of muscle groups, dorsiflexion against resistance, and plantar flexion against resistance).

2. Development or extension of abnormal neurologic signs indicates the need to reevaluate the therapeutic regimen.

3. Supervise maintenance of body alignment, observing the following guidelines:
• During side-lying, keep the bed flat and one or both lower extremities flexed.
• When the patient is supine, elevate the head of the bed 20 degrees to 45 degrees and flex the knees at least 45 degrees.
• Do not allow the patient to lie prone.

3. Positioning should not stress the back muscles or the vertebral column. Improper alignment may impair healing or extend injury.

4. Administer medications, as ordered, observing for therapeutic effectiveness and monitoring as follows:

• muscle relaxants—observe for excessive drowsiness, and alert the patient to use caution when beginning ambulation.

• anti-inflammatory drugs—if nonsteroidal drugs are used, observe for GI irritation or bleeding, and monitor for signs of hepatotoxicity; if steroids are used, watch for development of infection.

• analgesics—observe for adverse effects according to the particular medications used, and encourage discussion of long-term pain-control plans and alternative therapies.

4. Medication protocols may vary significantly, depending on the doctor's preference and on underlying conditions.

• Muscle relaxants reduce painful spasm and promote rest.

• Anti-inflammatory medications decrease edema and pressure on adjacent tissues and structures.

• Analgesics control pain and promote relaxation. Dependence may be a problem with long-term analgesic use, so early planning for alternatives is essential.

5. Assess lung sounds at least every 8 hours and report any abnormal findings. Supervise 10 deep breaths every 2 hours while the patient is awake. Encourage hourly use of the incentive spirometer, as ordered.

5. The bed acts as a splint, restricting thoracic movement. Reduced chest expansion contributes to the development of atelectasis, pneumonia, and other respiratory complications. Full expansion promotes optimal lung function.

6. Supervise quad sets, calf pumping, and circle motions of the ankle 10 times each, four times daily.

6. Immobility may cause thrombophlebitis or embolus formation from poor venous return. Exercise decreases venous stasis.

7. Apply elastic stockings, as ordered, until the patient is ambulatory. Remove them twice daily, then provide skin care:
• Bathe the patient once daily.
• Apply lotion without massaging the muscle.
• Inspect for and report any reddened areas.
• Keep the stockings wrinkle-free.

7. Elastic stockings are thought to assist venous return by supporting affected muscle groups.

8. Supervise repositioning at least every 2 hours, using the logrolling method to turn the patient. Use caution to prevent shearing of delicate skin.

8. Skin breakdown is prevented by periodically relieving pressure over bony prominences. Logrolling prevents twisting and strain on back muscles.

9. While the patient is on bed rest, maintain dietary intake high in bulk, fluids, and roughage and lower than usual in calories. Consult with the dietitian to develop a diet plan that incorporates patient preferences as much as possible.

9. Immobility reduces peristaltic movement, so intake may need to be altered to maintain the patient's normal bowel habits. Metabolic needs are lower when the patient is on bed rest; undesired weight gain can occur if caloric intake is not reduced. Incorporating preferred foods may increase compliance with restrictions.

10. Coordinate and supervise implementation of a progressive activity schedule, incorporating the doctor's medical recommendations and the physical therapist's expertise. Ensure that the patient participates in planning.

10. A gradual return to activity reduces the risk of reinjury during healing and allows muscle strength to increase to meet demands.

11. Instruct the patient about movements that may stretch or strain back muscles and the vertebral column, such as poor body mechanics when lifting, bending, pulling, or pushing; quick, jerky motions; and improper use of such implements as a broom, rake, or shovel.

11. These activities are under the patient's control. Taking precautions may help reduce or prevent stress to the injured back.

12. Instruct the patient about the effects of straining at stool, coughing, or sneezing. Advise splinting the abdomen with arms or pillows and assuming a recumbent position (if possible) during coughing or sneezing episodes.

12. These activities increase muscle stress and pain. Splinting the abdomen provides added back support.

13. If ordered, apply pelvic traction for 1 hour, with rest periods of 3 to 4 hours between sessions. Ensure that the belt fits snugly over the iliac crests and that the patient's torso aligns with the pull of traction. Avoid pressure on ropes or pulleys from bedding or equipment. Elevate the patient's knees and the head of the bed slightly, avoiding extreme angles. If traction increases pain, notify the doctor.

13. Short-term pelvic traction may relieve pressure on the affected nerve by counteracting muscle spasm. Long-term traction, however, tends to aggravate the condition. Proper application and positioning are essential for therapeutic benefit. Increased pain with traction indicates the need to reevaluate the therapy.

14. As ordered, apply moist heat for 20 minutes, four times daily.

14. Moist heat is more effective than dry heat in promoting muscle relaxation.

15. As ordered, instruct the patient in the correct application and use of a back brace or corset, emphasizing that such devices should be worn only for the prescribed amount of time.
    Teach the patient to apply the brace or corset while lying supine, to fasten it snugly and ensure that the belts or ties are not twisted, to inspect the skin for pressure points daily and report areas of discomfort, to wear low-heeled shoes with no-slip soles, and to avoid falls.

15. A back brace or corset usually is used for only a short time. Extended use may cause the muscles to weaken, reducing the support and strength needed to maintain a healthy back. Proper teaching prevents complications.

16. Additional individualized interventions: _____

16. Rationales: _____

Target outcome criteria*
Within 7 to 10 days of admission, the patient will:
• verbalize absence of pain at rest
• engage in prescribed movement without pain
• assume only recommended positions
• perform pulmonary hygiene measures regularly
• perform leg exercises regularly
• exhibit neurologic findings at the preinjury level.

By the time of discharge, the patient will:
• have clear lungs
• have intact skin without signs of breakdown
• have no signs or symptoms of thromboembolic phenomena
• have normal bowel elimination
• have weight at or slightly below the preinjury level
• list precautions to observe regarding medication therapy
• list movements to avoid
• apply corset or brace (if ordered) appropriately.

Nursing diagnosis: *Altered role performance related to bed rest, effects of medications, prolonged discomfort, and required alterations in activity*

NURSING PRIORITY: Promote a positive self-concept.

Interventions

1. Include the patient as a participant in care-planning conferences. Allow as many choices as possible within therapeutic guidelines. Encourage the patient's participation in designing and implementing goals and activities.

Rationales

1. Participation in planning and implementing health management activities helps reduce frustration from loss of usual roles and fosters an increased sense of independence and self-control.

---

*Because the degree of injury and response to therapy vary widely among patients with low back pain, outcome criteria must be developed for the individual patient.

2. Discuss positive and negative feelings the patient may experience: for example, about the sick role, the recovery or rehabilitation role, role expectations when well, the potential for being accused of malingering, and life-style changes for preventing further injury.

2. Exploring feelings experienced during long-term disability helps prepare the patient for potential problems and facilitates adjustment to life-style alterations. For example, sick and recovery roles may actually provide the patient with certain rewards, such as more time for family and hobbies. Identifying such factors early in care planning may help the patient find other ways to meet such needs after recovery.

3. Help the patient identify coping resources and refocus negative feelings, such as learning to see difficulties as challenges rather than obstacles.

3. Identifying resources and thinking positively promote a full commitment to recovery.

4. Avoid authoritarian attitudes.

4. "Taking over" by caregivers diminishes the patient's self-esteem.

5. As appropriate, refer the patient to the occupational therapy department for diversionary activities while physical activity is limited.

5. Suitable diversionary activities provide opportunities to meet goals and feel productive despite the disability. Such activities also may help promote relaxation and reduce boredom during prolonged bed rest.

6. With the patient, identify strategies to maintain motivation during rehabilitation. Consider using a reward system, breaking down long-term goals into short-term goals, and varying routines to maintain the patient's interest.

6. Maintaining motivation is a key factor in successful rehabilitation. The ability to plan motivation strategies reflects the patient's level of self-esteem and acceptance of responsibility.

7. Additional individualized interventions: _____

7. Rationales: _____

Target outcome criteria
Throughout the hospital stay, the patient will:
• participate actively in care planning
• participate in diversionary activities
• identify coping resources
• plan and use strategies to maintain motivation.

Nursing diagnosis: *Knowledge deficit related to recovery, rehabilitation, and long-term management of low back injury*

NURSING PRIORITY: Teach the patient and family about back care, assisting with adaptation to necessary changes.

Interventions

1. Provide information about the anatomy and physiology of the following: vertebrae, including their articulation; disks and how their positions relate to pressure; spinal cord and nerve branches and their sensory and motor functions; and the spinal canal and fluid.

Rationales

1. Knowledge of anatomy and physiology prepares the patient for further teaching about the therapeutic regimen.

2. Provide information about required life-style changes.

2. Teaching the patient about these changes promotes health and reduces or eliminates the possibility of reinjury.

Sitting recommendations:
• Don't sit for more than 20 minutes without changing position.

• Sitting greatly increases intervertebral pressure.

• Keep the knees higher than the hips, such as by using a footstool.

• This position reduces stress on the spinal column.

• Sit in a firm chair with a straight back.

• Soft or overstuffed chairs and sofas do not firmly support the spinal column.

Driving recommendations:
• Always wear seat belts.

• Tilt the front seat so the knees are higher than the hips.

• Change position frequently, keeping the buttocks tilted forward.

• Allow for frequent rest stops that include walking, standing, or lying down.

Standing and walking recommendations:
• Stand to perform as many tasks as possible, being careful not to stand in one position too long. If prolonged standing is required, shift body weight from one foot to the other, or elevate one foot on a stool.

• When turning, turn the feet first, and avoid quick, jerking motions.

• Avoid shoes with heels higher than ½" (1.3 cm).

Lifting recommendations:
• Use principles of body mechanics when lifting, such as squatting directly in front of the object to be lifted, holding it close to the body, and then rising to a standing position without bending the back. Do not keep legs straight while lifting and do not reach over furniture to perform such tasks as closing windows.

• Do not lift heavy objects.

Exercise recommendations:
• Perform the following exercises as prescribed, beginning with 5 repetitions once daily and increasing to 20 repetitions twice daily within a 4-week period: pelvic tilt, knee-chest exercises, gluteal setting, and modified sit-ups (keeping the knees bent, as prescribed).
　Begin and end all exercise sessions by applying heat to the low back for at least 10 minutes. If any of these exercises causes pain, or if pain is present before beginning exercise, stop the exercise program and notify the doctor.

3. Teach about correct posture. Have the patient stand against the wall with head, shoulders, and buttocks touching it and with one hand placed in the lumbar lordotic space between the back and the wall. Then demonstrate how contraction of the rectus abdominis and gluteus maximus muscles rotates the pelvis and decreases this space. Explain that the patient should use this posture when walking, standing, and sitting.

4. Discuss the most common causes of low back pain, particularly muscle spasm and pressure on the nerve root, which causes pain to radiate from the low back down the sciatic nerve.

5. Discuss how pressure can damage nerves and may affect the lower extremities' structure and function. Emphasize the importance of reporting muscle atrophy, lost or decreased reflexes, lost or decreased function, and sensory loss.

6. Discuss with family or loved ones their ideas and feelings concerning the patient's current and long-term health status.

• Seat belts help prevent serious trauma to the spinal column should a motor vehicle accident occur.

• This position decreases strain on back and shoulder muscles.

• This position decreases lumbar lordosis and reduces strain on the low back muscles and spinal column.

• Frequent rest stops relieve stress caused by sitting.

• Next to lying down, standing best reduces intervertebral pressure.

• The low back is vulnerable to injury from twisting movements.

• High heels shift the center of gravity and strain the vertebral column and back musculature.

• Bending from a forward position with the legs straight places unnecessary strain on the vertebral column and back musculature.

• Lifting heavy objects strains the back muscles.

• A regular prescribed exercise program will strengthen abdominal and back muscles. Heat application allows for maximum muscle extension and contraction and reduces muscle spasm.

3. Correct posture reduces stress on the lumbosacral spine and musculature.

4. Knowing the causes of low back pain may help the patient identify the pain's origin and determine relief strategies.

5. Early reporting of changes in lower-extremity function, sensation, or appearance may facilitate corrective intervention.

6. Support from family members or loved ones is essential to recovery and rehabilitation.

7. Additional individualized interventions: _____

7. Rationales: _____

Target outcome criteria
By the time of discharge, the patient will:
• demonstrate understanding of the back's structure and function
• demonstrate knowledge of and strategies for implementing specific life-style changes, as prescribed

• select appropriate pain relief strategies
• list specific significant neurologic changes to report
• perform the prescribed exercise regimen
• list precautions to take before activities.

Discharge planning

NURSING DISCHARGE CRITERIA
Upon the patient's discharge, documentation shows evidence of:
• absence of severe debilitating pain
• ability to control pain using oral medications
• initiation of physical therapy exercise program or plans for outpatient treatment program
• completion of diagnostic radiology work-up
• ability to perform ADLs independently or with minimal assistance
• ability to transfer and ambulate with minimal difficulty
• absence of pulmonary or cardiovascular complications
• absence of skin problems or breakdown
• adequate home support system or referral to home care if indicated by inadequate home support system or the patient's inability to provide self-care.

PATIENT-FAMILY TEACHING CHECKLIST
Document evidence that the patient and family demonstrate an understanding of:
___ nature of low back injury
___ signs and symptoms indicating delayed healing or reinjury
___ recommended daily exercise program
___ common feelings about life-style changes
___ plan for resuming activity
___ resources for support of life-style modification
___ role of family members or loved ones in rehabilitation program
___ proper posture, lifting techniques, and positioning to prevent reinjury
___ all discharge medications' purpose, dosage, administration schedule, and adverse effects requiring medical attention (usual discharge medications include analgesics and muscle relaxants)
___ date, time, and location of follow-up appointments
___ how to contact the doctor.

DOCUMENTATION CHECKLIST
Using outcome criteria as a guide, document:
___ clinical status on admission
___ significant changes in clinical status
___ pertinent diagnostic findings

___ pain relief measures
___ nutritional intake
___ elimination status
___ progressive activity program and progress
___ complications of immobility, if any
___ patient-family teaching
___ discharge planning.

ASSOCIATED PLANS OF CARE
Ineffective Individual Coping
Knowledge Deficit
Laminectomy
Pain

References
Carpenito, L. *Handbook of Nursing Diagnosis.* Philadelphia: J.B. Lippincott Co., 1990.
Carpenito, L. *Nursing Diagnosis: Application to Clinical Practice,* 3rd ed. Philadelphia: J.B. Lippincott Co., 1990.
Gordon, M. *Nursing Diagnosis: Process and Application,* 2nd ed. New York: McGraw-Hill Book Co., 1987.
Luckman, J., and Sorensen, K. *Medical-Surgical Nursing: A Psychophysiologic Approach,* 3rd ed. Philadelphia: W.B. Saunders Co., 1987.

Major Burns

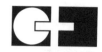

DRG information

DRGs involving burns may be assigned based on specific sites, percent of body surface burned, percent of third-degree burns, and surgical procedures. The following are examples of some DRG classifications for burns:

DRG 458 Nonextensive Burns With Skin Grafts.
Mean LOS = 15.8 days
Principal diagnoses include first-, second-, or third-degree burns of face, scalp, head, or neck (with or without loss of body part). Usually includes burns involving 10% to 49% of body surface, with 10% to 19% third-degree burns.

Additional DRG information: This diagnosis must be accompanied by one or more of the following principal procedures:
• graft (free skin, full-thickness, or split-thickness) to breast, hand, or other site
• heterograft or homograft to skin.

DRG 459 Nonextensive Burns With Wound Debridement and Other Operating Room Procedures.
Mean LOS = 10.9 days
Principal diagnoses include selected principal diagnoses listed under DRG 458.

Additional DRG information: This diagnosis must be accompanied by one or more of the following selected principal procedures:
• debridement of infection or burn
• amputation of penis or upper or lower limb
• revision of amputation stump
• closure of oral, bronchial, tracheal, thoracic, or gastric fistula
• reconstruction, repair, or plastic operations and reattachments of body parts or organs.

Introduction
DEFINITION AND TIME FOCUS

A burn is a traumatic skin injury caused by exposure to heat, chemicals, or electricity. A burn's severity depends on its depth and the body surface area affected. Partial-thickness burns can be superficial (first-degree), involving only the epidermis, or deep (second-degree), involving the epidermal and dermal layers of the skin. Because some epithelial tissue, such as the hair follicles, is uninjured, the skin can regenerate. Full-thickness burns (third and fourth-degree) involve the epidermis, dermis, subcutaneous tissues, and, sometimes, underlying muscle, tendon, and bone. Full-thickness burns require skin grafting to heal.

The total body surface area (TBSA) burned is estimated using the Rule of Nines or the Lund and Browder chart. Both the burn's depth and area are used to determine the initial treatment and if admission to a burn unit is necessary. Treatment in a burn unit is in-

dicated for patients with a partial thickness burn involving more than 25% of TBSA; a full-thickness burn involving more than 10% of TBSA; burns complicated by trauma, chronic illness, or inhalation or electrical injuries; or burns affecting such special areas as the face, eyes, ears, hands, feet, or the perineum. Children under age 2 and adults over age 60 also should be treated in a burn unit.

Minor burns can be treated in the emergency department or in the doctor's office. Patients with moderate burns without complications can be treated in a general critical care setting. This plan focuses on the patient admitted for treatment of superficial and deep partial-thickness burns involving more than 25% of TBSA.

ETIOLOGY AND PRECIPITATING FACTORS
• occupational exposure to causes of burns, such as fuels, chemicals, electricity, or hot substances
• home exposure to causes of burns, such as stoves, electricity, heaters, chemicals, matches, or cigarettes
• outdoor exposure to causes of burns, such as ultraviolet light, lightning, barbecues, or flammable liquids
• high-risk populations, such as young children, older adults, drug or alcohol abusers, chronically ill or debilitated patients, or those working in high-risk jobs

Focused assessment guidelines
NURSING HISTORY (Functional health pattern findings)

Health perception—health management pattern
• may report a high occupational risk for burns
• may report a high-risk activity that caused the burn
• may report chronic illness or debilitation

Nutritional-metabolic pattern
• may report thirst
• may report nausea, vomiting, and loss of appetite
• may report feelings of abdominal fullness

Elimination pattern
• may report decreased or absent urination

Activity-exercise pattern
• may report pain and stiffness when moving involved area
• may report difficulty breathing at rest and during movement

Cognitive-perceptual pattern
• may report pain
• may repeatedly verbalize the circumstances of the burn, or may report confusion and loss of memory about burn incident

Self-perception—self-concept pattern
• may express fear of loss of body part or disfigurement
• may express fear of dying

Role-relationship pattern
• may express concern about whereabouts and condition of others involved in the burn incident
• may express fear about maintaining role in family and in relationships
• may express concern over effects of injury on family
• may express fear about not being able to work again

Sexuality-reproductive pattern
• may express fear about future sexual performance
• may express fear about lack of sexual attractiveness because of injury

Coping—stress tolerance pattern
• initially may express lack of concern about burn
• may express fear and anxiety
• may express being overwhelmed by burn

Value-belief pattern
• may express need to see member of clergy

PHYSICAL FINDINGS
Note: Physical findings may vary depending on the burn's type, depth, surface area, and location.

Pulmonary
• tachypnea, dyspnea, shortness of breath on exertion
• with an inhalation injury, soot in nostrils or sputum
• stridor
• wheezing
• hoarse voice
• diminished breath sounds
• mucosal edema, vesicles, redness

Cardiovascular
• tachycardia
• hypotension
• arrhythmias
• pale, clammy, diaphoretic, or cool skin
• with an electrical injury, cardiac arrest with ventricular fibrillation, chest pain, or cardiac irritability

Neurologic
• agitation
• memory loss
• confusion
• headache
• mentation changes

Gastrointestinal
• decreased or absent bowel sounds
• distention
• vomiting
• dry mouth and mucous membranes

Genitourinary
• oliguria or anuria
• cloudy or tea-colored urine

Musculoskeletal
• pain and stiffness on movement of affected areas
• with an electrical injury, tetany and bone fractures caused by tetany or fall

Integumentary
• with a superficial partial-thickness burn, bright red to pink color, glistening blisters, blanching on pressure, and pain
• with a deep partial-thickness burn, pink to white color, blanching, pain, sensitive to pressure, and blisters
• with a full-thickness burn, white, gray, brown, or black skin color; eschar (coagulated and necrotic tissue) formation; no pain or pressure sensations; no blanching; dry, easily pulled out hair
• massive edema
• hypothermia
• shivering

DIAGNOSTIC STUDIES
• complete blood count—determines red blood cell count, hemoglobin level, and hematocrit, reflecting any blood loss or destruction and indicating the blood's oxygen-carrying ability. The white blood cell (WBC) count reflects the ability of the WBCs to respond to the inflammatory process. Baseline data and serial evaluations may reflect the seriousness of the fluid shifts and cell destruction accompanying major burns.
• serum electrolyte level—monitors fluid, electrolyte, and acid-base status. Hyperkalemia occurs initially because of the release of potassium into the serum during cell destruction and the hemoconcentration caused by fluid shifts into the interstitium. Hypokalemia may occur during the second day after injury as electrolytes are excreted into the urine. Other electrolytes may be low during the initial period after injury because of the massive shifts of fluid and electrolytes into the interstitium.
• blood glucose level—monitors the effect of the catabolic burn state on sugar metabolism and insulin production
• blood urea nitrogen and creatinine levels—monitor the adequacy of kidney function; acute tubular necrosis is a common complication after major tissue destruction
• clotting time (prothrombin time and partial thromboplastin time)—may reflect coagulation problems associated with major tissue destruction
• serum proteins (albumin and globulin) and serum osmolality—may reflect movement of intravascular colloids in and out of the interstitium.

• arterial blood gas (ABG) values—monitor oxygenation, ventilation, and acid-base status, especially with a suspected inhalation injury. Initially, they reveal respiratory alkalosis, reflecting hyperventilation; later, metabolic acidosis, reflecting hypoxemia and shock.
• carboxyhemoglobin level—may be elevated, confirming carbon monoxide poisoning and smoke inhalation
• urinalysis, specific gravity, urine electrolytes, and urine myoglobin levels—monitor kidney status; total urine output monitors hydration status
• blood and tissue cultures—provide baseline data and monitor infections
• chest X-ray—usually normal at first; in 1 to 2 days, may reveal atelectasis or pulmonary edema
• electrocardiogram—may reveal arrhythmias
• ventilation-perfusion pulmonary scan—may reveal areas of nonventilation and nonperfusion
• bronchoscopy—may reveal abnormalities of the bronchial tree such as redness, blistering, edema, or soot
• tissue biopsies and cultures—may reveal excessive wound contamination

POTENTIAL COMPLICATIONS
• hypovolemic shock
• cardiac arrhythmias
• cardiac arrest
• respiratory arrest
• atelectasis, pneumonia
• pulmonary edema
• infection, sepsis, septic shock
• acute tubular necrosis
• acute renal failure
• conversion of partial-thickness burns to full-thickness burns
• contractures
• loss of mobility and function
• scarring
• social and emotional isolation
• hematologic disorders

Nursing diagnosis: High risk for injury: continuing tissue injury related to continued exposure to heat or chemicals

NURSING PRIORITY: Stop the burn from expanding.

Interventions

1. Remove any jewelry, belts, coins, or other metal objects from the patient and then immediately flush the burn with cool water for 10 to 15 minutes. Document your actions.

2. For a chemical burn, quickly remove the patient's clothes, brush off dry chemicals, and flush the burns with large amounts of water. Observe the site for chemical residues. After flushing, use a neutralizer, if appropriate, on any remaining chemicals; consult a burn center or poison control center for the appropriate agent. Assess the site hourly and as needed for continuing damage, such as spreading redness, blistering, or loss of sensation. Document your findings.

3. Temporarily cover the flushed burn with a clean or sterile dressing or sheet while other interventions continue.

4. Additional individualized interventions: _____

Rationales

1. Metal items retain heat and permit continued thermal burning. Immediate flushing with cool water will cool the tissue and may limit the damage. Prolonged flushing or using ice water may cause such complications as arrhythmias, hypothermia, or shock.

2. Clothes may contain chemical residues and should be removed to prevent further injury. Thorough flushing with water will remove most chemicals. Neutralization may be helpful, but flushing is a higher initial priority than finding an appropriate neutralizer. Some chemicals, such as alkalies, may continue to cause damage even when neutralized, making ongoing assessments necessary.

3. Covering the burn may limit contamination and decrease pain from air exposure. Further burn care, such as debridement and application of topical antibiotics, has a low priority as compared with stabilization of airway, breathing, and circulation.

4. Rationales: _____

Target outcome criteria
Within the first hour after admission, the patient will:
• display minimal or no continuing tissue damage, such as additional areas of redness, blistering, or sensation loss
• manifest no signs of chemical residue on skin.

Collaborative problem: *High risk for hypoxemia related to airway burns and carbon monoxide inhalation*

NURSING PRIORITY: Promote ventilation and gas exchange.

Interventions

1. Maintain a patent airway. Anticipate the need for endotracheal intubation and mechanical ventilation.

2. Assess the patient's respiratory status on admission, then every 15 minutes until stable, then every 1 to 2 hours. Monitor respiratory rate; chest movements; use of accessory muscles; signs of anxiety or restlessness; color; breath sounds; adventitious sounds such as crackles, gurgles, or wheezes; hoarseness when speaking; and soot around the nostrils. Notify the doctor and document findings. Be prepared to assist with chest wall escharotomy, if necessary.

3. Monitor ABG values initially and then every shift and as needed for changes in respiratory status. Monitor initial and serial carboxyhemoglobin levels. Notify doctor of and document any abnormalities.

4. Provide 100% humidified oxygen therapy, as needed and ordered, especially for smoke inhalation or respiratory distress. Document oxygen administration.

5. Obtain initial and serial chest X-rays, as ordered.

6. Encourage deep-breathing and coughing exercises every hour and as needed. Assist with incentive spirometer use. Document pulmonary hygiene measures.

7. Administer bronchodilators every 4 to 8 hours, if ordered. Document their use.

8. Assess the amount, color, and consistency of sputum, including the presence of soot, every shift. Notify the doctor and document your findings.

9. Assist with bronchoscopy.

Rationales

1. Airway burns or inhalation of hot air can cause laryngospasms, progressive edema, and rapid airway occlusion up to 8 hours after the burn. Intubation is usually performed before progressive edema occludes the airway.

2. Abnormal findings, including hoarseness, crackles, wheezes, gurgles, signs of hypoxemia, restlessness, and soot around the nostrils, may indicate an inhalation injury and impending respiratory failure. Circumferential chest burns can restrict chest wall expansion and require escharotomy to allow ventilation.

3. ABG values reflect general oxygenation and acid-base levels. Low oxygen and high carbon dioxide levels may indicate a need for oxygen therapy or mechanical ventilation. Carbon monoxide interferes with oxygen transport because of its strong affinity for hemoglobin. Carboxyhemoglobin levels reflect the amount of abnormal hemoglobin present.

4. Oxygen therapy may be required during the initial post-injury period to maintain desirable ABG levels, help eliminate carbon monoxide, and assist burn healing.

5. Pulmonary involvement may not appear on X-ray for up to 24 hours.

6. Regular deep-breathing and coughing exercises promote lung expansion, mobilize secretions, and prevent atelectasis. Incentive spirometry encourages deep inspiratory efforts that expand the alveoli more effectively than forceful expiratory efforts.

7. Bronchodilators may interrupt bronchospasms and counteract the narrowing effect of airway edema.

8. Soot in the sputum may confirm an inhalation injury. Excessive sputum may indicate an infection.

9. Bronchoscopy is used diagnostically to locate soot in smaller airways, airway burns, and pulmonary inflammation. It also is used therapeutically to remove soot and secretions, minimizing the risk of later infection and atelectasis.

10. After stabilization, assist with intermittent positive-pressure breathing (IPPB) therapy every 4 hours, if ordered. Document all treatments.

10. IPPB therapy promotes lung expansion by the deep delivery of bronchodilators and positive-pressure breaths.

11. Additional individualized interventions: _____

11. Rationales: _____

Target outcome criteria
Within 24 hours of admission, the patient will:
• display no signs of respiratory distress
• display improving breath sounds

• have moist mucous membranes.

Collaborative problem: *Hypovolemia related to movement of vascular fluids to the interstitium and water evaporation from burns*

NURSING PRIORITY: Maintain vascular fluid volume.

Interventions

1. On admission, place one or two large-bore I.V. lines in large veins in the arms, using aseptic technique. Document your actions.

2. Collaborate with the doctor on fluid replacement therapy. Administer fluids, as ordered, and document their use.

• On admission, assess the patient's fluid needs. Use the Rule of Nines or the Lund and Browder chart to determine the TBSA burned; use a fluid replacement formula, preferably the Parkland formula (4 ml Ringer's lactate × kg body weight × % TBSA), to determine the volume of fluid needed in the first 24 hours after injury.

• Give crystalloid fluid replacements during the first 24 hours after injury. According to the Parkland formula, administer half the volume in the first 8 hours, a quarter in the next 8 hours, and a quarter in the last 8 hours.

• After 24 to 48 hours, administer colloids and dextrose in water solutions.

3. Assess adequacy of fluid replacement every 1 to 2 hours and as needed, including vital signs, urine output, urine specific gravity, mentation, weight, serum electrolytes and osmolality, and hematocrit. Document your findings.

4. Assess serum electrolyte levels and administer replacements, as ordered. Document your actions. See Appendix C, "Fluid and Electrolyte Imbalances," for general assessments and interventions.

Rationales

1. Large I.V. access lines are needed to give the large amounts of fluids required during the fluid resuscitation period.

2. Appropriate fluid therapy is critical to the patient's survival.

• Fluid replacement formulas, in conjunction with the TBSA burned, estimate the fluid replacement needed every 24 hours. Numerous fluid replacement formulas are available. The American College of Surgeons and the American Burn Association recommend the Parkland formula.

• Large amounts of crystalloid fluids are needed to replace the massive amounts of vascular fluids that leak into the interstitium during the first 24 hours, a result of inflammation and increased capillary permeability.

• After the capillary membranes stabilize, colloids such as plasma can be administered to replace colloid losses. Dextrose in water solutions are also given to replace evaporative fluid loss and as a maintenance solution.

3. Normal vital signs, urine output (50 to 100 ml/hour), specific gravity and osmolality, mental status, serum electrolyte levels, and hematocrit all reflect adequate fluid replacement. Diuresis commonly begins on the third day after injury. A weight loss of less than 2% a day during this time reflects adequate fluid replacement.

4. During the first 24 to 48 hours, electrolytes follow the fluid shifts into the interstitium, reducing the amounts available in the intravascular areas. Electrolyte replacement may be necessary except for potassium, whose serum levels increase because of cell destruction during the immediate postburn period. Careful monitoring guides electrolyte replacement. The "Fluid and Electrolyte Imbalances" appendix includes general assessments and interventions for electrolyte imbalances.

5. After fluid resuscitation is complete and the patient's gastrointestinal function returns, begin enteral feedings and remove the I.V. lines. Document your actions.

6. Additional individualized interventions: _____

_____

5. Enteral feedings should begin as soon as possible to decrease the risk of infection at the I.V. insertion sites.

6. Rationales: _____

_____

Target outcome criteria
Within 24 hours of admission, the patient will:
• manifest normal vital signs
• have a urine output of 50 to 100 ml/hour
• stay within normal ranges for urine specific gravity, serum electrolytes, serum osmolality, and hematocrit
• have no observable changes in mentation.

Within 48 to 72 hours of admission, the patient will manifest a weight loss of no more than 2% a day.

Collaborative problem: High risk for peripheral ischemia related to circumferential eschar formation on arms and legs, compartment syndrome, or vascular disruption

NURSING PRIORITY: Maintain adequate tissue perfusion.

Interventions

1. When possible, elevate burned areas, but not above the level of the heart.

2. Assess tissue perfusion distal to the burn site every 1 to 2 hours, noting color, temperature, capillary refill, pulses, sensation, function, and pain. Notify the doctor of and document any abnormalities.

3. Assist the doctor in performing an escharotomy, if necessary. Assess the escharotomy site for bleeding and circulation return. Apply dressings to the site. Document your actions.

4. If ordered, apply proteolytic enzymes, such as sutilains (Travase), to eschar. Assess and document their effect.

5. Additional individualized interventions: _____

_____

Rationales

1. Elevation may decrease edema by using gravity to optimize venous return.

2. As eschar hardens, it may constrict circulation, particularly if it is circumferential. The patient with arm or leg burns also is at great risk for compartment syndrome, in which edema increases pressure in a fascial compartment and compresses nerves, blood vessels, and muscle. Early recognition of impaired circulation allows early intervention and minimizes the risk of permanent damage.

3. Incisions across areas of eschar formation release tissue tension and allow circulation to return to constricted areas. Assessment provides for early identification and correction of complications.

4. Proteolytic enzymes selectively digest necrotic tissue. By softening the eschar, they decrease its constricting effects.

5. Rationales: _____

_____

Target outcome criteria
Within 1 to 2 days of admission, the patient will:
• display signs of adequate tissue perfusion distal to the burned area, such as pink color, good capillary refill, warmth, sensation, function, and minimal pain
• display minimal bleeding or other complications at eschar site.

Nursing diagnosis: *High risk for burn infection related to loss of protective integument, exposure to contamination, decreased perfusion, and impaired immunologic response*

NURSING PRIORITIES: (a) Protect the burn and (b) prevent or minimize infection.

Interventions

1. Explain the purpose and methods of burn care to the patient and family.

2. Use strict aseptic technique, including cap, mask, gown, and sterile gloves, during all burn care. Wash the burn once or twice daily with a mild soap or normal saline solution. A hydrotherapy tub, shower stretcher, or basins at the bedside may be used. Use a gentle circular scrubbing motion. Debride with scissors if necessary. Shave hair over involved areas, except for the eyebrows. Rinse with water. Document your actions.

3. During washing and debridement, assess the burn for color, drainage, size, odor, elevations or depressions, and pain. Document your findings.

4. Apply topical antibiotics, if ordered, after washing and debridement, typically silver nitrate, mafenide acetate (Sulfamylon), silver sulfadiazine (Silvadene), or povidone-iodine (Betadine). Use aseptic technique including mask, cap, gown, and sterile gloves. Cover the burn with gauze or stretch bandages after applying antibiotics. Monitor for medication-related complications such as pain, leukopenia, tissue damage, or electrolyte depletion. If signs of medication-related complications occur, notify the doctor and document your findings.

5. Leave partial-thickness burns exposed to air, if ordered. Document scab formation and condition of the burn.

6. Monitor temporary wound covers, such as biologic, biosynthetic, or synthetic dressings, if used. Change as needed, observing for infection and excessive exudate. Remove excess liquid, as necessary. Document your actions.

7. Maintain patient warmth during washing, debridement, and dressing changes. Limit procedures to 30 minutes or less. Document the procedure and the patient's tolerance.

8. Assist in obtaining needle biopsy cultures from burns, as ordered. Document the procedure.

9. Assess for signs of sepsis, including increased pulse rate, respiratory rate and temperature, decreased blood pressure, decreased urine output, and mentation changes, every 2 to 4 hours and as needed. Notify the doctor of and document abnormal findings.

Rationales

1. Understanding the purpose of wound care may help the patient cope with the inevitable pain such care causes, while understanding the general methods may decrease fear of the unknown. Involving family members in teaching and care, when appropriate, acknowledges their learning needs and the importance of their emotional support to the patient.

2. To reduce the risk of infection, strict aseptic technique must be used when the burn is uncovered. Regular washing and debridement removes dead tissue and stimulates the development of granulation tissue, which serves as the base for skin grafts. Shaving excess hair removes a medium for bacterial growth. Eyebrows are not shaved because they may not grow back, leaving the patient with an odd facial appearance.

3. Regular assessment may identify early signs of infection and allow timely treatment.

4. Topical antibiotics are commonly used to prevent massive bacterial colonization of burns from the patient's skin flora or contaminants. Strict aseptic technique reduces the risk of infection. Monitoring for adverse effects or complications of antibiotic therapy helps avoid further compromise of the patient's status.

5. Partial-thickness burns may heal in a week without complications when left exposed to air.

6. Temporary wound covers used early in treatment prevent infection and evaporative losses and promote granulation tissue development. The dressings are left in place for varying amounts of time. Usually, excessive exudate should be removed to enhance the dressing's adherence.

7. Evaporative water loss during procedures may increase the risks of volume deficit, electrolyte loss, and shock.

8. Needle biopsy cultures are more accurate monitors of wound infection than surface cultures. Early detection of wound infection allows timely treatment and may prevent sepsis.

9. Loss of the skin barrier, frequent manipulation of the burn wounds, and the general catabolic state place the patient at high risk for sepsis. Early recognition and treatment may prevent irreversible sepsis and septic shock, a major cause of death in burn patients.

10. Administer tetanus toxoid on admission, as ordered. Administer tetanus immunoglobulin in another site, if tetanus toxoid has not been given during the preceding 10 years. Document their administration.

10. Burns are at high risk for anaerobic infections, including tetanus. Tetanus toxoid stimulates antibody production. Tetanus immunoglobulin provides protection until tetanus antibodies develop. Using different sites prevents inactivation of the immunoglobulin.

11. Give I.V. antibiotics, as ordered, if major wound sepsis occurs. Observe for secondary infections of the mouth, GI tract, and the genitalia. Monitor for resistance to topical and systemic antibiotics. Document your findings.

11. I.V. antibiotics usually are given only for major wound sepsis because areas of eschar have poor circulation and are better treated with topical antibiotics. Secondary infections may result from overgrowth of normally suppressed pathogens. Development of resistant strains of microorganisms is a common result of long-term topical antibiotic use.

12. Additional individualized interventions: _____

_____

12. Rationales: _____

_____

Target outcome criteria
Within 1 week of admission, the patient will:
• display clean and healing superficial burns, including scab formation
• display development of red granulation tissue over deeper partial-thickness wounds that are also free from odor, purulent drainage, and elevations or depressions

• display no complications of topical antibiotic use, such as pain, leukopenia, tissue damage, electrolyte or fluid loss, or secondary infections
• display intact wound covers
• manifest vital signs, WBC count, urine output, and mentation within normal ranges.

Nursing diagnosis: *Pain related to tissue destruction and exposure of nerves in partially destroyed tissue*

NURSING PRIORITY: Relieve pain.

Interventions

1. See the "Pain" plan, page 69.

2. Administer I.V. analgesics 10 to 20 minutes before burn cleaning, debridement, and dressing changes. Medicate frequently and liberally within the ordered parameters. Document administration and degree of pain relief achieved.

3. Decrease anxiety and fear by explaining procedures and treatments thoroughly. Document teaching. Refer to the "Knowledge Deficit" plan, page 56, and the "Ineffective Individual Coping" plan, page 51.

4. Additional individualized interventions: _____

_____

Rationales

1. The "Pain" plan includes general assessments and interventions for a patient with pain. This plan contains additional information specific to the burn patient.

2. Burn care is excruciatingly painful and may need to be repeated several times daily. Anticipation increases the patient's perceived pain. Frequent and liberal analgesic administration may prevent the pain from reaching intolerable levels. Addiction to pain medication is rare in burn patients. The I.V. route is preferred because massive edema and inflammation reduce medication absorption through the subcutaneous and intramuscular routes.

3. Fear of the unknown, helplessness, and powerlessness may increase pain. Burn care is complex and long term. Thorough teaching and emotional support may allay fear of the unknown and provide the patient some sense of control over treatment, which may lessen the pain experience. The "Knowledge Deficit" and "Ineffective Individual Coping" plans contain general assessments and interventions applicable to any patient.

4. Rationales: _____

_____

Target outcome criterion
Within 1 to 2 days of admission, the patient will experience minimal pain during burn care.

Nursing diagnosis: *High risk for impaired skin integrity related to nonadherence of graft and impaired donor site healing*

NURSING PRIORITY: Optimize burn healing.

Interventions

1. Apply homografts or heterografts in single sheets to freshly cleaned burns, as ordered, using aseptic technique. Trim to prevent overlapping. Smooth the graft, removing wrinkles and air. Apply thin gauze (with or without antibiotic ointment) over the graft, as ordered. Apply a dressing over the gauze. Protect the site from movement or trauma. Document your actions.

2. After surgery for autografting, immobilize the graft and protect it from injury for at least 48 hours. Keep the large, bulky dressings in place. Use a bed cradle. Prevent prolonged pressure over the graft. Elevate the graft site to the highest position possible. Use splints and elastic bandages over graft sites, particularly when the patient walks. Discontinue activities, such as hydrotherapy or active physical therapy, for several days after grafting. Document your actions.

3. Protect the donor site from infection or trauma. If outer dressings are used, keep them in place by using splints and limiting exercise for several days. Leave the inner gauze dressing in place until it falls off, usually in 2 to 3 weeks. Use a heat lamp or hair dryer to dry the site for 15 to 20 minutes four times daily or as ordered. Leave the site exposed to air, as ordered. Document treatments and condition of the site every shift.

4. Observe the homograft, heterograft, or autograft for signs of adherence; monitor all grafts and donor sites for signs of infection. Report immediately any redness, exudate, blood under the graft, swelling, separation, drainage, foul odor, or increased temperature, pulse rate, or respirations. Document your findings.

5. Apply moist warm compresses to the donor site, if ordered, for 20 to 30 minutes four times a day. Document your actions.

6. Apply topical antibiotics to the burn and donor site and administer systemic antibiotics intravenously, if ordered. Document your actions.

7. Additional individualized interventions: _____

Rationales

1. Homografts and heterografts are temporary biological dressings that protect burns and stimulate formation of granulation tissue until autografts can be applied. Removing wrinkles and air pockets promotes adherence. Gauze and dressings protect the graft. Freshly grafted sites must be protected from accidental dislodgment until circulation has been established with underlying tissue.

2. The graft must be immobilized and protected from trauma and movement for several days to prevent dislodgment and promote circulation until it adheres. Large dressings provide protective padding. A bed cradle prevents pressure from bed linens. Elevation limits edema. Splints and elastic bandages provide support, maintain dressing placement, prevent excessive movement of the graft site, and allow some activity. Excessive moisture or exercise may dislodge the graft in the first days after grafting.

3. The donor site must be protected to prevent its conversion from a partial-thickness wound to a deeper-thickness wound. Using dressings and splints and limiting exercise may protect the site and promote tissue regeneration. The inner gauze is left in place to stabilize and cover the site during tissue regeneration; early removal could traumatize the new tissue. Heat increases circulation and promotes healing. Air exposure promotes drying and scab formation.

4. Regular assessment may permit early detection of graft rejection or wound sepsis.

5. Warmth and moisture may increase circulation and promote epithelization.

6. As previously described, topical antibiotics are commonly used to prevent wound sepsis from the patient's skin flora. Systemic antibiotics are used when major wound sepsis occurs.

7. Rationales: _____

Target outcome criteria
Within 2 to 5 days after grafting, the patient will:
• display an intact and healing graft without redness, swelling, exudate formation, bleeding, or foul odor
• display a dry and healed donor site
• manifest normal vital signs
• display no signs of wound sepsis
• maintain activity limitations.

Nursing diagnosis: *Nutritional deficit related to increased metabolic needs of burn healing*

NURSING PRIORITY: Provide adequate nutrition to promote burn healing.

Interventions

1. Refer to the "Nutritional Deficit" plan, page 63.

2. Upon the patient's admission, insert a nasogastric tube and withhold food and fluids until bowel sounds return. Provide I.V. fluids and total parenteral nutrition continuously, as ordered. Assess patient tolerance, including weights, intake and output, edema, and blood glucose, electrolyte, and protein levels. Document your findings.

3. After bowel function returns, provide a high-calorie, high-protein diet with vitamin supplements, as ordered. Provide high-calorie liquids, such as milk-shakes or prepared liquid diet supplements, instead of water. Take the patient's food preferences into consideration whenever possible. Document daily intake.

4. Additional individualized interventions: _____

Rationales

1. The "Nutritional Deficit" plan contains general assessments and interventions for a patient with a nutritional deficit. This section provides additional information pertinent to the burn patient.

2. A burn commonly causes paralytic ileus, which prevents oral intake for 2 to 4 days. Nutritional requirements are met intravenously during this time. Regular assessments monitor the adequacy of fluid and nutrient intake.

3. A high-calorie, high-protein diet (between 5,000 and 6,000 calories daily) may be required to meet the increased metabolic needs for tissue healing. All intake must help meet these increased needs, so milk-shakes are preferable to water. Because the burn patient commonly experiences loss of appetite, offering favorite foods may improve intake. Extra vitamins are needed to meet tissue-healing needs.

4. Rationales: _____

Target outcome criteria
Within 1 week of admission, the patient will:
• display minimal or no signs of nutritional deficit
• manifest expected wound healing
• display no more than a 10% weight loss.

Nursing diagnosis: *Impaired physical mobility related to prescribed position and movement limitations*

NURSING PRIORITY: Maintain mobility within range of limitations.

Interventions

1. Implement measures in the "Impaired Physical Mobility" plan, page 36, as appropriate.

2. Provide active and passive range-of-motion (ROM) exercises to arms and legs with a healing graft every 2 hours and as needed. Document patient tolerance.

Rationales

1. The "Impaired Physical Mobility" plan covers general information about this problem. This plan provides additional information pertinent to burn patients.

2. ROM exercises prevent contractures and promote circulation, healing, and a sense of well-being.

3. Promote self-care within the patient's limitations.

3. Self-care increases the patient's activity level and promotes a sense of well-being and control over the environment.

4. Provide protective devices, such as splints and dressings, during exercise, as ordered. Document their use.

4. Protective devices allow mobility while maintaining the integrity of the graft site.

5. Position body parts in anatomic and functional alignment. Document your actions.

5. Anatomic and functional alignment prevents contracture formation and promotes eventual return to normal activities.

6. Provide pain medication, as needed and ordered. Document its administration.

6. Pain relief encourages movement and activity.

7. Additional individualized interventions: _____

7. Rationales: _____

Target outcome criteria
Within 2 weeks of admission, the patient will:
• have no contractures
• manifest anatomic and functional positions of arms and legs

• perform ROM and other exercises
• experience minimal pain during activities.

Nursing diagnosis: *Body-image disturbance related to extensive burns and potential scarring*

NURSING PRIORITY: Promote adjustment to body changes.

Interventions

1. Refer to the "Ineffective Individual Coping" plan, page 51, and the "Grieving" plan, page 31.

Rationales

1. The extensive emotional adjustments necessary to recover from the burn may severely tax the patient's and family's coping abilities. Grieving for lost appearance or the function of body parts is a necessary first step in emotional recovery. The plans listed provide multiple interventions helpful to recovery.

2. Encourage verbalization of feelings about the burn, potential scarring, and loss of function. Document concerns.

2. Verbalization of concerns decreases anxiety and fear and encourages self-appraisal to determine realistic goals.

3. Provide information about procedures and expected results. Document teaching and the patient's response.

3. Knowledge of procedures and expected results decreases fear of the unknown and encourages patient participation and cooperation during recovery.

4. Encourage realistic goals.

4. Focusing on realistic goals, such as small, obtainable daily goals, may prevent disappointment and despair during recovery.

5. Additional individualized interventions: _____

5. Rationales: _____

Target outcome criteria
Throughout the recovery period, the patient will:
• express fears and concerns openly
• set small, realistic goals for recovery

• participate in recovery.

Discharge planning
NURSING DISCHARGE CRITERIA
Upon the patient's discharge, documentation shows evidence of:
• stable vital signs and monitoring parameters
• healing graft and donor sites
• absence of wound or systemic sepsis
• stable fluid and electrolyte status
• renal status within normal limits
• adequate nutrition and fluid intake
• ability to perform ROM and other exercises
• anatomic and functional positions of arms and legs
• absence of such complications as shock, cardiac arrhythmias, renal failure, contractures, or bleeding
• minimal edema.

PATIENT-FAMILY TEACHING CHECKLIST
Document evidence that the patient and family demonstrate an understanding of:
___ grafting and wound care procedures, including expected course of healing
___ signs and symptoms of such complications as shock, bleeding, infection, and graft rejection
___ importance of ROM exercises and anatomic and functional positioning of affected arms and legs
___ nutritional needs
___ comfort measures for pain
___ protective measures, such as splints and dressings, for wounds
___ long-term recovery goals.

DOCUMENTATION CHECKLIST
Using outcome criteria as a guide, document:
___ clinical status on admission
___ significant changes in status
___ pertinent diagnostic test findings
___ status of graft and donor sites
___ complications, such as shock, arrhythmias, sepsis, renal failure, or contractures
___ oxygen therapy
___ ROM and other exercises
___ tolerance of tubbing, debridement, and wound care
___ pain and effect of medication
___ mental and emotional status
___ patient-family teaching
___ discharge planning.

ASSOCIATED PLANS OF CARE
Impaired Physical Mobility
Ineffective Individual Coping
Knowledge Deficit
Nutritional Deficit
Pain

References
Bayley, E. "Wound Healing in Patients with Burns," *Nursing Clinics of North America* 25(1):205-22, January, 1990.

Beare, P., and Myers, J., eds. *Principles and Practice of Adult Health Nursing.* St. Louis: C.V. Mosby Co., 1990.

Dossey, B.M., Guzetta, C.E., and Kenner, C.V., *Critical Care Nursing: Body–Mind–Spirit,* 3rd ed. Philadelphia: J.B. Lippincott Co., 1992.

Kinney, M., Packa, D., and Dunbar, S. *AACN'S Clinical Reference for Critical-Care Nursing.* New York: McGraw-Hill Book Co., 1988.

Martin, L. "Nursing Implications of Today's Burn Care Technique," *RN* 52(5):26-33, May 1989.

McKenry, L., and Salerno, E. *Mosby's Pharmacology in Nursing,* 17th ed. St. Louis: C.V. Mosby Co., 1989.

Patrick, M., Woods, S., Craven, R., Rokosky, J., and Bruno, P. *Medical-Surgical Nursing: Pathophysiological Concepts,* 2nd ed. Philadelphia: J.B. Lippincott Co., 1991.

Phipps, W., Long, B., Woods, N., and Cassmeyer, V., eds. *Medical-Surgical Nursing: Concepts and Clinical Practice,* 4th ed. St. Louis: Mosby-YearBook, 1991.

Thompson, J., McFarland, G., Hirsch, J., Tucker, S. and Bowers, A. *Mosby's Manual of Clinical Nursing,* 2nd ed. St. Louis: C.V. Mosby Co., 1989.

MUSCULOSKELETAL AND INTEGUMENTARY DISORDERS

Multiple Trauma

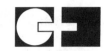

DRG information

DRG 444 Multiple Trauma. Age 17 +. With Complication or Comorbidity (CC).
Mean LOS = 5.1 days
Principal diagnoses include:
• traumatic amputation of extremities
• crushing injuries of various sites (external)
• injuries to blood vessels of various sites (internal)
• open wounds complicated by delayed treatment, delayed healing, or primary infection.
DRG 445 Multiple Trauma. Age 17 +. Without CC.
Mean LOS = 3.6 days
Principal diagnoses include selected principal diagnoses listed under DRG 444. The distinction is that DRG 445 excludes complications or comorbidities.
DRG 446 Multiple Trauma. Age 0 to 17.
Mean LOS = 2.4 days
Principal diagnoses include selected principal diagnoses listed under DRG 444. The distinction is that DRG 446 excludes patients greater than 17 years.
DRG 486 Other Operating Room Procedures for Multiple Significant Trauma.
Mean LOS = 12.5 days
DRG 487 Other Multiple Significant Trauma.
Mean LOS = 7.6 days
Additional DRG information: The documentation of all injuries sustained and procedures (surgical and non-surgical) performed is paramount to receiving maximum reimbursement for multiple trauma patients: for example, a bedside excisional debridement could alter the DRG, as could the documentation of injuries from different significant trauma body site categories.

Introduction
DEFINITION AND TIME FOCUS
Multiple trauma results from accidental or intentional injury to more than one body part, organ, or system. Trauma usually can be described as either blunt or penetrating, depending on whether the skin is broken.

This plan focuses on the first few days after trauma — the critical-care phase. It assumes that the patient has been moved from the field to the emergency department for stabilization, to surgery where essential repairs have been accomplished, and then to the unit. If the patient is not already stable, plan and implement appropriate cardiopulmonary support and cervical spine protection, and provide preoperative care based on institution policies. Although every possible complication cannot be included, this plan reviews major complications in detail and refers to other plans where appropriate. Long-term rehabilitation is not covered here, but prevention of long-term disability — the focus of nursing care — is discussed. The plan refers to special equipment used to care for the trauma patient, but no endorsement of a specific product or manufacturer is implied.

ETIOLOGY AND PRECIPITATING FACTORS
• chemical impairment of mentation and judgment, such as by alcohol, narcotics, cocaine, or other street drugs
• suicide attempts
• assaults
• falls
• industrial accidents
• motor vehicle accidents
• pedestrian-vehicle collisions
• sports injuries
• underlying physical problems, such as acute myocardial infarction or cerebrovascular accident
• major psychiatric disorders
• recent personal stress

Focused assessment guidelines
NURSING HISTORY (Functional health pattern findings)

Health perception — health management pattern
• likely to be a male age 15 to 35; about 75% of trauma patients are male

Nutritional-metabolic pattern
• usually well-nourished

Activity-exercise pattern
• may have a history of athletic competition

Cognitive-perceptual pattern
• complains of pain, if conscious
• is likely to report or display confusion, anxiety, or amnesia, if conscious

Coping — stress tolerance pattern
• may be undergoing a situational or maturational life crisis
• may have a history of psychiatric problems

PHYSICAL FINDINGS
Note: Alcohol, drugs, anxiety, restlessness, decreased level of consciousness (LOC), or altered sensory function commonly interfere with accurate assessment. Serial observations and analysis of trends in findings are critical. Physical findings vary with the particular trauma present.

Cardiovascular
- hypotension and tachycardia (if shock is present)
- hypertension and tachycardia (if shock is absent)
- diminished or absent pulse (if trauma is to an extremity)
- arrhythmias
- jugular venous distention (if cardiac tamponade is present)
- muffled heart sounds (if cardiac tamponade is present)
- capillary refill time greater than 3 seconds (if shock or vascular disruption is present)

Pulmonary
- tachypnea
- shallow respirations
- paradoxical chest movement (if flail chest is present)
- crepitus and ecchymoses (if chest trauma is present)

Gastrointestinal
- Cullen's sign (ecchymoses around umbilicus) and Grey-Turner's sign (ecchymoses in flanks) if intra-abdominal or retroperitoneal bleeding present (a late sign)

Neurologic
- decreased LOC
- rhinorrhea or otorrhea (if cerebrospinal fluid leak is present)
- pupillary changes
- sensory or motor impairment (if the trauma is to the head, the spinal cord, or an extremity)

Integumentary
- abrasions
- lacerations
- ecchymoses
- road burns
- Battle's sign (ecchymoses over mastoid area) and raccoon's eyes (periorbital ecchymoses) if basilar skull fracture or facial fracture is present
- pallor, mottling, or cyanosis
- cool, cold, or clammy skin

Musculoskeletal
- fractures
- amputations

DIAGNOSTIC STUDIES
- complete blood count — commonly reveals decreased hemoglobin and hematocrit values secondary to hemorrhage; white blood cell count may be elevated
- serum electrolytes — monitors fluid and electrolyte status
- blood urea nitrogen and serum creatinine levels — may be elevated secondary to decreased renal perfusion in shock
- lactate levels — may be elevated, reflecting anaerobic metabolism in shock; high initial levels are associated with low probability of survival
- serum bilirubin — assesses hepatic damage
- cardiac isoenzymes — determine acute myocardial infarction, a common cause of trauma, or cardiac injury
- arterial blood gas (ABG) levels — vary, depending on cardiopulmonary status; generally, respiratory alkalosis occurs if tachypnea is present; respiratory acidosis occurs if respiratory depression is present; metabolic acidosis occurs if shock is present
- coagulation panel — monitors for disseminated intravascular coagulation
- serum aspartate transaminase, alanine transaminase, and lactic dehydrogenase levels — monitor for liver damage
- anteroposterior, odontoid, and lateral cervical spine (C-spine) radiography — an essential procedure to visualize C1 to C7; can detect spinal injury or "clear" the C-spine of fractures
- 12-lead electrocardiography (ECG) — can help evaluate myocardial infarction or contusion, arrhythmias, electrolyte imbalance, or antiarrhythmic agent effects
- chest X-ray — can detect fractured ribs, widened mediastinum, pneumothorax, hemothorax, or other life-threatening chest injuries; a chest X-ray can also confirm placement of an endotracheal tube and central lines and monitor for adult respiratory distress syndrome, pneumonia, and other complications
- anteroposterior pelvic X-ray, including both hips — can detect pelvic ring disruption or hip dislocation
- diagnostic peritoneal lavage — may reveal blood, feces, bile, or amylase, indicating abdominal injury
- excretory urogram, cystogram, or ureterogram — used to identify the size, location, and filling of the renal pelvis, ureters, and urethra
- computed tomography (CT) scan — can visualize injuries to the head, neck, spine, abdomen, and kidneys
- arteriography — determines vessel integrity
- radionuclide scanning and sonography — assists in the identification of organ structure and function; especially useful in suspected chest, abdominal, or pelvic injuries

POTENTIAL COMPLICATIONS
- infection or sepsis
- pulmonary embolism
- atelectasis or pneumonia
- adult respiratory distress syndrome
- disseminated intravascular coagulation
- renal failure
- cardiac failure
- liver failure
- increased intracranial pressure
- paralysis
- fat embolism
- compartmental syndrome
- malnutrition
- multisystem organ failure
- post-traumatic stress disorder

Collaborative problem: *High risk for hypoxemia related to pulmonary injury, head injury, shock, or other factors*

NURSING PRIORITY: Maintain optimal airway, ventilation, and oxygenation.

Interventions

1. Maintain a patent airway. Maintain C-spine precautions until radiologic or tomographic findings have ruled out ligamentous injury or fracture.

2. Monitor ventilatory status. Observe respiratory rate, rhythm, effort of breathing, and tidal volume. Monitor trends in ABG values. Prepare for intubation and mechanical ventilation, as ordered, particularly if the patient has flail chest, pulmonary contusion, or shock. Refer to the "Mechanical Ventilation" plan, page 227.

3. Provide supplemental oxygen, as ordered.

4. Obtain serial chest X-rays at least daily, as ordered.

5. Additional individualized interventions: _____

Rationales

1. Although airway patency will have been evaluated before unit admission, trauma to the head, face, neck, or torso can compromise a previously patent airway at any time. Although C-spine clearance usually is done before unit admission, general precautions may still be required while awaiting the official radiologic reading. The C6 and C7 vertebrae may be difficult to clear in a patient with large shoulders, and CT scan may be required.

2. If the patient's condition deteriorates, ventilatory status may change abruptly. Deterioration also may be insidious (for example, if the patient tires), so close monitoring is essential. The "Mechanical Ventilation" plan presents comprehensive information on indications for, types of, and nursing care for mechanical ventilation.

3. All multiple trauma patients need supplemental oxygenation. Hypoxemia involves many factors and may result from pulmonary injury, depressed LOC, decreased cardiac output, ischemia, acidosis, and other factors. Supplemental oxygen elevates arterial oxygen tension, ensuring that the blood reaching the tissues provides the maximum amount of oxygen possible.

4. Serial chest X-rays can detect complications in time for corrective action.

5. Rationales: _____

Target outcome criteria
According to individual readiness, the patient will:
• display ABG levels within normal limits
• have clear breath sounds bilaterally
• have clear lung fields on chest X-ray.

Collaborative problem: *High risk for shock related to hypovolemia, cardiac injury, spinal cord injury, or sepsis*

NURSING PRIORITIES: (a) Monitor for shock, and (b) restore circulating blood volume and tissue perfusion if shock occurs.

Interventions

1. Implement measures in the "Hypovolemic Shock" plan, page 346, as appropriate, such as monitoring LOC, vital signs, urinary output, ECG pattern, hemodynamic measurements, and laboratory values; maintaining patency of two large-bore I.V. lines; and administering fluids and positive inotropic agents, as ordered.

Rationales

1. The "Hypovolemic Shock" plan covers assessment and interventions for this potential problem in detail. This plan provides additional information specific to the trauma patient.

2. Implement autotransfusion, when possible. Follow the manufacturer's directions for citration, if used, and reinfusion.

2. The patient's blood, when captured in drainage, is an ideal source of blood replacement because it decreases the possibility of transfusion reactions and infection. Citration may be used to prevent the retrieved blood from coagulating in the autotransfusor.

3. Monitor continually for new or ongoing bleeding.

3. Commonly, restoration of adequate blood pressure reverses peripheral vasoconstriction and dislodges fragile clots, so additional bleeding becomes apparent.

4. Collaborate with the doctor to adjust blood replacement needs according to the sites of suspected or obvious bleeding and estimated amount lost.

4. Rough guidelines exist for the amount of blood loss to expect with particular injuries, such as for the following closed orthopedic injuries: humerus, 1 to 2 units; ulna-radius, ½ to 1 unit; pelvis, 2 to 12 units; tibia-fibula, ½ to 4 units; and ankle, ½ to 2 units. With open injuries, an estimated 1 to 3 additional units may be lost per site. Such guidelines, when used with clinical findings, help determine appropriate blood replacement.

5. Warm I.V. fluids before administration.

5. The volume of fluid required in a major trauma resuscitation is so massive that infusing room temperature solutions and cold blood products may cause hypothermia and shivering. Shivering requires an extraordinary energy expenditure the patient can ill afford.

6. Additional individualized interventions: _____

6. Rationales: _____

Target outcome criteria
Within 24 hours of the onset of therapy, the patient will:
• have an adequate circulating volume, as manifested by normal vital signs; warm, dry skin; urine output within normal limits; and strong, bilaterally equal peripheral pulses
• have a core temperature within normal limits.

Collaborative problem: *High risk for undetected injury related to mechanism of injury*

NURSING PRIORITIES: (a) Correlate the mechanism of injury with the patient's clinical presentation, and (b) remain alert for new signs of injury.

Interventions

BLUNT HEAD TRAUMA

1. Implement measures in the "Increased Intracranial Pressure" plan, page 134, as appropriate.

Rationales

1. Brain damage may not reflect velocity and duration of the injuring force because a contracoup injury may be worse than the coup injury to the head. Preadmission health status, the specific injury, and immediate detection and treatment of increased intracranial pressure are critical to survival. The "Increased Intracranial Pressure" plan discusses these problems in detail.

2. Monitor LOC, pupillary reactions, motor function, and sensory function. Alert the doctor immediately to any signs of neurologic deterioration.

2. Brain damage may not be apparent until days or weeks after injury. Signs of acute subdural hematoma usually appear within 24 hours of injury. An epidural hematoma, usually from arterial bleeding secondary to blows to the temple that tear the middle meningeal artery, is life-threatening and requires immediate surgical evacuation. Signs of concussion usually reverse within 24 hours, while those from contusion may persist for several days. Failure to recover within the expected time may indicate ongoing pathology or previously undetected injury and requires medical evaluation.

3. Additional individualized interventions: _____

3. Rationales: _____

BLUNT CHEST TRAUMA

1. Notify the doctor promptly of the onset of subcutaneous emphysema in the chest or neck, gastric contents in tracheal secretions, severe chest pain, deteriorating ABG values, or dyspnea.

1. These signs may indicate tracheal disruption or esophageal or bronchial tears. The trachea, esophagus, and bronchi are attached to other body structures by "stalks" that are prone to tearing from direct impact, deceleration, and shearing or rotary forces associated with blunt trauma.

2. Monitor for indicators of cardiac tamponade, such as rising central venous pressure, falling blood pressure, neck-vein distention, or muffled heart sounds. Notify the doctor immediately and prepare for pericardiocentesis.

2. When the chest strikes the steering wheel in a motor vehicle accident, for example, the heart is compressed between the sternum and vertebrae. The abrupt increase in intracardiac pressure may cause cardiac rupture. Damage may also occur to great vessels, especially to the vena cava and pulmonary veins, which are thought to have different deceleration rates than the atria. Cardiac damage may occur even without thoracic injury, if a lap belt compresses the abdomen and the knees strike the dashboard. Abdominal and leg compression creates a "hydraulic ram" effect, displacing abdominal viscera and blood upward, increasing intracardiac pressure, and causing cardiac damage.

3. Monitor for signs of cardiac contusion, including tachycardia, chest pain, arrhythmias, elevated pulmonary capillary wedge pressure, and indicators of heart failure. Obtain serial ECGs, cardiac enzymes, and a Doppler echocardiogram during the diagnostic phase, as ordered. Provide care, as ordered, depending on the contusion's effect on the patient.

3. Cardiac contusion may result from horizontal or vertical deceleration, compression, or shock wave damage in a gunshot wound to the chest or abdomen. Some controversy exists over management of cardiac contusion. Recent studies show little risk for most patients. If an ECG and Doppler echocardiogram do not reveal electrical or mechanical dysfunction, this disorder need not be considered critical. If function is impaired or arrhythmias threaten cardiac output, however, treatment should be similar to that for acute myocardial infarction.

4. Monitor for signs of pulmonary contusion, such as dyspnea, increasing pulmonary secretions (usually bloody), increasing inspiratory pressure while on a volume ventilator, and hypoxemia. Follow serial ABG measurements and chest X-ray results.

4. Pulmonary insufficiency from contusions increases within the first several hours after injury. Contusion creates swelling, a natural inflammatory process, and a capillary leak, which is worsened by the aggressive fluid resuscitation necessary for the multiple trauma patient.

5. Additional individualized interventions: _____

5. Rationales: _____

BLUNT ABDOMINAL TRAUMA

1. Report changes in abdominal pain, tenderness, rebound tenderness, absent bowel sounds, and increased abdominal distention.

1. Lap belt restraints may produce intraperitoneal, retroperitoneal, or pelvic disruption, resulting in life-threatening hemorrhage. These acceleration-deceleration injuries may not appear immediately after injury but hours or even days later.

2. Maintain placement and patency of gastric and urinary catheters, as ordered. Avoid nasogastric tube placement if facial fractures or cribriform plate injury is suspected. Avoid urinary catheter insertion if blood is present at the urinary meatus; notify the doctor.

3. Additional individualized interventions: _____

_____

BLUNT SPINAL CORD INJURY

1. Perform and document a motor and sensory examination every shift.

2. Additional individualized interventions: _____

_____

PENETRATING WOUNDS

1. With bullet wounds, observe the wound edge for necrosis and distal tissue for perfusion. Also inspect carefully for other wounds.

2. With stab wounds, observe distal vascular supply and tissue integrity, and assess signs of underlying organ function. Assume underlying vessel, tissue, and organ damage until proven otherwise.

3. Additional individualized interventions: _____

_____

ALL INJURIES

1. Assess and report to the doctor if the apparent mechanism of injury and observed injuries do not match.

2. Additional individualized interventions: _____

_____

2. A gastric catheter decompresses the stomach and helps detect gastric bleeding; a urinary catheter does the same for the bladder. Attempts to insert a nasogastric tube when facial fractures or cribriform plate injury is present may result in catheter placement into the brain. Bleeding at the urinary meatus may indicate urethral transection and requires medical evaluation.

3. Rationales: _____

_____

1. Mechanisms of spinal cord injury include horizontal loading, vertical loading, and acceleration or deceleration. Horizontal loading is lateral cord motion, such as when the patient hits the ground after being ejected from an automobile. Vertical loading results in cord compression, such as with a vertical fall or diving injury. Acceleration or deceleration injuries are common in falls.

2. Rationales: _____

_____

1. Bullet wounds usually are explored surgically because of the erratic path the bullet may take as it moves through tissue and because the bullet's kinetic energy (which depends on its mass and velocity) creates a much larger internal wound than the surface may indicate.

2. Depending on the length of the weapon and the direction of penetration, body areas other than that of the surface wound may be injured. For example, an abdominal stab wound may penetrate the diaphragm and involve the chest cavity, or a buttock stab wound may enter the abdomen. A high index of suspicion is critical.

3. Rationales: _____

_____

1. Inconsistencies between the apparent mechanism of injury and pattern of observed injuries may indicate previously undetected mechanisms of injury or abuse.

2. Rationales: _____

_____

Target outcome criterion
Throughout the unit stay, the patient will have previously unapparent injuries detected and treated promptly.

Nursing diagnosis: *Impaired physical mobility related to orthopedic injury*

NURSING PRIORITIES: (a) Restore maximum mobility, (b) strengthen muscle groups involved in weight bearing and range of motion, and (c) prevent orthopedic complications.

Interventions

1. Implement measures in the "Impaired Physical Mobility" plan, page 36, as appropriate.

2. Elevate casted extremities. Check neurovascular function every 1 to 2 hours. Report to the doctor altered sensation, increased pain, decreased ability to move fingers or toes, and capillary refill time greater than 3 seconds.

3. Observe uncasted extremities for crepitus, deformity, swelling, discoloration, pain, paralysis, pulse loss, and muscle spasms. If present, splint the extremity and notify the doctor.

4. If reimplantation is planned for a severed body part, maintain the part in a sealed plastic bag on ice; do not soak, wrap, or pack in ice. Prepare the patient for reimplantation surgery.

5. Maintain traction and immobilization of all C-spine injuries and all other unstable spinal fractures. Besides halo traction, methods include using Gardner-Wells, Barton-Cone, or Crutchfield tongs.

6. Prevent skin breakdown and other hazards of immobility by obtaining turning orders and restrictions, as appropriate, instituting a program of diligent side-to-side turning, at least every 2 hours as ordered, or using trauma beds. Trauma beds include:
• Roto Rest bed

• air bag beds (avoid these for the patient in spinal traction)

• Stryker Wedge Frame and CircOlectric beds.

7. Apply, monitor, and maintain continuous passive range-of-motion or sequential compression devices, if ordered.

8. Additional individualized interventions: _____

Rationales

1. The "Impaired Physical Mobility" plan presents comprehensive information on the hazards of immobility and their prevention. This plan provides additional information pertinent to the trauma patient.

2. Extremities in casts commonly swell from tissue edema; elevation decreases the amount of swelling. Altered sensation, increased pain, limited movement, and prolonged capillary refill time indicate that the swelling is causing neurovascular compromise. Unrecognized damage can threaten limb survival or function.

3. Occasionally, injuries may be missed during resuscitation, especially if other life-threatening injuries require immediate surgery.

4. Several hours may elapse before reimplantation. Maintaining the body part as described preserves viability.

5. Maintaining traction prevents further injury to the spinal cord. Although C-spine injuries require immediate treatment along with other life-threatening injuries, treatment of thoracolumbar injuries can be deferred until the patient is stable.

6. Skin breakdown, thromboembolism, and other complications of immobility may threaten life or markedly prolong recovery. Preventive methods depend on the injury and degree of activity allowed.

• A Roto Rest bed cycles automatically and continuously to 90-degree positions and has been used with various injuries, including C-spine fractures. A patient on a ventilator can be cared for easily on this bed.

• Various air bag beds are available. Benefits include side-to-side turning, bacterial filtration, and prevention of skin breakdown. Because of the potential for deflation with air bag beds, they are contraindicated for the patient with an unstable spine. A Roto Rest bed is better suited for the patient in spinal traction.

• Although these beds facilitate turning, they do not automatically change the patient's position and thus require more nursing supervision. They are no longer recommended.

7. These devices are designed to maintain leg range of motion and prevent deep venous stasis and thromboembolism.

8. Rationales: _____

Target outcome criterion
By the third day after traumatic injury, the patient will
have no new evidence of skin breakdown or other
complications of immobility.

Nursing diagnosis: *High risk for post-trauma response related to overwhelming psychological assault from sudden, unexpected injury*

NURSING PRIORITY: Facilitate effective coping.

Interventions

1. Refer to the "Ineffective Individual Coping" plan, page 51, the "Grieving" plan, page 31, and the "Dying" plan, page 11.

2. Observe for indications that the patient is reexperiencing the traumatic incident, such as flashbacks, intrusive thoughts, nightmares, guilt over survival, and excessive talking about the event. Also observe for indications of psychic numbing, such as confusion, amnesia, limited affect, misinterpretation of reality, and poor impulse control.

3. Encourage the patient to discuss feelings and reach out to others for help in coping with them. Explicitly acknowledge the intense feelings involved and the difficulty in coping with them.

4. Reassure the patient about being safe now. Praise behaviors contributing to survival, if appropriate.

5. Support the family and help them understand the patient's response.

6. With the patient's and family's consent, call in counseling professionals, such as a spiritual advisor, social worker, or trauma stress specialist. Refer the patient and family to a trauma support group, if available.

7. Additional individualized interventions: _____

Rationales

1. These plans contain helpful interventions for any trauma patient and the family. This plan provides additional specific information.

2. These signs and symptoms characterize the post-traumatic response that may follow a sudden event over which the victim felt powerless, such as a motor vehicle accident, natural disaster, or act of violence.

3. Retelling the incident and verbalizing feelings are important steps toward psychic integration of the experience. Reaching out to others provides comfort and reestablishes psychological security. By recognizing the powerful feelings involved and acknowledging the patient's difficulty in coping with the experience, the nurse conveys respect and establishes rapport and trust.

4. The post-traumatic syndrome can be so intense that the patient becomes absorbed in reexperiencing the terrifying incident. Reassurance helps reorient the patient to reality and brings closure to the terrifying incident. Praise for survival behaviors helps restore a sense of control.

5. Distress at seeing the patient upset may cause the family to shut off verbalizations, crying, and other expressions of emotion. Although well intentioned, such blocking may ultimately interfere with the patient's ability to integrate the experience.

6. Counseling professionals offer special skills that may facilitate coping. Calling them in without consent, however, may reinforce the powerless feeling the patient experienced during the traumatic incident.

7. Rationales: _____

Target outcome criteria
According to individual readiness, the patient will:
• discuss feelings about the traumatic incident
• learn to cope with flashbacks and other signs of the post-traumatic response.

Nursing diagnosis: *Potential for injury: complications related to impaired immunologic defenses, hypermetabolic state, stress, and other factors*

NURSING PRIORITY: Prevent or minimize complications.

Interventions

1. Identify and minimize potential sources of infection. For example, use strict aseptic technique when opening invasive lines; provide care at the insertion site of skeletal pins, wires, and tongs, as ordered; and administer antibiotics, as ordered. If a cerebrospinal fluid leak is present, avoid suctioning and packing the nose or ears, and tell the patient to avoid nose blowing. Ideally, remove and replace I.V. lines and urinary catheters within 24 hours of insertion in the field or emergency department.

2. Verify that tetanus prophylaxis was administered, if needed.

3. Provide adequate nutrition within 24 hours of admission, as ordered. Refer to the "Nutritional Deficit" plan, page 63, for details.

4. Prevent stress ulcers by administering antacids, titrated to gastric pH, and histamine antagonists or anticholinergic agents, as ordered. Monitor gastric drainage for occult blood.

5. Monitor for signs and symptoms of compartmental syndrome, such as unrelievable pain, muscle tension, and neurovascular compromise. If any of these signs and symptoms are present, alert the doctor and assist with measurement of compartmental pressure or transfer to surgery for fasciotomy.

6. Monitor for signs and symptoms of myoglobinuric renal failure, such as decreased urine output and elevated specific gravity. Notify the doctor and obtain plasma creatine phosphokinase (CPK) and urine myoglobin levels, as ordered. If myoglobinuria is present, administer fluids and mannitol, as ordered.

Rationales

1. Breach of the skin barrier, ischemia and necrotic tissue, inadequate inflammatory response, chronic disease, large numbers of invasive procedures, malnutrition, and pharmacologic agents contribute to the high risk of infection for the trauma patient. The measures listed prevent or treat infection. Lines and catheters placed hurriedly tend to become contaminated and serve as a wick for infection. Early replacement minimizes the infection risk.

2. Although tetanus prophylaxis usually is accomplished in the emergency department, it may have been overlooked if life-threatening injuries required immediate surgery.

3. Adequate nutrition is critically important to recovery because trauma induces a hypermetabolic response. Commonly, paralytic ileus or facial, airway, esophageal, chest, or abdominal injuries preclude oral nutrition. If these injuries are substantial, a jejunostomy tube is placed during the initial chest or abdominal surgery. If the enteral route is unavailable, parenteral nutrition should be started. Nutritional goals include achieving positive nitrogen balance and preventing complications from inadequate nutrition, such as sepsis, delayed wound healing, and multiple organ failure. The "Nutritional Deficit" plan discusses this potential complication in detail.

4. The trauma patient is at increased risk for stress ulcers. Prevention is the best therapy. The medications indicated reduce the secretion and acidity of gastric fluids, and gastric drainage monitoring can detect incipient stress ulcers.

5. Compartmental syndrome, also called low-velocity crush syndrome, results from excessive pressure within a fascial compartment caused by swollen tissue or blood confined within the compartment. Soft tissue injury, burns, pneumatic antishock garment use, and tight casts or dressings increase the risk of compartmental syndrome. Neurovascular compromise results and, if the pressure is not relieved by fasciotomy, the end result may be nerve damage or paralysis.

6. Myoglobinuria reflects myoglobin release from muscle damage associated with crush injury or compartmental syndrome. When circulation is restored to the damaged tissue, a flood of myoglobin enters the central circulation. Myoglobinuria peaks about 3 hours after circulation is restored and may persist for as long as 12 hours after the ischemic event. If myoglobin precipitates in the renal tubules, it may cause acute renal failure. Elevated plasma CPK and urine myoglobin levels confirm the diagnosis. Fluid administration and osmotic diuresis maintain renal tubular flow and lessen the risk of myoglobin clogging the renal tubules.

7. If musculoskeletal, soft tissue, burn, arterial, or multisystem trauma is present, observe for signs of fat embolism, such as sudden onset of respiratory distress, tachypnea, tachycardia, decreased LOC, and personality changes. If any of these signs or symptoms are present, alert the doctor.

7. Fat embolism results from mobilization of fat globules (for example, fat escaping from a fractured bone) or altered fat metabolism. The signs and symptoms from fat globules lodging in the lungs, brain, and kidneys usually occur 24 to 48 hours after injury. The early signs listed may be followed by petechiae (which appear 2 to 4 days after injury), retinal changes, and hematuria. Untreated, fat embolism may result in adult respiratory distress syndrome. Treatment is controversial but usually includes mechanical ventilation with positive end-expiratory pressure and possibly corticosteroids.

8. If death is imminent, consult with the doctor, family, and organ transplant team about possible organ donation.

8. Because trauma commonly involves young, previously healthy people, the trauma patient may be a suitable organ donor. Although contemplating the end of a loved one's life is naturally distressing, donating the patient's organs may bring meaning and comfort to the family.

9. Additional individualized interventions: _____

9. Rationales: _____

Target outcome criteria
Throughout the hospital stay, the patient will:
• receive care designed to prevent complications
• receive prompt treatment for complications that do occur.

If death is imminent and the patient is a suitable donor, the family will be approached about organ donation.

Discharge planning

NURSING DISCHARGE CRITERIA
Upon the patient's discharge, documentation shows evidence of:
• stable vital signs
• stable laboratory values
• absence of major complications, such as sepsis, renal failure, and increased intracranial pressure.

PATIENT-FAMILY TEACHING CHECKLIST
Document evidence that the patient and family demonstrate an understanding of:
___ extent of injuries
___ prognosis
___ treatments
___ pain management
___ post-trauma response
___ coping resources
___ organ donation process, if appropriate.

DOCUMENTATION CHECKLIST
Using outcome criteria as a guide, document:
___ clinical status on admission
___ significant changes in status
___ pertinent laboratory and diagnostic test findings
___ airway and ventilation support
___ fluid administration
___ medication administration
___ nutritional support
___ emotional support
___ measures to prevent or treat complications
___ patient-family teaching
___ discharge planning.

ASSOCIATED PLANS OF CARE
Acute Renal Failure
Adult Respiratory Distress Syndrome
Disseminated Intravascular Coagulation
Dying
Grieving
Hypovolemic Shock
Impaired Physical Mobility
Increased Intracranial Pressure
Ineffective Individual Coping
Knowledge Deficit
Mechanical Ventilation
Nutritional Deficit
Pain
Sensory-Perceptual Alteration

References

Alspach, J., ed. *Core Curriculum for Critical Care Nursing,* 4th ed. Philadelphia: W.B. Saunders Co., 1991.

Cardona, V., et al., eds. *Trauma Nursing: From Resuscitation Through Rehabilitation.* Philadelphia: W.B. Saunders Co., 1988.

Chmielewski, C., and Zellers, L. "Continuous Arteriovenous Hemofiltration in the Patient with Hepatorenal Syndrome," *Critical Care Nursing Clinics of North America* 2(1):115-22, March 1990.

Foreman, M., ed. "Gerontologic Considerations," *Critical Care Nursing Quarterly* 12(1):1-89, June 1989.

Hoyt, N. "Host Defense Mechanisms and Compromises in the Trauma Patient," *Critical Care Nursing Clinics of North America* 1(4):735-65, December 1989.

Innerarity, S. "Electrolyte Emergencies in the Critically Ill Renal Patient," *Critical Care Nursing Clinics of North America* 2(1):89-99, March 1990.

Rea, R., ed. *Trauma Nursing Core Course Instructor Manual.* Chicago: Emergency Nurses Association, 1987.

Richardson, D., et al. *Trauma: Clinical Care and Pathophysiology.* Chicago: Yearbook Medical Pubs., 1987.

Smith, M. "Renal Trauma, Adult and Pediatric Considerations," *Critical Care Nursing Clinics of North America* 2(1):66-77, March 1990.

"Standards and Guidelines for Cardiopulmonary Resuscitation (CPR) and Emergency Cardiac Care (ECC)," *Journal of the American Medical Association* 255(21):2979-84, June 6, 1986.

Strange, J. *Shock Trauma Care Plans.* Springhouse, Pa.: Springhouse Corp., 1987.

Trunkey, D., and Lewis, F. *Current Therapy of Trauma,* 3rd ed. St. Louis: Mosby-Year Book, 1991.

Osteomyelitis

DRG information
DRG 238 Osteomyelitis.
     Mean LOS = 10.4 days
     Principal diagnoses include:
       • acute osteomyelitis
       • chronic osteomyelitis
       • unspecified osteomyelitis.

Introduction
DEFINITION AND TIME FOCUS
Osteomyelitis is a bone infection that may be classified as primary, secondary, or chronic. *Primary osteomyelitis* occurs from compound fractures, penetrating wounds, or surgery. *Secondary osteomyelitis* may be hematogenous (bloodborne) or may represent extension of nearby infections (especially pressure ulcers). *Chronic osteomyelitis,* a persistent bone infection manifested by draining sinus tracts, is rare.

    This plan focuses on the patient receiving nonsurgical treatment of osteomyelitis for which postdischarge antibiotic therapy is anticipated.

ETIOLOGY AND PRECIPITATING FACTORS
• bone infection (either bloodborne or from an open wound) with sufficient numbers of pathogenic bacteria, most commonly *Staphylococcus aureus*
• sufficient bone and soft-tissue trauma and hematoma to provide growth media for the infecting agent
• implantation of foreign material (joint replacements, methyl methacrylate, or metallic internal fixation devices) that may impair the body's ability to control bacterial growth
• infection near bone or joints

Focused assessment guidelines
NURSING HISTORY (Functional health pattern findings)

Health perception — health management pattern
• may display lack of knowledge about basic health care practices, especially hand washing and signs and symptoms of infection
• commonly has a history of unreported local infection
• may have unreported systemic indicators of infection, such as fever, malaise, weakness, irritability, anorexia, and generalized sepsis (rare)
• may report a recent upper respiratory tract infection, urinary tract infection, otitis media, impetigo, tonsillitis, or dental procedure
• may have a history of disinterest in learning about care of an immobilization device or devices (for example, cast, splint, external fixator, or brace) needed previously

Activity-exercise pattern
• may complain of weakness and fatigue

Cognitive-perceptual pattern
• may report pain in affected limb, increasing with movement

Sleep-rest pattern
• may report night sweats
• may complain that pain affects sleep

PHYSICAL FINDINGS
General
• emotional irritability

Cardiovascular
• tachycardia

Integumentary
• localized edema and erythema in infection area
• localized tenderness in infection area
• draining wound, with either serous or gross purulent drainage (may not be present in all patients)
• diaphoresis and flushing with fever
• chronically draining sinus tracts (rare)

Musculoskeletal
• pseudoparalysis (inability to move joints adjacent to area of osteomyelitis because of anticipated pain)
• muscle spasm in infected extremity

DIAGNOSTIC STUDIES
• wound aspirate or bone biopsy of sequestrum (involved bone) — demonstrates the infecting organism
• complete blood count — reveals leukocytosis and, after prolonged infection, anemia related to associated decrease in erythropoietin production and reduced red blood cell life span
• erythrocyte sedimentation rate — elevated; degree of elevation relates to extent of infection
• blood cultures — may reveal infecting organism when shaking chills and temperature spikes are associated with osteomyelitis
• X-rays of involved bones — may eventually show evidence of osteonecrosis and new bone formation
• radioisotope scanning — may reveal areas of increased vascularity, indicating infection
• sinograms of draining sinus tracts — may outline involved areas of chronic osteomyelitis
• computed tomography scan — may reveal changes indicating osteonecrosis
• magnetic resonance imaging — may reveal soft tissue inflammation

POTENTIAL COMPLICATIONS
• chronic osteomyelitis
• sepsis
• dysfunctional limb
• refractory, life-threatening infection requiring amputation
• pathologic fractures
• nonunion of existing fractures

Nursing diagnosis: *Pain related to inflammation*

NURSING PRIORITY: Relieve pain.

Interventions

1. See the "Pain" plan, page 69.

2. Clearly identify and document the source and degree of pain. Aid the patient in rating pain, using a scale of 1 to 10 (1 = minor pain, 10 = severe pain).

3. Medicate the patient with narcotics and nonsteroidal anti-inflammatory drugs (NSAIDs), as ordered, and carefully document their effectiveness. Monitor for adverse reactions.

4. Instruct the patient in nonpharmacologic pain control methods, including relaxation, enhanced relaxation, guided imagery, distraction (verbal, auditory, visual, or tactile), rhythmic breathing, cutaneous stimulation (such as with oil of wintergreen), massage, transcutaneous electrical nerve stimulation, use of heat and cold, and biofeedback. Document methods that the patient finds helpful.

5. Elevate and support the affected extremity.

6. Schedule necessary activity of the involved extremity to coincide with the peak effectiveness of analgesics or anti-inflammatory agents.

7. Instruct the patient to report increasing or uncontrolled pain, and explain why.

8. Use adjunctive devices (such as a bed cradle, antirotation boots, or a mechanical bed) to aid in pain control.

9. Maintain traction and support devices (such as a cast, a splint, or internal fixators), as ordered.

10. Additional individualized interventions: _____

Rationales

1. General interventions for pain are detailed in this plan.

2. Continuing or increasing severe pain may indicate increasing inflammation.

3. Bone pain is usually severe.

4. Nonpharmacologic pain control allows self-control of pain without medication adverse reactions. Ice, for example, not only acts as a tactile distraction and stimulates large-diameter cutaneous sensory neurons, decreasing deeper pain sensation (the gate control theory), but also causes vasoconstriction, thus reducing edema that contributes to pain.

5. Elevation enhances venous return to reduce inflammatory edema; supportive positioning protects against muscle strain and spasm.

6. Timing activity with the peak of medication action decreases discomfort while allowing necessary mobility.

7. Increasing or uncontrolled pain may indicate worsening osteomyelitis, ineffective therapy, or both.

8. Reducing direct pressure, rotational force, and discomfort from turning may help control pain in some circumstances.

9. Immobilization and external support devices aid fracture healing, protect the infected bone from excessive stress, and decrease pain.

10. Rationales: _____

Target outcome criteria

Within 1 day of admission, the patient will:
• show no indications of uncontrolled pain, such as facial grimacing, tachycardia, increased blood pressure, or groaning
• verbalize pain control
• rate pain severity, on a scale of 1 to 10, as decreased since admission.

Within 2 days of admission, the patient will:
• verbalize or demonstrate an understanding of at least two personally effective nonpharmacologic methods of pain control
• verbalize an understanding of the need to report increasing or uncontrolled pain.

Nursing diagnosis: *High risk for recurrent or spreading infection related to knowledge deficit*

NURSING PRIORITY: Teach the patient to recognize local and systemic indicators of infection.

Interventions

1. Instruct about signs and symptoms of local infection (erythema, edema, localized tenderness, serous or purulent discharge, and local warmth) and systemic infection (fever, malaise, weakness, and irritability). Teach the need to report limited range of motion as a possible indication of spreading infection. Stress the need to report these findings promptly.

2. Evaluate learning by having the patient list the signs and symptoms of infection, preferably in writing. Document learning. See the "Knowledge Deficit" plan, page 56.

3. Provide the patient with a written list of local and systemic signs and symptoms of infection for periodic review. Document the material provided.

4. When necessary, establish continuity through community health nurse referrals for continued education or evaluation of learning.

5. Additional individualized interventions: _____

_____

Rationales

1. Prompt reporting of these signs and symptoms ensures early identification and treatment of infection.

2. Having the patient list signs and symptoms provides feedback about learning and an opportunity to identify omissions and correct misconceptions. The "Knowledge Deficit" plan contains further details related to patient teaching.

3. Readily accessible review materials help the patient retain new knowledge.

4. Some patients will not benefit from the patient education provided and will require continued instruction or appropriate follow-up care.

5. Rationales: _____

_____

Target outcome criteria

Within 2 days of admission, the patient will:
• be able to list local and systemic signs and symptoms of infection
• verbalize an understanding of the need to alert health care providers promptly if infection occurs.

By the time of discharge, the patient will have arranged for appropriate follow-up care by a public health or visiting nurse (if appropriate).

Nursing diagnosis: *High risk for injury related to use of antibiotics with high potential for toxic effects*

NURSING PRIORITY: Prevent or minimize toxic effects of antibiotic therapy.

Interventions

1. Teach the patient about antibiotic administration, especially monitoring for significant antibiotic adverse effects. See *Minimizing adverse effects of antibiotic therapy.*

2. Instruct the patient to report any adverse effects promptly.

3. Additional individualized interventions: _____

Rationales

1. A patient's knowledgeable participation in self-care while in the hospital improves the quality of care, allows for rapid identification of complications, and prepares the patient for self-care after discharge.

2. Prompt identification and notification reduce the potential for long-term complications.

3. Rationales: _____

MINIMIZING ADVERSE EFFECTS OF ANTIBIOTIC THERAPY

The following chart lists common antibiotics and appropriate interventions.

Drugs	Nursing considerations
aminoglycosides (gentamicin, neomycin, streptomycin, and tobramycin)	• Teach the potential for ototoxicity (as shown by high-frequency hearing loss [for example, decreased ability to hear a ticking wristwatch], tinnitus, vertigo, and dizziness); superimposed infections (especially fungal infections of mucous membranes or from indwelling vascular access catheters); and nephrotoxicity (as shown by oliguria, polyuria, abnormal specific gravity, and rapid weight gain). • Explain the rationale for baseline and weekly audiograms and serum creatinine and blood urea nitrogen (BUN) studies. • Monitor and document fluid intake and output and urine specific gravity while the patient is hospitalized. Report oliguria, polyuria, and specific gravity extremes (less than 1.010 and greater than 1.030). When appropriate, instruct the patient about continuing this monitoring after discharge. • Weigh the patient twice weekly and document. Instruct about twice weekly weight measurement after discharge. Report weight gain exceeding 3 lb (1.4 kg). • Teach the patient to closely monitor mucous membranes for indications of fungal infection (redness, tenderness, cheesy white discharge, black or furry tongue, fever, nausea, and diarrhea) and the need to report any that occur.
penicillins (ampicillin, carbenicillin, cyclacillin, methicillin, and oxacillin)	• Teach the potential for anemia (as shown by weakness, paleness, and malaise), hypersensitivity reactions (as shown by asthmatic reactions, erythematous-maculopapular rash, urticaria, and anaphylaxis), and overgrowth of nonsusceptible organisms leading to opportunistic infection (as shown by fever, chills, and continuing or increasing indications of infection or inflammation).
cephalosporins (cefamandole, cefazolin, cefoxitin, cephalothin, cephapirin, and cephradine)	• Teach the potential for opportunistic infections (as shown by fever, chills, and continuing or increasing indications of infection or inflammation), photosensitivity (unusual skin sensitivity to sunlight), and, in the patient with suspected renal or hepatic disease, nephrotoxicity (as shown by oliguria, polyuria, abnormal specific gravity, and rapid weight gain) and hepatotoxicity (as shown by jaundice, icteric sclera, dark brown urine, and pale, pasty stools). • Explain the rationale for baseline and weekly measurement of serum creatinine, BUN, lactic dehydrogenase, serum aspartate aminotransferase and serum alanine aminotransferase levels. • Monitor and instruct the patient about nephrotoxicity and weight gain, as discussed under "aminoglycosides" above. • When oral medications are used, teach the patient to avoid concurrent intake of iron products or dairy foods because they decrease cephalosporin absorption. • Instruct the patient to avoid direct sunlight and to use sunblocking agents when sun exposure is unavoidable.

MINIMIZING ADVERSE EFFECTS OF ANTIBIOTIC THERAPY *(continued)*

Drugs	Nursing considerations
sulfonamides (sulfadiazine, sulfamethoxazole, sulfamethoxydiazine, sulfamethoxypyridazine, sulfapyridine, and sulfisoxazole)	• Teach the potential for nephrotoxicity (as shown by polyuria, oliguria, abnormal specific gravity, and rapid weight gain), agranulocytosis (as shown by fever and lesions of the mucous membranes, gastrointestinal tract, and skin), crystalluria (as shown by evidence of renal calculi—hematuria, pyuria, frequency, urgency, retention, and pain in the flank, lower back, perineum, thighs, groin, labia, or scrotum), and hemorrhagic tendencies (as shown by epistaxis, bleeding gums, prolonged bleeding from wounds, ecchymoses, melena, hematuria, hemoptysis, and hematemesis from disruption of intestinal flora and synthesis of vitamin K). • Explain the rationale for baseline and weekly measurement of serum creatinine, BUN, and granulocyte levels. • Monitor and instruct the patient about nephrotoxicity and weight gain, as discussed under "aminoglycosides" above. • Instruct the patient taking oral sulfonamides to drink 8 oz of fluid with each dose. Encourage total fluid intake of at least 8 8-oz glasses daily.
fluoroquinolones (enoxacin and ciprofloxacin)	• Teach the potential for adverse reactions (such as nausea, vomiting, diarrhea, abdominal discomfort, dizziness, headaches, insomnia, slit lamp eye changes, and skin disorders). Nausea associated with enoxacin may be decreased by taking the medication within one hour of a meal. • Teach the potential for drug interactions, especially when taking theophylline, because these agents slow the clearance of theophylline and increase its potential for toxicity. Under the doctor's supervision, the theophylline dosage may need to be decreased. Similarly, concurrent use of antacids may decrease absorption of fluoroquinolones. • Explain the need to take ciprofloxacin two hours after meals and to drink plenty of fluids while taking this agent. • Monitor for and instruct the patient about nephrotoxicity and weight gain, as discussed under "aminoglycosides" above.
I.V. antibiotics	• When indwelling vascular access catheters are used for antibiotic administration, closely monitor the insertion sites for inflammation or irritation that does not respond to treatment with topical antibiotics. Teach the patient to monitor for this complication and promptly report it to the health care provider. • Teach close monitoring of wounds for indications of unresolving or increasing inflammation or infection (which are evidence of opportunistic infection).
Any oral antibiotic	• Instruct the patient about the need to take medication as ordered. Although some antibiotic therapy (such as with fluoroquinolones) may be administered orally, this does not decrease the need to ensure that medications are administered on schedule to provide adequate serum drug levels.

Target outcome criteria

Within 2 days after initiation of therapy, the patient will:
• (with aminoglycoside therapy) list signs and symptoms of ototoxicity, nephrotoxicity, and superimposed infections
• (with penicillin therapy) list signs and symptoms of anemia, hypersensitivity reaction, and opportunistic infections
• (with cephalosporin therapy) list signs and symptoms of photosensitivity, hepatotoxicity, nephrotoxicity, and opportunistic infections
• (with sulfonamide therapy) list signs and symptoms of nephrotoxicity, agranulocytosis, crystalluria, and hemorrhagic tendencies

• (with fluoroquinolone therapy) list the signs and symptoms of nephrotoxicity and potential drug interactions
• verbalize the importance of rapidly reporting signs and symptoms of untoward effects.

By the time of discharge, the patient will:
• demonstrate the ability to perform monitoring procedures as needed for specific antibiotics
• have arranged for necessary follow-up care (if appropriate).

Nursing diagnosis: *Disuse syndrome related to prolonged infection, pain, and immobilization*

NURSING PRIORITY: Help the patient regain or exceed usual activity level.

Interventions	Rationales
1. Assess and document the patient's baseline activity level, including muscle strength and ability to perform activities of daily living (ADLs).	1. Adequate baseline information allows determination of individualized goals.
2. Document activity goals set in collaboration with the patient.	2. Involving the patient in planning increases the potential for success. Goals provide focus.
3. Teach the patient about the need to maintain muscle strength and endurance while immobilized. Provide instruction in isotonic and isometric exercises that can be accomplished within the patient's activity limitations.	3. Maintenance exercise programs decrease loss of muscle strength and endurance during immobilization by maintaining adequate blood flow to muscle and by stressing bone to ensure continued balance in bone remodeling.
4. Have the patient demonstrate the exercises, and evaluate and document the patient's learning. Establish and monitor an exercise regimen throughout the hospital stay. Help the patient establish a home exercise program as well, and ensure community health care follow-up after discharge, when needed.	4. Return demonstration of exercises allows effective evaluation of patient learning. Monitoring the exercise regimen ensures that the patient will maintain strength and endurance.
5. Provide abundant positive reinforcement. Develop goals of increasing strength (increasing increments of resistance or weight) and endurance (increasing numbers or repetitions or longer exercise periods), when feasible.	5. Positive reinforcement helps establish health-promoting behaviors. Isometric and isotonic exercises performed within activity restrictions may increase strength and endurance in unaffected body areas.
6. Provide written materials on exercises for review as needed. Document the materials provided.	6. Written materials increase understanding of exercises and the potential for doing exercises as required.
7. Additional individualized interventions: _____	7. Rationales: _____

Target outcome criteria
Within 2 days of admission, the patient will verbalize an understanding of the need for exercise, list exercise goals, and demonstrate the exercise regimen.

By the time of discharge, the patient will independently perform exercises and verbalize an understanding of their necessity when mobility is restricted.

Discharge planning
NURSING DISCHARGE CRITERIA
Upon the patient's discharge, documentation shows evidence of:
• wound drainage within expected parameters, with little or no purulent or bloody drainage
• stable vital signs
• absence of fever
• absence of pulmonary or cardiovascular complications
• no erythema, edema, or tenderness at wound site
• no loss of range of motion in joints adjacent to the infection
• ability to control pain using oral medications
• stabilizing weight and adequate nutritional intake
• ability to perform ADLs at usual level
• ability to transfer, ambulate, and perform prescribed exercise regimen at usual level or with minimal assistance
• ability to perform wound care and dressing changes as prescribed, with minimal assistance
• hemoglobin and blood cultures within normal parameters
• white blood cell count within expected parameters
• normal bowel and bladder function
• adequate home support system or referral to home care if indicated by inadequate home support system or inability to perform self-care.

If the patient is discharged with an indwelling vascular access catheter, documentation also shows:
• evidence of automatic referral to home care or arrangements for short-term stay in a nursing home (depending on the patient's home support system and ability to care for catheter and administer medications independently)
• knowledge of where to obtain additional supplies
• knowledge of signs and symptoms indicating catheter dysfunction or infection
• ability to follow prescribed medication regimen and I.V. administration technique
• ability to monitor weight and follow instructions for oral intake, as directed
• knowledge of signs and symptoms indicating fungal or other systemic infection.

PATIENT-FAMILY TEACHING CHECKLIST
Document evidence that the patient and family demonstrate an understanding of:
___ disease and implications
___ hand washing techniques
___ dressing changes, pin site care, cast care, or care of braces or splints, as appropriate
___ nonpharmacologic pain control interventions
___ use of elevation and supportive positioning
___ range-of-motion exercise of the affected extremity, as appropriate
___ dietary requirements
___ all discharge medications' purpose, dosage, administration schedule, precautions, and adverse effects requiring medical attention (usual discharge medications include antibiotics, analgesics, and NSAIDs)
___ need to report increasing or uncontrolled pain
___ care of indwelling vascular access catheters
___ self-administration of I.V. antibiotics
___ vascular access complications
___ patient exercise regimen
___ how to obtain clarification of instructions or further information
___ date, time, and place of follow-up appointments
___ referral agencies and medical supply resources
___ how to contact the doctor.

DOCUMENTATION CHECKLIST
Using outcome criteria as a guide, document:
___ clinical status on admission
___ significant changes in status
___ pertinent laboratory and diagnostic test findings
___ baseline information on muscle strength, ADLs performed, endurance, and collaborative goals established with the patient
___ source and degree of pain, especially if persistent or increasing
___ effective pain relief measures
___ daily or biweekly measurement of weight, intake, output, and urine specific gravity, when appropriate

___ appearance of indwelling vascular access catheter site, and catheter care
___ patient-family teaching
___ discharge planning.

ASSOCIATED PLANS OF CARE
Chronic Renal Failure
Ineffective Individual Coping
Knowledge Deficit
Pain
Surgical Intervention
Urolithiasis

References
Carpenito, L. *Handbook of Nursing Diagnosis,* 4th ed. Philadelphia: J.B. Lippincott Co., 1991.
Hoyt, N.J. "Infections Following Orthopaedic Injury," *Orthopaedic Nursing* 5(5):15-24, September-October 1986.
Martin, M. "Oral Antibiotics for Treatment of Patients with Chronic Osteomyelitis," *Orthopaedic Nursing* 8(3):35-38, May-June 1989.
McKenry, L., and Salerno, E. *Mosby's Pharmacology in Nursing.* St. Louis: C.V. Mosby Co., 1989.
Phipps, W., Long, B., Woods, N., and Cassmeyer, V. *Medical Surgical Nursing: Concepts and Clinical Practice,* 4th ed. St. Louis: Mosby-Year Book, 1991.
Pozzi, M., and Peck, N. "An Option for the Patient with Chronic Osteomyelitis: Home Intravenous Antibiotic Therapy," *Orthopaedic Nursing* 5(5):9-14, 54, September-October 1986.
Swearingen, P.L. *Manual of Nursing Therapeutics,* 2nd ed. St. Louis: Mosby-Year Book, 1990.

Radical Neck Dissection

DRG information

DRG 076 Other Respiratory System Operating Room (O.R.) Procedures. With Complication or Comorbidity (CC).
Mean LOS = 10.5 days
DRG 077 Other Respiratory System O.R. Procedures. Without CC.
Mean LOS = 4.6 days
Principal diagnoses include:
• excision of regional lymph nodes
• excision or repair of larynx
• tracheostomy.
DRG 400 Lymphoma or Leukemia with Major O.R. Procedure.
Mean LOS = 10.1 days
Principal diagnoses include:
• malignant neoplasm of lymph nodes
• lymphosarcoma.

Additional DRG information: Radical neck dissection has a number of alternative DRGs. The DRG assigned depends on the cause for the surgery (where the cancer is located), not on its extent (tracheostomy or laryngectomy) or how radical a dissection is performed.

Introduction
DEFINITION AND TIME FOCUS

Radical neck dissection (RND) is a surgical procedure performed for cancers of the head and neck. Normally, RND involves the surgical removal of:
• lymph nodes in the neck
• lymphatic vessels
• the sternocleidomastoid muscle
• the internal jugular vein
• the spinal accessory nerve (innervates the trapezius muscle)
• the submandibular salivary gland
• the tail of the parotid gland.

When RND is combined with removal of a tumor located in the mouth, pharynx, or larynx (a common occurrence), a tracheostomy is usually created. If a total laryngectomy is performed, the tracheostomy will be permanent, and the opening between the trachea and the pharynx will be surgically closed. A patient who does not require total laryngectomy may have a temporary tracheostomy until surgical or radiation-related edema subsides. After surgery, the patient is commonly admitted to the intensive care unit (ICU) initially. This clinical plan focuses on preoperative and postoperative care for the patient undergoing RND.

ETIOLOGY AND PRECIPITATING FACTORS

RND is performed to remove:
• primary malignant tumors of the mouth, pharynx, or larynx
• skin lesions (melanomas).
    Risk factors associated with these cancers include:
• heavy use of alcohol and cigarettes (oral and laryngeal cancer)
• pipe or cigar smoking (oral cancer)
• tobacco chewing (oral cancer)
• exposure to nickel or wood dust or woodworking chemicals (nasopharyngeal cancer)
• fair complexion and long-term or frequent sun exposure (melanoma).

Focused assessment guidelines
NURSING HISTORY (Functional health pattern findings)

Health perception — health management pattern
• history of heavy cigarette smoking, alcohol abuse, or both
• may have had radiation or chemotherapy (for head and neck cancer)
• may have history of previous head or neck cancer

Nutritional-metabolic pattern
• may report weight loss
• may report dysphagia, sore throat, or difficulty chewing
• may report no appetite
• may have a history of skin lesions (basal cell)

Sleep-rest pattern
• may report fatigue

Cognitive-perceptual pattern
• may report change in taste sensation
• may report neck pain (rare)

Self-perception — self-concept pattern
• views self as strong, active, and easy-going, or may be passive
• may report voice change

Role-relationship pattern
• may describe self as independent of others
• may be head of household
• may have a history of sporadic employment related to alcoholism

Coping—stress tolerance pattern
- may have delayed seeking treatment (denial)
- may tend to avoid issues requiring a decision
- may have only spouse or friend as major support system

Value-belief pattern
- views disease as life-threatening
- wants to have surgery in order to return to usual activities
- with melanoma, may have difficulty accepting seriousness of disease and need for radical surgery

PHYSICAL FINDINGS
Pulmonary
- productive cough or wheezing
- hoarseness
- difficulty breathing

Gastrointestinal
- nonhealing ulcer in oral cavity
- may be edentulous or have poor oral hygiene

Neurologic
- otalgia (ear pain)

Integumentary
- melanoma

Musculoskeletal
- lump on neck

DIAGNOSTIC STUDIES
- blood studies, including complete blood count and electrolyte determinations—establishes preoperative baseline; findings usually within normal limits; decreased albumin levels indicate altered nutrition; elevated or depressed white blood cell count may indicate immune system's response to the disease or stage of recovery from radiation therapy or chemotherapy
- liver function test—rules out liver disease before surgery
- chest X-ray—may show metastasis or pulmonary disease
- head and neck X-rays or computed tomography (CT) scan—identify location and extent of tumor and metastasis to sinuses, neck, or brain
- panendoscopy and biopsy—define tumor type and extension of tumor
- barium swallow—if dysphagia is present, defines involvement of pharynx, epiglottis, or esophagus
- lymphoscintigraphy (for melanoma)—identifies involved lymph nodes and drainage pathways
- laryngogram—if hoarseness is present, defines area of involvement in larynx and extent of airway obstruction
- abdominal CT scan—may demonstrate metastasis to abdominal organs
- upper or lower GI series—may demonstrate metastasis to esophagus or digestive system

POTENTIAL COMPLICATIONS
- airway obstruction
- carotid artery rupture
- cutaneous or tracheoesophageal fistula formation

Nursing diagnosis: *Preoperative knowledge deficit related to unfamiliar diagnosis and surgical procedure*

NURSING PRIORITY: Supplement the patient's and family's knowledge of impending surgery.

Interventions

1. See the "Knowledge Deficit" and "Surgical Intervention" plans, pages 56 and 81 respectively.

2. On admission, assess the patient's knowledge base. Encourage questions. Help the patient and family to identify concerns and methods to cope with them. As appropriate, explain and illustrate the signs and symptoms of head and neck cancer, the planned treatment, and the expected postoperative outcomes. After surgery, the patient can expect a bulky neck dressing, ICU care until stable, a nasogastric tube, intubation or tracheostomy, skin catheters, and skin graft and donor sites. Document the patient's and family's level of understanding and their response.

Rationales

1. These plans contain general interventions for the patient undergoing surgery who has a knowledge deficit.

2. Knowledge of expected events decreases anxiety and gives a sense of control. Providing information helps the patient and family focus questions on topics they do not understand. Individuals differ in the amount of detail desired: some may want only minimal descriptions while others may request to see pictures or equipment. Airway management after surgery varies, but most patients have a temporary tracheostomy until edema subsides. The temporary tracheostomy is usually closed within 2 weeks after surgery, depending on the patient's status. If the patient will be undergoing radiation therapy, the tracheostomy may be maintained longer. The patient undergoing total laryngectomy will have a permanent tracheostomy.

3. Additional individualized interventions: _____

3. Rationales: _____

Target outcome criteria
Before surgery, the patient will:
• state the reason for surgery and expected outcomes
• exhibit a decreased anxiety level.

Before surgery, the family members will describe their greatest concern and at least one way they will deal with it.

Nursing diagnosis: *Ineffective individual coping: avoidance related to inaccurate perception of health status*

NURSING PRIORITY: Promote accurate perception of health status and available resources for health promotion.

Interventions

1. On admission, determine the time between initial symptoms and when treatment was sought. Explain the common signs and symptoms. Allow expression of guilt, resentment, and regret if treatment was delayed because of denial or avoidance. Emphasize that treatment *is* occurring now.

2. Evaluate for alcohol dependence. As part of the admission interview, question the patient specifically, directly, and matter-of-factly about alcohol consumption patterns, noting the time of the last drink. Observe for periorbital edema and ecchymoses or abrasions in various stages of healing. Be alert to any excessive use of such toiletries as mouthwash.

3. Assess for signs and symptoms of alcohol withdrawal delirium, as follows:
• mild (4 to 16 hours after the last drink) — tremors, agitation, tachycardia, vomiting, hypertension, diarrhea
• moderate (1 to 3 days later) — profuse diaphoresis, seizures, hallucinations, incontinence
• severe (variable onset, usually about 72 hours after the last drink) — delirium tremens, hyperthermia, violent behavior, extreme blood pressure changes, disorientation.
    Notify the doctor if withdrawal is suspected, and institute sedative therapy, as ordered, along with any other medical measures.

4. After surgery, teach risk factors for head and neck cancer, and document the patient's level of understanding.

5. Before discharge, offer resources available for smoking cessation and alcohol rehabilitation, and document the plan for follow-up.

6. Additional individualized interventions: _____

Rationales

1. If the time between which symptoms appeared and the patient sought help is lengthy, denial may be the patient's primary coping method. Initial symptoms commonly are mild and may be easily ignored. Verbalization decreases unnecessary guilt if treatment was delayed.

2. Alcohol dependence is a typical finding in this patient group and must be identified for early assessment and treatment of withdrawal symptoms. Specific questions may unmask hidden alcoholism; although these patients tend to underestimate their consumption, they usually can and will accurately identify the time of their last drink. Periorbital edema suggests fluid retention, possibly related to excessive alcohol consumption. Lesions in various stages may be a sign of frequent falls because of intoxication. The patient may attempt to fend off withdrawal symptoms by using alcohol-laden toiletries while in the hospital.

3. Severe alcohol withdrawal delirium is a potentially life-threatening occurrence that may be prevented with early intervention. Sedation (usually with benzodiazepines) may prevent the syndrome's progression. Untreated, severe alcohol withdrawal delirium may result in myocardial infarction, cerebrovascular accident, or other serious complications.

4. A review of risk factors provides a baseline for discussion and planning to eliminate known risks.

5. Major life-style changes require support and follow-up. Smoking and alcohol intake are major risk factors for the recurrence of head and neck cancer.

6. Rationales: _____

> **Target outcome criterion**
> By the time of discharge, the patient will state one action to decrease the risk of recurrence of head and neck cancer.

Nursing diagnosis: *Altered role performance related to muscle weakness and job disruption*

NURSING PRIORITY: Advise the patient of available resources for job adjustment.

Interventions

1. Before surgery, assess the physical requirements of the patient's job, especially noting any heavy lifting or use of shoulder muscles. Have the patient and family discuss work options with the patient's employer. Involve a social worker or vocational rehabilitation specialist.

2. Before discharge, document a plan for alternative employment or disability follow-up.

3. Additional individualized interventions: _____

_____

Rationales

1. The patient may be unaware of surgery's effect on job performance. Planning minimizes postoperative distress about changed abilities or activity restrictions. A social worker or vocational rehabilitation specialist may offer new options.

2. Financial concerns and the need for job security may be major obstacles to compliance with the total treatment plan if not addressed before discharge.

3. Rationales: _____

_____

> **Target outcome criteria**
> Before surgery, the patient will express minimal anxiety about work and finances.
>
> By the time of discharge, the patient will state a plan for vocational rehabilitation.

Nursing diagnosis: *High risk for ineffective airway clearance related to edema and excessively thick secretions*

NURSING PRIORITIES: (a) Prevent airway obstruction and (b) facilitate secretion removal.

Interventions

1. In the immediate postoperative period, assess and document upper airway patency, the presence and consistency of secretions, and the patient's ability to clear the airway.

2. If a tracheostomy is present, provide humidification and oxygen, as ordered. Suction the patient according to amount and consistency of secretions, possibly as often as every hour in the first 24 hours after surgery.

3. Assess the wound site for increasing edema, reevaluating upper airway patency and documenting changes at least hourly for the first 24 hours after surgery. Note and report any choking sensation, sense of apprehension, change in respiratory rate or depth, and increased upper airway sounds or tracheal shift.

Rationales

1. The effects of surgery and intubation alter airway patency and secretion consistency. Patients vary in their ability to expectorate secretions.

2. A tracheostomy bypasses the normal humidification function of the nose, so the patient requires supplemental humidity to liquefy secretions. The need for suctioning varies, depending on the duration of intubation, preoperative lung status, and the patient's response to the tracheostomy.

3. Early signs of upper airway obstruction are subtle and progressive and may be related to pressure on the trachea from increasing edema at the wound site. If edema compromises the airway, immediate medical intervention is required.

4. If the patient has a permanent tracheostomy, teach the patient and at least one family member the skills necessary for home care. Include the following points:
• need for adequate humidification
• suctioning
• tube cleaning
• emergency reinsertion of the tube if it dislodges
• stoma covering
• need to cover the stoma when showering
• need to carry medical alert identification.

4. Skill at tracheostomy care reduces the patient's and family's anxiety and increases their confidence in coping with the life-style changes the surgery creates. Suctioning and cleaning are necessary to maintain airway patency. An emergency plan for tube dislodgment may help avert panic if this complication occurs. A stoma covering prevents aspiration of dust or insects, and covering the stoma during showers and avoiding water sports prevents aspiration of water. Medical alert identification will help emergency medical personnel quickly establish an appropriate airway if the patient suffers a cardiac arrest or airway compromise.

5. Additional individualized interventions: _____

_____

5. Rationales: _____

_____

Target outcome criteria
Throughout the postoperative period, the patient will maintain airway patency.

Within 48 hours after surgery, the patient will effectively clear the airway with minimal assistance.

By the time of discharge, the patient and family will:
• demonstrate the correct technique for suctioning and cleaning the tube
• verbalize a plan for emergency airway maintenance.

By the time of discharge, the patient will:
• identify ways to avoid aspiration
• verbalize the intent to obtain medical alert identification.

Nursing diagnosis: *Impaired swallowing related to decreased strength of muscles involved in mastication or to edema, tracheostomy tube, or esophageal sutures**

NURSING PRIORITIES: (a) Prevent aspiration and (b) promote adequate food intake.

Interventions

1. Teach the patient to use oral suction equipment, and keep it at the bedside continuously.

2. Be present during meals, and teach the patient to use the "supraglottic swallow" (if the patient has a tracheostomy); eat soft foods in frequent, small feedings (if the patient underwent total laryngectomy); and place food in the area of the mouth unaffected by surgery. Encourage persistence in swallowing, and document progress.

3. Additional individualized interventions: _____

_____

Rationales

1. An increase in the amount of secretions is common after RND and difficult to handle if swallowing is impaired. Saliva flows continually; the ability to suction secretions decreases the patient's anxiety and minimizes the risk of choking.

2. The "supraglottic swallow" protects the airway and decreases the potential for aspiration. The sequence is usually cough, take a breath, take food, swallow, cough, swallow, and breathe. Soft foods and frequent feedings gradually stretch the esophageal incision site and encourage muscle relaxation. Swallowing success is increased when the patient can control food in the mouth; inspecting the mouth after swallowing indicates areas of weakness and helps determine the optimal site for food placement. Initial attempts may be unsuccessful and discouraging unless support is given. New techniques require practice to be effective.

3. Rationales: _____

_____

---

*This diagnosis applies to the patient who has had combined surgery, including RND.

Target outcome criteria
Throughout the postoperative period, the patient will:
• exhibit no aspiration
• use suction equipment effectively.

By the time of discharge, the patient will:
• control oral secretions without using suction
• use a modified eating technique effectively.

Nursing diagnosis: *High risk for injury related to impaired tissue integrity and sensory alterations (decreased sense of temperature, touch, and hearing on side of surgery)*

NURSING PRIORITIES: (a) Prevent injury and (b) maintain sensory function.

Interventions	Rationales
1. See the "Skin Grafts" plan, page 508.	1. This plan contains interventions for skin graft care.
2. Maintain continuous suction on drainage catheters: the recommended level is 100 to 120 mm Hg. When the patient ambulates, use a portable drainage collector. Interrupt suction, using universal precautions, to assess the system's patency every 1 to 2 hours for the first 48 hours, then every 4 hours until drains are removed.	2. Negative pressure is required to remove clots and fluid from the surgical wound. Inadequate suction may cause drain blockage and result in excessive edema, airway obstruction, or both.
3. Observe and document wound drainage every 8 hours. Report abnormalities, especially any sudden increase in the amount of drainage. Instruct the patient and family on the importance of careful observation.	3. A dramatic increase in bloody drainage may indicate impending carotid artery rupture. This is most likely in the immediate postoperative period, or later if infection or fistula formation occurs near the carotid artery. An increase in clear fluid or a change to milky drainage may indicate infection or fistula formation. Typically, drainage is less than 100 ml every 8 hours for the first 2 days, then less than 20 ml every 8 hours on succeeding days.
4. If infection or a fistula occurs, determine the need for placing the patient on carotid artery rupture precautions. These vary among institutions but always include avoidance of coughing, sudden head movements, and Valsalva's maneuver. Ensure that supplies are placed at the bedside as follows: • towels, packing, and dressings • hemostats and clamps • gowns and gloves • suture materials • a light source • a laryngoscope, cuffed endotracheal and tracheostomy tubes, and a 10 ml syringe • suction equipment.	4. The carotid artery may be exposed if surrounding tissues are damaged by infection or if fistula formation delays healing. Artery rupture is a life-threatening complication requiring immediate medical intervention. Keeping needed supplies at the bedside facilitates prompt intervention if rupture occurs.
5. If carotid rupture occurs, stay with the patient, call for help, apply direct pressure if the hemorrhage site is visible, and maintain airway patency by orotracheal suctioning if hemoptysis is present.	5. Most patients remain awake during carotid artery rupture. External pressure on a visible site controls the hemorrhage temporarily until help arrives. The trachea is a common pathway for internal hemorrhage.
6. Inspect and document changes at the wound site, especially noting redness, pallor, and increasing edema. Report abnormalities.	6. Redness or pallor may indicate tension on the area, requiring arm, shoulder, or neck repositioning or adjustment of tracheostomy ties or the oxygen collar. Increasing edema may indicate inadequate or blocked drainage tubes.
7. Clean the suture line, as ordered, and document changes. Usual care involves removing crust with hydrogen peroxide and sterile swabs three or four times daily, followed by a thin application of bactericidal ointment to the suture line.	7. Cleaning facilitates healing and decreases the potential for infection. Controversy continues, however, regarding the relative effectiveness of available bactericidal preparations.

8. Assess for and document any hearing loss on the side of surgery. If so, speak to the patient on the unaffected side. Do not shout. Use active listening skills at the bedside.

8. Edema may temporarily block the ear canal. Shouting may intimidate or annoy the patient. Standing near the patient when speaking or listening facilitates communication.

9. Support the patient's shoulder and arm at all times. Begin range-of-motion exercises, as ordered.

9. Proper body alignment promotes healing and decreases tension on the surgical site. Innervation to the muscle is lost, but muscle mass remains and requires exercise to prevent atrophy.

10. Teach the patient to protect the surgical site when performing ADLs. Also teach the male patient to look at the neck when shaving rather than depending on touch. Emphasize the importance of testing food temperatures before eating. Discourage the use of heat for relief of shoulder pain.

10. Numbness increases the risk of accidental injury while shaving and eating. Heat should not be used to treat shoulder pain because temperature awareness in that area is impaired after surgery.

11. Additional individualized interventions: _____

11. Rationales: _____

Target outcome criteria
Within 5 days after surgery, the patient will:
• exhibit less than 20 ml of drainage every 8 hours
• exhibit decreased redness, no pallor, no increased edema, and minimal areas of crusting at the wound site.

Throughout the postoperative period, the patient will:
• support the shoulder and arm effectively
• receive immediate intervention if the carotid artery ruptures.

By the time of discharge, the patient will:
• protect the wound site effectively during ADLs
• identify areas of numbness and state protective measures for each area.

Nursing diagnosis: *Pain related to edema, intubation, and the surgical wound*

NURSING PRIORITY: Relieve postoperative pain.

Interventions

1. See the "Pain" plan, page 69.

2. For headache, administer medication as ordered and document promptly. Keep the head of the bed elevated at all times.

3. For a sore throat, administer mouth care before meals, and offer fluids every 1 to 2 hours.

4. For shoulder pain, support the arm and shoulder at all times; teach the patient support methods; and administer medication promptly, as ordered, at the onset of pain and before ambulation or activities of daily living (ADLs). Document all measures taken.

5. Additional individualized interventions: _____

Rationales

1. This plan contains general interventions for pain management.

2. Edema related to loss of lymphatics and the jugular vein can cause postoperative headache. The semi-upright position facilitates fluid drainage and decreases pressure.

3. Fluids bathe the oral mucosa and stimulate salivary flow.

4. Adequate support decreases tension on the wound site and maintains body alignment. Analgesics decrease pain, facilitating resumption of therapeutic activity.

5. Rationales: _____

Target outcome criteria
Throughout the postoperative period, the patient will:
• verbalize absence or relief of pain
• exhibit relaxed posture and facial expression.

Nursing diagnosis: *Nutritional deficit related to anorexia and impaired swallowing*

NURSING PRIORITY: Optimize nutritional intake.

Interventions

1. On admission, document the patient's height, weight, weight loss, intake pattern, and food consistency tolerances. See the "Nutritional Deficit" plan, page 63.

2. Consult a dietitian for a thorough nutritional assessment to calculate calorie and protein requirements.

3. Monitor and document intake at each meal. Assess and document changes in chewing and swallowing ability. Supplement the diet as needed. Administer enteral feedings, as ordered, and document the patient's response.

4. Weigh the patient twice weekly, and document.

5. Administer mouth care or an analgesic, as ordered, before meals.

6. Additional individualized interventions: _____

Rationales

1. Weight and weight loss help establish the patient's current nutritional status. Intake patterns and food consistency tolerances provide a focus for dietary planning. The "Nutritional Deficit" plan provides further details.

2. Nutritional requirements are increased in disease and during treatment. The dietitian's expertise helps meet individual patient needs.

3. To achieve the required calorie and protein intake, additional feedings are often necessary. Changes in chewing and swallowing ability require dietary modifications. Individual patients respond differently to enteral feedings, and frequent adjustment is required.

4. Weight changes indicate progress or the need for adjustment to meet body requirements.

5. Good oral hygiene enhances food appeal when appetite is poor. Analgesics may be indicated if pain keeps the patient from eating.

6. Rationales: _____

Target outcome criteria
Throughout the postoperative period, the patient will:
• experience no further weight loss
• have nutritional intake meeting calculated calorie and protein requirements.

Nursing diagnosis: *Altered oral mucous membrane related to intake restrictions and nasogastric tube*

NURSING PRIORITIES: (a) Minimize mucous membrane damage and (b) promote healing.

Interventions

1. While the patient is restricted from taking food or fluids, provide mouth care every 2 hours, as ordered.

2. After oral intake is resumed, provide mouth care after meals and at bedtime.

Rationales

1. Mouth care stimulates saliva flow and removes pooled secretions, which foster bacterial growth. Usually, care involves half-strength hydrogen peroxide and normal saline solution.

2. Food trapped in the altered oral cavity serves as a medium for bacterial growth and must be removed to prevent infection.

3. If oral suture lines are present, perform mouth care using a power spray, according to protocol and as ordered. Document the appearance of the oral cavity, and note changes.

3. Crusting requires the pressure of a power spray for adequate removal.

4. Additional individualized interventions: _____

4. Rationales: _____

Target outcome criteria
Throughout the postoperative period, the patient will:
• exhibit pink and moist mucous membranes
• exhibit no signs and symptoms of infection.

Nursing diagnosis: *Impaired verbal communication related to oral surgery and tracheostomy**

NURSING PRIORITIES: (a) Maximize communication and (b) minimize patient frustration.

Interventions

1. Before surgery, help the patient select postoperative methods of communication. Document the methods chosen; options include:
• pencil and paper on a clipboard
• a "magic slate"
• a communication board or set of cards with pictures of commonly needed items
• an electrolarynx device (for later postoperative stages).

2. After surgery, tag the call system "patient cannot talk." Explain to the patient and family that the patient can still use the call system.

3. Address the patient in a normal conversational tone.

4. Allow the patient using a communication device to finish writing before replying.

5. Obtain a speech therapy consultation, as ordered.

6. Teach the patient with a tracheostomy to cover the opening when speaking, according to protocol or as ordered.

7. Additional individualized interventions: _____

Rationales

1. Using alternative communication methods of the patient's choosing decreases anxiety and facilitates communication. The patient may prefer pencil and paper because the "magic slate" may be associated with childlike feelings of helplessness. The patient can help prepare a communication board or picture cards before surgery, increasing self-control. An electrolaryngeal device for the patient undergoing laryngectomy usually is not used until 5 to 7 days after surgery, so another method will be needed initially.

2. This alerts the secretary or nurse that the patient's call must be attended to quickly. The patient is assured that personal needs will be met.

3. Inability to speak does not necessarily indicate deafness.

4. This prevents incorrect second-guessing and allows the patient to express feelings adequately.

5. Speech therapy exercises improve speech clarity.

6. This prevents air leakage around the trachea, improving speech clarity and volume.

7. Rationales: _____

Target outcome criteria
Throughout the hospital stay, the patient will:
• maintain communication
• experience minimal frustration with communication.

---

*This diagnosis applies to the patient who has had combined surgery, including RND.

Nursing diagnosis: *Bathing and hygiene or dressing and grooming self-care deficits related to muscle weakness, pain, and uncompensated neuromuscular impairment*

NURSING PRIORITIES: (a) Maximize the patient's self-care ability and (b) encourage the use of affected muscles.

Interventions

1. After surgery, demonstrate methods to compensate for loss of function, such as using the unaffected arm and shoulder to bathe, comb hair, and dress by putting clothing on the affected side first.

2. Administer an analgesic, as ordered, before activities.

3. Teach strengthening exercises, as ordered, and document progress. Refer the patient to a physical therapist for an ongoing activity plan.

4. Additional individualized interventions: _____

Rationales

1. Initial weakness may discourage the patient from using the unaffected arm and shoulder to the fullest advantage.

2. This encourages arm use without pain.

3. The muscle can be trained to tense, offsetting some of the shoulder drop that occurs with lost innervation. The physical therapist's expertise helps in planning rehabilitation.

4. Rationales: _____

Target outcome criterion
Within 5 days after surgery, the patient will be able to bathe and dress with minimal help.

Nursing diagnosis: *Family coping: potential for growth related to successful management of situational crisis (prolonged treatment for head and neck cancer)*

NURSING PRIORITY: Support the family.

Interventions

1. Assess and document the family's reactions to and feelings about the patient's illness, care, and future needs. Allow the family time and space away from the patient to verbalize their feelings and concerns.

2. Discuss with the patient and family the dietary, activity, and life-style modifications needed as a result of surgery or any future treatment, such as radiation therapy or chemotherapy. Document the course of action the patient and family choose.

3. After surgery, teach the patient and family skills needed after discharge, such as preparing a high-calorie, high-protein diet; enteral feeding; changing dressings (if a fistula develops); performing special mouth care, as ordered; and providing tracheostomy care and suctioning. Discuss signs and symptoms of possible complications and a plan of action should complications occur. If a tracheostomy is present, provide referral for home care follow-up.

4. Arrange for a person who has undergone similar surgery to visit, if the patient desires. Document the patient's and family's response to the visit.

Rationales

1. Verbalization facilitates the family's ability to identify strengths and plan for the patient's postoperative care.

2. Planning decreases anxiety surrounding discharge home. Typically, the initial symptoms of head and neck cancer require changes in diet. Family members may have already made these changes and identified others; in this case, the family may simply need reassurance that plans are appropriate.

3. Instruction, demonstration, and practice of home-care skills enable the patient and family to effectively meet needs after discharge. Familiarity with procedures increases self-care abilities and the confidence of both the patient and family. Explanation of potential problems and possible solutions relieves anxiety and encourages early assessment and prompt treatment of complications.

4. A peer can identify common problems and helpful solutions, and act as a positive role model, benefiting both the patient and family.

5. Initiate and document referral to appropriate community resource groups, such as home health care, a cancer support group, a smoking cessation group, or an alcoholism support group.

5. Support groups strengthen and expand the patient's and family's coping resources.

6. Additional individualized interventions: _____

6. Rationales: _____

Target outcome criteria

By the time of discharge, family members will:
• state the plan for support after discharge
• demonstrate skills needed for home care — dietary management, wound care, and mouth care

• verbalize plans for required life-style modifications related to current or future treatments
• identify the most common complication and state the plan of action should this complication occur.

Nursing diagnosis: *Body-image disturbance related to change in physical appearance and to functional limitations*

NURSING PRIORITY: Encourage acceptance of change and limitations.

Interventions

1. See the "Grieving" and "Ineffective Individual Coping" plans, pages 31 and 51 respectively.

2. After surgery, demonstrate acceptance by looking directly at the patient when speaking and giving care.

3. Discuss and document family reactions to appearance changes and the level of acceptance the patient needs.

4. By the second postoperative day, help the patient to ambulate outside the room.

5. Prepare the patient for the wound's appearance, and discuss the healing process.

6. Prepare the patient for possible social rejection after discharge. Discuss and document feelings and responses.

7. Encourage prescribed exercises to strengthen the shoulder muscle.

8. Additional individualized interventions: _____

Rationales

1. These plans contain interventions helpful in coping with potential body-image disturbance.

2. The patient can sense nonverbal communication. An initial positive response to the patient's changed appearance strengthens self-esteem.

3. Awareness of patient needs helps the family give adequate support.

4. Early ambulation outside the room encourages adjustment to changes.

5. Initial appearance is distorted until healing is complete. Preparing the patient in advance minimizes distress over the wound's appearance.

6. Acquaintances may have limited experience with facial surgery, and the patient should be prepared for their responses. Discussion of possible reactions may help minimize the painfulness of such encounters.

7. The muscle can be strengthened to offset shoulder drop.

8. Rationales: _____

Target outcome criteria

Within 2 days after surgery, family members will show beginning acceptance of the patient's appearance and give positive support.

By the time of discharge, the patient will:
• show beginning acceptance of body changes and limitations
• verbalize a method for dealing with rejection.

Discharge planning

NURSING DISCHARGE CRITERIA

Upon the patient's discharge, documentation shows evidence of:
• stable vital signs
• absence of fever
• absence of life-threatening dysphagia
• absence of pulmonary and cardiovascular complications
• hemoglobin and white blood cell levels within normal parameters
• a healing wound with drainage amount within expected parameters and no evidence of bloody or purulent drainage
• completion of a diagnostic workup for evidence of cancer
• ability to tolerate adequate oral nutrition
• ability to perform wound care, dressing changes, and exercise program independently or with minimal assistance
• ability to perform ADLs and ambulate at usual level
• ability to control pain using oral medications
• adequate home support system or referral to home care if indicated by patient's inability to perform ADLs, ambulate, and care for wound as directed.

Additional information to be documented if the patient has undergone a laryngectomy or a tracheotomy:
• ability to communicate adequately
• ability to perform tracheostomy care independently or with minimal assistance
• ability to perform emergency tracheostomy care if the entire tracheostomy apparatus dislodges
• automatic referral to home care or nursing home care if indicated by inadequate home support system and patient's inability to perform tracheostomy care.

PATIENT-FAMILY TEACHING CHECKLIST

Document evidence that the patient and family demonstrate an understanding of:
___ extent of disease and surgery, and implications
___ caloric requirements and dietary modifications
___ wound care
___ mouth care
___ schedule for resuming activities and returning to work
___ common changes in feelings after RND
___ signs and symptoms of disease recurrence
___ all discharge medications' purpose, dose, administration schedule, and adverse effects requiring medical attention (usual discharge medications include an analgesic and an antibiotic)
___ date, time, and location of follow-up appointments
___ how to contact the doctor
___ need for smoking-cessation program or alcoholism rehabilitation, as needed
___ community resources for speech rehabilitation, physical therapy, and support
___ when and how to seek emergency medical care.

DOCUMENTATION CHECKLIST

Using outcome criteria as a guide, document:
___ clinical status on admission
___ significant changes in status
___ pertinent laboratory and diagnostic test findings
___ pain relief measures
___ wound appearance and drainage
___ mouth care and wound care
___ nutritional intake
___ patient-family teaching
___ discharge planning.

ASSOCIATED PLANS OF CARE

Dying
Grieving
Ineffective Family Coping
Ineffective Individual Coping
Knowledge Deficit
Nutritional Deficit
Pain
Skin Grafts
Surgical Intervention

References

Carpenito, L. *Nursing Diagnosis: Application to Clinical Practice,* 4th ed. Philadelphia: J.B. Lippincott Co., 1991.

Griffin, C., and Lockhart, J. "Learning to Swallow Again," *American Journal of Nursing* 87(3):314-17, March 1987.

Schwartz, S., and Yuska, C. "Common Patient Care Issues Following Surgery for Head and Neck Cancer," *Seminars in Oncology Nursing* 5(3):191-94, August 1989.

Sigler, B. "Nursing Care for Head and Neck Tumor Patients," in *Comprehensive Management of Head and Neck Tumors.* Edited by Thawley, S., et al. Philadelphia: W.B. Saunders Co., 1987.

Thompson, J., et al., eds. *Mosby's Manual of Clinical Nursing,* 2nd ed. St. Louis: C.V. Mosby Co., 1989.

Tweed, S. "Identifying the Alcoholic Client," *Nursing Clinics of North America* 24(1):13-32, March 1989.

MUSCULOSKELETAL AND INTEGUMENTARY DISORDERS

Skin Grafts

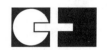

DRG information

DRG 263 Skin Grafts or Debridement for Skin Ulcer or
Cellulitis. With Complication or Comorbidity
(CC).
Mean LOS = 16.0 days
DRG 264 Skin Grafts or Debridement for Skin Ulcer or
Cellulitis. Without CC.
Mean LOS = 9.2 days
DRG 439 Skin Grafts for Injuries.
Mean LOS = 7.2 days

Introduction
DEFINITION AND TIME FOCUS
Skin grafting is the process of covering damaged tissue, such as burns or pressure ulcers, with healthy skin transplants. The skin transplants may be autografts from the patient's body, homografts from another person, or heterografts from a different species (such as porcine grafts). Grafts vary in thickness, depending on the extent of the wound, the availability of donor sites, the mobility and vascularity of the area to be covered, and the desired cosmetic results. The usual types are:
• split-thickness grafts — epidermis and part of the dermis, varying from thin to thick, meshed or nonmeshed; thinner grafts are used for large, hidden areas, thicker grafts for large, visible areas
• full-thickness grafts — epidermis and dermis, used for visible, mobile areas such as the eyelids and hands
• flap grafts — autografts of skin and subcutaneous tissue where part of the flap is left attached to the donor site, used for large areas with a poor blood supply.

This plan focuses on the patient with any large, open skin wound who is admitted for preoperative wound preparation and skin grafting with a split-thickness autograft.

ETIOLOGY AND PRECIPITATING FACTORS
• burns of sufficient extent or depth to require grafting for protection and healing
• large pressure ulcers, particularly over bony, avascular areas, that cannot heal effectively through normal epithelialization and granulation from the wound edges inward
• major trauma, such as avulsion of an extremity, that may require grafting for protection and to preserve function

Focused assessment guidelines
NURSING HISTORY (Functional health pattern findings)
Note: Because skin grafts are performed for disparate reasons, such as burns, pressure ulcers, and trauma, a typical presenting picture does not exist. However, the nurse must assess all patients undergoing skin grafting for preoperative preparedness to ensure optimal outcomes; therefore, this section presents preoperative assessment guidelines instead.

Health perception — health management pattern
• Determine the purpose for grafting, including the cause and extent of the injury; the grafting procedure; expectations for successful graft adherence; and the potential for return of function as the basis for care, patient teaching, and discharge planning.
• Determine the patient's perceptions regarding potential disfigurement and its impact on health status and life-style.

Nutritional-metabolic pattern
• Assess typical nutritional intake for adequate fluids, calories, proteins, and vitamins.
• Assess nutritional status for signs of nutritional deficiency, such as weight loss and poor skin and hair condition, that may increase the risk of graft loss and infection.
• Assess for general conditions that may contribute to poor healing, such as general debilitation, immobility, age, prolonged bed rest, skin and circulatory problems, and inability to perform activities of daily living (ADLs).
• Assess the graft site for the presence of healthy granulation tissue and the absence of necrotic areas, drainage, and odor. Grafts will adhere only to healthy granulated tissue.

Elimination pattern
• Assess for elimination problems, such as frequent bowel and bladder incontinence, that may contribute to skin breakdown and poor healing.

Activity-exercise pattern
• Assess normal activity and exercise habits to determine the patient's potential for adjusting to position and activity limitations.
• Establish a baseline assessment of present musculoskeletal and neurologic functions for comparison to potential postoperative changes in function and sensation.

Sleep-rest pattern
• Assess normal sleep patterns to guide postoperative management of pain and rest.

Cognitive-perceptual pattern
• Determine the patient's readiness for treatment by assessing understanding of the injury's extent, the prognosis for return of function, the surgical procedure, and rehabilitation phases during the hospital stay and home care.

Self-perception—self-concept pattern
• Assess the patient's usual self-perception—self-concept pattern to determine ability to adapt positively during the hospital stay and recovery at home.
• Assess the impact of body changes on the patient's feelings of self-worth.

Role-relationship pattern
• Assess the patient's concerns regarding the impact of current or potential disfigurement on relationships with family and others.
• Assess family members' and friends' ability to support the patient.

Sexuality-reproductive pattern
• Assess the patient's concerns regarding alterations in physical attractiveness, ability to feel sensations, and ability to perform sexually. (Note: Grafted tissue may have decreased touch sensation.)

Coping—stress tolerance pattern
• Assess for anxiety, anger, and depression related to changes in body image and potentially permanent disfigurement. (Note: Regression is a common coping pattern for the patient with large wounds needing grafting.)

Value-belief pattern
• Assess the effect of cultural and value-belief systems on the patient's response to illness.

PHYSICAL FINDINGS*
Cardiovascular
• poor capillary refill

Neurologic
• diminished sensation, including pain response, over wound
• increased pain response around wound edges

Integumentary
• fragile skin
• poor skin turgor
• ulcerated area (damage may extend to subcutaneous tissue, underlying fat, and muscle; tissue may be reddened, draining, and necrotic)

Musculoskeletal
• limited mobility
• limited range of motion (ROM)

DIAGNOSTIC STUDIES
• culture and sensitivity testing of wound drainage—may indicate infecting organism and help determine the most desirable antibiotic treatment
• white blood cell count—may be elevated in presence of inflammation and infection
• complete blood count—may show a low hematocrit, which may affect tissue healing
• clotting time—may be prolonged, affecting tissue healing
• serum protein (albumin and globulin) and fat (cholesterol and triglycerides) levels—may be depressed in poor nutritional status
• postoperative tissue biopsy—may show infection or indicate degree of graft success
• ultrasound—may determine size of wound, particularly if deep

POTENTIAL COMPLICATIONS
• nonadherence of graft
• infection
• contractures
• hypertrophic scar formation at donor or recipient site

Collaborative problem: *High risk for nonadherence of graft related to inadequate wound preparation*

NURSING PRIORITY: Prepare the wound properly for grafting.

Interventions

1. Assess and document wound condition on admission and at least every shift. Indicate the wound's size, color, and depth and the presence or absence of odor, drainage, necrotic tissue, and swelling.

Rationales

1. Initial documentation provides baseline data concerning wound condition. Regular assessment and documentation provide data on the pattern of healing.

---

*The physical findings listed here are wound related.

2. Change dressings every shift, as ordered, using good hand washing and sterile technique. Use wet-to-dry dressings.

3. Clean the wound and surrounding skin with soap and water, as ordered, every shift. Apply topical agents such as povidone-iodine (Betadine), as ordered, according to recommended guidelines.

4. Irrigate the wound with sterile water every shift, as ordered.

5. Apply hydrophilic agents such as dextranomer (Debrisan) every shift, as ordered.

6. Apply enzymes such as fibrinolysin and desoxyribonuclease (Elase) to the wound every shift, as ordered. Apply only to the wound, protecting healthy tissue with an ointment such as zinc oxide.

7. Assist the doctor, as needed, with surgical debridement of necrotic tissue.

8. Apply barrier dressings such as Op-Site, if ordered, every 3 to 4 days or as needed for leakage.

9. Change the patient's position every 2 hours, protecting the affected area from pressure by using rubber rings, extra padding, or special positioning.

10. Additional individualized interventions: _____

2. Conscientious attention to technique helps prevent infection. Wet-to-dry dressings aid healing by debriding the wound, keeping the tissue moist, and applying antiseptics.

3. Cleaning the skin prevents bacterial colonization and spread. Topical microbicidal agents such as povidone-iodine may help prevent infections.

4. Wound irrigation with large amounts of sterile water removes drainage, debriding agents, and contaminants.

5. Hydrophilic agents absorb drainage and aid in wound debridement.

6. Enzymes soften necrotic tissue by fibrinolytic action, breaking up clots and exudates. Although enzymes act primarily on necrotic tissue, healthy tissue may be irritated unless protected.

7. Removal of necrotic tissue speeds healing and granulation tissue development.

8. Barrier dressings maintain a moist environment, which promotes granulation tissue formation.

9. Position changes promote circulation and prevent tissue damage from prolonged pressure.

10. Rationales: _____

Target outcome criteria
Within 2 days of admission, the patient will:
• exhibit signs of wound healing
• exhibit no redness over pressure points.

Collaborative problem: High risk for nonadherence of graft related to postoperative exudate or blood accumulation, movement, or infection

NURSING PRIORITIES: (a) Maintain graft integrity and (b) promote graft healing.

Interventions

1. Maintain movement restrictions for 3 days or as ordered. Use splints, restraints, pillows, or other devices to maintain the desired position.

2. Elevate the grafted area, if possible, for 1 week after surgery.

3. Continuously protect the graft from injury, using splints or bed cradles.

Rationales

1. Movement of the tissue under the graft may dislodge it. Adherence will be evident several days after surgery, although 2 to 3 weeks are needed for vascularization.

2. Elevation prevents swelling, which could cause graft separation.

3. Jarring or pressure may dislodge the graft.

4. Assist the doctor during initial removal of inner dressings and graft inspection, usually 1 to 2 days after surgery. Document findings. Thereafter, carefully assess the graft every 8 hours and document its appearance. Report immediately any swelling, redness, and exudate or blood under the graft.

4. Initial dressing removal must be done with utmost care to prevent separating the graft from the underlying tissue. Regular inspections allow prompt treatment of complications. Any substance, such as exudate or blood, coming between the graft and underlying tissue may cause separation. Swelling or redness may indicate infection, which can dislodge the graft. The doctor must carefully remove any drainage by aspiration or by rolling an applicator toward a nicked area.

5. Maintain dressings continuously, as ordered. Report unusual drainage or dislodged dressings.

5. Various dressings — including petroleum gauze, nonadhesive gauze, coarse mesh gauze, and moist saline-soaked gauze — are used to maintain gentle pressure on the graft. Drainage or dislodged dressings may prevent adherence.

6. Apply moist, warm compresses for 20 to 30 minutes four times daily, as ordered.

6. Warmth and moisture increase circulation and enhance epithelial tissue formation and blood supply to the graft.

7. Administer topical or systemic antibiotics, or both, as ordered.

7. Antibiotics may be used to prevent or treat graft infection.

8. Additional individualized interventions: _____

8. Rationales: _____

Target outcome criteria
Within 2 days after surgery, the patient will:
• exhibit an intact graft
• exhibit a graft free from injury
• maintain position
• maintain activity limitations
• keep the dressing intact.

Within 2 weeks after surgery, the patient will:
• exhibit a graft free from infection, swelling, and exudate or blood accumulation
• exhibit graft adherence and blood supply formation.

Nursing diagnosis: *High risk for infection of donor site related to surgical excision of half of the skin layer*

NURSING PRIORITY: Promote healing of the donor site.

Interventions

1. Maintain dressings over the donor site for 1 to 2 days. Document your actions. Then replace the outer layers or remove them and leave the inner layer exposed, as ordered. Leave the inner dressing in place until it falls off spontaneously.

2. Promote drying by leaving the donor site exposed to air or by cautiously applying heat from a heat lamp or hair dryer for 15 to 30 minutes four times daily or as ordered.

3. Promote air circulation to the donor site by using a cradle to keep bedding and clothing away from the site.

4. If infection occurs, apply wet antiseptic dressings such as acetic acid four times daily, as ordered.

5. After healing (usually in 2 to 3 weeks), apply lotion to the site four times daily or as ordered.

Rationales

1. Dressings are left over the site until serum dries. The inner dressing is either a nonadherent dressing, such as Xeroform, or fine mesh gauze; it is left in place until it falls off (usually 2 to 3 weeks).

2. Drying, such as from evaporation or heat, enhances serum formation and helps prevent infection. (Note: Skin at the donor site is sensitive to excess heat.)

3. Air circulation aids drying and healing.

4. Antiseptic dressings decrease microorganism growth and aid healing.

5. Lotions keep the skin soft and help prevent scarring.

6. Additional individualized interventions: _____

6. Rationales: _____

Target outcome criteria

Within 2 days after surgery, the patient will exhibit a dry, infection-free donor site.

Within 2 weeks after surgery, the patient will:
• exhibit a reepithelialized donor site
• exhibit soft and unscarred skin.

Nursing diagnosis: *Impaired physical mobility related to position and movement limitations*

NURSING PRIORITY: Promote maintenance of muscle tone and skin integrity.

Interventions

1. Provide active and passive ROM exercises to unaffected areas every 2 hours, as ordered.

2. Promote self-care according to the patient's tolerance and the doctor's orders.

3. Apply splints and other devices, as ordered, either continuously or as needed during activities or ambulation.

4. Provide relief as needed for discomfort or pain. See the "Pain" plan, page 69.

5. Additional individualized interventions: _____

Rationales

1. ROM exercises promote muscle tone, circulation, and a feeling of well-being; they also help prevent contractures.

2. Self-care enhances feelings of independence and control over the course of recovery.

3. Protective devices allow some mobility while protecting the graft site.

4. The patient will experience pain from the graft and donor sites and discomfort from immobility. Relief from pain or discomfort encourages movement, as allowed, and aids healing by promoting a sense of well-being. The "Pain" plan contains general interventions for pain management.

5. Rationales: _____

Target outcome criteria

Within 8 hours after surgery, the patient will:
• have no uncontrolled pain or discomfort
• exhibit an intact graft

• perform ADLs, position changes, ROM exercises, and other activities as allowed.

Nursing diagnosis: *Nutritional deficit related to increased metabolic needs secondary to tissue healing*

NURSING PRIORITY: Provide adequate calories and protein to promote tissue healing.

Interventions

1. Assess and document nutritional status daily, including weight; condition of skin, hair, and mucous membranes; and wound healing. Note baseline serum total protein findings.

2. Provide a high-calorie, high-protein diet along with vitamin supplements. Document calorie intake and fluid intake and output daily.

Rationales

1. Baseline and ongoing assessment data help guide dietary intake.

2. A diet high in calories, protein, and vitamins aids tissue healing. Maintaining fluid balance is necessary for supple skin.

3. Additional individualized interventions: _____

3. Rationales: _____

Target outcome criteria
Within 1 week after surgery, the patient will:
• exhibit no signs or symptoms of inadequate nutritional intake
• exhibit a healing wound.

Nursing diagnosis: *Body-image disturbance related to wound and potential scarring*

NURSING PRIORITY: Optimize adjustment to body changes.

Interventions	Rationales
1. Allow expression of fears and concerns related to wounds and scarring. Document patient concerns. Encourage continuity of discussion by all health team members on all shifts by documenting the patient's current psychological status on the plan of care.	1. Sharing concerns releases tension and opens discussion, which may lead to more realistic self-appraisal of body changes.
2. Provide information about the expected stages of graft healing during nursing care and as needed.	2. Knowing what to expect decreases fear of the unknown and allows the patient to participate in assessment of healing. Initially, the area will be reddened, swollen, and different in appearance from surrounding tissue. After 6 months, the area will be more normal in appearance as swelling decreases and color matches other tissue.
3. Additional individualized interventions: _____	3. Rationales: _____

Target outcome criteria
Within 8 hours after surgery, the patient will:
• verbalize freedom from anxiety about the wound and healing, on request
• express appropriate expectations regarding healing.

Nursing diagnosis: *Knowledge deficit related to home care of donor and graft sites*

NURSING PRIORITY: Provide information to optimize long-term healing of donor and graft sites.

Interventions	Rationales
1. See the "Knowledge Deficit" plan, page 56.	1. The "Knowledge Deficit" plan contains general interventions related to patient teaching.
2. Teach the patient and family the following care measures:	2. These measures provide the following benefits:
• Apply topical ointments such as corticosteroids (as ordered) and skin softeners (lanolin and mineral oil) to the donor and graft sites.	• Corticosteroids prevent inflammation, which can compromise circulation and healing. Grafted tissue may lack lubricating glands and may dry more readily.

• Maintain pressure and protective dressings as ordered.

• Avoid sun exposure by wearing protective clothing and using sunscreen lotions until the graft heals completely (usually in 6 to 12 months).

• Maintain activity and position limitations as ordered.

• Perform ROM exercises and maintain a positioning program, as ordered, until the tissue heals and matures in 6 to 12 months.

• Maintain a diet high in calories, protein, and vitamins.

• Avoid smoking. Attend a smoking cessation program, if needed.

• Assess the donor and graft sites daily for healing progress and absence of such complications as redness or other discolorations, swelling, drainage, bad odor, pain, and excessive warmth.

3. Additional individualized interventions: _____

_____

• Pressure dressings inhibit excessive scar formation. Protective dressings may be necessary because new tissue is very sensitive and easily injured.

• New tissue lacks melanin-producing cells and is more susceptible to sunburn. Melanin-producing cells may regenerate in 6 to 12 months.

• Premature or excessive activity may dislodge the graft.

• ROM exercises and positioning extend the affected area and prevent contractures.

• Additional calories, protein, and vitamins are necessary for tissue healing because the stresses of an open wound, surgery, and hospitalization create a catabolic state.

• Smoking decreases blood flow and oxygen supply to peripheral tissues, thus inhibiting healing.

• Healing tissue should be warm, flat, only slightly more reddened than the surrounding tissue, and flexible, and it should have a capillary refill time of less than 3 seconds. Such signs and symptoms as redness, swelling, and pain may indicate an infection, which could prevent permanent graft adherence.

3. Rationales: _____

_____

Target outcome criteria
By the time of discharge, the patient will:
• demonstrate ointment and dressing application
• describe specific activity and position limitations
• explain skin protection methods
• identify diet requirements

• describe appropriate graft and donor site appearance
• list two risk factors for poor healing
• list four signs of complications.

Discharge planning

NURSING DISCHARGE CRITERIA

Upon the patient's discharge, documentation shows evidence of:
• healing and intact donor and graft sites with no evidence of abnormal drainage or swelling
• ability to control pain using oral medications
• stable vital signs
• absence of fever
• absence of pulmonary or cardiovascular complications
• hemoglobin level and white blood cell count within normal parameters
• ability to perform proper graft and donor-site care independently or with minimal assistance
• ability to tolerate adequate nutritional intake
• absence of hospital-acquired contractures
• ability to verbalize and demonstrate activity and position limitations
• absence of bowel and bladder dysfunction
• ability to perform ADLs, transfers, and ambulation at usual level with minimal assistance

• an adequate home support system or referral to home care or a nursing home if indicated by an inadequate home support system, inability to perform ADLs, or inability to care for graft and donor sites independently.

Additional information: The patient undergoing skin grafts for pressure ulcers is commonly disabled, not independently mobile, and dependent on others for care. Because of this, the patient is considered a "vulnerable adult." Any patient with pressure ulcers should automatically be referred to the social services department so that the ulcers' cause can be investigated. Most states have an automatic reporting mechanism for vulnerable adults, and nurses should be aware of this.

The patient with this diagnosis commonly lives in a nursing home, in which case the nursing home staff should be contacted to ascertain their ability to care for the patient during convalescence. Important questions to consider include: Does the nursing home have adequate staff to care for the patient? Does the nursing home have access to a special mattress or bed that promotes healing? What is the charge for such equipment? Where can the patient be discharged if the nursing home cannot provide adequate care or supply needed equipment?

Under Medicare, the cost of special equipment — such as a Clinitron bed — is covered in an acute-care setting but is not covered in a nursing home at the per diem rate. This creates a problem if the patient is discharged to a nursing home that cannot supply the necessary equipment. Another issue to consider is whether the patient meets Medicare's criteria for extended care benefits. Many patients who undergo skin grafting are eligible for care in extended care facilities upon discharge. If the patient lives at home with a capable, willing caregiver, obtaining and paying for equipment and supplies must be addressed. All of these issues must be considered early in the hospital stay to prevent a delay in discharge. Although these are all nursing considerations, the social services department will probably address them, which is why a social services referral should be automatic.

PATIENT-FAMILY TEACHING CHECKLIST
Document evidence that the patient and family demonstrate an understanding of:
___ care of the graft and donor sites
___ signs and symptoms of complications
___ activity and position limitations
___ all discharge medications' purpose, dosage, administration schedule, and adverse effects requiring medical attention (usual discharge medications include topical ointments, such as corticosteroids, and skin softeners, such as lanolin or mineral oil)
___ recommended dietary modifications
___ date, time, and location of follow-up appointments
___ how to contact the doctor.

DOCUMENTATION CHECKLIST
Using outcome criteria as a guide, document:
___ clinical status on admission
___ significant changes in status
___ pertinent laboratory and diagnostic test findings
___ wound condition (donor and graft sites)
___ pain episodes
___ pain relief measures
___ activity and position limitations
___ resumption of ADLs
___ nutritional intake
___ psychological adjustment
___ patient-family teaching
___ discharge planning.

ASSOCIATED PLANS OF CARE
Grieving
Ineffective Family Coping
Ineffective Individual Coping
Knowledge Deficit
Pain
Surgical Intervention

References

Beare, P.G., and Myers, J.L., eds. *Principles and Practice of Adult Health Nursing.* St. Louis: C.V. Mosby Co., 1990.

Dossey, B.M., Guzetta, C.E., and Kenner, C.V. *Critical Care Nursing: Body–Mind–Spirit,* 3rd ed. Philadelphia: J.B. Lippincott Co., 1992.

McKenry, L.M., and Salerno, E. *Mosby's Pharmacology in Nursing,* 17th ed. St. Louis: C.V. Mosby Co., 1989.

Patrick, M.L., Woods, S.L., Craven, R.F., Rokosky, J.S., and Bruno, P.M. *Medical-Surgical Nursing: Pathophysiological Concepts,* 2nd ed. Philadelphia: J.B. Lippincott Co., 1991.

Phipps, W.J., Long, B.C., Woods, N.F., and Cassmeyer, V.L., eds. *Medical-Surgical Nursing: Concepts and Clinical Practice,* 4th ed. St. Louis: Mosby-Year Book, 1991.

Reese, J.L. "Nursing Interventions for Wound Healing in Plastic and Reconstructive Surgery," *Nursing Clinics of North America* 25(1):223-33, March 1990.

Thompson, J.M., McFarland, G.K., Hirsch, J.E., Tucker, S.M., and Bowers, A.C. *Mosby's Manual of Clinical Nursing,* 2nd ed. St. Louis: C.V. Mosby Co., 1989.

MUSCULOSKELETAL AND INTEGUMENTARY DISORDERS

Total Joint Replacement in a Lower Extremity

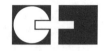

DRG information

DRG 209 Major Joint and Limb Reattachment Procedure.
Mean LOS = 10.6 days

DRG 471 Bilateral or Multiple Major Joint Procedures of the Lower Extremity.
Mean LOS = 14.2 days

Additional DRG information: These DRGs have been significant money losers because of the cost of surgical components and the rehabilitation time. Although the surgeon may inform the patient before surgery about transfer to a nursing home or extended care facility (ECF), most patients want to stay in the hospital until they feel ready to go home. Nurses can help prepare the patient for an early discharge and transfer.

Introduction
DEFINITION AND TIME FOCUS

Total joint replacement involves the surgical implantation of a prosthesis, which replaces the damaged articulating surfaces of the joint. Joint damage may result from debilitating arthritis or from traumatic degenerative bone disease. In the lower extremity, total joint replacement entails removing the damaged tissues, including bone, synovium, and cartilage. An acrylic cement may be used to attach a metallic prosthesis, which replaces the femoral head or the femoral condyle, or a polyethylene prosthesis, which replaces the acetabulum or tibial plateau. Porous, coated metal implants have been developed that allow bone to grow into the joint area; this method may be used instead of the acrylic cement.

This plan focuses on preoperative and postoperative care of the patient admitted for total hip or knee replacement.

ETIOLOGY AND PRECIPITATING FACTORS

• factors contributing to joint debilitation, including arthritis, infection, trauma, and obesity
• causes of degenerative joint incongruity, including hormonal imbalance, instability related to dysplasia, calcium deficiency from menopause, and physiologic changes from aging
• femoral head irregularities from Legg-Calvé-Perthes disease or avascular necrosis

Focused assessment guidelines
NURSING HISTORY (Functional health pattern findings)

Health perception—health management pattern
• may demonstrate decreased motivation to carry out a previously prescribed rehabilitation program for an injured or painful joint
• may report a history of misconceptions about care of injured or painful joint—for example, may report exercise during acute pain episodes or inappropriate use of mobility aids
• may have accompanying problems, such as obesity, excessive involvement in sports, neurologic deficits, arthritis, or evidence of osteoporosis
• may have a history of problems with or surgical procedures involving this or other joints
• may report need for specific aids (such as a knee immobilizer) to prevent falls or further damage
• may report short- or long-term use of prescribed corticosteroids

Nutritional-metabolic pattern
• may report inadequate nutrient intake before admission, indicating poor tissue state for wound healing

Elimination pattern
• may report constipation (related to decreased mobility)

Activity-exercise pattern
• may report inability to ambulate, sit up, change position, move extremities, or get in and out of bed
• may report inability to tolerate an exercise program because of unusual fatigue and weakness before or after exercise
• may report some soreness over bony prominences
• may report a history of unusual swelling around affected joint
• may report decreased ability to perform activities of daily living (ADLs)
• may report decreased leisure activity related to joint problems

Sleep-rest pattern
• may report ineffective rest and sleep patterns, with frequent waking because of pain or stiffness
• may report stiffness after sleep or periods of rest

Cognitive-perceptual pattern
• reports pain, stiffness, or both, usually chronic and associated with movement or weight bearing
• may report lack of knowledge about the specific joint condition, causes of the condition, aggravating factors, ways this procedure will change the condition, stages of recovery and rehabilitation, and personal responsibility during recovery and rehabilitation
• may display poor recognition of needs related to healing of affected joint, especially concerning nutrition needed for healing and limitations on ADLs and planned exercise

Role-relationship pattern
• may describe inadequate support system during planned rehabilitation program

Coping — stress tolerance pattern
• may report concern about recovery of full function in affected joint

PHYSICAL FINDINGS
Note: Physical findings vary, depending on the joint involved and the nature and extent of the injury or disease.

Cardiovascular
• normal peripheral pulses in affected extremity

Neurologic
• decreased bilateral patellar and Achilles reflexes

Musculoskeletal
• pain on active or passive range-of-motion (ROM) exercise of affected joint
• limited ROM or contracture of affected joint
• varus, valgus, or flexion deformity of knees
• decreased leg strength
• shortening of affected limb
• impaired gait
• joint enlargement, inflammation, or tenderness
• distorted posture from pain or effort to maintain balance
• crepitation on movement

Integumentary
• ischemic blanching or redness over bony prominences

DIAGNOSTIC STUDIES*
• serum electrolytes — may show hypokalemia from corticosteroid use
• fasting blood glucose — may show hyperglycemia from corticosteroid use
• bilateral X-ray of hip or knee joints — demonstrates extent of degenerative changes
• chest X-ray — may demonstrate presence of lung disease, indicating that the patient is a poor surgical risk during anesthesia and the first 3 to 5 postoperative days

POTENTIAL COMPLICATIONS
• hemorrhage
• thrombophlebitis
• infection (systemic, wound, or joint)
• disarticulation of prosthesis
• pulmonary embolus
• atelectasis
• pneumonia
• neurovascular damage in the extremity
• fat embolism
• osteomyelitis

Collaborative problem: *High risk for postoperative complications (hypovolemic shock, neurovascular damage, or thromboembolic phenomena) related to surgical trauma, bleeding, edema, improper positioning, or immobility*

NURSING PRIORITY: Prevent or promptly detect complications.

Interventions

1. For hypovolemic shock, implement these measures:

• See the "Surgical Intervention" plan, page 81.

Rationales

1. Both usual postoperative factors and the unique nature of joint replacement place the patient at risk for hypovolemic shock.

• The "Surgical Intervention" plan contains general interventions related to postoperative shock. This plan presents information pertinent to the patient undergoing hip or knee replacement.

---

*Laboratory findings are usually nonspecific for the disease.

• Maintain patency of the wound drainage device (such as a Hemovac). Assess, measure, and record the amount of drainage every 8 hours or as needed to maintain continuous suction. Monitor the amount of bleeding, and report unusual increases.

2. For neurovascular damage, implement these measures:

• Perform neurovascular checks every hour for the first 4 hours after the patient's return from surgery, then every 2 hours for 12 hours, and then every 4 hours until ambulatory. Assess pedal pulses, capillary refill time, toe temperature, skin color, foot sensation, and ability to move the toes and dorsiflex the ankle. Compare findings to the other extremity as well as to earlier findings. Once the patient is ambulatory, reassess at least daily.

• Notify the doctor immediately if pedal pulses are absent or unequal bilaterally; if capillary refill time is greater than 3 seconds; if the patient has cold toes, pale skin, foot numbness, tingling, or pain; or if the patient cannot move the toes.

• Maintain positioning as recommended. See the "Impaired physical mobility" nursing diagnosis in this plan for further details.

• Apply ice packs to the affected joint for 24 to 48 hours after surgery, if ordered.

• Maintain patency of the drainage device as previously described.

3. For thromboembolic phenomena, implement these measures:

• Instruct and coach preoperative exercises for calves, quadriceps, gluteals, and ankles. After surgery, supervise performance of exercises 5 to 10 times hourly while the patient is awake.

• Monitor for signs of thromboembolism, assessing daily for calf pain, a positive Homan's sign, redness, and swelling. See the "Surgical Intervention" and "Thrombophlebitis" plans, pages 81 and 361 respectively, for details.

• Apply elastic stockings to both legs (to the affected extremity only after the dressing is removed). Remove twice daily for 1 hour. Check the skin for signs of pressure.

• Monitor for signs of fat embolism daily. Immediately report sudden onset of dyspnea, tachycardia, pallor or cyanosis, or pleuritic pain. See the "Surgical Intervention" plan for details.

• Administer prophylactic anticoagulants (aspirin, heparin, or warfarin [Coumadin]), as ordered. Monitor clotting studies and report findings outside the recommended therapeutic range. Observe for (and advise the patient and family to report) melena, petechiae, epistaxis, hematuria, ecchymoses, or other unusual bleeding.

• The hip area is highly vascular. Also, the patient may be taking an anticoagulant to prevent thromboembolism. Initial drainage may be frankly bloody but should become serosanguineous within a few hours. A typical amount is 300 to 500 ml in the first 24 hours after surgery, decreasing to 100 ml within 48 hours. The drainage device usually is removed by the fifth postoperative day.

2. Altered neurovascular status may be associated with trauma to the nerves or blood vessels as a result of surgery, joint dislocation, edema, improper positioning, or excessive tightness of abduction pillow straps.

• Early detection of neurovascular damage facilitates prompt intervention to correct the underlying cause and minimize the chance of permanent damage.

• Early medical intervention can prevent permanent damage in the affected extremity.

• Proper positioning is critical to prevent prosthesis dislocation, which can trap and irreparably damage nerves or blood vessels.

• Ice packs promote vasoconstriction, thereby decreasing inflammation, edema, and bleeding.

• Drainage must be maintained because fluid accumulation could exert pressure on nearby nerves and vessels.

3. The patient undergoing total joint replacement is at particular risk for thrombophlebitis, embolism, and fat embolism because of immobility-induced venous stasis and possible surgical trauma to veins.

• Practice before surgery enhances the patient's ability to perform exercises later. These exercises are designed to promote venous return, minimizing the risk of thromboembolic phenomena.

• Calf pain, redness, or swelling may indicate thrombus formation. The "Surgical Intervention" plan contains general interventions related to various thrombotic and embolic phenomena. The "Thrombophlebitis" plan provides additional details on assessing for this complication.

• Elastic support stockings may promote venous return by redirecting flow from superficial veins to deeper veins.

• The patient undergoing total joint replacement is at particular risk for fat embolism because of bone marrow release from surgical disruption of flat (pelvic) or long bones.

• Prophylactic anticoagulants may reduce the risk of thrombophlebitis or thromboembolism. However, the patient must be monitored carefully because anticoagulant use may cause uncontrolled bleeding.

4. Additional individualized interventions: _____

4. Rationales: _____

Target outcome criteria

For hypovolemic shock
Within 2 hours after surgery, the patient will:
• exhibit blood pressure and pulse rate within normal limits
• exhibit drainage changing from frank bleeding to serosanguineous.

Within 1 day after surgery, the patient will:
• exhibit drainage less than 500 ml/day
• exhibit serosanguineous drainage.

Within 2 days after surgery, the patient will exhibit drainage less than 100 ml/day.

For neurovascular damage
Throughout the hospital stay, the patient will:
• exhibit bilaterally equal pedal pulses and toe temperature
• exhibit capillary refill time less than 3 seconds
• have no foot numbness or tingling
• be able to move the toes spontaneously and dorsiflex the ankle.

For thromboembolic phenomena
Within 3 days after surgery, the patient will exhibit no signs or symptoms of fat embolism:
• be alert and oriented
• experience no respiratory distress
• exhibit no petechiae
• have a PO_2 level of 80 to 100 mm Hg.

Throughout the hospital stay, the patient will exhibit no signs or symptoms of thromboembolism:
• present bilaterally clear breath sounds
• exhibit vital signs within normal limits
• experience no calf pain on foot dorsiflexion (negative Homan's sign).

Nursing diagnosis: *Impaired physical mobility related to hip or knee surgery*

NURSING PRIORITIES: (a) Maintain proper alignment of the affected extremity to prevent dislocation of the prosthesis, (b) increase mobility in the extremity through implementation of the rehabilitation plan, and (c) educate the patient concerning rehabilitation needs.

Interventions

1. Before surgery, instruct the patient about the correct postoperative positioning of the affected extremity:
• hip—maintain flexion of the hip joint at a 45-degree angle or less. Do not rotate the hip joint externally. Do not adduct the hip joint (do not cross the legs). .
• knee—do not flex or hyperextend the leg. Maintain the leg slightly elevated from the hip, using a pillow or continuous passive motion machine as ordered, typically for 48 to 72 hours.

2. Before surgery, teach the patient how to use the appropriate walking device (walker or crutches). Provide practice with the device, if possible.

3. After surgery, maintain the patient on bed rest as ordered, usually for 24 to 72 hours. Place the affected joint in the prescribed position (usually in the neutral position), using traction, rolls, splints, pillows, or derotation boots, as ordered and appropriate. Observe position and activity precautions, as noted above.

4. At least every 8 hours, observe for shortening of the extremity, a sudden increase in pain, a bulge over the femoral head on the affected side (in hip replacement), and decreased neurovascular status of the affected extremity. Report any such findings to the doctor immediately.

Rationales

1. Preoperative teaching provides information that helps the patient maintain proper positioning of the joint after surgery. The positions described help prevent prosthesis dislocation.

2. Preoperative instruction and practice, if possible, allow the patient to feel more secure when using the device.

3. The affected joint must be stabilized to prevent dislocation. Excessive flexion, internal rotation, or adduction will cause postoperative hip dislocation. Knee elevation helps reduce swelling and pain.

4. These signs indicate prosthesis dislocation, a common occurrence in hip replacement that requires immediate attention.

5. Supervise position changes at least every 2 hours. Have the patient use a trapeze and either shift weight in bed or turn to the unaffected side. Assist only as necessary.

5. Self-propelled movement helps the patient maintain muscle tone and reduces the risk of skin breakdown.

6. Implement a planned and progressive daily ambulation schedule, as ordered, 1 to 3 days after surgery. Use either crutches or a walker to allow weight bearing as recommended. Coordinate this activity with the physical therapy program.

6. Progressive daily ambulation promotes the patient's return to increased physical activity and self-care.

7. Ensure that unaffected joints are put through at least ten repetitions of full ROM exercises, three to four times daily.

7. ROM exercises of unaffected joints must be maintained during periods of decreased activity. Arthritic joints lose function more rapidly when activity is restricted.

8. Help the patient maintain preferred rest and sleep routines. Use back rubs, other skin care measures, positioning, and ordered medications, as necessary.

8. Uninterrupted periods of full relaxation and deep sleep help maintain the energy needed for remobilization of the affected joint.

9. Collaborate with the health care team to design an appropriate rehabilitation plan that includes:
• muscle-strengthening activities until maximum potential strength is reached
• increasing ROM of the affected joint until full ROM is attained
• return to occupational and leisure activities.

9. An effective rehabilitation plan requires input from the doctor, physical therapist, occupational therapist, and professionals from other appropriate disciplines to maximize the patient's rehabilitation potential.

10. Identify, with the patient, the specific methods that will be used to implement the plan.

10. For a rehabilitation program to be successful, the patient must agree to the plan and be able to describe its implementation.

11. Additional individualized interventions: _____

11. Rationales: _____

Target outcome criteria
By the time of discharge, the patient will:
• maintain mobility of unaffected joints equal to or greater than preoperative level
• perform self-care activities at or above the preoperative level
• verbalize an understanding of the rehabilitation plan.

By the time of discharge, the patient with a hip replacement will:
• walk with an assistive device and partial weight bearing on the affected side, as tolerated
• observe ROM restrictions — flexion of the affected joint limited to 90 degrees during the rehabilitation phase.

By the time of discharge, the patient with a knee replacement will:
• ambulate with an assistive device and light weight bearing, as tolerated
• wear a knee immobilizer until independent straight leg-raising is demonstrated.

Nursing diagnosis: *Impaired skin integrity related to surgery*

NURSING PRIORITIES: (a) Promote wound healing and (b) prevent infection.

Interventions

1. Maintain the patency of the drainage device, as previously described. Avoid contaminating the drainage port when emptying the device.

Rationales

1. Adequate suction with a self-controlled vacuum must be maintained to prevent blood collection in the joint — an excellent medium for bacterial growth. Contamination of the device may lead to wound infection.

2. Do not administer injections in the affected extremity. Teach the patient to take precautions to minimize the risk of injury.

3. Assess daily for signs of infection: fever, chills, purulent drainage, incisional swelling, redness, and increasing tenderness. Teach the patient which signs and symptoms to report.

4. Additional individualized interventions: _____

_____

2. Any break in the skin may predispose the patient to infection.

3. Infection is devastating to a patient with total joint replacement because the joint cannot be saved once infection and prosthetic loss occur.

4. Rationales: _____

_____

Target outcome criteria

By the time of discharge, the patient will:
• exhibit no bleeding
• exhibit no signs of infection
• exhibit warm and dry skin
• exhibit wound healing
• list signs and symptoms to report.

Discharge planning

NURSING DISCHARGE CRITERIA

Upon the patient's discharge, documentation shows evidence of:
• absence of fever
• vital signs within acceptable limits
• absence of signs and symptoms of infection at the incision
• absence of contractures or skin breakdown
• administration of oral anticoagulant medication for at least the previous 48 to 72 hours and partial thromboplastin time within acceptable parameters
• ability to control pain using oral medications
• absence of bowel or bladder dysfunction
• absence of pulmonary or cardiovascular complications
• ability to perform ADLs independently or with minimal assistance
• adherence to hip flexion and adduction restrictions when transferring and ambulating
• adherence to weight-bearing restrictions when transferring or ambulating
• ability to transfer and ambulate independently or with minimal assistance, using appropriate assistive devices
• ability to tolerate adequate nutritional intake
• absence of signs and symptoms of prosthesis dislocation
• adequate home support system or referral to home care or nursing home if indicated by an inadequate home support system; inability to perform ADLs, transfers, and ambulation independently; or inability to adhere to flexion or weight-bearing restrictions
• demonstration of maximum hospital rehabilitation benefit.

Additional information: One of the peer review organization criteria used when reviewing total joint replacement is whether the patient received maximum hospital benefit. The major criteria are whether the patient had a physical therapy evaluation and whether discharge planning was appropriate. The discharge would be deemed premature if a rehabilitation program had not been designed and if the patient showed evidence of medical instability.

Discharge planning for a patient who undergoes total hip or knee replacement should include automatic referral to the social services department. Most patients cannot function at their usual level after this procedure, especially if it is bilateral. Documentation should indicate plans for long-term rehabilitation. The nurse is not necessarily responsible for this documentation; the physical therapist, occupational therapist, or discharge planner–social worker may provide it.

After discharge, many patients are eligible for care in a nursing home or ECF until they can ambulate 50′ to 80′ (15 to 24 m) independently or with minimal assistance. Because the discharge plan commonly includes early discharge with transfer to an ECF, early referral to the social services department is essential to allow adequate time to find an opening at an appropriate facility.

PATIENT-FAMILY TEACHING CHECKLIST

Document evidence that the patient and family demonstrate an understanding of:
___ implications of joint replacement
___ rationale for continued use of antiembolism stockings

___ all discharge medications' purpose, dosage, administration schedule, and adverse effects requiring medical attention (discharge medications typically include analgesics, antibiotics, anti-inflammatories, and anticoagulants)

___ need for laboratory and medical follow-up if discharged on warfarin

___ schedule for progressive ambulation and weight bearing

___ additional activity restrictions

___ signs and symptoms of infection, bleeding, and dislocation

___ use of self-help devices, such as a raised toilet seat

___ appropriate resources for posthospitalization care

___ diet to promote healing

___ wound care

___ date, time, and location of follow-up appointments

___ how to contact the doctor.

DOCUMENTATION CHECKLIST
Using outcome criteria as a guide, document:

___ clinical status on admission

___ significant changes in status

___ preoperative and postoperative teaching

___ position of affected extremity

___ exercises and ROM achieved

___ neurovascular checks

___ calf pain

___ wound drainage

___ progressive ambulation

___ pain relief measures

___ patient-family teaching

___ discharge planning and referrals

___ presence or absence of disabling fatigue

___ nutritional intake.

ASSOCIATED PLANS OF CARE
Ineffective Individual Coping
Knowledge Deficit
Pain
Surgical Intervention

References

Beare, P., and Myers, J. *Principles and Practice of Adult Health Nursing.* St. Louis: C.V. Mosby Co., 1990.

Carpenito, L. *Nursing Diagnosis: Application to Clinical Practice,* 4th ed. Philadelphia: J.B. Lippincott Co., 1992.

Gordon, M. *Nursing Diagnosis: Process and Application,* 2nd ed. New York: McGraw-Hill Book Co., 1987.

Luckman, J., and Sorenson, K.C. *Medical-Surgical Nursing.* Philadelphia: W.B. Saunders Co., 1987.

Phipps, W., et al. *Medical-Surgical Nursing: Concepts and Clinical Practice,* 4th ed. St. Louis: Mosby-Year Book, 1991.

Thompson, J., et al. *Mosby's Manual of Clinical Nursing,* 2nd ed. St. Louis: C.V. Mosby Co., 1989.

Ziegler, Shirley, et al. *Nursing Process, Nursing Diagnosis, and Nursing Knowledge.* East Norwalk, Conn.: Appleton & Lange, 1986.

Diabetes Mellitus

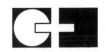

DRG information
DRG 294 Diabetes. Age 35 + .
    Mean LOS = 5.9 days
DRG 295 Diabetes. Ages 0 to 35.
    Mean LOS = 4.4 days
    Principal diagnoses for DRGs 294 and 295
    include:
    • diabetes mellitus (DM) without complica-
    tion
    • DM with coma
    • DM with ketoacidosis
    • DM with other manifestations
    • DM with unspecified complications
    • glycosuria.

Introduction
DEFINITION AND TIME FOCUS
DM is a chronic metabolic disorder in which an absolute or relative lack of endogenous insulin causes abnormal metabolism of carbohydrates, proteins, and
fats. The clinical hallmark of diabetes is hyperglycemia. Altered glucose metabolism provokes a pattern of
associated acute and chronic complications. This plan
focuses on the two most common types of diabetes,
Type I (insulin-dependent DM) and Type II (non-insulin-dependent DM), their diagnosis, and initiation of a
treatment and management regimen.
    Note: Although Type II is commonly called non-
insulin-dependent DM, these patients may require insulin as part of their management plan, either initially
or later in the course of the disease.

ETIOLOGY AND PRECIPITATING FACTORS
Type I (10% to 15% of cases; primary defect is inadequate or absent insulin production)
• genetic predisposition, probably related to genes of
human leukocyte antigen affecting immune system
• destruction of beta (insulin-producing) cells in pancreas, possibly related to the body's autoimmune response
• islet-cell antibodies
• viral infections
Type II (approximately 80% to 90% of cases; primary
defect is inadequate insulin production and insulin resistance)
• genetic predisposition, not yet as clearly implicated
as in Type I, leading to diminished endogenous insulin
secretion and action
• obesity (in 80% to 90% of patients at diagnosis)
• sedentary life-style
• possibly other environmental factors

Focused assessment guidelines
NURSING HISTORY (Functional health pattern findings)
Note: Type I DM is commonly diagnosed when the patient presents in diabetic ketoacidosis (DKA); Type II
is commonly diagnosed on routine examination or
when the patient seeks treatment for one of the many
associated symptoms. Many medications may be associated with impaired glucose tolerance, including steroids, some diuretics, oral contraceptives, anticonvulsants, and psychoactive medications. The doctor who
suspects diabetes should ensure that medication-related factors are identified and ruled out before making the diagnosis.

Health perception—health management pattern
Type I
• family history of diabetes
• weight loss
• usually under age 30
• acute onset of symptoms (flulike syndrome)
Type II
• family history of diabetes
• usually overweight
• usually over age 40
• gradual onset of symptoms
• may complain of multiple minor symptoms

Nutritional-metabolic pattern
Type I
• increased thirst (polydipsia)
• increased appetite (polyphagia)
• ketosis
• nausea (occasionally)
Type II
• may have polydipsia and polyphagia
• may give history of diet high in refined carbohydrates and calories

Elimination pattern
Type I
• typically complains of polyuria
• may have constipation or diarrhea
Type II
• typically complains of nocturia
• may complain of polyuria
• may have constipation or diarrhea
• may be taking diuretics for another condition

Activity-exercise pattern
Type I
- may complain of sudden weakness
- may complain of increased fatigue or sleepiness

Type II
- may complain of gradually increasing weakness and fatigability
- may give history of lack of regular exercise

Sleep-rest pattern
Type I
- sleep disturbance related to nocturia

Type II
- may complain of nocturia
- may complain of drowsiness after meals

Cognitive-perceptual pattern
Type I
- may report dizziness or orthostatic hypotension
- may complain of abdominal pain

Type II
- may complain of pruritus, acute or recurrent urinary tract infections (UTIs), or recurrent vaginitis
- may report poorly healing skin infections
- may complain of myopia or blurred vision
- may complain of muscle cramping
- may complain of abdominal pain
- may complain of numbness, pain, or tingling in extremities

PHYSICAL FINDINGS
Cardiovascular
- tachycardia
- postural hypotension
- syncope

Pulmonary
- deep, rapid (Kussmaul's) respirations (in DKA)

Gastrointestinal
- abdominal distention
- decreased bowel sounds
- abdominal tenderness
- diarrhea or constipation

Integumentary
- poorly healing skin wounds
- skin infections
- warm, flushed, dry skin (in DKA)

Neurologic
- irritability
- drowsiness
- confusion
- coma (in DKA)

Genitourinary
- vaginal discharge
- vaginal infections
- perineal irritation
- impotence

DIAGNOSTIC STUDIES*
- random serum glucose test — a level greater than or equal to 200 mg/dl plus classic signs and symptoms confirms DM
- fasting serum glucose test — elevation greater than 140 mg/dl on more than one occasion confirms DM
- urinalysis — reveals glycosuria and (in Type I) ketonuria
- glucose tolerance test — confirms DM if levels are greater than or equal to 200 mg/dl for at least two sample values (at 2 hours and at one other time between 0 and 2 hours after glucose load)
- blood insulin level — Type I, absent or minimal; Type II, low, normal, or high
- plasma proinsulin level — normal to elevated in Type II
- plasma C-peptide level — Type I, absent; Type II, normal to elevated
- arterial blood gas levels — may reveal metabolic acidosis, particularly common in Type I, with compensatory respiratory alkalosis
- electrolyte panel — may be normal or may reveal hyponatremia or hyperkalemia associated with dehydration or DKA (Type I); needed to establish baseline
- blood urea nitrogen level — may be normal or elevated (in DKA or in presence of renal involvement)
- thyroid function studies — may be ordered to rule out coexisting thyroid dysfunction, which could increase need for insulin and contribute to hyperglycemia (thyroid disorders more common in Type I)
- electrocardiography — commonly ordered to establish baseline and to rule out underlying cardiac disorders
- chest X-ray — needed to establish baseline

POTENTIAL COMPLICATIONS
- coma related to DKA, hypoglycemia, or hyperosmolar hyperglycemic nonketotic syndrome (HHNKS)
- renal failure (nephropathy)
- conditions related to degenerative vascular disease: accelerated atherosclerosis, cerebrovascular accident, myocardial infarction, thrombophlebitis, peripheral vascular disease
- retinopathy, blindness, or cataracts
- neuropathies, autonomic and especially peripheral
- microangiopathies

---

*Laboratory values listed apply to nonpregnant adults; for values in children and pregnant women, see Kneisl and Ames (1986).

Collaborative problem: *Hyperglycemia related to inadequate endogenous insulin (Type I DM) or inadequate endogenous insulin and insulin resistance (Type II DM)*

NURSING PRIORITY: Prevent or minimize complications when establishing treatment regimen to control altered glucose metabolism.

Interventions

1. Administer insulin (I.V., I.M., or subcutaneously [S.C.]) or oral hypoglycemics.

• Monitor fingerstick blood glucose levels according to unit protocol, typically every 6 hours. Always check the blood glucose level before giving hypoglycemic medications. Follow established protocol for withholding the dose based on normal values. Also monitor urine ketone levels according to protocol.

• Be aware of differences in peak action and duration of action for various hypoglycemic medications:

—Rapid-acting insulins (Regular, Semilente) peak between 2 and 6 hours; intermediate-acting insulins (NPH, Lente) peak between 6 and 12 hours; long-acting insulins (Ultralente, PZI) peak between 10 and 30 hours; and other human and semisynthetic insulins peak between 2 and 15 hours.

—Oral hypoglycemics peak on the average between 3 and 4 hours.

2. Establish and maintain an I.V. fluid infusion (usually normal saline solution). Monitor for dry mucous membranes, poor skin turgor, cracked lips, abdominal pain, elevated urine specific gravity, elevated hematocrit, and other signs of dehydration. Keep an accurate intake and output record. Document daily weight.

Rationales

1. Insulin increases cellular glucose uptake and decreases gluconeogenesis. Exogenous insulin is essential for controlling Type I DM and may also be used in Type II DM. In initial treatment of Type I or II, especially if DKA is present, I.V. infusion of regular insulin may be ordered concurrently with aggressive fluid replacement. The I.V. route is preferred because it offers the fastest absorption rate, but too-rapid lowering of blood glucose without adequate fluid replacement may cause vascular collapse or cerebral edema. Alternatively, the slower-acting I.M. route may be used. Circulatory insufficiency can make insulin uptake from S.C. sites unpredictable; however, it is the route of choice for ongoing therapy. Oral hypoglycemics are indicated only in Type II DM because their effectiveness depends on endogenous insulin.

• In the initial diagnosis and treatment of DM, frequent assessment of glucose levels is essential for monitoring the patient's response. Checking the glucose level and withholding the dose if the level is acceptable prevents medication-induced hypoglycemia. Protocols for withholding doses vary depending on the hypoglycemic ordered and patient status. Urine ketones assist in monitoring the body's use of fats for energy (usually occurs with inadequate insulin levels) and need for insulin therapy.

• Awareness of these characteristics helps the nurse correlate onset and duration of signs and symptoms with peaks and troughs in serum drug levels.

—Insulins differ according to onset, peak, and duration of action. The type of insulin, timing of injections, and individual response influence when a reaction is most likely to occur. With insulins given in the morning, a reaction from a short-acting insulin is most likely between breakfast and lunch; an intermediate-acting insulin, between midafternoon and dinner; and a long-acting insulin, between 2 a.m. and 7 a.m.

—Because duration of action is more prolonged with oral agents, a single daily or divided dose is usually sufficient for control. Reactions are most likely to coincide with peak action.

2. Hyperglycemia causes dehydration through hyperosmolality: Water is drawn from the cells into the vascular system and then into the urine in an attempt to maintain homeostasis. Normal saline is the preferred solution to prevent further elevation of blood glucose (and to replace sodium in DKA). Accurate intake and output documentation and daily weights are essential for assessing fluid status and for early detection of inadequate renal function. Daily weight is a gross indicator of general fluid and nutritional status.

ENDOCRINE DISORDERS

3. Observe for signs of medication-induced hypoglycemia: pallor, confusion, diaphoresis, headache, weakness, shallow respirations, irritability, and restlessness or stupor. Reactions are most likely to coincide with peak insulin effect or late or missed meals, depending on the type of insulin and the patient's response. If a reaction occurs, notify the doctor, measure blood glucose level, and treat immediately with I.V. glucose, glucagon, or oral glucose, depending upon protocol and the patient's responsiveness. Once the patient is stable, use the episode as an example for teaching.

4. Observe for signs of DKA (in Type I DM only):
• early—nausea; fatigue; polyuria; dry, flushed skin; dry mucous membranes; thirst; and tachycardia
• late—vomiting, poor skin turgor, lethargy, Kussmaul's respirations, acetone breath, hypotension, and abdominal pain.
    If the patient's condition suggests DKA, notify the doctor immediately. Obtain a blood glucose level (usually 300 to 800 mg/dl), and check urine ketones (typically positive). Treat according to protocol (usually rapid hypotonic or isotonic I.V. fluid replacement, I.V. insulin, and—as hyperglycemia and dehydration resolve—potassium replacement; ensure that the patient has had some urine output before adding potassium to I.V. fluids). Once the patient is stable, use the episode as an example for teaching. See the "Diabetic Ketoacidosis" plan, page 531, for details.

5. Observe for signs of HHNKS (in Type II DM): lethargy or stupor, fatigue, drowsiness, confusion, coma, seizures, intense thirst, and very dry mucous membranes. If the patient's condition suggests HHNKS, notify the doctor immediately. Obtain a blood glucose level (typically over 800 mg/dl), check urine ketones (usually negative), and obtain a serum osmolality level, as ordered (characteristically over 350 mOsm/kg). Treat according to protocol, typically vigorous hypotonic fluid replacement, low-dose insulin, and potassium repletion. Once the patient is stable, use the episode as an example for teaching. Refer to the "Hyperosmolar Hyperglycemic Nonketotic Syndrome" plan, page 539, for further details.

6. Additional individualized interventions: _____

3. Insulin reactions can occur with relative suddenness. If the newly diagnosed diabetic patient is unaware of the symptoms' significance and does not seek treatment, a hypoglycemic reaction may be life-threatening.

4. Inadequate pharmacologic control, increased dietary intake, infection, stress, or the interaction of other factors may cause DKA in Type I DM. Hyperglycemia causes osmotic diuresis, which provokes compensatory mechanisms to maintain blood volume and pressure. In DKA, incomplete breakdown of fatty acids leads to accumulation of ketones in the bloodstream in addition to high (unusable) glucose levels. This leads to a state of metabolic acidosis, usually with a compensatory respiratory alkalosis. I.V. fluids correct dehydration and insulin facilitates glucose metabolism. As hyperglycemia and dehydration resolve, potassium shifting from the plasma back into the cells may unmask hypokalemia related to urinary potassium loss. The "Diabetic Ketoacidosis" plan contains comprehensive information on managing this complication.

5. HHNKS, a complication that occurs over days to weeks, develops most commonly in the older and infirm Type II diabetic patient who does not recognize (or does not react to) fluid loss. It usually is caused by infection or massive fluid loss. The pathophysiology includes severe hyperglycemia and profound dehydration in the absence of ketosis. Perhaps because of pancreatic exhaustion, not enough insulin is produced to metabolize glucose, so glucose accumulates. However, enough insulin is produced to prevent adipose tissue breakdown, so ketosis does not occur. Blood glucose and osmolality levels are much more elevated in HHNKS than in DKA.
    Hypotonic fluids help reverse high serum osmolality; vigorous replacement is necessary because of the extent of dehydration. The patient with HHNKS may be more sensitive to insulin than the patient with DKA. Urinary potassium loss may require earlier replacement in HHNKS than in DKA. The "Hyperosmolar Hyperglycemic Nonketotic Syndrome" plan contains detailed guidance on managing this complication.

6. Rationales: _____

Target outcome criteria
Within 2 hours of admission, the patient will:
• have an improved blood glucose level
• be awake and alert
• present vital signs within normal limits.

Within 24 to 48 hours of admission, the patient will:
• show no signs of dehydration
• have controlled blood glucose levels
• have no hypoglycemia, or have promptly treated hypoglycemic episodes with no associated complications
• have no ketones in urine (if recovering from DKA).

Nursing diagnosis: *Knowledge deficit related to newly diagnosed complex chronic disease*

NURSING PRIORITY: Coordinate self-care teaching with establishment of a diabetes control regimen.

Interventions

1. See the "Knowledge Deficit" plan, page 56.

2. Emphasize that DM control involves coordinating many aspects of daily living with prescribed interventions. Teach the significance of insulin or oral hypoglycemics for disease control. Demonstrate injection techniques, and observe patient performance. Rotate sites for S.C. injections every 7 to 10 days (abdominal sites are preferred over arms or legs). Document site rotation. Link medication needs to other factors, such as diet and exercise. Ensure that the patient and family are aware of signs and treatment of hypoglycemia as well as the protocol for managing persistent hyperglycemia, DKA (for Type I DM), and HHNKS (for Type II DM). Involve family members in all teaching. Use the patient's symptomatic episodes as teaching tools. Where possible, link changes in habits to the prevention of complications.

3. Involve the patient, family, and dietitian in planning a therapeutic diet. Reinforce nutritional guidelines. Encourage supervised weight loss if the patient is overweight. Ensure the patient has written exchange lists and diet guidelines before discharge. Provide referral for further questions and special situations (such as "sick day" management, pregnancy, dining out, exercise, use of alcohol, or complications).

4. For Type I DM only, teach blood glucose and urine ketone testing methods for home use. Observe patient demonstrations for accuracy of testing, interpretation of results, and documentation. Provide target glucose ranges. Be aware that the patient may think "the lower the better" regarding blood glucose; ensure that the patient understands the body's need for glucose in regulated amounts. Encourage the patient to keep a daily record of glucose monitoring. At least annually, evaluate the patient's technique and provide revised target glucose ranges, if necessary.

5. Emphasize the importance of regular activity and exercise and of maintaining the same level of activity from day to day.

6. Teach or review "sick day" management techniques: testing blood glucose and urine ketones more often, increasing fluids, continuing to take diabetes medication, contacting the doctor early in illness, and postponing exercise.

Rationales

1. This plan provides guidelines for patient teaching.

2. Patient understanding is essential for home management of DM. A patient may mistakenly believe that attention to a single factor (for example, medication) will control the disorder. Compliance may increase if the patient links control with personal preventive efforts. Observing the patient's injection technique and providing opportunities for supervised practice help ensure accuracy. Rotating injection sites (after using same site for 7 to 10 days) minimizes lipodystrophy and helps prevent scar tissue formation; documentation serves as a reminder. Insulin absorption is fastest from abdominal sites (followed by arm sites, then leg sites) and abdominal sites are minimally affected by exercise. The need for medication increases with stress, infection, and higher caloric intake but may decrease with excessive activity, decreased caloric intake, or vomiting. Awareness of hyperglycemia and hypoglycemia (signs and symptoms, possible causes, treatment, and prevention) decreases patient anxiety and increases self-control; using the patient's personal experiences as teaching tools helps the patient identify and recognize personal responses to the disease.

3. Involving the patient and family with dietary planning helps ensure compliance at home. Diet is specific for each patient. For the patient with Type II DM, diet alone or diet with weight loss may be sufficient to control hyperglycemia. Written materials help minimize misunderstanding. Referral ensures an ongoing source of dietary information. The registered dietitian is an important member of the health care team and the best professional to provide nutrition counseling. The nurse's role typically is to provide reinforcement and support.

4. Successful home management of DM requires that the patient perform self-monitoring to ensure that the prescribed regimen of medication, diet, and exercise remains appropriate to needs. Stressors (or disease progression) may change body requirements; blood and urine testing alerts the patient to such changes and helps avert complications. Misconceptions about the disease may have disastrous consequences. Keeping a record of glucose levels helps identify trends. Periodic evaluation helps detect errors in the testing methods and ensures that target glucose ranges reflect the patient's current needs.

5. Exercise stimulates carbohydrate metabolism, lowers blood pressure, aids in weight control, and may help avert or minimize circulatory complications by increasing levels of high-density lipoproteins. Increases or decreases in activity may necessitate dietary or medication changes.

6. Unless managed carefully, even minor illnesses can quickly lead to such diabetic emergencies as hyperglycemia, hypoglycemia, DKA, or HHNKS.

ENDOCRINE DISORDERS

7. Tell the patient to be aware of increased susceptibility to infections; discuss ways to avoid exposure. Review signs of infection: redness, swelling, exudate, and fever. Emphasize the importance of prompt, appropriate treatment of even minor injuries to avoid serious complications.

7. A compromised state of health may make the diabetic patient more susceptible to some infections; also, healing may be impaired or prolonged because of associated vascular insufficiency. Awareness of signs of infection may help ensure prompt treatment. Because of impaired healing from DM, even minor cuts or scratches may develop into gangrenous lesions. Infection also affects medication and dietary needs.

8. Discuss ways to prevent the vascular complications of DM:

8. DM is characterized by degenerative vascular changes that predispose the patient to infections, ulcerations, and gangrene, particularly of the legs and feet.

• Teach the patient how to perform foot care, skin care, leg exercises, and to assess circulatory status; observe return demonstration of all techniques. If the patient smokes, emphasize the importance of quitting. Ensure that the patient and family receive a written foot care plan.

• Careful skin care may help avert serious problems. Leg exercises may help develop collateral circulation and promote venous return. Nicotine causes vasoconstriction and contributes to circulatory impairment; additionally, smoking greatly increases the risk of significant heart disease. Written instructions help ensure full compliance.

• Discuss potential eye complications of DM. Help the patient understand the significance of careful disease control (especially glucose and blood pressure) in preventing or slowing diabetic retinopathy. Emphasize the importance of early reporting of vision changes and annual ophthalmologic evaluation.

• The retina consumes oxygen at a higher rate than other body tissues; thus, it is sensitive to the effects of vascular degeneration (microangiopathy) associated with DM. These effects may eventually lead to retinopathy, retinal detachment, and blindness. Although some treatment is available, the most effective deterrent to blindness is careful disease control. Early reporting of vision changes may permit palliative treatment.

• Teach the symptoms of UTI and renal impairment — flank pain, fever, dysuria, pyuria, frequency, urgency, and oliguria — and emphasize the importance of prompt treatment. Emphasize the importance of an annual kidney function evaluation (24-hour urine collection for protein and creatinine). Help the patient understand the importance of glucose and blood pressure control in preventing nephropathy.

• Glycosuria predisposes the patient to UTIs; recurrent severe UTIs or pyelonephritis may increase the likelihood of renal failure. Nephropathy is a long-term complication related to vascular changes in the small vessels of the glomerulus. Proteinuria is the hallmark of changes in renal function.

9. Discuss the implications of diabetic neuropathy (autonomic and peripheral). Explain peripheral symptoms, such as paresthesias, pain, and sensory loss. Emphasize the importance of foot care. Instruct the patient and family to report urine retention or incontinence, orthostatic hypotension, decreased perspiration, diarrhea, or impotence.

9. Gradual degeneration of peripheral nerves may cause paresthesias and pain, followed by loss of sensation, particularly in the legs and feet; the patient may thus be unaware of injuries. The signs listed may indicate autonomic nerve dysfunction; if so, the patient may not exhibit the usual signs of hypoglycemia.

10. Additional individualized interventions: _____

10. Rationales: _____

Target outcome criteria
Within 48 hours of diagnosis, the patient will:
• initiate diet planning with dietitian
• observe and practice injection technique (if insulin is ordered)
• practice blood glucose and urine ketone testing (Type I DM only).

By the time of discharge, the patient will:
• demonstrate proficiency in injection technique
• produce evidence of site rotation documentation
• discuss disease management in relation to medication, diet, exercise, and stress
• demonstrate proper foot care
• discuss hypoglycemia and appropriate treatment
• discuss hyperglycemia and appropriate treatment
• plan adequate diet for 3-day period
• perform and interpret blood glucose and urine ketone tests accurately.

Nursing diagnosis: *High risk for altered health maintenance related to lack of material resources, lack of support, or ineffective coping*

NURSING PRIORITY: Optimize health maintenance.

Interventions

1. Assess the patient's resources, including financial management capabilities and family support system.

2. Involve the family in all teaching and planning.

3. Arrange appropriate follow-up home health visits before the patient's discharge.

4. Link the patient and family with community resources and mutual support groups.

5. Encourage verbalization of feelings, and support healthy coping behaviors. See the "Ineffective Individual Coping" plan, page 51.

6. Additional individualized interventions: _____

Rationales

1. Independent home management of DM requires the ability to organize activities in a relatively stable setting. Patients are commonly admitted to the hospital "out of control" because of poor financial management and lack of a support system.

2. Family members may help reinforce teaching and encourage compliance.

3. Transferring new knowledge and skills for disease management from the hospital to the home may be difficult. Home visits allow assessment of environmental factors that may contribute to noncompliance.

4. Diagnosis of DM commonly involves major patient reeducation and life-style changes. Community or mutual support groups can offer ongoing education and support. Because hospitalization for DM is less frequent than in the past, or of short duration, outpatient diabetes education programs are essential.

5. As with the diagnosis of any serious chronic disease, the patient with DM may experience denial, anger, grief, and other emotions as part of a normal response. Expression of feelings is a necessary prelude to acceptance of the disease and active, responsible management. Supporting healthy coping behaviors helps maintain the patient's independence and sense of self-control—both essential for compliance. The "Ineffective Individual Coping" plan contains detailed interventions related to this problem.

6. Rationales: _____

Target outcome criteria

By the time of discharge, the patient will:
• verbalize understanding of need for life-style changes
• ask appropriate questions
• verbalize feelings about diagnosis
• participate actively in disease control planning

• have resource deficits resolved or appropriate referrals completed
• have a home visit or outpatient follow-up appointments scheduled.

ENDOCRINE DISORDERS

Discharge planning

NURSING DISCHARGE CRITERIA

Upon the patient's discharge, documentation shows evidence of:
- blood glucose level less than 200 mg/dl
- ability to manage medication administration
- ability to understand and follow dietary regimen
- ability to follow and perform exercise regimen
- ability to perform foot and skin care
- ability to perform and interpret results of blood glucose and urine ketone testing (Type I DM only)
- adequate home support system
- referral to home care or outpatient services for reinforcement of teaching or if home support is unavailable*
- no signs of infection
- stable vital signs
- ability to describe emergency measures for managing hyperglycemia and hypoglycemia.

PATIENT-FAMILY TEACHING CHECKLIST

Document evidence that the patient and family demonstrate an understanding of:
___ disease and implications
___ for all medications: purpose, dosage, administration schedule, and adverse effects requiring medical attention (usual discharge medications include insulin or oral hypoglycemics)
___ blood glucose and urine ketone testing (Type I DM only)
___ interrelationship of diet, exercise, and other factors in disease management
___ hypoglycemia (signs and symptoms, possible causes, treatment, and prevention)
___ hyperglycemia (signs and symptoms, possible causes, treatment, and prevention)
___ diet management
___ exercise regimen
___ foot care
___ signs of infection and appropriate treatment
___ signs and implications of neuropathy
___ symptoms of retinopathy and need to report them
___ signs and symptoms of urinary and renal complications and need to report them
___ community resources
___ when and how to access emergency medical treatment
___ date, time, and location of follow-up appointments
___ how to contact the doctor
___ written materials, insulin, and syringes, as provided.

DOCUMENTATION CHECKLIST

Using outcome criteria as a guide, document:
___ clinical status on admission
___ significant changes in status
___ pertinent laboratory and diagnostic test findings
___ episodes of hyperglycemia and hypoglycemia
___ dietary intake and planning
___ activity and exercise regimen
___ medication therapy
___ I.V. line patency
___ patient-family teaching
___ discharge planning and availability of community resources.

ASSOCIATED PLANS OF CARE

Chronic Renal Failure
Diabetic Ketoacidosis
Grieving
Hyperosmolar Hyperglycemic Nonketotic Syndrome
Hypoglycemia
Ineffective Individual Coping
Knowledge Deficit
Retinal Detachment
Thrombophlebitis

References

Galloway, J., et al., eds. *Diabetes Mellitus,* 9th ed. Indianapolis: Eli Lilly and Co., 1988.

Guthrie, D., ed. *Diabetes Education: A Core Curriculum for Health Professionals.* Chicago: American Association of Diabetes Educators, 1988.

Kneisl, C., and Ames, S. *Adult Health Nursing: A Biopsychosocial Approach.* Reading, Mass.: Addison-Wesley Publishing Co., 1986.

Luckmann, J., and Sorensen, K. *Medical-Surgical Nursing: A Psychophysiologic Approach,* 3rd ed. Philadelphia: W.B. Saunders Co., 1987.

Milchvich, S., and Dunn-Long, B. *Diabetes Mellitus: A Practical Handbook,* 5th ed. Palo Alto: Bull Publishing Co., 1990.

Rorden, J. *Nurses as Health Teachers: A Practical Guide.* Philadelphia: W.B. Saunders Co., 1987.

Thompson, J., et al. *Manual of Clinical Nursing,* 2nd ed. St. Louis: C.V. Mosby Co., 1989.

---

*Because patients with DM are rarely admitted to the hospital unless the disease is out of control or is causing complications, always consider a referral to home care or an outpatient or community diabetes program to reinforce hospital teaching and to allow further observation.

Diabetic Ketoacidosis

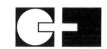

DRG information
DRG 294 Diabetes. Age 35 + .
     Mean LOS = 5.9 days
DRG 295 Diabetes. Age 0 to 35.
     Mean LOS = 4.4 days

Introduction
DEFINITION AND TIME FOCUS
Diabetic ketoacidosis (DKA) is a life-threatening endocrine emergency in which an acute or absolute insulin deficiency produces metabolic acidosis. Clinical hallmarks include hyperglycemia, dehydration, ketosis, and electrolyte imbalance. DKA is most commonly seen in Type I (insulin-dependent) diabetes and may be present at the time of diagnosis.

Diabetes mellitus (DM), the disease of insulin deficiency, alters the metabolism of carbohydrates, fats, and proteins, resulting in various physiologic derangements that may become life-threatening. Insulin, an anabolic hormone secreted by pancreatic islet cells, facilitates glucose transport across cell membranes. It thus promotes glucose uptake, metabolism, and storage (as glycogen). Insulin also promotes fatty acid synthesis and amino acid transport while inhibiting excessive breakdown of fats and proteins. In Type I DM, the basic defect is thought to be inadequate or absent insulin secretion, while in Type II (non-insulin-dependent) DM, inadequate insulin secretion or insulin resistance or both are thought to be responsible.

This plan focuses on the critically ill diabetic patient admitted with ketoacidosis.

ETIOLOGY AND PRECIPITATING FACTORS
• usually occurs only in Type I DM
• mortality rate reported at 3% to 12%
• most common causes include newly diagnosed Type I DM, incorrect exogenous insulin dosage (omitted or decreased), and stressful states (such as acute illness, infection, myocardial infarction, or trauma)
• occasionally, no cause is identified

Focused assessment guidelines
NURSING HISTORY (Functional health pattern findings)

Health perception — health management pattern
• newly diagnosed or known history of Type I DM
• in known Type I DM, insulin, diet, and exercise used to control blood glucose level
• onset of symptoms usually over hours to days
• family history of diabetes uncommon

Nutritional-metabolic pattern
• may complain of anorexia, nausea, abdominal pain, and vomiting
• reports or displays increased thirst (polydipsia)
• reports or displays increased hunger (polyphagia)
• may report weight loss

Elimination pattern
• commonly complains of excessive urination (polyuria) and nighttime urination (nocturia)
• may have diarrhea or constipation

Activity-exercise pattern
• may complain of weakness, fatigue, or lethargy

Sleep-rest pattern
• may report disturbed sleep (from nocturia)

Cognitive-perceptual pattern
• may report or display dizziness or confusion
• may have blurred vision
• may complain of abdominal pain or cramps

PHYSICAL FINDINGS
Cardiovascular
• postural (orthostatic) hypotension
• weak, rapid pulse
• low to normal blood pressure
• hyperthermia
• capillary refill time greater than 3 seconds

Pulmonary
• deep, rapid (Kussmaul's) respirations
• ketotic, acetone breath odor
• dyspnea, tachypnea

Gastrointestinal
• abdominal distention
• decreased bowel sounds
• abdominal tenderness or pain (may mimic acute appendicitis)
• dry mucous membranes

Integumentary
• dry skin and mucous membranes
• warm, flushed skin, especially on face
• poor or decreased skin turgor
• sunken or soft eyes
• may have skin infections or poorly healing skin wounds

Neurologic

- lethargy, stupor, or coma
- fatigue, drowsiness, disorientation, or confusion
- seizures
- normal, decreased, or absent reflexes

Genitourinary

- polyuria initially; oliguria and anuria may follow
- may have underlying renal involvement (in chronic Type I DM)

Musculoskeletal

- weakness
- decreased or absent deep tendon reflexes

DIAGNOSTIC STUDIES

- serum glucose—elevated (300 to 800 mg/dl or higher)
- arterial blood gas (ABG) levels—may reveal mild to severe metabolic acidosis with respiratory compensation (pH less than 7.35 and bicarbonate less than 10 mEq/liter)
- electrolyte panel—levels may be low, normal, or elevated depending on severity of dehydration and DKA; hyponatremia and hyperkalemia common
- blood urea nitrogen and creatinine—may be normal or elevated depending on severity of dehydration and DKA and presence of underlying renal disease

- serum amylase—rules out pancreatitis
- osmolality—usually less than 350 mOsm/kg
- complete blood count and white blood cell count—may be elevated in presence of infection; hemoglobin and hematocrit may be elevated secondary to dehydration
- ketones—positive in urine and serum
- electrocardiography—used to rule out myocardial infarction; T wave abnormalities seen with hyperkalemia
- chest X-ray—rules out infection
- anion gap $(Na + K) - (Cl + CO_2)$—elevated, usually over 12 mEq/liter, indicating excessive metabolic acid production
- cardiac enzymes—rule out myocardial infarction
- blood, urine, sputum cultures—detect infection's source

POTENTIAL COMPLICATIONS*

- coma and death if DKA untreated
- fluid overload
- hypoglycemia if DKA overtreated
- hypovolemic shock

Collaborative problem: *Hypovolemia related to osmotic diuresis or vomiting, or both*

NURSING PRIORITY: Restore fluid volume rapidly.

Interventions

1. Monitor for signs and symptoms of dehydration and shock, such as tachycardia; hypotension; weak peripheral pulses; capillary refill time greater than 3 seconds; warm, dry, flushed skin; poor skin turgor; and polyuria or oliguria. Continuously monitor blood pressure and cardiac rate and rhythm.

Rationales

1. In DKA, the blood glucose level is elevated because of decreased cellular uptake and use of glucose. The resulting hyperglycemia increases serum osmolality and triggers a fluid shift from the intracellular to the extracellular space, producing intracellular dehydration. Compensatory renal glucose spillage, a powerful control mechanism to prevent excessive hyperglycemia, produces intense, obligatory osmotic diuresis resulting in extracellular dehydration. Eventually, severe dehydration decreases glomerular filtration. The resulting oliguria aggravates hyperglycemia and hyperosmolality. Signs and symptoms indicate the severity of the deficit and the adequacy of fluid replacement. As volume is restored, signs and symptoms should gradually resolve; failure to do so indicates inadequate fluid replacement or continuing fluid losses.

---

*Keep in mind that long-term complications of DM (such as retinopathy, neuropathy, nephropathy, cardiovascular disease, and peripheral vascular disease) will influence nursing interventions and treatment strategies.

2. Observe for signs and symptoms of electrolyte imbalances (see Appendix C, "Fluid and Electrolyte Imbalances," for details):
• hyperkalemia in the first 1 to 4 hours of treatment

• hypokalemia after 1 to 4 hours of treatment

• hyponatremia early in treatment

• hypernatremia later in treatment

• anion gap greater than 12.

3. Monitor serum osmolality and electrolyte values, as ordered. Report abnormal values to the doctor.

4. On admission, establish and maintain one or more I.V. lines in large peripheral veins.

5. Monitor intake and output (I&O) and urine specific gravity meticulously. Weigh the patient daily, and document findings. Insert an indwelling urinary (Foley) catheter, as ordered.

6. Administer I.V. solutions, as ordered. Replacement may include 4 to 9 liters in the first 24 hours, typically:

• normal saline solution, 1 to 2 liters in the first 2 hours

• 0.45% sodium chloride, after the first few hours, or 0.45% sodium chloride with 5% dextrose in water when blood glucose level reaches 250 mg/dl or urine glucose level is less than 1%

2. Electrolyte status may change rapidly, so monitor closely to identify any imbalances.

• Buffering of excess hydrogen ions released in acidosis displaces intracellular potassium into the serum.
• Renal excretion of potassium accelerates because of hyperkalemia, and the high serum level masks the resulting total body potassium deficit. As therapy reduces acidosis, potassium ions move into the cells from the serum, unmasking the underlying deficit.

• Diuresis and ketone excretion cause hyponatremia from urinary sodium losses.

• As metabolic control is restored, the kidneys begin to conserve sodium. This sodium retention, added to sodium administration in I.V. fluids, may produce hypernatremia.

• Anion gap is a laboratory calculation of the difference between unmeasured anions and cations in the blood. An elevated level indicates abnormal production of metabolic acids, including the ketone bodies produced in DKA. The normal anion gap is less than 12.

3. Laboratory values provide objective data on the type and degree of physiologic derangements present. In addition, serum osmolality values guide fluid replacement, while electrolyte values guide electrolyte repletion.

4. Dehydration is the most immediately life-threatening aspect of DKA. In addition, the body must be adequately hydrated for insulin to be effective. Large veins permit rapid administration of the large amounts of fluid necessary to reverse severe dehydration.

5. I&O, specific gravity, and weight records reflect the degree of fluid imbalance and effectiveness of therapy. Initially, output greatly exceeds intake, unless severe dehydration and oliguria are present. As the patient is rehydrated, fluid losses continue for the first several hours until glycosuria and osmotic diuresis are controlled. An indwelling catheter facilitates accurate measurement of urinary fluid loss. An indwelling catheter is rarely used in a conscious patient.

6. The selection of I.V. fluid depends on the patient's blood glucose and electrolyte levels, whereas the amount depends on the existing fluid deficit and ongoing fluid losses. The average fluid deficit on admission ranges from 4 to 9 liters. Volume repletion is essential in reversing hypovolemia and allowing continued renal glucose excretion, an important compensatory mechanism in restoring glucose levels to normal.
• Normal saline solution replaces lost volume and sodium without increasing blood glucose.
• As the serum sodium level returns to normal, the saline concentration of I.V. solutions is reduced to prevent sodium overload. A solution containing glucose may be used as the blood glucose level returns to normal to prevent hypoglycemia.

ENDOCRINE DISORDERS

• plasma volume expanders, such as albumin, if dehydration is severe (administer only after normal saline solution administration is underway).

• Usually, normal saline administration is sufficient to reverse volume depletion. Although rarely used, plasma volume expanders may be necessary in severe dehydration. If they are administered before normal saline solution, however, their hypertonicity increases cellular dehydration.

7. Administer therapy for electrolyte imbalances, as ordered.

7. Hyperkalemia, hyponatremia, and hypernatremia usually resolve with appropriate fluid administration and control of hyperglycemia. Hypokalemia usually requires I.V. administration of supplemental potassium. Do not add potassium until urine output is established. Potassium replacement usually includes potassium chloride alternated with potassium phosphate.

8. For at least 24 hours after rapid fluid repletion, observe for signs and symptoms of pulmonary edema, such as crackles, dyspnea, cough, or frothy sputum. If any are present, alert the doctor immediately.

8. Rapid fluid repletion causes hemodilution. Lowered plasma oncotic pressure may allow fluid to leak into the pulmonary interstitial space, producing pulmonary edema. Pulmonary edema requires prompt aggressive medical intervention.

9. Additional individualized interventions: _____

9. Rationales: _____

Target outcome criteria
Within 12 hours after the onset of therapy, the patient will:
• have blood pressure and cardiac rate and rhythm within normal limits
• display adequate peripheral perfusion, as manifested by strong peripheral pulses and capillary refill time less than 3 seconds.

Within 24 hours after the onset of therapy, the patient will:
• have urine output of 60 to 100 ml/hour
• have a balanced I&O
• have normal skin turgor, mucous membrane moisture, and other clinical signs of adequate hydration
• show no signs or symptoms of electrolyte imbalances
• have a normal anion gap (less than 12).

Collaborative problem: *Hyperglycemia related to decreased cellular glucose uptake and use*

NURSING PRIORITY: Restore glucose control gradually.

Interventions

1. Assess blood glucose levels on admission and as ordered. Perform bedside fingerstick monitoring of blood glucose every hour until normal, then every 6 hours; then before meals and at bedtime; or as ordered.

Rationales

1. Blood glucose levels are the most direct indicators of deranged glucose metabolism and are used to determine therapy. As glomerular filtration of glucose exceeds the transport maximum, glucose spills into the urine. Because blood glucose levels are much more accurate than urine glucose levels, bedside fingersticks are the favored monitoring method. The goal is to reduce the glucose level approximately 100 mg/dl an hour.

2. Assess blood ketone level on admission and as ordered. Perform bedside urine monitoring every void until ketone level is low, then every 6 hours or before meals and at bedtime.

2. When carbohydrate metabolism is impaired, the body uses fat as a fuel source. Lipolysis produces free fatty acids, which when oxidized produce ketone bodies. Blood ketone levels directly reflect the degree of ketogenesis. The body initially compensates by buffering ketoacids with bicarbonate. When ketoacid production exceeds buffering, ketoacids accumulate in the blood, producing acidosis. Some of the excess ketoacids are excreted in the urine (largely as sodium salts). Urine ketone levels measure ketone excretion. Urine ketones may be positive for 24 to 48 hours after DKA resolves.

3. Administer insulin, as ordered, typically a continuous I.V. infusion of regular insulin. Occasionally, boluses of regular insulin may be given by intravenous, intramuscular, or subcutaneous injection in conjunction with the I.V. infusion.

3. Exogenous insulin controls gluconeogenesis and keto-genesis and increases cellular glucose uptake. In profound dehydration, medication absorption may be erratic, so the intravenous route is most reliable (keep in mind that a small amount of insulin may bind to I.V. tubing and bottles). The optimal dose and type of I.V. administration are controversial. High-dose insulin therapy, although effective, increases the risks of hypoglycemia and cerebral edema from lowering the blood glucose level too rapidly. Low-dose therapy, although equally effective in many cases, carries the risk of undertreatment. Periodic boluses may allow swings in blood glucose level; the goal is to lower the glucose level only 100 mg/dl/hour. Continuous infusion allows delivery of low dosage. Remember, intravenous insulin absorption is greater than intramuscular absorption, which in turn is greater than subcutaneous absorption.

4. Alert the doctor when the blood glucose level reaches 250 mg/dl.

4. As metabolic control is reestablished, the blood glucose level may drop precipitously from the combined effects of therapy and continuing glycosuria. At 250 mg/dl, the I.V. infusion should be changed from normal saline solution to one containing glucose, or the insulin dose should be decreased to avoid hypoglycemia.

5. Observe for signs and symptoms of medication-induced hypoglycemia, such as headache, confusion, irritability, restlessness, trembling, pallor, diaphoresis, and stupor. If these signs and symptoms are present, notify the doctor, obtain a bedside fingerstick blood glucose level without delay, and treat immediately with food, oral glucose gel, or I.V. glucose or glucagon, depending upon unit protocol and the patient's level of consciousness (LOC).

5. The brain depends on glucose almost exclusively for energy. Hypoglycemia produces dramatic cerebral dysfunction and a profound stress response. The longer hypoglycemia persists, the greater the chance of transient or permanent neurologic damage. Hypoglycemic reactions may be fatal if left untreated. Mild reactions should be treated with protein and carbohydrates (such as milk and crackers). Simple sugars should be reserved for severe reactions.

6. Additional individualized interventions: _____

6. Rationales: _____

Target outcome criteria

Within 2 hours of the onset of therapy, the patient will display a blood glucose level returning to normal.

Within 24 hours of the onset of therapy, the patient will:
• display a blood glucose level less than 250 mg/dl
• have a small or negative urine ketone level.

Nursing diagnosis: *Sensory-perceptual alteration related to cerebral dehydration, decreased perfusion, hypoxemia, or acidosis*

NURSING PRIORITIES: (a) Ensure patient safety and (b) monitor return to the patient's usual LOC.

Interventions

1. Implement standard safety precautions, such as keeping side rails up, for the critically ill patient.

Rationales

1. A decreased LOC makes the patient unable to guard against accidental injury.

2. Monitor LOC constantly. Alert the doctor if LOC does not return to normal within 2 hours of the onset of therapy.

2. Decreased LOC in early DKA may result from hyperosmolality, marked cellular dehydration from osmotic diuresis, altered cellular function from anaerobic metabolism, or acidotic cerebrospinal fluid. Persistently decreased or worsening LOC may result from cerebral edema caused by a precipitous lowering of the blood glucose level. A substantial difference between blood glucose concentration and the concentration of glucose metabolites in the brain creates an osmotic gradient, drawing water into the brain and producing cerebral edema. LOC should return to normal with therapy; failure to do so suggests another disorder and requires further medical evaluation.

3. Additional individualized interventions: _____

_____

3. Rationales: _____

_____

Target outcome criterion
Within 24 hours of the onset of therapy, the patient will display a normal LOC.

Collaborative problem: *Acidosis related to altered LOC, ketosis, and decreased tissue perfusion*

NURSING PRIORITIES: (a) Maintain optimal ventilation and oxygenation, and (b) restore normal acid-base balance.

Interventions

1. Maintain a patent airway.

2. Monitor respiratory status every hour, including:

• respiratory rate and depth

• breath odor
• breath sounds.

3. Anticipate intubation and mechanical ventilation if increasing respiratory distress is present.

4. Administer oxygen, as ordered.

5. Monitor ABG levels, as ordered.

6. Administer I.V. sodium bicarbonate, as ordered, typically if pH is less than 7.1 or bicarbonate is less than 10 mEq/liter.

Rationales

1. Decreased LOC increases risk of aspiration.

2. Serial assessments allow timely detection of respiratory abnormalities.
• The body responds to ketoacidosis, a form of metabolic acidosis, by increasing the rate and depth of ventilation to blow off carbon dioxide and induce a compensatory respiratory alkalosis. The presence of Kussmaul's respirations indicates severe acidosis.
• Acetone breath indicates respiratory excretion of ketones.
• Breath sounds indicate the adequacy of ventilation. Abnormal sounds may suggest pneumonia (an infection that can cause DKA) or fluid overload.

3. Although rarely needed, these measures may be necessary to maintain airway patency and ventilatory adequacy.

4. Acidosis impairs oxygen delivery to tissues. Hypoxia provokes anaerobic metabolism, which produces lactic acid and further worsens the metabolic acidosis. Supplemental oxygen elevates arterial oxygen tension, reducing the need for anaerobic metabolism.

5. ABG levels document the type and degree of acid-base imbalances present and the effectiveness of therapy for DKA. Abnormalities normally resolve with fluid and electrolyte replacement and insulin therapy.

6. These parameters indicate severe acidosis. Bicarbonate administration replenishes bicarbonate ions, which buffer excess hydrogen ions, thus returning pH to normal. Use of I.V. sodium bicarbonate is uncommon.

7. While the patient is acutely ill, withhold food and fluids, even if the patient is extremely thirsty. Auscultate bowel sounds every 8 hours. Insert a gastric tube, as ordered, and connect to suction. Remove the gastric tube and allow oral intake of food and fluids only after LOC and bowel sounds return to normal.

7. Intense thirst is a compensatory mechanism for dehydration, but oral fluid intake can be dangerous. Because hyperglycemia decreases bowel motility, abdominal pain, nausea, and vomiting are common. Vomiting increases the risk of aspiration. Bowel sounds reflect gastrointestinal motility. Allowing oral intake only after bowel sounds and LOC are normal reduces the risk of aspiration. Use of gastric tubes is rare, unless the patient is unconscious.

8. Additional individualized interventions: _____

8. Rationales: _____

Target outcome criteria

Within 24 hours of the onset of therapy, the patient will:
• breathe at a rate of 12 to 24 respirations/minute
• display eupnea.

Within 36 hours of the onset of therapy, the patient will:
• have ABG levels within normal limits
• have normal bowel sounds
• be able to take oral food and fluids safely.

Nursing diagnosis: *Knowledge deficit related to complex disease and therapy*

NURSING PRIORITY: Identify and meet immediate learning needs.

Interventions

1. Refer to the "Knowledge Deficit" plan, page 56.

2. When the patient's condition allows, determine learning needs. Ascertain whether DM is a new or previously identified diagnosis. If the patient is a known diabetic, assess for possible causes of DKA, for example, a missed insulin dose or undetected infection.

3. When the patient's condition allows, begin a teaching program that reviews principles of "sick day" management, including:
• continuing to take insulin or oral hypoglycemic agents
• changing diet to frequent small meals of soft or liquid foods
• contacting the doctor early in the illness
• checking blood glucose every 1 to 4 hours
• checking urine ketones every void
• increasing sugar-free fluids to more than 4 oz (120 ml) per hour
• postponing exercise.

4. Use the patient's symptomatic episode as a teaching tool. Involve the family members in all teaching sessions.

5. As appropriate, initiate teaching about the cause of diabetes, signs and symptoms, significance of insulin, injection techniques, factors affecting medication needs (such as food intake and exercise), therapeutic diet, blood and urine testing, importance of consistent level of daily exercise, increased susceptibility to infections, recognition and management of hyperglycemic and hypoglycemic episodes, and long-range complications, such as neuropathy and retinopathy. Refer to the "Diabetes Mellitus" plan, page 523.

Rationales

1. The "Knowledge Deficit" plan provides general guidelines for patient teaching.

2. Learning needs vary depending upon whether the patient is a new or known diabetic. If the patient is newly diagnosed, extensive teaching is necessary. With a known diabetic, DKA episodes are usually preventable, and instruction may focus on unmet learning needs or areas needing reinforcement.

3. Although teaching is crucial to successful management of DM, physiologic needs take precedence in the critically ill patient. Extensive teaching may need to be deferred until after the patient's condition stabilizes. Understanding principles of "sick day" management may avert future crises.

4. The immediacy of the DKA episode makes it a powerful teaching tool for actively involving the patient and family.

5. Although the patient's and family's knowledge of all these topics is essential for ongoing home management of DM, only initial teaching is feasible for the critically ill patient. The "Diabetes Mellitus" plan contains detailed information on these topics.

6. Document learning needs and teaching. When the patient is discharged, communicate learning needs and arrange for teaching to continue on an outpatient basis.

6. The patient's condition, extensiveness of learning needs, and the hectic unit atmosphere may mean that the patient is likely to be discharged before learning is complete. Documentation and communication enhance continuity of care.

7. Additional individualized interventions: _____

7. Rationales: _____

Target outcome criteria
By the time of discharge, the patient and family will:
• identify learning needs
• show beginning involvement in learning, if appropriate.

Discharge planning
NURSING DISCHARGE CRITERIA
Upon the patient's discharge, documentation shows evidence of:
• stable vital signs within normal limits
• blood glucose level within normal limits without I.V. insulin
• return to premorbid LOC — ideally, alert and oriented
• ABG and anion gap levels within normal limits
• patient's active participation in self-care.

PATIENT-FAMILY TEACHING CHECKLIST
Document evidence that the patient and family demonstrate an understanding of initial teaching related to:
___ sick day management
___ cause and implications of DM
___ causes of DKA, including signs and symptoms and appropriate responses
___ significance of insulin
___ signs, symptoms, and interventions for hyperglycemia and hypoglycemia
___ dietary management
___ exercise plan
___ blood glucose and urine ketone testing
___ plan for completing unmet learning needs, including use of community and outpatient resources.

DOCUMENTATION CHECKLIST
Using outcome criteria as a guide, document:
___ clinical status on admission
___ significant changes in status
___ pertinent diagnostic test findings
___ I.V. fluid therapy
___ pharmacologic intervention
___ oxygen administration
___ patient-family teaching
___ discharge planning.

ASSOCIATED PLANS OF CARE
Acute Renal Failure
Diabetes Mellitus
Hyperosmolar Hyperglycemic Nonketotic Syndrome
Hypoglycemia
Hypovolemic Shock
Knowledge Deficit
Sensory-Perceptual Alteration

References
Davidoff, F. "Diabetic Emergencies," in *Critical Care Nursing: A Holistic Approach*, 5th ed. Edited by Hudak, C., Gallo, B., and Benz, J. Philadelphia: J.B. Lippincott Co., 1990.

Galloway, J., et al., eds. *Diabetes Mellitus*, 9th ed. Indianapolis: Eli Lilly and Co., 1988.

Guthrie, D., ed. *Diabetes Education: A Core Curriculum for Health Professionals*. Chicago: American Association of Diabetes Educators, 1988.

Huzar, J. "Diabetes Now: Preventing Acute Complications," *RN Magazine*, 52(8):34-40, August 1989.

Tueller, B. "Endocrine-Metabolic Imbalances," in *Nursing the Critically Ill Adult*, 3rd ed. Edited by Holloway, N. Menlo Park, Calif.: Addison-Wesley Publishing Co., 1988.

Zimmerman, B. "Managing the Diabetic During Critical Illness," *The Journal of Critical Illness*, 5(7): 774-80, 1990.

Hyperosmolar Hyperglycemic Nonketotic Syndrome

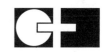

DRG information
DRG 294 Diabetes. Age 35 + .
     Mean LOS = 5.9 days
DRG 295 Diabetes. Age 0 to 35.
     Mean LOS = 4.4 days

Introduction
DEFINITION AND TIME FOCUS
Hyperosmolar hyperglycemic nonketotic syndrome (HHNKS) is an endocrine emergency with a mortality rate as high as 50%, if left untreated. Like diabetic ketoacidosis (DKA), it produces profound hyperglycemia and dehydration, but unlike DKA, ketosis and acidosis are absent. It presents a diagnostic puzzle because its clinical picture is similar to both DKA and cerebrovascular accident (CVA). It may occur in Type I (insulin-dependent) or Type II (non-insulin-dependent) diabetes mellitus (DM) but is more common in Type II and may be present at the time of diagnosis.

    The basic defect in HHNKS is a relative insulin deficiency in which enough insulin is secreted to prevent ketoacidosis but not enough to prevent hyperglycemia. Failure to recognize or respond to the thirst mechanism, which signals developing dehydration, exacerbates the problem. A precipitating factor (such as infection, new diagnosis of DM, CVA, or myocardial infarction) also is common. Clinical hallmarks include hyperglycemia, dehydration, hyperosmolality, and electrolyte imbalance without ketosis. This plan focuses on the critically ill patient admitted with HHNKS.

ETIOLOGY AND PRECIPITATING FACTORS
• usually only occurs in Type II DM, but up to 50% of episodes occur in persons with no previous history of DM
• acute illness (such as myocardial infarction or cerebrovascular accident)
• treatments (such as dialysis or total parenteral nutrition)
• infection (such as pneumonia or urinary tract infection)
• surgery
• newly diagnosed DM
• drugs (such as steroids, thiazides, or beta blockers)
• loss of thirst mechanism

Focused assessment guidelines
NURSING HISTORY (Functional health pattern findings)

Health perception–health management pattern
Note: History typically is obtained from a family member or friend because the patient's level of consciousness is decreased.
• newly diagnosed or known history of Type II DM
• family history of DM common
• more common in older patients (over age 50)
• slow onset of symptoms, typically over days to weeks

Nutritional-metabolic pattern
• increased thirst (polydipsia) or loss of thirst mechanism
• anorexia
• weight loss

Elimination pattern
• may complain of polyuria, nocturia, and incontinence
• may have diarrhea or constipation

Activity-exercise pattern
• may complain of weakness, fatigue, or lethargy

Sleep-rest pattern
• sleep disturbance related to nocturia

Cognitive-perceptual pattern
• may report dizziness or orthostatic hypotension
• confusion
• may have blurred vision
• decreased or altered sensorium

PHYSICAL FINDINGS
Neurologic
• lethargy or stupor
• fatigue, drowsiness, disorientation, or confusion
• seizures
• normal, decreased, or absent reflexes

Pulmonary
• tachypnea or dyspnea
• absence of Kussmaul's respirations (differential finding from DKA)
• absence of acetone breath (differential finding from DKA)

Cardiovascular
- tachycardia
- postural hypotension
- may have other cardiovascular disease (such as hypertension or congestive heart failure)
- hyperthermia
- capillary refill time greater than 3 seconds

Renal
- polyuria (early stage)
- oliguria (late stage)
- nocturia
- incontinence

Integumentary
- dry skin and mucous membranes
- poor skin turgor
- warm, flushed skin
- sunken or soft eyes
- may have skin infections or poorly healing wounds

Gastrointestinal
- abdominal distention
- decreased bowel sounds

DIAGNOSTIC STUDIES
- serum glucose levels—usually greater than 800 mg/dl, may be as high as 3,000 mg/dl
- arterial blood gases—usually normal
- electrolyte panel—levels may be low, normal, or elevated depending on severity of dehydration and HHNKS

- blood urea nitrogen (BUN) and creatinine—may be normal to elevated depending on severity of dehydration and DKA, and presence of underlying renal disease
- urine ketones—usually negative
- serum osmolality—usually greater than 350 mOsm/kg
- complete blood count and white blood cell count—may be elevated in presence of infection
- hemoglobin and hematocrit values—may be elevated secondary to dehydration
- electrocardiography—may reveal underlying cardiac disorder or arrhythmias
- chest X-ray—needed to establish baseline and rule out infection
- anion gap—normal
- blood, urine, and sputum cultures—used to detect infection's source

POTENTIAL COMPLICATIONS*
- fluid overload, congestive heart failure, or pulmonary edema
- disseminated intravascular coagulation
- hypoglycemia (if HHNKS overtreated)
- hypovolemic shock
- cerebral edema
- coma and death if untreated

Collaborative problem: *Hypovolemia related to osmotic diuresis*

NURSING PRIORITY: Restore fluid volume.

Interventions

1. Monitor for signs and symptoms of dehydration and shock, such as tachycardia; hypotension; weak peripheral pulses; capillary refill time greater than 3 seconds; warm, dry, flushed skin; poor skin turgor; polyuria or oliguria; increased hematocrit; increased urine specific gravity; and increased serum osmolality. Monitor blood pressure and cardiac rate and rhythm continuously.

Rationales

1. Impaired insulin release or peripheral insulin resistance causes hyperglycemia, which in turn causes hyperosmolality. To compensate for the hyperosmolality, fluid shifts from the intracellular to the extracellular space, dehydrating cells. Renal glucose spillage, an important compensatory mechanism for hyperglycemia, triggers an intense osmotic diuresis. This diuresis causes obligatory fluid and electrolyte losses, reflected in an elevated hematocrit and increased serum osmolality. Severe hypovolemia decreases glomerular filtration, aggravating the hyperglycemia and hyperosmolality and eventually producing oliguria and increased specific gravity. Fluid loss is usually greater in HHNKS than in DKA, so signs of dehydration may be severe. As volume is restored, signs and symptoms should resolve gradually; failure to do so indicates inadequate fluid replacement or continuing losses.

---

*Diabetes-related complications may be present and include retinopathy, neuropathy, nephropathy, cardiovascular disease, and peripheral vascular disease. These complications will influence nursing interventions and treatment strategies.

2. Observe for signs and symptoms of electrolyte imbalances, particularly hypernatremia and hypokalemia (see Appendix C, "Fluid and Electrolyte Imbalances," for details). Monitor serum electrolyte levels, as ordered, and report abnormal values to the doctor. Administer electrolyte replacements, as ordered.

2. Electrolyte status may change rapidly in response to fluid shifts, so close observation for signs and symptoms of imbalances is essential. Hypernatremia results from the large water deficit. In contrast to DKA, where acidosis causes hyperkalemia that commonly masks a low total body potassium, urinary losses in HHNKS result in hypokalemia. Hypernatremia usually resolves with fluid administration, while hypokalemia usually requires earlier potassium replacement than with DKA. Potassium doses depend on serum potassium levels.

3. Monitor serum osmolality, as ordered. Report levels greater than 295 mOsm/kg.

3. Laboratory values document the extent of hyperosmolality, which usually is more marked than in DKA because of the failure of the thirst mechanism and the intense osmotic diuresis. Values greater than 320 mOsm/kg indicate severe hyperosmolality.

4. Implement standard measures for hypovolemia, as ordered. Maintain patency of one or more I.V. lines, insert an indwelling urinary (Foley) catheter, and monitor intake and output and daily weights. Refer to the "Diabetic Ketoacidosis" plan, page 531, for details.

4. These measures are the same as with DKA. The "Diabetic Ketoacidosis" plan describes these interventions and associated rationales in detail. Because HHNKS is seen more commonly in older patients, an indwelling urinary catheter is useful; it is necessary in the unconscious patient.

5. Administer I.V. solutions, as ordered, typically 6 to 8 liters in the first 12 hours:

• normal saline solution if serum sodium level is less than 130 mEq/liter

• 0.45% saline solution if serum sodium level is greater than 145 mEq/liter

• dextrose in water when blood glucose levels reach 250 mg/dl or serum osmolality reaches 300 mOsm/kg.

5. Aggressive fluid repletion is necessary because of the severity of dehydration in HHNKS.

• A very low serum sodium level reflects large urinary sodium losses. Isotonic saline solution replaces sodium and replenishes volume.

• An elevated serum sodium level reflects decreased glomerular filtration and avid sodium retention in severe hypovolemia. Hypotonic fluid provides free water to reverse hyperosmolality.

• As blood glucose or serum osmolality approaches normal, changing to a glucose-containing solution prevents hypoglycemia.

6. During fluid replacement, monitor closely for signs and symptoms of fluid overload, including crackles, S_3 heart sound, neck-vein distention, dyspnea, or persistently depressed level of consciousness. If any indicators are present, notify the doctor.

6. Because the patient with HHNKS usually is older and has significant preexisting disease, the risk for congestive heart failure, pulmonary edema, or cerebral edema is higher than in DKA. These signs and symptoms require prompt nursing intervention and medical evaluation.

7. Additional individualized interventions: _____

7. Rationales: _____

Target outcome criteria
Within 24 hours of the onset of therapy, the patient will:
• have blood pressure, cardiac rate and rhythm, and peripheral perfusion within normal limits
• display a urine output of 60 to 100 ml/hour

• manifest serum osmolality levels within normal limits
• manifest serum electrolyte levels within normal limits.

ENDOCRINE DISORDERS

Collaborative problem: *Hyperglycemia related to inadequate insulin secretion or peripheral insulin resistance, or both*

NURSING PRIORITY: Lower blood glucose.

Interventions

1. Implement measures for this problem contained in the "Diabetic Ketoacidosis" plan, page 531, but with the following modifications:

• Administer low-dose insulin judiciously, as ordered.

• Monitor very closely for medication-induced hypoglycemia.

2. If the patient developed HHNKS while on high-carbohydrate enteral nutrition or hyperosmolar dialysis, consult with the doctor about revising orders for these therapies.

3. Additional individualized interventions: _____

Rationales

1. Care for hyperglycemia is similar in both HHNKS and DKA, but with different emphasis on two points.

• Because some endogenous insulin is produced, the patient with HHNKS is more sensitive to exogenous insulin than a patient with DKA, and lower insulin doses are usually needed.

• Because the patient with HHNKS retains some control of glucose metabolism, the risk for developing hypoglycemia in response to measures that lower blood glucose is high.

2. Modifying or discontinuing these causes of HHNKS removes an unnecessary glucose load for the patient.

3. Rationales: _____

> **Target outcome criterion**
> Within 24 hours of the onset of therapy, the
> patient will display a blood glucose level less than 250
> mg/dl.

Nursing diagnosis: *Sensory-perceptual alteration related to cerebral dehydration, decreased perfusion, hypoxemia, glucose deprivation, or cerebral edema during rapid rehydration*

NURSING PRIORITIES: (a) Restore the patient's level of consciousness, and (b) protect the patient from injury.

Interventions

1. Evaluate neurologic status every 1 to 4 hours, as indicated by the rapidity of other changes in the patient's condition. Alert the doctor to deepening coma or other indications of deteriorating neurologic functioning.

2. Institute seizure precautions. Promptly report any seizures to the doctor.

3. Additional individualized interventions: _____

Rationales

1. Neurologic changes, which are characteristic of this disorder, correlate closely with the degree of hyperosmolality. Deteriorating neurologic function may indicate serious pathophysiologic derangements, other previously undetected disorders, or inadequate therapy, and it requires medical evaluation.

2. Seizures occur commonly with HHNKS, as a result of cerebral dehydration, cerebral edema (during rehydration), or glucose deprivation (if hypoglycemia occurs).

3. Rationales: _____

Target outcome criterion
Within 24 hours, the patient will display usual neurologic status; ideally, alert, oriented, and able to move all extremities.

Nursing diagnosis: *Knowledge deficit related to complex disease*

NURSING PRIORITY: Teach the patient and family to avoid recurrence of HHNKS, if appropriate.

Interventions

1. Identify cause of HHNKS. If it is DM, implement measures contained in the "Diabetic Ketoacidosis" plan (with the exception of ketone testing), page 531, as appropriate.

2. Additional individualized interventions: _____
_____

Rationales

1. The "Diabetic Ketoacidosis" plan details measures that also apply to teaching some HHNKS patients. It is pertinent to patients with uncontrolled DM in whom HHNKS may recur. It is inappropriate when HHNKS results from high-carbohydrate nutrition or hyperosmolar dialysis; in those instances, HHNKS should not recur once the cause has been removed.

2. Rationales: _____
_____

Target outcome criteria
By the time of discharge, the patient and family will:
• identify learning needs, if appropriate
• show beginning involvement in learning, if appropriate.

Discharge planning

NURSING DISCHARGE CRITERIA
Upon the patient's discharge, documentation shows evidence of:
• stable vital signs within normal limits
• blood glucose level within normal limits without I.V. insulin
• return to usual level of consciousness
• arterial blood gas levels within normal limits
• electrolyte levels within normal limits.

PATIENT-FAMILY TEACHING CHECKLIST
Document evidence that the patient and family demonstrate an understanding of:
__ cause and significance of HHNKS
__ methods to decrease risk, if appropriate.

If the patient has DM, also document understanding of the following items:
__ oral hypoglycemic agents and insulin, if appropriate
__ hyperglycemia and hypoglycemia (signs and symptoms, possible causes, treatment, and prevention)
__ dietary plan
__ exercise and activity plan
__ blood glucose testing
__ learning needs at time of discharge
__ community resources.

DOCUMENTATION CHECKLIST
Using outcome criteria as a guide, document:
__ clinical status on admission
__ significant changes in status
__ pertinent laboratory and diagnostic test findings
__ I.V. fluid therapy
__ pharmacologic intervention
__ patient-family teaching
__ discharge planning.

ASSOCIATED PLANS OF CARE
Acute Renal Failure
Diabetic Ketoacidosis
Disseminated Intravascular Coagulation
Hypovolemic Shock
Knowledge Deficit

References
Galloway, J., et al., eds. *Diabetes Mellitus*, 9th edition. Indianapolis, Ind.: Eli Lilly and Co., 1988.
Guthrie, D., ed. *Diabetes Education: A Core Curriculum for Health Professionals.* Chicago: American Association of Diabetes Educators, 1988.
Tueller, B. "Hyperosmolar Hyperglycemic Nonketotic Coma," in *Nursing the Critically Ill Adult*, 3rd ed. Edited by Holloway, N. Menlo Park, Calif.: Addison-Wesley Publishing Co., 1988.

ENDOCRINE DISORDERS

ENDOCRINE DISORDERS
Hypoglycemia

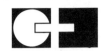

DRG information
DRG 296 Nutritional and Miscellaneous Metabolic
Disorders. Age 17 + . With Complication or
Comorbidity (CC).
Mean LOS = 6.1 days
DRG 297 Nutritional and Miscellaneous Metabolic
Disorders. Without CC.
Mean LOS = 4.1 days
DRG 298 Nutritional and Miscellaneous Metabolic
Disorders. Age 0 to 17.
Mean LOS = 3.2 days

Introduction
DEFINITION AND TIME FOCUS
Diabetes mellitus (DM) is a chronic metabolic condition involving an absolute (as in Type I DM) or relative (as in Type II DM) lack of endogenous insulin. A
delicate balance of diet, medicine (insulin or oral hypoglycemics), and exercise is needed to achieve glucose
homeostasis. Alterations in glucose metabolism can
provoke acute complications. This plan focuses on one
of the most common acute complications of DM: hypoglycemia. Hypoglycemia (also called low blood sugar,
insulin reaction, and insulin shock) occurs when the
serum glucose level falls below 50 mg/dl (normal is 55
to 115 mg/dl). It can be life threatening if left untreated. Usually, hypoglycemia is an acute complication of Type I (insulin-dependent) DM, with a
prevalence ranging from 4% to 26%, and is seen more
commonly with attempts to establish normoglycemia to
prevent, delay, or reverse chronic complications of DM.
It also can occur in Type II (non-insulin-dependent)
DM, especially with use of the oral agent chlorprop-
amide (Diabinese), but is less common.

ETIOLOGY AND PRECIPITATING FACTORS
• excessive or unplanned exercise (common)
• delayed or missed meal (common)
• very tight serum glucose control (common)
• inappropriate insulin regimen (common)
• too much insulin or oral hypoglycemic medicine (common)
• renal failure (common)
• alcohol use (common)
• underlying renal disease (nephropathy)
• pancreatic tumor (rare)

Focused assessment guidelines
NURSING HISTORY (Functional health pattern findings)

Health perception—health management pattern
• may report history of diabetes
• may use oral hypoglycemics or insulin, along with
diet and exercise, to control diabetes

Nutritional-metabolic pattern
• may report feeling hungry
• may complain of nausea

Elimination pattern
• may report increased perspiration

Activity-exercise pattern
• may complain of weakness
• may report lethargy
• may report feeling faint

Sleep-rest pattern
• may report bizarre dreams or nightmares
• may experience restless sleep
• may note difficulty waking in the morning

Cognitive-perceptual pattern
• may complain of lack of concentration
• may report blurred vision

PHYSICAL FINDINGS
Cardiovascular
• tachycardia
• palpitations
• syncope

Integumentary
• pallor
• flushing
• sweating (diaphoresis)

Neurologic
• irritability and mood swings
• confusion or uncontrollable behavior
• seizures
• glazed stare

Musculoskeletal
• weakness

DIAGNOSTIC STUDIES
• random serum glucose level—less than 50 mg/dl

POTENTIAL COMPLICATIONS*
• rebound hyperglycemia (if hypoglycemia overtreated)
• irreversible coma or brain damage, or death, if hypoglycemia untreated

---

Nursing diagnosis: *High risk for injury related to inappropriate exogenous insulin use, lack of food, or excessive exercise*

NURSING PRIORITY: Restore glucose level to normal.

Interventions

1. Observe for signs and symptoms of hypoglycemia constantly:
• adrenergic signs and symptoms (anxiety, tremor, nervousness, flushing, numbness, weakness, hunger, nausea, pallor, irritability, sweating, palpitations)
• neuroglycopenic signs and symptoms (moderate: headache, mental dullness, confusion, fatigue; or severe: senile dementia, glazed stare, bizarre dreams, difficulty waking, nightmares, coma, seizures).
Document findings.

2. Document suspected hypoglycemia with bedside glucose fingerstick or serum glucose, following hospital protocol.

3. Treat hypoglycemia promptly:

• If the patient is alert and the glucose level is less than 60 mg/dl (or below normal level specified by your institution), give a simple carbohydrate, such as glucose gel, by mouth. For mild symptoms, give 10 to 20 g; for moderate symptoms, 20 to 30 g. Follow with a complex carbohydrate and protein snack, such as one-half glass of milk with two graham crackers or four soda crackers (unless a meal will be eaten within an hour).

• If the patient is alert and the glucose level is greater than 80 mg/dl, do not treat. Check on and reassure the patient frequently.

Rationales

1. With hypoglycemia, adrenergic signs and symptoms occur first because low blood glucose stimulates the sympathetic nervous system to release catecholamines. In mild hypoglycemia, these may be the only signs and symptoms that occur. If hypoglycemia remains untreated, neuroglycopenic symptoms emerge because of starvation of cerebral neurons, which are only able to use glucose for energy. Symptoms may be moderate or severe. In long-standing Type I DM, many patients have "hypoglycemia unawareness," where they experience none of the usual symptoms of hypoglycemia until they suddenly lose consciousness. This is a dangerous and life-threatening situation.

2. Most institutions request a serum glucose level if the fingerstick glucose is less than 50 mg/dl and before treatment. A patient may complain of symptoms of hypoglycemia when the glucose level is normal or elevated. Symptoms may occur with a normal glucose level if the glucose level is quickly lowered or if the patient has had a high glucose level recently brought under control.

3. Prompt treatment reduces the risk of injury.

• Glucose gel or liquids containing simple sugars provide a measured amount of simple, quick-acting glucose. Using fruit juice is no longer recommended because it provides a variable amount of fructose, a concentrated form of glucose that is absorbed very rapidly and may cause rebound hyperglycemia. Other concentrated forms of glucose such as sugared soda or candy also cause an unreliable rise in blood glucose and may cause rebound hyperglycemia. Carbohydrates and protein cause a gradual rise in the glucose level to prevent recurrence of hypoglycemia.

• This is a normal glucose level. The goal of diabetes management is to keep the glucose level as near to normal as possible to prevent, reverse, or delay DM-related complications.

---

*Chronic complications of DM may be present, including retinopathy, neuropathy, nephropathy, cardiovascular disease, or peripheral vascular disease. These complications will influence nursing interventions and treatment strategies.

ENDOCRINE DISORDERS

• If the patient is unconscious with a glucose level less than 60 mg/dl, ensure airway patency, check pulse rate, and administer 50% dextrose (25 g by I.V. push) or glucagon (1 mg I.M. or subcutaneously), according to protocol.

• The patient with DM may also have cardiac disease, so it is important to recognize that unconsciousness may not be related to hypoglycemia. The patient's airway and pulse should be assessed immediately to detect emergency cardiac conditions. The unconscious hypoglycemic patient usually suffers from severe hypoglycemia. Because of the effect of glucose deprivation on cerebral neurons, immediate measures must be taken to reverse the hypoglycemic state. I.V. dextrose supplies glucose most rapidly. Glucagon administration stimulates glycogenolysis, the release of glucose from liver glycogen stores. Never give an unconscious patient liquids by mouth because of the risk of aspiration.

4. Recheck the glucose level 15 minutes after treatment. Repeat treatment if glucose level remains low. If the patient was unconscious, give a protein and carbohydrate snack when fully awake.

4. Blood glucose may drop again rapidly. Rechecking may indicate the need for further treatment. Carbohydrates and protein will cause a sustained rise in blood glucose.

5. If hypoglycemia occurs frequently, consult the doctor.

5. The patient's medication, diet, and activity regimens may need adjustment.

6. Additional individualized interventions: _____

6. Rationales: _____

Target outcome criteria
Within 15 minutes of the onset of treatment, the patient will:
• have a serum glucose level greater than 80 mg/dl
• be alert, oriented, and able to communicate.

Nursing diagnosis: *Knowledge deficit related to complex disease.*

NURSING PRIORITY: Teach the patient and family how to avoid and appropriately manage hypoglycemia.

Interventions

1. Once the hypoglycemic episode is over, use it as a learning experience. Involve family members in all teaching sessions. Help them to identify the causes of hypoglycemia, if possible.

Rationales

1. The patient needs to realize that occasional episodes of hypoglycemia can and will happen. By being prepared, the patient and family will be able to alleviate symptoms quickly. Common causes of hypoglycemia usually involve too much insulin or oral hypoglycemic, missed or delayed meals and snacks, or excessive exercise. In the hospital, the patient who can take nothing by mouth because of tests, procedures, surgery, or nausea and vomiting is also at risk for hypoglycemia. Identifying causes may help the patient avoid future episodes.

2. Review the signs and symptoms of hypoglycemia with the patient and family. If possible, have patient identify personal signs and symptoms.

2. Each patient responds individually to hypoglycemia. Symptoms may be mild to severe. Some patients have no symptoms. Early identification of symptoms promotes quick treatment and possibly a less severe hypoglycemic episode.

3. Discuss appropriate treatment strategies for hypoglycemia with the patient and family:
• If symptoms are mild and the blood glucose level is less than 60 mg/dl, eat a carbohydrate and protein snack.
• If symptoms are severe, eat a simple sugar.
• If the patient is unconscious, a family member should administer glucagon and call for emergency medical assistance.

3. A protein and carbohydrate snack causes a gradual rise in the glucose level. Because the goal of management is a normal glucose level, rebound hyperglycemia can occur if the patient eats too much food or uses simple sugars. If the episode occurs close to a meal, the patient may elect to eat a little earlier as treatment. Family members may need one-on-one teaching before administering glucagon.

4. Review strategies to prevent hypoglycemia with the patient and family. Encourage the patient to:
• wear a medical identification bracelet and carry a medical identification card
• have a source of food available at all times at home, in the car, at work, and any other place the patient frequents
• monitor glucose level regularly and record results
• work closely with the doctor and health care team if a pattern of hypoglycemia develops.

5. Additional individual interventions: _____

_____

4. Carrying and wearing medical identification will alert others to the potential for hypoglycemia if the patient is unable to speak. Having food available at all times ensures quick treatment of hypoglycemia. Regularly monitoring glucose level and recording the results helps identify patterns of hypoglycemia. These records should be reviewed at each outpatient visit. Correct insulin administration is essential for optimal effectiveness.

5. Rationales: _____

_____

Target outcome criteria
By the time of discharge, the patient and family will be able to:
• recognize that hypoglycemia is possible
• state signs and symptoms, possible causes, treatment, and preventive strategies related to hypoglycemia.

Discharge planning
NURSING DISCHARGE CRITERIA
Upon the patient's discharge, documentation shows evidence of:
• stable vital signs within normal limits
• blood glucose level within normal limits without I.V. glucose
• return to usual level of consciousness.

PATIENT-FAMILY TEACHING CHECKLIST
Document evidence that the patient and family demonstrate an understanding of:
__ cause and significance of hypoglycemia
__ signs and symptoms
__ preventive measures
__ treatment strategies
__ proper use of insulin or oral agents
__ dietary management
__ exercise and activity plan
__ blood glucose monitoring
__ urine ketone testing (for Type I DM only)
__ chronic complications related to DM
__ learning needs at time of discharge
__ community resources.

DOCUMENTATION CHECKLIST
Using outcome criteria as a guide, document:
__ clinical status on admission
__ significant changes in status
__ pertinent laboratory and diagnostic test findings
__ I.V. fluid therapy
__ pharmacologic intervention
__ patient-family teaching
__ discharge planning.

ASSOCIATED PLANS OF CARE
Diabetic Ketoacidosis
Hyperosmolar Hyperglycemic Nonketotic Syndrome
Hypovolemic Shock
Knowledge Deficit

References
Galloway, J., et al., eds. *Diabetes Mellitus*, 9th ed. Indianapolis, Ind.: Eli Lilly and Co., 1988.

Guthrie, D., ed. *Diabetes Education: A Core Curriculum for Health Professionals.* Chicago: American Association of Diabetes Educators, 1988.

Huzar, J. "Diabetes Now: Preventing Acute Complications," *RN Magazine* 52(8):34-40, August 1989.

Kevil, T. "Hypoglycemia," in *Decision Making in Critical Care Nursing.* Edited by Williams, S. Toronto: B.C. Decker, 1991.

Schultz, J. "Current Diabetes Care: An Update," *NURSEWEEK* 4(11):8-11, June 24, 1991.

Tueller, B. "Endocrine-Metabolic Imbalances," in *Nursing the Critically Ill Adult,* 3rd ed. Edited by Holloway, N. Menlo Park, Calif.: Addison-Wesley Publishing Co., 1988.

ENDOCRINE DISORDERS

RENAL DISORDERS
Acute Renal Failure

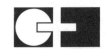

DRG information
DRG 316 Renal Failure.

> Mean LOS = 6.4 days
> Principal diagnoses include:
> - chronic or unspecified renal failure
> - acute renal failure (unspecified, with renal cortical necrosis, renal medullary necrosis, or tubular necrosis, or with other specified pathologic lesion in kidney)
> - oliguria or anuria.

Additional DRG information: Renal failure accompanied by any operative procedure will not be classified under DRG 316.

DRG 317 Admit for Renal Dialysis.

> Mean LOS = 2.2 days
> Principal diagnoses include aftercare involving intermittent dialysis.

Additional DRG information: Renal failure without intermittent dialysis is coded differently from renal failure with intermittent dialysis. For the latter, the principal diagnosis is actually "Admission for Dialysis"; renal failure becomes a secondary diagnosis.

Introduction
DEFINITION AND TIME FOCUS
Acute renal failure (ARF) is a sudden cessation or decrease in renal function. In ARF, the kidneys cannot maintain fluid and electrolyte balance or filter metabolic waste products. ARF disrupts all body systems and may cause problems in cardiac, respiratory, gastrointestinal, neurologic, musculoskeletal, integumentary, genitourinary, and endocrine-metabolic functions. The mortality rate can be high depending on the cause, the patient's age, and related physical problems.

Most ARF patients who recover progress through three stages: oliguria, diuresis, and recovery. The oliguric stage lasts about 2 weeks (a shorter period represents a better prognosis). The diuretic stage may last several weeks. The recovery stage may last up to a year, with initial rapid improvement and a continuing slow return to near-normal function. In some cases, patients have nonoliguric ARF with increasing azotemia and urine volumes for 12 days and a return to normal in another 12 days. If the patient does not recover, long-term hemodialysis, peritoneal dialysis, continuous arteriovenous hemofiltration, or kidney transplantation is necessary.

This plan focuses on the patient admitted for treatment of ARF, including identification of its cause and support of body systems until the kidneys begin to recover, or evaluation for dialysis or transplantation.

ETIOLOGY AND PRECIPITATING FACTORS
- prerenal problems leading to decreased renal perfusion, such as hemorrhage, all forms of shock, excessive vomiting or diarrhea, heart failure or other causes of decreased cardiac output, burns, excessive diuresis, third-spacing of fluids, hypotension, vasodilation, or obstruction of the aorta or renal arteries
- renal (parenchymal) problems leading to destruction of kidney tissue, such as acute tubular necrosis from ischemia or nephrotoxins, glomerulonephritis, emboli, allergic inflammation, or infections
- postrenal problems leading to obstruction of urine flow, such as calculi, prostate enlargement, tumors, or retroperitoneal fibrosis
- preexisting multisystem problems increase risk of ARF, especially in an older patient

Focused assessment guidelines
NURSING HISTORY (Functional health pattern findings)

Health perception — health management pattern
- may report decreased amount and frequency of urination
- may report headaches, swelling of feet and ankles, and palpitations
- may report a recent high-risk episode, such as infection; cardiac, aortic, or biliary surgery; trauma; ingestion of aspirin, antibiotics, or other drugs; exposure to toxins; or an allergic response to food, drugs, or blood transfusions
- may have a history of urinary tract infections, diabetes mellitus, hypertension, kidney disease, or cardiac or liver problems
- may report pain around the flank or costal margin areas

Nutritional-metabolic pattern
- may report loss of appetite, nausea
- may report a weight gain or loss
- may report an odd taste in mouth
- may report increased saliva or a dry mouth

Elimination pattern
- may report decreased or absent urination
- may report a change in urine color and smell
- may report abdominal cramps, a feeling of fullness, diarrhea, or constipation
- may report pruritus

Activity-exercise pattern
• may report difficulty in breathing at rest and during exercise
• may report weakness and fatigue
• may report muscle cramps

Sleep-rest pattern
• may report longer sleep periods than usual

Cognitive-perceptual pattern
• may report periods of dizziness
• may report memory loss and inability to concentrate

Role-relationship pattern
• may have job-related exposure to nephrotoxic chemicals, such as carbon tetrachloride, dyes, fungicides, pesticides, or heavy metals

Sexuality-reproductive pattern
• may report loss of sexual drive, impotence, or loss of menstruation

Coping—stress tolerance pattern
• may report increased irritability and decreased ability to handle stress

PHYSICAL FINDINGS
Note: Physical findings may vary, depending on the cause, type, and stage of ARF.

Genitourinary
• oliguria (less than 400 ml/day)
• less commonly, anuria (less than 50 ml/day) or high urine output (1 to 2 liters/day in nonoliguric ARF)
• abnormal urine color, clarity, or smell (such as red or brown color, cloudiness, or foul smell)

Neurologic
• lethargy, apathy
• tremors, seizures
• memory loss, confusion
• coma

Cardiovascular
• arrhythmias
• bounding, rapid pulse; normal or high blood pressure; and distended neck veins (with hypervolemia)
• tachycardia, low blood pressure, or orthostatic hypotension (with hypovolemia)
• pericardial-type chest pain (mild to severe pain that may increase with movement or decrease with leaning forward)
• anemia

Pulmonary
• rapid respirations, dyspnea, or crackles (with hypervolemia)
• tachypnea (with hypovolemia)
• Kussmaul's respirations (with acidosis)

Gastrointestinal
• moist tongue and increased saliva (with hypervolemia)
• dry tongue and mucous membranes (with hypovolemia)
• vomiting
• diarrhea
• stomatitis

Musculoskeletal
• muscle spasms (tetany)
• weakness
• asterixis

Integumentary
• moist, warm skin and pitting edema over bony areas (with hypervolemia)
• decreased skin turgor and dry skin (with hypovolemia)
• bruises
• thin, brittle hair and nails
• pallor

DIAGNOSTIC STUDIES
• 24-hour urine output and serum creatinine and blood urea nitrogen (BUN) levels—monitor the kidneys' ability to excrete fluid and waste products. Oliguric ARF is characterized by oliguria and rising BUN and creatinine levels. Patients with nonoliguric ARF exhibit a urine output of 1 to 2 liters/day and rising BUN and creatinine levels. The diuretic stage is characterized by increasing urine output (2 to 3 liters/day), indicating returning glomerular filtration. BUN and creatinine levels remain high during this stage because the kidneys cannot concentrate the urine effectively. As the kidneys regain concentrating ability during the recovery stage, the BUN and creatinine levels begin to fall and stabilize at normal or near normal levels depending upon the residual damage to the kidneys.
• serum electrolyte panel—monitors fluid, electrolyte, and acid-base status. Elevated potassium, sodium, and phosphate levels; decreased calcium level; and a decreased pH level indicate poor renal function.
• urinalysis—monitors renal excretion and concentration abilities. Sodium and potassium concentrations may vary, depending on the cause and type of ARF. Casts, crystals, hematuria, and proteinuria may be present. White blood cells (WBCs) may indicate infection. With prerenal conditions, specific gravity and osmolality may be high; with renal conditions, they may be constant at 1.010 and approximately 300 mOsm/kg respectively.
• creatinine clearance—reflects glomerular filtration rate (GFR) and is an accurate indication of renal function. A decrease indicates a poor GFR. A value of 50 to 84 ml/minute indicates mild failure; 10 to 49 ml/minute, moderate failure; and less than 10 ml/minute, severe failure.

RENAL DISORDERS

• fractional sodium excretion or renal failure index—compares the clearance of sodium to the clearance of creatinine; indexes greater than 1 may indicate non-functioning tubules
• urine-plasma creatinine concentration ratios and urine-plasma urea concentration ratios—reflect the kidneys' ability to save water and excrete wastes. Values vary depending upon the cause and type of ARF. In prerenal failure, ratios are high, reflecting kidney conservation of sodium and water; in acute tubular insufficiency, the kidneys' inability to perform these functions results in low urine-plasma ratios.
• BUN-creatinine ratio—reflects GFR and tubular function. In prerenal failure, the ratio is high (usually greater than 20:1), reflecting increased tubular reabsorption of urea. In acute tubular insufficiency, the ratio remains approximately 10:1, reflecting increased reabsorption of both urea and creatinine by the damaged tubules.
• complete blood count (CBC)—may reveal low red blood cell (RBC) count, hemoglobin, and hematocrit, reflecting anemia. An elevated WBC count may reflect infection.
• coagulation studies—may be abnormal if disseminated intravascular coagulation causes ARF
• renal concentration tests—may show the kidneys' inability to concentrate solutes in urine
• electrocardiography (ECG)—may show arrhythmias or high peaked T waves, flattened P waves, and widened QRS complexes associated with high potassium levels
• kidney-ureter-bladder X-rays—show size, structure, and position of kidneys, ureters, and bladder. The kidneys may be normal or enlarged in ARF. Changes in bladder or ureters suggest postrenal ARF.

• computed tomography scan—shows cross-sectional views of renal structures
• ultrasound scan—may show internal and external abnormalities in kidney size and shape
• I.V. or retrograde pyelogram—may show obstruction, constriction, or masses
• renal biopsy—may help differentiate among parenchymal kidney diseases
• renal angiography—may show renal artery abnormalities, cysts, or tumors
• radionuclide tests (renal scan and renogram)—may show abnormal distributions of radioactive compounds, indicating structural abnormalities or impaired perfusion or uptake
• cystoscopy—may show urethra and bladder abnormalities

POTENTIAL COMPLICATIONS
Note: Most complications result from the uremic syndrome—the accumulation of waste products in the blood. Some complications result from the kidneys' inability to maintain the normal hormonal functions of stimulating RBC production, regulating calcium absorption, and controlling the renin-angiotensin system.
• infection (sepsis is the most dangerous complication of ARF)
• stress ulcer
• heart failure
• pericarditis
• pneumonitis
• encephalopathy
• peripheral neuropathy
• coagulation defects
• pathologic fractures from bone demineralization
• gastrointestinal bleeding

Collaborative problem: *Electrolyte imbalance related to decreased electrolyte excretion, excessive electrolyte intake, or metabolic acidosis*

NURSING PRIORITY: Prevent complications of electrolyte imbalance.

Interventions

1. Monitor and document electrolyte levels every 8 to 12 hours and as needed, as ordered, particularly potassium, phosphate, calcium, and magnesium. See Appendix C, "Fluid and Electrolyte Imbalances," for general assessment parameters and interventions for abnormal electrolyte levels.

2. Continuously monitor the ECG and document your findings. See Appendix A, "Monitoring Standards." Note and promptly report peaked, high T waves; prolonged PR interval; or a widened QRS complex.

Rationales

1. The kidneys' inability to regulate electrolyte excretion and reabsorption may result in high potassium and phosphate levels, a low calcium level, and a high or low magnesium level. These levels can change quickly and result in such complications as cardiac arrhythmias, muscle response changes, mentation changes, skin irritation, and even death. General assessment parameters and interventions are included in the "Fluid and Electrolyte Imbalances" appendix.

2. Electrolyte abnormalities can trigger arrhythmias and cardiac arrest. The "Monitoring Standards" appendix contains general assessments for arrhythmias. The signs listed indicate hyperkalemia severe enough to cause a cardiac emergency.

3. If hyperkalemia is present, administer and document the following, as ordered:

• I.V. glucose (50%) and insulin solution

• I.V. calcium chloride or calcium gluconate

• cation-exchange resins, such as sodium polystyrene sulfonate (Kayexalate) with sorbitol, orally or rectally (do not give oral doses with fruit juices)

• I.V. sodium bicarbonate solution.

4. Limit dietary and drug intake of potassium; for example, avoid juices high in potassium and drugs such as potassium penicillin (Pentids) or potassium-containing antacids.

5. Give aluminum hydroxide antacid (Amphojel) with meals and every 4 hours, as ordered. Document administration.

6. Give calcium and vitamin supplements as needed and ordered. Document their administration.

7. Limit intake of magnesium, as from magnesium-containing antacids.

8. Give sodium chloride I.V., as needed and ordered. Document its administration.

9. Additional individualized interventions: _____

_____

3. The kidneys' inability to excrete the potassium released into the serum by normal cellular metabolism results in dangerously high potassium levels.

• Glucose and insulin may transport potassium into cells temporarily, thus lowering serum potassium in an emergency.

• Calcium competes with potassium for entry into heart cells, thus decreasing the dangerous effect of hyperkalemia on cardiac rhythm.

• Sodium polystyrene sulfonate removes potassium at the rate of 1 mEq/g of drug by exchanging it for sodium in the bowel. Sorbitol helps remove the exchanged and bound potassium from the bowel by acting as an osmotic diarrheic. Fruit juices may bind with sodium polystyrene sulfonate and decrease its effectiveness.

• ARF causes metabolic acidosis, which may increase the release of potassium from cells in exchange for hydrogen ions. Sodium bicarbonate corrects acidosis by combining with hydrogen ions, allowing potassium to move back into the cells.

4. When the kidneys cannot excrete potassium, excess intake can push serum potassium to dangerously high levels.

5. The kidneys cannot excrete the phosphates released from normal cellular metabolism or from dietary phosphate intake. Aluminum hydroxide binds with phosphate in the bowels and prevents absorption into the bloodstream, thus decreasing hyperphosphatemia.

6. The kidneys' inability to stimulate the absorption of calcium in the bowel results in hypocalcemia and bone demineralization. High phosphate levels also cause hypocalcemia. Calcium and vitamin D supplements increase the serum calcium levels, helping to prevent bone demineralization and other adverse effects of hypocalcemia.

7. The kidneys cannot excrete magnesium.

8. Usually, sodium intake is restricted to prevent fluid overload. However, major losses through vomiting, diarrhea, and wound drainage may create a need for sodium replacement.

9. Rationales: _____

_____

Target outcome criteria
Within 8 hours after treatment for hyperkalemia, the patient will:
• have a serum potassium level within normal limits
• show no signs of hyperkalemia on ECG
• have arterial blood gas (ABG) levels within normal limits.

Within 24 hours of admission and then continuously, the patient will:
• have serum electrolyte levels within expected limits
• have normal sinus rhythm.

Nursing diagnosis: *Fluid volume excess related to sodium and water retention*

NURSING PRIORITIES: (a) Maintain adequate hydration, and (b) prevent fluid overload.

Interventions

1. See Appendix C, "Fluid and Electrolyte Imbalances."

2. Assess for signs of fluid overload and document findings.

• Assess vital signs, lung sounds, and peripheral edema every 4 hours, or more frequently if appropriate. Assess weight and CBC, especially hematocrit, daily. If invasive hemodynamic monitoring lines are present, measure central venous pressure (CVP), pulmonary artery pressures, pulmonary capillary wedge pressure (PCWP), and mean arterial pressure (MAP) every 1 to 2 hours. Measure cardiac output, as ordered, typically every 12 hours.

• Report the following promptly: high blood pressure, rapid pulse, rapid respirations, high hemodynamic parameters, crackles or gurgles, peripheral edema, increasing daily weight, or low hematocrit.

• Also report the following promptly: low hemodynamic monitoring parameters, rapid pulse, low blood pressure, dry skin and mucous membranes, poor skin turgor, decreased weight, or high hematocrit.

3. Measure and document intake and output (I&O) every 8 hours.

4. Restrict fluid intake to measured losses plus 400 ml/day, unless fluid or weight losses are excessive. Correlate the I&O record with daily weights. Consult the doctor about increasing fluid replacement if excessive fluid losses are present or if weight loss exceeds 1 lb (0.5 kg) per day. Document fluid administration.

5. Give I.V. infusions continuously through an infusion pump, as ordered.

6. Provide hard candies, ice chips, and mouth care every 2 hours as needed and ordered. Document your actions.

7. Give diuretics, such as mannitol, furosemide (Lasix), or ethacrynic acid (Edecrin), as needed and ordered. Document administration and results. Administer vasodilators, as ordered, such as low-dose dopamine (Intropin).

8. Additional individualized interventions: _____

Rationales

1. Appendix C contains general information on fluid and electrolyte imbalances. This plan presents additional information specific to ARF.

2. Inability to maintain normal fluid homeostasis results in fluid overload during the oliguric stage and potential dehydration during the diuretic stage.

• Regular assessment of indicated parameters provides for early detection of imbalances.

• Prompt medical intervention is necessary to resolve imbalances. These signs indicate fluid overload. A low hematocrit may reflect hemodilution from overhydration.

• These signs reflect a low circulating fluid volume. High hematocrit may reflect hemoconcentration.

3. A careful comparison of I&O is necessary to prevent fluid overload or dehydration.

4. Because the kidneys cannot eliminate excess fluids, intake must be restricted to replacement of lost fluids. The additional 400 ml represents insensible fluid losses (through lungs, skin, and stool). Although such losses are estimated at 400 ml/day, excess losses from high temperatures, wound drainage, diarrhea, or vomiting may require increasing this amount. Daily weight may help guide fluid replacement because the ARF patient usually loses ¾ lb (0.3 kg) to 1 lb/day from catabolism. A loss of more than 1 lb/day may indicate a need for additional fluids.

5. The patient with ARF is susceptible to fluid overload. An infusion pump prevents accidental administration of fluid boluses.

6. Fluid restrictions cause dry mouth and thirst. These measures aid mouth comfort by stimulating salivation and removing debris during fluid restriction.

7. Diuretics may be given initially in prerenal conditions to increase fluid volume through the kidneys in an attempt to prevent ARF. However, diuretics may cause ARF in marginally functioning kidneys and are not effective in nonfunctioning kidneys. Vasodilators expand the vascular bed, lessening vascular congestion and the risk of pulmonary edema. Low-dose dopamine causes dopaminergic stimulation of renal blood vessels, thus increasing renal perfusion.

8. Rationales: _____

Target outcome criteria
By the time of discharge, the patient will:
- have normal vital signs and hemodynamic readings within normal parameters
- have clear lungs
- display minimal or absent peripheral edema
- manifest normal skin turgor
- have moist and clean mucous membranes
- maintain a steady weight.

Nursing diagnosis: *High risk for injury: complications related to uremic syndrome*

NURSING PRIORITIES: (a) Assess for signs and symptoms of uremia, (b) monitor for complications, and (c) prevent injuries.

Interventions

1. See Appendix B, "Acid-Base Imbalances."

2. Monitor BUN, creatinine, uric acid, and pH levels once daily or as needed and ordered. Monitor ABG levels once daily or as needed and ordered. Document your findings.

3. Assess for and document signs and symptoms of uremia every 2 to 4 hours and as needed. Note headache, mentation changes, fatigue, confusion, lethargy, pruritus, uremic frost, stomatitis, nausea and vomiting, ammonia breath odor, weight loss, muscle wasting, Kussmaul's respirations, seizures, or coma. Report significant findings to the doctor.

4. Give sodium bicarbonate I.V. as needed and ordered, typically if the plasma bicarbonate level is 10 to 15 mEq/liter or less. Document administration.

5. Assess the hemodialysis access site (shunt or catheter), if present, every 2 hours for patency, warmth, color, thrill, and bruit. Check circulation above and below the access site. Do not use the access site for I.V. infusions or to draw blood. Do not take blood pressures on an arm or leg with an access site. Inject heparinized normal saline solution every 12 hours to maintain patency. Keep alligator clamps attached to the dressings. Document access site status and report abnormalities promptly to the doctor.

6. Assess the peritoneal dialysis access catheter site, if present, every 24 hours and as needed for signs and symptoms of infection, including redness, swelling, excess warmth, and drainage. Also assess for general signs and symptoms of infection, including fever, malaise, abdominal pain, and cloudy drainage. Maintain surgical aseptic technique when manipulating the site, changing dressings, or adding medication to the dialysate.

7. Prepare the patient for dialysis, as needed and ordered, when potassium, BUN, and creatinine levels, and other parameters indicate worsening uremia, usually every 1 to 3 days.

Rationales

1. Appendix B contains general information on acid-base imbalances. This plan presents additional information specific to ARF.

2. Accumulation of the metabolic waste products in the blood and increasing acidosis reflect worsening failure and may indicate the need for dialysis.

3. Uremia affects every system and may cause subtle changes as the condition worsens. Careful assessments are valuable in determining the need for dialysis and gauging its frequency.

4. Acidosis is commonly treated by dialysis, but severe cases may be treated with sodium bicarbonate.

5. The access site must remain patent because of the limited number of large vessels available for dialysis. Early discovery of a clotted shunt or catheter may allow clot removal and salvaging of the site. Using the site for purposes other than dialysis increases the risk of infection and loss of the site. Regular heparinization prevents clotting. Alligator clamps should be available to clamp the shunt or catheters in the event of accidental disconnection.

6. The patient undergoing peritoneal dialysis is at high risk for peritonitis, a life-threatening complication. Early detection of infection permits aggressive intervention and increases the likelihood of its success.

7. Both hemodialysis and peritoneal dialysis remove serum waste products and excess fluids and electrolytes, allowing a more homeostatic metabolic state.

RENAL DISORDERS

8. Monitor drug administration and blood levels continually. Assess potential nephrotoxicity, electrolyte content, dosage, and timing with dialysis.

8. Renal dysfunction may decrease drug excretion, resulting in excessive blood levels and varying durations of drug effects. Certain drugs, including antibiotics, may be nephrotoxic and may worsen kidney damage. Drugs containing electrolytes should be limited to prevent undesirable effects. Dialysis may remove some drugs from the blood, so drug administration should be timed with dialysis treatments. Monitoring blood levels provides accurate guidelines for drug therapy.

9. Monitor hematocrit and hemoglobin level daily for signs of anemia. Give packed RBCs, folic acid, and iron supplements as needed and ordered. Document your findings and actions.

9. Erythropoietin, a hormone manufactured by the kidneys, normally stimulates RBC production. Diminished erythropoietin production in ARF results in anemia. Folic acid and iron supplements stimulate RBC production and may correct the anemia. Administering packed cells instead of whole blood provides oxygen-carrying RBCs without exacerbating fluid overload.

10. Assess continually for signs and symptoms of hemorrhage, including changes in vital signs, CBC, and coagulation panel. If present, alert the doctor immediately. Give vitamin K, packed RBCs, and other blood components as needed and ordered, and document their use. See the "Gastrointestinal Hemorrhage" plan, page 394.

10. Uremic syndrome places the patient at high risk for stress ulcers and coagulation problems. General interventions for the patient with GI bleeding are included in the "Gastrointestinal Hemorrhage" plan.

11. Assess daily for signs and symptoms of pericarditis, including tachycardia, fever, friction rub, and pleuritic pain that is relieved by sitting forward. If these indicators are present:

11. About 20% of patients with ARF develop pericarditis (inflammation of the pericardial sac).

• Notify the doctor. Administer steroids or nonsteroidal anti-inflammatory agents, as ordered. Document their use.

• Untreated, pericarditis can lead to pericardial effusion and cardiac tamponade. The medications listed relieve inflammation.

• Monitor every 4 hours for indicators of pericardial effusion and a small cardiac tamponade: weak peripheral pulses, pulsus paradoxus greater than 10 mm Hg, or a decreased level of consciousness. If present, alert the doctor immediately.

• Pericardial effusion can range from mild to major. Mild effusion produces a small cardiac tamponade and mildly decreased cardiac output. Increased dialysis may be used to remove the uremic toxins causing mild effusion.

• Monitor continually for indicators of a large cardiac tamponade: distended neck veins, profound hypotension, and rapid loss of consciousness. Summon immediate medical assistance and prepare for emergency pericardial aspiration.

• A large cardiac tamponade—a medical emergency—compromises cardiac output severely. Immediate removal of pericardial fluid is necessary to allow ventricular filling and prevent cardiac arrest.

12. Additional individualized interventions: _____

12. Rationales: _____

Target outcome criteria
Immediately at the start of dialysis, the patient will:
• have a patent dialysis shunt or catheter
• display no signs of infection
• manifest no signs of hemorrhage.

Within 3 days of admission, the patient will:
• have a normal blood pressure
• display strong, regular peripheral pulses
• show a level of consciousness within normal limits
• manifest a normal temperature.

Within 7 days of admission, the patient will:
• have BUN, creatinine, uric acid, and pH values within expected limits
• display ABG levels within normal limits
• manifest no signs or symptoms of uremia
• maintain therapeutic drug levels
• have a hemoglobin level and hematocrit within expected limits
• display no signs of pericarditis.

Nursing diagnosis: *High risk for infection related to decreased immune response and skin changes secondary to uremia*

NURSING PRIORITY: Assess for and prevent infection.

Interventions

1. Assess continually for signs of infection, such as increased temperature, redness, swelling, warmth, and drainage. Document findings and report them to the doctor.

2. Continually protect the patient from cross-contamination by practicing medical and surgical asepsis.

3. Give antibiotics every 4 to 12 hours, as ordered, and document their use. Follow the guidelines for drug administration in the "High risk for injury" nursing diagnosis above.

4. Provide site care and dressing changes for central and peripheral I.V. lines, catheters, and dialysis shunts every 12 to 48 hours, according to policy. Assess and document condition of skin and puncture sites; document date and care given.

5. Provide skin care at frequent intervals. Use preventive measures such as position changes, range-of-motion exercises, massage, wrinkle-free linens, and protective pads and mattresses. Document skin condition and nursing care given. See the "Impaired Physical Mobility" plan, page 36.

6. Avoid continuous invasive procedures, such as indwelling urinary (Foley) catheterization. Catheterize intermittently, as needed and as ordered.

7. Collect urine, blood, and secretion specimens for culture and sensitivity laboratory tests, as needed and ordered. Document your actions.

8. Additional individualized interventions: _____

_____

Rationales

1. Uremic syndrome suppresses normal cell metabolism and immune response, resulting in an increased risk for infection, a major cause of death for ARF patients. Continuous assessment is necessary to identify infection and to begin early treatment, reducing the risk of life-threatening sepsis and septicemia.

2. Careful hand washing and using aseptic technique during procedures and when handling equipment may prevent infection.

3. Antibiotics are a potent weapon against infection; however, many are nephrotoxic. Because the kidneys may be unable to excrete antibiotics normally, lower-than-normal doses may be needed. Coordination with dialysis is important to minimize drug removal and maintain therapeutic blood levels.

4. Site care may prevent the accumulation of secretions that could serve as growth media for infective organisms, while regular assessment may allow the early identification of infection. Careful documentation of site care promotes continuity of care.

5. Skin integrity is compromised in the patient with ARF and uremia because of altered metabolism and the accumulation of fluid and waste products in the tissues. Frequent skin care may counteract the increased risk of skin breakdown and infection. The "Impaired Physical Mobility" plan provides further detail on preventing skin breakdown.

6. Continuous invasive procedures provide reservoirs for infective organisms in a patient already at high risk for infection.

7. Careful monitoring of body secretions for infection may allow timely and appropriate treatment if needed.

8. Rationales: _____

_____

Target outcome criteria
Within 72 hours of admission and then continuously, the patient will:
- have a normal temperature
- have noncontaminated access sites for lines and catheters
- have negative cultures
- if taking antibiotics, have a therapeutic blood level.

RENAL DISORDERS

Nursing diagnosis: *Nutritional deficit related to anorexia, nausea and vomiting, and restricted dietary intake*

NURSING PRIORITIES: (a) Maintain nutritional status, and (b) minimize protein catabolism.

Interventions	Rationales
1. See the "Nutritional Deficit" plan, page 63.	1. General assessments and interventions are included in the "Nutritional Deficit" plan. This nursing diagnosis focuses on information specific to ARF.
2. Administer medication to control nausea and vomiting, as needed and as ordered. Document administration and patient response. Provide small, frequent meals. Document dietary intake.	2. The patient with ARF commonly experiences nausea and vomiting because of uremia's effects on the GI system. Medication and smaller servings enhance tolerance to the diet.
3. Collaborate with the doctor and nutritionist to design a high-carbohydrate diet that provides small quantities of high-quality proteins (containing essential amino acids); limits fluids, potassium, and sodium; and includes vitamin supplements.	3. A high-carbohydrate diet provides calories for energy while sparing proteins and preventing protein catabolism. Because the kidneys cannot excrete the waste products of protein metabolism, proteins are limited to easily used high-quality proteins. The kidneys cannot regulate water balance, thus fluids are limited. Electrolytes, such as potassium, are limited because the kidneys cannot excrete them. Sodium is limited to prevent volume overload. Dialysis may remove vitamins, requiring administration of supplements.
4. Additional individualized interventions: _____	4. Rationales: _____

Target outcome criteria
Upon discharge, the patient will:
• be free from nausea and vomiting
• display only limited weight loss, muscle wasting, or edema

• display a pattern of regular and adequate meals
• verbalize having enough energy for activities of daily living.

Nursing diagnosis: *Knowledge deficit related to complexity and life-threatening nature of ARF and dialysis*

NURSING PRIORITY: Provide information on ARF and dialysis, as appropriate.

Interventions	Rationales
1. See the "Knowledge Deficit" plan, page 56.	1. General interventions appropriate for any patient are included in the "Knowledge Deficit" plan.
2. Provide, as appropriate, the following information: • the common stages of ARF • medications • signs and symptoms that should be reported to the nurse, such as dizziness and nausea • procedures, including hemodialysis or peritoneal dialysis • dietary modifications • activity restrictions.	2. The acutely ill patient may not be receptive to extensive teaching. However, if appropriate, teaching may decrease anxiety and enhance recovery.
3. Additional individualized interventions: _____	3. Rationales: _____

Target outcome criteria
According to individual readiness, the patient will be able to relate:
• signs and symptoms, such as headache, nausea, and vomiting, to be reported to the nurse
• rationale for treatments, including dialysis, dietary modifications, and activity restrictions.

Discharge planning
NURSING DISCHARGE CRITERIA
Upon the patient's discharge, documentation shows evidence of:
• stable vital signs and monitoring parameters
• absence of infection, hemorrhage, and major complications in all systems
• stabilized fluid and electrolyte status, including limited edema and appropriate potassium, calcium, sodium, phosphate, and magnesium levels
• stabilized BUN, creatinine, uric acid, and pH levels
• intact and healing dialysis access site
• stable nutritional status including a positive nitrogen balance and minimal weight loss
• therapeutic drug levels.

PATIENT-FAMILY TEACHING CHECKLIST
Document evidence that the patient and family demonstrate an understanding of:
___ common stages of ARF and patient's current stage
___ fluid and diet regimen, including limitations of protein, electrolytes, and fluids
___ rest and activity schedule
___ medications, including action and adverse effects
___ dialysis treatment if appropriate, including schedule and adverse effects
___ signs and symptoms, including fever, pain, nausea, vomiting, and dizziness, to report to the nurse.

DOCUMENTATION CHECKLIST
Using outcome criteria as a guide, document:
___ clinical status on admission
___ significant changes in status
___ pertinent laboratory and diagnostic test findings, including serum drug levels
___ dialysis access site condition and care
___ urine characteristics and quantity, if appropriate
___ I&O
___ weights
___ diet tolerance
___ activity tolerance
___ mentation status
___ skin status
___ pertinent procedures including dialysis.

ASSOCIATED PLANS OF CARE
Gastrointestinal Hemorrhage
Knowledge Deficit
Nutritional Deficit

References
Baer, C. "Acute Renal Failure: Recognizing and Reversing its Deadly Course," *Nursing* 20(6):34-40, 1990.

Beare, P., and Myers, J., eds. *Principles and Practice of Adult Health Nursing.* St Louis: C.V. Mosby Co., 1990.

Dossey, B.M., Guzetta, C.E., and Kenner, C.V. *Critical Care Nursing: Body–Mind–Spirit.* Philadelphia: J.B. Lippincott, Co., 1992.

Kinney, M., Packa, D., and Dunbar, S. *AACN'S Clinical Reference for Critical-Care Nursing,* 2nd ed. New York: McGraw-Hill Book Co., 1987.

McKenry, L., and Salerno, E. *Mosby's Pharmacology in Nursing,* 17th ed. St. Louis: C.V. Mosby Co., 1989.

Patrick, M., Woods, S., Craven, R., Rokosky, J., and Bruno, P. *Medical-Surgical Nursing: Pathophysiological Concepts,* 2nd ed. Philadelphia: J.B. Lippincott Co., 1991.

Phipps, W., Long, B., Woods, N., and Cassmeyer, V., eds. *Medical-Surgical Nursing: Concepts and Clinical Practice,* 4th ed. St. Louis: Mosby-Year Book, 1991.

Thompson, J., McFarland, G., Hirsch, J., Tucker, S., and Bowers, A. *Mosby's Manual of Clinical Nursing,* 2nd ed. St. Louis: C.V. Mosby Co., 1989.

RENAL DISORDERS

Chronic Renal Failure

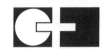

DRG information

DRG 316 Renal Failure.
   Mean LOS = 6.4 days
   Principal diagnoses include chronic renal
   failure.
DRG 317 Admit for Renal Dialysis.
   Mean LOS = 2.2 days
DRG 315 Other Kidney and Urinary Tract Operating
   Room Procedures.
   Mean LOS = 7.5 days
   Principal diagnoses include arteriovenostomy
   for renal dialysis.

Introduction
DEFINITION AND TIME FOCUS

Chronic renal failure (CRF) is a progressive, irreversible decrease in kidney function to the point where homeostasis can no longer be maintained. Usually slow and insidious, CRF eventually has consequences in all organ systems and physiologic processes. The final stage of CRF, when more than 90% of kidney function is permanently lost, is called end-stage renal disease (ESRD). During ESRD, chronic abnormalities occur, and patient survival depends on maintenance dialysis or kidney transplantation. This plan focuses on the ESRD patient receiving maintenance hemodialysis or peritoneal dialysis, who has been admitted for evaluation of the systemic consequences of CRF and the effectiveness of therapy.

ETIOLOGY AND PRECIPITATING FACTORS

• untreated acute renal failure or poor response to treatment (for example, acute tubular necrosis)
• diabetes mellitus (DM) leading to diabetic nephropathy
• severe hypertension leading to hypertensive nephropathy
• lupus erythematosus leading to lupus nephritis
• recurrent glomerulonephritis, typically related to chronic streptococcal infection
• pyelonephritis
• polycystic kidney disease
• chronic use of nephrotoxic drugs
• frequent lower urinary tract infections (UTIs) with eventual kidney involvement
• neoplasms (metastatic or primary)
• developmental and congenital disorders
• complications of pregnancy (for example, eclampsia, UTI, hemorrhage, or abruptio placentae)
• sarcoidosis
• amyloidosis
• Goodpasture's syndrome (autoimmune disease involving basement membrane of glomerular capillaries)

Focused assessment guidelines
NURSING HISTORY (Functional health pattern findings)

Health perception – health management pattern
• signs and symptoms that cause the patient to seek health care vary widely and may include decreased urinary output, edema, extreme fatigue, depression, loss of interest in environment, impotence, and flank pain
• commonly has a history of acute or chronic renal problems and may be receiving treatment for acute renal failure, chronic renal insufficiency, hypertension, DM, generalized arteriosclerosis and atherosclerosis, lupus erythematosus, or other systemic diseases involving the kidneys

Nutritional-metabolic pattern
• typically reports anorexia, nausea, and vomiting
• may report weight loss related to decreased intake of nutrients or weight gain related to fluid retention
• may report unpleasant taste in mouth

Elimination pattern
• if in an early stage of CRF, may report polyuria and nocturia
• if in advanced stage of CRF, may report oliguria (with polycystic kidney disease, urinary output may be normal, or polyuria may occur)
• may report diarrhea alternating with constipation

Activity-exercise pattern
• typically reports fatigue, malaise, and decreased energy level

Sleep-rest pattern
• may report extreme somnolence or insomnia and restlessness
• may report sleep often interrupted by muscle cramps and leg pain

Cognitive-perceptual pattern
• may report shortened attention span
• may report memory loss
• may report decreased ability to perform abstract reasoning or mathematical calculations
• may report loss of interest in environment

Self-perception – self-concept pattern
• may report depression or frequent mood swings
• may report altered self-concept and body image
• may report decreased self-esteem
• may report reduced level of independence and self-care
• may report sense of powerlessness and hopelessness

Role-relationship pattern
• may be unable to work
• may be unable to maintain spousal and parental roles
• may report decrease in social contacts and activities

Sexuality-reproductive pattern
• female may report amenorrhea, infertility, decreased libido, and decreased or absent sexual expression
• male may report impotence, decreased libido, and decreased or absent sexual expression

Coping—stress tolerance pattern
• may describe ineffective individual and family coping patterns in response to changes caused by chronic catastrophic disease and its treatment
• may exhibit defense mechanisms (for example, denial, projection, displacement, or rationalization)

Value-belief pattern
• may express loss of confidence in health care providers
• may question lifelong religious and philosophical values and beliefs or may intensify beliefs and derive support from them

PHYSICAL FINDINGS
Integumentary
• rough, dry skin
• bronze-gray, pallid skin color
• pruritus
• ecchymoses
• poor skin mobility and turgor (skin mobility is the ease with which it can be lifted between the fingers; turgor is the speed with which it resumes position)
• excoriation
• signs and symptoms of inflammation
• thin, brittle nails
• coarse and thinning hair

Cardiovascular
• hypertension, or hypotension (uncommon)
• orthostatic hypotension
• pitting edema of feet, legs, fingers, and hands
• periorbital edema
• sacral edema
• engorged neck veins
• arrhythmias
• pericardial friction rub (with pericarditis)
• paradoxical pulse (with pericardial effusion or tamponade)
• palpitations

Pulmonary
• crackles
• shortness of breath
• coughing
• thick, tenacious sputum
• deep, rapid respirations (with acidosis)

Gastrointestinal
• smell of urine and ammonia on the breath
• gum ulcerations and bleeding
• dry, cracked, bleeding mucous membranes and tongue
• vomiting
• bleeding from GI tract
• constipation or diarrhea
• weight loss related to decreased intake of nutrients masked by fluid retention (peripheral edema), leading to increase in overall body weight; after the patient receives appropriate treatment (fluid restriction and dialysis), excess fluid is decreased and weight loss is especially evident
• liver enlargement
• ascites

Neurologic
• malaise, weakness, and fatigue
• confusion and disorientation
• memory loss
• slowing of thought processes
• changes in sensorium (somnolence, stupor, or coma)
• seizures
• changes in behavior (irritability, withdrawal, depression, psychosis, or delusions)
• numbness and burning of soles of feet
• decreased sensory perception
• muscle cramps
• restlessness of legs
• diminished deep tendon reflexes
• positive Chvostek's and Trousseau's signs (rare)

Musculoskeletal
• muscle cramps (especially in the legs)
• loss of muscle strength
• limited range of motion in joints
• bone fractures
• lumps (calcium-phosphate deposits) in skin, soft tissues, and joints
• footdrop with motor nerve involvement

Reproductive
• amenorrhea (in females)
• atrophy of testicles (in males)
• gynecomastia

DIAGNOSTIC STUDIES
• blood urea nitrogen (BUN) levels—elevated
• serum creatinine levels—elevated (see *Creatinine ranges in renal failure*, page 560)
• creatinine clearance—decreased by more than 90% in ESRD (see *Creatinine ranges in renal failure*, page 560)
• serum electrolyte levels—hypernatremia (common), hyperkalemia, hyperphosphatemia, hypocalcemia, elevated calcium-phosphate product, hypermagnesemia
• venous CO_2 (comparable to arterial HCO_3) levels—decreased

CREATININE RANGES IN RENAL FAILURE

Renal function	Serum creatinine (approximate mg/100 ml)	Creatinine clearance (ml/min)
Normal	1.0 to 1.4	85 to 150
Mild failure	1.5 to 2.0	50 to 84
Moderate failure	2.1 to 6.5	10 to 49
Severe failure	>6.5	<10
End-stage failure	>12	0

Data from Lancaster (1984)

• arterial blood gas levels — acid-base imbalance, typically metabolic acidosis
• hemoglobin and hematocrit values — decreased (hemoglobin usually 6 to 8 mg, hematocrit usually 20% to 25%)
• red blood cell (RBC) count — decreased
• serum albumin and total protein levels — commonly decreased
• alkaline phosphatase levels — may be elevated
• white blood cell count — may be elevated
• urinalysis — of minimal diagnostic value in ESRD
• renal biopsy — indicates the nature and extent of renal disease; necessary to diagnose CRF's cause

• radionuclide tests (renal scan and renogram) — may show abnormal renal structure and function
• renal arteriogram — may identify narrowed, stenosed, missing, or misplaced blood vessels
• plain X-ray of kidneys, ureters, and bladder — may indicate gross structural abnormalities
• ultrasonography — may indicate gross structural abnormalities
• computed tomography scan — may show renal masses, abnormal filling of the collecting system, or vascular disorders
   Note: Because CRF commonly coexists with other systemic diseases and because it affects all organ systems and physiologic processes, numerous additional laboratory tests and diagnostic procedures are commonly required to assess the other diseases and systemic consequences of CRF.

POTENTIAL COMPLICATIONS
• uncontrollable hypertension
• hyperkalemia and related cardiac electrical conduction deficits
• pericarditis, pericardial effusion, or pericardial tamponade
• pulmonary edema
• congestive heart failure
• osteodystrophy
• metastatic calcium-phosphate calcifications
• aluminum intoxication
• profound neurologic impairment
• profound psychosocial disequilibrium
• abnormal protein, lipid, and carbohydrate metabolism
• accelerated atherosclerosis
• anemia

Collaborative problem: *High risk for hyperkalemia related to decreased renal excretion, metabolic acidosis, excessive dietary intake, blood transfusion, catabolism, and noncompliance with therapeutic regimen*

NURSING PRIORITY: (a) Implement measures to prevent or treat hyperkalemia, and (b) monitor their effectiveness.

Interventions

1. Monitor serum potassium daily, and notify the doctor if the level exceeds 5.5 mEq/liter.

2. Assess and report signs and symptoms of hyperkalemia — slow, irregular pulse; muscle weakness and flaccidity; diarrhea; and electrocardiographic (ECG) changes (tall, tented T wave; ST segment depression; prolonged PR interval; wide QRS complex; or cardiac standstill, indicating extreme hyperkalemia).

Rationales

1. Hyperkalemia causes adverse and even lethal physiologic effects.

2. Cardiovascular signs and symptoms are the most important physiologic indicators of the effects of hyperkalemia.

3. Implement measures to prevent or treat metabolic acidosis, as ordered, such as administering alkaline medications (for example, sodium bicarbonate) and maintenance dialysis.

3. In the acidotic state, hydrogen ions move into the cell to compensate for the acidosis; potassium ions move out of the cell and into the plasma to maintain electrochemical neutrality.

4. If blood transfusions are necessary, administer fresh packed RBCs during dialysis, as ordered.

4. In fresh blood, fewer RBCs have hemolyzed and released potassium as compared with stored blood. Dialysis removes excess potassium.

5. Decrease catabolism by encouraging the patient to consume prescribed amounts of dietary protein and carbohydrates, by treating infections, and by decreasing fever.

5. Catabolism causes release of intracellular potassium into the plasma. Appropriate intake of dietary protein reduces breakdown of the body's cells. Infections and fever increase the metabolic rate and can lead to a catabolic state.

6. Encourage compliance with the therapeutic regimen.

6. Dietary noncompliance can result in excessive potassium intake; noncompliance with the dialysis regimen causes hyperkalemia from decreased removal of potassium.

7. Implement and evaluate therapy for hyperkalemia, as ordered:

- sodium bicarbonate I.V.

- hypertonic glucose and insulin I.V.

- calcium lactate or calcium gluconate I.V.

- cation-exchange resin (such as Kayexalate)

- dialysis.

7. Rationales for hyperkalemia therapy include the following:

- Sodium bicarbonate helps correct acidosis and causes potassium to shift from the plasma back into the cells.
- Hypertonic glucose and insulin cause potassium to move from the extracellular to the intracellular space.
- Calcium antagonizes potassium and reduces its potentially deleterious effects on the cardiac conduction system.
- This medication exchanges sodium for potassium and increases potassium excretion through the intestines.
- Dialysis rapidly and efficiently removes potassium from the blood.

8. Monitor serial serum potassium levels and ECG readings for signs of hypokalemia during treatment.

8. Overtreatment of hyperkalemia may result in hypokalemia.

9. Additional individualized interventions: _____

9. Rationales: _____

Target outcome criteria
Within 2 hours after treatment is initiated, the patient will:
- maintain serum potassium levels within a range of 3.5 to 5.5 mEq/liter
- exhibit no signs of hyperkalemia on ECG
- have an arterial pH of 7.35 to 7.45 and a venous CO_2 of 22 to 25 mEq/liter (or as defined as acceptable for the patient).

By the time of discharge, the patient will demonstrate ability to plan a 3-day diet incorporating potassium restrictions and other dietary requirements.

Collaborative problem: *High risk for pericarditis, pericardial effusion, and pericardial tamponade related to uremia or inadequate dialysis*

NURSING PRIORITY: Detect complications and intervene promptly to maintain hemodynamic status.

Interventions

1. Assess for signs and symptoms of pericarditis daily: fever, chest pain, and pericardial friction rub. Report their occurrence to the doctor.

Rationales

1. Of CRF patients on dialysis, 30% to 50% develop uremic pericarditis; the classic triad of fever, chest pain, and pericardial friction rub is the hallmark of this condition.

2. If signs and symptoms of pericarditis are present, collaborate with the nephrology team to assess the adequacy of dialysis and increase frequency as necessary and as ordered.

3. If signs and symptoms of pericarditis are present, assess for signs and symptoms of pericardial effusion and tamponade every 4 hours, as follows:
• Palpate peripheral pulses for rate, quality, waxing, and waning.
• Assess for paradoxical pulse greater than 10 mm Hg.
• Assess for peripheral edema.
• Assess for decrease in sensorium.
• Assess for profound hypotension, narrow pulse pressure, weak or absent peripheral pulses, cold and poorly perfused extremities, rapid decrease in sensorium, and bulging neck veins (signs of rapidly occurring large tamponade).

4. If tamponade develops, prepare the patient for emergency pericardial aspiration.

5. Encourage compliance with the therapeutic regimen.

6. Additional individualized interventions: _____

_____

2. Inadequate dialysis, with subsequent uremic toxin accumulation, is one cause of pericarditis; intense dialysis therapy is the usual treatment.

3. Pericardial effusion is a common complication of pericarditis that can lead to tamponade, a life-threatening condition. Signs and symptoms vary from mild compromise of cardiac output with small effusion to severely compromised hemodynamic status in tamponade.
   To assess paradoxical pulse, place a blood pressure cuff on the patient's arm and instruct the patient to breathe normally. Inflate the cuff above the systolic level. Slowly deflate the cuff and note the systolic pressure on expiration. Wait, reinflate the cuff, and deflate it again, this time noting the systolic pressure on inspiration. The difference between the two readings is the paradoxical pulse. A paradoxical pulse of 10 mm Hg or less indicates a normal blood pressure response to inspiration. A value greater than 10 mm Hg indicates an exaggerated response to inspiration typical of cardiac tamponade.

4. The mortality rate in tamponade is 95%. Immediate aspiration of fluid from the pericardial cavity is essential to restore cardiac function and hemodynamic status.

5. Dialysis removes uremic toxins that can cause pericarditis. Dialysis combined with fluid restriction reduces the risk of effusion.

6. Rationales: _____

_____

Target outcome criteria
With adequate treatment, the patient will exhibit relief of pericarditis, maintenance of hemodynamic status, and prevention of complications as evidenced by:
• blood pressure within defined parameters
• strong, regular peripheral pulses
• normal heart sounds (strong, readily audible apical impulse without friction rub)
• normal temperature

• maintenance of alert and oriented (or usual) mental status
• maintenance of usual respiratory status
• absent or decreased peripheral edema
• ECG without evidence of pericarditis
• maintenance of usual energy level.

Collaborative problem: *Hypertension related to sodium and water retention and malfunction of the renin-angiotensin-aldosterone system*

NURSING PRIORITY: Implement the therapeutic regimen and patient teaching to control hypertension.

Interventions

1. Administer antihypertensive medications, as ordered, and assess for desired and adverse effects. Reassure the patient that some adverse effects may decrease once the body adjusts to the medication.

Rationales

1. Antihypertensive medications are an essential part of treatment for CRF. Antihypertensives act by vasodilation, beta-adrenergic blocking, or angiotensin blocking. Reassurance helps prevent noncompliance from initial adverse effects.

2. Measure blood pressure at various times of the day with the patient supine, sitting, and standing. Record blood pressure readings on a flow sheet to correlate the influence of time of day, positioning, medications, diet, and weight. Teach the patient to measure blood pressure and pulse rate.

2. Blood pressure measurements commonly vary throughout the day and in relation to medication administration, diet, weight, and positioning. Excessive doses of antihypertensives or dehydration can cause orthostatic hypotension.

3. Teach the patient how to avoid orthostatic hypotension by changing position slowly, such as sitting for 5 minutes when changing from a supine to a standing position.

3. Orthostatic hypotension may cause falls and injuries. Medication noncompliance may result if the patient is unable to prevent orthostatic hypotension.

4. Encourage compliance with therapy.

4. Dialysis removes sodium and water and controls vascular volume; diet restrictions prevent excessive sodium and fluid intake.

5. Instruct the patient to report any changes that may indicate fluid overload, hypertensive encephalopathy, or vision changes. These include periorbital, sacral, or peripheral edema; headaches; seizures; and blurred vision.

5. These signs and symptoms may indicate poor control of hypertension and the need to alter therapy.

6. Recognize the significance of funduscopic changes reported on medical or nursing examination: arteriovenous nicking, exudates, hemorrhages, and papilledema.

6. These conditions suggest uncontrolled hypertension and the need to reevaluate the therapeutic regimen.

7. Additional individualized interventions: _____

7. Rationales: _____

Target outcome criteria
Throughout the hospital stay, the patient will:
• exhibit blood pressure within defined limits
• show no hypertensive complications.

By the time of discharge, the patient will demonstrate ability to measure blood pressure and pulse rate.

Collaborative problem: *Anemia related to decreased life span of RBCs in CRF, bleeding, decreased production of erythropoietin and RBCs, and blood loss during hemodialysis*

NURSING PRIORITIES: (a) Stabilize the RBC count and (b) maximize tissue perfusion.

Interventions

1. Assess daily the degree of anemia (as reflected by hemoglobin level, hematocrit, and RBC count) and its physiologic effects, such as fatigue, pallor, dyspnea, palpitations, ecchymoses, and tachycardia.

2. Administer the following as ordered, and assess for desired and adverse effects: iron and folic acid supplements, androgens, vitamin B complex, vitamin C, and epoietin alfa (Epogen). Do not administer folic acid and vitamins during dialysis or iron with phosphate binders.

3. Assist the patient to develop an activity and exercise schedule, with regular rest periods, to avoid undue fatigue.

Rationales

1. The severity of anemia and its physiologic effects vary. The therapeutic plan is based on anemia's effects on the individual patient.

2. Iron, folic acid, and vitamins are required for RBC production, but are commonly deficient in the CRF patient's diet. Androgens help stabilize the RBC count. Like endogenous erythropoietin, epoietin alfa (erythropoietin produced through recombinant DNA techniques) stimulates red blood cell production. However, the patient's iron stores must be adequate for epoietin alfa to be effective. Dialysis removes folic acid and vitamins. Phosphate binders decrease iron absorption.

3. Decreased hemoglobin decreases tissue oxygenation and increases fatigue. A carefully developed activity and exercise plan can lessen fatigue and allow the patient to perform activities of daily living (ADLs).

4. Avoid taking unnecessary blood specimens.

4. Frequent collection of blood specimens worsens anemia.

5. Instruct the patient how to prevent bleeding: using a soft toothbrush, avoiding vigorous nose blowing, preventing constipation, and avoiding contact sports.

5. Bleeding from any site worsens anemia.

6. Administer blood transfusions as indicated and ordered.

6. Blood transfusions are administered only when the patient becomes symptomatic with low hematocrit; frequent blood transfusions suppress RBC production even further. Fresh packed RBCs are administered during dialysis, as noted previously.

7. Additional individualized interventions: _____

7. Rationales: _____

Target outcome criteria
Throughout the hospital stay, the patient will:
• maintain a stable hematocrit within a defined range, usually 20% to 25%
• exhibit symptomatic relief of the effects of anemia
• verbalize ways to protect self from trauma
• perform ADLs without undue fatigue.

Collaborative problem: *High risk for osteodystrophy and metastatic calcifications related to hyperphosphatemia, hypocalcemia, abnormal vitamin D metabolism, hyperparathyroidism, and elevated aluminum levels*

NURSING PRIORITY: Minimize bone demineralization and metastatic calcifications.

Interventions

1. Administer phosphate binders, calcium supplements, and vitamin D supplements, as ordered, and assess their effects:
• Weekly, monitor serum levels of calcium, phosphate, alkaline phosphatase, aluminum, and calcium-phosphate product; report abnormal findings to the doctor.
• Monitor X-rays for bone fractures and joint deposits.
• Weekly, palpate joints for enlargement, swelling, and tenderness.
• Weekly, inspect the patient's gait, range of motion in joints, and muscle strength.

Rationales

1. In renal failure, the decreased glomerular filtration rate causes phosphate retention and hyperphosphatemia; plasma calcium levels decrease to compensate. Decreased vitamin D metabolism by the kidneys decreases calcium absorption from the GI tract. The decrease in plasma calcium levels stimulates production of parathyroid hormone, which causes reabsorption of calcium and phosphate from the bones and eventual bone demineralization.

As plasma calcium and phosphate levels rise, the plasma calcium phosphate product level also rises; the excess calcium phosphate is deposited as metastatic calcifications in joints, soft tissue, eyes, heart, and brain. These metastatic calcifications decrease function of the involved organs. Administering phosphate binders, such as aluminum hydroxide (Amphojel), aluminum carbonate (Basaljel), or calcium carbonate (Phos-ex), with meals binds phosphate in the GI tract and decreases its absorption. Calcium and vitamin D supplements help support normal plasma calcium levels.

Excess aluminum (absorbed from phosphate binders and from high levels of aluminum in water used to prepare dialysate) is deposited into the bones and exacerbates osteodystrophy.

2. With the patient, develop an activity and exercise schedule to avoid immobilization.

2. Immobilization increases bone demineralization.

3. Daily, question the patient about signs and symptoms of hypocalcemia: numbness, tingling, and twitching of fingertips and toes; carpopedal spasms; seizures; and confusion.

3. Hypocalcemia causes nervous system irritability and alters nerve conduction. The signs and symptoms listed indicate tetany, hypocalcemia's most obvious manifestation.

4. Monitor each ECG (or ECG report) for prolonged QT interval, irritable arrhythmias, and atrioventricular conduction defects.

4. Hypocalcemia can alter normal cardiac electrical conduction.

5. Daily, assess for positive Chvostek's and Trousseau's signs. See Appendix C, "Fluid and Electrolyte Imbalances," for details.

5. Positive Chvostek's and Trousseau's signs indicate hypocalcemia.

6. Encourage the patient to comply with therapy.

6. Dialysis, medications, and diet work together to maintain acceptable calcium-phosphate balance.

7. Additional individualized interventions: _____

7. Rationales: _____

Target outcome criteria

Throughout the hospital stay, the patient will:
• exhibit serum calcium, phosphorus, alkaline phosphatase, aluminum, and calcium-phosphate product levels within an acceptable range
• exhibit minimal bone demineralization on bone scan

• exhibit minimal calcium-phosphate deposits
• show no signs or symptoms of hypocalcemia
• maintain a safe, painless level of activity.

Nursing diagnosis: *High risk for nutritional deficit related to anorexia, nausea, vomiting, diarrhea, restricted dietary intake, GI inflammation with poor absorption, and altered metabolism of proteins, lipids, and carbohydrates*

NURSING PRIORITY: Maintain acceptable nutritional status.

Interventions

1. Assess nutritional status on admission by determining weight in relation to height and body build; serum albumin, protein, cholesterol, and transferrin values; triceps skinfold thickness; degree of weakness and fatigue; dietary intake; and history of anorexia, nausea, vomiting, and diarrhea.

2. Weigh the patient daily, comparing actual and ideal body weights. Be sure to consider the effect of excess fluid on actual weight by comparing the current weight with nonedematous weight (500 ml fluid = 1 lb body weight). Teach the patient to measure weight under consistent conditions, to maintain a weight record, and to maintain an intake and output record.

3. Encourage the patient to eat the maximum amount of nutrients allowed. Encourage compliance with the dialysis regimen.

4. Encourage intake of foods high in calories from carbohydrates and low in protein, potassium, sodium, and water. Provide related teaching, including planning of food and fluid intake.

5. As necessary, consult with a dietitian to find ways to include the patient's preferences in the prescribed diet.

6. Implement interventions to reduce nausea and vomiting, diarrhea or constipation, and stomatitis.

Rationales

1. A baseline assessment is necessary to monitor progress and the need to modify the patient's diet.

2. Achieving ideal body weight is the goal. If the patient is at less than ideal body weight, additional calories may be added to the diet; if above ideal body weight, calorie restriction may be necessary.

3. Diet and dialysis must complement each other to minimize toxin accumulation and maintain fluid and electrolyte and acid-base balance.

4. High-carbohydrate foods provide calories for energy and allow storage of dietary proteins. Restriction of potassium, sodium, and water is necessary to prevent electrolyte imbalances and volume overload. Protein is restricted to control the degree of uremia.

5. Including preferred foods makes the diet more palatable and increases dietary compliance.

6. These conditions commonly result in anorexia or decreased GI absorption of nutrients.

7. Monitor BUN, serum creatinine, sodium, potassium, albumin, and total protein levels as indicators of dietary adequacy and compliance with dietary restrictions. (Consult with the doctor regarding appropriate laboratory values for the patient.)

7. BUN levels may be elevated from excessive dietary protein; serum creatinine levels may be elevated from inadequate dietary protein and subsequent muscle breakdown; serum albumin levels are decreased in the malnourished patient; serum sodium and potassium levels are elevated by excessive intake. Appropriate laboratory values vary depending on the type of dialysis and other therapeutic measures, and so must be determined for the individual patient.

8. Additional individualized interventions: _____

8. Rationales: _____

Target outcome criteria
During the hospital stay, the patient will:
• maintain weight within 2 lb (5 kg) of ideal body weight
• exhibit BUN, serum sodium, potassium, albumin, and total protein levels within acceptable limits
• maintain pre-illness pattern of elimination.

By the time of discharge, the patient will:
• plan a 3-day dietary intake (including fluid)
• demonstrate ability to weigh self and to maintain weight and intake and output records.

Nursing diagnosis: *High risk for altered oral mucous membrane and unpleasant taste related to accumulation of urea and ammonia*

NURSING PRIORITY: (a) Maintain intact oral mucous membrane and (b) relieve unpleasant taste.

Interventions

1. On admission, inspect oral mucous membrane for ulcers and bleeding.

2. Teach the patient an appropriate mouth care regimen that includes rinsing with a pleasant-tasting or dilute vinegar mouthwash as needed, using a soft toothbrush to clean teeth at least twice daily, sucking sour candies or lemon wedges as needed, and drinking cool liquids (within fluid restrictions).

3. Encourage the patient to comply with therapy.

4. Additional individualized interventions: _____

Rationales

1. Early detection and treatment can lessen consequences of severe stomatitis. (Excessive uremic toxins cause stomatitis.)

2. Mouthwash decreases unpleasant taste and halitosis. Vinegar achieves the same results by neutralizing ammonia. A soft toothbrush reduces the risk of bleeding, and frequent mouth care decreases bacterial growth and the chance of infection. Sour candies or lemon wedges improve taste in the mouth while decreasing thirst.

3. Dialysis removes uremic toxins, which are partly responsible for stomatitis.

4. Rationales: _____

Target outcome criteria
Throughout the hospital stay, the patient will:
• present clean, moist oral mucous membrane without ulcers, bleeding, or signs of infection
• report pleasant taste and sensation in mouth.

Collaborative problem: *High risk for peripheral neuropathy related to effects of uremia, fluid and electrolyte imbalances, and acid-base imbalances on the peripheral nervous system*

NURSING PRIORITY: Ameliorate effects of peripheral neuropathy.

Interventions

1. On admission, have a physical therapist assess muscle strength, gait, and degree of neuromuscular impairment.

2. In collaboration with a physical therapist, help the patient develop an activity and exercise regimen.

3. Guard against leg and foot trauma.

4. Administer analgesics as ordered and indicated; observe for desired effects.

5. Encourage the patient to comply with therapy.

6. Additional individualized interventions: _____

Rationales

1. A baseline assessment is essential for devising an individualized activity and exercise schedule.

2. Regular activity and exercise prevent the hazards of immobility.

3. With decreased peripheral sensation, the patient may be unaware of impending trauma.

4. Analgesics may be necessary for severe pain; if the medication ordered is excreted by the kidneys, observe for toxic effects.

5. Dialysis removes uremic toxins and improves fluid and electrolyte and acid-base balance.

6. Rationales: _____

Target outcome criterion
Throughout the hospital stay, the patient will ambulate and carry out ADLs safely and comfortably.

Nursing diagnosis: *High risk for impaired skin integrity related to decreased activity of oil and sweat glands, scratching, capillary fragility, abnormal blood clotting, anemia, retention of pigments, and calcium phosphate deposits on the skin*

NURSING PRIORITIES: (a) Maintain intact skin and (b) relieve dryness and itching.

Interventions

1. On admission and twice daily, assess skin for color, turgor, ecchymoses, texture, and edema.

2. Keep the skin clean while relieving dryness and itching using superfatted soap, oatmeal baths, and bath oils; apply lotion daily and as needed, especially while the skin is still moist after bathing.

3. Keep the patient's nails trimmed.

4. Monitor serum calcium and phosphorus levels weekly.

5. Administer phosphate binders, as ordered.

6. Administer antipruritic medications as indicated and ordered; assess effects.

Rationales

1. A baseline assessment is essential for developing an individualized skin care plan. Regular follow-up assessments allow modification as necessary.

2. These measures help relieve dry skin. Applying lotion immediately after bathing helps the skin retain moisture. Itching decreases when the skin is kept moist; decreased itching prevents scratching and subsequent skin excoriation.

3. Trimming prevents excoriation from scratching.

4. Excess calcium phosphate deposited in the skin causes dryness and itching.

5. These medications decrease serum phosphate levels and thus lessen irritating deposits in the skin.

6. These medications are indicated in severe pruritus when other measures are not effective.

RENAL DISORDERS

7. Encourage the patient to comply with therapy.

7. Dialysis removes uremic toxins that dry and irritate the skin and helps normalize serum calcium and phosphorus levels.

8. Additional individualized interventions: _____

8. Rationales: _____

Target outcome criteria
Throughout the hospital stay, the patient will:
• present intact, clean, infection-free skin
• exhibit relief from dryness and itching.

Nursing diagnosis: *High risk for altered thought processes related to the effects of uremic toxins, acidosis, fluid and electrolyte imbalances, and hypoxia on the central nervous system*

NURSING PRIORITY: Protect the patient from neurologic complications.

Interventions

1. On admission and daily, assess the patient's thought processes. With assistance from the family, compare current findings with premorbid intellectual status.

2. Alter communication methods as needed.

3. Minimize environmental stimuli. Alter the environment as needed to ensure the patient's safety.

4. Do not administer opiates or barbiturates.

5. Encourage the patient to comply with therapy.

6. Additional individualized interventions: _____

Rationales

1. The premorbid status provides guidelines for establishing realistic goals. Ongoing assessment allows prompt detection of any changes and modification of treatment as needed.

2. The patient will typically require short periods of simple communication, responding best to direct questions.

3. Excessive environmental stimuli may cause sensory overload and disorientation. The patient usually functions best in a consistently quiet, organized environment that is free from hazards.

4. Opiates and barbiturates have an increased half-life in renal failure. Mental status worsens as a result.

5. Dietary restrictions and dialysis are essential to control uremic toxin buildup and fluid and electrolyte and acid-base balance, and to reduce the risk of adverse effects on the central nervous system.

6. Rationales: _____

Target outcome criteria
By the time of discharge, the patient will:
• show improved memory and reasoning ability
• show an increased interest in ADLs

• present no neurologic complications such as seizures and encephalopathy.

Nursing diagnosis: *High risk for noncompliance related to knowledge deficit; lack of resources; adverse effects of diet, dialysis, and medications; denial; and poor relationships with health care providers*

NURSING PRIORITY: Help the patient make informed choices about compliance and noncompliance.

Interventions	Rationales
1. Clarify the patient's understanding of the therapeutic regimen and the consequences of noncompliance.	1. In many cases, noncompliance results from the patient's lack of understanding about the nature of the disease and the objectives of therapy.
2. Assess for physiologic, psychological, social, and cultural factors that could contribute to noncompliance. Explore ways to alter treatment to fit the patient's social and cultural beliefs.	2. Many patients deny that they have a chronic, irreversible illness. Compliance is more likely if treatment is congruent with the patient's beliefs.
3. Teach the patient about the therapeutic regimen, including medications, common problems related to CRF and their management, and plans for follow-up care. Clarify areas of misunderstanding in relation to the disease and therapeutic regimen. Allow the patient to make as many informed decisions and choices from as many alternatives as possible.	3. The patient is more likely to comply if encouraged to participate in decision making and allowed maximum independence. Thus, each patient requires an individualized plan of care that considers physiologic, psychosocial, and cultural factors and the patient's desires.
4. Additional individualized interventions: _____	4. Rationales: _____

Target outcome criteria

Throughout the hospital stay, the patient will:
• verbalize knowledge of the therapeutic regimen
• verbalize willingness to follow the therapeutic regimen or a realistic treatment alternative more in keeping with personal beliefs and life-style.

By the time of discharge, the patient will:
• explain the cause and implications of the disease
• name each medication and its dosage, interval, desired effects, and adverse effects
• describe associated problems, how to manage them, and when to report them
• explain the plan for follow-up care.

Nursing diagnosis: *High risk for sexual dysfunction related to the effects of uremia on the endocrine and nervous systems and to the psychosocial impact of CRF and its treatment*

NURSING PRIORITY: Help the patient and spouse (or partner) achieve satisfying sexual expression.

Interventions	Rationales
1. Discuss with the patient and spouse (or partner) the meaning of sexuality and reproduction to them, how changes in sexual functioning affect masculine and feminine roles, and mutual goals for their sexual functioning.	1. Sexuality and reproduction assume different levels of significance at various stages of maturity and at various times during CRF. Sex drive varies from person to person; therefore, sexuality and reproduction are very personal experiences. Sexual dysfunction affects sex role in many ways, based on past experiences and future expectations. Thus, the nurse must explore sexuality with the couple to establish baseline data and to determine their mutual goals.
2. Evaluate the couple's receptiveness to learning, and discuss alternative methods of sexual expression.	2. If impotence or decreased libido is present or if intercourse causes fatigue, and if the couple is receptive to experimentation, then fellatio, cunnilingus, or mutual masturbation may provide sexual gratification.

3. Emphasize the importance of giving and receiving love and affection as alternatives to intercourse.

3. Sexual intercourse and orgasm are not necessarily the goal of all meaningful intimate interactions: love and affection are also important in strengthening a relationship.

4. Consult with the doctor about the appropriateness of a penile prosthesis for a male patient, if indicated.

4. If a male patient cannot achieve or maintain an erection, a penile prosthesis may provide a means for successful intercourse.

5. Additional individualized interventions: _____

5. Rationales: _____

Target outcome criteria
Throughout the hospital stay, the patient will:
• express concerns about sexual and reproductive functioning with spouse or partner
• express satisfaction with sexual relationship with spouse or partner.

Nursing diagnosis: *Knowledge deficit related to vascular access care*

NURSING PRIORITY: Teach the patient about care and precautions related to vascular access.*

Interventions

1. Emphasize the patient's crucial role in protecting the vascular access.

Rationales

1. The vascular access is essential for hemodialysis. Loss of access may disrupt the dialysis schedule and require surgery.
   Various vascular access methods may be used. The most common is the internal arteriovenous (AV) fistula, an internal surgical anastomosis of an artery and vein. It usually is placed in the nondominant forearm and requires 2 to 3 months for the venous wall to thicken and the fistula to distend. The major complications are occlusion and postdialysis bleeding.
   An AV shunt is the connection of an artery and vein using two pieces of soft pliable plastic (Silastic) tubing and a polytetrafluorethylene (Teflon) connector to form an external loop. An AV shunt may be used while an internal fistula matures. The external AV shunt is rarely used because of its many complications, which include clotting, infection, and accidental separation.

2. Whether the patient has an AV shunt or an AV fistula, explain these activity restrictions for the affected extremity:
• Do not wear constrictive clothing or jewelry.
• Do not carry heavy objects.
• Do not allow blood pressure measurements.
• Do not allow venipunctures for I.V. fluids or laboratory blood specimens.
• Do not lie on the access.

2. These activities threaten the integrity of the vascular access and may cause occlusion, dislodgment, or infection.

---

*If the patient is receiving peritoneal dialysis, consult the "Peritoneal Dialysis" plan, page 587.

3. If the patient has an internal AV fistula, teach these additional measures:
- Assess patency daily by feeling for pulsation at the anastomosis site.

- If pulsation is absent, contact a nephrology professional immediately.
- If a pressure dressing is applied after dialysis, remove it after 4 hours.

- Check needle insertion sites for bleeding for 4 hours after dialysis, or longer if bleeding occurs.

4. If the patient has an external shunt, teach these additional measures:
- Check shunt patency every 4 hours by examining the shunt for the presence of bright red blood and by feeling above the venous side of the shunt for a thrill.

- If blood in the shunt has separated into serum and fibrin strands or if a thrill is absent, contact a nephrology nurse or nephrologist immediately.
- Perform daily AV shunt care according to the dialysis unit protocol.
- At the time of AV shunt care, check insertion sites for redness, swelling, or drainage. Report any of these signs to the doctor.
- After AV shunt care, apply a sterile dressing and wrap gauze securely (but not tightly) around the extremity. Clip two bulldog clamps to the edge of the gauze dressing.
- Do not pull on the tubing.

- If the shunt separates, use bulldog clamps to clamp the arterial side of the shunt first and then the venous side; reconnect the tubing and remove the clamps. Notify the doctor.
- If the shunt dislodges, apply firm pressure about ¾" (2 cm) above the exit site. If bleeding is minimal and stops, notify nephrologist about dislodgment. If bleeding is profuse or continues, go immediately to the emergency department.

5. Additional individualized interventions: _____

_____

3. These interventions apply only to an internal fistula.

- Because the fistula is internal, patency cannot be determined visually. Pulsation is caused by the surge of arterial blood into the vein to which the artery has been anastomosed.

- Loss of pulsation implies impending loss of patency. A clotted fistula may require surgery.
- Direct pressure on the venipuncture sites is necessary to control bleeding. Usually 10 minutes of firm finger pressure is sufficient, but at times a pressure dressing may be applied. If left on too long, a pressure dressing may cause occlusion.
- Because the patient is heparinized during hemodialysis, bleeding may occur after dialysis.

4. These interventions apply only to an external shunt.

- The shunt is wrapped with a gauze dressing between dialyses, with a small loop left accessible under the edge of the dressing. The presence of bright red blood and a thrill confirm shunt patency.
- A clot must be removed immediately to salvage the vascular access. Only a doctor or a specially trained nurse should remove a clot.
- Details of shunt care vary among institutions. Follow your institution's recommended protocol.
- These are signs of infection, a common problem. Unless treated promptly, site infection may lead to septicemia and the loss of the AV shunt.
- The dressing protects the tubing from separating or being dislodged. Bulldog clamps must be immediately accessible at all times in case of shunt separation.
- Pulling on the tubing can cause skin erosion and accidental separation or dislodgment of the shunt. If a shunt separates, the patient can bleed to death within a few minutes.
- Because arterial pressure is higher than venous pressure, more blood can be lost from the arterial side of the shunt. Immediately clamping both lines minimizes blood loss and facilitates reconnection.
- Usually, the elasticity of blood vessels allows them to seal the openings remaining after shunt dislodgment. If bleeding is profuse or continues, however, sutures may be required.

5. Rationales: _____

_____

RENAL DISORDERS

Target outcome criteria
Throughout the hospital stay, the patient will:
- describe all protective measures appropriate to the particular vascular access
- correctly demonstrate the procedure for checking shunt or fistula patency
- describe specific measures to control bleeding

- state how to contact a nephrology professional
- demonstrate daily care for an external AV shunt, if appropriate
- state three signs of infection related to an AV shunt.

Discharge planning

NURSING DISCHARGE CRITERIA

Upon the patient's discharge, documentation shows evidence of:
- ability to perform care of the shunt or fistula
- vital signs within expected parameters
- stable nutritional status
- intact skin
- ability to control pain using oral medications
- acceptable hemoglobin levels
- absence of pulmonary complications
- absence of cardiovascular complications
- ability to comply with and tolerate diet and fluid restrictions
- weight within expected parameters
- home support adequate to ensure compliance with therapy or appropriate referrals made for follow-up care
- appropriate activity tolerance
- absence of fever and other signs of infection
- ability to manage ADLs.

PATIENT-FAMILY TEACHING CHECKLIST

Document evidence that the patient and family demonstrate an understanding of:
___ cause and implications of renal failure
___ purpose of dialysis
___ all discharge medications' purpose, dosage, administration schedule, desired effects, and adverse effects (usual discharge medications include antihypertensives, phosphate binders, calcium, vitamin D, folic acid, iron, vitamins B and C, and others, depending on patient's response to the disease)
___ recommended diet and fluid modifications
___ common problems related to CRF and their management
___ care of the shunt or fistula (if receiving hemodialysis)
___ how to obtain and record weights
___ how to measure and record blood pressure and pulse rate
___ how to maintain an intake and output record
___ problems to report to health care provider
___ financial and community resources to assist with treatment of CRF
___ dialysis schedule, location of dialysis facility, and day and time of appointments
___ resources for counseling
___ how to contact the doctor or nephrology nurse.

DOCUMENTATION CHECKLIST

Using outcome criteria as a guide, document:
___ clinical status on admission
___ significant changes in status
___ pertinent laboratory and diagnostic test findings
___ response to medication
___ physical and psychological response to dialysis
___ nutritional intake
___ activity and exercise tolerance
___ ability to perform self-care
___ compliance with therapy
___ patient-family teaching
___ postdischarge referrals and plans for long-term and follow-up care.

ASSOCIATED PLANS OF CARE

Anemia
Dying
Grieving
Ineffective Individual Coping
Knowledge Deficit
Pain
Peritoneal Dialysis

References

Kneisl, C.R., and Ames, S.A. *Adult Health Nursing: A Biopsychosocial Approach.* Reading, Mass.: Addison-Wesley Publishing Co., 1986.

Lancaster, L.E., ed. *Core Curriculum for Nephrology Nursing,* 2nd ed. Pitman, N.J.: American Nephrology Nurse's Association, 1991.

Lancaster, L.E. "Renal Failure: Pathophysiology, Assessment, and Intervention," *Critical Care Nursing* 2(1):38-40, January/February 1982.

Lancaster, L.E., ed. *The Patient With End Stage Renal Disease,* 2nd ed. New York: John Wiley & Sons, 1984.

Richard, C.J. *Comprehensive Nephrology Nursing.* Boston: Little, Brown & Co., 1986.

Ileal Conduit Urinary Diversion

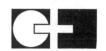

DRG information

DRG 303 Kidney, Ureter, and Major Bladder Procedure
for Neoplasm.
Mean LOS = 11.9 days
DRG 304 Kidney, Ureter, and Major Bladder Procedure
for Non-neoplasm. With Complication or Comorbidity (CC).
Mean LOS = 10.3 days
DRG 305 Kidney, Ureter, and Major Bladder Procedure
for Non-neoplasm. Without CC.
Mean LOS = 5.5 days

Introduction
DEFINITION AND TIME FOCUS

An ileal conduit urinary diversion, also known as a
urostomy or Bricker procedure, is the most common
urinary diversion procedure for adults. It is usually
performed with a cystectomy and involves isolating a
6″ to 8″ (15 to 20 cm) segment of the terminal ileum,
with its mesentery intact, then reanastomosing the GI
tract. The proximal end of the isolated ileal segment is
sutured closed, and the distal end of the ileal segment
is brought out through the right lower abdominal quadrant and everted to form a stoma. The ureters are implanted into the body of the ileal segment, which then
becomes a conduit for urine. Other segments of the
small or large intestine can be used as conduits for
urinary diversion, especially if the ileum has been
damaged by radiation. Ileal conduit urinary diversion
is most commonly performed for transitional cell cancer of the bladder; however, in rare instances, it may
also be done for other conditions requiring total cystectomy, such as severe trauma to the bladder or persistent, severe urinary tract infections. This plan
focuses on the immediate preoperative and postoperative care of a patient undergoing ileal conduit diversion for transitional cell cancer of the bladder.

ETIOLOGY AND PRECIPITATING FACTORS

• transitional cell carcinoma of the bladder requiring
cystectomy—that is, lesions unresponsive to conservative treatment, lesions at or near the bladder neck in
the female, or deep infiltrating tumors that may involve the lymphatic system

Focused assessment guidelines
NURSING HISTORY (Functional health pattern findings)

Health perception—health management pattern
• may report sudden onset of gross painless hematuria;
may be intermittent

• may have been under treatment for transitional cell
carcinoma of the bladder (being followed by cystoscopy
every 3 to 6 months)
• may have history of intravesical instillations of chemotherapeutic agents, such as thiotepa (Thiotepa), mitomycin C (Mutamycin), or doxorubicin (Adriamycin),
after transurethral resection of a bladder tumor, or
may have received intravesical Bacillus Calmette-Guérin (BCG; TheraCys) as prophylactic treatment
against tumor recurrence
• may have received preoperative radiation therapy to
shrink the tumor and reduce spread at the time of surgery.
• may have received limited information from physician about upcoming urinary diversion surgery and its
effects on activities of daily living (ADLs)
• if 50 to 70 years old and male, at increased risk
• may be cigarette smoker (increases risk of bladder
cancer)

Elimination pattern
• may have a history of urinary urgency or frequency
for 3 to 8 months before diagnosis of transitional cell
carcinoma of bladder
• may currently have cystitis as an adverse effect of
intravesical chemotherapy

Sleep-rest pattern
• may report sleep disturbances from nocturia

Self-perception—self-concept pattern
• typically expresses negative feelings about self along
with anger; disappointment; fear of pain, mutilation,
and loss of control; and distaste for altered bodily
functions

Role-relationship pattern
• may have occupational exposure to dust and fumes
from dyes, rubber, leather, leather products, paint, or
organic chemicals (increases risk of bladder cancer)
• usually concerned about spouse's or partner's adjustment to ostomy and possibility that ostomy may
change that person's feelings toward the patient

Coping—stress tolerance pattern
• if diagnosis of bladder cancer is recent, patient may
focus concerns on cancer treatment, and not on the
creation of an ostomy

Value-belief pattern
• may have delayed seeking medical attention because
of fear combined with embarrassment over the intimate nature of problem

PHYSICAL FINDINGS

Note: Transitional cell carcinoma may be asymptomatic except for the following genitourinary symptoms.

Genitourinary

• gross hematuria
• urgency, frequency, and dysuria unrelieved by antibiotics

DIAGNOSTIC STUDIES

• complete blood count — drop in hematocrit and hemoglobin may indicate internal bleeding; elevated white blood cell count may signify beginning of infection or abscess
• electrolyte panel — monitors fluid status and acid-base balance
• serum creatinine, and blood urea nitrogen levels — used to monitor renal function
• preoperative intravenous pyelogram (IVP) — helpful in evaluating upper urinary tract functioning: size and location of kidneys, filling of the renal pelvis, and outline of ureters
• postoperative conduitogram or loopogram — assesses length and emptying ability of the conduit along with the presence or absence of stricture, reflux, angulation, or obstruction
• X-ray of kidneys, ureter, and bladder — indicates structural changes in the urinary tract along with presence or absence of stool or gas in GI tract

POTENTIAL COMPLICATIONS

• peritonitis
• leakage at point of GI anastomosis
• leakage at proximal end of the conduit
• ureteral leakage
• abscess formation
• thrombophlebitis
• stoma necrosis
• ureteral obstruction from edema or mucus
• wound dehiscence
• small-bowel obstruction
• pneumonia
• ileus
• atelectasis
• wound infection
• mucocutaneous separation around stoma

Nursing diagnosis: *Knowledge deficit related to an ileal conduit*

NURSING PRIORITY: Prepare the patient physically and emotionally for upcoming urinary tract alterations.

Interventions

1. Assess what the patient already knows about the upcoming cystectomy and creation of an ileal conduit from information the doctor has provided or from someone who has had an ostomy.

2. Assess the patient's ability to learn. Check occupation, level of education, and hobbies, and note if the patient may have difficulty learning.

3. Assess the patient's manual dexterity and visual acuity, and determine if any sensory deficits are present. Enlist the help of a family member, if possible and appropriate. Allow the patient to see and handle a pouch at eye level before surgery.

4. Inquire about the patient's past and recent fluid intake habits, especially quantity and preferred types of fluids.

5. Describe construction of the conduit, the rationale for bowel preparation, and normal stoma characteristics.

Rationales

1. The patient may have received limited or confusing information from the doctor. If the patient has known anyone with an ostomy, impressions gained from that person will strongly influence personal expectations of surgery and adaptation to the ostomy.

2. Learning difficulties, especially reduced reading ability, will affect the strategy and literature used to teach ostomy care.

3. Degree of dexterity will affect the patient's ability to care for the stoma and apply a pouch effectively. If the patient cannot care for the stoma, a family member is the best substitute. Handling the pouch before surgery increases later adaptation.

4. Inadequate fluid intake may cause odor problems from urine concentration and peristomal skin problems from dehydration.

5. The patient should know that an ileal conduit is not a substitute bladder. Bowel preparation usually consists of 2 to 3 days of clear liquids by mouth only, a bowel-cleansing oral liquid, and erythromycin (Erythrocin) and neomycin (Mycifradin) by mouth.

6. Anticipate problems with pouch use. Assess the patient for allergies or sensitivity to tape or adhesives.

6. Any allergy to these products suggests a need to patch-test the patient for sensitivity before selecting ostomy equipment.

7. Request a doctor's order for an enterostomal (ET) nurse to mark the stoma site before surgery. This mark should place stoma away from old scars, dimples, the umbilicus, belt line, fat folds, and skin creases, and within the rectus muscle in a spot the patient can see. The stoma may be placed above the umbilicus in an obese or wheelchair-bound patient.

7. The stoma should be marked where the pouch will have an optimal seal, giving the patient some sense of control. Placing the stoma within the rectus muscle reduces the risk of hernia or prolapse. To achieve independence, the patient must be able to see the stoma.

8. If the patient is male, discuss what effect the cystectomy may have on sexual functioning. Promise future help in this area if the patient needs it.

8. Informed legal consent includes the male patient's understanding that erectile dysfunction can be expected along with ejaculatory incompetence. It is important to give the patient "permission" to discuss sexual concerns.

9. Additional individualized interventions: _____

9. Rationales: _____

Target outcome criterion
Before surgery, the patient will verbalize understanding of upcoming surgery and its expected effects on ADLs.

Collaborative problem: *High risk for postoperative peritonitis related to GI or genitourinary anastomosis breakdown or leakage*

NURSING PRIORITY: Prevent and assess for signs of peritonitis.

Interventions

1. Monitor and document nasogastric (NG) tube patency, NG output, abdominal pain and distention, bowel sounds, and appearance of and drainage from the abdominal incision.

2. Evaluate for signs of GI anastomosis leakage and peritonitis, such as paralytic ileus and abdominal pain with muscle rigidity, vomiting, and leukocytosis.

3. Monitor for signs of urine leakage. Assess carefully for pouch leakage to allow for accurate output measurement. Document characteristics of urine output and presence of ureteral stents or catheters. When changing pouch (if necessary because of leakage), observe that urine is dripping from *each* stent. Also note abdominal wound drainage, abdominal tenderness or distention, bowel sounds, and temperature.

4. Additional individualized interventions: _____

Rationales

1. Adynamic ileus usually resolves within 72 hours after surgery. Changes in NG output, rapid abdominal distention, and crampy pain with hyperactive and tinkling bowel sounds may indicate small-bowel obstruction. Obstruction increases pressure on newly anastomosed sites.

2. A GI anastomosis is weakest until the fourth day after surgery. Leakage of intestinal secretions may result in peritonitis. I.V. fluids, electrolyte replacement, intestinal decompression, and massive doses of antibiotics are indicated if peritonitis is present.

3. Urine should be blood-tinged for only 1 to 2 days after surgery. Improper pouch fit or application can cause ongoing stomal bleeding. Ureteral stents prevent ureteral obstruction from edema or mucus; it is normal for urine to flow out around the stents. Signs of urine leakage may include a sudden decrease in urine output with a corresponding increase in drainage from the wound or a drain. Abdominal distention, an increase in abdominal pain, prolonged ileus, and fever may also indicate urine leakage. Small leaks may seal themselves within 8 to 12 hours; otherwise, surgery is needed.

4. Rationales: _____

> **Target outcome criteria**
> Within 1 to 2 days after surgery, the patient will:
> • have stabilized urine output
> • have no gross hematuria.
>
> Within 4 to 5 days after surgery, the patient will:
> • pass flatus
> • have normal bowel sounds
> • be afebrile
> • show no signs of peritonitis.

Collaborative problem: *High risk for stomal ischemia and necrosis related to vascular compromise of conduit*

NURSING PRIORITY: Monitor stoma viability.

Interventions

1. Apply a disposable transparent urinary pouch, as ordered, and attach the pouch to a bedside drainage bag.

2. Observe the stoma for color changes every 4 hours and as needed.

3. Report color change of stoma (to purple, brown, or black) immediately to the doctor.

4. To differentiate superficial ischemia from necrosis, insert a small, lubricated test tube about ½″(1.3 cm) into the stoma, then shine a flashlight into the lumen of the test tube. Observe for red, moist mucosa indicating that the body of conduit is viable.

5. Additional individualized interventions: _____

Rationales

1. A transparent pouch with continual bedside drainage allows visualization of the stoma.

2. Color changes reflect adequacy of perfusion. Stoma should stay red or pink.

3. Color changes may imply ischemia leading to a necrotic, nonviable stoma. A necrotic stoma can develop from tension on the mesentery, possibly from abdominal distention; from twisting of the conduit during surgery; or from arterial or venous insufficiency. A necrotic stoma requires surgery.

4. If the inner lumen of conduit is viable, the stoma may be showing only minimal ischemia from edema; the stoma may then change color and appear viable. A dusky stoma may slough its outer layer during the next 5 to 7 days.

5. Rationales: _____

> **Target outcome criterion**
> Within 12 to 24 hours after surgery, the patient will have a viable stoma with red, moist mucosa or a dusky stoma with a viable conduit.

Collaborative problem: *High risk for stoma retraction and mucocutaneous separation related to peristomal trauma or tension on the intestinal mesentery*

NURSING PRIORITIES: (a) Monitor the mucocutaneous border, (b) minimize the risk of separation, and (c) encourage healing.

Interventions

1. Apply a pouch with an antireflux valve, as ordered.

2. If compatible with the pouch barrier, use a skin sealant under the pouch to protect and waterproof peristomal skin.

Rationales

1. An antireflux valve promotes healing by preventing urine from pooling on the stoma and mucocutaneous border.

2. Protecting and waterproofing the peristomal skin by routinely applying a skin sealant encourages healing of the mucocutaneous border and minimizes trauma when removing the pouch.

3. If mucocutaneous separation occurs, protect the separated area and take measures to encourage granulation. Fill the mucocutaneous separation with karaya powder, then apply stoma adhesive paste and a properly sized skin barrier and pouch. Notify the surgeon of the separation.

3. Mucocutaneous separation does not usually require surgery. The measures described increase the rate of healing and provide additional support for the stoma. If, however, the stoma retracts through the fascia into the peritoneum, peritonitis may develop and surgery is essential.

4. Additional individualized interventions: _____

4. Rationales: _____

Target outcome criterion
By 5 to 7 days after surgery, the patient will have a healed mucocutaneous border around a budded stoma.

Nursing diagnosis: *Altered urinary elimination related to creation of an ileal conduit*

NURSING PRIORITIES: (a) Protect peristomal skin and contain urine, and (b) teach the patient the conduit's function and purpose.

Interventions

1. Maintain a good pouch seal, and protect peristomal skin with sealants.

2. Review the construction and function of the conduit, assuring the patient of GI tract continuity. Use diagrams and pictures.

3. Describe and show normal urine and stoma characteristics. Explain the following: The conduit and stoma are made from the GI tract, so they have the same red, moist lining as the mouth. The stoma has no sensory nerve endings, so it is insensitive to pain. Without a sphincter, voluntary control of urination is gone. The stoma is very vascular and may bleed when cleaned. The GI tract makes mucus, so mucus in the urine is to be expected.

4. Additional individualized interventions: _____

Rationales

1. Urine can irritate and macerate the skin after prolonged contact.

2. Reviewing preoperative teaching after surgery reinforces information the patient may have forgotten or misunderstood. The patient should understand the nature of the surgery and its anatomical effects. The patient may mistakenly expect the ileal conduit to act as a substitute bladder.

3. The patient needs to know what is now normal. Blood in the urine can result from stomal bleeding. Urine will flow fairly frequently from the stoma. There will be a greater amount of mucus in the urine during the early postoperative period, when oral intake is low, or when a urinary infection is present. The patient may mistake mucus for pus.

4. Rationales: _____

Target outcome criteria
Within 3 days after surgery, the patient will:
• have intact skin around the stoma
• describe normal stoma and urine characteristics.

RENAL DISORDERS

Nursing diagnosis: *Body-image disturbance related to urinary diversion*

NURSING PRIORITIES: (a) Minimize damage to self-concept and (b) promote a healthy body image.

Interventions	Rationales
1. Encourage the patient to express feelings and beliefs about the diagnosis, surgery, and stoma.	1. The patient may feel fear or isolation or may harbor misconceptions. Expression of feelings is the first step in the coping process.
2. Allow for privacy when teaching ostomy care.	2. Privacy encourages the patient to ask questions and facilitates learning.
3. Have the patient empty the pouch in the bathroom.	3. Mimicking normal bathroom behavior minimizes feelings of being handicapped or different.
4. Suggest a visit from a United Ostomy Association (UOA) visitor (may also be helpful before surgery). The local chapter will be listed in the telephone directory's white pages.	4. The UOA provides the patient with fellowship, information, and support from others with ostomies. Seeing a well-adjusted person with an ostomy can encourage hope and provide a positive role model for the patient.
5. Show an accepting, tolerant attitude when performing or teaching ostomy care. Explain that wearing gloves is necessary to comply with universal precautions.	5. The nurse's acceptance and tolerance reassure the patient and facilitate advancement to complete self-care. The patient may perceive the nurse's gloves as a sign of unacceptance of or disgust for the new stoma.
6. Additional individualized interventions: _____	6. Rationales: _____

Target outcome criteria
Within 2 to 4 days after surgery, the patient will:
- verbalize feelings about the ostomy
- demonstrate ability to empty pouch in bathroom

- express confidence about ability to care for self.

Nursing diagnosis: *Knowledge deficit related to care of the ileal conduit*

NURSING PRIORITY: Encourage independence in caring for the ileal conduit.

Interventions	Rationales
1. Instruct the patient how to empty the pouch when it is one-third to one-half full. Demonstrate the emptying procedure using a pouch the patient is not wearing. (A female can sit on the toilet to empty; a male can stand.)	1. Emptying is usually taught first because it is done most often. A too-full pouch may pull away and have to be changed. Opening and closing the spout is easier to practice on a pouch the patient can hold out and see. Mimicking normal toileting behavior facilitates the patient's adjustment.
2. Demonstrate the use and care of the nighttime bedside drainage bag. Run tubing from the drainage bag down the patient's pajama leg, or attach it to the leg with a hook-and-loop closure (Velcro) strap. Attach the pouch, with urine in it, to the drainage bag. Explain that the drainage bag is easily cleaned with white vinegar and water or a commercial cleaner.	2. A bedside drainage bag prevents pouch overfilling and leakage at night. Attaching a partially filled pouch prevents suction vacuum, which can lead to overfilling and leakage. Cleaning keeps the drainage bag free from odor and urine sediment or crystals.

3. Encourage the patient to change the pouch by giving step-by-step written instructions, teaching the use of wicks, having the patient practice on a stoma model, explaining that the patient should clean urine and mucus from stoma and skin with warm water only, using a mirror if necessary to help the patient see the underside of the stoma, and having the patient apply the pouch while standing.

3. Written instructions promote continuity of care. Wicks (rolled-up gauze or tampons) are placed on the stoma to absorb urine and keep the peristomal skin dry so the pouch can seal. Practicing on a stoma model decreases fear and allows for repetition. Water is used for cleaning because soap can leave a film on the skin and disrupt the pouch seal. The patient needs to monitor the condition of the peristomal skin during each pouch change. Standing minimizes abdominal creases, which predispose the pouch to leakage.

4. Teach the patient how to treat minor peristomal skin irritations using karaya powder and a skin sealant. Explain that momentary stinging may result if karaya powder or sealant is applied to denuded skin, but they should be used to prevent more serious peristomal skin complications.

4. Routinely applying a skin sealant before pouch application protects skin from adhesives and urine. Treating minor skin irritations with karaya powder and sealant minimizes the risk of serious complications requiring surgery. Intact, healthy skin increases a pouch's wearing time and prevents unexpected leaks.

5. Explain fluid intake requirements. Demonstrate pH testing of urine. Check pH routinely on the first few drops of urine in a freshly changed pouch. Warn against touching nitrazine paper to the skin or stoma. Explain why the patient should not drink more than 3 or 4 glasses of citrus juice or milk per day.

5. Normal urine is acidic in a well-hydrated adult. Touching nitrazine paper to the skin or stoma will yield inaccurate results. The patient may need to drink 10 to 12 glasses of fluid daily to keep urine acidic; drinking large amounts of citrus juice or milk will negate this effect and make urine alkaline. Alkaline urine predisposes the patient to foul-smelling urine, urinary infections, peristomal skin irritations, stomal stenosis, increased mucus production from the conduit, urine crystals and calculi, and pyelonephritis.

6. List recommended ways to control urine odor through diet. Explain that pouches are odor-proof except during emptying and changing.

6. Increased urine odor is associated with eating fish, eggs, asparagus, onions, and spicy foods.

7. Define routine follow-up care, and explain the rationale for it.

7. The patient will see the urologist routinely every 6 to 12 months. Routine follow-up includes urine culture and sensitivity testing to rule out or detect infection, plus IVP or a renal scan to check upper urinary tract function and evaluate for recurrent tumor. The stoma and skin should be checked and pouch problems evaluated.

8. Address any special concerns the patient has about living with an ostomy. Consult an ET nurse for specialized ostomy care.

8. ET nurses are specially trained to teach, counsel, and help rehabilitate the ostomy patient. They are knowledgeable about the newest pouch supplies and can assist the patient in coping with problems of daily living.

9. Additional individualized concerns: _____

9. Rationales: _____

RENAL DISORDERS

Target outcome criteria
Within 5 days after surgery, the patient will display learning readiness, such as looking at the stoma or holding wicks.

By the time of discharge, the patient will have changed the pouch two or three times with minimal assistance from the nurse.

Nursing diagnosis: *High risk for sexual dysfunction: male erectile dysfunction related to cystectomy and possible ejaculatory incompetence with prostatectomy*

NURSING PRIORITIES: (a) Help the patient maximize remaining sexual function and (b) provide information or referrals as needed.

Interventions

1. Assess the patient's readiness to discuss sexual matters. If the patient is not ready, arrange for outpatient follow-up.

2. Describe the separate nerve pathways for sexual excitement, erection, ejaculation, and orgasm. Explain which ones may be affected by surgery and why.

3. If indicated, mention alternatives such as a penile prosthesis or external devices that aid erection. Refer the patient to the urologist or ET nurse for details.

4. Additional individualized interventions: _____

Rationales

1. The patient may deny interest in resumption of sexual activity at first, while learning to cope with the ostomy and the diagnosis of cancer.

2. Cystectomy may only affect the patient's ability to experience erection or ejaculation.

3. The patient may need specific suggestions for resumption of fulfilling sexual activity. A urologist may surgically implant a penile prosthesis. The ET nurse can counsel the patient on alternatives, help obtain information on external devices, and suggest ways to minimize the ostomy's presence during sex.

4. Rationales: _____

Target outcome criterion
During the postoperative teaching phase, the patient will ask questions about sexual matters or agree to appropriate referrals.

Discharge planning
NURSING DISCHARGE CRITERIA
Upon the patient's discharge, documentation shows evidence of:
• a viable stoma
• stable vital signs
• stable nutritional status
• absence of pulmonary or cardiovascular complications
• adequate support system for postdischarge assistance and ability to perform stoma care
• referral to home care if indicated by lack of a home support system or inability to perform ADLs and stoma care
• absence of fever
• ability to control pain using oral analgesics
• no need for I.V. support (discontinued for at least 24 hours before discharge)
• bowel sounds
• healing incision with no redness or other sign of infection
• ability to ambulate at preoperative level.

PATIENT-FAMILY TEACHING CHECKLIST
Document evidence that the patient and family demonstrate an understanding of:
___ extent of tumor and resection
___ nature of urinary diversion and its construction
___ incision care (if not healed)
___ procedure for emptying and changing pouch
___ use and cleaning of bedside drainage system
___ treatment of minor peristomal skin irritations
___ written list of supplies and suppliers, with doctor's prescription to facilitate insurance payment
___ chemotherapy (if needed) and its expected adverse effects
___ availability of support groups such as UOA and the American Cancer Society (list their telephone numbers)
___ amount and types of fluids preferred, along with any dietary considerations, such as avoiding odor-causing foods
___ signs and symptoms to report to the doctor, such as fever, flank pain, or hematuria
___ concerns to report to the ET nurse, such as pouch problems and skin or stoma problems

___ signs and symptoms of urinary tract infection
___ considerations in resuming sexual activity
___ date and time of follow-up appointments
___ how to contact the doctor
___ how to contact the ET nurse.

DOCUMENTATION CHECKLIST
Using outcome criteria as a guide, document:
___ clinical status on admission
___ significant changes in status
___ pertinent laboratory and diagnostic test findings
___ preoperative marking of stoma site
___ preoperative teaching
___ bowel preparation
___ UOA visitor recommendation (if appropriate)
___ stoma viability
___ mucocutaneous border and sutures
___ urine characteristics
___ patient's response to ostomy
___ fluid intake and output
___ presence of stents
___ GI status
___ incision status
___ patient's progress in learning ostomy care
___ patient-family teaching
___ discharge planning.

ASSOCIATED PLANS OF CARE
Grieving
Ineffective Family Coping
Ineffective Individual Coping
Knowledge Deficit
Surgical Intervention

References

Cancer Response System, *Facts and Figures.* June, 1990. 1-800-ACS-2345. (periodically updated computer printout from American Cancer Society)

Cohen, A. "Body Image in the Person with a Stoma," *Journal of Enterostomal Therapy* 18(2):68-71, March-April 1991.

Dobkin, K.A. "Nursing Care of a Patient with Urinary Diversion," *Journal of Urological Nursing* 4:4, October-November-December 1985.

Dudas, S. "Rehabilitation of the Patient with Cancer," *Journal of Enterostomal Therapy* 18(2):61-67, March-April 1991.

LaGasse, J. "Ostomy Teaching Protocol," *Ostomy/Wound Management* 31:23-28, November-December 1990.

Smith, D., and Babaian, J. "Patient Adjustment to an Ileal Conduit after Radical Cystectomy," *Journal of Enterostomal Therapy* 16(6):244-46, November-December 1989.

RENAL DISORDERS

RENAL DISORDERS
Nephrectomy

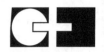

DRG information
DRG 303 Kidney, Ureter, and Major Bladder Procedures
for Neoplasm.
Mean LOS = 11.9 days
DRG 304 Kidney, Ureter, and Major Bladder Procedures
for Non-neoplasms. With Complication or
Comorbidity (CC).
Mean LOS = 10.3 days
DRG 305 Kidney, Ureter, and Major Bladder Procedures
for Non-neoplasms. Without CC.
Mean LOS = 5.5 days

Introduction
DEFINITION AND TIME FOCUS
Kidney removal may be necessary for various reasons.
The reason for the excision dictates the surgical approach. The flank or lumbar approach, the traditional
approach through the retroperitoneum, is indicated in
inflammatory renal disease, calculi, perinephric abscess, hydronephrosis, and renal cystic disease. The
transabdominal approach allows easy access to the
renal vessels, as is required in renal tumors, trauma,
or renal vascular disease. Either approach is acceptable to remove a kidney for transplantation.

This plan focuses on the immediate pre- and postoperative care for the patient undergoing nephrectomy.
Refer to the "Surgical Intervention" plan, page 81, for
more detailed information on preoperative and postoperative care.

ETIOLOGY AND PRECIPITATING FACTORS
The primary reasons for nephrectomy include, but are
not limited to:
• renal tumors
• obstructive uropathy (intrinsic or extrinsic), including renal calculi, vascular lesions (such as abdominal
aortic aneurysm), pelvic disorders (such as endometriosis), GI disorders (such as Crohn's disease), retroperitoneal disorders (such as tumor or abscess), or effects
of radiation therapy
• blunt or penetrating trauma
• kidney donation.

Focused assessment guidelines
NURSING HISTORY (Functional health pattern findings)

Health perception – health management patterns
• if older, may have history of concomitant health problems (such as diabetes mellitus, hypertension, hyperparathyroidism, or vascular disease) that contributed
to need for nephrectomy

• may express concerns or fears about maintaining
normal kidney function after surgery
• may express concerns about diet and activity restrictions and need for adjuvant therapies after surgery
• may have history of contact with nephrotoxic substances

Activity-exercise pattern
• may report fatigue

Nutritional-metabolic pattern
• may report anorexia, nausea or vomiting, or weight
loss

Self-perception – self-concept pattern
• may report anxiety or depression

PHYSICAL FINDINGS
Cardiovascular
• hypertension
• tachycardia
• edema or ecchymosis at injury site (with trauma)
• hypotension (rare)

Pulmonary
• tachypnea
• congestion (rarely)

Genitourinary
• dysuria
• hematuria
• oliguria
• polyuria

Musculoskeletal
• pain with movement
• ecchymosis
• muscle spasm (rarely)

Integumentary
• diaphoresis
• pallor (with significant blood loss)

DIAGNOSTIC STUDIES
Note: Diagnostic studies, performed before surgery,
may reveal no significant abnormalities initially, unless related to a coexisting condition.
• complete blood count—establishes baseline; may reveal preexisting disorder (such as anemia) or extent
of blood loss from injury; white blood cell count may
be elevated in response to injury
• blood typing and cross-matching—allows blood replacement during surgery

• chemistry panel—establishes baseline and reveals imbalances that may be related to renal dysfunction or that may affect care during surgery (such as potassium imbalances that may cause cardiac irritability during anesthesia); blood urea nitrogen and creatinine levels evaluate renal function
• prothrombin time and partial thromboplastin time—establishes baseline; some patients (older, obese, or with prosthetic valves) may receive anticoagulant therapy after surgery to minimize the risk of thromboembolism complications
• urinalysis—establishes baseline and evaluates renal function
• chest X-ray—rules out preexisting conditions that may affect care during surgery

• 12-lead electrocardiography (ECG)—establishes baseline and identifies preexisting cardiac abnormalities; may indicate cardiac contusion in patient with blunt chest trauma

POTENTIAL COMPLICATIONS
• shock
• hemorrhage
• pulmonary embolism
• thrombophlebitis
• atelectasis
• pneumonia
• wound infection, dehiscence, and evisceration
• paralytic ileus
• acute renal failure

Nursing diagnosis: *Knowledge deficit related to perioperative procedures*

NURSING PRIORITY: Prepare the patient for perioperative procedures.

Interventions

1. See the "Knowledge Deficit" plan, page 56.

2. See the "Surgical Intervention" plan, page 81.

3. Tell the patient where the incision will be made (flank or abdomen), whether to expect a chest tube (for a flank incision) or a drain (for an abdominal incision), and the potential effects of positioning during surgery.

4. Additional individualized interventions: _____

Rationales

1. General interventions related to patient teaching are included in the "Knowledge Deficit" plan.

2. General interventions related to perioperative procedures are included in the "Surgical Intervention" plan.

3. Knowing what to expect decreases the patient's anxiety and increases the likelihood of compliance after surgery.

4. Rationales: _____

Target outcome criteria
Before surgery, the patient will:
• verbalize understanding of perioperative procedures
• demonstrate ability to perform coughing and deep-breathing exercises, use the incentive spirometer, splint the incision, and perform leg exercises.

Nursing diagnosis: *Pain related to tissue injury, edema, or spasm after surgery*

NURSING PRIORITY: Prevent or reduce pain.

Interventions

1. See the "Pain" plan, page 69.

2. Teach the patient about postoperative analgesia administration (injection, patient-controlled analgesia pump, or epidural infusion), potential adverse effects, and the importance of requesting medication before pain becomes severe.

Rationales

1. The "Pain" plan contains general interventions regarding pain management.

2. The patient is more likely to comply with postoperative care if pain is controlled.

3. Additional individualized interventions: _____

3. Rationales: _____

Target outcome criteria
Within 1 hour of pain onset, the patient will:
- verbalize increased comfort
- display a relaxed posture and facial expression

- have vital signs within normal limits.

Collaborative problem: *High risk for fluid and electrolyte imbalance related to decreased renal reserve and third-space fluid shifting immediately after surgery*

NURSING PRIORITY: Prevent fluid and electrolyte imbalance.

Interventions

1. See Appendix C, "Fluid and Electrolyte Imbalances."

2. Preserve and protect the remaining kidney.

- Maintain adequate hydration. Monitor urine output, color, and specific gravity, as ordered.

- Avoid or minimize use of nephrotoxic agents, such as aminoglycoside antibiotics and chemotherapeutic agents.

- Instruct the patient regarding the importance of discharge recommendations, such as avoiding heavy lifting for up to 8 weeks, and recommended life-style changes, such as limiting vigorous or contact sports and wearing a seatbelt when in a car. Emphasize the need to report symptoms of kidney infection promptly.

3. Additional individualized interventions: _____

Rationales

1. The "Fluid and Electrolyte Imbalances" appendix contains detailed information on these imbalances.

2. Removal of one kidney makes preservation of remaining renal function imperative.

- Appropriate hydration preserves renal function and promotes efficient removal of metabolic wastes.

- Nephrotoxic agents can damage the remaining kidney.

- The patient who understands activity restrictions and life-style modifications is more likely to comply with them. Restricting activities for several weeks protects the healing surgical site. Limiting contact sports and wearing seatbelts reduces the risk of renal trauma, while prompt treatment of infection reduces the risk of compromise or loss of renal function and the resulting need for dialysis.

3. Rationales: _____

Target outcome criteria
Within 1 day after surgery, the patient will:
- have normal urine output
- have adequate I.V. or oral fluid intake
- exhibit normal electrolyte levels.

By the time of discharge, the patient will state discharge recommendations and intention to adhere to them.

Collaborative problem: *High risk for atelectasis related to anesthesia, immobility, pain, presence of chest tube, and location of incision*

NURSING PRIORITIES: (a) Maintain adequate oxygenation and (b) prevent pulmonary complications.

Interventions

1. Implement interventions listed under "High risk for postoperative atelectasis" in the "Surgical Intervention" plan, page 83. As needed, check pulmonary status frequently, help the patient to perform incentive spirometry, encourage frequent position changes, and promote early and progressive ambulation.

Rationales

1. In addition to the risk of atelectasis inherent to general anesthesia, the patient with a lumbar or flank incision is at increased risk because the intercostal muscles must be spread and the twelfth rib may be removed. The resulting pain limits deep inspiration. If not detected and treated aggressively, atelectasis can lead to pneumonia. The "Surgical Intervention" plan contains measures to prevent this complication.

2. Additional individualized interventions: _____

2. Rationales: _____

Target outcome criteria
After surgery, the patient will:
• maintain a respiratory rate of 10 to 20 breaths/minute
• have unlabored, deep respirations

• manifest audible, clear breath sounds in all lobes.

Collaborative problem: *High risk for postoperative paralytic ileus or intestinal obstruction related to surgical manipulation, anesthesia, and immobility*

NURSING PRIORITY: Promptly detect abnormal GI function.

Interventions

1. Implement measures listed under "High risk for postoperative paralytic ileus" in the "Surgical Intervention" plan, page 88. As appropriate, assess the abdomen frequently, monitor nasogastric tube drainage, administer fluids, provide a diet appropriate to peristaltic activity, and encourage early and frequent ambulation.

2. Additional individualized interventions: _____

Rationales

1. Bowel manipulation during nephrectomy increases the risk of paralytic ileus, the most common GI complication. Significant manipulation increases the risk of intestinal obstruction. The "Surgical Intervention" plan details related interventions and their rationales.

2. Rationales: _____

Target outcome criteria
By the time of discharge, the patient will:
• have normal, active bowel sounds
• tolerate a normal diet

• have regular bowel movements.

Discharge planning
NURSING DISCHARGE CRITERIA
Upon the patient's discharge, documentation shows evidence of:
• stable vital signs
• absence of cardiovascular or pulmonary complications
• absence of fever
• healing wound without signs of infection (swelling, inflammation, tenderness, or drainage)
• ability to tolerate oral intake
• ability to ambulate and perform activities of daily living same as before surgery
• ability to void and have bowel movements same as before surgery
• ability to control pain using oral medications
• adequate home support system or referral to home health agency or nursing home, if indicated.

PATIENT-FAMILY TEACHING CHECKLIST
Document evidence that the patient and family demonstrate an understanding of:
___ plan for resuming normal activity, with restrictions
___ dietary recommendations
___ wound care
___ signs of wound infection or other complications
___ all discharge medications' purpose, dosage, administration, and adverse effects requiring medical attention (discharge medications may include analgesics and antibiotics)
___ necessary home care and referrals for follow-up care
___ when and how to contact the doctor
___ date, time, and place of follow-up appointments.

RENAL DISORDERS

DOCUMENTATION CHECKLIST

Using outcome criteria as a guide, document:

___ clinical status on admission

___ preoperative assessment and treatment

___ preoperative teaching and its effectiveness

___ preoperative checklist (usually includes documentation of operative consent; pertinent laboratory test results; skin preparation; voiding on call from the operating room; and removal of nail polish, jewelry, dentures, glasses, hearing aids, and prostheses — check hospital's specific requirements)

___ postoperative assessment and treatment

___ amount and character of drainage on dressing and through drains

___ patency of I.V. lines, nasogastric tube, indwelling urinary (Foley) catheter, and drains

___ pulmonary hygiene

___ pain relief measures

___ activity tolerance

___ nutritional intake and tolerance

___ fluid intake and output

___ bladder and bowel function

___ pertinent laboratory findings

___ patient-family teaching

___ discharge planning.

ASSOCIATED PLANS OF CARE

Knowledge Deficit

Pain

Surgical Intervention

References

Genitourinary Problems. NurseReview. Springhouse, Pa.: Springhouse Corp., 1989.

Guyton, A. *Textbook of Medical Physiology,* 8th ed. Philadelphia: W.B. Saunders Co., 1991.

Kniesl, C., and Amos, S. *Adult Health Nursing: A Biopsychosocial Approach.* Reading, Mass.: Addison-Wesley Publishing Co., 1986.

Luckmann, J., and Sorenson, K. *Medical-Surgical Nursing: A Psychophysiological Approach,* 3rd ed. Philadelphia: W.B. Saunders Co., 1987.

Schwartz, S. *Principles of Surgery,* 5th ed. New York: McGraw-Hill Book Company, 1989.

Peritoneal Dialysis

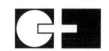

DRG information

DRG 316 Renal Failure.
   Mean LOS = 6.4 days
   Principal diagnoses include:
   • acute renal failure
   • chronic renal failure.
DRG 449 Poisoning and Toxic Effects of Drugs. Age
   17 +. With Complication or Comorbidity
   (CC).
   Mean LOS = 4.3 days
   Principal diagnoses include drug overdose.
DRG 450 Poisoning and Toxic Effects of Drugs. Age
   17 +. Without CC.
   Mean LOS = 2.6 days
DRG 451 Poisoning and Toxic Effects of Drugs. Age 0
   to 17.
   Mean LOS = 3.8 days
DRG 205 Disorders of the Liver except Malignancy,
   Cirrhosis, and Alcoholic Hepatitis. With CC.
   Mean LOS = 6.7 days
   Principal diagnoses include hepatic coma.
DRG 206 Disorders of the Liver except Malignancy,
   Cirrhosis, and Alcoholic Hepatitis. Without
   CC.
   Mean LOS = 3.8 days
Additional DRG information: Peritoneal dialysis is used
to treat numerous disorders. Therefore, the diagnosis
necessitating its use determines the DRG assigned.
Examples of diagnoses for peritoneal dialysis are
listed above.

Introduction
DEFINITION AND TIME FOCUS

Peritoneal dialysis (PD) indirectly removes excess
water, solutes, and toxins from the blood by using the
peritoneal membrane as a dialyzing membrane. Solution (dialysate) is instilled into the peritoneal cavity
through a catheter and remains for a prescribed period
of time, usually 15 minutes to 4 hours. During that
time (dwell time), substances in the blood and in the
dialysate equalize across the membrane, moving from
areas of higher concentration to areas of lower concentration. The solution is then allowed to flow out (drain
time), removing excess water and waste products. PD
is contraindicated with:
• recent abdominal, retroperitoneal, or chest surgery
• abdominal drains
• preexisting peritonitis
• diaphragmatic tears
• paralytic ileus

• diffuse bowel disease
• respiratory insufficiency.
This plan focuses on the patient receiving PD for the
first time and then regularly (at least three times
weekly).

ETIOLOGY AND PRECIPITATING FACTORS

PD is indicated to treat chronic renal failure, acute
renal failure, drug overdose, and hepatic coma. The
patient awaiting hemodialysis whose vascular access
device is not yet operable may receive PD temporarily.
Because PD is not a diagnosis but a procedure, this
plan does not address specific illnesses. Refer to plans
for specific disorders for more information.

Focused assessment guidelines
NURSING HISTORY (Functional health pattern findings)

Health perception — health management pattern
• may have a history of chronic or acute renal failure
• may have inadequate or exhausted venous access
• may be under treatment for diabetes mellitus
• may have a history of drug overdose or drug intolerance
• may have a history of a clotting disorder or cardiovascular disease

Nutritional-metabolic pattern
• may report anorexia, nausea, or vomiting
• may report weight loss or diet intolerance

Elimination pattern
• may report diminished urine output
• may report constipation

Role-relationship pattern
• may report inability to work or maintain usual roles
because of chronic, disabling illness, treatment regimen, or both

Self-perception — self-concept pattern
• may verbalize decreased sense of self-worth

Coping — stress tolerance pattern
• may express denial, anger, or depression over condition and needed treatment

Activity-exercise pattern
• may report fatigue
• may report shortness of breath or other signs of exercise intolerance

Value-belief pattern
• may report religious or personal beliefs that do not allow blood transfusions

PHYSICAL FINDINGS*
Cardiovascular
• hypertension
• periorbital, ankle, or sacral edema

Pulmonary
• crackles
• dyspnea

Gastrointestinal
• nausea
• anorexia
• hiccoughs
• constipation
• stomatitis

Neurologic
• lethargy
• confusion
• shortened attention span
• restlessness

Integumentary
• fragile skin
• dry, flaky skin
• yellow-gray skin hue
• ecchymoses or purpura
• poor skin turgor

Musculoskeletal
• impaired mobility
• bone deformities

DIAGNOSTIC STUDIES
• creatinine clearance—determines glomerular filtration rate, which directly reflects renal function
  — normal, 85 to 150 ml/minute
  — mild renal failure, 50 to 84 ml/minute
  — moderate renal failure, 10 to 49 ml/minute
  — severe renal failure, less than 10 ml/minute
  — end-stage renal failure, 0 ml/minute
• serum creatinine levels—determine renal function (normal is 1.0 to 1.4 mg/dl; elevation indicates renal impairment; see the "Chronic Renal Failure" plan, page 558)
• arterial blood gas (ABG) levels—determine acid-base abnormalities (normal pH is 7.35 to 7.45; the patient in renal failure is usually acidotic)
• serum electrolyte levels—usually show hyperkalemia (greater than 5 mEq/liter)
• sodium level—may be low (less than 120 mEq/liter) because of kidney's inability to conserve sodium
• phosphate and calcium levels—commonly show hypocalcemia and hyperphosphatemia
• blood urea nitrogen levels—elevated in renal failure, reduced in severe liver damage
• complete blood count—hemoglobin level may be reduced from decreased erythropoietin production
• erythrocyte sedimentation rate—increased if infection present
• serum drug levels—determine degree of drug overdose
• culture and sensitivity of PD drainage—identifies causative organism and appropriate antibiotic for peritoneal infection
• chest X-ray—rules out congestive heart failure

POTENTIAL COMPLICATIONS
• peritonitis
• respiratory distress
• cardiac arrhythmias
• hypovolemia or hypervolemia
• hyperglycemia
• electrolyte imbalance
• bowel or bladder perforation

Nursing diagnosis: *High risk for injury: bleeding, perforation, or ileus related to catheter insertion or irritation from dialysate*

NURSING PRIORITY: Prevent or promptly detect and report injuries related to PD.

Interventions

1. Have the patient void before catheter insertion.

Rationales

1. The catheter is inserted with a trocar near the bladder. Bladder distention increases the risk of perforation.

---

*Physical findings related to renal failure.

2. During dialysate infusion, observe for indications of bladder or bowel perforation, such as an extreme urge to urinate or defecate; large urine output; fecal color, odor, or material in returned dialysate; and liquid or watery stools. If any occur, stop the infusion and notify the doctor immediately.

3. Report persistently blood-tinged dialysate.

4. Auscultate bowel sounds every 4 hours.

5. Inspect and palpate the abdomen every 8 hours between dialysate infusions.

6. Monitor the patient's appetite and sense of well-being.

7. Encourage ambulation.

8. Apply warm compresses to the abdomen.

9. Additional individualized interventions: ＿＿＿＿＿＿＿＿

___

2. Bowel or bladder perforation may lead to severe peritonitis unless detected. Surgical repair and prompt antibiotic therapy are indicated. The signs listed appear when dialysate leaks into the bladder or bowel.

3. Slight bleeding may be normal after catheter insertion, but the fluid should clear rapidly. Persistent bleeding or gross blood in the return flow requires prompt evaluation.

4. Diminished or absent bowel sounds may suggest ileus or bowel obstruction from bowel injury or irritation from catheter placement or dialysate.

5. Abdominal distention and tenderness may indicate ileus.

6. Anorexia, nausea, vomiting, and malaise can be signs and symptoms of ileus.

7. Ambulation stimulates peristalsis.

8. Heat increases peristalsis.

9. Rationales: ＿＿＿＿＿＿＿＿＿＿＿＿＿＿＿＿

___

Target outcome criteria
After catheter insertion, the patient will:
• have no unusual urge to void or defecate
• produce the usual amount of urine and stool
• have dialysate returns free from fecal material or blood.

Throughout the hospital stay, the patient will:
• have normal bowel sounds
• maintain a normal bowel elimination pattern
• show no abdominal distention and tenderness.

Nursing diagnosis: *High risk for ineffective breathing pattern related to elevation of diaphragm during PD exchanges and reduced mobility*

NURSING PRIORITY: Prevent respiratory distress and pulmonary complications during PD exchanges.

Interventions

1. Elevate the head of the bed during exchanges.

2. Administer oxygen, as ordered.

3. Assess for possible causes of pain or discomfort. Administer analgesics, as ordered.

4. Encourage deep-breathing and coughing exercises during PD exchanges, hourly while awake. Teach and promote hourly incentive spirometer use, as ordered.

5. Auscultate the patient's lungs every hour, assessing for and reporting crackles or other abnormal findings.

Rationales

1. Elevating the head of the bed minimizes pressure on the diaphragm and allows fuller chest expansion.

2. Hypoventilation related to pressure on the diaphragm reduces arterial PO_2 levels.

3. Pain may prevent effective breathing. Rapid inflow of dialysate, patient position, and air in the system can all cause discomfort; possible causes should be investigated before analgesics are given.

4. Good pulmonary hygiene helps prevent fluid accumulation in the lungs and air passages by promoting full chest expansion and preventing collapse of alveoli.

5. Crackles suggest pulmonary complications related to fluid retention.

6. Turn and reposition the patient at least every hour.

6. Changing position promotes full chest excursion and optimal drainage of dialysate.

7. Perform chest percussion every 2 hours.

7. Percussion helps loosen secretions.

8. Additional individualized interventions: _____

8. Rationales: _____

Target outcome criteria
During PD treatment, the patient will:
- show no dyspnea
- have minimal or no crackles
- perform pulmonary hygiene measures effectively.

Collaborative problem: *High risk for altered fluid and electrolyte balance related to dialysis and underlying disease or disorder*

NURSING PRIORITY: Maintain normal fluid and electrolyte balance.

Interventions

1. See Appendix C, "Fluid and Electrolyte Imbalances." Closely monitor vital signs, observing for tachycardia or orthostatic changes.

2. Monitor serum potassium levels, as ordered, to help determine appropriate additions to the dialysate.

3. Maintain accurate fluid intake and output records. Notify the doctor if the fluid return deficit exceeds 500 ml.

4. Additional individualized interventions: _____

Rationales

1. The "Fluid and Electrolyte Imbalances" appendix provides detailed information on the fluid and electrolyte disturbances seen in the patient receiving PD.

2. Dialysate normally contains no potassium. This is desirable for the hyperkalemic patient, but it may cause hypokalemia in others.

3. Normally, return should be equal to or slightly greater than the amount infused. A persistent deficit that is not corrected by position changes may indicate fluid retention.

4. Rationales: _____

Target outcome criteria
During PD exchanges, the patient will:
- show no distended neck veins
- have a decrease in peripheral edema
- have blood pressure within the normal range
- have a dialysate deficit less than 500 ml.

Nursing diagnosis: *High risk for infection related to invasive procedure*

NURSING PRIORITY: Prevent infection.

Interventions

1. Use strict aseptic technique for all aspects of PD, including daily dressing changes.

2. Maintain a sterile, closed system during exchanges.

Rationales

1. Introduction of pathogens through the catheter may cause peritonitis.

2. Airborne bacteria can cause infection if introduced into the peritoneal cavity.

3. Observe for and report leakage around the catheter.

3. Further securing the catheter at the entry site and reducing the amount or rapidity of the infusion may control leakage. Moisture around the catheter provides a pathway for microorganisms and increases the risk of infection.

4. Observe the catheter site for redness, exudate, and edema.

4. These are signs of infection.

5. Observe the outflow for cloudiness, sediment, and odor. Observe the patient for signs of peritonitis, such as abdominal pain, guarding, rigidity, and rebound tenderness.

5. Fluid appearance and odor may indicate peritonitis. Physical signs result from peritoneal inflammation.

6. Take and record the patient's temperature at least every 8 hours.

6. Temperature elevation is a sign of infection.

7. Administer systemic or local antibiotics, as ordered. Add antibiotics to the dialysate using the two-needle technique (one needle used to draw up the medication, another to inject it into the dialysate).

7. Antibiotics prevent the growth and reproduction of bacteria. The two-needle technique reduces the risk of contamination.

8. Additional individualized interventions: _____

8. Rationales: _____

Target outcome criteria
By the time of discharge, the patient will:
• be afebrile for 24 hours
• have no exudate, edema, redness, or leakage at the catheter site
• show no signs of peritonitis
• have clear return drainage.

Nursing diagnosis: *Pain related to dialysate temperature or to rapid inflow of dialysate*

NURSING PRIORITY: Minimize discomfort during fluid exchanges.

Interventions

1. Warm the dialysate to body temperature before beginning the infusion.

2. Change the patient's position every 1 to 2 hours.

3. Slow the infusion rate by lowering the bottle and by clamping the tubing as needed.

4. Prevent air from entering the catheter.

5. Notify the doctor if pain persists.

6. See the "Pain" plan, page 69.

7. Additional individualized interventions: _____

Rationales

1. Cold dialysate causes vasoconstriction (which interferes with circulation to the peritoneal membrane) and discomfort.

2. Frequent position changes improve dialysate drainage.

3. Reducing bottle height decreases the infusion rate and reduces pressure during fill time.

4. Air introduced into the abdominal cavity causes distention and pain, sometimes referred to the shoulder area. Air in the tubing may also create an air lock, preventing adequate dialysate flow.

5. Persistent pain may indicate peritonitis.

6. The "Pain" plan contains further details related to pain management.

7. Rationales: _____

RENAL DISORDERS

Target outcome criterion
During PD treatment, the patient will verbalize absence
or minimal amount of abdominal discomfort.

Nursing diagnosis: *Nutritional deficit related to anorexia, abdominal distention, stomatitis, or nausea*

NURSING PRIORITY: Promote adequate nutritional intake.

Interventions

1. With the dietitian and patient, plan a menu that incorporates personal preferences, increased nutrient needs, and any restrictions related to the underlying disorder.

2. Offer snacks and supplements between meals, providing plenty of high-protein foods unless contraindicated. Avoid foods high in potassium if hyperkalemia is a problem. See the "Chronic Renal Failure" plan, page 558, for more information.

3. Encourage frequent oral hygiene.

4. Offer small, frequent meals.

5. Avoid manipulating equipment or emptying drainage bags at mealtime.

6. Drain the peritoneal cavity before meals. If possible, allow 1 to 2 hours between a meal and the next dialysate infusion.

7. If the patient cannot tolerate adequate oral intake, discuss enteral or parenteral feedings with both the patient and doctor.

8. Additional individualized interventions: _____

Rationales

1. The dietitian's expertise may be helpful in selecting food for optimal nutritional value. When the patient's appetite is decreased, considering individual preferences is essential to promote adequate intake.

2. PD can cause weekly protein losses of 30 to 70 g. The adult dialysis patient requires 45 to 50 kcal/kg daily. Hyperkalemia is common in renal failure. The "Chronic Renal Failure" plan contains specific interventions related to diet planning.

3. Good oral hygiene decreases unpleasant odors and tastes in the mouth that can decrease appetite.

4. Large amounts of food may seem overwhelming and unappetizing. The patient may complain of being too full to eat because of pressure from peritoneal fluid.

5. Unpleasant sights and odors may cause nausea and vomiting.

6. Draining peritoneal fluid decreases intra-abdominal pressure and may enable the patient to eat and retain food more easily.

7. During acute illness, enteral or parenteral nutrition may be indicated.

8. Rationales: _____

Target outcome criteria
During PD, the patient will:
• participate in dietary planning
• perform oral hygiene before and after meals
• eat adequate amounts of protein-rich foods.

By the time of discharge, the patient will:
• retain food for at least 12 hours
• tolerate oral intake of at least 0.5 g/kg of ideal weight daily and 45 to 50 kcal/kg/day.

Discharge planning
NURSING DISCHARGE CRITERIA
Upon the patient's discharge, documentation shows evidence of:
- vital signs stable and within expected parameters
- electrolyte, ABG, and hemoglobin levels within acceptable parameters
- absence of drainage, redness, and edema at catheter site
- absence of cardiovascular and pulmonary complications
- absent or minimal peripheral edema
- ability to tolerate adequate nutritional intake, as ordered
- absence of abdominal distention and tenderness
- absence of nausea and vomiting
- normal bowel and bladder function
- stabilizing weight
- ability to control pain using oral medications
- ability to ambulate and perform activities of daily living independently or with minimal assistance
- adequate home support system or referral to home care or a nursing home as indicated by inadequate home support system, frequency of and tolerance to PD, and inability to care for self.

Additional information: For long-term PD, the patient typically receives treatments at home with the assistance of home-care nurses. The number of treatments needed and the patient's ability to perform treatments at home are essential in determining where the patient will be discharged. Long-term PD treatments create financial problems for most patients. For this reason, a referral to the social services department should be an automatic part of discharge planning.

PATIENT-FAMILY TEACHING CHECKLIST
Document evidence that the patient and family demonstrate an understanding of:
— renal failure (pathophysiology, signs and symptoms, and implications)
— concepts of PD treatment
— importance of aseptic technique during treatment
— dietary modifications (sodium restrictions and high protein intake)
— all discharge medications' purpose, dosage, administration schedule, and adverse effects requiring medical attention (discharge medications vary, depending on underlying disorder)
— catheter care between treatments
— activity restrictions (usually only contact sports and swimming are prohibited)
— importance of a daily weight record
— changes in condition to report to the doctor
— date, time, and location of next treatment
— community resources
— how to get help in an emergency.

DOCUMENTATION CHECKLIST
Using outcome criteria as a guide, document:
— clinical status at beginning of treatment, including vital signs and weight
— significant changes in clinical status
— appearance of catheter site
— time each exchange begins and ends
— fluid intake and output
— color, odor, and character of dialysate return
— care of catheter site
— weight at end of treatment
— nutritional intake
— pertinent laboratory and diagnostic test findings
— bowel status
— patient-family teaching
— discharge planning.

ASSOCIATED PLANS OF CARE
Acute Renal Failure
Chronic Renal Failure
Knowledge Deficit
Liver Failure
Pain
Total Parenteral Nutrition

References
Alfaro, R. *Applying Nursing Diagnosis and Nursing Process.* Philadelphia: J.B. Lippincott Co., 1990.
The Lippincott Manual of Nursing Practice, 5th ed. Philadelphia: J.B. Lippincott Co., 1991.
Richard, C. *Comprehensive Nephrology Nursing.* Boston: Little, Brown & Co., 1986.

RENAL DISORDERS

Urolithiasis

DRG information

DRG 323 Urinary Stones. With Complication or Comorbidity (CC) or Treatment with Extracorporeal Shock-wave Lithotripsy.
Mean LOS = 2.9 days
DRG 324 Urinary Stones. Without CC.
Mean LOS = 2.2 days
DRG 304 Kidney, Ureter, and Bladder Procedures for Non-neoplasm. With CC.
Mean LOS = 10.3 days
DRG 305 Kidney, Ureter, and Bladder Procedures for Non-neoplasm. Without CC.
Mean LOS = 5.5 days
DRG 310 Transurethral Procedures. With CC.
Mean LOS = 4.1 days

Introduction
DEFINITION AND TIME FOCUS

Urolithiasis is the formation of mineral crystals (renal calculi or stones) around organic matter in the urinary tract. Calcium oxalate and calcium phosphate calculi are the most common. Calculi in the renal pelvis usually cause no symptoms until they pass into a ureter, where they commonly obstruct urine flow and cause severe pain, bleeding, and infection. This plan focuses on the patient admitted for treatment of upper urinary tract calculi by percutaneous nephrolithotomy with ultrasonic lithotripsy. In this procedure, a nephroscope is passed through a small incision into the kidney. The calculi are then fragmented with ultrasonic waves, flushed, and aspirated by suction or grasped and removed with forceps or special baskets.

ETIOLOGY AND PRECIPITATING FACTORS

• urinary tract infection (UTI), which increases the alkalinity of the urine and causes calcium and other substances to precipitate and form renal calculi
• immobility, dehydration, and urine obstruction or stasis, increasing likelihood that calculus-forming substances will precipitate
• metabolic or dietary changes, such as hyperthyroidism; bone disease; corticosteroid use; excessive vitamin A and D intake; diet high in calcium or purine; or other factors increasing calcium, phosphorus, uric acid, and other calculus-forming substances in the blood or urine
• more common in males ages 30 to 50 years

Focused assessment guidelines
NURSING HISTORY (Functional health pattern findings)

Health perception—health management pattern
• typically complains of severe pain: if calculi are in the pelvis, reports dull constant pain, usually over costovertebral angle; if in a ureter, reports intermittent, excruciating pain radiating anteriorly down to vulva (female) or testes (male); in some cases, may not report pain or may report abdominal pain
• may have history of UTI or previous calculus formation and treatment (a history of calculi increases the risk of recurrence)

Nutritional-metabolic pattern
• may report nausea, vomiting, diarrhea, and abdominal discomfort
• may report diet high in calcium (milk, cheese, beans, nuts, cocoa), purine (fish, fowl, meat, organ meat), oxalate (spinach, parsley, rhubarb, cocoa, instant coffee, tea), or vitamins A and D
• may report decreased fluid intake

Elimination pattern
• may report history of UTI or urinary tract obstruction
• may report blood in urine (hematuria)
• may report cloudy, odorous urine (indicates infection); painful, urgent, and frequent urination; and decreasing urine output

Activity-exercise pattern
• may report sedentary occupation or recent increased need for bed rest

Cognitive-perceptual pattern
• may report difficulty understanding metabolic influences on calculus formation and the new treatment options available (percutaneous ultrasonic lithotripsy and extracorporeal shock-wave lithotripsy)

Role-relationship pattern
• may report family history of renal calculi, gout, or other renal problems

Sexuality-reproductive pattern
• may describe sexual dysfunction related to UTI and pain

Coping—stress tolerance pattern
- may appear anxious and in obvious distress

PHYSICAL FINDINGS
Genitourinary
- calculi in urine
- costovertebral tenderness
- hematuria
- pyuria
- oliguria
- urinary frequency

Gastrointestinal
- vomiting
- abdominal tenderness
- diarrhea
- abdominal distention
- absent bowel sounds

Integumentary
- warm, flushed skin or chills and fever
- pallor
- diaphoresis

DIAGNOSTIC STUDIES
- urinalysis—commonly shows red blood cells, white blood cells (WBCs), crystals, casts, minerals, and pH changes; urine culture commonly shows presence of bacteria
- 24-hour urine study—commonly shows high levels of calcium, phosphorus, uric acid, creatinine, oxalate, or cystine

- nitroprusside urine test—may show cystine levels above 300 mg/day
- blood studies—may show high serum levels of calcium, protein, electrolytes, uric acid, phosphates, blood urea nitrogen, creatinine, or WBCs
- serum and urine creatinine tests—may show renal dysfunction (creatinine levels high in serum, low in urine)
- kidney-ureter-bladder X-ray—commonly shows calcium calculi and gross anatomical changes, such as distortions or enlargement (uric acid calculi cannot be visualized)
- intravenous urography (intravenous pyelogram IVP)—commonly shows anatomical abnormalities, obstruction, and outlines of radiopaque calculi
- computed tomography scan, with or without dye—commonly shows calculi, masses, or other abnormalities
- cystoscopy—commonly shows obstruction or other problems

POTENTIAL COMPLICATIONS*
- bleeding (may be acute or delayed for 1 to 2 weeks)
- sepsis
- renal pelvis perforation and loss of irrigating fluid into retroperitoneal area
- nonremovable calculi
- loss of calculus fragments into retroperitoneum

Nursing diagnosis: *Pain related to procedural manipulation, incision, and passage of calculus fragments*

NURSING PRIORITY: Relieve pain.

Interventions

1. See the "Pain" plan, page 69.

2. Assess and document pain episodes.

3. Medicate with analgesics and antispasmodics, as ordered. Narcotic analgesics are usually necessary.

4. Apply heat to painful areas, as ordered, for 15 to 20 minutes every 2 hours as needed.

5. Administer antiemetics as ordered and needed.

Rationales

1. General interventions for pain are included in that plan.

2. Pain may indicate calculus movement. Persistent pain may indicate obstruction or perforation. Sudden absence of pain may indicate calculus passage. Increased ureteral pressure may cause abdominal pain from extravasation of urine into perirenal spaces.

3. These medications reduce pain, relax tense muscles, and reduce reflex spasms. Narcotic analgesics are warranted because of the pain's severity.

4. Heat relaxes tense muscles and diminishes reflex spasms.

5. Nausea and vomiting are commonly associated with renal pain from shared nerve pathways.

*Rarely occur after percutaneous ultrasonic lithotripsy.

RENAL DISORDERS

6. Encourage activity, as allowed. (The patient with an indwelling ureteral catheter may be on bed rest to prevent dislodgment.)

6. Activity prevents urine stasis, helps retard calculi formation, aids passage of calculus fragments, and promotes return of urinary tract function.

7. Additional individualized interventions: _____

_____

7. Rationales: _____

_____

Target outcome criteria
Within 1 to 2 hours of the procedure, the patient will:
• experience pain relief
• show a relaxed facial expression and posture

• have no nausea or vomiting.

Nursing diagnosis: *High risk for altered urinary elimination patterns: dysuria, oliguria, pyuria, or frequency related to calculus fragment passage, obstruction, hematuria, or infection*

NURSING PRIORITIES: (a) Prevent urinary tract complications and (b) promote return of normal urinary function.

Interventions

1. Measure each voiding and note urine characteristics. Monitor fluid intake and output every 4 to 8 hours, more frequently if the patient is oliguric. Alert the doctor if urine output is less than 30 ml/hour.

2. Monitor the patency of an indwelling ureteral catheter or indwelling urinary (Foley) catheter every hour.

3. Strain all urine for calculi and calculus fragments. Send any calculi for laboratory analysis. Notify the doctor of calculi passage and document your observations.

4. Observe for signs of ureteral obstruction (increased flank pain and oliguria) or urethral obstruction (bladder distention and suprapubic pain), and report any that occur.

5. Observe for signs of dehydration, such as dry skin and mucous membranes, thirst, poor skin turgor, low urine output, decreased blood pressure, tachycardia, and weight loss.

6. Encourage intake of 12 to 17 8-oz glasses (3,000 to 4,000 ml) of fluid daily. Document intake.

Rationales

1. Urine characteristics may indicate such complications as infection (cloudy, odorous urine) and hemorrhage. Some hematuria is expected for 1 to 2 days after surgery, but bright red blood may indicate hemorrhage. Adequate fluid intake is necessary to flush calculi through the kidneys, prevent further calculus formation, and prevent tissue damage. Adequate urine output indicates proper kidney function. Calculi may increase the frequency and urgency of urination as they near the ureterovesical junction.

2. If present, a ureteral catheter aids passage of calculus fragments and prevents obstruction of urine flow. A patent urinary catheter aids in monitoring urine output and assessing calculus passage. Calculus fragments can easily obstruct catheters.

3. The type and amount of calculi passed may influence the treatment used to prevent recurrence.

4. Calculi are most likely to lodge in a ureter or the urethra.

5. Dehydration concentrates urine, increasing the risk of calculus formation and infection.

6. Fluids enhance passage of calculus fragments and help prevent obstruction and infection.

7. Give antibiotics every 4 to 8 hours, as ordered.

7. UTI is a major predisposing factor for urolithiasis. UTI provides organic material and alkalizes urine, precipitating minerals and causing calculi formation. Antibiotics are commonly given to prevent infection and recurrence.

8. Monitor and document vital signs every 2 to 4 hours, as ordered.

8. Changes in vital signs may indicate infection or other complications. Fever is common.

9. As ordered, irrigate the catheter with acid or alkaline solutions, depending on calculus composition.

9. Catheter irrigations with acid or alkaline solutions promote acidification or alkalinization of the urine and help prevent further calculus formation.

10. Additional individualized interventions: _____

10. Rationales: _____

Target outcome criteria
Within 3 days of surgery, the patient will:
• have urine that is normal in appearance and quantity
• have no infection
• have no hematuria
• show a reduced amount of calculus fragments in the urine

• have catheters removed without problems
• show adequate hydration
• have normal vital signs.

Nursing diagnosis: *Knowledge deficit related to potential causes of calculus formation*

NURSING PRIORITY: Promote understanding of the medical regimen to prevent calculi recurrence.

Interventions

1. See the "Knowledge Deficit" plan, page 56.

2. Provide information, reinforcing as necessary, and document teaching regarding:
• dietary limitations for calcium calculi (dairy products and green leafy vegetables), uric acid calculi (meats, legumes, and whole grains), and oxalate calculi (chocolate, caffeinated beverages, beets, and spinach)

• need for regular activity

• need for adequate fluid intake

• need to maintain desired urine pH with medications and regular urine pH testing, according to the doctor's recommendations

• need to monitor and treat metabolic and other conditions (such as gout) that predispose the patient to calculus formation

• signs and symptoms of recurrence, such as pain, hematuria, oliguria.

3. Additional individualized interventions: _____

Rationales

1. The "Knowledge Deficit" plan contains general information on patient teaching.

2. The patient needs accurate information to comply with the preventive regimen.
• Limiting foods rich in calculus-forming substances may inhibit recurrence. (A dietitian can provide details about specific diets, which vary considerably.)

• Activity decreases urine stasis and the risk of calculus formation.
• Fluids flush calculus fragments and help prevent recurrence.

• Depending on their composition, calculi may form in either acid or alkaline urine. The goal of treatment is to prevent calculus formation by maintaining the urine at the desired pH using appropriate medications.
• Treating underlying conditions, such as gout (uric acid accumulation), is necessary to prevent calculus formation.

• The incidence of recurrence is high.

3. Rationales: _____

RENAL DISORDERS

> **Target outcome criteria**
> By the time of discharge, the patient will:
> • verbalize dietary restrictions, the need for increased fluid intake, the recommended activity level, the need to monitor such metabolic problems as gout, and the signs and symptoms of recurrence
> • demonstrate accurate testing and interpretation of urine pH.

Discharge planning

NURSING DISCHARGE CRITERIA

Upon the patient's discharge, documentation shows evidence of:
• absence of gross hematuria
• absence of fever
• healing incision with no redness or other signs of infection
• absence of pulmonary or cardiovascular complications
• ability to tolerate and follow dietary and fluid regimen
• ability to perform activities of daily living independently
• ability to ambulate same as before hospitalization
• ability to perform pH monitoring
• ability to control pain using oral medications
• absence of infection or appropriate antibiotic prescribed
• stable vital signs
• absence of indwelling ureteral or urinary catheter or, if urinary catheter is present, ability to perform appropriate catheter care
• referral to home care if catheter is in place or if the patient's home support system is inadequate.

PATIENT-FAMILY TEACHING CHECKLIST

Document evidence that the patient and family demonstrate an understanding of:
___ care of incisions, drains, or catheters
___ activity precautions
___ dietary modifications
___ desired fluid intake
___ all discharge medications' purpose, dosage, administration schedule, and adverse effects requiring medical attention; usual medications include ascorbic acid (to increase urine acidity), ammonium chloride (for phosphate calculi), sodium or potassium phosphate (to decrease urine calcium for calcium calculi), sodium bicarbonate, acetazolamide (Diamox) and allopurinol (Lopurin) (for uric acid calculi), and antibiotics
___ signs and symptoms of recurring calculi
___ urine pH testing
___ need for follow-up laboratory tests
___ need for follow-up visits with the doctor
___ need for follow-up diagnostic tests
___ date, time, and location of next appointment
___ how to contact the doctor.

DOCUMENTATION CHECKLIST

Using outcome criteria as a guide, document:
___ clinical status on admission
___ significant changes in status
___ pertinent laboratory and diagnostic test findings
___ renal pain episodes
___ pain relief measures
___ passage of renal calculi fragments
___ fluid intake
___ urine output and characteristics
___ other therapies
___ nutritional intake
___ patient-family teaching
___ discharge planning.

ASSOCIATED PLANS OF CARE

Knowledge Deficit
Pain
Surgical Intervention

References

Beare, P.G., and Myers, J.L., eds. *Principles and Practice of Adult Health Nursing.* St. Louis: C.V. Mosby Co., 1990.

Brown, S.M. "Quantitative Measurement of Anxiety in Patients Undergoing Surgery for Renal Calculus Disease," *Journal of Advanced Nursing* 15(8):962-70, August 1990.

Patrick, M.L., Woods, S.L., Craven, R.F., Rokosky, J.S., and Bruno P.M. *Medical-Surgical Nursing: Pathophysiological Concepts,* 2nd ed. Philadelphia: J.B. Lippincott Co., 1991.

Phipps, W.J., Long, B.C., Woods, N.F., and Cassmeyer, V.L., eds. *Medical-Surgical Nursing: Concepts and Clinical Practice,* 4th ed. St. Louis: Mosby-Year Book, 1991.

Reilly, N.J. "The New Wave in Lithotripsy: Implications for Nursing," *RN* 51(3):44-49, 1988.

Thompson, J.M., McFarland, G.K., Hirsch, J.E., Tucker, S.M., and Bowers, A.C. *Mosby's Manual of Clinical Nursing,* 2nd ed. St. Louis: C.V. Mosby Co., 1989.

Acquired Immunodeficiency Syndrome

DRG information

DRG 488 HIV With Extensive Operating Room Procedure.
  Mean LOS = 18.8 days
DRG 489 HIV With Major Related Condition.
  Mean LOS = 10.2 days
DRG 490 HIV With or Without Other Related Condition.
  Mean LOS = 5.9 days
Additional DRG information: To ensure maximum reimbursement, document all complications of acquired immunodeficiency syndrome.

Introduction
DEFINITION AND TIME FOCUS

Acquired immunodeficiency syndrome (AIDS) is a progressive, incurable disorder of cell-mediated and humoral immunity caused by the human immunodeficiency virus (HIV), a retrovirus previously referred to as the human T-lymphotropic virus type III (HTLV-III) or the lymphadenopathy-associated virus (LAV). HIV is a ribonucleic acid (RNA) virus that selectively infects human cells marked with a CD4 surface antigen and, when stimulated, rapidly produces additional HIV, destroying and killing the human cell. Although T4 lymphocytes are most commonly infected, any cell with the CD4 surface antigen is vulnerable to infection, including monocytes, macrophages, bone marrow progenitors, and glial, gut, and epithelial cells. HIV infection renders the patient immunodeficient and susceptible to opportunistic infections, unusual cancers, and other characteristic abnormalities.

Since it first described AIDS in 1981, the Centers for Disease Control (CDC) has modified its case surveillance definition, classifying HIV infection according to four groups:
• Group I—patients who develop acute illness 3 to 6 weeks after primary infection and have nonspecific flu-like signs and symptoms
• Group II—asymptomatic patients
• Group III—patients with persistent generalized lymphadenopathy with no other symptoms
• Group IV—patients with full-blown AIDS, as evidenced by other symptoms or opportunistic diseases.

Group IV is further divided into five disease subgroups:
• Subgroup A—constitutional diseases
• Subgroup B—neurologic diseases
• Subgroup C—secondary infectious diseases
• Subgroup D—secondary cancers
• Subgroup E—other diseases.

The CDC defines AIDS as an illness characterized by laboratory evidence of HIV infection, coexisting with one indicator disease or more (see *Diagnostic criteria for AIDS*, page 600).

Two disorders commonly linked with AIDS are *Pneumocystis carinii* pneumonia (PCP) and Kaposi's sarcoma (KS). PCP, the most common opportunistic infection present at diagnosis, is a protozoal pneumonia. KS is a malignant neoplasm that begins as reddish or purplish skin lesions with variable distribution that may gradually spread, involving internal organs, mucous membranes, and lymph nodes. Various other conditions may present with AIDS, including infections related to cytomegalovirus (CMV), *Mycobacterium avium, M. intracellulare, Cryptococcus, Candida,* herpesvirus, and *Salmonella.*

AIDS currently has no cure and the prognosis for long-term survival is very poor, although survival varies significantly depending on the patient's overall health status, the availability of effective and prompt treatment for specific conditions, the patient's response to such treatment, and other factors. In acute episodes, early detection increases the likelihood of a favorable outcome. This plan focuses on the patient admitted for diagnosis and treatment of one or more AIDS-related conditions.

ETIOLOGY AND PRECIPITATING FACTORS
• multiple sexual partners, anal and vaginal intercourse, and other situations where sexual transmission of the virus is possible or normal protective barriers are reduced
• I.V. drug use, multiple blood transfusions (especially before 1985), and other situations allowing exposure to HIV-contaminated blood
• high-risk groups include homosexual and bisexual men, I.V. drug users, recipients of contaminated blood or blood products, sexual partners of those considered at high risk, and neonates born to mothers who were HIV-positive during pregnancy

Focused assessment guidelines
NURSING HISTORY (Functional health pattern findings)

Health perception—health management pattern
• may be asymptomatic or report mononucleosis-like symptoms for 3 to 6 weeks after initial exposure
• may report weeks to months of fatigue, malaise, low-grade fever, drenching night sweats, anorexia, sore throat, upper respiratory disorder that lingers, cough, or shortness of breath

DIAGNOSTIC CRITERIA FOR A.I.D.S.

According to the CDC (1987), a patient who tests positive for HIV infection and has one or more of the following diseases is diagnosed as having AIDS.

Viruses
- Herpes simplex virus that causes a mucocutaneous infection of more than 1 month; or bronchitis, pneumonitis, or esophagitis
- Cytomegalovirus in an organ other than the liver, spleen, or lymph nodes
- Papovavirus, such as progressive multifocal leukoencephalopathy

Bacteria
- Mycobacteria that cause disease outside the lungs, skin, or cervical or hilar lymph nodes
- Salmonella infection that causes recurrent, nontyphoidal septicemia

Fungi
- Candidal infection that causes disease in the esophagus, trachea, bronchi, or lungs
- Cryptococcosis that causes extrapulmonary disease
- Histoplasmosis or coccidioidomycosis that causes disease outside the lungs and cervical and hilar lymph nodes

Source: *Diseases*, Springhouse Corporation, 1993

Protozoa
- *Pneumocystis carinii* pneumonia
- Toxoplasmosis of the brain
- Cryptosporidiosis or isosporiasis that causes diarrhea for more than 1 month

Cancer
- Kaposi's sarcoma
- Primary lymphoma of the brain
- Other malignant lymphomas, such as B cell or unknown immunologic phenotype, small noncleaved lymphoma, and immunoblastic lymphoma

Other
- Wasting syndrome that causes unexplained weight loss of more than 10% and diarrhea or fever that lasts for more than 1 month
- Dementia that causes cognitive or motor dysfunction and interferes with work or activities of daily living

---

- may have a history of recurrent infections, amebiasis, or herpes simplex infections
- may have known exposure to HIV
- may identify self as being at high risk, such as a male homosexual or bisexual, I.V. drug user, or recipient of blood products
- may have a history of multiple blood transfusions
- may be the sexual partner of someone at high risk

Nutritional-metabolic pattern
- likely to report anorexia or dysphagia
- commonly reports weight loss greater than 10 lb (4.5 kg) in 1 month
- commonly reports episodic oral candidiasis (thrush), which may interfere with eating and taste

Elimination pattern
- commonly reports persistent diarrhea, even with treatment
- may report incontinence (from myopathy)

Activity-exercise pattern
- commonly reports severe exertional shortness of breath (with pulmonary involvement)
- may report dry mouth
- likely to display lack of energy and malaise
- may report leg weakness (from myopathy)

Sleep-rest pattern
- commonly reports drenching night sweats
- may describe erratic sleep patterns because of other symptoms

Cognitive-perceptual pattern
- may exhibit or describe forgetfulness, depression, mental dullness or lability, difficulty concentrating, or other changes in mental status
- may report headache
- may complain of pain from tumor invasion, fever, or neurogenic causes

Role-relationship pattern
- may report close friends or sexual partners who have died from AIDS
- commonly expresses anxiety over potential loss of social contact if diagnosis becomes known to others, or expresses distress over actual losses

Sexuality-reproductive pattern
- may report sexual activity with multiple partners
- commonly reports previous infection with other sexually transmitted diseases

Coping—stress tolerance pattern
- typically a young to middle-age, previously healthy person who reports little experience with illness or death
- may have delayed seeking medical attention until symptoms became severe because of fear, denial, lack of information, or low self-esteem
- commonly expresses extreme anxiety regarding diagnosis, current status, and prognosis
- may exhibit denial as initial coping behavior
- commonly displays signs of depression
- may express suicidal thoughts

Value-belief pattern
• may believe that illness is punishment for previous behavior

PHYSICAL FINDINGS
Pulmonary
• shortness of breath
• dry cough
• crackles

Gastrointestinal
• diarrhea
• hepatomegaly
• splenomegaly
• diffuse abdominal tenderness
• thrush
• mucosal lesions
• hairy leukoplakia on tongue

Neurologic
• anxiety
• decreased mental acuity (as shown by slowed speech or impaired memory)
• tendency to not initiate conversation
• impaired sense of position or vibration
• weakness
• paresthesias or paralysis
• hyperreflexia
• retinal abnormalities
• diffuse retinal hemorrhage or exudates
• positive Babinski's sign

Integumentary
• drenching night sweats
• in KS, reddish or purplish lesions varying in size from a few millimeters to a few centimeters across; may be macules or papules, usually appearing first on the head and neck or mucous membranes
• dermatitis
• lymphadenopathy
• herpes zoster or simplex
• anal warts
• diffuse dry skin
• butterfly rash on nose or cheeks
• tinea
• edema (with advanced KS)
• hypersensitivity to light touch

Musculoskeletal
• weakness
• pain
• stiff neck

DIAGNOSTIC STUDIES
• enzyme-linked immunosorbent assay (ELISA) — identifies HIV antibody (In the asymptomatic person, the ELISA is not diagnostic for AIDS: an individual may have a positive test without subsequently developing signs or symptoms. In addition, the ELISA may be falsely negative if performed too soon after exposure to the virus, or falsely negative or falsely positive if the person has had influenza or another viral illness recently. A positive ELISA in a patient who exhibits one or more indicator diseases such as PCP, KS, emaciation, or dementia can be considered diagnostic. Consult current CDC guidelines.)
• Western blot assay — uses electrophoretically marked proteins to distinguish and differentiate antibodies; used with ELISA to confirm diagnosis

The following laboratory findings represent characteristic values in patients with AIDS but are not specific to or diagnostic of AIDS:
• complete blood count (CBC) — reveals leukocytopenia and anemia
• total T-cell count — reduced; T4 cell count commonly less than 400/mm^3
• T4 T-cell to T8 T-cell (T4 to T8) ratio — low; decrease depends on patient's status, usually less than 1.0 (T4 T-cells also are known as helper or inducer T-cells; T8 T-cells also are known as cytotoxic or suppressor T-cells)
• immunoglobulin levels — usually elevated, especially IgG and IgA
• platelet count — shows thrombocytopenia
• skin test antigen studies — reveal anergy
• aspartate aminotransferase level — may be elevated (associated with hepatitis)
• lactic dehydrogenase level — may be elevated in PCP
• serum cholesterol level — may be low
• serum iron level — may be low
• hepatitis screen — may demonstrate carrier state or active disease (positive hepatitis-B surface antigen in serum)
• stool examination for ova and parasites — may reveal parasites or infection (such as cryptosporidiosis or salmonellosis)
• serum albumin and protein levels — may be low in emaciation
• blood urea nitrogen (BUN) level — may be elevated in emaciation

The following diagnostic procedures may be ordered for patients with AIDS:
• bronchoscopy — to diagnose PCP or other disorders, by transbronchial lung biopsy (to examine tissue) or by bronchoalveolar lavage to obtain a specimen containing PCP cysts
• chest X-ray — may reveal diffuse interstitial infiltrates (associated with PCP); however, may not be diagnostic even in active PCP
• open-lung biopsy — may provide definitive diagnosis of KS-related pulmonary symptoms or evidence of CMV infection
• culture of lesions — may demonstrate *Candida* or other organisms
• biopsy of lesions — may demonstrate KS, toxoplasmosis, or other complications
• gallium scan — may show radio-labeled gallium accumulation in white blood cells of infected areas; used to help establish early diagnosis of PCP, although test is nonspecific

• blood cultures—may identify pathogen if bacteremia is present
• lumbar puncture—results vary; may reveal cryptococcal meningitis; culture of spinal fluid may reveal HIV; results may be inconclusive for CMV infection
• sputum test for acid-fast bacillus—may indicate *Mycobacterium*
• computed tomography scan or magnetic resonance imaging (MRI)—may identify lesions for later biopsy; MRI may be the only means to detect progressive multifocal leukoencephalopathy
• bone marrow aspiration—may reveal hypoplasia

POTENTIAL COMPLICATIONS
• Burkitt's lymphoma
• toxoplasmosis
• multifocal leukoencephalopathy
• cryptococcal meningitis
• *Candida* meningitis
• herpes simplex
• cryptosporidiosis
• CMV infection
• diffuse organ infection
• disseminated bacterial infection
• hemorrhage
• encephalopathy
• tuberculosis
• *Mycobacterium avium* or *M. intracellulare* infection
• dementia

Collaborative problem: *High risk for infection related to immunosuppression (low T4 lymphocyte count or low T4 to T8 ratio)*

NURSING PRIORITIES: (a) Prevent or promptly treat new infections and (b) minimize effects of associated hyperthermia.

Interventions

1. Implement CDC and institution precautions for the immunosuppressed patient, including meticulous handwashing before entering the patient's room and after leaving, providing only cooked foods, prohibiting standing water in the room (such as in flower vases), protecting the patient from visitors with infections, and preventing the patient from handling live flowers or plants.

2. Monitor vital signs, including temperature, at least every 4 hours. Report fever onset or temperature spikes immediately.

3. Monitor CBC daily and report increasing leukopenia or neutropenia.

Rationales

1. The immunosuppressed patient is at risk for infection from any source, even those considered benign to a healthy person, such as raw fruits and vegetables. Such precautions minimize the patient's exposure to infectious organisms. Handwashing is the primary infection control measure for any patient. Gloves are recommended along with protective gowns and eye wear, as indicated, to guard against exposure to HIV-contaminated blood or secretions. (See *Protecting the health care provider from HIV infection* for more information on infection control.) Raw produce may harbor gram-negative bacilli; standing water provides a medium for microorganisms, particularly *Pseudomonas*. Visitors may transmit organisms through direct contact or airborne bacteria. Plants and soil may harbor fungi.

2. Fever is the body's response to pyrogens released from invading microorganisms. The increase in metabolic rate is accompanied by a corresponding increase in the heart and respiratory rates. In the severely immunocompromised patient, however, the usual response mechanisms may fail, and sepsis may occur in the absence of fever. For this reason, careful, frequent observation to detect subtle changes in the patient's condition is essential.

3. These changes indicate further compromise of the body's ability to resist or fight infection.

PROTECTING THE HEALTH CARE PROVIDER FROM H.I.V. INFECTION

Because the following is not a patient problem, it is presented separate from the rest of the plan.

Collaborative problem: *High risk for infection of health care provider because of exposure to infected waste, blood, body fluids, and needle stick injury*

NURSING PRIORITY: Prevent exposure to HIV and other infectious diseases and respond to any known exposures.

Interventions

1. Participate in inservice programs on current universal blood and body fluid precautions and body substance isolation.

2. If a needle stick injury or exposure to infected waste, blood, or body fluid occurs, follow hospital policies and procedures, such as:
• washing the wound thoroughly and reporting the incident to the nursing supervisor
• receiving confidential counseling, including updated information on confidential testing and treatment.

Rationales

1. The CDC recommends these techniques to prevent the spread of HIV, hepatitis, and other contagious diseases.

2. The risk of seroconversion from a needle stick is 0.4%. The CDC recommends testing initially and then at 6 weeks, 12 weeks, and 6 months. Research shows that zidovudine may help prevent seroconversion if treatment starts within 1 hour after exposure.

Target outcome criteria
After appropriate education, the health care provider will implement necessary precautions to prevent HIV exposure.

After HIV exposure, the health care provider will receive appropriate confidential counseling with the options of testing and treatment.

---

4. Monitor potential sites of infection daily. Check I.V. and injection sites, mucous membranes (including the rectum and vagina), and any wounds or skin breaks for changes in color, texture, or sensation; swelling; pain; induration; purulent drainage; or other abnormalities. If the patient is alert, discuss the importance of ongoing monitoring and early reporting of signs and symptoms of infection to medical personnel.

5. Be alert for signs and symptoms of neurologic infection, including stiff neck, headache, visual or motor abnormalities, memory impairment, and altered level of consciousness. Compare new findings with baseline neurologic or mental status findings, and report abnormalities to the doctor immediately. Consult with the doctor about the need for a lumbar puncture or MRI series.

6. Monitor for evidence of new pulmonary infections, checking lung sounds at least every 8 hours. Report crackles, decreased breath sounds, or other abnormal findings promptly.

4. The skin is one of the body's most important barriers against infection, and any break in the skin provides an entry point for microorganisms. Classic signs and symptoms of infection may be masked or delayed in the immunocompromised patient, so regular, careful observation for any changes is essential. For example, dysphagia may indicate esophagitis, while white patches in the mouth may signal candidiasis (both are common in AIDS). Any suspicious area warrants prompt investigation because even benign microorganisms can cause life-threatening illness in a patient with AIDS.

5. Neurologic abnormalities are common in AIDS, with approximately 40% of patients experiencing some neurologic involvement during the course of the disease. About 10% of patients seek initial medical attention because of neurologic symptoms from the HIV infection or a secondary infection. Encephalitis, the most common neurologic complication, may be caused by various microorganisms, including CMV and *Toxoplasma gondii*. Progressive multifocal leukoencephalopathy, another common finding, is usually detectable only by MRI scanning. Early detection and treatment of neurologic infection is crucial; once such involvement is advanced, the patient's prognosis is poor.

6. The most common AIDS-related pulmonary infection is PCP, but others—including tuberculosis—may occur. Although the effectiveness of current pharmacologic treatment for PCP is related to individual response, prompt treatment of other pulmonary infections may be lifesaving for the immunocompromised patient.

HEMATOLOGIC AND IMMUNOLOGIC DISORDERS

7. Obtain cultures, as ordered, from blood, stool, urine, sputum, or wound drainage. Evaluate sensitivity results and verify appropriateness of antibiotic therapy.

8. Administer antibiotics and anti-infectives, as ordered. The following medications are used commonly to treat AIDS-related infections, but others may be used.

• co-trimoxazole (Bactrim, Septra): Observe for and report adverse effects, such as rash, leukopenia, sore throat, purpura, jaundice, or signs of renal failure. Discontinue drug if rash occurs.
• pentamidine isethionate (Pentam): Observe for and report any adverse effects, such as leukopenia, hypotension, hypoglycemia, and sterile abscesses at injection sites. If administered by I.V. infusion, give over 45 to 90 minutes.
• pyrimethamine with sulfadoxine (Fansidar) or pyrimethamine (Daraprim): Observe for and report leukopenia, rash, purpura, or pruritus. Administer folic acid supplements, as ordered, and observe for glossitis.

9. If antiviral treatments are ordered, such as with zidovudine (Retrovir, AZT), didanosine (Videx), or dideoxycytidine (ddC), provide patient teaching and make appropriate interventions. (Consult current guidelines, as recommendations may change with further study.)

• Acetaminophen (Tylenol), aspirin, indomethacin (Indocin), probenecid (Benemid), cimetidine (Tagamet), lorazepam (Ativan), or ranitidine (Zantac) should be used cautiously during zidovudine therapy. Consult the doctor before administering any other medications, including over-the-counter medications.
• Obtain laboratory tests, as ordered (usually T-cell count, liver and kidney function tests, and CBC initially and at least every 2 weeks for several months). Transfusions may be required if toxicity develops.

• Observe for and report any adverse reactions to zidovudine, such as headache, abdominal discomfort, anxiety, rash, or itching, or to ddC or didanosine, such as seizures, irritability, difficulty sleeping, pancreatitis, or neuropathy.
10. If fever is present, administer acetaminophen, as ordered. Consult the doctor about alternating doses of acetaminophen with aspirin, naproxen (Naprosyn), or ibuprofen (Motrin) for persistent fever. Check platelet count and bleeding time before giving aspirin or ibuprofen, and withhold medication if clotting is prolonged.

7. If a new infection is suspected, immediate cultures will identify causative organisms. Sensitivity results guide antibiotic therapy.

8. Depending on the organism, therapy may involve several drugs simultaneously. Antibiotics may also be ordered prophylactically. Effectiveness varies, particularly in a second episode of PCP, which has a mortality rate of approximately 75%. If CMV is also involved, the mortality rate is higher.

• Co-trimoxazole is the antibiotic of choice for PCP. The drug also fights infections caused by *Shigella, Proteus, Klebsiella, Enterobacter,* and other bacteria. Skin rash may be an early sign of a severe or life-threatening reaction.
• Pentamidine is used to treat PCP and may be administered I.M., I.V., or by aerosol. Slow I.V. administration reduces the risk of hypotension.

• Pyrimethamine is indicated in toxoplasmosis. Because pyrimethamine is a folic acid inhibitor, folic acid supplements are recommended. Rash may be an early sign of a severe drug reaction. Glossitis may indicate folic acid deficiency.

9. Zidovudine is an antiviral agent that has shown promise against HIV in early studies. Made from thymidine, a component of deoxyribonucleic acid, the drug appears to block reproduction of the virus, probably by interfering with reverse transcriptase. Early studies also revealed increases in T4 cell counts, restored sensitivity to skin test antigens, fever reduction, and improved neurologic status. While zidovudine may improve overall status, it does *not* kill the virus, cure AIDS, or prevent transmission. Didanosine, approved in October 1991, has similar properties to zidovudine; ddC is still under investigation, as are combination therapies with the three antiviral medications.

• These medications may impair zidovudine metabolism, resulting in toxicity.

• To qualify for zidovudine therapy, the patient must have PCP or a T-cell count less than 500/mm^3. Because zidovudine may cause severe neutropenia, anemia, or other blood dyscrasias, periodic monitoring is essential. Neutrophil counts of 1,000/mm^3 or less may indicate the need for dosage reduction or temporary discontinuation of therapy.

• Because no long-term studies have been completed, the reactions listed are based on results from a small, controlled trial group. Any new symptom, or worsening of an existing symptom, should be investigated promptly.

10. Acetaminophen, aspirin, and ibuprofen inhibit the effects of pyrogens on the thermoregulatory center, thereby reducing fever. Aspirin and acetaminophen may impair zidovudine metabolism, resulting in toxicity; alternating antipyretics may avoid this effect. Aspirin and ibuprofen may decrease platelet adhesion, prolonging clotting time.

11. Institute the following measures for fever, as ordered and appropriate: administering antipyretics, using a hypothermia blanket, monitoring for signs of dehydration, and replacing fluids as needed. See Appendix C, "Fluid and Electrolyte Imbalances."

11. A hypothermia blanket may be necessary to reduce body temperature if aspirin and acetaminophen are ineffective or contraindicated. Prolonged fever increases the metabolic rate and promotes diaphoresis, contributing to dehydration and electrolyte imbalances. The "Fluid and Electrolyte Imbalances" appendix contains detailed information on these imbalances.

12. Additional individualized interventions: _____

12. Rationales: _____

Target outcome criteria
Throughout the hospital stay, the patient will:
• receive continuous protection against infection
• receive prompt treatment for new infections
• display no unanticipated medication adverse effects
• exhibit no signs or symptoms of dehydration.

Nursing diagnosis: *High risk for ineffective individual coping related to life-threatening illness, potential loss of usual roles, decisions regarding treatment, or poor prognosis for long-term survival*

NURSING PRIORITY: Promote positive coping behaviors.

Interventions

1. Assess for excessive anxiety. Note signs and symptoms, such as poor eye contact, agitation, or restlessness.

2. Introduce yourself and other staff members. Provide continuity of caregivers; minimize use of unfamiliar staff whenever possible. Demonstrate acceptance: use touch, make eye contact, and listen actively.

3. Implement measures to promote physical relaxation, as indicated, including progressive relaxation or controlled breathing techniques, therapeutic use of heat or massage, environmental modifications (such as reducing noise, heat, light, and other stimuli), physical therapy, and providing familiar articles brought from home.

4. Encourage verbalization of feelings. Anticipate fear, guilt, and anger, and accept such expressions as normal. If uncomfortable discussing explicit issues, arrange for another nurse to care for the patient. Whenever possible, refer the patient at the time of diagnosis to a mental health professional who can provide ongoing counseling.

Rationales

1. Prolonged or excessive anxiety may have negative psychological and physiologic effects. Anxiety interferes with the ability to learn, make decisions, and mobilize resources. Anxiety also increases sympathetic nervous system activity, increasing metabolic and cardiac demands and placing further stress on the body.

2. Consistency in staffing facilitates development of trust. Unfamiliar staff members may increase the patient's anxiety. Demonstrating acceptance promotes a therapeutic relationship. Patients with AIDS commonly report "feeling like lepers"; touch reduces this sense of isolation.

3. The patient may be unaware of physical tension and its contribution to anxiety. Physical relaxation promotes restoration of psychological equilibrium.

4. The diagnosis of AIDS carries an enormous psychosocial impact that may overwhelm the patient initially. The patient is typically unable to use usual defenses and resources; for example, denial may be impossible because of the media's coverage of AIDS, and friends or family may abandon the patient once the diagnosis is confirmed. If the disease was contracted through sexual contact, the patient may experience guilt over unresolved issues, anxiety or anger toward previous partners, or ambivalence about past or future desires or behaviors. The diagnosis requires that the patient immediately rethink relationships and commonly involves a loss of intimacy at a time when the patient needs support. Multiple referrals may lead to fragmented care; consistency in follow-up promotes optimal use of resources.

HEMATOLOGIC AND IMMUNOLOGIC DISORDERS

5. Identify and discuss unhealthy coping behaviors. Teach the patient about the effects of alcohol or drug abuse on immune function.

5. The patient may use alcohol or illegal drugs to avoid painful realities. If the disease was contracted through I.V. drug use, the underlying dependency must be addressed when planning care. Alcohol and drug abuse can compromise immune activity.

6. Help the patient identify and list specific fears and concerns contributing to anxiety. Focus on modifiable factors.

6. Anxiety increases when fears seem overwhelming and all encompassing. Identifying specific concerns helps quantify feelings and allows the patient to begin planning a coping strategy. Focusing on modifiable factors may increase the patient's sense of control.

7. Help the patient identify and activate resources, considering inner strengths, coping ability, and such external supports as friends, family, and a spiritual advisor. See the "Ineffective Individual Coping" plan, page 51.

7. Initial anxiety may be so overwhelming that the patient is unable to mobilize usual coping methods. The "Ineffective Individual Coping" plan provides specific interventions for the patient experiencing anxiety.

8. Acknowledge the unknowns of AIDS. Answer questions honestly and accurately. Accept the patient's response to losses. See the "Dying" and "Grieving" plans, pages 11 and 31 respectively.

8. Acknowledging unknowns reassures the patient that the caregiver understands and is sensitive to the profound changes AIDS implies. Reminding the patient that emotional reactions are a normal response to a realistic threat may reduce anxiety and facilitate coping. The "Grieving" and "Dying" plans provide further interventions related to psychosocial adjustment to illness and the losses illness entails.

9. Additional individualized interventions: _____

9. Rationales: _____

Target outcome criteria
Throughout the hospital stay, the patient will:
• use positive coping behaviors
• display awareness of legal rights and available support, if appropriate to condition
• have opportunities to address issues of grieving and dying

• identify specific personal stressors
• identify resources and begin mobilizing them.

Collaborative problem: *High risk for hypoxemia related to ventilation-perfusion imbalance, pneumonia, and weakness*

NURSING PRIORITY: Promote oxygenation.

Interventions

1. Assess continually for signs of hypoxemia, such as tachycardia, restlessness, anxiety, tachypnea, irritability, and pallor or cyanosis. Monitor oxygenation with an oximeter or take arterial blood gas (ABG) measurements, as ordered and needed for increasing dyspnea or inadequate respiratory effort. Report abnormal findings immediately, and prepare the patient for ventilatory support, as condition indicates.

2. Administer oxygen therapy via nasal cannula, face mask, nonrebreather mask, or continuous positive airway pressure mask according to unit protocol or as ordered.

Rationales

1. PCP causes hard cysts to form in the interstitial spaces of the lungs, displacing surfactant and decreasing diffusion across the alveolar-capillary membrane. As arterial PO_2 levels decrease, the sympathetic nervous system attempts to compensate by increasing the heart rate. Progressive deterioration in ventilatory status may lead to respiratory failure—a common cause of death in AIDS-related illness. Ventilatory support may be required to maintain oxygenation. However, arterial PO_2 levels in patients with PCP and AIDS tend to be higher than those in patients with PCP alone and are sometimes even within normal range.

2. Supplemental oxygen elevates arterial oxygen content and decreases hypoxia.

3. Perform airway clearance measures, as needed:
• If the patient is cooperative, teach coughing and deep breathing exercises, and encourage hourly use of the incentive spirometer, as ordered.
• If the patient is uncooperative, perform artificial sighing and coughing with a hand-held resuscitation bag hourly. Suction as needed if the patient is unable to cough effectively, as indicated by noisy respirations or gurgles auscultated over the large airways. Use supplemental oxygen before, during, and after airway clearance procedures.

3. The patient may be unable to clear the airway effectively because of general debilitation and weakness. Deep-breathing helps expand the lungs fully and prevents areas of atelectasis associated with pneumonia and bed rest. Incentive spirometry and coughing also promote lung expansion; however, exercise caution because coughing and positive-pressure breathing may cause alveolar rupture secondary to decreased surfactant in PCP. All airway clearance procedures may reduce PO_2 levels. Supplemental oxygen may be provided through nasal prongs during suctioning.

4. Observe for complications of bronchoscopy; report any bleeding, anxiety, or unusual findings.

4. Irritation from the bronchoscope may cause bleeding, further decreasing oxygenation and threatening airway patency.

5. Evaluate and document the following every 8 hours and as needed: presence or absence of an effective cough, sputum character and color, respiratory effort, skin color, breath sounds, and activity tolerance. Be alert for changes in level of consciousness, and report promptly any that occur.

5. Careful serial observations of respiratory status are essential to detect subtle changes that may indicate the need to reevaluate therapy. The patient with PCP may require multiple antibiotics if other infections occur simultaneously. Changes in level of consciousness may signal impending respiratory failure.

6. If narcotic analgesics are used to control pain, be alert for signs of respiratory depression after analgesic administration. Report an excessively slowed respiratory rate, frequent sighing, decreased alertness, or any other indications of inadequate respiratory effort.

6. Narcotics cause central nervous system depression and may impair respiratory center function.

7. Assist with self-care activities as needed (see the "Impaired physical mobility" nursing diagnosis in this plan). Teach energy conservation measures, such as using a shower chair, organizing activities and grouping procedures, using large muscles, avoiding activities that involve raising the arms over the head, and scheduling rest periods between activities.

7. Because activity increases oxygen demand, hypoxemia may worsen with exertion. Sitting requires less energy than standing. Organizing and grouping procedures reduce unnecessary exertion. Raising the arms over the head rapidly causes fatigue; large-muscle groups are more efficient.

8. Additional individualized interventions: _____

8. Rationales: _____

Target outcome criteria
Within 2 days of admission, the patient will:
• exhibit decreased dyspnea
• exhibit oximeter or ABG measurements improved from baseline

• cough and deep-breathe effectively
• initiate a plan for energy conservation.

Nursing diagnosis: *Sensory-perceptual alteration related to neurologic involvement*

NURSING PRIORITY: Minimize effects of neurologic changes.

Interventions

1. Assess the patient's mental and neurologic status on admission and at least daily thereafter, including level of consciousness, orientation, long-term and recent memory, ability to follow directions and think abstractly, speech, pupillary responses, and strength and sensation in arms and legs.

Rationales

1. Baseline and ongoing mental and neurologic assessments allow early detection of neurologic involvement, a common and usually ominous finding in the patient with AIDS. Neurologic manifestations occur in approximately 40% of patients with AIDS and include confusion, emotional lability, memory loss, and mental dullness.

2. Evaluate the patient's emotional state, considering the effects of depression, anxiety, grief, or other emotions on mental status findings. Also be alert to the possibility that medications may cause confusion, memory impairment, or other unusual findings.

2. Emotional responses and medication adverse effects may contribute to reduced alertness, confusion, withdrawal, hyperactivity, anxiety, or other mental status changes.

3. Assess for possible visual impairment by using an eye chart, if possible. If the patient has significant visual impairment, prevent injury by placing items within easy reach and ensuring that side rails are always up.

3. CMV infection of the optic nerve can cause blindness. Vision changes may be particularly frightening and difficult for the patient to accept. Precautionary interventions, particularly if confusion is also a factor, reduce the risk of injury.

4. If confusion is present, provide cues for reorientation, such as identifying yourself when entering the room, putting identifying signs on doors and objects, providing a large calendar and clock, discussing the day's events, and encouraging frequent visits, if possible, from family and friends.

4. Reorientation may help decrease anxiety, reduce the risk of injury, and facilitate coping.

5. Explain neurologic symptoms to the patient and to family and friends. Emphasize supportive behaviors, such as using humor, changing the subject if repetitive or irrational behaviors are present, providing gentle reminders of appropriate behavior, and listening actively.

5. Explanations may help the patient feel less isolated and anxious about mentation changes. Family members and friends may be more supportive if they understand that mentation changes may be related to disease progression.

6. Provide a safe and supportive environment, instituting safety measures appropriate to the patient's deficits.

6. Confusion, disorientation, and loss of function are emotionally devastating. Because the disoriented patient is at increased risk for injury, safety measures must be instituted.

7. Observe for involuntary movements, paresthesias, numbness, pain, weakness, and atrophy of extremities. Consult the doctor regarding treatment, if needed, and institute measures to protect the extremities if sensation is impaired.

7. Distal symmetrical sensorimotor neuropathy is a common peripheral nerve complication in AIDS. The cause is unknown. Although a relatively benign condition, it may cause significant discomfort. Treatment may include heat, range-of-motion exercises, and electrical stimulation.

8. Additional individualized interventions: _____

8. Rationales: _____

Target outcome criteria
Throughout the hospital stay, the patient will:
• use cues for reorientation
• take appropriate precautions to prevent injury

• acknowledge limitations appropriate to neurologic deficits.

Nursing diagnosis: *Social isolation related to communicable disease, associated social stigma, and fear of infection from social contact*

NURSING PRIORITY: Minimize feelings of social isolation.

Interventions

1. Assess the patient's support system, such as family, spouse (or partner), and friends. Ask the patient and others in the support system about any recent losses in their lives, any recent change in the patient's living situation, and attitudes of family and friends toward the disease.

Rationales

1. The patient's and others' lack of accurate knowledge, as well as the social stigma associated with AIDS, may diminish the patient's social contacts. In addition, the patient may isolate self from fear of contracting infections from others. Assessing the patient's social support system helps identify resources and may allow the nurse to correct misconceptions about the disease.

2. Provide opportunities for the patient and family to express their feelings.

3. Provide an atmosphere of acceptance. Encourage staff, family, and friends to touch and hug the patient.

4. Teach family and friends about ways the AIDS virus is *not* transmitted, including the following: toilet seats and bathroom fixtures, swimming pools, dishes, furniture, handshakes, hugging, social (dry) kissing and other nonsexual physical gestures of affection, pets (although pets may carry microorganisms threatening to the patient), doorknobs, or casual social contact.

Saliva, tears, and coughing are considered unlikely sources of transmission. If an opportunistic infection is present, family members should observe the usual precautions, including handwashing, good health habits, and avoiding contact with contaminated secretions. Provide written materials to reinforce these points.

5. Provide the patient and family with telephone numbers of available resources for counseling, support, and information. Check with the local public health department for resources in your area. The following numbers may also be helpful:
• Centers for Disease Control (CDC), Atlanta: 1-800-342-AIDS
• CDC Information: 1-800-342-7514
• AIDS Foundation, San Francisco: 1-415-864-4376
• National Gay Task Force, New York: 1-800-221-7044.
Refer the patient to the social services department for help with financial concerns.

6. Additional individualized interventions: _____

_____

2. Expressing feelings helps decrease the sense of isolation.

3. Physical contact decreases feelings of isolation and demonstrates caring. Family and friends may need gentle reminders that such contact does not transmit the virus. The nurse can be a good role model for family and friends.

4. The "worried well" (those who are healthy but worried about contracting AIDS) may be torn between their desire to support the patient and their concern for personal health. Education may help reduce their conflicts and encourage normal interaction with the patient. The AIDS virus does not survive on inanimate objects and is killed by soap and hot water. Opportunistic infections can be transmitted to others, but healthy individuals are at no greater risk than usual. Written materials reinforce oral teaching and provide a source for future reference.

5. Ongoing support is essential for the AIDS patient and the family throughout the illness. Support groups offer understanding, practical advice, and the latest information on new developments, which may surpass the support clinicians can provide. In addition, such groups may provide enriching relationships that enhance the patient's ability to cope with the disease. Referral to a social services department is essential because treatment is expensive and the patient may have special housing needs.

6. Rationales: _____

_____

Target outcome criteria
Throughout the hospital stay, the patient will:
• verbalize feelings related to social losses
• express and receive affection

• contact support and resource persons, as appropriate.

Nursing diagnosis: *Impaired physical mobility related to fatigue, weakness, hypoxemia, depression, altered sleep patterns, medication adverse effects, and orthostatic hypotension*

NURSING PRIORITIES: (a) Promote maximum physical mobility and (b) prevent complications associated with decreased mobility.

Interventions

1. Provide standard nursing care for decreased mobility. Refer to the "Impaired Physical Mobility" plan, page 36.

2. Assess the need for sedatives, administer medications as ordered, and monitor their effects.

Rationales

1. The "Impaired Physical Mobility" plan provides general nursing interventions for this condition. This plan supplies additional information specific to the AIDS patient.

2. Anxiety and worry commonly interrupt sleep in the patient with AIDS. Rest is essential for healing.

3. Encourage the patient experiencing weakness or orthostatic hypotension to use the call light, ask for assistance when standing and walking, and leave belongings within reach.

4. Assist with activities of daily living (ADLs) as necessary. Anticipate the patient's needs.

5. Additional individualized interventions: _____

3. The patient may have never been this weak or dizzy before and may need reminders to ask for assistance.

4. The patient may never have been sick or hospitalized before and may feel uncomfortable asking for help.

5. Rationales: _____

Target outcome criteria
Throughout the hospital stay, the patient will:
• appear rested
• verbalize adequacy of rest
• call for assistance as appropriate
• experience no falls or other injuries related to weakness

• engage in physical activity as tolerated
• develop no complications from impaired mobility.

Nursing diagnosis: *Nutritional deficit related to nausea, vomiting, diarrhea, anorexia, medication adverse reactions, or decreased nutrient absorption secondary to the disease*

NURSING PRIORITY: Promote adequate nutritional intake.

Interventions

1. Provide typical assessments and interventions for nutritional status. Refer to the "Nutritional Deficit" plan, page 63, for information.

2. Administer antiemetics, as ordered, if nausea and vomiting are present.

3. Consult the doctor about nasogastric (NG) feedings or total parenteral nutrition (TPN) if the patient is unable to tolerate adequate oral intake or has severe chronic diarrhea. See the "Total Parenteral Nutrition" plan, page 411, for further information.

4. Additional individualized interventions: _____

Rationales

1. The "Nutritional Deficit" plan discusses general interventions for this condition. This plan contains additional information pertinent to AIDS.

2. Chemotherapeutic agents administered for infections commonly cause nausea and vomiting. Antiemetics block stimulation of the vomiting center.

3. NG feedings provide nutrients without as many associated complications as TPN. However, severe diarrhea from cryptosporidiosis, salmonellosis, or intestinal KS lesions may reduce GI absorption, making TPN necessary.

4. Rationales: _____

Target outcome criteria
Throughout the hospital stay, the patient will maintain adequate oral intake of food *or* tolerate enteral or parenteral feedings without complications.

By the time of discharge, the patient will:
• exhibit BUN values decreased since admission
• take food orally without excessive nausea or vomiting *or* verbalize and demonstrate understanding of outpatient or home TPN therapy, if appropriate.

Nursing diagnosis: *High risk for fluid volume deficit related to chronic, persistent diarrhea associated with opportunistic infection*

NURSING PRIORITY: Maintain optimal fluid status.

Interventions

1. See Appendix C, "Fluid and Electrolyte Imbalances."

2. Additional individualized interventions: _____

Rationales

1. Diarrhea is one of the most problematic symptoms for the AIDS patient. Various microorganisms contribute to the problem, while rectal mucosal lesions, hemorrhoids, and nutritional deficit exacerbate it further. Fever increases the potential for dehydration. The "Fluid and Electrolyte Imbalances" appendix provides further guidelines for monitoring fluid and electrolyte status and intervening to maintain optimal hydration and metabolic balance.

2. Rationales: _____

Target outcome criterion
Throughout the hospital stay, the patient will maintain normal fluid and electrolyte status, or receive prompt corrective measures if imbalances occur.

Nursing diagnosis: *Altered oral mucous membrane related to infections or masses*

NURSING PRIORITY: Reduce discomfort and prevent further damage to the mucous membrane.

Interventions

1. Assess the patient's mouth at least twice daily for signs and symptoms of thrush, lesions, or bleeding.

2. Ensure that the patient receives or completes mouth care after meals and at bedtime. Provide the following instructions:
• Use a soft toothbrush or swabs.
• Use dilute hydrogen peroxide or toothpaste.

3. Apply lubricant to the lips as needed.

4. Obtain cultures from suspicious oral lesions, as ordered.

5. Avoid using alcohol, lemon-glycerin swabs, and commercial mouthwashes.

6. Assess for and report any inflammation or ulceration of the oral mucosa and any leukoplakia, pain, dysphagia, or voice changes.

7. Additional individualized interventions: _____

Rationales

1. Candidiasis is extremely common in AIDS and has even been considered a harbinger of the disease. Lesions may occur as a medication adverse effect or from changes in normal oral flora.

2. Mouth care helps reduce the risk of infection by maintaining circulation to the mucous membrane and by decreasing bacteria in the mouth. Vigorous brushing is discouraged because it may cause bleeding and injure the mucous membrane, providing a place of entry for pathogens.

3. Lubricant helps prevent dry and cracked lips.

4. Culture results guide therapy.

5. These products contain alcohol, which may dry and irritate mucous membranes.

6. Stomatitis, pharyngitis, and esophagitis are common AIDS-related infections. Initial symptoms include inflammation of the mucous membranes, voice changes, and difficulty swallowing (if the inflammation involves the esophagus or larynx).

7. Rationales: _____

HEMATOLOGIC AND IMMUNOLOGIC DISORDERS

> **Target outcome criteria**
> Throughout the hospital stay, the patient will:
> • perform or receive oral care at least four times daily
> • have oral mucous membrane lesions (if present) treated promptly.

Nursing diagnosis: *High risk for impaired skin integrity related to effects of immobility, disease, medications, or poor nutritional status*

NURSING PRIORITY: Prevent skin breakdown.

Interventions

1. Implement usual measures to detect and prevent skin breakdown, such as inspection, frequent turning, and skin care.

2. If a pressure ulcer develops, institute therapeutic treatment, as ordered. This may include:

• cleaning or debridement agents (according to hospital protocol or the doctor's recommendations)

• topical antibiotics

• blow-drying after bathing or treatments (follow hospital policy)

• positioning to avoid pressure on the lesion, using foam or other padding as needed.

3. If the patient is receiving I.V. or I.M. pentamidine isethionate for PCP, rotate injection sites and monitor them carefully for sterile abscesses.

4. Observe for urticaria, maculopapular rash, or pruritus.

5. Provide appropriate patient teaching related to the above measures.

6. Additional individualized interventions: _____

Rationales

1. Immunosuppression makes effective treatment of pressure ulcers difficult. Preventive care is essential.

2. Prompt treatment is essential to prevent further complications.

• Agent selection depends on the patient's status and the doctor's preference. Half-strength povidone-iodine solution (Betadine) is commonly used.

• The choice of prophylactic antibiotic (which varies) should be reevaluated if infection develops.

• A blow dryer may be useful for certain areas, such as the rectum.

• Additional pressure leads to further tissue breakdown.

3. Pentamidine is an irritating drug, and sterile abscesses are a common adverse effect.

4. Medications commonly used to treat opportunistic infections (such as co-trimoxazole, ethambutol [Myambutol], and pyrimethamine) may cause skin irritation. Additionally, HIV infection itself may result in skin abnormalities.

5. For the able patient, such knowledge promotes self-care and a sense of increased control and self-esteem. For the patient unable to perform self-care, such knowledge promotes understanding of frequent interventions.

6. Rationales: _____

> **Target outcome criterion**
> Throughout the hospital stay, the patient will present clean, dry, and intact skin, or if breakdown occurs, receive appropriate treatment.

Nursing diagnosis: *High risk for sexual dysfunction related to fatigue, depression, fear of rejection, and fear of disease transmission*

NURSING PRIORITIES: (a) Promote a positive sexual self-concept and (b) teach safer sex practices.

Interventions

1. Determine if the patient is currently involved in a sexual relationship by asking direct questions in a nonjudgmental manner. If you are uncomfortable discussing sexuality, refer the patient to another professional or an AIDS counselor.

2. Encourage open discussion and sharing of feelings between the patient and spouse (or partner). Provide accurate information.

3. Encourage expression of affection and nonsexual touching, such as hugging, massage, and holding hands.

4. Discuss safer sex practices. Refer to current CDC guidelines for detailed, up-to-date recommendations. Teach the patient and spouse (or partner) to observe the following guidelines:
• Engage in a mutually monogamous relationship.

• Avoid exchange of blood or body fluids, including swallowing semen.
• Use sexual techniques that do not involve exchange of body fluids, such as mutual masturbation and fantasy.
• Avoid sex practices classified as "unsafe," such as intercourse without a condom, oral sex without a condom, and inserting objects into the rectum.
• Maintain safe sexual practices throughout lifespan.

5. Additional individualized interventions: _____

Rationales

1. Because the disease may be transmitted through sexual contact, assessing sexual relationships is essential. Many patients with AIDS are abandoned by their partners after diagnosis. If the patient is a homosexual, the high incidence of AIDS among homosexual males may add to the anxiety of both the patient and spouse (or partner). This is especially true if the patient's sexual orientation is not known or accepted by family or friends.

2. Sharing of feelings may help the couple maintain closeness and offer mutual support. Accurate information helps dispel fears based on misunderstandings about AIDS.

3. Liberal use of touch reduces feelings of shame and abandonment.

4. Safer sex guidelines may help reduce the likelihood of disease transmission. CDC guidelines are revised frequently, so nurses should consult current information before providing specific teaching.
• Multiple sexual contacts are associated with an increased risk of HIV transmission.
• The virus is transmitted through such exchanges.

• Alternative techniques may provide sexual satisfaction without the risk of disease transmission.

• Unsafe practices are associated with disease transmission.

• Even after AIDS education and years of safe sexual practices, the patient may relapse to unsafe behaviors.

5. Rationales: _____

Target outcome criteria
By the time of discharge, the patient will:
• list safer sex measures
• exchange affection with loved ones

• share sexual concerns with spouse or partner, if present.

Nursing diagnosis: *Knowledge deficit related to symptoms of disease progression, risk factors, transmission of disease, home care, and treatment options*

NURSING PRIORITY: Provide the patient and family with complete and accurate information.

Interventions

1. See the "Knowledge Deficit" plan, page 56.

Rationales

1. The "Knowledge Deficit" plan contains detailed interventions for patient and family teaching. This plan contains additional information pertinent to AIDS.

2. Teach the patient and loved ones about infection prevention measures, including:

• regular cleaning of bathrooms and kitchen

• avoiding crowds and persons with known or suspected infections; using good handwashing techniques

• avoiding touching fish tanks, animal waste, or birdcages

• consulting the doctor before obtaining pets

• avoiding raw fruits and vegetables and unpasteurized milk

• smoking cessation, as indicated

• consulting the doctor about vaccines

• following dietary recommendations, including high-protein, high-calorie intake

• eliminating sources of standing water

• practicing good health habits, such as getting adequate rest and regular exercise, and avoiding steroids or recreational drugs that may further decrease immune function.

3. Discuss symptoms that may indicate AIDS-related complications. These include night sweats, chest pain, shortness of breath, swollen glands, persistent fever, weight loss, diarrhea, weakness, purplish blotches on the skin, white patches or ulcerations in the mouth, difficulty swallowing, dry cough, headache, confusion, easy bruising, and skin lesions. Emphasize the importance of promptly reporting symptoms to health care providers.

4. Review with the family recommendations for home care and waste disposal:
• Wash hands thoroughly before touching the patient and after contact with blood or secretions.
• Use 1:10 bleach-in-water solution for cleaning blood spills and washing soiled bedding, medical equipment, bedpans or commodes, and soiled surfaces.
• Dispose of contaminated waste carefully. Flush body fluids, blood, and used tissues down the toilet. Place needles in a puncture-proof container; when full, seal the container and dispose of it in the trash. Double-bag non-flushable items soiled with secretions in plastic bags, tie closed, and dispose of in the trash.
• Use masks only when suctioning or performing other measures that may allow direct contact with secretions, or to protect the patient from the caregiver's infection.
• Wear gloves only when handling body fluids or blood.
• Wash dishes and utensils in hot, soapy water. Avoid sharing utensils or glassware.

5. Teach the patient and loved ones how the AIDS virus may be spread: by sexual activity or by direct contact of an infected person's blood or body fluids with the broken skin or mucous membrane of an uninfected person. Discuss such precautionary measures as:

• notifying other health care providers (such as the dentist) of the patient's AIDS status

• avoiding sharing needles and personal toiletry items (such as razors and toothbrushes)

2. Infection control is essential to minimize the risk of further complications.
• Moisture in bathrooms and kitchen may facilitate fungal growth.
• Immunosuppression renders the patient extremely susceptible to infections.
• Animal waste harbors microorganisms.
• Pets may carry intestinal protozoa.
• These may be sources of microorganisms.

• Smoking increases the incidence of respiratory infections.
• The immunosuppressed patient may not be able to manufacture appropriate antibodies and may develop the disease the vaccine would normally protect against.
• Malnutrition predisposes the patient to infection.

• Standing water provides a medium for microbial growth.
• Overall health maintenance maximizes immune response.

3. Early reporting of new symptoms, and prompt treatment of complications, may prolong active life.

4. Thorough, specific teaching reduces anxiety for family members and promotes safe and effective care. Current evidence does not suggest any danger of HIV transmission from casual contact. The CDC recommends that caregivers use blood and body fluid precautions.

5. Awareness of transmission factors may help the patient avoid spreading the disease to others.

• This allows health care providers to observe appropriate precautions to protect both the patient and themselves.
• Sharing these items may permit transmission of the virus.

• avoiding donating blood or organs

• preventing pregnancy

• safer sex practices (see the "High risk for sexual dysfunction" nursing diagnosis in this plan for details).

6. Provide information regarding the patient's legal rights, including privacy and confidentiality of medical records, laws protecting against discrimination in housing and employment, and the right to choose treatment and participate in research studies. If unable to provide such information yourself, refer the patient to an AIDS support group or other resources as appropriate.

7. Encourage the patient to explore treatment options with the doctor, including new or experimental medications and alternatives to traditional medicine (such as acupuncture, visualization, nutritional therapy, and stress control).

8. Additional individualized interventions: _____

_____

• The virus has been transmitted through blood transfusions and transplanted organs.

• The virus has a 20% to 30% chance of being transmitted to the fetus.

• Sexual activity is a major method of HIV transmission.

6. Because of the widespread fear of AIDS, the patient may encounter discrimination. Knowledge of legal rights and options may help prevent further losses.

7. At this time, no cure for AIDS exists; however, new or alternative therapies may offer as-yet-undocumented benefits. In addition, such therapies may offer the patient hope, energy, and an increased sense of wellness.

8. Rationales: _____

_____

Target outcome criteria
By the time of discharge, the patient will:
• list precautionary measures to avoid infections
• list symptoms that may indicate infections or other complications
• discuss appropriate home care and waste disposal guidelines

• list precautions to prevent disease transmission
• verbalize awareness of legal rights.

Discharge planning
NURSING DISCHARGE CRITERIA
Upon the patient's discharge, documentation shows evidence of:
• stable vital signs
• absence of cardiovascular and pulmonary symptoms
• absence of skin breakdown
• stabilizing weight
• ability to tolerate adequate nutritional intake
• ability to control pain and nausea using oral medications
• ability to transfer, ambulate, and perform ADLs independently or with minimal assistance
• absence of bowel or bladder dysfunction
• mentation indicating an ability for continued independent self-care
• adequate home support system or referral to home care or hospice if indicated by disease stage, inadequate home support system, or inability to manage ADLs and care independently.

PATIENT-FAMILY TEACHING CHECKLIST
Document evidence that the patient and family demonstrate an understanding of:
___ disease and its implications
___ all discharge medications (may include antibiotics or other chemotherapeutics)
___ community resources available for emotional support, financial counseling, grief counseling, and individual and family counseling
___ treatment options, including investigational studies
___ resources for long-term care or terminal care, such as a hospice
___ signs and symptoms of opportunistic infection or complications
___ ways to prevent HIV transmission
___ ways to decrease risk of new infection
___ symptoms to report to the health care provider
___ importance of keeping follow-up appointments
___ how to contact the doctor
___ legal rights and resources.

HEMATOLOGIC AND IMMUNOLOGIC DISORDERS

DOCUMENTATION CHECKLIST

Using outcome criteria as a guide, document:

___ clinical status on admission

___ significant changes in status

___ pertinent laboratory and diagnostic test findings

___ occurrence of opportunistic infections

___ treatment decisions

___ nutritional program and support

___ breathing patterns

___ sleep patterns

___ emotional coping

___ support from family and friends

___ patient-family teaching

___ discharge planning.

ASSOCIATED PLANS OF CARE

Dying

Grieving

Impaired Physical Mobility

Ineffective Family Coping

Ineffective Individual Coping

Lymphoma

Nutritional Deficit

Pain

Pneumonia

Total Parenteral Nutrition

References

Berger, J. "Neurologic Complications of HIV Infection," *Postgraduate Medicine* 81(1):72-79, January 1987.

Centers for Disease Control. "Public Health Service Statement on Management of Occupational Exposure to Human Immunodeficiency Virus, Including Considerations Regarding Zidovudine Postexposure Use," *Morbidity and Mortality Weekly Report* 39(RR-1):1-14, 1990.

Centers for Disease Control. "Update: Universal Precautions for Prevention of Transmission of Human Immunodeficiency Virus, Hepatitis B Virus, and Other Bloodborne Pathogens in Health-Care Settings," *Morbidity and Mortality Weekly Report* 37(24): 377-82, 387-88, 1988.

Cohen, P., Sande, M. and Volberding, P., eds. *The AIDS Knowledge Base.* Waltham, Mass.: Medical Publishing Group, 1990.

Flaskerud, J., and Ungvarski, P. *HIV/AIDS: A Guide to Nursing Care,* 2nd ed. Philadelphia: W.B. Saunders Co., 1992.

Gee, G., and Moran, T.A. *Current Concepts in AIDS Care: A Guide for Nurses and Nurse Practitioners.* Baltimore: Williams & Wilkins, 1988.

Halliburton, P. "Impaired Immunocompetence," in *Pathophysiological Phenomena in Nursing: Response to Illness.* Edited by Carrieri, V.K., et al. Philadelphia: W.B. Saunders Co., 1986.

Hopkins, C. "AIDS: Implementation of Universal Blood and Body Fluid Precautions," *Infectious Disease Clinics of North America,* 3(4):747-62, December 1989.

Hutman, S. "Dr. Gottlieb Reviews the VII International Conference on AIDS," *AIDS Patient Care* 5(5):227-230, October 1991.

Lewis, A. *Nursing Care of the Patient with AIDS/ARC.* Rockville, MD: Aspen Publishers, 1988.

Mathewson, H. *"Pneumocystis carinii* Pneumonia: Chemotherapy and Prophylaxis," *Respiratory Care* 34(5):360-62, May 1989.

Minkoff, H.L. "AIDS in Pregnancy," *Current Problems in Obstetrics, Gynecology, and Fertility* 12(6):206-35, 1989.

Redenius, W., and Dodd, S. "Clinical Update," *RNAIDS-LINE,* Summer 1990.

Sande, M.A. and Volberding, P.A. *Medical Management of AIDS,* 2nd ed. Philadelphia: W.B. Saunders Co., 1990.

Smeltzer, S.C., and Whipple, B. "Women and HIV Infection," *Image* 23(4):249-256, Winter 1991.

Stall, R., Ekstrand, M., Pollack, L., and Coates, T. "Relapse From Safer Sex: The Next Challenge for AIDS Prevention Efforts," *Journal of Acquired Immune Deficiency Syndrome* 3(12):1181-87, December 1990.

HEMATOLOGIC AND IMMUNOLOGIC DISORDERS

Anemia

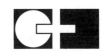

DRG information

DRG 395 Red Blood Cell Disorder. Age 17 + .
  Mean LOS = 4.6 days
  Principal diagnoses include:
  • acquired hemolytic anemia
  • iron-deficiency anemia
  • aplastic anemia
  • other.
DRG 396 Red Blood Cell Disorder. Age 0 to 17.
  Mean LOS = 2.1 days

Introduction
DEFINITION AND TIME FOCUS

Anemia is not a disease but a laboratory diagnosis
comprising a constellation of physiologic symptoms.
These symptoms result from an inadequate number of
circulating red blood cells (RBCs) or from a decreased
hemoglobin level. The primary function of the RBC is
to carry oxygen from the lungs to the tissues; anemia
reduces the blood's oxygen-carrying capacity and produces signs and symptoms of tissue hypoxia.
  Anemia occurs in three situations:
• life-threatening conditions, such as massive hemorrhage or bone marrow depression requiring strict isolation
• life-threatening complications, such as arrhythmias,
angina, or pulmonary edema
• as a complication of another disease, such as lymphoma.
  Anemia may be classified by cause or by RBC mor-
phology; both are discussed in the appropriate sections
below. This plan focuses on the newly diagnosed anemic patient with hemorrhagic or dietary deficiency
anemia, the most common types. The principles of
care can be generalized to other types of anemia but
would be supplemented with condition-specific care,
such as discontinuing medication (in toxic hemolytic
reactions) or offering genetic counseling (in sickle-cell
disease).

ETIOLOGY AND PRECIPITATING FACTORS

• excessive bleeding (acute or chronic)
• decreased RBC production, caused by:
  —dietary deficiencies of iron, folic acid, or vitamin B_{12}
  —damaged bone marrow (aplastic anemia) from
  medications, such as chloramphenicol (Chloromycetin) or sulfonamides; from chemotherapy with alkylating and antimetabolite agents; or from
  radiation
  —impaired production of erythropoietin (in kidney
  disease)

  —defective hemoglobin synthesis (as in sickle-cell
  disease and thalassemia)
  —decreased metabolic oxygen demand (as in hypothyroidism)
• increased RBC destruction (hemolytic anemia),
caused by:
  —hereditary disorders (such as sprue, sickle-cell
  disease, or thalassemia)
  —autoimmune hemolytic reactions (such as from
  transfusions or lupus erythematosus)
  —toxic drug reactions (such as from penicillin,
  methyldopa [Aldomet], quinine [Quindan], quinidine
  [Duraquin], or sulfonamides)
  —trauma (such as burns and crush injuries)
  —systemic diseases (such as Hodgkin's disease and
  lymphomas)

Focused assessment guidelines
NURSING HISTORY (Functional health pattern findings)

Note: Not all of the following signs and symptoms are
present in all anemias. Because of the many types of
anemias, symptoms vary widely. The symptoms also
vary with the anemia's severity. The patient with mild
anemia (hemoglobin greater than 10 g/dl) is usually
asymptomatic at rest but is symptomatic with exertion. The patient with moderate anemia (hemoglobin 6
to 10 g/dl) is chronically fatigued as well as symptomatic on exertion. The patient with severe anemia
(hemoglobin less than 6 g/dl) is exhausted, cold, and
symptomatic even at rest.

Health-perception—health-management pattern
• typically reports fatigue, headaches, dizziness, irritability, or sensation of being cold
• may report history of bleeding (such as from ulcers or
hemorrhoids), renal disease, liver disease, cancer, chronic
infections, or (especially in older patients) angina
• may report current or recent use of medications (see
list above) that affect RBC production (rare)
• may report recent exposure to a chemical or a myelo-
toxic substance (such as benzene or a benzene deriva-
tive) or to large doses of radiation (rare)
• may report family history of a disease such as
sickle-cell anemia, thalassemia major, or hereditary
spherocytosis (all rare)

Activity-exercise pattern
• reports fatigue, decreasing activity tolerance, weakness, shortness of breath, palpitations, or claudication

Cognitive-perceptual pattern
• may report dizziness, headache, numbness, or tingling of fingers and toes

Nutritional-metabolic pattern
• may report weight loss, anorexia, nausea, indigestion, pruritus, or soreness of mouth, esophagus, or tongue (all rare)

Elimination pattern
• may report tarry stools, constipation, diarrhea, or flatulence (all rare)
• may report brown, hazy urine (rare)
• may report gross blood in excretions (rare)

Sexuality-reproductive pattern
• may report loss of libido, irregular menstruation or amenorrhea (if female), or impotence (if male)

PHYSICAL FINDINGS
Cardiovascular
• tachycardia
• cardiac enlargement (less common)
• murmurs (less common)
• dependent edema (less common)
• vascular bruits (less common)
• bounding arterial pulses (less common)

Pulmonary
• dyspnea on exertion
• tachypnea
• orthopnea (less common than other signs)

Integumentary
• pallor of skin and mucous membranes
• diaphoresis
• delayed wound healing
• purpura (less common than other signs)
• jaundice (less common than other signs)
• spider angiomas (less common than other signs)

DIAGNOSTIC STUDIES
• hemoglobin level — may be decreased with iron-deficiency, pernicious, hemolytic, and hemorrhagic anemias
• hematocrit value — may be low
• RBC count — may be below normal
• microscopic evaluation of peripheral blood (performed by a hematologist) — reveals size, shape, color, and number of RBCs; useful in diagnosing the specific type of anemia

    Note: The morphologic classification of anemias is based on structural changes seen in RBCs, which are classified by size and hemoglobin content:
    — Normocytic (normal size) and normochromic (normal color) RBCs are associated with anemias of sudden blood loss; pregnancy; chronic disease such as cancer, kidney disease, or chronic infection; and some hemolytic anemias.

    — Macrocytic (abnormally large) and normochromic RBCs are associated with pernicious anemia, folic acid anemia, vitamin B_{12} deficiency, and some hemolytic anemias.
    — Microcytic (abnormally small) and normochromic RBCs are associated with anemias of chronic disease.
    — Microcytic and hypochromic (pale-colored) RBCs are associated with iron-deficiency anemia and thalassemia.

• erythrocyte indices — use the RBC count and hematocrit and hemoglobin values to define the size, hemoglobin weight, and hemoglobin concentration of a typical RBC; mean corpuscular volume (MCV) gives the average cell size; mean corpuscular hemoglobin (MCH) gives the average hemoglobin weight; and mean corpuscular hemoglobin concentration (MCHC) identifies the average hemoglobin volume. Low MCV and MCHC indicate microcytic, hypochromic anemia (such as iron-deficiency anemia and thalassemia); a high MCV suggests macrocytic anemia (such as folic acid anemia or vitamin B_{12} deficiency).
• reticulocyte count — if low, may indicate hypoplastic or pernicious anemia; if high, may indicate bone marrow response to anemia resulting from blood loss or hemolysis
• erythrocyte fragility test — if low, may indicate thalassemia, iron-deficiency anemia, or sickle-cell disease; if high, may indicate spherocytosis (hereditary disorders associated with autoimmune hemolytic anemia)
• direct Coombs' test — positive response may indicate autoimmune hemolytic anemia (idiopathic, drug-induced, or caused by an underlying disease such as cancer or lupus erythematosus)
• hemoglobin electrophoresis — identifies hemoglobin types by measuring the degree of negative charge
• sickle-cell test — identifies sickle-cell disease and trait (hemoglobin electrophoresis is then needed to differentiate the two disorders)
• serum iron and total iron-binding capacity (TIBC) levels — serum iron level decrease and TIBC increase indicate iron-deficiency anemia
• serum folic acid levels — low levels may indicate megaloblastic anemia
• serum vitamin B_{12} levels — low levels could indicate inadequate dietary intake of vitamin B_{12} or a malabsorption disorder
• bone marrow aspiration and biopsy — histologic examination and differential count with erythroid-to-myeloid ratio useful for differential diagnosis of aplastic, hypoplastic, or pernicious anemia
• liver-spleen scan — can detect splenomegaly associated with hereditary spherocytosis
• chest X-ray — may show cardiac enlargement

POTENTIAL COMPLICATIONS
• hemorrhagic shock
• angina pectoris
• congestive heart failure
• pulmonary edema
• renal damage
• arrhythmias

Collaborative problem: *Hypoxemia related to decreased oxygen-carrying capacity of RBCs*

NURSING PRIORITY: Prevent or promptly relieve hypoxemia.

Interventions

1. Elevate the head of the bed.

2. Monitor for and report signs of hypoxemia, such as restlessness, irritability, and confusion. Observe oral mucosa, fingernail beds, palmar creases, and conjunctivae for pallor or cyanosis.

3. Monitor respirations before and after activity. Assess lung sounds at least every 8 hours and report crackles, gurgles, or decreased breath sounds to the doctor promptly.

4. Monitor the patient's pulse, noting strength and rate. Report a pulse that does not fall within normal limits for the patient.

5. Note chest pain or palpitations.

6. Monitor arterial blood gas (ABG) measurements as ordered, and report results to the doctor.

7. Administer oxygen, as ordered.

8. Administer whole blood or packed RBCs, as ordered.

9. Monitor hemoglobin level and hematocrit value.

Rationales

1. This position allows for greater lung expansion, promoting alveolar gas exchange.

2. Baseline and serial assessments of these signs of hypoxemia help individualize care. Neurologic signs reflect cerebral ischemia. Skin color changes are observed best in unpigmented sites. Because cyanosis indicates the presence of 5 g/dl or more of desaturated hemoglobin and hemoglobin levels may be so depressed that the patient cannot accumulate 5 g/dl of desaturated hemoglobin without decompensating, cyanosis may be absent or a very late sign.

3. Dyspnea and tachypnea may be present in mild to moderate anemia. The exact cause of dyspnea is unclear. One hypothesis suggests that decreased oxygen pressure plays an important role. Congestive heart failure may develop with severe anemia if the heart is unable to handle the increased cardiac output necessary to compensate for the lower oxygen saturation of the blood.

4. To compensate for the decreased hemoglobin level, cardiac rate and output increase. Pulse weakness, threadiness, and rapidity are more pronounced as anemia becomes more severe.

5. Angina pectoris may develop in severe anemia from ischemia of the heart muscle. Palpitations reflect increased myocardial irritability secondary to hypoxemia.

6. ABG measurements document the degree of hypoxemia. Inadequate hemoglobin saturation decreases the oxygen-carrying capacity of the blood.

7. Supplemental oxygen helps prevent tissue hypoxia by elevating the arterial oxygen content.

8. Transfusions elevate the RBC count, hemoglobin level, and hematocrit value. An increased hemoglobin level improves arterial oxygen content, lessening signs and symptoms of hypoxemia.

9. These tests provide objective evidence of the degree of anemia and the efficacy of treatment.

HEMATOLOGIC AND IMMUNOLOGIC DISORDERS

10. Maintain a warm room temperature. Provide extra blankets if the patient desires.

10. The body compensates for chronic hypoxemia by lowering the metabolic rate and shunting blood to vital organs, making the patient more sensitive to cold. A cold room temperature induces vasoconstriction, which further impairs the release of oxygen to tissues.

11. Additional individualized interventions: _____

11. Rationales: _____

Target outcome criteria*

Throughout the hospital stay, the patient will:
- display vital signs within normal limits
- have no palpitations or chest pain
- maintain usual mental status
- have ABG meaurements within normal limits
- show normal skin color
- have clear lung sounds
- maintain acceptable hemoglobin and hematocrit values (as determined by the doctor)
- have no complaints of feeling cold.

Nursing diagnosis: *Nutritional deficit related to stomatitis, glossitis, anorexia, fatigue, lack of knowledge, or sociocultural factors*

NURSING PRIORITY: Maintain adequate nutritional intake.

Interventions

1. Provide mouth care before and after meals, or assist the patient in performing mouth care. (Using a soft or sponge toothbrush minimizes trauma to the gums.)

2. Observe for soreness of the tongue, mouth, and esophagus.

3. Recommend a bland diet (avoidance of hot, spicy, or acidic foods).

4. Serve six small meals a day, providing foods that appeal to the patient and meet specific dietary needs. Consult the dietitian for a specific diet. Specific needs vary with the type of anemia and may include the following:
- for iron deficiency — red meat, organ meats, green vegetables, and enriched breads and cereals
- for vitamin B_{12} deficiency — meat, chicken, liver, shellfish, dairy products, and egg yolks
- for folic acid deficiency — green and leafy vegetables, fruits, meats, and whole-grain breads and cereals
- for vitamin C deficiency — citrus fruits and juices.

Rationales

1. A patient with pernicious anemia or severe iron-deficiency anemia may have a sore mouth, tongue, or esophagus. Mouth care soothes and refreshes irritated tissues and can stimulate the patient's appetite. Frequent mouth care also decreases bacterial growth, thereby decreasing the risk of infection.

2. Stomatitis and glossitis may be present in pernicious anemia.

3. Spicy and acidic foods can further irritate the mouth, tongue, and esophagus. Hot foods have stronger odors than cold foods and may not appeal to the patient with a poor appetite.

4. Small portions require less energy to consume and digest. Large meals shunt blood to the GI tract, further contributing to fatigue. Foods that appeal to the patient are more likely to be eaten. The dietitian is best qualified to plan a diet that meets the patient's needs.

---

*Note: The expected outcomes for a patient with newly diagnosed anemia vary, depending upon the type of anemia, its severity, its chronicity, the treatment selected, and the underlying disease. Therefore, these outcome criteria are general; more specific outcomes may need to be determined for each patient.

5. Administer vitamins and minerals, as ordered (for example, iron preparations, vitamin B_{12}, folic acid, and vitamin C). Use the Z-track method to administer intramuscular iron. If parenteral iron is ordered, a test dose must be given to screen for allergies. Be alert for adverse effects of parenteral iron. If oral iron is prescribed, monitor the patient and teach these precautions:
• Take iron with meals.
• Avoid taking iron with dairy products, eggs, coffee, tea, or antacids.
• Increase vitamin C intake.
• If iron is in liquid form, dilute it, drink it through a straw, and rinse the mouth afterward.

5. Iron, vitamin B_{12}, and folic acid are needed to synthesize hemoglobin. The patient taking either folic acid or vitamin B_{12} may have allergic symptoms of wheezing and itching. Possible adverse reactions to parenteral iron can include tachycardia, muscle pain, chest pain, backache, headache, chills, dizziness, fever and nausea. The Z-track method minimizes leakage of iron into surrounding tissues (thus minimizing pain) or out through the injection site (thus minimizing medication loss and tissue staining). Precautions for oral iron maximize absorption and minimize gastric distress and tooth staining. Vitamin C promotes iron absorption and influences folic acid metabolism.

6. Teach the patient the importance of a well-balanced diet, including specific dietary needs. Emphasize the importance of adequate intake. Relate dietary recommendations to the patient's signs and symptoms.

6. Lack of knowledge can contribute to poor dietary intake. Stressing the importance of diet may enlist the patient's cooperation despite fatigue or discomfort. Using personal examples makes recommendations more meaningful.

7. Document the patient's food intake.

7. Accurate documentation helps determine daily calorie needs.

8. Weigh the patient daily or as ordered.

8. The patient's weight can be used as part of the ongoing nutritional assessment and can help monitor fluid status.

9. If the patient's nutritional needs are not met by dietary intake, consult the doctor about enteral or parenteral feeding.

9. Tube feedings or total parenteral nutrition may be indicated to improve nutritional status.

10. Before discharge:
• assess the patient's understanding of the importance of proper nutrition
• evaluate the patient's ability to obtain the prescribed diet and medications
• make referrals to social services or community agencies as indicated.

10. Poor nutrition may result from ignorance, poverty, or limited ability to shop for food, as in the debilitated older person who depends on public transportation.

11. Additional individualized interventions: _____

11. Rationales: _____

Target outcome criteria
By the time of discharge, the patient will:
• show signs of improving nutritional deficiencies (manifested by improved hematocrit value and hemoglobin, serum albumin, and folic acid levels)
• have less tongue, mouth, and esophagus soreness
• increase weight toward normal for age, height, and body type

• have increased energy level
• follow recommended diet
• verbalize ability to obtain recommended diet after discharge or have appropriate referrals made.

Nursing diagnosis: *High risk for impaired skin integrity related to tissue hypoxia, decreased mobility, and bed rest*

NURSING PRIORITY: Maintain skin integrity.

Interventions	Rationales
1. Assess the patient's skin, including bony prominences, for redness and induration at every position change.	1. Mechanical pressure and decreased hemoglobin availability increase the risk of tissue hypoxia and cell damage. Abnormally red skin, especially over a pressure point, may indicate reactive hyperemia after relief of pressure-induced ischemia. Induration results from cellular changes that occur with ischemia.
2. Keep the skin clean and dry; keep the bed linen dry and wrinkle-free.	2. The skin is the first line of defense against infection. Moisture provides a good medium for bacterial growth and can lead to maceration. Wrinkle-free linens distribute pressure evenly over the skin.
3. Reposition the patient at least every 2 hours. Apply lotion to and massage pressure points. Increase the frequency of position changes if redness or induration occurs. Avoid weight-bearing on reddened areas.	3. Hypoxemia increases the risk of tissue breakdown. Frequent turning relieves pressure and reestablishes blood flow. Massaging pressure points with lotion keeps the skin soft and increases circulation. Redness results from reactive hyperemia when pressure is relieved. Weight-bearing on reddened areas may worsen ischemia.
4. Teach active range-of-motion (ROM) exercises, and instruct the patient to do them hourly while awake, if tolerated. (If the patient cannot tolerate active ROM exercises, substitute passive ones.)	4. Movement stimulates circulation and maintains muscle tone and joint mobility.
5. Assess the patient's need for a pressure-relieving device, such as a foam mattress or alternating pressure mattress, and obtain the device if indicated. (A doctor's order may be required to ensure insurance reimbursement.)	5. Pressure-relieving devices eliminate, change, or decrease the amount of pressure on the skin, improving or maintaining circulation.
6. Additional individualized interventions: _____	6. Rationales: _____

> **Target outcome criterion**
> Throughout the hospital stay, the patient will maintain skin integrity.

Nursing diagnosis: *Self-care deficit related to weakness and fatigue*

NURSING PRIORITY: Increase the patient's independence in activities of daily living (ADLs) while minimizing weakness and fatigue.

Interventions	Rationales
1. Provide rest periods between activities and an environment that promotes rest. Get a description of the patient's room at home, and try to simulate it if possible. Teach the importance of rest.	1. Rest decreases oxygen demand. Simulating features of the patient's room at home contributes to relaxation.
2. Assess the patient's normal ADLs, and offer help in prioritizing them.	2. Initially, the patient may need to limit activities to a few. Involving the patient in selecting these activities gives a sense of self-control.

3. Help the patient ambulate. Observe for and teach signs of activity intolerance, such as dizziness, fainting, shortness of breath, chest pain, and worsened fatigue. Monitor orthostatic vital signs.

3. Orthostatic hypotension may aggravate cerebral ischemia or cardiac ischemia. The patient may need encouragement to change position slowly and to pace activities according to tolerance.

4. Allow as much self-care as possible, and assist as needed.

4. Self-care encourages independence and helps promote and maintain self-esteem.

5. Place personal items (such as a water pitcher and tissues) within the patient's reach.

5. Placing personal items within the patient's reach encourages independence while conserving energy.

6. Additional individualized interventions: _____

6. Rationales: _____

Target outcome criteria
By the time of discharge, the patient will:
• perform simple ADLs, such as eating, washing face and hands, and toileting, independently without complaints of fatigue
• identify priority tasks on which to expend energy.

Nursing diagnosis: *Hopelessness related to chronic fatigue, activity intolerance, and lack of independence*

NURSING PRIORITY: Provide emotional support and guidance in solving practical problems.

Interventions

1. Actively listen while the patient expresses personal feelings and frustrations.

2. Identify and assess the patient's personal resources. Assist with problem solving.

3. Provide information about available community agencies and the services provided by each. With the patient's consent, make appropriate referrals.

4. Additional individualized interventions: _____

Rationales

1. Active listening provides empathic support.

2. The patient's participation in identifying personal resources represents a significant step in actively coping with problems.

3. The patient may require help to meet basic needs. Community assistance may be available for preparing meals, performing light household duties, assisting with ADLs, and counseling.

4. Rationales: _____

Target outcome criteria
By the time of discharge, the patient will:
• identify personal support systems
• identify community resources.

Discharge planning

NURSING DISCHARGE CRITERIA

Upon the patient's discharge, documentation shows evidence of:
• stable vital signs
• absence of fever
• hemoglobin and hematocrit values within acceptable parameters
• ABG measurements within normal parameters
• absence of cardiovascular and pulmonary complications, such as dyspnea and angina
• ability to tolerate adequate nutritional intake
• stabilizing weight
• ability to obtain recommended diet
• ability to perform ADLs and ambulate the same as or better than before hospitalization
• adequate home support system or referral to home care (as indicated by lack of home support system, inability to follow diet and medication regimen, or inability to perform ADLs and tolerate moderate activities).
Note: State professional review organizations (PROs) have specific parameters for acceptable hemoglobin levels upon discharge. Parameters vary by state. A hospital can receive a citation for discharging a patient whose hemoglobin is less than 10 g/dl, especially if the patient is readmitted within 15 days of discharge. Therefore, the patient's blood work results should be examined closely at discharge, and any abnormal findings should appear in the discharge summary.

PATIENT-FAMILY TEACHING CHECKLIST

Document evidence that the patient and family demonstrate an understanding of:
___ type of anemia and implications
___ all discharge medications' purpose, dosage, administration schedule, and adverse effects requiring medical attention
___ special dietary needs
___ community resources
___ signs and symptoms indicating need for medical attention
___ dates, times, and location of follow-up appointments
___ how to contact the doctor.

DOCUMENTATION CHECKLIST

Using outcome criteria as a guide, document:
___ clinical status on admission
___ significant changes in clinical status
___ pertinent laboratory and diagnostic test findings
___ nutritional intake
___ activity tolerance
___ patient-family teaching
___ discharge planning.

ASSOCIATED PLANS OF CARE

Geriatric Considerations
Ineffective Individual Coping
Knowledge Deficit
Pain

References

Carpenito, L. *Nursing Diagnosis: Application to Clinical Practice,* 4th ed. Philadelphia: J.B. Lippincott Co., 1991.

Carrieri, V., Lindsey, A., and West, C. *Pathophysiological Phenomena in Nursing.* Philadelphia: W.B. Saunders Co., 1986.

Cerrato, P. "Does Your Patient Need More Iron?" *RN* 53(7):63-66, July 1990.

Diagnostics, 2nd ed. Nurse's Reference Library. Springhouse, Pa.: Springhouse Corp., 1986.

Froberg, J. "The Anemias: Causes and Courses of Action," *RN* 52(1):24-29, January, 1989.

Griffin, J. *Hematology and Immunology: Concepts for Nursing.* East Norwalk, Conn.: Appleton & Lange, 1986.

Luckmann, J., and Sorensen, K. *Medical-Surgical Nursing: A Psychophysiological Approach,* 3rd ed. Philadelphia: W.B. Saunders Co., 1987.

Thompson, J., et al. *Mosby's Manual of Clinical Nursing,* 2nd ed. St. Louis: C.V. Mosby Co., 1989.

Disseminated Intravascular Coagulation

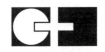

DRG information

DRG 397 Coagulation Disorders.

Mean LOS = 5.5 days

Principal diagnoses include all types of coagulation defects or disorders, including disseminated intravascular coagulation.

Introduction

DEFINITION AND TIME FOCUS

Disseminated intravascular coagulation (DIC) is a complex, acquired hematologic disorder characterized by a paradoxical blend of coagulation and hemorrhage. One or more procoagulants—such as bacterial toxins, exposure of collagen in damaged blood vessel walls, or tissue fragments—provoke uncontrolled microcirculatory coagulation through the intrinsic clotting pathway, extrinsic clotting pathway, or both.

The explosive production of thrombin causes widespread microcirculatory deposition of fibrin and rapid consumption of clotting factors. It also triggers the body's fibrinolytic system, a homeostatic mechanism that limits coagulation. Fibrin split products, a byproduct of fibrinolysis, exacerbate bleeding because they function as anticoagulants. Because of the anticoagulants and the scarcity of clotting factors, the patient cannot form stable clots and bleeding occurs throughout the body. This plan focuses on the patient in the critical care unit with acute DIC.

ETIOLOGY AND PRECIPITATING FACTORS

- shock
- septicemia
- neoplasms
- transfusion reactions or other hemolytic conditions
- trauma, lengthy cardiopulmonary bypass operations, or other tissue injury
- liver disease

Focused assessment guidelines

NURSING HISTORY (Functional health pattern findings)

Health perception–health management pattern

Patient reports are relatively unimportant in diagnosis of DIC. Usually, the patient is too ill from the primary disorder to be aware of or report subjective manifestations. Even if the patient is alert, the widespread manifestations of DIC may cause variable, nonspecific symptoms.

Nutritional-metabolic pattern

- may complain of nausea or vomiting

Activity-exercise pattern

- may report dyspnea
- may report fatigue

Cognitive-perceptual pattern

- may report confusion

PHYSICAL FINDINGS

Physical findings are quite variable, depending on the underlying disorder, degree of organ involvement, and stage of DIC.

Cardiovascular

- blood oozing from multiple sites, such as I.V. insertion sites, incisions, and nasal mucosa around endotracheal or nasogastric tubes
- repeated episodes of minor bleeding
- frank hemorrhage
- hypotension

Integumentary

- acral cyanosis (irregularly shaped, patchy cyanosis of fingers, toes, or ears), considered diagnostic of DIC
- petechiae
- purpura
- ecchymoses
- hematomas

Pulmonary

- tachypnea
- epistaxis

Gastrointestinal

- hematemesis
- melena

Neurologic

- coma
- seizures

Renal

- hematuria

DIAGNOSTIC STUDIES

Note: DIC is a laboratory diagnosis based on a characteristic pattern of abnormal values.

- prothrombin time—prolonged, indicating dysfunction of the extrinsic clotting pathway

• partial thromboplastin time—prolonged, indicating dysfunction of the intrinsic clotting pathway
• fibrinogen level—decreased because of fibrinogen consumption
• platelet count—diminished because of platelet consumption
• fibrin split products—increased because of fibrinolysis
• antithrombin III levels—decreased, indicating consumption by excessive thrombin formation

• D-dimer—increased, indicating excessive breakdown of fibrin bonds; highly predictive of DIC
• peripheral blood smear—reveals large platelets, reflecting rapid platelet usage, and red blood cell fragments, reflecting damage during red blood cell passage through fibrin webs

POTENTIAL COMPLICATIONS
• organ necrosis

Collaborative problem: *High risk for hemorrhage related to consumption of clotting factors, increased fibrinolysis, and presence of endogenous anticoagulants*

NURSING PRIORITY: Control clotting and bleeding.

Interventions

1. Collaborate with the doctor to identify and treat the cause of DIC; for example, administer I.V. fluids to correct hypovolemia or antibiotics to combat sepsis, as ordered.

2. Monitor the presence and degree of hemorrhage. Observe for persistent oozing of blood at multiple sites, petechiae, purpura, ecchymoses, and hemorrhagic gingivitis. Note bleeding from wounds, drains, and chest tubes. In the female patient, check for vaginal bleeding. Test all drainage for occult blood.

3. Monitor coagulation panel, as ordered.

4. Administer heparin, if ordered. Monitor the activated partial thromboplastin time (APTT), as ordered, and report values exceeding two times normal.

5. Administer transfusion therapy, as ordered, typically fresh whole blood, fresh frozen plasma, platelet concentrate, or cryoprecipitate.

6. Maintain a normal blood pressure by giving fluid and medications, as ordered.

7. Monitor for fluid overload. Observe for crackles, neck vein distention, or increased pulmonary artery (PA) and wedge pressures. If indicated, collaborate with the doctor to reduce fluid volume, such as by administering diuretics.

Rationales

1. Removing or controlling the underlying cause of DIC is essential to effective treatment.

2. The presence and degree of bleeding provides a rough indicator of the severity of DIC.

3. Coagulation values document the degree of DIC. They may be abnormal even if the patient does not show clinical signs of the disorder.

4. Heparin disrupts the vicious cycle of clotting and bleeding in DIC. Although it cannot lyse existing clots, it can prevent further clot formation. Heparin therapy during intense bleeding is controversial; however, it may be indicated when signs of thrombosis are present and blood component therapy is underway. Heparin inhibits thrombin (therefore limiting platelet aggregation and conversion of fibrinogen to fibrin) and factor X (therefore blocking both intrinsic and extrinsic pathways that lead to thrombin formation). Monitoring the APTT allows the doctor to adjust the heparin dose to maintain a therapeutic blood level.

5. Transfusion therapy replaces depleted clotting factors. Some doctors order it only after initiating heparinization, theorizing that replacing factors before interrupting the clotting cycle will only potentiate DIC.

6. Both hypotension and hypertension are detrimental to the DIC patient. Hypotension contributes to the disease, while hypertension can dislodge precarious blood clots and initiate fresh bleeding.

7. The patient with DIC usually receives large amounts of fluid and frequent transfusions in an attempt to maintain optimal blood volume and cardiac output. Also, pulmonary capillary fragility increases the risk of interstitial edema. Untreated, fluid overload can progress to pulmonary edema.

8. Additional individualized interventions: _____

8. Rationales: _____

Target outcome criteria
Within 72 hours of the onset of bleeding, the patient will:
• have no further episodes of oozing or frank hemorrhage
• exhibit vital signs within normal limits

• exhibit coagulation laboratory values within normal limits.

Collaborative problem: *Ischemia related to microcirculatory thrombosis*

NURSING PRIORITY: Restore tissue perfusion.

Interventions

1. Assess status of organ systems at least every 4 hours, including:
• neurologic function, such as level of consciousness, pupils, and sensorimotor function of the arms and legs
• cardiovascular function, such as pulse rate and volume, blood pressure, electrocardiogram pattern, and PA and wedge pressures
• gastrointestinal function, such as bowel sounds and abdominal girth.

2. Monitor renal function closely. Document hourly urine output, noting and reporting any decreasing trend. Summarize fluid intake and output every 8 hours, noting and reporting any undesirable fluid retention.

3. As ordered, implement measures (such as fluid administration) to treat the underlying cause of tissue ischemia.

4. Additional individualized interventions: _____

Rationales

1. Tissue ischemia and necrosis can occur in any body system from the widespread deposition of thrombi in the microcirculation. In addition, hypotension activates the complement system, resulting in increased vascular permeability and blood cell lysis, and the kallikrein system, resulting in increased vascular permeability and vasodilation. The net results are arteriolar vasoconstriction, capillary dilation, and arteriovenous shunting. Stagnant blood accumulates in the dilated, bypassed capillaries and becomes acidotic, further damaging tissue and contributing to clotting.

2. The renal system is most likely to suffer from thrombosis, resulting in acute tubular necrosis. Decreasing hourly urine outputs or oliguria may reflect this development. Because oliguria may also reflect other factors common in DIC, such as hypotension, cardiac failure, or hypovolemia, it must be interpreted in the context of the patient's overall condition.

3. Tissue ischemia is best treated by attacking its causes, such as hypovolemia.

4. Rationales: _____

Target outcome criteria
Within 72 hours, the patient will:
• produce hourly urine outputs exceeding 60 ml/hour
• exhibit a balanced fluid intake and output

• display normal vital signs.

Collaborative problem: *High risk for hypoxemia related to increased pulmonary shunting, anemia, and acidosis*

NURSING PRIORITY: Optimize oxygenation.

Interventions

1. Monitor arterial blood gas (ABG) values, as ordered, for hypoxemia and acidosis.

2. Assess physical indicators of pulmonary status at least every 4 hours. Note increasing respiratory rate, abnormal respiratory rhythm, and crackles or other abnormal lung sounds. Observe nail beds and buccal mucosa for pallor and central cyanosis.

3. Administer supplemental oxygen, positive end-expiratory pressure (PEEP), or mechanical ventilation, as ordered.

4. Additional individualized interventions: _____

Rationales

1. Ischemic damage to the pulmonary parenchyma increases pulmonary shunting, impairing oxygen uptake in the lungs. Red blood cell destruction produces a hemolytic anemia. These factors lessen arterial oxygen content. Also, acidosis and decreased tissue perfusion impair oxygen delivery to the tissues.

2. Respiratory rate accelerates to compensate for hypoxemia. Rhythm changes may reflect medullary hypoxemia. Adventitious lung sounds may reflect alveolar accumulation of fluid as the heart fails from ischemia. Pallor and cyanosis reflect arterial oxygen desaturation.

3. Supplemental oxygen alone may be insufficient to raise low arterial oxygen content from pulmonary shunting. PEEP and mechanical ventilation may be necessary to improve functional residual capacity enough to combat hypoxemia.

4. Rationales: _____

Target outcome criteria
Within 72 hours, the patient will:
• have ABG values within normal limits
• display a eupneic respiratory pattern

• have a respiratory rate between 18 and 24 breaths/minute
• display pink nail beds and buccal mucosa.

Nursing diagnosis: *Impaired skin integrity related to capillary fragility*

NURSING PRIORITY: Prevent further bleeding.

Interventions

1. Avoid needle punctures, whenever possible. If a needle puncture is essential, use the smallest gauge needle possible and apply pressure to the site for 10 minutes afterward. Whenever possible, administer medications I.V., as ordered.

2. Handle the patient very gently. Be particularly careful to avoid disturbing healing areas.

3. Use cushioning and pressure-relieving devices, such as sheepskin. Pad the bed rails.

4. Provide gentle mouth care with swabs and diluted mouthwash.

5. Additional individualized interventions: _____

Rationales

1. These measures may help reduce hematoma formation. In addition, because of poor tissue perfusion, medication deposited I.M. may be absorbed erratically, if at all. Administering medications I.V. promotes absorption and avoids creating a puncture site from which the patient may bleed.

2. Gentle handling minimizes skin trauma. Being particularly careful around healing sites minimizes the risk of dislodging unstable clots.

3. Such action minimizes the risk of hematoma development from extreme capillary fragility.

4. A toothbrush may damage fragile capillaries and result in gingival bleeding.

5. Rationales: _____

Target outcome criterion
Within 72 hours of onset of DIC, the patient will have no new hematoma formation.

Nursing diagnosis: *Pain related to tissue ischemia, hematomas, or bleeding into organ or joint capsules*

NURSING PRIORITY: Relieve pain.

Interventions

1. Assess for pain frequently. Use various pain-relieving measures, such as ice packs for hematomas or soothing music. Promote rest and provide emotional support. Consult the "Pain" plan, page 69, for details.

2. Administer pain medications I.V.

3. Additional individualized interventions: _____

Rationales

1. The "Pain" plan contains additional interventions for any patient in pain. This plan contains interventions specific to DIC. Soothing music helps relieve tension and lessen pain perception.

2. DIC may cause erratic absorption of I.M. medications.

3. Rationales: _____

Target outcome criteria
Within 1 hour of pain onset, the patient will:
• have a relaxed facial expression and body posture
• if able to communicate, indicate that pain is relieved.

Discharge planning

NURSING DISCHARGE CRITERIA
Upon the patient's discharge, documentation shows evidence of:
• stable vital signs
• laboratory coagulation panel within normal limits
• no bleeding episodes for at least 24 hours.

PATIENT-FAMILY TEACHING CHECKLIST
Document evidence that the patient and family demonstrate an understanding of:
___ basic pathophysiology and implications of DIC
___ rationale for therapy
___ pain relief measures.

DOCUMENTATION CHECKLIST
Using outcome criteria as a guide, document:
___ clinical status on admission
___ significant changes in status
___ pertinent diagnostic test findings
___ bleeding episodes
___ transfusion and fluid replacement therapy
___ pain relief measures
___ patient-family teaching
___ discharge planning.

ASSOCIATED PLANS OF CARE
Acute Renal Failure
Adult Respiratory Distress Syndrome
Cardiac Surgery
Hypovolemic Shock
Impaired Physical Mobility
Ineffective Individual Coping
Liver Failure
Major Burns
Mechanical Ventilation
Multiple Trauma
Nutritional Deficit
Pain

References
Bang, N. "Diagnosis and Management of Thrombosis," in *Textbook of Critical Care,* 2nd ed. Edited by Shoemaker, W., et al. Philadelphia: W.B. Saunders Co., 1988.

Holloway, N. *Nursing the Critically Ill Adult,* 4th ed. Menlo Park, Calif.: Addison-Wesley Publishing Company, 1993.

HEMATOLOGIC AND IMMUNOLOGIC DISORDERS

Leukemia

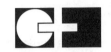

DRG information

DRG 403   Lymphoma or Nonacute Leukemia. With
Complication or Comorbidity (CC).
Mean LOS = 8.2 days

DRG 404   Lymphoma or Nonacute Leukemia. Without
CC.
Mean LOS = 4.3 days

DRG 405   Acute Leukemia without Major Operating
Room (OR) Procedure. Age 0 to 17.
Mean LOS = 4.9 days

DRG 473   Acute Leukemia without Major OR Procedure. Age 17 +.
Mean LOS = 9.9 days

DRG 409*   Radiotherapy.
Mean LOS = 6.7 days

DRG 410*   Chemotherapy.
Mean LOS = 2.7 days

Introduction
DEFINITION AND TIME FOCUS
Leukemia is the proliferation and accumulation of abnormal blood cells in the bone marrow or lymph tissue.
The malignant cells prevent normal hematopoiesis in
the blood marrow, and migrate to other organs and tissues, causing the disease's symptoms. The leukemias
may be classified according to several criteria, such as
the cell and tissue type involved, the duration and
course of the disease, or the number of leukocytes in
the blood and bone marrow.

Leukemia is classified as *acute* if the bone marrow
is infiltrated with undifferentiated, immature cells
(blasts) and as *chronic* if the cells are primarily differentiated and mature. The most common types of leukemia involve abnormalities of white blood cells (WBCs),
specifically granulocytes and lymphocytes.

Acute monoblastic leukemia is characterized by increased monoblasts (monocyte precursors). Adults
with monoblastic leukemia have a poor prognosis, surviving about 1 year.

Acute myeloblastic (granulocytic) leukemia (AML) involves uncontrolled proliferation of myeloblasts, the
precursors of granulocytes. The incidence of AML increases with age. The overall prognosis is poor, with a
high mortality rate from infection and hemorrhage,
usually within 1 year.

In *acute lymphoblastic leukemia* (ALL), immature
lymphocytes proliferate in the bone marrow. ALL is
primarily a children's disease, with peak incidence between ages 2 and 4. Approximately 50% to 60% of patients survive 5 years.

Chronic granulocytic leukemia shows abnormal development of granulocytes in the bone marrow, blood and
tissues. An initial chronic phase is followed by an
acute phase known as the blastic crisis. Chronic granulocytic leukemia occurs most commonly in patients
age 30 to 50. Patients survive 2 to 4 years after the
initial phase but live only 3 to 6 months once the blastic crisis phase starts.

Chronic lymphocytic leukemia is the production and
accumulation of functionally inactive but long-lived
and mature-appearing lymphocytes. Patients (usually
age 50 to 70) typically survive 2 to 10 years.

This plan focuses on the adult patient admitted for
diagnosis and treatment of leukemia.

ETIOLOGY AND PRECIPITATING FACTORS
The exact cause of leukemia is not known. Possible
causes include:
• exposure to carcinogenic chemicals, such as benzene,
alkylating agents, or chloramphenicol
• ionizing radiation
• viruses such as the Epstein-Barr virus
• famial tendency, congenital disorders such as Down's
syndrome, chromosomal abnormalities, ataxia-telangi-
ectasia, and congenital immune deficiencies.

Focused assessment guidelines
NURSING HISTORY (Functional health pattern findings)

Health perception—health management pattern
• usually reports gradual or sudden onset of fever, fatigue, weakness and lassitude, or headache
• may relate evidence of bleeding tendencies, such as
gingival bleeding, purpura, petechiae, ecchymoses and
easy bruising, epistaxis, and prolonged menstruation
• may report being a monozygotic (identical) twin
• may relate a positive family history for leukemia or
chromosomal abnormalities
• may relate exposure to carcinogenic agents or ionizing radiation

Nutritional-metabolic pattern
• reports nausea, anorexia, or weight loss
• may complain of sore throat or dysphagia

Elimination pattern
• may report blood in urine
• may report tarry stools

---

*These DRGs are used for the patient with leukemia admitted for either radiation or chemotherapy treatment.

Activity-exercise pattern
- reports fatigue and weakness
- may report dyspnea and palpitations on exertion
- may report diminished activity because of bone and joint pain
- may report abnormal bruising after minor trauma

Sleep-rest pattern
- reports increased desire or need for sleep and rest

Cognitive-perceptual pattern
- may complain of discomfort from mouth ulcers; abdominal, bone, and joint pain; and chills

Role-relationship pattern
- may verbalize difficulty in maintaining role function because of fatigue

Sexuality-reproductive pattern
- may have decreased libido secondary to extreme fatigue
- may report menorrhagia, if female

Coping – stress tolerance pattern
- may initially deny diagnosis

Value-belief system
- may view diagnosis of cancer as punishment
- may have a passive, fatalistic philosophy of life and death

PHYSICAL FINDINGS
General
- elevated temperature
- fatigued appearance

Cardiovascular
- tachycardia
- systolic ejection murmur

Respiratory
- labored breathing
- rapid breathing
- wheezing
- gurgles
- decreased breath sounds
- nosebleeds

Gastrointestinal
- gingival hypertrophy or bleeding
- mouth ulcers
- hepatosplenomegaly
- increased abdominal girth
- vomiting
- oral or rectal mucosal ulceration

Neurologic
- confusion
- visual changes

Integumentary
- pallor
- purpura
- petechiae
- pale mucous membranes
- ecchymoses
- erythema
- rash
- poor turgor

Genitourinary
- hematuria

Lymphoreticular
- lymphadenopathy

Musculoskeletal
- joint swelling
- decreased exercise tolerance

DIAGNOSTIC STUDIES
- complete blood count (CBC) – reflects bone marrow suppression by WBC infiltration
    - WBC count usually greater than 50,000/mm^3 but may be low
    - differential shows increased number of lymphocytes or increased number of polymorphonuclear cells
    - red blood cell (RBC), hemoglobin, and hematocrit values below normal; platelet count very low, may be less than 50,000/mm^3
- prothrombin time and partial thromboplastin time – may be prolonged
- histochemistry – specific chemistry tests for leukemia show Sudan black, peroxidase, or muramidase positive
- uric acid and lactic dehydrogenase levels – elevated in acute leukemia; may indicate extensive bone marrow infiltration
- liver enzyme levels – may be elevated, showing hepatic infiltration
- leukocyte alkaline phosphatase levels – may be decreased
- blood cultures – may show general sepsis
- urinalysis – may show bacteria and WBCs (indicating infection) or RBCs (indicating bleeding)
- blood urea nitrogen (BUN) and creatinine levels – may be elevated in renal infiltration and failure
- bone marrow aspiration – shows domination by leukemia blast cells of the affected cell line, may show abnormalities specific to leukemia, such as Auer bodies, Philadelphia chromosome; shows decreased RBC levels and decreased platelet formation
- lumbar puncture – may detect central nervous system (CNS) infiltration and meningeal irritation
- liver-spleen scan – shows hepatosplenomegaly and enlarged abdominal lymph nodes
- chest X-ray – may show lung infiltration, infection, or mediastinal adenopathy
- computed tomography scan – may show enlarged lymph nodes or areas of consolidation

POTENTIAL COMPLICATIONS
- infection, including sepsis
- hemorrhage, especially of the CNS
- immunosuppression
- meningeal irritation
- cardiotoxicity secondary to chemotherapy

- hyperuricemia
- mouth ulcers
- constipation or diarrhea secondary to chemotherapy
- arrhythmias secondary to electrolyte imbalance
- malnutrition, including protein-calorie imbalances

Nursing diagnosis: *High risk for infection related to incompetent bone marrow and immunosuppressive effects of chemotherapy treatment*

NURSING PRIORITIES: (a) Recognize early signs of infection and (b) minimize local and systemic infection.

Interventions

1. Assess the CBC, noting a WBC count below 2,000/mm^3 and any sudden rise or fall in neutrophil level.

2. Place the patient in a private room or in protective isolation, according to protocol and the patient's condition. Maintain the immediate environment free from bacterial contamination, disinfect or sterilize equipment, keep equipment at the bedside, and do not use such items for other patients. Prohibit visitors or staff with known infections, such as a cold or influenza, from the room.

3. Monitor, report, and document any sign or symptom of infection: temperature above 100.4° F (38° C) lasting longer than 24 hours; chills; pulse above 100 beats/minute; crackles or gurgles; cloudy, foul-smelling urine; urgency or burning upon urination; redness; swelling; drainage from any orifice; perineal, rectal, or vaginal pain or discharge; and painful skin lesions.

4. Monitor and record fluid intake and output. Encourage fluid intake of up to 12 8-oz glasses (3,000 ml) daily, unless contraindicated.

5. Use strict aseptic technique when starting an I.V. Consult your hospital's policy manual for frequency of I.V. site and tubing changes.

6. Provide a low-bacteria diet. Avoid raw fruits and vegetables, and use only cooked and processed or pasteurized foods.

7. Take measures to prevent respiratory tract infections. Instruct the patient to turn, cough, deep-breathe, and use the incentive spirometer every 2 hours. Document respiratory assessment every 4 hours.

8. Avoid invasive procedures, such as urinary catheterization, injections, and venipunctures, when possible. Examine the sites of earlier invasive procedures (such as bone marrow aspiration or venipuncture) for signs of inflammation.

Rationales

1. A decreased WBC count places the patient at increased risk for infection. Such a decrease results from both the disease and from chemotherapy. A sudden change in the neutrophil level indicates impending infection. Infection is a major cause of morbidity and mortality in the immunosuppressed patient.

2. The patient must be protected from potential sources of infection.

3. An elevated temperature unrelated to drug or blood product administration indicates infection in about 80% of patients with leukemia. The immunosuppressed patient is unable to mount a normal response to infection, so an infection that would be harmless in a patient with a normal WBC count can cause septicemia in the leukopenic patient. Early treatment of any infection is essential to prevent complications and death.

4. Adequate fluid balance is essential to prevent dehydration from fever and fluid shift in septic shock.

5. Strict aseptic technique and frequent site and tubing changes minimize the risk of bacterial contamination.

6. These measures minimize potential sources of bacterial contamination from food.

7. Immobility promotes stasis of respiratory secretions, increasing the risk of pneumonia and atelectasis.

8. Any invasive procedure is a potential source of bacterial invasion. Take care to minimize trauma to the skin because of impaired healing abilities.

9. Provide meticulous skin care, paying close attention to any alteration in skin integrity. Wash the skin at least twice daily with antibacterial solutions. Monitor and document skin condition every shift.

9. The skin is the body's first line of defense against infection. Any break in skin integrity is a source of potentially lethal bacterial contamination. The leukemic patient is as susceptible to infection from normal flora as from outside contamination. Frequent skin care minimizes the possibility of superficial skin breakdown and resultant infection.

10. Avoid trauma to the rectal mucosa; take the patient's temperature orally, and prevent constipation by ensuring adequate hydration and administering stool softeners, as ordered.

10. Damage to rectal mucosa from frequent rectal temperatures or hard, dry stools may cause rectal abscesses.

11. Observe for and report clinical signs of septicemia, such as tachycardia, hyperventilation, hypotension, or subtle mental changes. Obtain cultures and institute I.V. antibiotic therapy with cephalosporins (as ordered) within 1 hour of identifying signs and symptoms. Monitor fibrin degradation products (FDP) levels if the patient is septicemic.

11. Septicemia may occur without fever. Symptoms reflect initial stages of insufficient tissue perfusion. Prompt recognition and treatment of septic shock are crucial to prevent irreversible hypovolemia and decreased cardiac output. The septicemic patient is at increased risk for disseminated intravascular coagulation (DIC). Elevated FDP levels are seen in DIC.

12. Reduce fever higher than 100° F (38° C). Administer acetaminophen (Tylenol) 650 mg every 4 hours, as ordered. Use tepid sponge baths, remove unnecessary clothing and linens, and apply a hypothermia blanket, as ordered. Prevent chilling and encourage oral fluid intake.

12. Several measures may be necessary to reduce fever to a manageable level in the immunosuppressed patient. Untreated, high temperatures contribute to fluid imbalance, discomfort, and CNS complications.

13. Prepare the patient for granulocyte transfusion if the WBC count is consistently below 500/mm³ and the patient has signs of infection. Infuse granulocytes slowly over 2 to 4 hours, as ordered. Observe for and document signs of a serious transfusion reaction, such as hypotension, allergic response, or wheezing. Discontinue the transfusion and notify the doctor immediately if a reaction occurs.

13. Granulocyte transfusions are usually effective in the patient with granulocytopenia and progressive infections that do not respond to antibiotics or in the patient whose bone marrow does not recover after chemotherapy.
   Shaking chills and temperature elevations are not serious reactions to a WBC transfusion and should not prompt discontinuation of this critically important treatment.

14. Additional individualized interventions: _____

14. Rationales: _____

Target outcome criteria
Within 8 hours of admission, the patient will:
• have potential sites of infection identified and monitored
• present a temperature below 100° F
• exhibit pulse and respirations within normal limits.

Within 1 day of admission, the patient will increase fluid intake to at least 8 8-oz glasses (2,000 ml) daily.

Within 3 days of admission, the patient will:
• exhibit no septicemia
• exhibit no dysuria
• have normal lung sounds.

Within 7 days of admission, the patient will:
• have intact oral mucous membranes
• have no skin or rectal abscesses
• exhibit a stable WBC count
• maintain normal temperature
• display negative urine, vaginal, blood, and sputum cultures.

HEMATOLOGIC AND IMMUNOLOGIC DISORDERS

Collaborative problem: *High risk for hemorrhage related to incompetent bone marrow and the immunosuppressive effects of chemotherapy*

NURSING PRIORITY: Minimize the potential for life-threatening hemorrhage.

Interventions

1. Monitor, report, and document signs and symptoms of bleeding problems:
• platelet count less than 50,000/mm³
• petechiae, especially on distal portions of upper and lower extremities
• ecchymotic areas
• bleeding gums
• prolonged oozing from minor cuts or scratches
• frank or occult blood in urine, stool, emesis, or sputum
• prolonged heavy menstruation
• decline in hematocrit and hemoglobin values
• narrowing pulse pressure with increased pulse rate
• restlessness, confusion, or lethargy.

2. Implement measures to prevent bleeding during invasive procedures:

• Use the smallest gauge needle possible when performing venipuncture or giving injections. Apply firm, direct pressure to the injection site for 3 to 5 minutes after the injection. If bleeding does not stop after 5 minutes, apply a sandbag to the site and notify the doctor.

• Monitor and document the condition of old puncture sites (such as from venipuncture, lumbar puncture, or I.V. infusion).

3. Provide a soft, bland diet, avoiding foods that are thermally, mechanically, or chemically irritating. Use only a soft-bristle or sponge toothbrush and an alcohol-free mouthwash (such as normal saline) every 4 to 8 hours.

4. Administer docusate sodium (Colace) or another stool softener daily, as ordered. Monitor and document the frequency of bowel movements. Avoid using enemas, suppositories, harsh laxatives, and rectal thermometers.

5. Instruct the patient to avoid activities that may cause bleeding, such as forcefully blowing the nose; using a straight-edged razor; wearing tight, restrictive clothing; and cutting nails.

6. Prepare the patient for a platelet transfusion, as ordered, when platelet counts drop below 20,000/mm³. Obtain baseline vital signs before initiating the transfusion. Use a 19-G butterfly needle, infusing each unit over approximately 10 minutes. Observe, report, and document signs of transfusion reactions: nausea, vomiting, fever, chills, urticaria, or wheezing. Discontinue the transfusion immediately if symptoms develop, keep the vein open with normal saline, and notify the doctor. Be prepared to administer diphenhydramine (Benadryl), hydrocortisone (SoluCortef), or acetaminophen.

7. Monitor hemoglobin and hematocrit values and test stools, urine, and sputum for occult blood, noting and reporting positive findings.

Rationales

1. Normal platelet levels are required to maintain vascular integrity, platelet plug formation, and stabilized clotting. A decrease leads to local or systemic hemorrhage. With a platelet count of less than 20,000/mm³, the patient is prone to spontaneous life-threatening bleeding. The patient with leukemia is prone to platelet deficiency because of the proliferation of WBCs, which interfere with normal platelet production, and because of the immunosuppressive effects of drug treatment.

2. Even minor invasive procedures can cause excessive bleeding, especially when the platelet count falls below 50,000/mm³.

• The patient with thrombocytopenia may continue to bleed excessively even after minor invasive procedures. Firm pressure minimizes further blood loss and hematoma formation. Pressure dressings may be necessary if bleeding continues.

• Spontaneous bleeding from old puncture sites may occur at platelet levels below 20,000/mm³.

3. The oral mucous membrane is very delicate in the leukemic patient and prone to hemorrhage with even minor irritation. Minimizing irritation decreases bleeding and promotes comfort.

4. Constipation and straining during defecation must be avoided to prevent trauma to the rectal mucosa as well as increased intracranial pressure, which could cause spontaneous CNS bleeding. Rectal bleeding may develop with minimal trauma.

5. The patient may be unaware that some common actions can be dangerous when platelet counts are severely decreased.

6. Platelet transfusions reduce the risk of hemorrhage. Although small-gauge needles are preferred for most venipunctures to minimize trauma, a 19-G needle is preferred for blood transfusions to prevent clogging. Because it is not always possible to remove all RBCs and antibodies from the serum, the possibility of a transfusion reaction always exists, especially for a patient receiving multiple transfusions. If a transfusion reaction occurs, the doctor must evaluate the patient. If the signs and symptoms are adequately controlled by diphenhydramine and acetaminophen, the remaining platelets can be transfused.

7. Decreasing hemoglobin and hematocrit values indicate hemorrhage. Occult bleeding must be detected and monitored to prevent hypovolemia.

8. Avoid administering aspirin, anticoagulants, indomethacin (Indocin), and medications containing alcohol. Give phenothiazines cautiously.

8. These medications induce or prolong bleeding.

9. Force fluid intake of 8 to 12 8-oz glasses (2,000 to 3,000 ml) daily, if tolerated. Check for elevated uric acid levels and acidic urine. Administer acetazolamide (Diamox), sodium bicarbonate, and allopurinol (Lopurin), as ordered. Monitor and record fluid intake and output. Provide appropriate patient teaching for measures to be continued after discharge.

9. Hyperuricemia can result from rapid chemotherapy-induced leukemic cell lysis. Proper hydration and medication therapy are essential to prevent obstruction of the renal pelvis and ducts and subsequent renal failure. Acetazolamide is a diuretic, sodium bicarbonate maintains alkaline urine pH, and allopurinol inhibits uric acid synthesis.

10. Additional individualized interventions: _____

10. Rationales: _____

Target outcome criteria
Within 1 day of admission, the patient will:
• exhibit a platelet count above 50,000/mm³
• exhibit normal blood pressure and pulse rate.

Within 3 days of admission, the patient will:
• exhibit no frank bleeding in stool, urine, emesis, or sputum
• present minimal extension of ecchymoses
• present minimal bleeding from puncture sites, gums, and nose
• have stable or improved hemoglobin, hematocrit, and platelet values
• exhibit minimal or no restlessness, confusion, lethargy, or other CNS symptoms.

Nursing diagnosis: *Activity intolerance from fatigue secondary to rapid destruction of leukemic cells; tissue hypoxia secondary to anemia; and depressed nutritional status*

NURSING PRIORITIES: (a) Minimize energy-depleting activities, (b) maximize energy resources, and (c) decrease tissue hypoxia.

Interventions

1. Assess, monitor, and document the cause, pattern, and impact of fatigue on the patient's ability to engage in activities of daily living (ADLs).

2. Monitor and document the degree of anemia present. Assess for pallor, weakness, dizziness, headache, and dyspnea. Evaluate and report hemoglobin, hematocrit, and RBC values, especially a significant or consistent drop in hemoglobin (below 8 g/dl) or hematocrit (below 25%). Prepare for a blood transfusion, as ordered.

3. Monitor and document vital signs before, during, and after blood transfusion. Use a 19-G or larger needle and tubing with a standard blood filter. Use standard Y tubing with normal saline solution.

4. Infuse blood slowly (20 drops/minute) for 15 minutes. Complete the transfusion within 1½ to 2 hours if the patient's condition remains stable.

Rationales

1. Causes of fatigue in the patient with leukemia commonly have an additive effect. To treat the problem effectively, the nurse must use a holistic approach.

2. The degree of anemia significantly affects the level of fatigue. Decreased RBC levels, and the resulting decrease in the blood's oxygen carrying ability, cause severe weakness, exhaustion, and inability to mobilize energy. The values given indicate severe anemia and require therapy with blood transfusions.

3. Knowledge of baseline and ongoing vital signs is imperative to monitor for signs and symptoms of transfusion reaction. A large needle allows a suitable flow rate and prevents clumping and destruction of RBCs. The filter screens fibrin clots and particulate matter. Normal saline is the only solution suitable for use with RBCs, because dextrose solutions cause hemolysis.

4. Blood is administered slowly during the first 15 minutes because transfusion reactions typically occur during this time. A slow rate minimizes the volume of cells transfused. However, blood should be transfused within 4 hours after leaving the blood bank, to prevent bacterial proliferation and RBC hemolysis.

5. Stop the transfusion at the first sign of a transfusion reaction: fever, chills, headache, low back pain, urticaria, wheezing, or hypotension. Keep the vein open with normal saline, and notify the doctor.

5. Transfusion reactions must be recognized immediately to prevent death or organ damage.

6. Implement measures to improve activity tolerance, such as the following:
• Provide uninterrupted rest periods before and after meals, procedures, and diagnostic tests.
• Instruct the patient to sit rather than stand when performing hygiene and daily care.
• Limit the number of visitors.
• Minimize environmental activity and noise.
• Assist the patient with activities.
• Keep supplies and personal articles within easy reach.

6. Quiet, restful periods before and after meals, procedures such as chemotherapy, and diagnostic procedures help increase activity tolerance and promote a rested feeling. Conserving energy and improving activity tolerance usually help the patient participate more actively in care and treatment.

7. Assess, report, and document the patient's tolerance for progressive activity. Stop activity if the patient's pulse rate increases more than 20 beats/minute above the resting rate, if the blood pressure increases more than 40 mm Hg systolic or 20 mm Hg diastolic, or if dyspnea, chest pain, dizziness, or syncope occurs.

7. The patient's response should guide any plan of progressive activity. Changes in baseline vital signs indicate that the patient is being pushed beyond therapeutic levels and activity should be stopped.

8. Reassure the patient that fatigue is an expected effect of chemotherapy.

8. The patient may fear that fatigue is related to extension of the disease. The patient should be reassured that fatigue is common after chemotherapy and does not necessarily reflect disease extension.

9. Additional individualized interventions: _____

9. Rationales: _____

Target outcome criteria
Within 1 day of admission, the patient will exhibit no adverse effects or toxic effects of blood transfusion, such as elevated temperature or urticaria.

Within 3 days of admission, the patient will:
• show improved ability to participate in self-care, bathing, and hygiene measures
• sleep 1 hour before and after treatments
• sleep 8 hours at night
• ambulate 20% farther each day
• participate in diversional activities, such as reading, doing puzzles, and watching television
• maintain hemoglobin level at 8 g/dl or higher
• maintain hematocrit value at 25% or higher.

Nursing diagnosis: *Nutritional deficit related to anorexia, nausea, vomiting, taste perception changes, and alterations in cellular metabolism secondary to disease and chemotherapy*

NURSING PRIORITIES: (a) Maximize oral intake of foods and fluids, and (b) minimize catabolism and protein and vitamin deficiencies.

Interventions

1. Provide standard nursing care related to nutritional deficit. Refer to the "Nutritional Deficit" plan, page 63, for details.

2. Provide high-calorie, high-protein snacks, such as milkshakes, puddings, and eggnog.

Rationales

1. The "Nutritional Deficit" plan presents general nursing care for this problem. This plan presents additional information related to leukemia.

2. Protein-calorie malnutrition is common in leukemia. Increased protein intake facilitates repair and regeneration of cells, and increased calories help fight the body's tendency toward cancer-induced catabolism.

3. Provide nutritional supplements between meals, as ordered. Serve them cold in a glass or other container, not in the can. Observe for and document undesirable adverse effects, such as gastric distention, cramping, or diarrhea.

4. When nausea or vomiting is present, administer antiemetics (such as phenothiazines, sedatives, or antihistamines), as ordered, 1 to 2 hours before chemotherapy and every 4 to 6 hours thereafter, for at least 12 to 24 hours. Monitor, report, and document the effectiveness of medications.

5. Additional individualized interventions: _____

3. Oral supplements are high in protein and are a valuable supplement to nutritious food. Many patients experience a metallic taste secondary to leukemia, and the sight of the can may aggravate this feeling. The adverse effects listed result from the high osmolality of supplemental liquids.

4. Antiemetic medications block stimulation of the true vomiting center and the chemoreceptor trigger zone in the brain, thus decreasing nausea and vomiting and promoting relaxation. To maintain a therapeutic blood level, antiemetic medications must be administered around the clock rather than as needed.

5. Rationales: _____

Target outcome criteria
Within 3 days of admission, the patient will:
• exhibit no weight loss
• maintain serum electrolyte levels within normal limits
• tolerate nutritional supplements between meals
• maintain intake equal to output
• have no nausea or vomiting
• retain about 75% of food intake.

Nursing diagnosis: *Altered oral mucous membrane related to decreased nutrition and immunosuppression secondary to disease and cytotoxic effects of chemotherapy*

NURSING PRIORITIES: (a) Minimize pain and discomfort from stomatitis and (b) prevent further trauma to and infection of the oral mucous membrane.

Interventions

1. Assess for signs and symptoms of stomatitis, such as dry and ulcerated oral mucosa, pain, viscous saliva, or difficulty in swallowing. Document and report the condition of the oral mucous membrane—including the lips, tongue, and gums—on a scale of 1 to 4, with 1 being normal and 4 being ulcerated, bleeding, irritated, and infected. Also observe the amount and viscosity of saliva. Obtain a culture of suspicious lesions, noting the results.

2. Teach an appropriate mouth care regimen.

• If platelet levels are above 40,000/mm³ and leukocyte levels above 1,500/mm³, recommend the following: brush the teeth with a soft, nylon-bristle toothbrush 30 minutes after meals and every 4 hours while awake. Place the brush at a 45-degree angle between the gums and the teeth, and move it in short horizontal strokes. Floss between teeth twice daily.

• If platelet or leukocyte levels are below the parameters specified, recommend rinsing only (using water or saline) until the values return to safer levels.

3. Provide hydrogen peroxide and water solution (1:2 or 1:4), baking soda and water (1 tsp to 500 ml), or normal saline to rinse the mouth during and after brushing.

Rationales

1. Stomatitis is both a sign of decreased immunocompetence and an adverse effect of chemotherapy that develops 7 to 10 days after treatment begins. Objective assessment is imperative for early identification of stomatitis so that appropriate therapy can be instituted.

2. Preventing accumulation of food debris and bacteria is essential to preventing breakdown of the oral mucous membrane.
• Take care to observe specified laboratory values, because even this regimen will cause severe bleeding if platelet counts are low. If the WBC count is low, mouth care could cause local infection.

• For the patient with low platelet or leukocyte levels, this regimen removes debris while minimizing the risks of bleeding or infection.

3. Commercial mouthwashes contain alcohol, which dry and irritate the oral mucosa.

4. Administer lidocaine (Xylocaine) viscous solution as needed, 1 tsp swished in the mouth every 3 to 4 hours, or acetaminophen with codeine elixir as needed, as ordered.

4. Lidocaine is a topical anesthetic that relieves pain from mouth ulcers. Acetaminophen with codeine works systemically to control pain, and the elixir is easily swallowed.

5. Lubricate lips with petrolatum or water-soluble lubricant (K-Y Lubricating Jelly), lip balm (ChapStick, Blistex), or mineral oil. Use gauze lubricated with petrolatum to protect the lips when the patient drinks from a cup or glass.

5. Severe dryness, sores, and ulcers on the lips cause pain when the patient drinks from a cup or glass. This pain further discourages the patient from drinking adequate fluids and maintaining an adequate fluid balance.

6. Encourage use of an artificial saliva product (Ora-Lub, Salivart, Xero-Lube).

6. Severe dryness of the oral mucous membrane increases the risk of tissue breakdown and impairs optimal nutritional intake. Artificial saliva supplements ease dryness, buffer acidity, and lubricate and soothe the mucous membrane.

7. Monitor, report, and document the appearance of white patches on the tongue and oral mucosa. Administer nystatin (Mycostatin) oral suspension or a gentian violet preparation, as ordered. Document the patient's response.

7. These white patches indicate yeast infection. (The immunosuppressed patient is prone to opportunistic infections such as candidiasis.) Prompt treatment of oral infection will prevent undue discomfort.

8. Apply a substrate of magnesium hydroxide (Milk of Magnesia) or a kaolin preparation (Kaopectate) with a swab or a gauze-covered tongue blade. (To prepare the substrate, allow the bottle to stand for several hours, then pour off the supernatant liquid.) Rinse with normal saline after 15 minutes.

8. Topical protective agents soothe irritated areas and promote healing.

9. Additional individualized interventions: _____

9. Rationales: _____

Target outcome criteria
Within 3 days of admission, the patient will:
• have no frank bleeding from gums
• show improved ability to swallow
• have decreased viscosity and improved amount of saliva.

Within 5 days of admission, the patient will:
• exhibit decreased number of open ulcers
• present negative cultures
• exhibit decreased number of white patches.

Nursing diagnosis: *High risk for ineffective individual coping related to uncertain prognosis and multiple disease- and treatment-induced losses*

NURSING PRIORITY: Promote healthy coping behavior.

Interventions

1. See the "Dying," "Grieving," and "Ineffective Individual Coping" plans, pages 11, 31, and 51 respectively.

Rationales

1. The patient with leukemia suffers multiple losses, and self-care ability, social contact, and energy level are reduced. Additionally, adverse effects from chemotherapy may cause body-image changes that are difficult to accept. Weakness, dependence on others, and an uncertain prognosis may create anxiety or contribute to depression. The plans listed provide specific interventions helpful in dealing with the psychosocial aspects of caring for a patient with leukemia.

2. Additional individualized interventions: _____

2. Rationales: _____

Target outcome criteria
Throughout the hospital stay, the patient will:
• use healthy coping behaviors
• verbalize feelings.

Discharge planning

NURSING DISCHARGE CRITERIA
Upon the patient's discharge, documentation shows evidence of:
• absence of fever
• absence of cardiovascular or pulmonary complications such as crackles, gurgles, arrhythmias, or atelectasis
• stabilizing weight
• WBC count greater than 2,000/mm³
• platelet count greater than 50,000/mm³
• hemoglobin level above 8 g/dl
• hematocrit value above 25%
• absence of signs and symptoms of infection
• ability to tolerate adequate nutritional intake
• absence of gingival bleeding and sores
• absence of hematuria or other bladder or bowel dysfunction
• ability to control pain using oral medications
• ability to perform ADLs, transfers, and ambulation independently or with minimal assistance
• adequate home support system or referral to home care or nursing home if indicated by an inadequate home support system or the patient's inability to perform ADLs, transfer, ambulate, and follow medication regimen.
Note: All patients with leukemia must be referred to the social service department. Leukemia is a financially draining disease, commonly requiring long-term and expensive treatment, so the patient is likely to have financial concerns. For terminal leukemia, refer the patient to a hospice.

PATIENT-FAMILY TEACHING CHECKLIST
Document evidence that the patient and family demonstrate an understanding of:
___ diagnosis and course of treatment
___ all discharge medications' purpose, dosage, administration schedule, and adverse effects requiring medical attention (usual chemotherapy medications include alkylating agents, such as busulfan [Myleran] and chlorambucil [Leukeran], antibiotics such as daunorubicin [Cerubidine] and doxorubicin [Adriamycin], antimetabolites such as methotrexate and 6-mercaptopurine [Purinethol], and plant alkaloids such as vincristine [Oncovin] and vinblastine [Velban])
___ ways of preventing and identifying infections
___ appropriate modifications of activity-rest patterns

___ ways of preventing, identifying, and reporting abnormal bleeding tendencies
___ techniques to control nausea, vomiting, and anorexia
___ recommended dietary modifications
___ techniques to prevent urinary calculi formation
___ appropriate oral hygiene techniques and procedures
___ signs and symptoms indicating relapse or exacerbation of disease
___ frequency of follow-up laboratory tests
___ schedule for future diagnostic tests, chemotherapy administration, and appointments with health care providers
___ how to contact the doctor
___ community resources for home management, lifestyle modifications, and support
___ emotional response to chronic or terminal illness
___ changes in family role patterns.

DOCUMENTATION CHECKLIST
Using outcome criteria as a guide, document:
___ clinical status on admission
___ significant changes in status, especially development of CNS symptoms and septicemia
___ pertinent laboratory and diagnostic test findings
___ response to chemotherapy treatments
___ management of chemotherapy adverse reactions
___ response to transfusions of RBCs, WBCs, or platelets
___ nutritional intake
___ fluid-electrolyte balance
___ activity-rest pattern
___ emotional coping patterns
___ condition of skin and mucous membranes
___ signs and symptoms of infection or bleeding tendencies
___ I.V. line patency and condition of veins
___ tolerance of diagnostic procedures
___ response to anti-infection measures.

ASSOCIATED PLANS OF CARE
Anemia
Dying
Grieving
Ineffective Individual Coping
Nutritional Deficit
Total Parenteral Nutrition

References

Burke, M., et al. *Cancer Chemotherapy: A Nursing Process Approach.* Boston: Jones & Bartlett Publishers, 1991.

Diseases, 2nd ed. Nurse's Reference Library. Springhouse, Pa.: Springhouse Corp., 1989.

Gordon, M. *Manual of Nursing Diagnoses: 1986-1987.* New York: McGraw-Hill Book Co., 1987.

Griffin, J. *Hematology and Immunology Concepts of Nursing.* East Norwalk, Conn.: Appleton-Century-Crofts, 1986.

Kneisl, C., and Ames, S. *Adult Health Nursing.* Reading, Mass.: Addison-Wesley Publishing Co., 1986.

Luckman, J., and Sorensen, K. *Medical-Surgical Nursing,* 3rd ed. Philadelphia: W.B. Saunders Co., 1987.

McIntire, S., and Cioppa, A. *Cancer Nursing: A Developmental Approach.* New York: John Wiley & Sons, 1986.

McNally, J.C., et al. *Guidelines for Oncology Nursing Practice,* 2nd ed. Philadelphia: W.B. Saunders Co., 1991.

Neoplastic Disorders. Nurse's Clinical Library. Springhouse, Pa.: Springhouse Corp., 1985.

Lymphoma

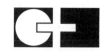

DRG information
DRG 400 Lymphoma or Leukemia with Major
  Operating Room (OR) Procedure.
  Mean LOS = 10.1 days
  Major OR procedures include biopsy, excision,
  or incision.
DRG 401 Lymphoma or Non-Acute Leukemia with
  Other OR Procedure. With Complication or
  Comorbidity (CC).
  Mean LOS = 10.2 days
DRG 402 Lymphoma or Non-Acute Leukemia with
  Other OR Procedure. Without CC.
  Mean LOS = 3.9 days
DRG 403 Lymphoma or Non-Acute Leukemia. With CC.
  Mean LOS = 8.2 days
DRG 404 Lymphoma or Non-Acute Leukemia. Without
  CC.
  Mean LOS = 4.3 days
Additional DRG information: After hospitalization for
the staging workup and initial course of therapy, the
patient would most likely receive ongoing chemother-
apy as an outpatient.

Introduction
DEFINITION AND TIME FOCUS
Lymphoma is the abnormal, malignant proliferation
and enlargement of lymph nodes, spleen, and other
lymphoid tissue, resulting in impaired cellular and humoral immunity, obstruction and infiltration of adjacent structures, and systemic involvement. Lymphomas
are classified as Hodgkin's (commonly called Hodgkin's
disease) or non-Hodgkin's.
  Hodgkin's disease is characterized by contiguous
node involvement. Extranodal spread at the time of diagnosis is uncommon. Staging is important in Hodgkin's disease, as in other cancers, because it helps
determine treatment and estimate prognosis. (See
Staging classification [Ann Arbor] for Hodgkin's disease,
page 642, for staging and treatment guidelines for
Hodgkin's disease.) Commonly, the disease is localized;
fever, weight loss, and night sweats (termed "B" symptoms in staging classification) are seen in about 40%
of patients at presentation. Hodgkin's disease occurs
most commonly between ages 15 and 35, with a second peak between ages 50 and 59.
  Non-Hodgkin's lymphomas comprise many histologic
variations. They are characterized by noncontiguous
nodal spread, commonly with extranodal involvement
in the GI tract, testes, central nervous system (CNS),
or bone marrow. The disease is usually disseminated;
"B" symptoms occur in only about 20% of patients.
Non-Hodgkin's lymphoma is three times more common
than Hodgkin's lymphoma in the United States and can

occur at any age, although peak incidence is between
ages 50 and 60.
  Both types of lymphoma are more common in
males than in females, and males tend to have a worse
prognosis.
  Hodgkin's and non-Hodgkin's lymphomas are considered together here because their clinical presenta-
tions, diagnostic workups, treatments, and nursing
management are similar. This plan focuses on the undiagnosed, symptomatic patient with lymphoma who is
admitted for a staging workup and initial therapy.

ETIOLOGY AND PRECIPITATING FACTORS
• viral etiology (suggested for some lymphomas; may
involve a herpeslike virus related to the Epstein-Barr
virus)
• family history (increased incidence among family
members suggests genetic and environmental factors)
• environmental exposure to certain herbicides (such
as phenoxyacetic acid) linked to increased risk of non-
Hodgkin's lymphoma

Focused assessment guidelines
NURSING HISTORY (Functional health pattern findings)

Health perception—health management pattern
• may report fever—highest in the afternoon; twice-
daily peaks greater than 101° F (38.3° C) are common
• may report drenching night sweats
• may report pruritus—more intense at night, worse
with bathing
• may report general malaise and fatigue
• may report painless, swollen lymph nodes (typically
in the cervical chain)

Nutritional-metabolic pattern
• may report unexplained weight loss
• may report anorexia
• may report pain in nodes immediately after drinking
alcohol (cause unknown)

Activity-exercise pattern
• may report general fatigue: "unable to do the things I
want to do"
• may report shortness of breath if ascites, pleural effusion, or anemia is present

Sleep-rest pattern
• may report sleep disturbances from night sweats

STAGING CLASSIFICATION (ANN ARBOR) FOR HODGKIN'S DISEASE

Stage	Description
I	Nodal involvement within one region
I E	Single extralymphatic organ or site
II	Nodal involvement within two or more regions, limited by the diaphragm
II E	Localized extranodal site and nodal involvement within one or more regions limited by the diaphragm
III	Nodal involvement of regions above and below the diaphragm
III E	With localized extralymphatic site
III S	With spleen involvement
III ES	Or both
IV	Diffuse or disseminated involvement of one or more extralymphatic organs or tissues, with or without lymph node involvement

E = extralymphatic involvement
S = spleen involvement
ES = both extralymphatic and spleen involvement

From: Carbone, P., et al. "Report of the Committee on Hodgkin's Disease Staging," *Cancer Research* 31:1860, 1971. Used with permission.

Self-perception — self-concept pattern
• may report fear regarding prognosis and progression of disease
• may report difficulty coping with changes in lifestyle, self-esteem, and body image

Cognitive-perceptual pattern
• may or may not want to know prognosis and expected progression of disease

Role-relationship pattern
• may report concern regarding role reversals at home and inability to fulfill previous roles

Sexuality-reproductive pattern
• may express concern regarding adverse effects of chemotherapy on fertility and sexual performance
• may report decreased libido from chemotherapy, radiation, or general fatigue

Coping — stress tolerance pattern
• may report increased anxiety

PHYSICAL FINDINGS
Lymphoreticular
• lymphadenopathy
• tonsillar enlargement
• edema and cyanosis of face and neck (rare)

Pulmonary
• shortness of breath (rare)
• cough (rare)
• stridor (rare)
• signs of pleural effusion (rare)

Gastrointestinal
• splenomegaly
• hepatomegaly
• ascites (uncommon)
• jaundice (rare)

DIAGNOSTIC STUDIES*
• complete blood count (CBC) and platelet count — may reveal neutrophilic leukocytosis and mild normochromic anemia, lymphopenia, or increased sedimentation rate
• serum alkaline phosphatase values — increased values indicate liver or bone involvement
• direct Coombs' (antiglobulin) test — detects autoimmune hemolytic anemia (more common in non-Hodgkin's lymphoma)
• immunoglobulin studies — may show overproduction of immunoglobulin by proliferating B-cell lymphocytes
• lymph node biopsy (performed on the most central node of the involved group) — Hodgkin's disease shows Reed-Sternberg cells, non-Hodgkin's lymphoma reveals destruction of lymph node architecture; normal cellular elements are replaced by increased lymphocytes and lymphoblasts
• intravenous pyelogram — detects unsuspected renal involvement and ureteral deviation and obstruction by involved nodes
• chest X-ray — with computed tomography (CT) scan, may reveal hilar lymphadenopathy; mediastinal masses in lymphoma usually appear as a dense rounded mass (occurring as commonly in the anterior mediastinum as in the middle mediastinum)
• lymphangiography — may show enlarged, foamy-looking nodes (number of nodes affected, unilateral or bilateral involvement, and extent of extranodal involvement help determine stage); less useful in non-Hodgkin's lymphoma because does not visualize mesenteric nodes, which are usually involved; occasionally, nodes are so enlarged they cannot be visualized
• abdominal CT scan — may detect intra-abdominal intrapelvic nodal involvement as well as liver involvement

---

*Extensive testing is necessary to diagnose and stage lymphoma.

• bone scan—used to detect bone involvement

• bone marrow aspirate and biopsy—elevated lymphocyte values indicate bone marrow involvement, more common in non-Hodgkin's lymphoma

• bilateral bone marrow biopsies—commonly performed because of spotty bone marrow involvement; chances of identifying bone marrow involvement are increased by 15% to 20% with bilateral procedure

• laparotomy and splenectomy—undertaken only if outcome will affect a therapeutic decision; may detect splenic involvement

POTENTIAL COMPLICATIONS

• intestinal obstruction and perforation
• ureteral obstruction
• sepsis (treatment-related)
• anemia
• thrombocytopenia (treatment-related)
• hyperuricemia (treatment-related)
• superior vena cava syndrome (airway occlusion related to edema from impaired superior vena cava drainage)
• spinal cord compression (rare)
• hypercalcemia (rare)
• sterility (treatment-related)
• secondary cancers (treatment-related)
• pleural, pericardial, or abdominal effusions

Collaborative problem: *High risk for respiratory compromise related to enlarged mediastinal nodes, pulmonary compression, and, for non-Hodgkin's lymphoma only, superior vena cava syndrome*

NURSING PRIORITY: Optimize alveolar ventilation.

Interventions

1. Position the patient comfortably when short of breath: elevate the upper torso at least 45 degrees, tilt the shoulders forward, support the arms away from the sides, and support the feet.

2. Teach and supervise therapeutic breathing techniques:
• pursed-lip breathing

• abdominal breathing.

3. Limit activity according to respiratory capabilities.

4. Plan activities to allow minimal energy expenditure and adequate rest periods: provide bed baths, assist the patient with meals as needed, and limit visitors.

5. Decrease anxiety associated with dyspnea: explain all procedures in a calm, supportive manner; provide a quiet environment to promote adequate rest; and use relaxation techniques, music, and other diversionary activities.

6. Control pain with analgesics, as ordered. Use nonpharmacologic pain control techniques as appropriate. See the "Pain" plan, page 69.

Rationales

1. This position promotes maximum aeration by taking weight off the shoulders and arms, allowing the accessory muscles to be used solely for breathing.

2. Breathing techniques minimize respiratory impairment.

• Pursed-lip breathing has two benefits: it creates back pressure, holding the airways open, and the prolonged expiration time slows the flow of air, preventing premature closure of the airways and allowing more complete emptying of the lungs.

• The abdominal muscles can aid the diaphragm during expiration. As the patient inhales, the abdominal muscles relax. During expiration, they contract and help the diaphragm move upward to expel air.

3. Decreased activity decreases the need for oxygen.

4. Fatigue is both a symptom of hypoxemia and a cause of increased dyspnea. As respiratory muscles tire, respiratory excursion and alveolar ventilation drop, worsening hypoxemia and reinforcing the vicious circle of fatigue and dyspnea.

5. Anxiety and fear increase the heart rate, increasing the need for oxygen.

6. Pain may be present if enlarged nodes are compressing adjacent structures or nerve roots. Pain control will help decrease anxiety, thereby reducing associated shortness of breath. The "Pain" plan contains specific information and detailed interventions.

HEMATOLOGIC AND IMMUNOLOGIC DISORDERS

7. Monitor for signs and symptoms of superior vena cava syndrome, as follows:
• early—neck vein distention (especially on arising), change in collar size, and headache
• advanced—progressive periorbital and facial edema, dizziness, cough, stridor, dysphagia, and dyspnea.

Report such findings to the doctor immediately, and transport the patient to the radiation therapy department, as ordered, if superior vena cava syndrome is identified.

After radiation therapy, assess for indications of improvement: reduced edema, increased ease in swallowing, and improved respiratory parameters.

7. In superior vena cava syndrome, enlarged nodes press on the superior vena cava, impairing normal venous drainage from the head and neck. The resulting progressive edema may lead to tracheal deviation and airway occlusion. Superior vena cava syndrome is considered an oncologic emergency. Radiation therapy is the treatment of choice: immediate therapy of 300 to 400 rads daily for 3 to 4 days, then a full course of 3,000 to 6,000 rads. In most patients, symptoms should decrease rapidly, usually within 48 to 72 hours.

8. Administer tranquilizers, as ordered.

8. Physiologic reactions to anxiety include stimulation of the autonomic nervous system, such as increased heart and respiratory rates. Tranquilizers relieve anxiety without inducing sleep. The benzodiazepines appear to depress the CNS at the limbic and subcortical levels of the brain, producing sedation and relaxing skeletal muscles.

9. Additional individualized interventions: _____

9. Rationales: _____

Target outcome criteria
Within 48 hours of admission, the patient will:
• demonstrate effective, regular use of breathing techniques
• verbalize pain relief

• tolerate increased activity level
• show relaxed posture and facial expression
• exhibit no head or neck cyanosis.

Collaborative problem: *High risk for sepsis related to leukopenia, lymphopenia from bone marrow involvement, chemotherapy, and radiation therapy effects*

NURSING PRIORITIES: (a) Maximize immunocompetence, and (b) prevent or promptly detect and treat superinfection.

Interventions

1. Prioritize patient care assignments. Care for the neutropenic patient first.

2. Observe good handwashing technique.

3. Monitor daily white blood cell (WBC) counts and differentials. Inform the patient and doctor of results.

Rationales

1. This minimizes the risk of cross-contamination by the caregiver.

2. The most important way to protect against infection is meticulous handwashing. Improper or infrequent handwashing is a well-known contributor to cross-contamination.

3. The degree of granulocytopenia indicates the patient's susceptibility to infection and is the most important factor in determining the risk of sepsis.

4. Take protective precautions when the patient's absolute granulocyte count is dangerously depressed, typically when less than 1,000/mm³. Protective measures should include:
- serving only cooked foods
- avoiding raw fruits and vegetables
- removing sources of standing water (such as vases of flowers)
- not handling live flowers or plants.

Institute further protective measures according to hospital protocol, as appropriate to the patient's condition.

5. Assess actual and potential infection sites at least every 8 hours, including the lungs, mouth, rectum, I.V. sites, vagina, and surgical incisions. Monitor urine culture results. Observe carefully for subtle changes in skin and mucous membrane color, texture, or sensation.

6. Screen and limit visitors. Prohibit visits by those with recent or current infections.

7. Institute an appropriate oral hygiene protocol. Monitor for oral herpes lesions and *Candida* stomatitis.

8. Avoid invasive measures, such as I.M. injections, enemas, rectal temperatures, suppositories, and indwelling urinary catheters whenever possible.

9. Measure the patient's temperature at least every 4 hours; if it is higher than 101.3° F (38.5° C) and the patient develops signs and symptoms of septic shock (tachycardia, tachypnea, restlessness, confusion, cough, decreased pulse pressure, and cool extremities), notify the doctor.

10. Obtain blood, urine, throat, and sputum cultures, using correct technique, as ordered. Ensure that cultures are obtained before antibiotic therapy begins.

11. Report all positive blood cultures, even if the patient is already taking antibiotics.

12. Administer antibiotics only after obtaining blood and urine cultures, ideally within 60 minutes of detecting sepsis. Give subsequent doses on time.

4. The risk of infection increases significantly when the absolute granulocyte count ranges from 500 to 1,000/mm³ and persists for more than a few days. The absolute granulocyte count indicates the number of mature WBCs (the cells most effective in fighting infection). To calculate the absolute granlulocyte count, add the percentage of polys (mature neurophils) to the percentage of bands (slightly immature neutrophils); multiply the result by the WBC count. Protective precautions may decrease the number of pathogenic organisms the immunosuppressed patient contacts. Raw fruits and vegetables are sources of gram-negative bacilli; live plants and soil are sources of fungi. Standing water may provide a medium for microorganisms, particularly *Pseudomonas.*

5. Early detection may prevent serious complications and spread of infection. In the immunocompromised patient, however, an altered inflammatory response complicates early detection. Classic signs and symptoms of infection (such as erythema, pus, and fever) may be masked in a neutropenic patient or in a patient taking steroids (a factor in many lymphoma protocols).

6. Minimizing the patient's exposure to microorganisms may help avert sepsis.

7. The patient with lymphoma is at increased risk for viral and fungal infections because of impaired cell-mediated immunity. (T lymphocytes protect against viruses, fungi, and parasites.)

8. Intact skin is the body's first line of defense. Sweat glands and sebaceous glands keep bacteria under control. Lysozymes, enzymes secreted by the sweat glands, attack the cell walls of bacteria. Sebum, secreted by the sebaceous glands, has antifungal and antibacterial properties. Skin and blood infections may occur when invasive measures damage the skin.

9. Septic shock (a medical emergency) is reversible in its early stages. Massive infection, usually from gram-negative bacteria, causes septic shock. As the body fights the infection, the bacteria die, releasing endotoxins that in turn impair cell metabolism and damage surrounding tissue. Lysozomal enzymes, bradykinin, and histamine cause peripheral vasodilation and increased capillary permeability, resulting in peripheral blood pooling, inadequate venous return, and severely reduced cardiac output.

10. Cultures must be uncontaminated to permit accurate diagnosis. Current culture results determine appropriate antibiotic therapy.

11. When specific organisms are identified, therapy should be modified according to antibiotic sensitivity.

12. Prompt, timely administration of antibiotics increases the survival rate in neutropenic patients. Therapeutic blood levels of medication must be maintained to treat sepsis effectively.

13. Additional individualized interventions: _____

13. Rationales: _____

_____

_____

Target outcome criteria
After a full course of antibiotic therapy (5 to 10 days) and return of adequate immunity, or 14 days after completion of the chemotherapy cycle, the patient will:
• be afebrile
• show no signs of systemic or localized infection.

Collaborative problem: *Pruritus related to histamine or leukopeptidase release from WBCs and to effects of radiation therapy*

NURSING PRIORITIES: (a) Relieve discomfort, and (b) prevent or minimize skin injury.

Interventions

1. Promote adequate hydration: 12 8-oz glasses (3,000 ml) of fluid daily, unless contraindicated.

2. Use emollient creams on the skin (if allowed during radiation therapy).

3. Provide tepid, cooling baths.

4. Keep the patient's fingernails short. Provide clean cotton gloves at night.

5. Use soap for sensitive or dry skin.

6. Administer antihistamines, antibiotics, tar extracts, or chemotherapeutic agents, as ordered.

7. Instruct the patient to avoid harsh cold and wind.

8. Remove excessive clothing or bedding; instruct the patient not to wear restrictive clothing.

9. Launder the patient's clothing with a nondetergent cleanser, and rinse thoroughly.

10. Additional individualized interventions: _____

_____

Rationales

1. Adequate hydration is essential to minimize skin dryness.

2. Emollient creams are oil-in-water emulsions. Water keeps the skin moist while the oil creates a film that slows normal evaporation.

3. Regular bathing helps protect the immunosuppressed patient from infection. Additionally, tepid water promotes vasoconstriction. Proteases are sensitive to heat, and the cutaneous nerve endings that mediate the scratch impulse are made more sensitive by vasodilation.

4. These measures may prevent damage to the skin if the patient cannot control scratching.

5. Soaps for sensitive skin have a large proportion of emollient oils and contain no detergents or dyes to strip the skin. They liquefy instantly and leave no irritating residue.

6. Antihistamines will help if the underlying cause of pruritus is increased histamine release. Tar extracts and topical steroids may inhibit protease release. If infection is the underlying cause, antibiotics are indicated. If a tumor is releasing enzymes, chemotherapy may shrink the tumor and proportionately reduce enzyme release.

7. Exposure to cold and wind dries the skin.

8. A cool environment promotes vasoconstriction. Restrictive clothing may irritate the skin.

9. These precautions help prevent chemical irritation of the skin.

10. Rationales: _____

_____

Target outcome criteria
Throughout the hospital stay, the patient will:
• present intact skin
• verbalize reduced discomfort
• list three self-care measures to minimize pruritus.

Collaborative problem: *High risk for hemorrhage related to decreased platelet count secondary to chemotherapy or radiation therapy effects*

NURSING PRIORITY: Maximize the patient's available protective mechanisms.

Interventions

1. Do not administer aspirin or aspirin-containing products.

2. Administer stool softeners, as ordered, and monitor the frequency of stools to detect constipation.

3. Avoid such invasive measures as I.M. injections, enemas, and rectal suppositories.

4. Use an electric razor when shaving the patient. Avoid activities with the potential for physical injury.

5. Administer steroids, as ordered, with milk products or antacids.

6. Maintain optimal nutritional status, encouraging protein intake.

7. Test all stool, emesis, and urine for occult blood.

8. Apply direct pressure to venipuncture sites for at least 5 minutes.

9. Administer platelet infusions, as ordered.

10. Use a soft-bristle toothbrush, and avoid flossing the patient's teeth.

11. Instruct the patient to avoid strenuous activity, Valsalva's maneuver, and lifting heavy objects.

12. Teach the patient self-protection measures related to the above interventions, such as avoiding aspirin, taking stool softeners, and using an electric razor.

13. Additional individualized interventions: _____

Rationales

1. The acetyl group in the aspirin compound inhibits platelet aggregation, thereby impairing fibrin strand formation. A single dose of aspirin produces an effect that remains for days, long after the aspirin has been metabolized and excreted.

2. Straining at stool produces excessive pressure on the anal orifice; the rectal area is highly vascular and can hemorrhage.

3. Intact skin reduces the risk of bleeding. A decreased platelet count means that even minor trauma may result in significant bleeding.

4. These measures minimize the risk of skin trauma.

5. Coating the stomach helps prevent gastric irritation.

6. Protein is needed to produce megakaryocytes, precursors of platelets.

7. Early detection of bleeding promotes early and effective treatment.

8. Decreased platelet levels prolong clot formation.

9. A platelet count below 20,000/mm^3 increases the risk of spontaneous hemorrhage. Active bleeding is an indication for platelet administration.

10. These measures decrease the risk of physical irritation to oral mucous membranes.

11. These activities increase intracranial pressure and may cause cerebrovascular hemorrhage.

12. The knowledgeable patient's active involvement in self-care minimizes the risk of hemorrhage, especially after discharge.

13. Rationales: _____

Target outcome criteria
Throughout the hospital stay, the patient will:
• have regular, soft, formed stools
• exhibit no uncontrolled bleeding.

Nursing diagnosis: *High risk for nutritional deficit related to anorexia, taste alterations, fatigue, nausea and vomiting, and altered oral mucous membrane*

NURSING PRIORITY: Promote adequate nutrition to enhance response to therapy and prevent complications.

Interventions

1. Arrange for a dietary consultation to address the patient's calorie and protein needs. Explore the patient's food preferences and attempt to obtain the foods requested. Explain prescribed dietary recommendations and help the patient set goals for meeting them.

2. Offer sandwiches and other cold foods.

3. Avoid giving liquids with meals.

4. Avoid offering favorite foods during peak periods of nausea and vomiting or while the patient is receiving chemotherapy.

5. Offer salty foods (such as broth or crackers) and tart foods (such as lemons or dill pickles) unless the patient has stomatitis.

6. Offer small, frequent meals, and encourage the patient to eat and drink slowly.

7. Avoid offering greasy foods.

8. Provide mouth care before meals and after vomiting episodes.

9. If taste alterations are present, consult with the dietary department and advise the patient to:
• use plastic utensils instead of metal silverware
• eat protein in the form of eggs, cheese, beans, and peanut butter instead of meat
• experiment with spices and flavorings to enhance taste sensation (such as mint, vanilla, lemon, and basil), unless contraindicated by stomatitis.

10. Advise the patient to increase intake of sugar and sweet foods.

Rationales

1. The dietitian's expertise may be helpful in planning a diet that meets the patient's needs while incorporating the patient's preferences. Including the patient in planning and goal-setting enhances compliance and promotes a sense of self-control.

2. The odor of hot foods commonly aggravates nausea.

3. Fluids contribute to gastric distention and may reduce intake of solid foods.

4. The patient can develop an aversion to foods served during periods of nausea and vomiting. During anorexic periods, favorite foods may supply the patient's only intake, so maintaining positive associations is essential.

5. These foods increase salivation and stimulate the taste buds. In the patient with stomatitis, however, salt and acidity will further irritate open mucous membranes.

6. Small meals and slow eating minimize gastric distention and help prevent early satiety.

7. High-fat foods decrease gastric emptying time, causing feelings of overfullness and distention.

8. Regular mouth care refreshes the mouth and enhances the flavor of foods.

9. The presence of actively dividing cells in the oral mucous membrane that excrete amino-acid-like substances enhances the bitter taste sensation. Large tumor mass also increases the degree and duration of any taste sensation. Beef and pork have high amino acid levels. A negative nitrogen balance also decreases the patient's threshold for the bitter taste sensation. Certain chemotherapy agents used in lymphoma protocols, specifically mechlorethamine (Mustargen), cyclophosphamide (Cytoxan), vincristine (Oncovin), and dacarbazine (DTIC-Dome) contribute further to taste alterations.

10. Taste alterations associated with the disease and chemotherapy commonly include decreased sensitivity to sweetness, although this is sometimes accompanied by an aversion to sweet foods. Increased sugar also boosts caloric intake.

11. Teach the patient how to use viscous lidocaine (Xylocaine) to reduce stomatitis pain (swish and swallow 15 ml 15 minutes before meals). If ineffective, try dyclonine (Dyclone).

11. A topical anesthetic decreases sensitivity to pain, enabling the patient to eat without discomfort.

12. Offer soft, moist foods, such as custards, ice cream, gelatins, cottage cheese, and ground meats with sauces and gravies.

12. Soft foods minimize mechanical irritation to the oral mucous membrane and are easier to swallow.

13. Encourage the patient to eat liquid and pudding supplements.

13. High-calorie supplements may compensate for decreased intake.

14. Consult the doctor regarding temporary enteral or parenteral feedings if other interventions are ineffective.

14. The patient may need a temporary alternative to oral nutrition to prevent severe malnutrition, which may affect the outcome of therapy.

15. Additional individualized interventions: _____

15. Rationales: _____

Target outcome criteria
Throughout the hospital stay, the patient will:
• participate in planning and implementing a dietary regimen
• maintain an adequate nutritional status to facilitate therapy.

Nursing diagnosis: *Knowledge deficit related to self-care of venous access device, including central venous catheter or subcutaneous port*

NURSING PRIORITY: Teach self-care techniques and measures for home management of the venous access device.

Interventions

1. Teach the patient the name of the catheter or port and its purpose and anatomical placement.

Rationales

1. Central venous catheters or subcutaneous ports may be used to administer chemotherapy. The patient who is knowledgeable about all aspects of care is better prepared to use good judgment in decision making and to teach others about care needs. Assuming greater responsibility for the device helps the patient develop an increased sense of control, easing incorporation of the device into the patient's body image.

2. Teach the patient how to change dressings at home (usually a clean, occlusive dressing changed when wet or soiled, or according to protocol). Have the patient demonstrate the proper technique before discharge; arrange for home care follow-up. If the patient has a subcutaneous port, explain that a dressing is not necessary because the device is completely under the skin.

2. Because the catheter exit site is a break in skin integrity, the risk of opportunistic infections increases. A clean occlusive dressing can decrease the potential for microbial contamination. The frequency of dressing changes varies among institutions.
    Anxiety may interfere with learning by decreasing the patient's ability to concentrate. Written materials and home care follow-up reinforce earlier learning and allow the patient to learn in a less-threatening environment.

3. Teach the patient to identify early signs and symptoms of local or generalized infection, such as redness, swelling, purulent drainage, fever, increased fatigue, and malaise.

3. Early detection of infection results in more timely and effective treatment.

4. Teach the patient the importance of proper irrigation technique, including frequency and solution used, as follows:
• for Hickman- or Broviac-type catheters — Irrigate daily with 2 ml of heparin solution, whether or not the catheter is in use.
• for Groshong-type catheters — Irrigate with 5 ml normal saline once a week when not in use.
• for subcutaneous ports — Irrigate with 5 ml of heparin solution once a month when not in use.

5. Inform the patient of potential complications and appropriate interventions, as follows:

• clot formation (catheter will not irrigate): Avoid forcing irrigation if resistance is felt. Contact the doctor.
• catheter damage (break or cut in catheter): For a Hickman-type catheter, clamp immediately with a toothless hemostat (send one home with the patient) and notify the doctor. For a Groshong-type catheter, wipe the proximal end clean and use a repair kit (send one home with the patient) to mend the distal portion or port.

• catheter displacement (catheter pulled out): Apply a pressure dressing and call the doctor. If bleeding is present, apply direct manual pressure until it stops.

6. Give the patient the names and telephone numbers of appropriate resource persons, such as the doctor, emergency squad, and the home-health nurse.

7. Additional individualized interventions: _____

_____

4. Although catheters and subcutaneous ports are in place continuously, chemotherapy administration is intermittent. Catheter or port patency must be maintained for the device to function. Proper technique decreases the risk of contamination.

5. Recognizing complications may prevent a potentially hazardous situation, such as infection, tissue damage, catheter migration, or loss of the device.
• Forcing irrigation may push a clot out the end of the catheter and into the circulatory system.
• A Hickman-type catheter may allow air to enter the vein when damaged. Immediate clamping stops any bleeding and prevents air influx. Groshong-type catheters have valvelike devices to prevent air influx; the patient can repair the catheter with the kit provided.

• Pressure controls bleeding if the catheter is accidentally removed.

6. A health care provider can speed resolution of a patient problem or concern. Knowing how and where to contact resource persons may help decrease anxiety and promote a sense of control.

7. Rationales: _____

_____

Target outcome criteria
By the time of discharge, the patient will:
• list signs of infection
• demonstrate dressing change and irrigation techniques as taught

• list three possible complications of a vascular access device and identify appropriate interventions for each.

Nursing diagnosis: *High risk for body-image or self-esteem disturbance related to effects of chemotherapy or radiation therapy*

NURSING PRIORITIES: (a) Prepare the patient for therapy, and (b) promote a positive self-concept.

Interventions

1. Inform the patient of anticipated adverse effects of chemotherapy or radiation that will affect body image and role performance. Suggest measures to prevent or lessen their impact (see *Suggestions for minimizing chemotherapeutic adverse effects*).

Rationales

1. Chemotherapy protocols for lymphoma are aggressive and cause numerous adverse effects. Radiation therapy may also cause severe adverse effects. Teaching the patient about specific preventive or palliative measures before therapy begins increases the patient's sense of control, decreases powerlessness, and promotes self-image.

SUGGESTIONS FOR MINIMIZING CHEMOTHERAPEUTIC ADVERSE EFFECTS

Alopecia
- Shampoo only one or two times weekly.
- Use a mild, protein shampoo.
- Avoid using an electric hair dryer or electric curlers.
- Avoid using hair spray or other drying products.
- Try a satin pillowcase to minimize tangling.
- Avoid excessive hair brushing or combing.
- Use a wide-toothed comb.
- Avoid using scalp hypothermia devices, which may reduce flow of medication to the head.

Weight gain
- Exercise regularly.
- Follow prescribed dietary guidelines.
- Select flattering, loose-fitting clothing.

Nausea and vomiting
- Avoid fatty, salty, or spicy foods.
- Use diversionary activities.
- Avoid eating or drinking for at least 1 hour before and after chemotherapy.
- Use a sedative that has an amnesic effect, such as lorazepam (Ativan), before chemotherapy, if prescribed.
- Suggest that family members avoid perfumes, aftershaves, and other aromatic toiletries.

Constipation
- Maintain a diet high in fiber, bulk, and fluids.
- Exercise regularly.
- Use stool softeners.

Diarrhea
- Try adding nutmeg to foods.
- Avoid milk or milk products (except yogurt, which may be helpful).
- Ensure adequate replacement of fluid and potassium.

Depression
- Understand that this is normal and usually temporary.
- Identify and use resources for emotional support.

Sore throat or dysphagia
- Observe self closely while eating for sore throat or difficulty swallowing.
- Eat soft foods.
- Use topical anesthetics as prescribed.

Dermatitis
- Avoid using deodorants, cosmetics, or creams, unless prescribed.
- Avoid hot baths or use of heat.

2. Inform the male patient of the availability of sperm banking before beginning chemotherapy.

3. Provide adequate time to discuss the patient's concerns and feelings. Strive to maintain a nonjudgmental attitude. See the "Grieving," "Ineffective Family Coping," and "Ineffective Individual Coping" plans, pages 31, 47, and 51 respectively.

4. Include the patient in decision making. Allow the patient to plan the day's events (within hospital limitations).

5. Instruct the patient and spouse (or partner) on specific sexual adverse effects of chemotherapy and radiation therapy: for example, decreased libido, decreased vaginal lubrication, and temporary impotence. Provide written material for specific interventions related to each. Encourage the couple to share concerns and ask questions. Refer them to the social services department or other resources for ongoing counseling and support, if needed.

6. Additional individualized interventions: _____

2. Because the peak incidence of Hodgkin's disease corresponds with peak childbearing years, fertility is a major concern. Chemotherapy may cause permanent sterility. For a male patient, sperm banking can help offset this adverse effect of treatment. The well-informed patient is able to base decisions on sound judgment after considering available options.

3. The patient is more likely to discuss personal concerns if a trusting relationship is developed. Judgmental responses that reflect the caregiver's personal biases may inhibit open discussion. These plans provide interventions helpful in addressing emotional needs.

4. Promoting maximum patient participation in care planning conveys respect and increases the patient's sense of control.

5. The couple may be comforted to know that many adverse effects of therapy are temporary. Fatigue, fear, anxiety, and lack of privacy may also contribute to problems. Many patients (and many health care professionals) are not well educated about sex or are uncomfortable discussing sexual problems. Written information is a less threatening but effective means of providing this information. Sharing concerns may reduce the couple's anxiety.

6. Rationales: _____

Target outcome criteria
Throughout the hospital stay, the patient will:
• verbalize feelings freely
• participate in decision making related to care.

By the time of discharge, the patient will:
• identify personal concerns that may affect self-concept
• identify personal or external resources to deal with concerns
• list measures to minimize effects of chemotherapy or radiation therapy.

Discharge planning
NURSING DISCHARGE CRITERIA
Upon the patient's discharge, documentation shows evidence of:
• stable vital signs
• absence of fever
• absence of cardiovascular or pulmonary complications
• ability to control pain using oral medications
• absence of bowel or bladder dysfunction
• WBC count within expected parameters
• absence of signs and symptoms of infection
• ability to tolerate adequate nutritional intake
• ability to perform activities of daily living and to ambulate independently or with minimal assistance
• ability to care appropriately for vascular access device, if present
• adequate home support system or referral to home care or a nursing home if indicated by inadequate home support system or the patient's inability to care for self.

PATIENT-FAMILY TEACHING CHECKLIST
Document evidence that the patient and family demonstrate an understanding of:
__ disease and its progression
__ signs and symptoms of infection and preventive measures
__ all discharge medications' purpose, dosage, administration schedule, and adverse effects requiring medical attention (usual discharge medications may include antineoplastics, analgesics, stool softeners, antiemetics, and others, depending on symptoms)
__ purpose and results of radiation therapy, schedule for future treatments, and management of anticipated adverse effects
__ maintenance of a vascular access device
__ indications for seeking emergency medical care
__ services available from local American Cancer Society chapter
__ availability of home health care and ancillary support services
__ date, time, and location of next scheduled appointment
__ how to contact the doctor.

DOCUMENTATION CHECKLIST
Using outcome criteria as a guide, document:
__ clinical status on admission
__ significant changes in clinical status
__ teaching about and response to diagnostic and staging workups
__ chemotherapy administration—I.V. line patency and site status, name of medication, dosage, and response (include teaching about protocol and the patient's response)
__ skin integrity over irradiated areas
__ transfusion therapy and response or reactions
__ nutritional status
__ status and maintenance of vascular access device
__ referrals initiated
__ patient-family teaching
__ discharge planning.

ASSOCIATED PLANS OF CARE
Dying
Grieving
Ineffective Family Coping
Ineffective Individual Coping
Knowledge Deficit
Nutritional Deficit

References
Brunner, L., and Suddarth, D. *The Lippincott Manual of Nursing Practice,* 5th ed. Philadelphia: J.B. Lippincott Co., 1991.

DeVita, V., et al. *Cancer: Principles and Practices of Oncology,* 3rd ed. Philadelphia: J.B. Lippincott Co., 1989.

Dodd, M. *Managing the Side Effects of Chemotherapy and Radiation Therapy.* Norwalk, Conn.: Appleton & Lange, 1987.

Gordon, M. *Nursing Diagnosis: Process and Application,* 2nd ed. New York: McGraw-Hill Book Co., 1987.

Groenwald, S., et al. *Cancer Nursing: Principles and Practices,* 2nd ed. Boston: Jones & Bartlett, 1990.

Holleb, A., Fink, D., and Murphy, G. *Textbook of Clinical Oncology.* Atlanta: American Cancer Society, 1991.

Otto, S. *Oncology Nursing.* St. Louis: Mosby-Year Book, 1991.

Tucker, R., and Rahr, V. "Nursing Care of the Patient with Non-Hodgkins Lymphoma: A Case Study," *Cancer Nursing,* 13(4):229-34, August 1990.

Hysterectomy

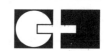

DRG information

DRG 353 Pelvic Evisceration, Radical Hysterectomy, and Radical Vulvectomy.
Mean LOS = 10.9 days

DRG 354 Uterine and Adnexa Procedure for Non-Ovarian, Adnexal Malignancy. With Complication or Comorbidity (CC).
Mean LOS = 7.6 days

DRG 355 Uterine and Adnexa Procedure for Non-Ovarian, Adnexal Malignancy. Without CC.
Mean LOS = 5.4 days

DRG 357 Uterine and Adnexa Procedures for Ovarian or Adnexal Malignancy.
Mean LOS = 10.6 days

DRG 358 Uterine and Adnexa Procedures for Non-Malignancy. With CC.
Mean LOS = 6.5 days

DRG 359 Uterine and Adnexa Procedures for Non-Malignancy. Without CC.
Mean LOS = 4.9 days

Introduction

DEFINITION AND TIME FOCUS

Hysterectomy is the surgical removal of the uterus. Several surgical variations exist. Subtotal hysterectomy, seldom performed, is the surgical removal of the corpus (body) of the uterus, leaving the cervical stump in place. Total hysterectomy is the surgical removal of the uterus and cervix. Total hysterectomy with bilateral salpingo-oophorectomy is the surgical removal of the uterus, cervix, uterine (Fallopian) tubes, and ovaries. (Salpingectomy is the surgical removal of the uterine tube or tubes; oophorectomy is the removal of an ovary or ovaries.) Radical hysterectomy is the surgical removal of the uterus, cervix, upper portion of the vagina, connective tissue, and lymph nodes.

All hysterectomy procedures result in permanent sterilization. If performed in conjunction with bilateral oophorectomy in the premenopausal woman, abrupt menopause results.

The surgical approach for a hysterectomy may be vaginal or abdominal. The vaginal approach is used for cervical cancer and uterine prolapse. The abdominal approach is commonly used for pelvic exploration for cancer or infection, removal of an enlarged uterus, or removal of tubes and ovaries.

This plan focuses on preoperative assessment and postoperative care for a patient undergoing total abdominal hysterectomy.

ETIOLOGY AND PRECIPITATING FACTORS

• recent diagnosis of cervical, endometrial, or ovarian cancer
• irreparable rupture or perforation of the uterus

• severe (life-threatening) pelvic infection
• myoma or nonmalignant tumor of the uterus
• history of endometriosis
• hemorrhage, metrorrhagia (dysfunctional uterine bleeding), postmenopausal bleeding, perimenopausal menometrorrhagia (excessive prolonged vaginal bleeding at irregular intervals), menorrhagia (excessive uterine bleeding occurring during regular menstruation), or postcoital bleeding with pelvic pain

Focused assessment guidelines
NURSING HISTORY (Functional health pattern findings)

Health perception—health management pattern
• may be postmenopausal with sudden uterine bleeding
• may have had abnormal Papanicolaou (Pap) smear results (if cervical or endometrial cancer is present)
• may have a history of prolonged postmenopausal estrogen replacement therapy (if endometrial cancer present)
• may have a history of prolonged, heavy, or painful menstruation (if uterine myoma, dysfunctional uterine bleeding, or endometrial cancer is present)
• may report a history of fibroids (myomas) in the uterus (if uterine myoma is present)

Nutritional-metabolic pattern
• may be obese

Elimination pattern
• may report a pattern of frequent urination related to presence and proximity of tumor

Activity-exercise pattern
• may report fatigue-related decrease in activity level if excessive vaginal bleeding has caused anemia

Sleep-rest pattern
• may report sleep disturbance related to nocturia
• may report sleep disturbance related to emotional stress of planned hospital stay and surgery

Cognitive-perceptual pattern
• may report a history of abdominal, pelvic, back, or leg pain
• may report fear of anticipated discomfort and pain from abdominal incision

Self-perception—self-concept pattern
• may express concerns about abdominal scar and removal of uterus
• may express concerns about femininity
• may express concerns about infertility

Role-relationship pattern
• may express concerns about spouse's or partner's acceptance of infertility

Sexuality-reproductive pattern
• may express concerns about resuming sexual intercourse after surgery

Value-belief pattern
• may have delayed seeking medical attention if perimenopausal (because irregular menses are normal during early menopause)

PHYSICAL FINDINGS
Gastrointestinal
• lower abdominal distention (with ovarian cancer)
• abdominal discomfort (with uterine myoma)
• adnexal mass (with ovarian cancer)

Genitourinary
• leukorrhea (with infection)
• vaginal bleeding (with uterine myoma)

Musculoskeletal
• leg edema (less common)

DIAGNOSTIC STUDIES
• hemoglobin level — may reveal decreased hemoglobin concentration, indicating anemia
• hematocrit — may reveal a decrease in volume percentage of red blood cells in whole blood, indicating blood loss

• white blood cell (WBC) count — may be elevated because of severe pelvic infection
• D&C (cervical dilatation and fractional curettage) and four-quadrant endometrial biopsy — provides endometrial tissue for a histopathologic study, which may reveal endometrial cancer
• wedge biopsy or conization biopsy of the cervix (removal of tissue for microscopic examination) — may reveal cervical cancer
• Pap smear (removal of exfoliated cervical cells) — may reveal cellular dysplasia
• colposcopy (visualization of the cervix with a colposcope) — may identify abnormal cell growth
• Schiller's test (staining of the cervix with iodine) — identifies abnormal cells
• ultrasound or computed tomography scan — may reveal size and location of mass

POTENTIAL COMPLICATIONS
• hemorrhagic shock
• peritonitis
• emboli
• pneumonia
• perforated bladder
• ligation of ureter
• wound infection
• atelectasis
• thrombophlebitis
• urine retention
• urinary tract infection

Collaborative problem: *High risk for thromboembolic and hemorrhagic complications related to immobility, venous stasis, pelvic congestion, or possible predisposing factors*

NURSING PRIORITY: Prevent or promptly treat thromboembolic and hemorrhagic complications.

Interventions

1. Monitor for signs of bleeding. Check vital signs and the surgical site according to standard postoperative protocol (see the "Surgical Intervention" plan, page 81, for details), and report tachycardia, dropping blood pressure, increasing drainage, restlessness, pallor, diaphoresis, or any other sign of hemorrhage immediately. Institute fluid replacement therapy, as ordered.

2. Institute measures to prevent and assess for thromboembolic phenomena: help the patient change position frequently, avoid using the knee gatch, tell the patient to avoid prolonged sitting, apply antiembolic hose, and assist the patient with range-of-motion exercises. See the "Surgical Intervention" and "Thrombophlebitis" plans, pages 81 and 361 respectively, for further details.

Rationales

1. The proximity of the surgical site to large vessels may increase the risk of significant postoperative bleeding. Additionally, a patient with a presurgical diagnosis of cancer may have clotting factor abnormalities that increase the risk of hemorrhage. Untreated, such bleeding rapidly progresses to hypovolemic shock; death may result. The "Surgical Intervention" plan provides further details about standard postoperative monitoring.

2. The postoperative patient is always at increased risk for thromboembolic complications because of circulatory disruption, immobility, and edema. The posthysterectomy patient may be at additional risk because of pelvic congestion. The "Surgical Intervention" and "Thrombophlebitis" plans contain further details regarding this potential postoperative problem.

3. Before discharge, instruct the patient to promptly report any bleeding and to avoid heavy lifting, prolonged sitting, and wearing constrictive clothes.

3. Postoperative hemorrhage may occur as late as 14 days after surgery. Avoiding activities that put stress on the operative site or cause venous stasis or pelvic congestion helps minimize the risk of bleeding or thromboembolic phenomena after discharge.

4. Additional individualized interventions: _____

4. Rationales: _____

Target outcome criteria
Throughout the hospital stay, the patient will:
• show no significant postoperative bleeding
• show no signs or symptoms of thromboembolic complications.

Nursing diagnosis: *High risk for postoperative infection related to abdominal incision, urinary tract proximity, contamination of peritoneal cavity, hypoventilation, anesthesia, or preoperative infection*

NURSING PRIORITY: Prevent or promptly detect and treat infection.

Interventions

1. Monitor for signs and symptoms of peritonitis, such as a significant increase in abdominal pain or a change in pain quality, abdominal rigidity or tenderness, nausea and vomiting, absent bowel sounds, or tachycardia. Report abnormal findings to the doctor immediately.

2. Implement standard postoperative nursing measures to prevent or detect other infections:

• atelectasis and pneumonia

• urinary tract infection (UTI)

• incisional infection.

See the "Surgical Intervention" plan, page 81, for further details.

3. Before discharge, teach the patient about signs and symptoms indicating infection, such as cough or respiratory congestion; urinary pain or burning, or cloudy urine; or redness, swelling, or purulent wound drainage. Emphasize the importance of promptly reporting such findings to the doctor.

4. Additional individualized interventions: _____

Rationales

1. The uterus is a peritoneal organ, so tissue oozing after its removal drains into the peritoneal cavity. Significant contamination from tissue, bleeding, or infection may result in potentially life-threatening peritonitis if not promptly treated.

2. The hysterectomy patient may be at increased risk for infection compared to other surgical patients because of the surgery site and the predisposing factors that may be involved.

• Ciliary depression from anesthesia, decreased mobility, and hypoventilation from abdominal incision pain contribute to stasis of pulmonary secretions, thus increasing the risk of infection.

• The urinary tract's proximity to the surgical area makes it prone to surgical trauma, edema, and resultant urine retention, which may predispose the patient to infection.

• Wound infection can be a complication of any surgery, but if the hysterectomy is performed because of cancer, the patient's immune response may be impaired, further increasing the risk.

Nursing measures related to these problems are standard postoperative interventions.

3. Prompt detection facilitates early treatment.

4. Rationales: _____

Target outcome criteria
Throughout the postoperative period, the patient will:
• show no signs of peritonitis
• perform pulmonary hygiene measures regularly
• show no signs of UTI
• have normal wound healing without evidence of infection.

Nursing diagnosis: *High risk for urine retention related to decreased bladder and urethral muscle tone from anesthesia and mechanical trauma*

NURSING PRIORITY: Promote optimal urinary elimination.

Interventions

1. Monitor for signs of urine retention after catheter removal, such as small, frequent voidings; bladder distention; intake greater than output; or restless behavior.

2. Implement measures to deal with retention, if it occurs. Encourage voiding. Obtain an order for catheterization if no voiding occurs within 8 hours after surgery. See the "Surgical Intervention" plan, page 81, for details.

3. Additional individualized interventions: _____

Rationales

1. Small, frequent voidings (less than 100 ml) may indicate urine retention, possibly related to edema, decreased muscle tone, or nerve damage to the bladder or urethra during surgery. Urine retention appears most commonly during the first 24 hours after surgery or catheter removal.

2. The "Surgical Intervention" plan contains specific information about this common postoperative problem.

3. Rationales: _____

Target outcome criteria
Within 8 hours after catheter removal, the patient will:
• void at least once
• produce adequate output (at least 100 ml per voiding)
• evidence clear, yellow urine.

Nursing diagnosis: *Pain related to abdominal incision and distention*

NURSING PRIORITY: Minimize and relieve abdominal pain.

Interventions

1. Implement measures for pain control. See the "Pain" and "Surgical Intervention" plans, pages 69 and 81 respectively.

2. Offer application of heat to the abdomen 48 hours after surgery, as ordered.

3. Additional individualized interventions: _____

Rationales

1. These plans contain measures applicable to any patient in pain.

2. Heat increases the elasticity of collagen tissue; lessens pain; relieves muscle spasms; helps resolve inflammatory infiltration, edema, and exudates; and increases blood flow. Heat applied less than 48 hours after surgery may cause undesirable edema.

3. Rationales: _____

Target outcome criteria
Within 1 hour of pain onset, the patient will verbalize reduction or relief of abdominal pain.

Within 3 days after surgery, the patient will:
• need analgesics less frequently or in lower doses
• pass flatus.

Nursing diagnosis: *High risk for body-image disturbance related to changes in body appearance and function as a result of surgery*

NURSING PRIORITY: Assist the patient in recognizing and accepting possible alteration in body appearance and function.

Interventions	Rationales
1. Assess the patient's level of understanding regarding hysterectomy and the recovery period.	1. Evaluating the patient's level of understanding allows the caregiver to individualize patient teaching according to the patient's preexisting knowledge base.
2. Acknowledge the patient's feelings of loss and dependency and fears of complications. Provide reassurance that these concerns are normal.	2. Loss of the uterus commonly triggers grief over lost fertility in young women and concerns about femininity. Acknowledgment validates the patient's feelings and encourages communication to alleviate fears and anxieties.
3. Provide opportunities, every shift, for the patient to discuss concerns about symptoms associated with recovery. Encourage discussion of possible fatigue, wound problems, discomfort, urinary problems, and weight gain. Clarify misconceptions of such posthysterectomy myths as growing fat and flabby, developing facial hair, becoming wrinkled or masculine in appearance, or becoming depressed and nervous.	3. Frequent, short teaching sessions enhance learning through repetition and by preventing information overload. Factual discussion prepares the patient to accept common symptoms. Such information does *not* act as a self-fulfilling prophecy. Clarifying misconceptions and myths reduces fears and anxiety during the recovery period.
4. Encourage the patient to discuss plans for recovery at home.	4. Such discussion allows the patient to make plans incorporating appropriate limitations in physical activities. It also demonstrates the patient's acceptance and understanding of physical abilities.
5. Additional individualized interventions: _____	5. Rationales: _____

Target outcome criteria
By the time of discharge, the patient will:
• verbalize understanding of body changes
• verbalize acceptance of possible alterations in body appearance and function.

Nursing diagnosis: *High risk for sexual dysfunction: decreased libido or dyspareunia related to fatigue, pain, grieving, altered body image, decreased estrogen levels, loss of vaginal sensations, sexual activity restrictions, or concerns about acceptance by spouse or partner*

NURSING PRIORITY: Facilitate healthy coping with sexual alterations.

Interventions	Rationales
1. Encourage the patient to explore perceptions of how surgery will affect sexual function. Listen sensitively.	1. Identifying current perceptions is the first step in coping with concerns. Sensitive listening allows the caregiver to identify appropriate and inappropriate perceptions.

2. Discuss the potential impact of surgery on sexuality by explaining:
• the predictability of temporarily decreased libido

2. Providing factual information clarifies misconceptions and reduces fears of sexual loss.
• Abdominal hysterectomy is major surgery that can have profound emotional implications. Fatigue, pain, and grieving may require so much coping energy that little remains for dealing with sexuality. The patient may need gentle "permission" to allow time to recover.

• the temporary nature of loss of vaginal sensations and of activity restrictions (sexual intercourse is discouraged for 4 to 6 weeks, then may be resumed gradually); also explain that return to full function is likely in approximately 4 months

• Vaginal sensory loss from surgical trauma resolves typically over a period of weeks to months. Activity restrictions allow time for tissues to heal.

• the rationale for avoiding douching during the recovery.

• Douching may increase the risk of infection or bleeding.

3. Explain that decreased libido and vaginal dryness may result from hormonal loss and that hormonal replacements are available.

3. The patient may not recognize that changes in sexual feelings and function can have a physiologic basis.

4. Suggest ways to ease sexual adjustment during the immediate postoperative period, such as holding hands, kissing, massage, and other methods of expressing love and sexuality.

4. Continued physical affection provides reassurance that a spouse's or partner's sexual interest continues after the hysterectomy.

5. Provide information and discuss options for conserving the patient's energy and preventing discomfort during return to sexual functioning, such as using a vaginal lubricant, scheduling sex for periods of peak energy, and avoiding positions that place pressure on the incision.

5. Sexual activity during the recovery period may be modified temporarily, but return to full sexual function is expected.

6. Encourage the patient and spouse or partner, if present, to share concerns and feelings with each other.

6. Mutual loving support is a positive factor in the couple's adjustment to sexual alterations.

7. Additional individualized interventions: _____

7. Rationales: _____

Target outcome criterion
By the time of discharge, the patient will verbalize strategies to manage temporary alteration in sexual functioning.

Discharge planning
NURSING DISCHARGE CRITERIA
Upon the patient's discharge, documentation shows evidence of:
• stable vital signs
• hemoglobin level and WBC count within normal parameters
• absence of cardiovascular and pulmonary complications
• bowel function same as before surgery
• absence of dysuria, hematuria, pyuria, burning, frequency, or urgency
• absence of fever

• absence of signs and symptoms of infection
• ability to control pain using oral medications
• ability to ambulate and perform activities of daily living (ADLs) same as before surgery
• healing surgical incision without redness, inflammation, or drainage
• ability to perform wound care independently or with minimal assistance
• ability to tolerate adequate nutritional intake
• adequate home support, or referral to home care if indicated by inadequate home support system or inability to perform ADLs and wound care.

PATIENT-FAMILY TEACHING CHECKLIST
Document evidence that the patient and family demonstrate an understanding of:
___ implications of total abdominal hysterectomy
___ all discharge medications' purpose, dosage, administration schedule, and adverse effects requiring medical attention
___ incision care (aseptic technique, dressing changes, irrigations, cleansing procedures, handwashing technique, and proper disposal of soiled dressings)
___ signs and symptoms of possible infection
___ dietary requirements and restrictions, if any
___ activity and exercise restrictions
___ date, time, and location of follow-up appointment
___ how to contact the doctor.

DOCUMENTATION CHECKLIST
Using outcome criteria as a guide, document:
___ clinical status on admission
___ postoperative clinical assessment
___ significant changes in status
___ appearance of incision and wound drainage
___ I.V. line patency and condition of site
___ assessment of pain and relief measures
___ nutritional intake
___ fluid intake and output
___ patient-family teaching
___ discharge planning.

ASSOCIATED PLANS OF CARE
Grieving
Ineffective Individual Coping
Knowledge Deficit
Pain
Surgical Intervention
Thrombophlebitis

References
Ames, S., and Kniesl, C. *Essentials of Adult Health Nursing.* Reading, Mass.: Addison-Wesley Publishing Co., 1988.

Brunner, L., and Suddarth, D. *Lippincott Manual of Nursing Practice,* 6th ed. Philadelphia: J.B. Lippincott Co., 1991.

Carpenito, L. *Nursing Diagnosis: Application to Clinical Practice,* 4th ed. Philadelphia: J.B. Lippincott Co., 1991.

Cohen, S., et al. "Another Look at Psychologic Complications of Hysterectomy," *Image* 21(1):51-53, Spring 1989.

Dulaney, P., et al. "A Comprehensive Education and Support Program for Women Experiencing Hysterectomies," *Journal of Obstetric Gynecologic and Neonatal Nursing,* 19(4):319-25, July-August 1990.

Gordon, M. *Manual of Nursing Diagnosis (1986-1987),* 2nd ed. New York: McGraw-Hill Book Co., 1987.

McNally, J., et al. *Guidelines for Cancer Nursing Practice,* 2nd ed. Philadelphia: W.B. Saunders Co., 1991.

Snyder, M. *Independent Nursing Interventions.* New York: John Wiley & Sons, 1985.

REPRODUCTIVE DISORDERS

REPRODUCTIVE DISORDERS
Mastectomy

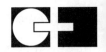

DRG information

DRG 257 Total Mastectomy for Malignancy with Complication or Comorbidity (CC).
Mean LOS = 5.0 days
Principal diagnoses include:
- carcinoma in situ, breast
- neoplasm, breast, malignant, secondary
- neoplasm, breast, uncertain behavior
- neoplasm, female or male breast, malignant (primary)
- neoplasm, skin, malignant, secondary

DRG 258 Total Mastectomy for Malignancy. Without CC.
Mean LOS = 4.0 days

DRG 259 Subtotal Mastectomy for Malignancy. With CC.
Mean LOS = 4.4 days

DRG 260 Subtotal Mastectomy for Malignancy. Without CC.
Mean LOS = 2.5 days

Introduction
DEFINITION AND TIME FOCUS

Mastectomy is the surgical removal of mammary tissue and, in some cases, the pectoral muscles. Although usually used to treat breast cancer, subcutaneous mastectomy (with preservation of chest muscles, skin, nipple, and areola) may be appropriate in male gynecomastia and severe fibrocystic breast disease requiring multiple biopsies. Subcutaneous mastectomy may also be performed to prevent breast cancer in women at increased risk. Mastectomy commonly is followed by chemotherapy or radiation therapy. However, if the tumor is large or the cancer is advanced (with skin or chest wall involvement), such treatments may be administered before surgery.

Breast tissue is affected by several cancers, including carcinoma of the secreting glands (ductal carcinoma), carcinoma of the glandular epithelium (breast adenomas), breast sarcomas, and lymphomas. Infiltrating intraductal carcinoma accounts for 80% of all breast cancers; it has a poor prognosis. Breast cancer is responsible for 36% of all new cancer cases and 18% of all cancer deaths in women; the high mortality rate has not changed significantly in 50 years.

The mastectomy performed depends on tumor size, nodal involvement, and evidence of metastasis. The patient's age and desire for breast reconstruction is also considered. Procedures include:
- lumpectomy — a complete excision of the tumor (usually followed by local irradiation to destroy microscopic cancer cells)
- partial (segmental) mastectomy — removal of tumor and adjacent tissue, leaving nipple, areola, and remaining breast tissue intact
- total (simple) mastectomy — removal of all breast and mammary tissue; pectoral muscles remain intact
- subcutaneous mastectomy — a variation of simple mastectomy in which the skin, nipple, areola, and chest muscles are preserved in preparation for breast reconstruction
- modified radical mastectomy (Patey method) — removal of all breast tissue, overlying skin, nipple and areola, minor pectoral muscle, and samples of adjacent and axillary lymph nodes
- radical mastectomy (Halsted method) — removal of tissue as in the modified radical mastectomy plus removal of the major pectoral muscle (rarely performed in the United States).

This plan focuses on the care of the female breast cancer patient before and after mastectomy.

ETIOLOGY AND PRECIPITATING FACTORS

Although the exact cause of breast cancer is unknown, risk factors have been identified.
Factors associated with the greatest risk:
- age — only 15% of cases occur before age 40; the greatest percentage occur between ages 45 and 60
- personal history of previous breast cancer
- family history of breast cancer — risk is 3 to 5 times higher if mother, sister, or daughter had the disease
- hormones — peak incidence between ages 45 and 49 probably related to ovarian estrogen problems; between ages 65 and 69, probably related to adrenal estrogen problems

Factors associated with increased risk:
- history of breast cancer in a maternal or paternal grandmother or aunt
- personal history of endometrial, ovarian, or colon cancer
- history of fibrocystic breast disease
- nulliparity
- birth of first child after age 30
- early onset of menstruation and late menopause
- estrogen replacement therapy
- culture — at increased risk if white in the upper socioeconomic levels of a Western society
- obesity
- diet high in animal fats
- daily alcohol consumption
- exposure to ionizing radiation — radon or naturally occurring nuclear fallout; excessive medical or dental X-rays; previous radiation therapy or fluoroscopy examinations (1% increase in risk per rad)

Focused assessment guidelines
NURSING HISTORY (Functional health pattern findings)

Health perception – health management pattern
• may report a painless, firm to hard lump or nodule that has indistinct boundaries and is not easily movable; may be found anywhere in breast tissue or axilla but most commonly in the left breast, upper outer quadrants, or just below the nipple
• may delay seeking treatment after tumor discovery
• may report focal, constant pain unrelated to menstrual cycle (advanced disease)
• may report spontaneous discharge of bloody, clear, or milky secretions from nipple or nipple inversion, retraction, elevation, ulceration, or scaliness (advanced disease)

Nutrition-metabolic pattern
• may report weight loss, anorexia, early satiety, and taste alterations, such as reduced sensitivity to sweetness or decreased desire for beef, pork, chocolate, coffee, and tomatoes (related to cancer or protein-calorie malnutrition)
• may report nausea, vomiting, stomatitis, and mucositis (related to chemotherapy or radiation therapy)

Elimination pattern
• may report constipation (related to anorexia, depression, immobility, or narcotic administration)
• may report diarrhea (related to increased bacterial growth from decreased GI tract motility)

Activity-exercise pattern
• may report general malaise
• may express weariness, weakness, or lack of physical energy
• may exhibit physical and emotional withdrawal related to depression
• may complain of shoulder and arm immobility related to pain

Sleep-rest pattern
• may report insomnia from pain, anxiety, or fear of cancer or the unknown
• may express increased desire for sleep (withdrawal behavior)

Self-perception – self-concept pattern
• may report grief related to perceived or actual loss
• may express body-image disturbance related to impending loss of breast or lymphedema
• may express guilt, anger, hostility, or denial related to diagnosis
• may equate breast loss with loss of femininity, desirability, and maternal instincts
• if alopecia is present, may report self-concept problem related to hair loss

Role-relationship pattern
• may exhibit hostility toward health care providers as a result of anger over role loss or sense of injustice
• may withdraw from family and friends to avoid anticipated rejection
• may report inability to assume family or work roles

Sexuality-reproductive pattern
• may express concern over need for additional surgery (hysterectomy with oophorectomy or adrenalectomy) if the tumor is estrogen receptive
• may report concern over adverse effects of androgenic drugs, including excessive facial hair (hirsutism), male pattern baldness, deepening voice, or increased libido

Coping – stress tolerance pattern
• anxiety, fear, restlessness, and depression related to unknown extent of tumor and resulting prognosis
• may express need for counseling
• may exhibit dependency
• may demonstrate extreme independence related to fears of becoming dependent or a burden to others
• may have financial, child care, and job concerns, especially if a single parent
• may demonstrate depression and despondency

Value-belief pattern
• may be socially conditioned to believe that personal worth and value are measured by the size and shape of breasts
• may assume a fatalistic attitude, equating cancer with death
• may perceive disease as punishment for past actions or indiscretions or fear passing cancer to the next generation
• may believe that external factors control personal life
• may feel forsaken by source of spiritual strength

PHYSICAL FINDINGS
Integumentary
• painless tumor, mass, lesion, thickening, or unusual growth in breast tissue
• palpable medial, supraclavicular, cervical or axillary nodes; isolated skin nodules; solitary, unilateral lesions; purplish color; heat and redness; ulcerations with secondary infection; or peau d'orange (skin of the orange) appearance resulting from lymphatic invasion and edema (advanced disease)
• alopecia (from chemotherapy)
• scalded skin syndrome (a debilitating condition in the immunosuppressed patient in which a *Staphylococcus aureus* infection produces epidermolytic toxins)

Hematologic
• hypercalcemia
• thromboembolic infarction related to hypercoagulability from cancer and tumor lysis

Cardiovascular
• hypertension related to effect of hypercalcemia on smooth muscle
• bradycardia or premature ventricular contractions caused by digitalis toxicity from increased calcium level
• compensatory tachycardia with decreasing blood pressure
• distended neck veins
• peripheral edema

Neurologic
• confusion, restlessness, or disorientation (resulting from serum calcium level above 15 mg/dl)
• muscle weakness and proximal myopathy
• diminished deep tendon reflexes

Renal
• polyuria or renal calculi, if hypercalcemia is present

Gastrointestinal
• polydipsia from polyuria
• nausea, vomiting, and anorexia as a result of hypercalcemia, chemotherapy, or radiation therapy

Musculoskeletal
• pathological fractures with bony metastases

DIAGNOSTIC STUDIES
• hemoglobin and hematocrit values — if low, may be related to anemia or blood loss during surgery; before surgery, the patient should donate 2 to 3 units of blood to maintain postoperative hemoglobin and hematocrit values and to aid healing
• serum calcium level — level above 11 mg/dl indicates hypercalcemia, a common complication of cancer
• serum phosphate level — hypophosphatemia is commonly associated with hypercalcemia
• platelet counts, prothrombin time (PT), and partial thromboplastin time (PTT) — a depressed platelet count, PT, and PTT may indicate disseminated intravascular coagulation (DIC)
• carcinoembryonic antigen titer — increases 75% with metastatic disease
• human chorionic gonadotropin — presence in blood or urine of nonpregnant females indicates cancer; declining amounts indicate treatment effectiveness
• serum ferritin level — may be low, indicating anemia
• serum albumin level — may be low from fluid shifting to interstitial spaces
• serum alkaline phosphatase level — if elevated, may indicate metastatic activity in bone and liver
• flow cytometry studies (cellular DNA content) — identify the 40% to 50% of patients at risk for recurrence

• estrogen receptor assay — estrogen-sensitive tumors are more susceptible to hormone therapy; non-estrogen-sensitive tumors have a low response rate to hormonal manipulation and a high recurrence rate
• mammography — may detect nonpalpable lesions (80% to 90% accurate)
• xeroradiography (a variation of mammography in which an aluminum plate with an electrically charged selenium layer is used in place of mammography film) — can detect breast cancers 1 to 2 years before the lesion is palpable
• thermography — measure heat emission (hot spots) from the breast tissue; cannot diagnose preclinical cancers
• magnetic resonance imaging — differentiates benign from malignant lesions; able to identify premalignant tissue changes; very accurate
• closed or open biopsy — differentiates between malignant and benign tumors
• liver and bone scans (indicated if liver chemistries are elevated) — may reveal metastatic disease
• electrocardiography (EGC) — T wave changes, bundle branch block, P wave notching, or other abnormalities may result from chemotherapy

POTENTIAL COMPLICATIONS
From breast cancer:
• hypercalcemia
• lymphedema
• hypophosphatemia
• thrombophlebitis
• DIC

From metastasis:
• pathological fractures
• obstructive uropathy
• metabolic acidosis (lactic acid increase)
• thrombocytopenia
• DIC
• superior vena cava syndrome
• spinal cord compression
• meningeal carcinomatosis
• intracerebral metastasis
• pleural effusion
• pulmonary embolism
• spontaneous pneumothorax

From metastasis or radiation therapy:
• inflammatory constrictive pericarditis
• pericardial effusion and tamponade
• scalded skin syndrome

From chemotherapy:
- alopecia
- anaphylaxis
- amyloidosis
- hyperuricemia
- gastrointestinal hemorrhage
- paralytic ileus
- cardiomyopathy or cardiotoxicity
- neurotoxicity

- pulmonary toxicity
- sepsis
- bone marrow suppression
- renal tubular necrosis

Other:
- reactive depression
- suicidal ideation

Collaborative problem: *Lymphedema related to interrupted lymph circulation from axillary node dissection during mastectomy*

NURSING PRIORITY: Prevent or minimize lymph stasis.

Interventions

1. Determine if the patient is to have a radical or modified radical mastectomy.

2. Before surgery, measure and record the circumference of each arm 2½″ (6 cm) above and below the elbow. After surgery, repeat measurement each morning until discharge.
- If lymphedema is noted, obtain an antiembolism sleeve for the patient to wear from morning to night (some patients wear the sleeve only at night).
- If lymphedema is severe, consult the doctor about using a mechanical pressure pump every 2 to 3 hours, as needed.

3. Immediately after mastectomy, position the affected arm on a pillow with the elbow higher than the shoulder, and the wrist and hand higher than the elbow.

4. Protect the affected arm from injury.

- Place the patient on an air mattress or sheepskin pad; pad the side rails.
- Keep the patient's fingernails short and smooth.
- Do not allow the patient to wear a name band, watch, or similar items on the affected arm.

5. Monitor laboratory data. Alert the doctor to deviations from these normal ranges:
- serum albumin level—3.5 to 5 g/dl
- serum sodium level—135 to 145 mEq/liter
- white blood cell (WBC) count—4,500 to 11,500 mm³.

6. Inspect the skin for color, translucency, temperature, or breakdown daily.

7. Check peripheral pulses daily.

8. Assess the arm for edema daily by pressing a thumb into the tissue for 5 to 10 seconds and observing for a depression after removing thumb.

Rationales

1. Radical mastectomy and modified radical mastectomy are the major cause of secondary lymphedema. During axillary node dissection, lymph channels are blocked or removed, shifting lymph fluid to soft tissue and decreasing lymphatic circulation.

2. Baseline measurements allow for later comparison. Lymphedema is present if the circumference of the affected arm is 1½″ (4 cm) larger than the unaffected arm.

- Compression of vein walls increases tissue perfusion and prevents venous stasis and edema.

- A mechanical pressure pump stimulates circulation more aggressively.

3. Positioning the arm above the apex of the heart facilitates lymph and blood movement by gravity flow.

4. Eliminating possible sources of trauma decreases the risk of infection.
- Padding cushions the affected arm.

- Short fingernails are less likely to damage the skin.
- Removing constricting bands prevents ischemia.

5. A low serum albumin level promotes lymphedema. A high serum sodium level promotes fluid retention. An abnormal WBC count may indicate infection (lymph node dissection increases the risk of infection).

6. Lymph stasis promotes infection and decreases arterial and venous circulation.

7. A pulse deficit may occur in the edematous arm.

8. Arm lymphedema usually presents as indurated (hardened) skin and, except in the early phase, is nonpitting.

9. Administer diuretics and salt-poor albumin, as indicated.

9. Diuretics promote fluid excretion. Albumin maintains osmotic pressure and prevents fluid shifting to the interstitial spaces of soft tissue.

10. Elevate and massage the affected arm daily with lotion, beginning at the wrist and advancing to the shoulder.

10. Elevation and compression increases lymph flow.

11. Administer pain medication 30 to 45 minutes before beginning exercises.

11. Pain relief promotes exercising.

12. Instruct the patient to elevate the affected arm for 30 to 45 minutes every 2 hours for 2 to 3 weeks after discharge, then 2 to 3 times daily for 6 weeks.

One day after surgery, have the patient perform the following exercises as often as the surgeon recommends:
• ball squeezing
• making a tight fist and then flexing and extending the fingers.

Two to three days after surgery, have the patient perform the following exercises as often as recommended:
• raising the affected arm to a 45-degree to 90-degree side angle
• walking the fingers up a wall to move the arm and shoulder
• bending over at the waist and letting the affected arm dangle, making small circular motions from the shoulder

At discharge, provide a copy of the American Cancer Society pamphlet "Reach to Recovery, Exercises After Mastectomy: Patient Guide."

Suggested post-discharge exercises include but are not limited to:
• rope pulley—Toss a rope over the top of a door. Sit with both legs bent at the knees and feet planted firmly on the floor. Hug both sides of the door with the knees. Holding the ends of the knotted rope, slowly raise the affected arm as far as comfortable by pulling down on the rope with the unaffected arm. Keeping the raised arm close to the head, reverse the motion; rest and repeat as tolerated.
• elbow pull—Stand with arms extended sideways at shoulder level. With bent elbows, clasp the fingers at the back of the neck and pull the elbows in toward each other until they touch. Relax, rest, and repeat as tolerated.

12. Exercise is essential to prevent muscle deformities, shortening, contractures, stiffness, and "frozen shoulder." Specific postoperative exercises depend on the extent of the surgery and whether skin grafting was necessary. Exercise regimens must have the surgeon's approval.

13. Refer the patient to Reach for Recovery or a similar support group.

13. Reach to Recovery volunteers have experienced breast cancer. Their "I've been there" approach aids the mastectomy patient's rehabilitation. They encourage the patient to use the affected arm and shoulder, and can facilitate psychological and emotional adaptation to the diagnosis of cancer, loss of a breast, and changes in body image and interpersonal relationships.

14. Teach the patient and family the signs and symptoms of lymphedema and when it is most likely to occur. Advise the patient to seek medical care if any of the following occur in the affected arm:
• pain
• tingling or tightness
• loss of sensation
• increased circumference
• muscle weakness.

14. The knowledgeable patient is more likely to obtain early treatment. Acute lymphedema occurs 4 to 6 weeks after surgery, can be transient, and is usually self-limiting; chronic lymphedema may occur weeks, months, or years after surgery.

15. Teach the patient how to maintain lymphatic circulation in the affected arm and prevent infection and injury. Reinforce teaching with written instructions.
• Use padded mitts around the oven, grill, or fireplace. Limit skin exposure to the sun and use a strong sunscreen when outdoors.
• Carry purses, packages, luggage, and other heavy objects on the unaffected side.
• Stop smoking.
• Avoid clothes with elastic or tight sleeves. Never allow blood pressure to be taken on the affected arm.
• Do not allow injections to be given in or blood to be drawn from the affected arm.

16. Additional individualized interventions: _____

_____

15. Maintaining effective lymphatic circulation and preventing infection and injury require the patient's active participation.
• These measure prevent burns.

• Carrying heavy items with the affected arm creates pressure that can lead to lymph stasis.
• Smoking constricts vessels.
• Tight sleeves and constricting bands impede lymph flow.

• Such measures prevent irritation and injury.

16. Rationales: _____

_____

Target outcome criteria
By the time of discharge, the patient will:
• list signs and symptoms of lymphedema
• demonstrate exercises to promote lymph circulation and minimize postoperative lymphedema

• display circumference equal in both arms
• remain free from infection and injury
• demonstrate increased mobility from ROM exercises.

Nursing diagnosis: *Body-image disturbance related to loss of a body part*

NURSING PRIORITY: Assist patient to cope with the loss of a breast.

Interventions

1. Provide empathetic emotional support. Encourage the patient to express feelings. Listen actively, use therapeutic touch, and be available to sit with the patient as needed. Also refer to the "Grieving" plan, page 31.

2. Assess the patient's feelings about the mastectomy.

3. Monitor the patient's comments about and willingness to look at and touch the incision site. Be alert for mood swings, continued tearfulness, expressions of overwhelming sadness, or withdrawal from family or friends.

4. Counsel the spouse or partner to hold and touch the patient.

5. Encourage the patient to wear make-up (if appropriate), nightgowns, and soft, front-closing brassieres (if dressings do not interfere).

Rationales

1. The patient is experiencing a time of intense personal crisis, and grieving is a normal part of emotional adjustment. Empathetic emotional support can facilitate healthy grieving and crisis resolution. The diagnosis of cancer, hospitalization, and surgery all present losses the patient may need to grieve for. The "Grieving" plan contains interventions helpful for any patient experiencing grief.

2. Attitudes, values, and beliefs influence physical and psychological adjustment.

3. Comments and behaviors can help the nurse assess the patient's level of acceptance.

4. The patient with a recent mastectomy has altered tactile perception over the operative site and over part of the upper arm. Touching creates intimacy and affirms that she is loved and lovable.

5. Some women adjust to breast surgery immediately; others need weeks or months. Attention to appearance may be a sign of recovering self-worth. The nurse's affirmation of the patient's continued femininity may bolster a shaky self-concept.

6. Offer to refer the patient to a mastectomy support group, a member of the clergy, a social worker, or a psychiatric or oncology clinical nurse specialist.

6. Other patients and professionals can help the patient accept an altered body image and return to wellness. However, such referrals should supplement nursing interventions, not substitute for the nurse's caring and empathy.

The American Cancer Society offers services to patients and their families, including "I Can Cope," an 8-week group program on learning how to live with cancer, and "Can Surmount," a support group facilitated by trained patients with cancer. Other local support groups facilitated by professionals also are available. Information about these services is available at all local offices of the American Cancer Society as well as through community hospitals.

7. Assess the patient's suitability for reconstructive surgery.

7. Contraindications to reconstructive breast surgery include inflammatory carcinomas, high dose radiation therapy, extensive systemic metastases, and unrealistic attitudes and expectations regarding the surgery's outcome.

8. If reconstruction is an option, support the patient in the decision making process.
• Encourage the patient to share thoughts and feelings related to breast reconstruction.
• Teach the patient about reconstruction procedures, the need for skin or muscle flap grafting, and the possibility of nipple and areolar reconstruction. Help the patient obtain information about the procedure's cost and the likelihood of insurance coverage. If possible, provide a copy of the American Cancer Society pamphlet "Breast Reconstruction Following Mastectomy from Cancer."
• Validate the patient's decision even if you believe it would not be appropriate for you.

8. The nurse can help the patient make an informed decision.
• Some patients immediately accept reconstruction, while others may believe a desire for reconstruction is vain.
• Reconstruction is an accepted option in the management of breast cancer. The patient should have the opportunity to talk and read about breast reconstruction.

• Clarifying and validating feelings conveys respect for the patient's values and beliefs.

9. If reconstruction is not an option or will be delayed, provide information about external breast prostheses when the patient asks about them.

9. Queries indicate emotional readiness to focus on this area. A breast prosthesis may boost the patient's self-esteem by providing a natural-appearing substitute for the lost breast.

10. After reconstruction, provide appropriate interventions to preserve the reconstructed breast.

• Assess the incision site. Note its appearance and the presence of any pain or tenderness to touch. Monitor WBC counts as ordered. If the suture line does not appear to be healing by primary intention, request a WBC count from the surgeon. Assess surgical drains daily.

• Be alert to pallor, cyanosis, coolness, or delayed capillary refill at the surgical site. If these signs occur, notify the doctor promptly. Protect the reconstructed breast from pressure. Assess the tightness of the dressing.

• Elevate the head of the bed to Fowler's or semi-Fowler's position.

• Monitor the patient's verbal comments and willingness to look at and touch the reconstructed breast.

• Provide psychological support. Encourage the patient to wear make-up (if appropriate), nightgowns, and soft, front-closing brassieres (if dressings do not interfere).

10. Loss of the reconstructed breast will provide a further blow to the patient's body image and jeopardize emotional recovery.

• Drainage, a darkening suture line, pain and tenderness to touch, and a WBC count over $11,000/mm^3$ indicate infection. Infection prolongs healing and promotes dependency on family members and health care professionals, which may result in decreased self-esteem and depression.

• These signs may indicate inadequate blood flow. If circulation is not restored, graft or implant rejection or flap necrosis may occur. Preventing pressure at the site promotes adequate blood flow.

• Elevating the head of the bed reduces edema and stress on the reconstructed breast.

• Comments and behaviors can help the nurse evaluate the patient's acceptance of the reconstructed breast.

• Some women adjust to a reconstructed breast immediately; others need weeks or months. Attention to appearance may be a sign of recovering self-worth. The nurse's affirmation of the patient's continued femininity may bolster a shaky self-concept.

• Counsel the patient's spouse or partner about the importance of expressing satisfaction with the reconstructed breast.

• Instruct the patient to begin daily, vigorous massage of the implant or graft 6 weeks after surgery.

• Educate the patient about the value of sharing information about reconstruction with other women.

• The spouse's or partner's attitude plays a powerful role in the patient's acceptance of the reconstructed breast.

• Massage helps prevent capsular contraction, maintain softness of the breast, and permit a more natural contour.

• If women are aware that reconstruction is an option, they may seek help when a lump or abnormality is first discovered, rather than delaying diagnosis and treatment for fear of disfigurement.

11. Encourage the patient to talk about sexual concerns. Suggestions to initiate conversation may include, "Tell me about any sexual concerns you might have as a result of your mastectomy." Or, "Some women have anxiety and fears about their sexual relationships following a mastectomy. Is there something you would like to discuss, or questions I might help you with? Or, "Some women have anxiety about their sexual relationships following this surgery. I will be happy to talk with you now, or later if you prefer. Here is my card with my phone number if you need to get in touch with me at another time."

11. Body image is intimately related to sexuality. Breast cancer patients require continuing education, support, and encouragement in dealing with the emotional trauma and sexual sequelae of treatment. Many patients will desire information but will not initiate the discussion with a physician or nurse. Such information is essential to emotional healing.

12. Maintain a hopeful and positive outlook when discussing sexuality. Clarify any misconceptions. Encourage the patient to talk with members of mastectomy support groups.

12. Maintaining a positive outlook conveys hope. Clarifying misconceptions (such as a mastectomy destroying sexual attractiveness) can gently challenge beliefs that otherwise might become self-fulfilling prophecies. Women who have "been there" may provide more credible reassurance than a health professional.

13. A few weeks after discharge, make a home call. Inquire about visits the patient has made away from home, and the resumption of social activities as well as physiological status. Reintroduce the subject of sexuality and ask about concerns the woman might have encountered since surgery.

13. Some patients remain at home to avoid their friends, and hesitate to resume social activities. Reasons for withdrawal may include fear of rejection by others. Fear of rejection from a spouse or significant other commonly manifests in withdrawal. Home calls provide an excellent opportunity for the nurse to ask questions about sex or sexuality and allow the patient to share any fears, concerns, or questions that might have arisen since discharge.

14. Additional individualized interventions: _____

14. Rationales: _____

_____

_____

Target outcome criteria
According to individual readiness, the patient will:
• be able to touch and look at the wound
• participate in decision making
• verbalize loss and work through the grief of an altered body image
• seek out community resources as necessary
• be able to talk about changes that impact sexuality with her partner

• if choosing reconstruction, experience no complications
• agree to share information about reconstruction with at least two friends or a group of women, if the patient desires.

Collaborative problem: *High risk for hypercalcemia related to abnormal calcium transport or skeletal metastases*

NURSING PRIORITY: Maintain normal serum calcium levels and prevent complications of hypercalcemia.

Interventions

1. Monitor for hypercalcemia (serum calcium level greater than 11 mg/dl). Early signs include nausea, vomiting, and anorexia.

2. Monitor blood pressure and heart rate every 2 hours.

3. Auscultate heart sounds and rhythms in four sites and record daily.

4. Assess ECG changes. Observe for prolonged PR intervals, lengthening QT intervals, lengthening and widening T waves, atrioventricular block, and asystole.

5. If the patient is receiving a digitalis glycoside, measure the apical pulse rate before administering; if below 60 beats/minute, withhold the drug and check with the doctor.

6. Assess the patient's level of consciousness every 4 to 8 hours. Assess for confusion, restlessness, disorientation, drowsiness, profound weakness, and personality changes. Orient to person, time, and place. Elevate and pad side rails, as indicated.

7. Document fluid intake and output every 2 hours to monitor fluid balance. Obtain baseline weight on admission. Weigh daily thereafter.

8. Assess amount and color of urine, and note specific gravity (normal range is 1.010 to 1.035).

9. Assess for flank pain and strain all urine for calculi.

10. Anticipate I.V. administration of saline, 250 to 300 ml/hour, and a loop diuretic such as furosemide (Lasix), 80 to 100 mg every 2 hours, as tolerated.

11. Anticipate administration of calcitonin (Calcimar), glucocorticoids, phosphates, plicamycin (Mithracin), or gallium nitrate (Ganite). Be alert to adverse reactions, which may include headache, anorexia, nausea and vomiting, hepatic and renal impairment, and hemorrhage from thrombocytopenia.

12. Apply an ice collar to the patient's neck if nauseated. Administer an antiemetic, if appropriate.

Rationales

1. Hypercalcemia, a metabolic complication, develops in 10% to 20% of all cancer patients; in breast cancer with metastasis, the incidence increases to 50%. Although the majority of patients with hypercalcemia have skeletal metastases, not all patients with metastases develop hypercalcemia.

2. Increased calcium levels can affect smooth muscle, causing hypertension.

3. Hypercalcemia may cause arrhythmias or extra heart sounds.

4. Changes in PR or QT intervals or T wave configuration indicate a serum calcium level of 16 mg/dl or more. Atrioventricular block and asystole may occur at serum calcium levels of 18 mg/dl.

5. Increased serum calcium levels enhance the action of digitalis drugs, possibly causing toxicity; the doctor may withhold the drug to prevent bradycardia, premature ventricular contractions, or paroxysmal atrial tachycardia.

6. If serum calcium levels are 15 mg/dl or more, central nervous system depression may alter mental status or thought processes, creating a risk for injury.

7. Effects of hypercalcemia include defective water conservation, leading to dehydration, sodium excretion, potassium wasting, and severe weight loss.

8. Hypercalcemia may interfere with antidiuretic hormone, limiting the kidney's ability to concentrate urine and resulting in polyuria.

9. Hypercalcemia may cause renal calculi to form.

10. Saline and furosemide diuresis usually causes calcium excretion, decreasing the serum calcium level.

11. These drugs may increase urinary calcium excretion and decrease intestinal calcium absorption by inhibiting bone resorption or inhibiting tumor production of prostaglandins.

12. Both hypercalcemia and the drugs used to treat it can cause nausea and vomiting through vagal nerve stimulation in the upper GI tract or through activation of the brain's chemoreceptor trigger zone. Vagal nerve stimulation produces vasodilation; an ice collar causes vasoconstriction, providing temporary relief from nausea. Antiemetics inhibit stimulation of the chemoreceptor trigger zone.

13. Provide mouth care every 4 hours, after vomiting, and before meals. Clean the teeth daily with baking soda and hydrogen peroxide or a similar solution.

13. Oral antiseptics refresh the mouth. Baking soda and hydrogen peroxide neutralize mouth acids.

14. Auscultate bowel sounds daily in four quadrants and record changes in pitch and frequency. Be alert to high pitched, diminished, or absent sounds. Increase fluid intake to 4 8-oz glasses (1,000 ml) every 8 hours, as tolerated.

14. Hypercalcemia depresses smooth muscle contractility, delays gastric emptying, and decreases intestinal motility, leading to constipation, obstipation, and paralytic ileus. Dehydration exacerbates obstipation and paralytic ileus.

15. Teach the patient and family signs and symptoms of hypercalcemia and appropriate interventions.

15. Hypercalcemia may recur.

16. If hypercalcemia does not respond to interventions, alert the family and help them prepare for the patient's death.

16. Uncontrollable hypercalcemia is a sign of impending death.

17. Additional individualized interventions: _____

17. Rationales: _____

Target outcome criteria
Within 48 hours, Ca^{++} levels of 12 mg/dl or more will decrease 2 to 4 mg/dl.

By the time of discharge, the patient with controllable hypercalcemia and family will verbalize signs and symptoms of blood calcium increase and appropriate interventions.

Discharge planning
NURSING DISCHARGE CRITERIA
Upon the patient's discharge, documentation shows evidence of:
• hemoglobin and hematocrit values within normal limits
• serum calcium and serum phosphate levels within normal limits
• platelet count, PT, and PTT within normal limits
• ferritin levels within normal limits
• serum albumin and serum globulin ratio normal (1.5:1)
• normal total protein values
• absent or low serum levels of carcinoembryonic antigen
• absence of human chorionic gonadotropin in serum or urine
• absence of metabolic complications
• absence of cardiac arrhythmias, and neuromuscular, renal, and gastrointestinal complications
• absence of secondary lymphedema
• arms equal in circumference
• radial pulses equal bilaterally
• affected arm free from injury
• ability to perform ROM exercises
• absence of "frozen shoulder"
• support from family and spouse or partner
• referral to other health care professionals, if indicated.

PATIENT-FAMILY TEACHING CHECKLIST
Document evidence that the patient and family demonstrate an understanding of:
___ nature of cancer and implications
___ signs and symptoms of oncologic emergencies
___ importance of support for the patient's decision regarding reconstructive surgery
___ signs and symptoms of graft rejection
___ activity recommendations and limitations
___ community or professional resources and support groups
___ need for follow-up appointments
___ need for long-term emotional support as a result of cancer diagnosis.

DOCUMENTATION CHECKLIST
Using outcome criteria as a guide, document:
___ clinical status on admission
___ presence of adequate support systems
___ patient-family teaching
___ activity and exercise tolerance and recommendations
___ discharge planning.

ASSOCIATED PLANS OF CARE
Dying
Grieving
Ineffective Family Coping
Ineffective Individual Coping
Lung Cancer
Pain
Surgical Intervention

References

Ashwanden, P., Belcher, A., Mattson, E.A., Moskowitz, R., and Riese, N. *Oncology Nursing—Advances, Treatments, and Trends into the 21st Century.* Gaithersburg, Md.: Aspen Publishing, 1990.

Auguste, L., Clancy, P., Cree, B., and Knauer, C. "Breast Cancer Surgery," in *Standards of Oncology Nursing Practice.* Edited by Brown, M., Kiss, M., Outlaw, E., and Viamontes, C. New York: John Wiley & Sons, 1986.

Beare, P., and Myers, J. *Principles and Practice of Adult Health Nursing.* St. Louis: C.V. Mosby Co., 1990.

Boring, C., Squires, T., and Tong, T. "Cancer Statistics 1991," *Ca—A Cancer Journal for Clinicians* 41(1):19-36, January-February 1991.

Danforth, D., and Lippman, M. "Surgical Treatments of Breast Cancer," in *Diagnosis and Management of Breast Cancer.* Edited by Lippmann, M., Lichter, A., and Danforth, D. Philadelphia: W.B. Saunders Co., 1988.

Eriksson, J. *Oncologic Nursing—A Study and Learning Tool.* Springhouse, Pa: Springhouse Corporation, 1990.

Goodman, C., and Harte, N. "Breast Cancer," in *Cancer Nursing—Principles and Practice,* 2nd ed. Edited by Groenwald, S., Frogge, M., Goodman, M., and Yarbro, C. Boston: Jones and Bartlett, 1990.

Holland, J., and Rowland, J. *Handbook of Psychooncology.* New York: Oxford Press, 1989.

Kline, P. "Suicidal Ideation," in *Critical Care Nursing of the Client with Cancer.* Edited by Chernecky, C., and Ramsey, P. Norwalk, Conn.: Appleton & Lange, 1984.

Lewis, B. "Breast Cancer," in *Cecil-Textbook of Medicine,* 18th ed. Edited by Wyngaarden, J., and Smith, L. Philadelphia: W.B. Saunders Co., 1988.

Purtilo, R. *Health Professional and Patient Interaction,* 4th ed. Philadelphia: W.B. Saunders, 1990.

Redfield, C., and Molbo, D. "Management of Persons with Problems of the Breast," In *Medical-Surgical Nursing: Concepts and Clinical Practice,* 4th ed. Edited by Phipps, W., Long, B., Woods, N., and Cassmeyer, V. St. Louis: Mosby-Year Book Co., 1991.

Spross, J. "Edema," in *Decision Making in Oncology Nursing.* Edited by Baird, S. Philadelphia: B.C. Decker, Inc., 1988.

Weinrich, S., and Weinrich, M. "Cancer Knowledge among Elderly Individuals," in *Enhancing the Role of Cancer Nursing.* Edited by Ash, C., and Jenkins, J. New York: Raven Press, 1990.

Prostatectomy

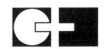

DRG information
DRG 334 Major Male Pelvic Procedure. With Complication or Comorbidity (CC).
Mean LOS = 9.4 days
DRG 335 Major Male Pelvic Procedure. Without CC.
Mean LOS = 7.9 days
DRG 336 Transurethral Prostatectomy. With CC.
Mean LOS = 5.3 days
DRG 337 Transurethral Prostatectomy. Without CC.
Mean LOS = 3.9 days

Introduction
DEFINITION AND TIME FOCUS
Prostatectomy is the surgical removal of the prostate, a gland (in males) located in line with the urethra and positioned between the bladder and rectum. There are three types of prostatectomies: a partial resection removes only enlarged tissue; a simple prostatectomy removes the prostate and its capsule; and a radical prostatectomy removes the prostate, its capsule, the seminal vesicles, and a portion of the bladder neck.

Four surgical approaches are used: transurethral, suprapubic, retropubic, and perineal (see *Surgical approaches to prostatectomy,* page 672). The surgery's extent and approach depends on the patient's general condition and the specific problem requiring treatment. The transurethral approach is suitable for a partial resection; the suprapubic for a simple prostatectomy; and the retropubic and the perineal for simple and radical prostatectomies.

Transurethral resection of the prostate (TURP), in which prostatic tissue is removed through the urethra, is performed most commonly. It is indicated for benign prostatic hypertrophy that can no longer be managed medically and for small cancerous lesions. Because this approach requires a lithotomy position, it is not suitable for the patient with a hip problem or prior surgery of the hip joint.

The suprapubic approach involves a lower abdominal suprapubic incision and then a bladder incision. It is indicated for prostatic obstruction and removal of bladder calculi or diverticula.

In the retropubic approach, the gland is entered directly through an abdominal incision, without an incision into the bladder. It is used to remove a gland too large for a TURP, to remove large cancerous lesions, and for the patient who cannot tolerate a lithotomy position.

With the perineal approach, an incision is made in the perineum, the area between the scrotum and anus. This approach is used for removal of a large gland when an abdominal approach is contraindicated, such as in an obese patient.

TURP usually has the shortest recovery period; the suprapubic approach, somewhat longer; and the retropubic and perineal approaches, the longest.

This plan focuses on preoperative and postoperative care for the patient undergoing prostatectomy.

ETIOLOGY AND PRECIPITATING FACTORS
• age — men aged 50 years and over usually experience some prostate enlargement
• benign prostatic hyperplasia — usually associated with hormonal changes of aging
• prostate cancer — unknown etiology, most common tumor is adenocarcinoma. Risk factors include:
— age (peak incidence averages at age 65)
— race (progresses faster in black men)
— marital status (lowest incidence in single men)
— occupation (increased incidence among workers employed in the rubber and cadmium industries)
— hormonal factors (altered androgen and estrogen metabolite levels may contribute)

Focused assessment guidelines
NURSING HISTORY (Functional health pattern findings)

Health perception — health management pattern
• may report preexisting cardiac or pulmonary disorders or diabetes
• may report preoperative urinary tract infection (UTI) and bladder outlet obstruction
• may report taking antibiotics for UTIs

Nutritional-metabolic pattern
• may report weight loss, nausea and vomiting, or anorexia (from impaired renal function because of obstruction or chronic UTI)

Elimination pattern
• may report urine retention, dysuria, frequency, hesitancy, nocturia, urgency, decreased stream, postvoid dribbling, urinary incontinence, or hematuria (rare)
• may report constipation or epigastric discomfort (from pressure of the bladder on the gastrointestinal tract)

Activity-exercise pattern
• may report decreased activity coinciding with pain
• may report fatigue and weakness from anorexia or nocturia, with associated sleep deprivation
• may report preexisting age-related cardiopulmonary disorders influencing exercise tolerance

SURGICAL APPROACHES TO PROSTATECTOMY

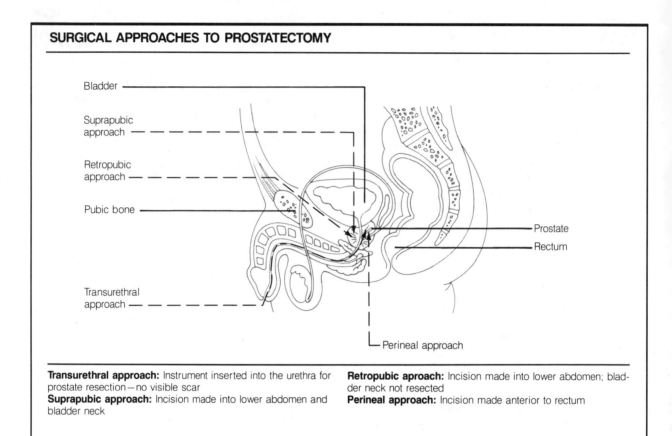

Bladder

Suprapubic approach

Retropubic approach

Pubic bone

Transurethral approach

Prostate

Rectum

Perineal approach

Transurethral approach: Instrument inserted into the urethra for prostate resection—no visible scar
Suprapubic approach: Incision made into lower abdomen and bladder neck

Retropubic aproach: Incision made into lower abdomen; bladder neck not resected
Perineal approach: Incision made anterior to rectum

Sleep-rest pattern
• may report sleep pattern disturbances from pain, nocturia, frequency, or urinary incontinence

Cognitive-perceptual pattern
• may report lack of knowledge about disease (benign prostatic hyperplasia or cancer) or surgical procedure and expected outcomes

Self-perception—self-concept pattern
• may express fears and anxieties about alterations in body image, retrograde ejaculation, or impotence from nerve transection or injury
• may express feelings of hopelessness, powerlessness, and lowered self-esteem associated with diagnosis of cancer

Role-relationship pattern
• may report disturbed role performance
• may express fear of social isolation associated with diagnosis of cancer
• may report experiences of family or friends who died from cancer or during surgery

Sexuality-reproductive pattern
• may report preexisting impotence as adverse effect of cardiac medications
• may discuss concerns about possible impotence
• spouse or sexual partner may express concerns about postoperative sexual performance

Coping—stress tolerance pattern
• may report fears and anxieties associated with diagnosis of cancer
• may appear depressed

Value-belief pattern
• may express disbelief (denial) about diagnosis of cancer
• may report increased reliance on spiritual support system as coping mechanism

PHYSICAL FINDINGS
Patients with localized prostatic cancer commonly have no symptoms; symptoms indicate advanced disease.

Genitourinary
- enlarged prostate on rectal examination
  - smooth, elastic, nonfixed gland suggests benign prostatic hyperplasia
  - hard, irregular, fixed nodule suggests cancer
- postvoid dribbling or incontinence
- urine retention
- hematuria (rare)

Cardiovascular
- peripheral edema (in renal failure or in hydroureteronephrosis from obstruction)

Pulmonary
- pulmonary edema (in renal failure or in hydroureteronephrosis from obstruction)

Musculoskeletal
- costovertebral angle tenderness (in renal failure)
- back pain or stiffness (with bony metastasis)

DIAGNOSTIC STUDIES
- white blood cell (WBC) count and sedimentation rate — increase with inflammation and infection*
- hemoglobin level, hematocrit, and platelet count — decrease with hemorrhage*
- prothrombin time (PT) and partial thromboplastin time (PTT) — increase with hemorrhage*
- blood typing and cross-matching — may be done in case transfusion is needed*
- acid phosphatase — increases in about 25% of patients with early prostatic cancer when total serum level is measured and in the majority of patients when specific enzymes are used
- prostate-specific antigen — increases in about 73% to 96% of patients with prostate cancer but may also be elevated in 55% to 80% of patients with benign prostatic hyperplasia; useful in monitoring patients for cancer metastasis after radical prostatectomy

- alkaline phosphatase level — increases when cancer metastasizes to bone
- blood urea nitrogen and creatinine levels — increase may indicate renal failure
- urinalysis — increase in WBCs suggests infection; increase in red blood cells indicates hematuria, which may delay surgery
- culture and sensitivity testing — defines microorganisms responsible for UTIs or other infections
- cystoscopy — evaluates degree of prostate gland fixation, especially when cancerous; evaluates bladder problems and allows direct assessment of obstruction
- prostate biopsy — provides differential diagnosis of cancer
- intravenous pyelogram — helps determine presence and severity of kidney obstruction
- chest X-ray — indicates lung status before surgery, may reveal lung metastasis
- electrocardiography — indicates preoperative cardiac status; used as baseline for comparison if changes occur
- bone scan — aids in detecting bony metastasis
- transrectal ultrasound — determines internal prostatic anatomy and its related pathology

POTENTIAL COMPLICATIONS
- hemorrhage
- hypovolemic or septic shock
- infection
- epididymitis
- rectal perforation during surgery
- pulmonary embolism
- atelectasis
- bowel incontinence with perineal prostatectomy (rare)

Collaborative problem: *High risk for hypovolemia related to prostatic or incisional bleeding after surgery†*

NURSING PRIORITY: Prevent or promptly detect internal or external bleeding.

Interventions

1. Monitor and document the amount of blood collecting on incisional dressings and in the urinary drainage system hourly for the first 12 to 24 hours after surgery, then every 4 hours. Typical drains and catheters include the following:
- for TURP, a urethral catheter
- for the suprapubic approach, a urethral catheter, a suprapubic tube, and an abdominal drain
- for the retropubic approach, a urethral catheter and an abdominal drain

Rationales

1. The amount of bleeding expected after surgery varies with the reason for and extent of the surgery. Heavy bleeding is expected for the first 24 hours after a TURP or a suprapubic or retropubic prostatectomy. Minimal bleeding is expected with the perineal approach.

   Blood loss from incisional drainage usually is minimal, while blood loss through the urinary catheter may range from minimal to life-threatening. Bright red blood indicates arterial bleeding; dark blood suggests venous bleeding.

---

*Preoperative values for these laboratory tests should be within normal limits.
†Although this and the following collaborative problems and nursing diagnoses apply to all types of prostatectomies, their relative importance varies with the specific surgical approach, as indicated in each problem.

• for the perineal approach, a urethral catheter and a perineal drain.
Observe the frequency of clots in the urine. Use universal precautions. Consult the surgeon concerning the amount of bleeding anticipated. Alert the surgeon if any of the following occur:
• bright red drainage
• persistent burgundy-colored drainage
• persistent clot formation.

Hemorrhage may occur with any surgical approach, but it is a particular problem with TURP. Venous bleeding during the early postoperative period is very common. If necessary, traction may be placed on the catheter for 6 to 8 hours.

Hemorrhage may occur with a suprapubic or perineal approach, but usually it is not a major problem. With the retropubic approach, the risk of hemorrhage usually is minimal because this approach affords better control of bleeding.

Blood volume loss may decrease cardiac output, arterial and venous blood pressure, and hemoglobin level, decreasing the blood's oxygen-carrying capacity. A blood volume loss of 20% or more can cause hypovolemic shock.

Expected removal times for urinary catheters are discussed later in this plan; abdominal drains are usually removed after 4 to 7 days (occasionally after 10 days with a radical perineal prostatectomy).

2. Evaluate and document pulse rate, blood pressure, respirations, skin color, and level of consciousness according to unit protocol—typically every 4 hours for 24 hours or until stable, then every 8 hours.

2. An increased pulse rate, a blood pressure 20 mm Hg below normal or 80 mm Hg or less, rapid and deep respirations, cold and clammy skin, pallor, and restlessness indicate shock.

3. Monitor hemoglobin level, hematocrit value, platelet count, and coagulation studies daily. Compare current values with preoperative values. Alert the doctor to abnormal values. Administer blood transfusions as ordered, using universal precautions.

3. A sudden decrease in hemoglobin level, hematocrit value, and platelet count or an increase in PT or PTT may indicate the need for a transfusion.

4. Consult the surgeon about applying traction to the catheter or preparing the patient for surgery if bleeding persists.

4. Applying traction pulls the catheter balloon against the bladder neck. The resulting pressure compresses bleeding vessels in the prostatic fossa. For prolonged or excessive bleeding, sutures or cauterization may be necessary.

5. Teach the patient to avoid straining during bowel movements. Avoid using rectal thermometers or tubes or giving enemas.

5. Straining to defecate or introducing objects into the rectum may cause bleeding, especially after the retropubic or perineal approach for radical prostatectomy.

6. Administer and document stool softeners and laxatives, as ordered. Use alternatives such as increased fiber, fluids, and prune juice in the diet. Monitor the frequency and consistency of bowel movements.

6. Preventing constipation is important to decrease the risk of bleeding or rectal tearing.

7. Teach the patient to avoid lifting heavy objects for 6 to 8 weeks after surgery to allow time for internal and external wound healing.

7. Undue strain on the abdominal and perineal muscles places stress on the bladder and prostate and may cause bleeding.

8. Additional individualized interventions: _____

8. Rationales: _____

Target outcome criteria
Within 24 hours after surgery, the patient will:
• show normal vital signs
• have normal laboratory values.

Within 3 days after surgery, the patient will:
• have regular bowel movements
• avoid straining the abdominal and perineal muscles.

Nursing diagnosis: *High risk for postoperative infection related to preoperative status or urinary catheter or abdominal drain placement*

NURSING PRIORITY: Prevent or promptly detect infection.

Interventions

1. Monitor and record vital signs according to unit protocol, typically every 4 hours for 24 hours or until stable, then every 8 hours. Notify the doctor of significant changes from the patient's baseline values.

2. Monitor the incision site daily for induration, erythema, and purulent or odorous drainage. Document all findings. Send drainage samples for culture and sensitivity testing, as ordered.

3. Monitor drains and catheters for patency, and irrigate as ordered, using universal precautions.

4. Provide and document meticulous urinary catheter care at least once daily. Send urine samples for culture and sensitivity testing, as ordered, using universal precautions.

5. Administer I.V. fluids, as ordered. Beginning on the first postoperative day, encourage oral fluid intake of 8 to 12 8-oz glasses (2,000 to 3,000 ml) daily (unless contraindicated) to maintain a urine output of at least 1,500 ml daily. Record fluid intake and output.

6. Encourage the patient to ambulate the day after surgery.

7. Administer and document prophylactic antibiotics, as ordered.

8. Additional individualized interventions: _____

Rationales

1. The risk of infection varies with the procedure used. The risk is high with the suprapubic approach, where a bladder incision can allow urine to leak into surrounding tissue. The presence of catheters or drains also increase the risk of infection. Sudden fever, chills, hypotension, and tachycardia are signs of septic shock, a particular risk after prostatectomy.

2. The skin is the first line of defense against infection. Testing drainage samples will identify the causative microorganism.

3. Catheter obstruction commonly occurs from blood clots at the tip of the indwelling urinary catheter. This may cause urine retention, stasis, and infection. Irrigation usually relieves obstruction.

4. Although questioned by some, most authorities believe that cleaning with soap and water is essential to prevent microbial growth. Analysis of urine samples will identify any microorganisms.

5. Adequate hydration promotes renal blood flow and flushes out bacteria in the urinary tract. The I.V. line is usually removed on the first postoperative day if the patient is tolerating oral fluids.

6. Immobility contributes to urinary stasis and creates a reservoir for microorganisms.

7. Antibiotics combat and control microbial growth. They are ordered prophylactically because of the high risk of infection with prostatectomy.

8. Rationales: _____

Target outcome criteria
Within 24 hours after surgery, the patient will:
• have no fever
• have no urinary clots
• ambulate.

Within 3 days after surgery, the patient will:
• present an incision free from inflammation, induration, bleeding, or purulent drainage
• have clear urine.

Nursing diagnosis: *Pain related to urethral stricture, catheter obstruction, bladder spasms, or surgical intervention*

NURSING PRIORITY: Relieve pain.

Interventions

1. See the "Pain" plan, page 69.

2. Observe for signs of bladder spasms, such as sharp intermittent pain, a sense of urgency, or urine around the catheter.

3. Irrigate, using universal precautions, and check the urinary catheter and tubing for kinks, blood clots, and mucus plugs, as needed.

4. Assess for incisional pain.

5. For severe or persistent pain, administer analgesics or antispasmodics, such as oxybutynin chloride (Ditropan). Administer medication at the pain's onset. Monitor vital signs before and after administering medication, and evaluate pain relief after 30 minutes.

6. Provide alternative pain relief measures and teach them to the patient. If appropriate, help the patient take a sitz bath and apply heat to the rectal area with a heat lamp after a perineal prostatectomy. Position the patient comfortably.

7. Additional individualized interventions: _____

Rationales

1. General interventions for pain management are included in the "Pain" plan. Measures specific to prostatectomy are covered below.

2. Bladder spasms occur when catheter placement or surgical manipulation irritate the bladder stretch receptors. Pain from bladder spasms can be severe in the transurethral and suprapubic approaches, in which the bladder is entered surgically. Spasm-induced pain is minimal with the retropubic and perineal approaches, because they do not involve a bladder incision.

3. Urine retention from catheter obstruction causes abdominal distention and pain, and may trigger bladder spasms. When the patient complains of suprapubic pain, this intervention usually is all that is needed.

4. Incisional pain usually is moderate with the suprapubic and retropubic approaches; with the perineal approach, it usually is mild.

5. Early medication administration prevents severe pain. Oxybutynin directly relaxes smooth muscle and inhibits acetylcholine's parasympathetic-stimulating action on the bladder.

6. Alternative pain relief measures may enhance relief in conjunction with analgesics. Heat application reduces inflammation. Proper positioning may decrease discomfort from the urinary catheter.

7. Rationales: _____

Target outcome criteria
Within 30 minutes after surgery, the patient will:
• have vital signs within normal limits
• have no urinary obstruction.

Within 1 hour after surgery, the patient will:
• have absence or relief of pain
• find a relaxed position in bed.

Nursing diagnosis: *High risk for urine retention related to urinary catheter obstruction*

NURSING PRIORITY: Prevent or minimize urine retention.

Interventions

1. Monitor and record continuous bladder irrigation, as ordered. Adjust the irrigating solution's flow rate, as ordered, to maintain pink-tinged urine.

Rationales

1. Continuous irrigation dilutes blood clots and decreases obstruction. Urine normally remains pink-tinged for 3 to 4 days.

2. If the patient is not on continuous bladder irrigation, irrigate the urinary catheter with 30 to 60 ml of normal saline solution every 3 to 4 hours or as needed and as ordered, using gentle pressure. Use aseptic technique and universal precautions.

2. Blood clots or mucus plugs may adhere to the tip of the catheter and obstruct urine flow. This occurs most commonly when continuous irrigation is not used.

3. Monitor and document fluid intake and output. Encourage fluid intake of 8 to 12 8-oz glasses (2,000 to 3,000 ml) daily.

3. Hydration increases urine flow. Urine output less than 60 ml/hour suggests obstruction or decreased renal perfusion.

4. Weigh the patient daily. Compare with preoperative weight, and document.

4. Increasing weight suggests urine retention.

5. Observe for suprapubic distention and discomfort every 4 hours while the patient is awake. If a suprapubic catheter is in place, monitor and record urine outflow. Use universal precautions.

5. Increased distention may signal urine retention. A suprapubic catheter is commonly placed after suprapubic prostatectomy or urethral trauma or stricture.

6. Additional individualized interventions: _____

6. Rationales: _____

Target outcome criteria
Within 24 hours after surgery, the patient will:
• have no urinary clots
• show approximately equal fluid intake and output
• have no suprapubic distention.

Within 48 hours after surgery, the patient will have stable weight.

Nursing diagnosis: *Urge incontinence related to urinary catheter removal, trauma to the bladder neck, or decrease in detrusor muscle or sphincter tone*

NURSING PRIORITY: Relieve or minimize incontinence.

Interventions

1. Before surgery, teach the patient to tighten buttock and perineal muscles for 5 to 10 seconds, then relax them, repeating 10 to 20 times/hour. Instruct the patient to perform this exercise before and after surgery.

Rationales

1. Urinary incontinence is more common with perineal incisions and takes longer to resolve. With a TURP, temporary incontinence results from trauma to the urinary sphincter. With the suprapubic approach, temporary incontinence may result from the bladder neck incision.
   Strengthening the bladder sphincter promotes bladder control after urinary catheter removal. Normal urinary function usually returns in 2 to 3 weeks, although complete urinary control may take as long as 6 months to return after a perineal incision.

2. Monitor and document the patient's urination pattern after catheter removal. Instruct the patient to void with each urge, but no more than once every 2 hours during the first 24 hours after surgery and no more than once every 4 hours subsequently.

2. Catheter removal occurs 3 to 5 days after TURP and as long as 12 days after other procedures. Voiding with each urge prevents urine retention, and spacing voidings aids in bladder retraining.

3. If a suprapubic catheter is present after the urethral catheter is removed, measure residual volume after each voiding, using universal precautions. Alert the doctor if the residual volume exceeds 50 ml.

3. When urethral and suprapubic catheters are present, the urethral catheter usually is removed on the first postoperative day to minimize the risk of stricture formation. The suprapubic catheter usually is clamped for 24 hours before removal 7 to 10 days after surgery. If the residual volume exceeds 50 ml, the catheter may be left in until complete emptying is achieved through the urethra.

4. Obtain one urine sample with each voiding during the first 24 hours after catheter removal, and note its color, amount, and specific gravity. Use universal precautions.

5. Provide absorbent incontinence pads. Keep the perineal area clean and dry.

6. Additional individualized interventions: _____

_____

4. Analysis of a urine specimen helps indicate renal function. Hematuria should gradually decrease, and volume should increase. Specific gravity reflects urine concentration.

5. Keeping the perineal area clean and dry promotes comfort and reduces the risk of infection.

6. Rationales: _____

_____

Target outcome criteria
Within 24 hours after surgery, the patient will:
• exercise perineal muscles
• void no more than once every 2 hours

• have no postvoid residual volume
• present a clean, dry perineal area.

Nursing diagnosis: *High risk for altered sexuality patterns: decreased libido related to fear of incontinence and decreased self-esteem; infertility related to retrograde ejaculation (from TURP and suprapubic prostatectomy); or impotence related to parasympathetic nerve damage (from radical prostatectomy)*

NURSING PRIORITY: Prevent or minimize impact of altered sexuality patterns.

Interventions

1. Teach the patient before surgery, and reinforce after surgery, the expected effects of prostatectomy on sexual functioning. Include the patient's spouse or partner in the discussion.

2. Encourage the patient and spouse or partner to verbalize feelings of loss, grief, anxiety, and fear.

3. Encourage the patient and spouse or partner to discuss feelings about and expectations of the sexual relationship.

4. Provide information about a penile prosthesis, if appropriate.

Rationales

1. Providing correct information may decrease threats to the patient's sexual self-esteem and body image by clarifying misconceptions. TURP and suprapubic prostatectomy will produce some degree of retrograde ejaculation secondary to opening of the bladder neck during surgery: seminal fluid flows into the bladder and is excreted in the urine. Retrograde ejaculation does not interfere with sexual activity but does cause infertility. Ejaculation should return to normal within a few months. Sexual function is unaffected by suprapubic prostatectomy; a patient with erectile capability can usually resume intercourse in 4 to 6 weeks. Impotence always results from a radical prostatectomy because perineal nerves are cut.

2. Loss of the prostate gland commonly causes feelings of loss and grief similar to those women experience after hysterectomy. The patient with prostate cancer may also fear transmitting cancer to his sexual partner.
    Some men feel that impotence and sterility make them less manly. Verbalizing these feelings decreases anxiety and may assist in identifying ways to deal with losses.

3. Promoting open communication between sexual partners may prevent misunderstandings, enhance the relationship, and increase the patient's feelings of self-worth.

4. A penile prosthesis restores erectile capacity and may increase the patient's feelings of self-worth and sexual self-esteem after radical prostatectomy, which causes impotence. The patient should be totally healed (2 to 3 months after prostatectomy) before pursuing prosthetic surgery.

5. Provide information and refer the patient for sexual counseling, as needed after surgery.

5. The patient may need a sexual counselor if the prostatectomy exacerbates preexisting sexual problems. Follow-up may be needed after discharge.

6. Additional individualized interventions: _____

6. Rationales: _____

Target outcome criteria
Within 24 hours before discharge, the patient will:
• identify impact of surgery or disease on sexuality
• express feelings about masculinity and changes in sexuality

• verbalize understanding of anticipated sexual capacity
• identify available community resources.

Nursing diagnosis: *Self-esteem disturbance related to incontinence, potential impotence, or sexual alterations*

NURSING PRIORITY: Maximize feelings of self-esteem.

Interventions

1. Encourage the patient to verbalize feelings about post-operative changes in body functioning and how these changes will affect life-style.

2. Assist the patient in identifying and using effective coping behaviors. If problems arise, see the "Ineffective Individual Coping" plan, page 51.

3. Encourage the patient to continue perineal and buttock exercises to decrease incontinence. Reassure the patient that incontinence is temporary. Instruct the patient to use absorbent pads to prevent embarrassment.

4. Compliment the patient on personal appearance. Instruct the spouse or partner and family to provide compliments and positive feedback to the patient.

5. Encourage the patient to participate in activities of daily living (ADLs) and in decisions affecting care.

6. Additional individualized interventions: _____

Rationales

1. As with sexual alterations discussed in the previous problem, verbalizing feelings about other changes in body function is the first step in identifying healthful coping methods.

2. Promoting positive coping behavior increases adaptation to change and also increases self-esteem.

3. Incontinence may cause the patient to avoid social activities and neglect self-care. See the "Urge incontinence" nursing diagnosis in this entry.

4. Knowledge that a person is perceived by others as attractive and sexually desirable fosters self-esteem. Positive feedback reinforces a positive self-image.

5. Participating in care activities fosters independence. Decision making increases self-control and self-confidence.

6. Rationales: _____

Target outcome criteria
By the time of discharge, the patient will:
• identify changes in social relationships
• identify effective coping behaviors
• express satisfaction with personal appearance

• express positive feelings of self-worth
• participate in daily care.

Discharge planning

NURSING DISCHARGE CRITERIA

Upon the patient's discharge, documentation shows evidence of:
- absence of urinary obstruction
- absence of urine retention
- urine output of at least 800 ml for the past 24 hours
- absence of gross hematuria or large clots
- absence of infection
- absence of pulmonary complications
- absence of cardiovascular complications (including thrombophlebitis)
- stable vital signs (oral temperature below 100° F [37.8° C] for the past 24 hours without antipyretics, and blood pressure within preoperative limits)
- ability to control pain using oral medications
- ability to perform ADLs independently
- ability to perform catheter care
- ability to tolerate diet
- adequate home support or referral to home health agency or extended care facility.

PATIENT-FAMILY TEACHING CHECKLIST

Document evidence that the patient and family demonstrate an understanding of:
___ surgical outcome and disease
___ all discharge medications' purpose, dosage, administration schedule, and adverse effects requiring medical attention (usual discharge medications include analgesics, antispasmotics if a urinary catheter is present, and antibiotics)
___ urinary catheter care techniques and supplies
___ signs and symptoms indicating obstruction, bleeding, or infection
___ supplies to manage incontinence
___ exercises to regain urinary control
___ common postoperative feelings
___ the appropriate activity level to prevent muscle straining
___ resumption of sexual activity and community resources for sexual counseling
___ community or interagency referral
___ need for consultation with an oncology specialist (if the diagnosis of cancer is confirmed)
___ availability of cancer support groups
___ date, time, and location of follow-up appointments
___ how to contact the doctor.

DOCUMENTATION CHECKLIST

Using outcome criteria as a guide, document:
___ clinical status on admission
___ significant changes in status after surgery
___ pertinent laboratory and diagnostic test findings
___ episodes of hemorrhage
___ transfusion with blood products
___ infection and treatment
___ fluid intake and output
___ urinary obstruction episodes
___ urine retention

___ urinary incontinence
___ patient-family teaching
___ discharge planning
___ community or interagency referral.

ASSOCIATED PLANS OF CARE

Grieving
Ineffective Family Coping
Ineffective Individual Coping
Pain
Surgical Intervention
Thrombophlebitis

References

Bachers, E. "Sexual Dysfunction After Treatment for Geniurinary Cancers," *Seminars in Oncology Nursing* 1(1):18-24, February 1985.

Drago, J. "The Role of New Modalities in the Early Detection and Diagnosis of Prostate Cancer," *CA — A Cancer Journal for Clinicians* 39(6):326-36, November-December, 1989.

Hogan, R. *Human Sexuality: A Nursing Perspective,* 2nd ed. East Norwalk, Conn.: Appleton & Lange, 1985.

Kneisl, C., and Ames, S. *Adult Health Nursing: A Biopsychosocial Approach.* Reading, Mass.: Addison-Wesley Publishing Co., 1986.

LaFollette, S. "Radical Retropubic Prostatectomy: Campbell and Walsh Techniques," *AORN Journal* 45(1):57-63, 66-69, January 1987.

Litwack, K., and House, D. "Practical Points in the Care of the Post-TURP Patient," *Journal of Post Anesthesia Nursing* 4(6):403-05, December 1989.

McNally, J., Stair, J., and Somerville, E. *Guidelines for Cancer Nursing Practice.* New York: Grune & Stratton, 1985.

Radioactive Implant for Cervical Cancer

DRG information

DRG 357 Uterine and Adnexa Procedures for Ovarian
or Adnexa Malignancy.
Mean LOS = 10.6 days
DRG 363 Dilation and Curettage (D&C), Conization,
and Radio-Implant for Malignancy.
Mean LOS = 3.3 days

Additional DRG information: Many patients now receive radioactive implants as outpatients, although in the past such patients were routinely hospitalized. A patient who receives an implant during removal of the malignant neoplasm is always hospitalized.

Introduction
DEFINITION AND TIME FOCUS

The primary treatment for cervical cancer, radiation therapy usually combines internal irradiation (given as inpatient therapy) with external irradiation (usually given as outpatient therapy). This plan focuses on inpatient management of the patient receiving a radioactive implant for cervical cancer. Cancers of the vagina and endometrium may also be treated in this manner with a similar nursing plan of care.

The implant may be inserted before, during, or after external radiation therapy. With the patient in the operating room and anesthetized, an applicator is inserted into the vagina. The stainless steel applicator consists of a central hollow tube, passed through the cervical os into the uterine cavity, and two hollow ovoids, placed in the vagina next to the cervix. After correct placement is confirmed by X-ray, the patient is brought back to the unit where the doctor threads the radioactive material (radium or cesium are most common) into the central cylinder and ovoids to radiate the cervix and the paracervical tissue, the usual area into which cervical cancer spreads.

The implant stays in place for 2 to 4 days. Computer calculations determine the radiation dose to the tumor and the dose absorbed by normal tissues, such as the bladder and rectum. After the dose has been delivered, the doctor removes the radioactive material and then the applicator. An analgesic or sedative may be required before removal.

ETIOLOGY AND PRECIPITATING FACTORS

Risk factors associated with the development of squamous cell carcinoma of the cervix include:
• early age of first intercourse
• multiple sexual partners
• multiparity
• history of herpes simplex virus II or human papilloma virus infection (condyloma or genital warts)

• cigarette smoking
• history of an abnormal Papanicolaou (Pap) smear.
Most of these risk factors are related to early or repeated exposure of the cervix to an oncogenic virus that is probably transmitted sexually.

Focused assessment guidelines
NURSING HISTORY (Functional health pattern findings)

Health perception — health management pattern
• reports abnormal vaginal bleeding, commonly occurring after intercourse or douching
• may have history of an abnormal Pap smear that was never adequately evaluated

Nutritional-metabolic pattern
• may report unexplained weight loss (not usually seen with early cancers)

Elimination pattern
• may report feelings of pelvic pressure with resulting constipation or frequent urination
• may report decreased urine output if the tumor has caused ureteral obstruction
• may report incontinence of stool or urine if rectovaginal or vesicovaginal fistulae are present

Activity-exercise pattern
• may report weakness or fatigue, especially if anemic from vaginal blood loss

Cognitive-perceptual pattern
• may report pelvic pain or pressure, sometimes experienced as low back pain
• may report leg or hip pain as the tumor encroaches on nerve roots

Self-perception — self-concept pattern
• may report anxiety or depression over the diagnosis of cancer and perceived threat of death

Role-relationship pattern
• may report isolation from family, friends, or co-workers

Sexuality-reproductive pattern
• may express fear of sexual intercourse because of bleeding or concern about transmitting cancer to partner
• may express grief related to loss of reproductive function

Coping—stress tolerance pattern
• may express feeling powerless and less able to cope with other stresses
• may express need for education and support from community resources

Value-belief pattern
• may express guilt over delaying early detection behaviors (regular Pap smears) or evaluation of early symptoms

PHYSICAL FINDINGS
Reproductive
• vaginal bleeding
• cervical tumor that may:
 —be exophytic (growing outward on the cervix) or endophytic (growing inside the endocervical canal, making the cervix barrel shaped)
 —extend down the vagina
 —extend to the pelvic side wall
 —invade the bladder or rectum

Gastrointestinal
• constipation
• passage of stool through vagina (rare)

Urinary
• frequent urination
• decreased urine output or anuria (rare)
• passage of urine through vagina (rare)

DIAGNOSTIC STUDIES*
• blood urea nitrogen and creatinine levels—may be elevated, indicating ureteral obstruction and diminished renal function
• hemoglobin and hematocrit values—may be lowered if vaginal bleeding has been heavy
• intravenous pyelogram—may show ureteral obstruction by pelvic tumor
• cystoscopy—may show bladder wall invasion by tumor
• barium enema or proctoscopy—may show extrinsic pressure by pelvic tumor or invasion into rectal wall
• lymphangiogram or computed tomography scan—may indicate spread of tumor outside the pelvis to para-aortic lymph nodes or other organs

POTENTIAL COMPLICATIONS
• deep-vein thrombosis or pulmonary embolus
• peritoneal perforation by the implant apparatus
• hemorrhage
• atelectasis or pneumonia

Nursing diagnosis: *High risk for injury related to dislodgment of the implant*

NURSING PRIORITY: Minimize risk of dislodgment and resulting perforation and peritonitis.

Interventions

1. Administer laxatives or enemas as ordered the night before the implant insertion. Document your actions.

2. Provide a low-residue diet with adequate fluid intake.

3. Administer medications as ordered to decrease peristalsis, such as diphenoxylate hydrochloride (Lomotil), loperamide hydrochloride (Imodium), or codeine.

4. Document the presence and position of the implant. When the patient returns from the operating room, place a small ink mark on the leg at the bottom of the applicator as a baseline indicator in case the applicator is dislodged. Also note the position of the handles on the applicator (vertical, horizontal, oblique).

5. Assess for signs and symptoms of perforation, including vaginal bleeding, abdominal pain or distention, fever, nausea, and vomiting. Notify the doctor immediately.

Rationales

1. Evacuating the lower colon minimizes the likelihood that stool will contaminate the field during the insertion procedure. Bowel movements or bedpan placement while the implant is in place may dislodge it or cause perforation by the implant apparatus.

2. Low-residue foods minimize bulk formation in the colon. Adequate oral fluid intake lessens the need for I.V. hydration.

3. Medications that slow bowel function induce the constipation necessary for optimal placement and effectiveness of the implant.

4. Accurate ongoing assessment of the implant's position detects dislodgment, which may lead to uterine perforation.

5. The uterine cavity may be perforated at the time of insertion or with considerable pelvic movement. Prompt medical intervention is required because perforation can lead to peritonitis.

---

*Initial laboratory data may reflect no significant abnormalities.

6. Document placement of an indwelling urinary catheter (may be done at the time of implant insertion) and connection to bedside drainage; record output.

6. Continuous urinary drainage allows the patient to keep the hips positioned as recommended and avoids the movement necessary for bedpan use. The catheter also helps decrease the risk of bladder injury during the procedure.

7. Raise the head of the bed slightly (usually no more than 45 degrees); place a trapeze bar over the bed. Limit side-to-side movement.

7. Because the implant apparatus may protrude slightly from the vagina, raising the patient's head more than 45 degrees may change the angle of her hips and could dislodge the implant. Changing the angle of her head will allow the patient to sleep, eat, or read more comfortably. A trapeze bar may allow the patient to move her upper body more easily. Side-to-side movement may dislodge the implant.

8. Encourage the patient to perform grooming and personal hygiene activities. Do not change bed linen unless necessary.

8. Self-care increases the patient's involvement and decreases the caregiver's radiation exposure. Changing linens may cause pelvic movement that could dislodge the implant.

9. After the implant is removed, administer (and document the use of) laxatives or enemas, begin regular diet, and discontinue constipating medications.

9. Normal bowel function is restored after the implant is removed so that the patient can be discharged with normal functions intact.

10. Additional individualized interventions: _____

10. Rationales: _____

Target outcome criteria
While the implant is in place, the patient will:
• have no bowel movements
• show no signs or symptoms of perforation.

After the implant is removed, the patient will have normal bowel movements.

Nursing diagnosis: *High risk for disuse syndrome related to imposed bed rest*

NURSING PRIORITY: Minimize risks of bed rest.

Interventions

1. Attach a footboard to the foot of the bed; teach foot and leg exercises, and encourage the patient to perform them every 2 hours to increase blood flow; and apply antiembolism stockings.

2. Assess for signs and symptoms of thromboembolic phenomena, including calf pain, redness, and warmth; positive Homan's sign; and sudden onset of chest pain and dyspnea. See the "Thrombophlebitis" plan, page 361, for details. Report abnormalities promptly.

3. Administer anticoagulants as prescribed; monitor for excessive bleeding around the implant.

4. Teach deep-breathing exercises and encourage the patient to perform them every 2 hours.

Rationales

1. Deep-vein thrombophlebitis or pulmonary embolism may occur in the patient on bed rest. The patient with gynecologic cancer is at increased risk from the pressure of the pelvic tumor on large vessels. Measures to decrease venous pooling lessen this risk.

2. These signs and symptoms reflect inflammation of the vein wall and clot formation. The "Thrombophlebitis" plan contains detailed information on thromboembolic phenomena.

3. Anticoagulants, such as heparin or warfarin (Coumadin), inhibit blood clotting, thus decreasing the risk of a thromboembolic event but increasing the risk of hemorrhage.

4. Bed rest contributes to poor lung expansion. Stasis of secretions leads to airway obstruction and atelectasis and provides a medium for bacterial growth. Deep-breathing exercises prevent pooling of secretions.

5. Assess for signs and symptoms of lung infection every shift, such as crackles, bronchial breath sounds, fever, productive cough, and pleuritic chest pain. Report abnormalities.

5. Systematic assessment improves the likelihood of prompt detection and treatment of developing infection.

6. Additional individualized interventions: _____

6. Rationales: _____

_____

_____

Target outcome criteria
While the implant is in place, the patient will:
• exercise lower extremities every 2 hours
• perform deep-breathing exercises every 2 hours.

Throughout the hospital stay, the patient will show no signs of pulmonary or vascular complications of bed rest.

Nursing diagnosis: *Social isolation related to implant radioactivity*

NURSING PRIORITY: Minimize feelings of social isolation while the radioactive implant is in place.

Interventions

1. Explain to the patient and family the reasons for isolation from other patients and the nursing staff. Limit time spent with the patient and remind the family to remain behind the lead shields as much as possible. Limit the number of visitors, and do not allow children or pregnant women into the room.

2. Organize patient care into multiple short interactions instead of spending a lot of time in the room. Arrange the room so that items are within the patient's reach. Check on the patient frequently from the door.

3. Encourage diversional activities such as reading, handwork, talking on the phone, or watching television.

4. Additional individualized interventions: _____

_____

Rationales

1. Time, distance, and lead shielding are the three components of safe care for a patient with a radioactive implant. The areas of lowest radiation levels are at the foot and the head of the bed, and the lead shields are placed at the patient's sides where the radiation dose is higher.

2. Limiting time spent near the implant, maximizing distance from the implant, and staying behind the lead shields when providing bedside care will protect the nurse from excessive radiation exposure. Because of the limited number of visitors permitted, the patient will welcome frequent contact with the nurse.

3. A patient with cancer commonly experiences social isolation. Add to this mandatory physical isolation, and the patient may feel disoriented, with lowered self-esteem. Performing meaningful activities will help the patient pass the time and lend some sense of normalcy to the situation. Support and encouragement from the nurse may boost the patient's spirits.

4. Rationales: _____

_____

Target outcome criteria
While the implant is in place, the patient will:
• encourage visitors' compliance with radiation safety principles
• verbalize understanding of why nursing time must be limited

• pass time with diversional activities.

Nursing diagnosis: *Altered sexuality patterns related to vaginal tissue changes or fear of radioactivity*

NURSING PRIORITY: Minimize the physical and psychosexual effects of a vaginal implant.

Interventions	Rationales
1. Allow the patient to explore concerns and fears about the radioactive implant and resumption of sexual activity. Reassure the patient that once the implant has been removed, the tissues do not retain any radioactivity and, therefore, cannot harm anyone.	1. The patient (and her partner) may be concerned with the risk of radiation exposure during intercourse.
2. Encourage intercourse (if the patient has a partner) or use of vaginal dilators when postimplant discomfort has abated (usually after 2 to 4 weeks).	2. Radiation can cause scarring, narrowing, or fibrosis of the vaginal tissues. Regular dilatation of the vagina through intercourse or the use of dilators will help minimize these effects. Vaginal flexibility facilitates vaginal examination and the taking of Pap smears to monitor the disease.
3. Discuss with the patient and spouse or partner (if present) fears and concerns related to pain and bleeding during intercourse. Encourage use of lubrication during intercourse.	3. Atrophy and the resulting dryness of the vaginal tissues can occur after radioactive implant insertion. Tissues may be thin and easily traumatized, leading to pain or bleeding. Lubrication with a water-soluble lubricant may make the patient and partner more comfortable. Do not recommend petroleum-based products; they are too thick and may cause greater irritation.
4. Additional individualized interventions: _____	4. Rationales: _____

Target outcome criteria
By the time of discharge, the patient will:
• verbalize understanding concerning potential problems after radioactive implant removal
• verbalize purpose and methods concerning maintenance of vaginal patency.

Discharge planning
NURSING DISCHARGE CRITERIA
Upon the patient's discharge, documentation shows evidence of:
• ability to perform activities of daily living (ADLs) independently
• ability to ambulate same as before surgery
• absence of dysuria
• stable vital signs
• absence of pulmonary or cardiovascular complications
• ability to have a bowel movement

• absence of infection
• ability to control pain with oral medications
• no need for I.V. support (preferably discontinued for at least 24 hours)
• hemoglobin level within expected parameters
• minimal vaginal discharge and absence of gross bleeding
• knowledge of how to contact a cancer support group
• adequate home support, or referral to home care if indicated by an inadequate home support system or inability to perform ADLs.

PATIENT-FAMILY TEACHING CHECKLIST
Document evidence that the patient and family demonstrate an understanding of:
___ the cancer and its implications
___ treatment administered
___ all discharge medications' purpose, dosage, administration schedule, and adverse effects requiring medical attention (generally, medications are not ordered routinely, but pain medication, antibiotics, or medications for constipation or diarrhea may be prescribed, depending on special problems)
___ need to call the doctor if abdominal pain or fever above 100° F (37.8° C) develops
___ the likelihood of weakness or fatigue for 7 to 10 days after discharge
___ likelihood of vulvovaginal discomfort for a few days
___ the possibility of some discharge (possibly bloody), for up to 2 weeks (Tell her to call the doctor if bleeding becomes heavy, requiring one or more pads every hour. Tampons are usually discouraged because of the increased risk of toxic shock syndrome.)
___ ability to resume intercourse after tenderness and discharge decrease
___ community resources for cancer education and support
___ date, time, and location of follow-up appointments
___ how to contact the doctor.

DOCUMENTATION CHECKLIST
Using outcome criteria as a guide, document:
___ clinical status on admission
___ significant changes in clinical status
___ pertinent laboratory and diagnostic test findings
___ preimplant patient teaching
___ results of preimplant laxatives or enemas
___ application of antiembolism hose and teaching of lower extremity exercises
___ function of indwelling urinary catheter
___ head of bed elevated no more than 45 degrees
___ correct placement of radioactive implant
___ nutritional intake
___ teaching of deep-breathing exercises
___ results of postimplant laxatives or enemas
___ patient-family teaching
___ discharge planning.

ASSOCIATED PLANS OF CARE
Grieving
Ineffective Family Coping
Ineffective Individual Coping
Knowledge Deficit
Pain

References
Hilderly, L.J. "Radiotherapy," in *Cancer Nursing: Principles and Practice.* Groenwald, Susan L., et al., eds. Boston: Jones & Bartlett Publishers, 1990.

Lowdermilk, D.L. "Nursing Care Update: Internal Radiation Therapy," *NAACOG's Clinical Issues in Perinatal and Women's Health Nursing* 1:4, 1990.

Piemme, J.A. "Radiation Therapy: Implants," in *Decision Making in Oncology Nursing.* Baird, S.B., ed. Toronto: B.C. Decker, Inc., 1988.

Shell, J., and Carter, J. "The Gynecological Implant Patient," *Seminars in Oncology Nursing* 3(1):54-66, February 1987.

Thompson, L.J. "Cancer of the Cervix," *Seminars in Oncology Nursing* 6(3):190-97, August 1990.

Section III

S elected condensed plans of care, arranged alphabetically, provide a database for quick review of problems, interventions, teaching, and documentation.

Abdominal Aortic Aneurysm Repair

NURSING DIAGNOSIS: *Knowledge deficit regarding preoperative and postoperative care related to aortic surgery*
Interventions
1. See the "Knowledge Deficit" plan, page 56.
2. See the "Surgical Intervention" plan, page 81.
3. Describe endotracheal intubation and mechanical ventilation.
4. Explain to the patient and family the need for close monitoring after surgery and the expected length of stay in the intensive care unit (ICU).
5. Explain the need for frequent vascular checks to assess graft patency and peripheral vascular status.
6. Explain activities that may prevent graft kinking or compression and postoperative edema of the lower extremities.
7. Additional individualized interventions: _____

COLLABORATIVE PROBLEM: *High risk for cardiac decompensation related to changes in intravascular volume, third space fluid shift, and increased systemic vascular resistance*
Interventions
1. After surgery, monitor the patient's vital signs according to unit protocol and nursing judgment (typically every 15 minutes until stable, then every hour for the first 24 hours, then every 2 hours until transfer to the medical-surgical unit, then every 4 hours).
2. Monitor hemodynamic parameters according to ICU protocol or doctor's orders until the pulmonary artery catheter is discontinued.
3. Continuously monitor heart rate and electrocardiogram for arrhythmias, particularly atrial fibrillation, until the patient is discharged to the general care floor.
4. Monitor effectiveness of antihypertensive or vasopressor medications, if prescribed.
5. Monitor for fluid and electrolyte imbalances.
6. Additional individualized interventions: _____

COLLABORATIVE PROBLEM: *High risk for hypercapnia, hypoxemia, or both related to endotracheal intubation, physiologic changes associated with aging, effects of general anesthesia, and presence of an abdominal incision*
Interventions
1. Assess vital signs on admission to the ICU and every hour for 24 hours, then every two hours until the patient returns to the medical-surgical unit, then every 4 hours.
2. See the "Mechanical Ventilation" plan, page 227.
3. Once the patient is extubated, provide supplemental oxygen, as ordered.
4. Administer analgesics for pain, as ordered.
5. Additional individualized interventions: _____

COLLABORATIVE PROBLEM: *High risk for bleeding related to extensive retroperitoneal dissection and vascular anastomosis*
Interventions
1. Monitor and document intake and output and vital signs every hour for 24 hours; monitor and document central venous pressure, pulmonary capillary wedge pressure, and laboratory values according to ICU protocols or doctor's orders.
2. Assess the dressings on admission to the unit and every hour for 4 hours, then every 4 hours.
3. Monitor and document the amount and character of nasogastric tube drainage every 2 hours for 24 hours, then every 4 hours.
4. Assess abdominal girth if retroperitoneal bleeding is suspected.
5. Additional individualized interventions: _____

NURSING DIAGNOSIS: *High risk for injury: complications related to surgical procedure and atherosclerosis*
Interventions
1. Monitor for decreased peripheral tissue perfusion: check peripheral pulses immediately upon admission and every hour for the first 24 hours, then every 4 hours until discharge.
2. Monitor for acute renal failure.
3. Monitor for signs and symptoms of bowel ischemia.
4. Monitor for signs and symptoms of spinal cord ischemia.
5. Monitor for intra-abdominal graft infection by noting temperature elevations, leukocytosis, or prolonged ileus.
6. Monitor for local wound infection by inspecting incision lines for erythema, edema, odor, and the amount and color of any drainage every 4 hours and as needed until discharge.
7. Additional individualized interventions: _____

NURSING DIAGNOSIS: *Pain related to surgical tissue trauma or ischemia*
Interventions
1. Assess patency and stability of the epidural catheter, if applicable. Monitor effectiveness of epidural analgesia as well as for adverse effects.
2. See the "Pain" plan, page 69.
3. Additional individualized interventions: _____

PATIENT-FAMILY TEACHING CHECKLIST
__ progressive activity and ambulation plan
__ incision care
__ signs and symptoms of wound infection or graft thrombosis
__ discharge medications' purpose, dosage, administration, and adverse effects
__ risk factors for atherosclerosis and their reduction
__ availability of community resources
__ date, time, and location of follow-up appointments

DOCUMENTATION CHECKLIST
___ clinical status on admission
___ significant changes in status
___ pertinent diagnostic test findings
___ presence or absence of peripheral pulses
___ pain relief measures
___ wound site appearance and amount, color, and consistency of any drainage
___ level of activity and the patient's response to progressive ambulation
___ patient-family teaching
___ discharge planning

ASSOCIATED PLANS OF CARE
Knowledge Deficit
Mechanical Ventilation
Pain
Surgical Intervention

Acquired Immunodeficiency Syndrome

COLLABORATIVE PROBLEM: *High risk for infection related to immunosuppression (low T4 lymphocyte count or low T4 to T8 ratio)*
Interventions
1. Institute Centers for Disease Control (CDC) and institution precautions for the immunosuppressed patient.
2. Monitor vital signs, including temperature, at least every 4 hours. Report fever onset or temperature spikes immediately.
3. Monitor complete blood count daily and report increasing leukopenia or neutropenia.
4. Monitor potential sites of infection daily.
5. Be alert for signs and symptoms of neurologic infection.
6. Monitor for evidence of new pulmonary infections, checking lung sounds at least every 8 hours.
7. Obtain cultures, as ordered, from blood, stool, urine, sputum, or wound drainage.
8. Administer antibiotics and anti-infectives, as ordered. Commonly used medications include co-trimoxazole (Bactrim, Septra), pentamidine isethionate (Pentam), pyrimethamine with sulfadoxine (Fansidar), and pyrimethamine (Daraprim).
9. If antiviral treatments are ordered, such as with zidovudine (Retrovir, AZT), didanosine (Videx), and dideoxycytidine (ddC), provide patient teaching (consult current guidelines, as recommendations may change with further study) and make appropriate interventions.
10. If fever is present, administer acetaminophen (Tylenol), as ordered. Consult the doctor about alternating doses of acetaminophen with aspirin, naproxen (Naprosyn) or ibuprofen (Motrin) for persistent fever. Check platelet count and bleeding time before giving aspirin or ibuprofen.
11. Institute fever control measures, as ordered.
12. Additional individualized interventions: _____

NURSING DIAGNOSIS: *High risk for ineffective individual coping related to life-threatening illness, potential loss of usual roles, decisions regarding treatment, or poor prognosis for long-term survival*
Interventions
1. Assess for excessive anxiety.
2. Introduce yourself and other staff members.
3. Implement measures to promote physical relaxation.
4. Encourage verbalization of feelings.
5. Identify and discuss unhealthy coping behaviors. Teach the patient about the effects of alcohol or drug abuse on immune function.
6. Help the patient identify and list specific fears and concerns contributing to anxiety.
7. Help the patient identify and activate resources.
8. Acknowledge the unknowns of acquired immunodeficiency syndrome (AIDS). Answer questions honestly and accurately. See the "Dying" and "Grieving" plans, pages 11 and 31 respectively.
9. Additional individualized interventions: _____

COLLABORATIVE PROBLEM: *High risk for hypoxemia related to ventilation-perfusion imbalance, pneumonia, and weakness*
Interventions
1. Assess continuously for signs of hypoxemia.
2. Administer oxygen therapy via nasal cannula, face mask, nonrebreather mask, or continuous positive airway pressure mask according to unit protocol or as ordered.
3. Perform airway clearance measures, as needed.
4. Observe for complications of bronchoscopy; report any bleeding, anxiety, or unusual findings.
5. Evaluate and document the following every 8 hours and as needed: presence or absence of an effective cough, sputum character and color, respiratory effort, skin color, breath sounds, and activity tolerance.
6. If narcotic analgesics are used to control pain, be alert for signs of respiratory depression after analgesic administration.
7. Assist with self-care activities as needed (see the "Impaired physical mobility" nursing diagnosis in this plan).
8. Additional individualized interventions: _____

NURSING DIAGNOSIS: *Sensory-perceptual alteration related to neurologic involvement*
Interventions
1. Assess the patient's mental and neurologic status on admission and at least daily thereafter.
2. Evaluate the patient's emotional state.
3. Assess for possible visual impairment by using an eye chart, if possible.
4. If confusion is present, provide cues for reorientation, such as identifying yourself when entering the room.
5. Explain neurologic symptoms to the patient and to family and friends.
6. Provide a safe and supportive environment, instituting safety measures appropriate to the patients deficits.
7. Observe for involuntary movements, paresthesias, numbness, pain, weakness, and atrophy of extremities.
8. Additional individualized interventions: _____

NURSING DIAGNOSIS: *Social isolation related to communicable disease, associated social stigma, and fear of infection from social contact*
Interventions
1. Assess the patient's support system.
2. Provide opportunities for the patient and family to express feelings.
3. Provide an atmosphere of acceptance.
4. Teach family and friends about ways the AIDS virus is *not* transmitted.
5. Provide the patient and family with telephone numbers of available resources for counseling, support, and information.
6. Additional individualized interventions: _____

NURSING DIAGNOSIS: *Impaired physical mobility related to fatigue, weakness, hypoxemia, depression, altered sleep patterns, medication adverse effects, and orthostatic hypotension*
Interventions
1. Provide standard nursing care for decreased mobility.
2. Assess the need for sedatives, administer medications as ordered, and monitor their effects.
3. Encourage the patient with weakness or orthostatic hypotension to use the call light, ask for assistance when standing and walking, and leave belongings within reach.
4. Assist with activities of daily living as necessary. Anticipate the patient's needs.
5. Additional individualized interventions: _____

NURSING DIAGNOSIS: *Nutritional deficit related to nausea, vomiting, diarrhea, anorexia, medication adverse reactions, or decreased nutrient absorption secondary to the disease*
Interventions
1. Provide typical assessments and interventions for nutritional status. Refer to the "Nutritional Deficit" plan, page 63, for information.
2. Administer antiemetics, as ordered, if nausea and vomiting are present.
3. Consult the doctor about nasogastric feedings or total parenteral nutrition if the patient is unable to tolerate adequate oral intake or has severe chronic diarrhea. See the "Total Parenteral Nutrition" plan, page 411, for further information.
4. Additional individualized interventions: _____

NURSING DIAGNOSIS: *High risk for fluid volume deficit related to chronic, persistent diarrhea associated with opportunistic infection*
Interventions
1. See Appendix C, "Fluid and Electrolyte Imbalances."
2. Additional individualized interventions: _____

NURSING DIAGNOSIS: *Altered oral mucous membrane related to infections or masses*
Interventions
1. Assess the patient's mouth at least twice daily for signs and symptoms of thrush, lesions, or bleeding.
2. Ensure that the patient receives or completes mouth care after meals and at bedtime.
3. Apply lubricant to the lips as needed.
4. Obtain cultures from suspicious oral lesions, as ordered.
5. Avoid using alcohol, lemon-glycerin swabs, and commercial mouthwashes.
6. Assess for and report any inflammation or ulceration of the oral mucosa and any leukoplakia, pain, dysphagia, or voice change.
7. Additional individualized interventions: _____

NURSING DIAGNOSIS: *High risk for impaired skin integrity related to effects of immobility, disease, medications, or poor nutritional status*
Interventions
1. Implement usual measures to detect and prevent skin breakdown, such as inspection, frequent turning, and skin care.
2. If a pressure ulcer develops, institute therapeutic treatment, as ordered.
3. If the patient is receiving I.V. or I.M. pentamidine isethionate for *Pneumocystis carinii* pneumonia, rotate injection sites and observe them carefully for sterile abscesses.
4. Observe for urticaria, maculopapular rash, or pruritus.
5. Provide appropriate patient teaching related to the above measures.
6. Additional individualized interventions: _____

NURSING DIAGNOSIS: *High risk for sexual dysfunction related to fatigue, depression, fear of rejection, and fear of disease transmission*
Interventions
1. Determine if the patient is currently involved in a sexual relationship by asking direct questions in a nonjudgmental manner.
2. Encourage open discussion and sharing of feelings between the patient and spouse (or partner).
3. Encourage expression of affection and nonsexual touching, such as hugging, massage, and holding hands.
4. Discuss safer sex practices. Refer to current CDC guidelines for detailed, up-to-date recommendations.
5. Additional individualized interventions: _____

NURSING DIAGNOSIS: *Knowledge deficit related to symptoms of disease progression, risk factors, transmission of disease, home care, and treatment options*
Interventions
1. See the "Knowledge Deficit" plan, page 56.

2. Teach the patient and family about infection prevention measures.
3. Discuss symptoms that may indicate AIDS-related complications.
4. Review with the family recommendations for home care and waste disposal.
5. Teach the patient and loved ones about how the AIDS virus may be spread.
6. Provide information regarding the patient's legal rights.
7. Encourage the patient to explore treatment options with the doctor.
8. Additional individualized interventions: _____

PATIENT-FAMILY TEACHING CHECKLIST
___ disease and its implications
___ all discharge medications (may include antibiotics or other chemotherapeutics)
___ community resources available for emotional support, financial counseling, grief counseling, and individual and family counseling
___ treatment options, including investigational studies
___ resources for long-term care or terminal care, such as a hospice
___ signs and symptoms of opportunistic infection or complications
___ ways to prevent human immunodeficiency virus transmission to others
___ ways to decrease risk of new infection
___ symptoms to report to the health care provider
___ importance of keeping follow-up appointments
___ how to contact the doctor
___ legal rights and resources

DOCUMENTATION CHECKLIST
___ clinical status on admission
___ significant changes in status
___ pertinent laboratory and diagnostic test findings
___ occurrence of opportunistic infections
___ treatment decisions
___ nutritional program and support
___ breathing patterns
___ sleep patterns
___ emotional coping
___ support from family and friends
___ patient-family teaching
___ discharge planning

ASSOCIATED PLANS OF CARE
Dying
Grieving
Impaired Physical Mobility
Ineffective Family Coping
Ineffective Individual Coping
Lymphoma
Nutritional Deficit
Pain
Pneumonia
Total Parenteral Nutrition

Acute Myocardial Infarction— Critical Care Unit Phase

COLLABORATIVE PROBLEM: *High risk for cardiogenic shock related to arrhythmias, impaired contractility, or thrombosis*
Interventions
1. Institute and document continuous electrocardiogram (ECG) monitoring on admission.
2. Record and analyze rhythm strips every 4 hours and as needed for significant variations.
3. Obtain serial 12-lead ECGs on admission, daily for 3 days, and as needed for chest pain.
4. Evaluate and document hourly or as needed: level of consciousness, pulse, blood pressure, heart sounds, breath sounds, urine output, skin color and temperature, and capillary refill time.
5. Establish and maintain a patent I.V. line. Document cumulative fluid intake and output hourly.
6. Administer heparin, warfarin sodium (Coumadin), or both, as ordered.
7. Prepare the patient for aggressive treatment measures, as ordered, which may include:
• thrombolytic therapy
• emergency coronary arteriography
• percutaneous transluminal coronary angioplasty
• coronary artery bypass surgery.
8. Additional individualized interventions: _____

COLLABORATIVE PROBLEM: *Hypoxemia related to ventilation-perfusion imbalance*
Interventions
1. Observe for signs and symptoms of hypoxemia. Monitor pulse oximetry or arterial blood gas values, as ordered.
2. Administer oxygen therapy according to medical protocol and nursing judgment.
3. If blood pressure is stable within normal limits, place the patient in semi-Fowler's position.
4. During the period of acute instability, place the patient on bed rest or chair rest. Once stabilized, increase activity as tolerated.
5. Provide adequate rest periods.
6. Additional individualized interventions: _____

COLLABORATIVE PROBLEM: *Chest pain related to myocardial ischemia*
Interventions
1. On admission, teach the patient to report any chest pain, chest tightness, heaviness, or burning immediately.
2. Monitor continually for signs and symptoms of chest pain.
3. Document pain episodes.
4. Administer medication promptly at the onset of pain.

5. During the initial period of cardiovascular instability, titrate morphine I.V. (if ordered) according to the level of pain and vital signs.
6. Remain with the patient until pain is relieved.
7. Position the patient comfortably. Use noninvasive pain relief measures and medications, as appropriate.
8. Additional individualized interventions: _____

_____

NURSING DIAGNOSIS: *High risk for ineffective individual coping related to fear of death, anxiety, denial, or depression*
Interventions
1. Implement measures in the "Ineffective Individual Coping" plan, page 51, as appropriate.
2. Administer tranquilizers, as ordered, typically a benzodiazepine.
3. Additional individualized interventions: _____

_____

NURSING DIAGNOSIS: *Constipation related to diet, bed rest, immobility, or medications*
Interventions
1. Encourage intake of the prescribed diet, which is usually low in calories, salt, and fat. Limit caffeine intake.
2. Supply a bedside commode when the patient's condition allows.
3. Administer stool softeners and laxatives judiciously, as ordered.
4. Provide privacy while the patient defecates.
5. Additional individualized interventions: _____

_____

NURSING DIAGNOSIS: *High risk for injury: complications related to myocardial ischemia, injury, necrosis, inflammation, or arrhythmias*
Interventions
1. Monitor constantly for general complications of acute myocardial infarction (AMI), including:

ARRHYTHMIAS
• Observe for ventricular arrhythmias.
• Observe for supraventricular arrhythmias.
• Administer antiarrhythmic agents, as ordered:
  —Class IA agents, such as procainamide hydrochloride (Pronestyl)
  —Class IB agents, such as lidocaine (Xylocaine)
  —Class II agents, such as propranolol (Inderal), metoprolol (Lopressor), and atenolol (Tenormin)
  —Class III agents, such as bretylium tosylate (Bretylol) and amiodarone (Cordarone)
  —Class IV agents, such as verapamil hydrochloride (Calan), nifedipine (Procardia), and diltiazem (Cardizem)
• Implement emergency measures as needed.

CONGESTIVE HEART FAILURE AND CARDIOGENIC SHOCK
• Implement measures in the "Cardiogenic Shock" and "Congestive Heart Failure" plans, pages 310 and 329 respectively.

INFARCT EXTENSION
• Monitor for new, increased, or persistent chest pain. Obtain a 12-lead ECG and administer pain medication, as ordered.
• Notify the doctor about pain as well as any indicators of new infarction reflected by 12-lead ECG.

PERICARDITIS
• Observe for pericardial chest pain, fever, tachycardia, and pericardial friction rub.
• Administer anti-inflammatory agents, as ordered.
• Monitor for indicators of pericardial effusion.
• Monitor for signs and symptoms of cardiac tamponade. If present, summon immediate medical assistance and prepare for emergency pericardial aspiration.

VENTRICULAR ANEURYSM
• Observe for signs and symptoms of ventricular aneurysm, which include those of congestive heart failure, thromboembolism, or persistent ectopy.
• Alert the doctor and prepare the patient for surgery, as ordered.

RUPTURE
• Monitor for signs and symptoms of papillary muscle rupture. Assist with treatment of cardiogenic shock or prepare the patient for surgery, as ordered.
• Observe for signs and symptoms of potential septal rupture. Initiate cardiopulmonary resuscitation, if necessary, and obtain immediate medical assistance. Implement measures to treat cardiogenic shock or prepare the patient for surgery, as ordered.
• Be alert for signs and symptoms of impending myocardial rupture. Notify the doctor immediately. Assist with emergency pericardiocentesis and treatment of cardiogenic shock, as ordered.

2. Monitor constantly for complications of particular types of AMI:

ANTERIOR, ANTEROSEPTAL, OR ANTEROLATERAL INFARCT
• Monitor for signs or symptoms of bundle branch block (BBB).
• Alert the doctor if you detect:
  —right BBB
  —left BBB
  —left anterior hemiblock or left posterior hemiblock.
• Observe closely for Mobitz II second-degree atrioventricular (AV) block or complete heart block. Prepare for prophylactic pacemaker insertion, as ordered.

INFERIOR INFARCT
• Monitor for sinus bradycardia and AV block.
• Observe for indicators of right ventricular (RV) infarct.
• If the patient is dehydrated on admission, watch for signs of RV infarction after I.V. hydration.
• When recording 12-lead ECGs on a patients with suspected inferior or posterior infarction, routinely record RV leads.
• If indicators of RV infarction appear, alert the doctor.

• If an RV infarction is confirmed, collaborate with the doctor to modify therapy.
  — Avoid administering diuretics. Administer fluid boluses, as ordered.
  — Administer inotropes and vasodilators judiciously, as ordered.
• Monitor hemodynamic parameters and clinical indicators of therapeutic effectiveness closely.
3. Additional individualized interventions: _____

NURSING DIAGNOSIS: *Knowledge deficit related to diagnostic procedures, therapeutic interventions, and long-range implications for life-style changes*
Interventions
1. Implement measures in the "Knowledge Deficit" plan, page 56, as appropriate.
2. Defer a formal rehabilitation and education program until the period of physiologic instability has passed. In the meantime:
• Establish rapport.
• Assess immediate learning needs.
• As appropriate, provide brief information.
• Note and document long-range learning needs.
3. Additional individualized interventions: _____

PATIENT-FAMILY TEACHING CHECKLIST
___ extent of infarction
___ activity restrictions
___ recommended dietary modifications
___ smoking-cessation program as needed
___ common emotional changes
___ community resources for life-style modification support and cardiac rehabilitation

DOCUMENTATION CHECKLIST
___ clinical status on admission
___ significant changes in status
___ pertinent diagnostic test findings
___ chest pain
___ pain relief measures
___ rhythm strip analyses
___ use of emergency protocols
___ hemodynamic trends and other data
___ I.V. line patency
___ oxygen therapy
___ other therapies
___ nutritional intake
___ patient-family teaching
___ discharge planning

ASSOCIATED PLANS OF CARE
Cardiogenic Shock
Congestive Heart Failure
Grieving
Impaired Physical Mobility
Ineffective Family Coping
Ineffective Individual Coping
Knowledge Deficit
Pain

Acute Myocardial Infarction— Stepdown Unit Phase

NURSING DIAGNOSIS: *Activity intolerance related to myocardial ischemia, decreased contractility, or arrhythmias*
Interventions
1. Using telemetry, continuously monitor heart rate, rhythm, and conduction.
2. Promote physical comfort and rest.
3. Prohibit smoking and intake of stimulants, such as coffee and other beverages that contain caffeine.
4. Encourage the patient to perform activities of daily living and diversional activities.
5. Implement the prescribed activity and exercise program.
6. Assess and document intolerance to activity or exercise, monitoring vital signs before, during, and after each session.
7. Stress the importance of avoiding Valsalva's maneuver and isometric exercises.
8. Provide supplemental oxygen, as ordered, using nursing judgment.
9. Administer vasodilators, as ordered, and monitor the patient's response. Also monitor for adverse effects, particularly hypotension.
10. Teach the patient to monitor pulse rate before and after activity or exercise.
11. Stress the importance of complying with the activity or exercise program and with rest requirements.
12. Encourage family members to support the patient's activity or exercise program.
13. Additional individualized interventions: _____

NURSING DIAGNOSIS: *High risk for ineffective individual coping related to anxiety, denial, or depression*
Interventions
1. Encourage verbalization of feelings.
2. Anticipate feelings of denial, shock, anger, anxiety, and depression.
3. Explain the grieving process to the patient and family.
4. Evaluate the meaning of the patient's altered body image and role responsibilities.
5. Assess daily for indicators of anxiety.
6. Assess daily for indicators of denial.
7. Assess daily for indicators of depression.
8. Additional individualized interventions: _____

NURSING DIAGNOSIS: *Altered sexuality pattern related to physical limitations secondary to cardiac ischemia and medications*
Interventions
1. Obtain a sexual history, including the incidence of chest pain during or after foreplay and intercourse.
2. Encourage the patient and spouse (or partner) to verbalize fears and anxieties. Provide time for joint and individual discussion.

3. Be aware of personal feelings about sexuality, making an appropriate referral if unable to counsel the couple effectively.
4. Provide printed material about acute myocardial infarction (AMI) and resumption of sexual activities.
5. Inform the patient that some medications can cause impotence or decrease libido.
6. Discuss ways to decrease the effects of sexual activity on the cardiovascular system, such as through medications and positioning.
7. Emphasize that sexual activity should be avoided after large meals or alcohol intake, in extreme temperatures, and under conditions of fatigue or increased stress.
8. As ordered, evaluate activity tolerance.
9. Teach symptoms that should be reported to the doctor if they occur during foreplay or intercourse.
10. Additional individualized interventions: _____

NURSING DIAGNOSIS: *Knowledge deficit related to newly diagnosed, complex disease and to unfamiliar therapy*
Interventions
1. Increase understanding of the disease.
2. Promote compliance with necessary dietary modifications.
3. Stress the importance of hypertension management.
4. Stress the importance of smoking cessation.
5. Promote stress reduction.
6. Additional individualized interventions: _____

PATIENT-FAMILY TEACHING CHECKLIST
___ the disease and its implications
___ measuring radial pulse rate accurately
___ all discharge medications' purpose, dosage, administration schedule, and adverse effects requiring medical attention (usual discharge medications include nitrates, beta blockers, antiarrhythmics, calcium antagonists, antihypertensives, and inotropic agents)
___ need for risk factor modification
___ prescribed diet
___ prescribed activity or exercise program
___ need for regularly scheduled rest periods
___ signs and symptoms to report to health care providers
___ need for follow-up care
___ when to resume sexual activity
___ availability of community resources
___ how to contact the doctor

DOCUMENTATION CHECKLIST
___ status on admission
___ significant changes in status
___ pertinent laboratory and diagnostic test findings
___ telemetry monitoring
___ chest pain
___ interventions for pain relief
___ dietary intake
___ medical therapies, including medications
___ emotional status
___ activity tolerance
___ patient-family teaching
___ discharge planning

ASSOCIATED PLANS OF CARE
Dying
Geriatric Considerations
Grieving
Ineffective Family Coping
Ineffective Individual Coping
Knowledge Deficit
Pain

Acute Renal Failure

COLLABORATIVE PROBLEM: *Electrolyte imbalance related to decreased electrolyte excretion, excessive intake, or metabolic acidosis*
Interventions
1. Monitor and document electrolyte levels every 8 to 12 hours and as needed, as ordered.
2. Continuously monitor electrocardiogram.
3. If hyperkalemia is present, implement the following measures, as ordered:
• I.V. glucose (50%) and insulin solution
• I.V. calcium chloride or calcium gluconate
• cation-exchange resins
• I.V. sodium bicarbonate solution.
4. Limit dietary and drug intake of potassium.
5. Give aluminum hydroxide antacid (Amphojel) with meals and every 4 hours, as ordered.
6. Give calcium and vitamin supplements as needed and ordered.
7. Limit magnesium intake, such as in antacids.
8. Give sodium chloride I.V., as needed and ordered.
9. Additional individualized interventions: _____

NURSING DIAGNOSIS: *Fluid volume excess related to sodium and water retention*
Interventions
1. See Appendix C, "Fluid and Electrolyte Imbalances."
2. Assess for signs of fluid overload.
• Assess the following every 1 to 2 hours: vital signs (blood pressure, pulse, respirations), central venous pressure (CVP), pulmonary artery wedge pressure (PAWP), pulmonary artery end-diastolic pressure (PAEDP), mean arterial pressure (MAP), adventitious lung sounds such as crackles or rhonchi, and peripheral edema. Measure cardiac output, as ordered, typically every 12 hours. Assess weight and complete blood count, especially hematocrit, daily.
• Report the following promptly: high blood pressure, rapid pulse rate, rapid respirations, high hemodynamic parameters (CVP, PAWP, PAEDP, MAP), crackles or gurgles, peripheral edema, increasing daily weight, or low hematocrit.
• Also report the following promptly: low hemodynamic monitoring parameters, rapid pulse rate, low blood pressure, dry skin and mucous membranes, poor skin turgor, decreased body weight, or a high hematocrit.
3. Measure intake and output levels every 2 hours.
4. Restrict fluid intake to measured losses plus 400 ml/day, unless fluid or weight losses are excessive. Consult the doctor about increasing the fluid replacement if excessive fluid losses occur or if weight loss exceeds 1 lb (0.5 kg) daily.

5. Give I.V. infusions continuously through an infusion pump, as ordered.

6. Provide hard candies, ice chips, and mouth care every 2 hours as needed and ordered.

7. Give diuretics, such as mannitol, furosemide (Lasix), or ethacrynic acid (Edecrin), as needed and as ordered. Administer vasodilators, as ordered.

8. Additional individualized interventions: _____

NURSING DIAGNOSIS: *High risk for injury: complications related to uremic syndrome*
Interventions

1. See Appendix B, "Acid-Base Imbalances."

2. Monitor blood urea nitrogen, creatinine, uric acid, and pH levels once daily (or as needed), as ordered. Monitor arterial blood gas values once daily or as needed and ordered.

3. Assess for signs and symptoms of uremia every 2 to 4 hours and as needed.

4. Give sodium bicarbonate I.V., as needed and ordered.

5. Assess the hemodialysis access site (shunt or catheter), if present, every 2 hours for patency, warmth, color, thrill, and bruit. Do not use the access site for I.V. infusions or blood withdrawal. Do not take blood pressures on an arm or leg with an access site. Keep alligator clamps attached to the dressings.

6. Assess the peritoneal dialysis access catheter site, if present, every 24 hours and as needed for signs and symptoms of infection.

7. Prepare the patient for dialysis every 1 to 3 days, as ordered.

8. Monitor drug administration and blood levels continually.

9. Monitor hematocrit and hemoglobin level daily for signs of anemia.

10. Assess continually for signs and symptoms of hemorrhage.

11. Assess daily for signs and symptoms of pericarditis. If indicators are present:
• Notify the doctor. Administer steroids or nonsteroidal anti-inflammatory agents, as ordered.
• Monitor every 4 hours for indicators of pericardial effusion and a small cardiac tamponade: weak peripheral pulses, pulsus paradoxus greater than 10 mm Hg, or a decreased level of consciousness. If present, alert the doctor immediately.
• Monitor continually for indicators of a large cardiac tamponade: distended neck veins, profound hypotension, and rapid loss of consciousness. If present, summon immediate medical assistance and prepare for emergency pericardial aspiration.

12. Additional individualized interventions: _____

NURSING DIAGNOSIS: *High risk for infection related to decreased immune response and skin changes secondary to uremia*
Interventions

1. Assess continually for signs of infection.

2. Continually protect patient from cross-contamination.

3. Give antibiotics every 4 to 12 hours, as ordered.

4. Provide site care and dressing changes for central and peripheral I.V. lines, catheters, and dialysis shunts every 12 to 48 hours.

5. Provide skin care at frequent intervals.

6. Avoid continuous invasive procedures.

7. Collect urine, blood, and secretion specimens as needed and ordered, for culture and sensitivity laboratory tests.

8. Additional individualized interventions: _____

NURSING DIAGNOSIS: *Nutritional deficit related to anorexia, nausea and vomiting, and restricted dietary intake*
Interventions

1. See the "Nutritional Deficit" plan, page 63.

2. Administer medication to control nausea and vomiting, as needed and ordered.

3. Collaborate with the doctor and nutritionist to provide a high-carbohydrate diet that provides small quantities of high-quality proteins (containing essential amino acids); limits fluids, potassium, and sodium; and includes vitamin supplements.

4. Additional individualized interventions: _____

NURSING DIAGNOSIS: *Knowledge deficit related to complexity and life-threatening nature of acute renal failure and dialysis*
Interventions

1. See the "Knowledge Deficit" plan, page 56.

2. Provide, as appropriate, the following information:
• the common stages of acute renal failure
• medications
• signs and symptoms that should be reported to the nurse, such as dizziness and nausea
• procedures, including hemodialysis or peritoneal dialysis
• dietary modifications
• activity restrictions.

3. Additional individualized interventions: _____

PATIENT-FAMILY TEACHING CHECKLIST

___ common stages of acute renal failure and patient's current stage

___ fluid and dietary regimen, including protein, electrolyte, and fluid limits

___ medications, including actions and adverse effects

___ dialysis treatment if appropriate, including schedule and adverse effects

___ signs and symptoms, including fever, pain, nausea and vomiting, and dizziness, to report to the nurse

CONDENSED PLANS OF CARE

DOCUMENTATION CHECKLIST
___ clinical status on admission
___ significant changes in status
___ pertinent laboratory and diagnostic test findings, including serum drug levels
___ dialysis access site condition and care
___ urine characteristics and quantity, if appropriate
___ intake and output levels
___ body weight
___ diet tolerance
___ activity tolerance
___ mentation status
___ skin status
___ pertinent procedures, including dialysis

ASSOCIATED PLANS OF CARE
Gastrointestinal Hemorrhage
Knowledge Deficit
Nutritional Deficit

Adult Respiratory Distress Syndrome

COLLABORATIVE PROBLEM: *Hypoxemia related to pulmonary shunt, interstitial edema, and alveolar edema*
Interventions
1. Monitor for clinical signs and symptoms:
• tachypnea
• progressive dyspnea
• abnormal breath sounds
• deteriorating level of consciousness.
2. Obtain chest X-ray daily, as ordered.
3. Obtain arterial blood gas values at least every 4 hours, as ordered. Note degree of hypoxemia and any acid-base imbalance.
4. Continuously monitor gas exchange status, as ordered, with a pulse oximeter or $S\bar{v}o_2$ catheter.
5. Prepare for endotracheal intubation, if necessary.
6. Implement mechanical ventilation, as ordered.
7. Implement positive end-expiratory pressure (PEEP), as ordered.
8. Monitor compliance.
9. Administer medications, as ordered:
• corticosteroids
• antibiotics.
10. Additional individualized interventions: _____

NURSING DIAGNOSIS: *High risk for injury: complications related to single or multiple organ failure*
Interventions
1. Maintain adequate cardiac output. Monitor pulmonary artery pressures, vital signs, electrocardiogram, and urine output.
2. Administer packed red blood cells, as ordered.
3. Administer crystalloid or colloid I.V. fluids, as ordered.

4. If necessary, obtain an order to institute gastric drainage.
5. Provide nutritional support, as ordered. See the "Nutritional Deficit" plan, page 63.
6. Monitor for signs and symptoms of infection. Institute aggressive treatment measures, as ordered.
7. Observe for signs of single or multiple organ failure.
8. Implement general supportive nursing measures to prevent complications of immobility. See the "Impaired Physical Mobility" plan, page 36.
9. Additional individualized interventions: _____

NURSING DIAGNOSIS: *High risk for ineffective individual and family coping related to abrupt onset of life-threatening illness*
Interventions
1. Implement the measures outlined in the "Ineffective Family Coping" plan, page 47, and the "Ineffective Individual Coping" plan, page 51.
2. Allow the family to interact with the patient.
3. Encourage the patient and family to verbalize feelings about treatments.
4. Provide an alternative means of communication for the patient.
5. Additional individualized interventions: _____

PATIENT-FAMILY TEACHING CHECKLIST
___ definition and pathophysiology of disease
___ probable cause
___ prognosis
___ rationale for mechanical ventilation, PEEP, and other therapies

DOCUMENTATION CHECKLIST
___ clinical status on admission
___ significant changes in status
___ pertinent diagnostic test findings
___ airway care
___ tolerance of ventilator and PEEP
___ response to medications
___ fluid therapy
___ nutritional support
___ nursing care to combat effects of immobility
___ psychological coping
___ patient-family teaching
___ discharge planning

ASSOCIATED PLANS OF CARE
Disseminated Intravascular Coagulation
Grieving
Impaired Physical Mobility
Ineffective Family Coping
Ineffective Individual Coping
Mechanical Ventilation
Multiple Trauma
Nutritional Deficit
Sensory-Perceptual Alteration

Alzheimer's Disease

COLLABORATIVE PROBLEM: *Impaired cognitive function related to degenerative loss of cerebral tissue*
Interventions
1. Assess the patient's present level of cognitive functioning.
2. Assign the patient to a room close to the nursing station.
3. Minimize hazards in the environment.
4. Maintain consistency in nursing routines.
5. Promote self-care independence.
6. Establish a therapeutic relationship.
7. Get the patient's attention. Give simple, specific instructions for accomplishing tasks.
8. Orient the patient to reality frequently and repetitively.
9. Administer medications, as ordered.
10. Use aids to improve language skills.
11. Minimize communication barriers.
12. Encourage social interaction.
13. Prevent excessive stimulation. Promote usual sleep-rest pattern.
14. Respond to the patient attentively and consistently.
15. Encourage reminiscence.
16. Prepare a patient identification card, bracelet, or name tag.
17. Additional individualized interventions: _____

NURSING DIAGNOSIS: *Nutritional deficit related to memory loss and inadequate food intake*
Interventions
1. Assess present nutritional status.
2. Offer a balanced diet, with small quantities of food given at regular and frequent intervals. Provide finger foods when possible.
3. Prepare the food tray in advance so that the patient may eat unassisted.
4. Provide time and privacy for eating.
5. Monitor and record daily weight.
6. Provide dietary information to the home caregiver.
7. Additional individualized interventions: _____

NURSING DIAGNOSIS: *High risk for injury related to wandering behavior, aphasia, agnosia, or hyperorality*
Interventions
1. Consider using a bell to alert caregivers when the patient is wandering.
2. Ensure that the patient is dressed appropriately for the temperature, including shoes that fit well.
3. Avoid using restraints.
4. Recommend safety measures to the family for home care.
5. Encourage a regular exercise program, as tolerated.
6. Observe for nonverbal cues to injury. Note repeated words or seemingly inappropriate statements. Alert the family to cues observed.
7. Additional individualized interventions: _____

NURSING DIAGNOSIS: *Constipation related to memory loss about toileting behaviors and to inadequate diet*
Interventions
1. Identify the bathroom location clearly.
2. Promote toileting at regular intervals.
3. Encourage a therapeutic diet with ample fluid and fiber.
4. Observe for nonverbal cues signaling the need for elimination.
5. Administer and document use of elimination aids, as ordered.
6. Monitor and document the frequency of elimination.
7. Additional individualized interventions: _____

NURSING DIAGNOSIS: *High risk for ineffective family coping related to progressive mental deterioration of the patient with Alzheimer's disease*
Interventions
1. Involve the family in all teaching. Use teaching as an opportunity to assess family roles, resources, and coping behavior.
2. Offer support, understanding, and reassurance to the family.
3. Involve a social worker or discharge planner in decisions regarding home care or nursing home placement.
4. Provide information regarding community resources, such as home care, financial and legal assistance, and an Alzheimer's support group. Encourage use of all available resources.
5. Additional individualized interventions: _____

PATIENT-FAMILY TEACHING CHECKLIST
___ diagnosis and disease process – for example, through literature from the Alzheimer's Association (70 East Lake Street, Suite 700, Chicago, IL 60601)
___ preparatory plans for adequate supervision and behavior management
___ approaches recommended to minimize environmental hazards
___ instructions for promoting self-care independence
___ recommended procedure for reorientation to home environment
___ need for identification bracelet or other medical alert device
___ all discharge medications' purpose, dosage, administration schedule, and adverse effects requiring medical attention
___ techniques for continued improvement of language skills
___ specific suggestions for meeting nutrition and elimination needs
___ available community resources
___ need for restoration of family equilibrium as roles change and patient dependence increases
___ probability of total patient regression
___ how to contact the doctor

DOCUMENTATION CHECKLIST
___ clinical status on admission, including level of cognitive function
___ planned approach to maintain patient safety, security, and orientation
___ laboratory data and diagnostic test findings
___ any change in the patient's behavioral response
___ level of communication and social interaction
___ dietary and elimination patterns
___ patient-family teaching
___ discharge planning

ASSOCIATED PLANS OF CARE
Geriatric Considerations
Grieving
Ineffective Family Coping
Ineffective Individual Coping
Knowledge Deficit

Angina Pectoris

NURSING DIAGNOSIS: *Chest pain related to myocardial ischemia*
Interventions
1. Assess and document chest pain episodes.
2. Assess the patient for nonverbal signs of chest pain.
3. Obtain a 12-lead electrocardiogram immediately during acute pain.
4. Administer sublingual nitroglycerin promptly at the onset of pain and document results.
5. Implement measures to improve myocardial oxygenation: institute oxygen therapy, place the patient on bed rest in semi- to high-Fowler's position, and minimize noise and distractions.
6. Stay with the patient during chest pain episodes.
7. Monitor and document the effects of beta blockers, calcium channel blockers, and vasodilators.
8. Establish and maintain I.V. access.
9. Additional individualized interventions: _____

COLLABORATIVE PROBLEM: *High risk for arrhythmias or acute myocardial infarction related to myocardial hypoxia and ischemia*
Interventions
1. Monitor, report, and document signs and symptoms of arrhythmias.
2. Administer antiarrhythmic medications as ordered, noting and documenting their effectiveness and adverse effects.
3. Decrease myocardial oxygen demands.
4. Monitor, report, and document signs and symptoms of inadequate tissue perfusion.
5. Monitor, report, and document signs and symptoms of developing myocardial infarction.
6. Additional individualized interventions: _____

NURSING DIAGNOSIS: *Activity intolerance related to development of chest pain upon exertion*
Interventions
1. Instruct the patient to stop immediately any activity that causes chest pain.
2. Instruct the patient to avoid Valsalva's maneuver.
3. Document activity tolerance and instruct the patient to increase activity gradually.
4. Promote physical rest and emotional comfort.
5. Additional individualized interventions: _____

NURSING DIAGNOSIS: *Altered health maintenance related to cardiovascular risk factors*
Interventions
1. Teach the patient about factors that may cause anginal attacks.
2. Instruct the patient to maintain a diet low in saturated fat and cholesterol and to achieve ideal body weight. Document current height and weight.
3. Provide six light meals per day.
4. Encourage avoidance of foods and beverages high in caffeine.
5. Discourage cigarette smoking.
6. Instruct the patient in stress-reduction techniques.
7. Start the patient on a cardiovascular fitness regimen when approved by the doctor.
8. Additional individualized interventions: _____

NURSING DIAGNOSIS: *Knowledge deficit related to unfamiliarity with diagnostic or therapeutic procedures*
Interventions
1. See the "Knowledge Deficit" plan, page 56.
2. Explain hospital protocol for cardiac catheterization to the patient and family.
3. Prepare the patient for percutaneous transluminal coronary angioplasty or coronary artery bypass graft surgery, if indicated.
4. For the patient undergoing coronary artery bypass graft surgery, see the "Cardiac Surgery" plan, page 299.
5. Additional individualized interventions: _____

PATIENT-FAMILY TEACHING CHECKLIST
___ angina's pathophysiology and implications
___ recommended modifications of risk factors (smoking, stress, obesity, lack of exercise, diet high in fat and cholesterol)
___ prescribed dietary modifications
___ resumption of daily activities
___ all discharge medications' purpose, dosage, administration schedule, adverse effects, and toxic effects (usual discharge medications include nitrates, beta blockers, calcium channel blockers, or antilipemic drugs)
___ common emotional adjustments

___ community resources for life-style and risk factor modification, such as stress- and weight-reduction groups, cardiac exercise programs, and smoking cessation programs

___ signs and symptoms indicating need for medical attention, such as chest pain unrelieved by three nitroglycerin tablets within 20 minutes, new pattern of anginal attacks, palpitations or skipped beats, syncope, dyspnea, or diaphoresis

___ date, time, and location of follow-up appointments

___ how to contact the doctor

DOCUMENTATION CHECKLIST

___ clinical status on admission
___ significant changes in status
___ chest pain episodes — precipitating, aggravating, and alleviating factors
___ pertinent laboratory and diagnostic test results
___ pain relief measures
___ oxygen therapy
___ I.V. therapy
___ use of protocols
___ nutritional intake
___ response to medications
___ emotional response to illness; coping skills
___ activity tolerance
___ patient-family teaching
___ discharge planning

ASSOCIATED PLANS OF CARE

Acute Myocardial Infarction — Stepdown Unit Phase
Ineffective Individual Coping
Knowledge Deficit
Pain

Cardiogenic Shock

COLLABORATIVE PROBLEM: *High risk for hypoxemia related to pulmonary congestion, decreased systemic perfusion, or both*
Interventions
1. Monitor pulmonary status as needed, typically every 15 minutes until stable and then every 2 hours.
2. Monitor arterial blood gas values as ordered, typically every 4 hours until stable or as needed. Obtain chest X-rays, as ordered.
3. If pulmonary congestion is present, place the patient in semi- or high-Fowler's position.
4. Administer supplemental oxygen, as ordered.
5. Monitor peripheral oxygen saturation continuously by pulse oximetry.
6. Suction as needed.
7. Assist with insertion of a pulmonary artery catheter, as ordered.
8. Monitor pulmonary artery pressure hourly, pulmonary capillary wedge pressure (PCWP) every 2 hours, and cardiac index (CI) every 4 hours, or as ordered. (CI equals cardiac output divided by body surface area, determined from a DuBois nomogram). Note both individual values and trends.

9. Determine the presence and severity of heart failure according to PCWP and CI.
10. Anticipate medical therapy consistent with Forrester subsets. Administer therapy as ordered.
• For patients with no signs of failure (Subset I), observe for its development.
• For patients with pulmonary congestion only (Subset II), administer medication, as ordered.
• If blood pressure is normal, administer diuretics.
• If blood pressure is elevated, administer vasodilators.
11. If administering morphine sulfate, observe for and report hypotension, nausea, and vomiting.
12. Alert the doctor immediately if the patient develops severe dyspnea, pink frothy sputum, marked neck-vein distention, or describes a sense of impending doom.
13. Additional individualized interventions: _____

COLLABORATIVE PROBLEM: *Inadequate cardiac output related to heart rate abnormalities or diminished contractility*
Interventions
1. Observe for signs and symptoms of decreased cardiac output.
2. Monitor the electrocardiogram continuously.
3. For patients with hypoperfusion only (Subset III):
• if heart rate is elevated, administer fluids. Document effectiveness and observe for adverse effects, especially fluid overload.
• if heart rate is depressed, assist with pacemaker insertion. Document effectiveness and observe for pacemaker malfunction.
4. For patients with pulmonary congestion and peripheral hypoperfusion (Subset IV), administer medications, as ordered.
• If blood pressure is depressed, administer positive inotropes, typically digitalis preparations, dopamine hydrochloride (Intropin), dobutamine hydrochloride (Dobutrex), or combined inotrope and vasodilator therapy, such as dopamine and sodium nitroprusside or amrinone (Inocor).
• If blood pressure is normal, administer vasodilators.
5. For patients in Subsets III and IV who do not respond to fluid and drug therapy, assist with intra-aortic balloon pump (IABP) counterpulsation.
6. Additional individualized interventions: _____

NURSING DIAGNOSIS: *Activity intolerance related to hypoxemia, weakness, or diminished cardiovascular reserve*
Interventions
1. Assess for signs and symptoms of activity intolerance.
2. Place the patient on complete bed rest; assist with activity, as needed.
3. Pace nursing care to promote rest.
4. When the patient's condition stabilizes, increase activity gradually, as ordered.
5. Additional individualized interventions: _____

PATIENT-FAMILY TEACHING CHECKLIST
___ cause and implications of cardiogenic shock
___ purpose of medications
___ rationales for other therapeutic interventions
___ need for continued treatment of underlying cause, including life-style modifications if appropriate

DOCUMENTATION CHECKLIST
___ clinical status on admission
___ significant changes in status
___ pertinent laboratory and diagnostic test findings
___ hemodynamic measurements
___ oxygen therapy
___ response to cardiac assist devices, such as a pacemaker or IABP
___ fluid therapy or restrictions
___ response to inotropes, vasodilators, or other drugs
___ dietary modifications
___ activity restrictions
___ patient-family teaching
___ discharge planning

ASSOCIATED PLANS OF CARE
Acute Myocardial Infarction—Critical Care Unit Phase
Hypovolemic Shock
Impaired Physical Mobility
Knowledge Deficit

Carotid Endarterectomy

COLLABORATIVE PROBLEM: *Blood pressure lability related to carotid sinus dysfunction, hypovolemia secondary to intraoperative or postoperative bleeding or fluid imbalance, acute myocardial infarction, or hypoxia*
Interventions
1. Assess blood pressure every 15 minutes for the first hour, then every hour or as needed for the first 24 hours after surgery.
2. Implement measures to control hypertension:
• Administer medication such as sodium nitroprusside (Nipride), as ordered.
• Administer pain medication as ordered.
• Provide a quiet, restful environment.
• Maintain activity restrictions as ordered.
• Maintain fluid restrictions as ordered.
3. Implement measures to control hypotension:
• Assess fluid intake and output every hour or as needed for the first 24 hours.
• If hypotension results from fluid loss, replace fluids as ordered.
• Assess for evidence of acute myocardial infarction.
• Administer vasopressors to maintain blood pressure within specified limits.
• Administer pain medications judiciously.
• Monitor incision and drainage system for bleeding and drainage.
4. Maintain oxygenation as ordered.
5. Additional individualized interventions: _____

COLLABORATIVE PROBLEM: *High risk for cerebral ischemia related to carotid artery clamping during surgery or vasospasm from clamping and manipulating cerebral vessels, hypovolemia secondary to blood loss, cerebral vessel compression from hematoma or edema, cerebral embolization from manipulation of the arteries, marked fluctuations in blood pressure, or thrombosis of the endarterectomy site*
Interventions
1. Assess level of consciousness, orientation, pupillary reaction, and motor and sensory function hourly or as needed for the first 24 hours.
2. Assess blood pressure, pulse, and respiratory rate hourly or as needed for the first 24 hour after surgery.
3. Assess for patency of the internal carotid artery by lightly palpating the superficial temporal and facial arteries hourly, or by monitoring vital signs.
4. Assess for signs of bleeding.
5. If bleeding is present, prepare the patient for corrective procedures.
6. Implement measures to promote adequate cerebral blood flow, as ordered:
• Detect and treat hypovolemia.
• Maintain drain patency.
• Change or reinforce dressing as necessary.
• Apply an ice pack at the incision line, as ordered.
• Support patient's head and neck during position changes and maintain body alignment.
• Administer corticosteroids, if ordered.
• Control hypertension with antihypertensive medications.
• Control hypotension with fluid replacement or vasopressors.
• Maintain activity restrictions.
7. Implement measures to minimize injury, if signs and symptoms of cerebral ischemia occur.
• Continue the measures above.
• Assess and report progression of signs and symptoms.
• Maintain the patient on bedrest with head of bed flat, unless contraindicated.
• Initiate seizure precautions.
• Provide emotional support to the patient and family.
8. Additional individualized interventions: _____

COLLABORATIVE PROBLEM: *Cranial nerve injury (particularly cranial nerves III, VII, IX, X, XII) related to surgical trauma or blood accumulation and edema in the surgical area*
Interventions
1. Assess cranial nerve function hourly for the first 24 hours after surgery or as needed.
2. Compare cranial nerve assessment to preoperative or recovery room baseline. Immediately report significant changes.
3. Implement measures to reduce edema or accumulation of fluid in the surgical area.
4. If nerve damage occurs, particularly to the facial, hypoglossal, vagus, or glossopharyngeal nerves, implement measures to prevent injury to the patient:
• Suction as needed.
• Withhold oral fluids and food until the gag reflex returns.

• Assess the patient's ability to chew and swallow before offering fluids or food.
• Place the patient in high-Fowler's position, unless contraindicated, during and after oral intake.
• Instill eyedrops or tape the eyelids shut if the patient's blink reflex is decreased or absent.
5. If the vagus or glossopharyngeal nerve is damaged (as shown by hoarseness, difficulty speaking clearly, or asymmetric movement of vocal cords), implement measures to facilitate communication. Pay close attention when the patient communicates.
6. If nerve damage does occur, provide emotional support to the patient and family.
7. Initiate appropriate referrals for follow-up care when cranial nerve damage persists.
8. Additional individualized interventions: _____

COLLABORATIVE PROBLEM: *High risk for acute myocardial infarction related to atherosclerosis and trauma of surgery*
Interventions
1. Assess for chest pain (see the "Acute Myocardial Infarction—Critical Care Unit Phase" plan, page 268). Also evaluate laboratory and diagnostic tests specific to cardiac function.
2. Assess blood pressure, pulse rate, and respiratory rate, as well as readings obtained from a pulmonary artery catheter (if used).
3. Administer nitroglycerin, as ordered, until preoperative cardiac medications can be resumed.
4. Implement the measures in the "Acute Myocardial Infarction—Critical Care Unit Phase" plan for the patient with myocardial infarction.
5. Additional individualized interventions: _____

COLLABORATIVE PROBLEM: *High risk for hypoxemia related to airway obstruction from tracheal compression or aspiration*
Interventions
1. Assess airway patency every 15 minutes for the first hour after surgery and then hourly, as needed, for 24 hours.
2. Assess oxygenation levels by continuous pulse oximetry or arterial blood gas levels, as needed. Also monitor ABG levels to assure that pH and partial pressure of arterial carbon dioxide also stay within normal limits. Document and report oxygen saturation below 95%, or as ordered, and arterial blood gas levels outside the prescribed limits.
3. If airway obstruction occurs, prepare to assist with endotracheal intubation or drainage of an incisional hematoma.
4. Assess for bleeding and hematoma formation.
5. Evaluate the patient's ability to swallow.
6. Assess for an intact gag reflex, ability to swallow and speak clearly with normal tones, and symmetrical movements of the vocal cords and soft palate.
7. Keep suctioning equipment at the bedside for oral, pharyngeal, or endotracheal suctioning as needed.

8. Implement measures to increase gas exchange and prevent hypoxemia.
9. Additional individualized interventions: _____

PATIENT-FAMILY TEACHING CHECKLIST
___ extent of surgery
___ extent of neurologic deficits, if any
___ rehabilitation, if needed
___ risk factors for atherosclerosis
___ need for life-style modifications
___ recommended dietary modifications
___ life-style modification programs, such as stress management classes, cardiovascular fitness, weight loss, smoking-cessation, and alcohol rehabilitation programs as needed
___ community resources for life-style modification support
___ all discharge medications' purpose, dosage, schedule, and adverse effects
___ signs and symptoms to report to health care provider

DOCUMENTATION CHECKLIST
___ clinical status on admission
___ significant changes in status, especially regarding motor, sensory, or visual deficits, or episodes of hypertension or hypotension
___ wound condition
___ pertinent laboratory and diagnostic test findings
___ episodes of headaches or seizures
___ respiratory support measures
___ pain relief measures
___ nutritional status
___ preoperative teaching
___ patient-family teaching
___ rehabilitation needs
___ discharge planning

ASSOCIATED PLANS OF CARE
Acute Myocardial Infarction—Critical Care Unit Phase
Cerebrovascular Accident
Increased Intracranial Pressure
Ineffective Individual Coping
Knowledge Deficit
Pain
Surgical Intervention

Cerebrovascular Accident

NURSING DIAGNOSIS: *High risk for ineffective airway clearance related to hemiplegic effects of a cerebrovascular accident (CVA)*
Interventions
1. Position the patient to keep the airway open.
2. If hemiplegia is present, position the patient on the affected side for shorter periods (less than 1 hour) than on the unaffected side (2 hours). Avoid positioning the hemiplegic arm over the abdomen.
3. Encourage coughing (except in the patient with a hemorrhagic CVA) and deep breathing. Suction as necessary.

4. Assess lung sounds at least every 4 hours.
5. Allow nothing by mouth until ability to swallow is evaluated. If the patient is able to swallow with minimum difficulty, assist and observe the patient's eating, as needed.
6. Additional individualized interventions: _____

COLLABORATIVE PROBLEM: *High risk for further cerebral injury related to interrupted blood flow (embolus, thrombus, or hemorrhage)*
Interventions
1. Assess neurologic status, checking level of consciousness, orientation, grips, leg strength, pupillary response, and vital signs every hour until neurologic status is stable.
2. Elevate the head of the bed slightly and provide supplemental oxygen as ordered.
3. If the CVA is occlusive:
• Administer anticoagulants, as ordered. Monitor prothrombin time and partial thromboplastin time, and check current results before giving each dose. Observe carefully for unusual bleeding, and report any that occurs.
• Administer antiplatelet aggregation medications, as ordered. Observe for gastric irritation.
• Administer medications to control blood pressure, as ordered. Be alert for signs of decreased cerebral perfusion and report immediately any that occur. Check blood pressure at least every 4 hours while the patient is awake.
4. If the CVA is hemorrhagic:
• Maintain the patient on complete bed rest for the first 24 hours to 1 week, as ordered. Minimize stress and external stimulation. Administer stool softeners or laxatives, as ordered.
• Administer medications to control blood pressure, as ordered. Report any signs of neurologic deterioration.
• Administer I.V. aminocaproic acid (Amicar), as ordered. Observe for and report hypotension, bradycardia, or signs of thrombus formation.
• Monitor the patient to maintain optimal fluid status, observing fluid restrictions, as ordered. Administer osmotic diuretics, as ordered. Monitor intake and output.
5. Additional individualized interventions: _____

NURSING DIAGNOSIS: *Impaired physical mobility related to damage to motor cortex or motor pathways*
Interventions
1. Maintain functional alignment in positioning the patient at rest. Support the affected arm when the patient is out of bed.
2. Provide passive (and active, if appropriate) range-of-motion exercises to all extremities at least four times a day. Collaborate with the physical therapist to plan a rehabilitation schedule with the patient and family.
3. When permitted, encourage the patient to do as much self-care as possible.
4. Apply antiembolism stockings, as ordered. Assess for signs of thromboembolic complications, and immediately report any that occur.
5. Protect the patient's skin.

6. Maintain adequate elimination. If the patient is catheterized, begin bladder retraining as soon as possible. If the patient is not catheterized, offer the bedpan every 2 hours. Observe urine and report any sign of infection. Monitor bowel movements. Reassure the patient that bowel and bladder control usually returns.
7. Additional individualized interventions: _____

NURSING DIAGNOSIS: *High risk for sensory-perceptual alteration related to cerebral injury*
Interventions
1. Establish closeness. Call the patient by name. Approach the patient's unaffected side.
2. Protect the patient from injury to the affected side.
3. If visual field deficits are present, remind the patient that frequent head-turning will widen the visual field.
4. Additional individualized interventions: _____

NURSING DIAGNOSIS: *High risk for impaired verbal communication related to cerebral injury*
Interventions
1. Assess communication ability.
2. Speak slowly and clearly, using short sentences.
3. Arrange referral to a speech therapist.
4. Reassure the patient that functional recovery is possible with patience and consistent rehabilitation efforts.
5. Additional individualized interventions: _____

NURSING DIAGNOSIS: *Knowledge deficit related to disease manifestations, the rehabilitation process, and ongoing home care*
Interventions
1. See the "Knowledge Deficit" plan, page 56.
2. Explain to the family that some emotional lability is commonly associated with cerebral injury.
3. Maintain an attitude of acceptance and understanding.
4. Instruct the patient and family about all medications to be taken at home.
5. If the patient is to be discharged home on anticoagulant therapy, provide thorough instructions about:
• medications' action, dosage, and schedule
• need for frequent follow-up laboratory testing
• signs of bleeding problems and the need to report them
• measures to control bleeding
• dietary considerations
• avoidance of aspirin and over-the-counter medications
• avoiding trauma
• the importance of wearing a medical alert tag and of notifying other health professionals about anticoagulant therapy.
6. Teach the importance of life-style modifications to minimize the risk of recurrence.
7. Teach the patient and family to recognize and report symptoms associated with transient ischemic attacks.

8. Teach the patient and family about:
- activity and positioning recommendations
- use of mobility aids such as slings, braces, and walkers
- airway maintenance and feeding considerations
- the bowel and bladder control program
- signs and symptoms of complications
- food and fluid intake recommendations
- skin care
- communication techniques
- coping with emotional lability.
9. Discuss with the family the advisability of learning cardiopulmonary resuscitation techniques.
10. Additional individualized interventions: _____

PATIENT-FAMILY TEACHING CHECKLIST
___ injury or disease process and implications
___ all discharge medications' purpose, dosage, administration schedule, and adverse effects requiring medical attention (discharge medications may include anticoagulants, antiplatelet aggregation medications, and antihypertensives)
___ need for follow-up laboratory tests (if indicated)
___ signs of cerebral impairment
___ signs of infection
___ signs of thromboembolic or other complications
___ activity and positioning recommendations and mobility aids
___ food and fluid intake recommendations
___ bowel and bladder control program
___ risk factors
___ safety measures
___ use of medical alert tag
___ advisability of cardiopulmonary resuscitation classes for the family
___ skin care
___ communication measures
___ verbal practice exercises
___ expected emotional lability and coping methods
___ community resources
___ when and how to use the emergency medical system
___ date, time, and location of follow-up appointment
___ home care arrangements

DOCUMENTATION CHECKLIST
___ clinical status on admission
___ significant changes in status
___ neurologic assessments
___ pertinent laboratory and diagnostic test findings
___ medication therapy
___ activity and positioning
___ food intake
___ fluid intake and output
___ bowel and bladder control measures
___ communication measures
___ patient-family teaching
___ discharge planning

ASSOCIATED PLANS OF CARE
Geriatric Considerations
Grieving
Impaired Physical Mobility
Ineffective Family Coping
Ineffective Individual Coping
Knowledge Deficit
Nutritional Deficit
Seizures
Thrombophlebitis

Cholecystectomy

COLLABORATIVE PROBLEM: *High risk for peritonitis related to possible preoperative perforation of the gallbladder*
Interventions
1. Monitor vital signs every 2 hours for 12 hours, then every 4 hours if stable. Document and report abnormalities.
2. Assess the abdomen during vital signs checks, noting bowel sounds, distention, firmness, and presence or absence of a mass in the right upper quadrant.
3. Note the location and character of pain during vital signs checks.
4. Maintain antibiotic therapy, as ordered.
5. Additional individualized interventions: _____

COLLABORATIVE PROBLEM: *High risk for hemorrhage related to decreased vitamin K absorption and decreased prothrombin synthesis*
Interventions
1. Monitor prothrombin time.
2. Administer vitamin K, as ordered.
3. Observe for bleeding.
4. Give injections using small-gauge needles.
5. Apply gentle pressure to injection sites instead of massaging them.
6. Additional individualized interventions: _____

NURSING DIAGNOSIS: *Pain related to gallbladder inflammation*
Interventions
1. See the "Pain" plan, page 69.
2. Administer medications, as ordered. These may include meperidine (Demerol), papaverine hydrochloride (Parabid), amyl nitrite, and nitroglycerin (Nitrostat).
3. Additional individualized interventions: _____

CONDENSED PLANS OF CARE

COLLABORATIVE PROBLEM: *High risk for postoperative infection related to obstruction or dislodgment of external biliary drainage tube*
Interventions
1. Monitor vital signs.
2. Assess the abdomen every shift for pain and rigidity.
3. Assess for signs of infection at the T-tube insertion site.
4. Assess for signs of T-tube obstruction.
5. Assess for signs of tube dislodgment.
6. Using sterile technique, connect the T-tube to a closed gravity drainage system and attach sufficient tubing.
7. Monitor the amount and character of any drainage.
8. Monitor stool color.
9. Place the patient in low Fowler's position upon return from surgery.
10. If the patient will be discharged with a T-tube in place, teach the patient and family how to care for the drainage system.
11. Additional individualized interventions: _____

NURSING DIAGNOSIS: *High risk for postoperative ineffective breathing pattern related to high abdominal incision and pain*
Interventions
1. Monitor respiratory rate and character every 4 hours.
2. Auscultate breath sounds once per shift.
3. Instruct and coach the patient about diaphragmatic breathing.
4. Assist the patient to use the incentive spirometer every hour when awake and every 2 hours at night.
5. Turn the patient every 2 hours.
6. Assess pain and administer pain medication, as needed, before activity.
7. Assist the patient to splint the incision while coughing.
8. Encourage the patient to increase ambulation progressively.
9. Additional individualized interventions: _____

NURSING DIAGNOSIS: *High risk for nutritional deficit related to preoperative nausea and vomiting, postoperative nothing-by-mouth status, nasogastric suction, altered lipid metabolism, and increased nutritional needs during healing*
Interventions
1. Maintain I.V. fluid replacement, as ordered. See Appendix C, "Fluid and Electrolyte Imbalances."
2. Once peristalsis returns, remove the nasogastric (NG) tube and encourage progressive resumption of dietary intake.
3. Clamp the T-tube during meals, as ordered.
4. Teach the patient and family about a fat-restricted diet, as ordered. Involve a dietitian.
5. Suggest small, frequent meals.
6. Instruct the patient to minimize alcohol intake.
7. Prepare the patient for the possibility of persistent flatulence.
8. Additional individualized interventions: _____

NURSING DIAGNOSIS: *High risk for altered oral mucous membrane related to nothing-by-mouth status and possible NG tube suction*
Interventions
1. Assess the oral mucous membrane once per shift.
2. Assist the patient with gentle mouth care at least twice daily or as needed.
3. Apply lubricant to the lips at least every 2 hours while the patient is awake.
4. Additional individualized interventions: _____

PATIENT-FAMILY TEACHING CHECKLIST
___ signs and symptoms of wound infection
___ dietary modifications (patient may be on a low-fat diet for up to 6 months; a nonrestrictive diet is resumed as soon as tolerated)
___ resumption of normal activities
___ resumption of sexual activity
___ all discharge medications' purpose, dosage, administration schedule, and adverse effects (postoperative patients may be discharged with oral analgesics)
___ if discharged with a T-tube, routine care and signs to report to the doctor
___ date, time, and location of follow-up appointment
___ how to contact the doctor

DOCUMENTATION CHECKLIST
___ clinical status on admission
___ significant changes in status
___ pertinent laboratory and diagnostic test findings
___ wound assessment
___ amount and character of T-tube drainage
___ pain relief measures
___ pulmonary hygiene measures
___ observations of oral mucous membrane
___ nutritional intake
___ gastrointestinal assessment
___ patient-family teaching
___ discharge planning

ASSOCIATED PLANS OF CARE
Knowledge Deficit
Pain
Pancreatitis
Surgical Intervention

Chronic Obstructive Pulmonary Disease

COLLABORATIVE PROBLEM: *Respiratory failure (PO$_2$ level less than 50 mm Hg, with or without PCO$_2$ level greater than 50 mm Hg) related to ventilation-perfusion imbalance*
Interventions
1. Obtain and report arterial blood gas (ABG) measurements.
2. Administer oxygen, as ordered.

3. Administer pharmacologic agents (bronchodilators, antibiotics, corticosteroids, and expectorants), as ordered. Monitor therapeutic levels, as indicated.

4. Perform bronchial hygiene measures, as ordered. Assess lung sounds. Report and document treatment effectiveness.

5. Maintain fluid intake at 8 to 12 8-oz glasses (2,000 to 3,000 ml) of water per day.

6. Monitor, document, and report signs of infection or further deterioration in respiratory status.

7. If possible, reduce or eliminate environmental irritants.

8. Additional individualized interventions: _____

NURSING DIAGNOSIS: *Ineffective breathing pattern related to emotional stimulation, fatigue, or blunting of respiratory drive*

Interventions

1. Reduce the work of breathing and lessen depletion of oxygen reserves.

2. Teach and help the patient to perform breathing exercises and coordinate breathing with activity.

3. Pace all activities.

4. Instruct the patient in breathing techniques to use when expressing feelings that create shortness of breath.

5. Avoid the use of sedatives or narcotics.

6. Additional individualized interventions: _____

NURSING DIAGNOSIS: *Nutritional deficit related to shortness of breath during and after meals and adverse reactions to medication*

Interventions

1. Use supplemental oxygen during mealtimes, as ordered.

2. Perform bronchial hygiene measures before meals. Provide mouth care. Remove secretions from the eating area.

3. Provide frequent, small meals.

4. Monitor the patient's weight and nutritional intake daily.

5. Obtain a dietary consultation as soon as the patient can take foods or fluids.

6. Additional individualized interventions: _____

NURSING DIAGNOSIS: *Activity intolerance related to shortness of breath, avoidance of physical activity with resultant muscle weakness, deconditioning, depression, and (possibly) exercise-related hypoxemia*

Interventions

1. Instruct the patient in breathing techniques to use when performing activities of daily living.

2. Administer oxygen during activity, as ordered.

3. Before recommending an activity level, assess for stable ABG measurements, fitness level, and factors contributing to inactivity.

4. Develop and implement a daily walking schedule, increasing time and distance as tolerated. Instruct the patient in ways to control shortness of breath when walking.

5. Before, during, and after walking, monitor the patient's response to exercise.

6. Additional individualized interventions: _____

NURSING DIAGNOSIS: *Sleep pattern disturbance related to bronchodilators' stimulant effect, shortness of breath, depression, and anxiety*

Interventions

1. Identify the patient's normal sleep pattern as well as the abnormal pattern.

2. Consult with the doctor about adjusting medications to optimize bronchodilation while minimizing stimulant effects.

3. Instruct the patient in performing bronchial hygiene before retiring and as needed for nocturnal dyspnea.

4. Administer oxygen therapy during the night, as ordered.

5. Monitor periods of sleeplessness, including degree of shortness of breath, pulse rate and rhythm, respiratory rate, and breath sounds.

6. Instruct the patient in relaxation techniques to be used at bedtime.

7. Additional individualized interventions: _____

NURSING DIAGNOSIS: *High risk for injury related to failure to recognize signs and symptoms indicating impending exacerbation*

Interventions

1. Teach the patient the signs and symptoms of impending exacerbation.

2. Emphasize the need to notify the doctor promptly if these symptoms occur, rather than altering the medication regimen without the doctor's knowledge.

3. Caution the patient to avoid overmedication.

4. Additional individualized interventions: _____

NURSING DIAGNOSIS: *Altered sexuality patterns related to shortness of breath, change in body image, deconditioning, change in relationship with spouse or partner, and adverse reactions to medications*

Interventions

1. Establish rapport with the patient and spouse (or partner). Discuss their feelings concerning changes in sexual functioning.

2. Help the patient learn or arrange therapies to optimize sexual function.

3. Additional individualized interventions: _____

PATIENT-FAMILY TEACHING CHECKLIST

___ practical energy conservation and breathing techniques

___ signs and symptoms of infection or exacerbation

CONDENSED PLANS OF CARE

___ all discharge medications' purpose, dosage, administration schedule, and adverse effects requiring medical attention (usual discharge medications include bronchodilators, corticosteroids, antibiotics, and expectorants)
___ bronchial hygiene measures
___ use, care, and cleaning of needed respiratory equipment
___ need for drinking 8 to 12 8-oz glasses of water per day
___ dietary restrictions
___ daily weight monitoring
___ avoiding exposure to infections and need for flu vaccination
___ avoiding lung irritants
___ exercise prescription
___ referrals to community agencies, as appropriate
___ date, time, and location of next appointment
___ how to contact the doctor

DOCUMENTATION CHECKLIST
___ clinical status on admission
___ significant changes in status
___ pertinent laboratory and diagnostic test findings, such as ABG levels
___ episodes of shortness of breath, including physical assessment parameters during each episode, treatment administered, and treatment outcome
___ respiratory status per shift
___ administration and outcome of therapies given
___ nutritional intake
___ fluid intake
___ exercise ability and activity level
___ patient-family teaching
___ discharge planning

ASSOCIATED PLANS OF CARE
Dying
Grieving
Ineffective Individual Coping
Knowledge Deficit
Pneumonia

Chronic Renal Failure

COLLABORATIVE PROBLEM: *High risk for hyperkalemia related to decreased renal excretion, metabolic acidosis, excessive dietary intake, blood transfusions, catabolism, and noncompliance with therapeutic regimen*
Interventions
1. Monitor serum potassium levels.
2. Assess for and report signs and symptoms of hyperkalemia.
3. Implement measures to prevent or treat metabolic acidosis, as ordered.
4. If blood transfusions are necessary, administer fresh-packed red blood cells (RBCs) during dialysis, as ordered.
5. Take measures to decrease catabolism.

6. Encourage compliance with the therapeutic regimen.
7. Implement and evaluate therapy for hyperkalemia.
8. Monitor serial serum potassium levels and electrocardiogram (ECG) for signs of hypokalemia during treatment.
9. Additional individualized interventions: _____

_____

COLLABORATIVE PROBLEM: *High risk for pericarditis, pericardial effusion, and pericardial tamponade related to uremia or inadequate dialysis*
Interventions
1. Assess for and report signs and symptoms of pericarditis.
2. Assess the adequacy of dialysis, and increase frequency as necessary and as ordered.
3. Assess for and report signs and symptoms of pericardial effusion and tamponade.
4. If tamponade develops, prepare the patient for emergency pericardial aspiration.
5. Encourage compliance with the therapeutic regimen.
6. Additional individualized interventions: _____

_____

COLLABORATIVE PROBLEM: *Hypertension related to sodium and water retention and malfunction of the renin-angiotensin-aldosterone system*
Interventions
1. Administer antihypertensive medications, as ordered, and assess for desired and adverse effects.
2. Measure and record blood pressure at various times of the day with the patient supine, sitting, and standing.
3. Teach the patient how to avoid orthostatic hypotension.
4. Encourage compliance with therapy.
5. Instruct the patient to report any changes that may indicate fluid overload.
6. Recognize the significance of funduscopic changes.
7. Additional individualized interventions: _____

_____

COLLABORATIVE PROBLEM: *Anemia related to decreased life span of RBCs in chronic renal failure (CRF), bleeding, decreased production of erythropoietin and RBCs, and blood loss during hemodialysis*
Interventions
1. Assess the degree of anemia and its physiologic effects.
2. Administer medications as ordered, and assess for desired and adverse effects.
3. Assist the patient to develop an activity and exercise schedule to avoid undue fatigue.
4. Avoid taking unnecessary blood specimens.
5. Instruct the patient how to prevent bleeding.
6. Administer blood transfusions as indicated and ordered.
7. Additional individualized interventions: _____

_____

COLLABORATIVE PROBLEM: *High risk for osteodystrophy and metastatic calcifications related to hyperphosphatemia, hypocalcemia, abnormal vitamin D metabolism, hyperparathyroidism, and elevated aluminum levels*

Interventions

1. Administer, and assess the effects of, phosphate binders, calcium supplements, and vitamin D supplements, as ordered.
• Weekly, monitor serum levels of calcium, phosphate, alkaline phosphatase, aluminum, and calcium-phosphate product; report abnormal findings.
• Monitor X-rays for bone fractures and joint deposits.
• Weekly, palpate joints for enlargement, swelling, and tenderness.
• Weekly, inspect the patient's gait, range of motion in joints, and muscle strength.
2. With the patient, develop an activity and exercise schedule to avoid immobilization.
3. Question the patient daily about signs and symptoms of hypocalcemia.
4. Monitor each ECG for prolonged QT interval, irritable arrhythmias, and atrioventricular conduction defects.
5. Assess daily for positive Chvostek's and Trousseau's signs.
6. Encourage the patient to comply with therapy.
7. Additional individualized interventions: _____

NURSING DIAGNOSIS: *High risk for nutritional deficit related to anorexia, nausea, vomiting, diarrhea, restricted dietary intake, GI inflammation with poor absorption, and altered metabolism of proteins, lipids, and carbohydrates*

Interventions

1. Assess nutritional status on admission.
2. Weigh the patient daily, comparing actual and ideal body weights.
3. Encourage the patient to eat the maximum amount of nutrients allowed. Encourage compliance with the dialysis regimen.
4. Encourage intake of foods high in calories from carbohydrates and low in protein, potassium, sodium, and water.
5. Consult with the dietitian to include the patient's preferences in the prescribed diet.
6. Implement interventions to reduce nausea and vomiting, diarrhea or constipation, and stomatitis.
7. Monitor indicators of dietary adequacy and compliance with dietary restrictions.
8. Additional individualized interventions: _____

NURSING DIAGNOSIS: *High risk for altered oral mucous membrane and unpleasant taste in mouth related to the accumulation of urea and ammonia*

Interventions

1. Inspect the oral mucous membrane on admission.
2. Teach the patient an appropriate mouth care regimen.
3. Encourage the patient to comply with therapy.
4. Additional individualized interventions: _____

COLLABORATIVE PROBLEM: *High risk for peripheral neuropathy related to effects of uremia, fluid and electrolyte imbalances, and acid-base imbalances on the peripheral nervous system*

Interventions

1. On admission, have a physical therapist assess muscle strength, gait, and degree of neuromuscular impairment.
2. Develop an activity and exercise regimen.
3. Guard against leg and foot trauma.
4. Administer analgesics, as ordered, and monitor effects.
5. Encourage the patient to comply with therapy.
6. Additional individualized interventions: _____

NURSING DIAGNOSIS: *High risk for impaired skin integrity related to decreased activity of oil and sweat glands, scratching, capillary fragility, abnormal blood clotting, anemia, retention of pigments, and deposition of calcium phosphate on the skin*

Interventions

1. Assess the skin for color, turgor, ecchymoses, texture, and edema.
2. Keep the skin clean while relieving dryness and itching; apply lotion, especially while skin is still moist after bathing.
3. Keep the patient's nails trimmed.
4. Monitor serum calcium and phosphorus levels weekly.
5. Administer phosphate binders, as ordered.
6. Administer antipruritic medications, as ordered.
7. Encourage the patient to comply with therapy.
8. Additional individualized interventions: _____

NURSING DIAGNOSIS: *High risk for altered thought processes related to the effects of uremic toxins, acidosis, fluid and electrolyte imbalances, and hypoxia on the central nervous system*

Interventions

1. On admission and daily, assess the patient's thought processes and compare them with premorbid intellectual status.
2. Alter communication methods as needed.
3. Minimize environmental stimuli. Alter the environment as needed.
4. Do not administer opiates or barbiturates.
5. Encourage the patient to comply with therapy.
6. Additional individualized interventions: _____

NURSING DIAGNOSIS: *High risk for noncompliance related to knowledge deficit; lack of resources; adverse effects of diet, dialysis, or medications; denial; and poor relationships with health care providers*

Interventions

1. Clarify the patient's understanding of the therapeutic regimen and the consequences of noncompliance.
2. Assess for factors that could contribute to noncompliance. Explore ways to alter the treatment regimen to fit the patient's social and cultural beliefs.

3. Teach the patient about areas of misunderstanding. Allow the patient to make as many decisions and choices from as many alternatives as possible.
4. Additional individualized interventions: _____

NURSING DIAGNOSIS: *High risk for sexual dysfunction related to the effects of uremia on the endocrine and nervous systems and to the psychosocial impact of CRF and its treatment*
Interventions
1. Discuss with the patient and spouse (or partner) the meaning of sexuality and reproduction to them, how changes in sexual functioning affect masculine and feminine roles, and mutual goals for their sexual functioning.
2. Discuss alternative methods of sexual expression.
3. Emphasize the importance of giving and receiving love and affection as alternatives to intercourse.
4. Consult with the doctor about the appropriateness of a penile prosthesis for a male patient.
5. Additional individualized interventions: _____

NURSING DIAGNOSIS: *Knowledge deficit related to vascular access care*
Interventions
1. Emphasize the importance of protecting the vascular access.
2. Whether the patient has a shunt or a fistula, explain measures to protect the affected extremity.
3. If the patient has an external shunt, teach these additional measures:
• Check shunt patency every 4 hours (look for blood and feel for thrill).
• If blood in the shunt has separated or a thrill is absent, contact a dialysis professional immediately.
• Perform daily shunt care.
• Observe the site for redness, swelling, or drainage.
• Keep bulldog clamps on the dressing.
• Do not pull on the tubing.
• If the shunt separates, clamp and reconnect it, then notify the doctor.
• If the shunt dislodges, apply firm pressure. If bleeding is minimal and stops, notify the nephrologist. If bleeding is profuse or continues, go to the emergency department.
4. If the patient has an internal fistula, teach these additional measures:
• Assess patency daily (feel for pulsations).
• If pulsation is absent, contact a nephrology professional immediately.
• If a pressure dressing is applied after dialysis, remove it after 4 hours.
• Check needle insertion sites for bleeding for 4 hours after dialysis.
5. Additional individualized interventions: _____

PATIENT-FAMILY TEACHING CHECKLIST
___ cause and implications of renal failure
___ purpose of dialysis

___ for all discharge medication: purpose, dosage, administration schedule, desired effects, and adverse effects (usual discharge medications include antihypertensives, phosphate binders, calcium, vitamin D, folic acid, iron, vitamins B and C, and others, depending on patient's response to the disease)
___ recommended diet and fluid modifications
___ common problems related to CRF and their management
___ care of the shunt and fistula (if receiving hemodialysis) or peritoneal catheter (if receiving peritoneal dialysis)
___ how to obtain and record weight
___ how to measure and record blood pressure and pulse
___ how to maintain an intake and output record
___ problems to report to health care provider
___ financial and community resources to assist with treatment of CRF
___ dialysis schedule, location of dialysis facility, and day and time of appointments
___ resources for counseling
___ how to contact doctor or nephrology nurse

DOCUMENTATION CHECKLIST
___ clinical status on admission
___ significant changes in status
___ pertinent laboratory and diagnostic test findings
___ response to medication
___ physical and psychological response to dialysis therapy
___ nutritional intake
___ activity and exercise tolerance
___ ability to perform self-care
___ compliance with therapy
___ patient-family teaching
___ postdischarge referrals and plans for long-term and follow-up care

ASSOCIATED PLANS OF CARE
Anemia
Dying
Grieving
Ineffective Individual Coping
Knowledge Deficit
Pain
Peritoneal Dialysis

Colostomy

COLLABORATIVE PROBLEM: *High risk for stomal necrosis related to the surgical procedure, bowel wall edema, or traction on the mesentery*
Interventions
1. Assess and document stoma color every 8 hours during the first 4 days after surgery.
2. If the stoma is ischemic or necrotic, check the viability of the proximal bowel.
3. Notify the doctor promptly if necrosis extends to the fascia level.

4. Implement measures to prevent or minimize abdominal distention.
5. Additional individualized interventions: _____

COLLABORATIVE PROBLEM: *High risk for stomal retraction related to mucocutaneous separation*
Interventions
1. Assess and document the integrity of the mucocutaneous suture line at each pouch change.
2. Initiate and document nutritional support measures for the patient at risk for nutritional deficiency.
3. Request vitamin A supplements for the patient receiving steroids.
4. For the patient with a loop colostomy stabilized by a rod or bridge, expect that the loop support will not be removed until the stoma granulates to the abdominal wall.
5. If mucocutaneous separation occurs, alter the pouch system to prevent fecal contamination of exposed subcutaneous tissue.
6. Additional individualized interventions: _____

NURSING DIAGNOSIS: *High risk for impaired skin integrity: peristomal skin breakdown related to fecal contamination of skin*
Interventions
1. Have an enterostomal therapy nurse mark the optimal stoma site before surgery, if possible.
2. Select a pouch system that matches the patient's abdominal contours.
3. Use pouching principles and products that will provide a secure pouch seal and protect the skin from stool and tape.
4. Change the pouch every 5 to 7 days and as needed if leakage, burning, or itching occurs.
5. Treat any denudation with absorptive powder and sealant or water.
6. Additional individualized interventions: _____

NURSING DIAGNOSIS: *Knowledge deficit related to unfamiliarity with altered bowel functioning involved in a descending or sigmoid colostomy*
Interventions
1. Assess the patient's candidacy for bowel function regulation by irrigation.
2. If the patient meets feasibility criteria, discuss management options.
3. Help the patient explore the options.
4. Establish a teaching plan based on the patient's decision.
5. Additional individualized interventions: _____

NURSING DIAGNOSIS: *High risk for body-image disturbance related to loss of control over fecal elimination*
Interventions
1. Teach the patient odor-control measures.
2. Teach the patient measures to reduce and control flatus.
3. Teach the patient how to conceal the pouch under clothing.
4. Discuss the normal emotional response to colostomy with the patient and family; include helpful coping strategies.
5. Offer information on the United Ostomy Association; arrange for an ostomy visitor if the patient wishes.
6. Discuss colostomy management during occupational, social, and sexual activity. Teach the patient to role-play difficult situations.
7. Additional individualized interventions: _____

NURSING DIAGNOSIS: *High risk for sexual dysfunction related to change in body image or damage to autonomic nerves (nerve damage applies only to the patient with a rectal resection, a particularly wide resection for cancer)*
Interventions
1. Discuss with patient (and spouse or partner, if possible) the importance of openness and honesty as well as the fact that both must adapt to the ostomy.
2. Teach the patient measures for securing and concealing the pouch during sexual activity.
3. For a female with a wide rectal resection, discuss the possible need for artificial lubrication.
4. For a male with a wide rectal resection, explain potential interference with erection and ejaculation; explain that no loss of sensation or orgasmic potential will occur; explore alternatives to intercourse as indicated; and reinforce the importance of intimacy.
5. Additional individualized interventions: _____

PATIENT-FAMILY TEACHING CHECKLIST
___ reason for colostomy
___ colostomy's impact on bowel function
___ normal stoma characteristics and function
___ pouch-emptying procedure
___ pouch-changing procedure
___ peristomal skin care
___ colostomy irrigation procedure (if applicable)
___ management of mucous fistula stoma (if applicable)
___ flatus and odor control
___ management of diarrhea and constipation
___ normal adaptation process and feelings after colostomy
___ community resources available for support
___ recommendations affecting resumption of preoperative life-style
___ potential alteration in sexual function (if applicable)
___ sources of colostomy supplies and reimbursement procedures for them

CONDENSED PLANS OF CARE

___ signs and symptoms to report to the doctor

___ need for follow-up appointment with the doctor (and enterostomal therapy nurse, if available)

___ how to contact the doctor

DOCUMENTATION CHECKLIST

___ clinical status on admission

___ significant changes in clinical status

___ GI tract function (bowel sounds, NG tube output, and colostomy output)

___ stoma color and status of mucocutaneous suture line

___ oral intake and tolerance

___ episodes of abdominal distention, nausea, and vomiting

___ incisional status (any signs of infection)

___ stoma location and abdominal contours

___ management plan, including pouching system selected (and decision about irrigation for patient with descending or sigmoid colostomy)

___ peristomal skin status

___ emotional response to colostomy and discussion of coping strategies

___ patient-family teaching

___ discharge planning

ASSOCIATED PLANS OF CARE

Grieving

Ineffective Family Coping

Ineffective Individual Coping

Knowledge Deficit

Pain

Surgical Intervention

Congestive Heart Failure

COLLABORATIVE PROBLEM: *Decreased cardiac output related to decreased contractility, altered heart rhythm, fluid volume overload, or increased afterload*

Interventions

1. Monitor and document heart rate and rhythm, heart sounds, blood pressure, pulse pressure, and the presence or absence of peripheral pulses.

2. Administer cardiac medications, as ordered, and document the patient's response. Observe for therapeutic and adverse effects.

3. Observe for signs and symptoms of hypoxemia. Ensure adequate oxygenation with proper positioning and administration of supplemental oxygen, as ordered.

4. Ensure adequate rest.

5. Monitor fluid status: obtain accurate daily weight, maintain accurate intake and output records, assess lung sounds, assess for dependent edema, and assess for dehydration.

6. Assess for increasing confusion.

7. Decrease the patient's fear and anxiety.

8. Additional individualized interventions: _____

NURSING DIAGNOSIS: *Fluid volume excess related to decreased myocardial contractility, decreased renal perfusion, or increased sodium and water retention*

Interventions

1. See Appendix C, "Fluid and Electrolyte Imbalances."

2. Monitor hourly fluid intake and output and 24-hour fluid balance. Weigh the patient daily.

3. Administer I.V. solutions, as ordered; avoid saline solutions.

4. If the patient is placed on fluid restriction, explain the rationale and establish a fluid intake schedule. Teach the patient how to record oral fluids and use microdrip tubing or an infusion pump to control I.V. intake.

5. Monitor serum creatinine and blood urea nitrogen levels.

6. Monitor serum sodium and potassium levels.

7. Additional individualized interventions: _____

NURSING DIAGNOSIS: *Activity intolerance related to bed rest and decreased cardiac output*

Interventions

1. Determine cardiac stability by evaluating blood pressure, heart rate and rhythm, and indicators of oxygenation.

2. When the patient is stable, institute a graduated activity program according to unit protocol.

3. Evaluate patient tolerance to new activities.

4. Alternate activity with rest periods.

5. Administer anticoagulants, as ordered.

6. Teach the patient how to avoid Valsalva's maneuver.

7. Additional individualized interventions: _____

NURSING DIAGNOSIS: *Nutritional deficit related to decreased appetite and unpalatability of low-sodium diet*

Interventions

1. Keep a daily record of caloric intake. Consult with the dietitian to identify caloric needs.

2. Assess the patient's food preferences, and plan meals to meet treatment requirements and patient needs.

3. Additional individualized interventions: _____

NURSING DIAGNOSIS: *Knowledge deficit related to complex disease process and treatment*

Interventions

1. Once the patient is stable, institute a structured teaching plan. See "Knowledge Deficit" plan, page 56.

2. Briefly explain the pathophysiology of heart failure.

3. Emphasize the patient's role in controlling the disease and the importance of medical follow-up.

4. Explain the rationale for dietary restrictions.

5. Explain the rationale for activity restrictions.

6. Teach about discharge medications.

7. Emphasize the importance of self-monitoring for signs and symptoms of increasing heart failure.

8. Discuss with the patient and family a plan for emergency care.
9. Review the plan for follow-up care.
10. Additional individualized interventions: _____

NURSING DIAGNOSIS: *High risk for noncompliance related to complicated treatment regimen, health beliefs, or negative relationship with caregivers*
Interventions
1. Observe for indicators of noncompliance.
2. Evaluate the extent and result of noncompliance.
3. Differentiate noncompliance from other problems.
4. Initiate discussion of the situation with the patient and family, involving a psychiatric clinician or other care team members as needed.
5. Express concern for the patient as a person.
6. Emphasize the seriousness of congestive heart failure (CHF) and the importance of self-care.
7. Discuss the following with the patient: life priorities, perception of prognosis, feelings about the illness's length, complexity of treatment, degree of confidence in caregivers, and health care beliefs.
8. Consider the patient's cultural and spiritual heritage.
9. Ask the patient about satisfaction with caregivers.
10. Validate conclusions about reasons for behavior with the patient and loved ones.
11. Collaborate with other caregivers to reevaluate the goals and implementation of care.
12. Search for alternative solutions.
13. Use creative negotiation strategies to set goals with the patient.
14. If the patient makes an informed choice not to follow the recommendations, and if negotiation is not possible:
• avoid punitive responses, and accept the decision
• keep open the option for treatment
• respect the patient's readiness to die, if present.
15. Additional individualized interventions: _____

PATIENT-FAMILY TEACHING CHECKLIST
___ cause and implications of CHF
___ signs and symptoms of increasing CHF
___ all discharge medications' purpose, dosage, administration schedule, and adverse effects requiring medical attention (usual discharge medications include inotropes, diuretics, vasodilators, and anticoagulants)
___ need for life-style modifications
___ dietary restrictions
___ activity restrictions
___ plan for follow-up care
___ plan for emergency care
___ how to contact the doctor

DOCUMENTATION CHECKLIST
___ clinical status on admission
___ significant changes in clinical status
___ pertinent laboratory and diagnostic test findings
___ fluid intake and output
___ nutritional intake

___ response to activity progression
___ response to illness and hospitalization
___ family's response to illness
___ patient-family teaching
___ discharge planning

ASSOCIATED PLANS OF CARE
Acute Myocardial Infarction – Critical Care Unit Phase
Acute Myocardial Infarction – Stepdown Unit Phase
Chronic Renal Failure
Dying
Grieving
Ineffective Individual Coping
Knowledge Deficit

Diabetes Mellitus

COLLABORATIVE PROBLEM: *Hyperglycemia related to inadequate endogenous insulin (Type I diabetes mellitus) or inadequate endogenous insulin and insulin resistance (Type II diabetes mellitus)*
Interventions
1. Administer insulin I.V., I.M., or subcutaneously, or oral hypoglycemics.
2. Establish and maintain an I.V. fluid infusion. Monitor for signs of dehydration. Keep an accurate intake and output record.
3. Monitor fingerstick blood glucose and urine ketone levels.
4. Observe for signs of hypoglycemia. If any occur, notify the doctor, obtain blood glucose measurements immediately, and treat immediately with I.V. glucose, glucagon, or oral glucose, depending on protocol and the patient's level of responsiveness.
5. In Type I diabetes mellitus (DM), observe for signs of diabetic ketoacidosis (DKA). If any occur, notify the doctor immediately, obtain blood glucose measurements immediately, and treat according to protocol.
6. In Type II DM, observe for signs of hyperosmolar hyperglycemic nonketotic syndrome (HHNKS). If suspected, notify the doctor immediately.
7. Additional individualized interventions: _____

NURSING DIAGNOSIS: *Knowledge deficit related to newly diagnosed complex chronic disease*
Interventions
1. See the "Knowledge Deficit" plan, page 56.
2. Teach the significance of insulin or oral hypoglycemics for disease control. Demonstrate injection techniques. Link medication needs to other factors, such as diet and exercise. Ensure that the patient and family are aware of signs and treatment of hypoglycemia and the protocol for managing persistent hyperglycemia, DKA, or HHNKS.
3. Involve the patient, family, and dietitian in planning a therapeutic diet.
4. Teach blood glucose or urine ketone testing methods for home use.

5. Emphasize the importance of regular activity and exercise and of maintaining the same level of activity from day to day.
6. Teach or review "sick day" management techniques.
7. Tell the patient to be aware of increased susceptibility to infections; discuss ways to avoid exposure.
8. Discuss vascular complications of DM.
• Teach the patient how to perform foot care, skin care, leg exercises, and to assess circulatory status; observe return demonstration of all techniques. If the patient smokes, emphasize the importance of quitting. Ensure that the patient and family receive a written foot care plan.
• Discuss potential eye complications of DM. Emphasize the importance of early reporting of vision changes.
• Teach the symptoms of urinary tract infection and renal impairment, and emphasize the importance of prompt treatment.
• Emphasize importance of annual kidney function evaluation.
9. Discuss the implications of diabetic neuropathy.
10. Additional individualized interventions: _____

NURSING DIAGNOSIS: *High risk for altered health maintenance related to lack of material resources, lack of support, or ineffective coping*
Interventions
1. Assess the patient's resources, including financial management capabilities and family support system.
2. Involve the family in all teaching and planning.
3. Arrange appropriate follow-up home health visits before discharge.
4. Link the patient and family with community resources and mutual support groups.
5. Encourage verbalization of feelings, and support healthy coping behaviors. See the "Ineffective Individual Coping" plan, page 51.
6. Additional individualized interventions: _____

PATIENT-FAMILY TEACHING CHECKLIST
___ disease and implications
___ for all medications: purpose, dosage, administration schedule, and adverse effects requiring medical attention (usual discharge medications include insulin or oral hypoglycemics)
___ blood glucose and urine ketone testing
___ interrelationship of diet, exercise, and other factors in disease management
___ hypoglycemia (signs and symptoms, possible causes, treatment, and prevention)
___ hyperglycemia (signs and symptoms, possible causes, treatment, and prevention)
___ diet management
___ exercise regimen
___ foot care
___ signs of infection and appropriate treatment
___ signs and implications of neuropathy
___ symptoms of retinopathy and need to report them
___ signs and symptoms of urinary or renal complications and need to report them

___ community resources
___ when and how to access emergency medical treatment
___ date, time, and location of follow-up appointments
___ how to contact the doctor
___ written materials, insulin, and syringes, as provided

DOCUMENTATION CHECKLIST
___ clinical status on admission
___ significant changes in status
___ pertinent laboratory and diagnostic test findings
___ episodes of hyperglycemia or hypoglycemia
___ dietary intake and planning
___ activity and exercise regimen
___ medication therapy
___ I.V. line patency
___ patient-family teaching
___ discharge planning and availability of community resources

ASSOCIATED PLANS OF CARE
Chronic Renal Failure
Diabetic Ketoacidosis
Grieving
Hyperosmolar Hyperglycemic Nonketotic Syndrome
Hypoglycemia
Ineffective Individual Coping
Knowledge Deficit
Retinal Detachment
Thrombophlebitis

Diabetic Ketoacidosis

COLLABORATIVE PROBLEM: *Hypovolemia related to osmotic diuresis or vomiting, or both*
Interventions
1. Monitor for signs and symptoms of dehydration and shock. Continuously monitor blood pressure and cardiac rate and rhythm.
2. Observe for signs and symptoms of electrolyte imbalances (see Appendix C, "Fluid and Electrolyte Imbalances" for details):
• hyperkalemia in the first 1 to 4 hours of treatment
• hypokalemia after 1 to 4 hours of treatment
• hyponatremia early in treatment
• hypernatremia later in treatment
• anion gap greater than 12.
3. Monitor serum osmolality and electrolyte values, as ordered.
4. On admission, establish and maintain one or more I.V. lines in large peripheral veins.
5. Monitor intake and output (I&O) and urine specific gravity meticulously. Weigh the patient daily, and document findings. Insert an indwelling urinary catheter, as ordered.
6. Administer I.V. solutions, as ordered, typically:
• normal saline solution, 1 to 2 liters in the first 2 hours
• 0.45% sodium chloride, after the first few hours, or 0.45% sodium chloride with 5% dextrose in water when blood glucose level reaches 250 mg/dl or urine glucose level is less than 1%

• plasma volume expanders, such as albumin, if dehydration is severe (administer only after normal saline solution administration is underway).

7. Administer therapy for electrolyte imbalances, as ordered.

8. For at least 24 hours after rapid fluid repletion, observe for signs and symptoms of pulmonary edema. If any are present, alert the doctor immediately.

9. Additional individualized interventions: _____

COLLABORATIVE PROBLEM: *Hyperglycemia related to decreased cellular glucose uptake and use*
Interventions
1. Assess blood glucose levels on admission and as ordered. Perform bedside fingerstick monitoring of blood glucose every hour until normal, then every 6 hours; then before meals and at bedtime; or as ordered.
2. Assess blood ketone level on admission and as ordered. Perform bedside urine monitoring every void until ketone level is low, then every 6 hours or before meals and at bedtime.
3. Administer insulin, as ordered.
4. Alert the doctor when the blood glucose level reaches 250 mg/dl.
5. Observe for signs and symptoms of medication-induced hypoglycemia.
6. Additional individualized interventions: _____

NURSING DIAGNOSIS: *Sensory-perceptual alteration related to cerebral dehydration, decreased perfusion, hypoxemia, or acidosis*
Interventions
1. Implement standard safety precautions.
2. Monitor level of consciousness (LOC) constantly.
3. Additional individualized interventions: _____

COLLABORATIVE PROBLEM: *Acidosis related to altered LOC, ketosis, and decreased tissue perfusion*
Interventions
1. Maintain a patent airway.
2. Monitor respiratory status hourly.
3. Anticipate intubation and mechanical ventilation if increasing respiratory distress is present.
4. Administer oxygen, as ordered.
5. Monitor arterial blood gas levels, as ordered.
6. Administer I.V. sodium bicarbonate, as ordered.
7. While the patient is acutely ill, withhold food and fluids, even if the patient is extremely thirsty. Auscultate bowel sounds every 8 hours. Insert a gastric tube, as ordered, and connect to suction.
8. Additional individualized interventions: _____

NURSING DIAGNOSIS: *Knowledge deficit related to complex disease and therapy*
Interventions
1. Refer to the "Knowledge Deficit" plan, page 56.
2. When the patient's condition allows, determine learning needs.
3. When the patient's condition allows, begin a teaching program.
4. Use the patient's symptomatic episode as a teaching tool. Involve the family members in all teaching sessions.
5. As appropriate, initiate teaching about diabetes. Refer to the "Diabetes Mellitus" plan, page 523.
6. Document learning needs and teaching.
7. Additional individualized interventions: _____

PATIENT-FAMILY TEACHING CHECKLIST
___ sick day management
___ cause and implications of diabetes mellitus
___ causes of diabetic ketoacidosis, including signs and symptoms and appropriate responses
___ significance of insulin
___ signs, symptoms, and interventions for hyperglycemia and hypoglycemia
___ dietary management
___ exercise plan
___ blood glucose and urine ketone testing
___ plan for completing unmet learning needs, including use of community and outpatient resources

DOCUMENTATION CHECKLIST
___ clinical status on admission
___ significant changes in status
___ pertinent diagnostic test findings
___ I.V. fluid therapy
___ pharmacologic intervention
___ oxygen administration
___ patient-family teaching
___ discharge planning

ASSOCIATED PLANS OF CARE
Acute Renal Failure
Diabetes Mellitus
Hyperosmolar Hyperglycemic Nonketotic Syndrome
Hypoglycemia
Hypovolemic Shock
Knowledge Deficit
Sensory-Perceptual Alteration

Disseminated Intravascular Coagulation

COLLABORATIVE PROBLEM: *High risk for hemorrhage related to consumption of clotting factors, increased fibrinolysis, and presence of endogenous anticoagulants*
Interventions
1. Collaborate with the doctor to identify and treat the cause of disseminated intravascular coagulation (DIC).

2. Monitor the presence and degree of hemorrhage.

3. Monitor coagulation panel, as ordered.

4. Administer heparin, if ordered. Monitor the activated partial thromboplastin time.

5. Administer transfusion therapy, as ordered.

6. Maintain a normal blood pressure by giving fluid and medications, as ordered.

7. Monitor for the development of fluid overload.

8. Additional individualized interventions: _____

_____

COLLABORATIVE PROBLEM: *Ischemia related to microcirculatory thrombosis*

1. Assess status of organ systems at least every 4 hours, including:
- neurologic function
- cardiovascular function
- gastrointestinal function.

2. Monitor renal function closely. Document hourly urine output.

3. As ordered, implement measures (such as fluid administration) to treat the underlying cause of tissue ischemia.

4. Additional individualized interventions: _____

_____

COLLABORATIVE PROBLEM: *High risk for hypoxemia related to increased pulmonary shunting, anemia, and acidosis*

Interventions

1. Monitor arterial blood gas levels, as ordered.

2. Assess physical indicators of pulmonary status at least every 4 hours.

3. Administer supplemental oxygen, positive end-expiratory pressure, or mechanical ventilation, as ordered.

4. Additional individualized interventions: _____

_____

NURSING DIAGNOSIS: *Impaired skin integrity related to capillary fragility*

Interventions

1. Avoid needle punctures, whenever possible. If necessary, use the smallest needle gauge possible and apply pressure afterward.

2. Handle the patient very gently.

3. Use cushioning and pressure-relieving devices.

4. Provide gentle mouth care.

5. Additional individualized interventions: _____

_____

NURSING DIAGNOSIS: *Pain related to tissue ischemia, hematomas, or bleeding into organ or joint capsules*

Interventions

1. Assess for pain frequently. Consult the "Pain" plan, page 69, for details.

2. Administer pain medications I.V.

3. Additional individualized interventions: _____

_____

PATIENT-FAMILY TEACHING CHECKLIST

___ basic pathophysiology and implications of DIC

___ rationale for therapy

___ pain relief measures

DOCUMENTATION CHECKLIST

___ clinical status on admission

___ significant changes in status

___ pertinent diagnostic test findings

___ bleeding episodes

___ transfusion and fluid replacement therapy

___ pain relief measures

___ patient-family teaching

___ discharge planning

ASSOCIATED PLANS OF CARE

Acute Renal Failure
Adult Respiratory Distress Syndrome
Cardiac Surgery
Hypovolemic Shock
Impaired Physical Mobility
Ineffective Individual Coping
Liver Failure
Major Burns
Mechanical Ventilation
Multiple Trauma
Nutritional Deficit
Pain

Duodenal Ulcer

COLLABORATIVE PROBLEM: *High risk for GI hemorrhage related to extension of duodenal ulcer into the submucosal layer of the intestinal lining*

Interventions

1. Observe for and report signs of GI hemorrhage.

2. Institute nasogastric intubation, if ordered.

3. Institute continuous saline lavage, if ordered.

4. If the patient is actively bleeding, check vital signs hourly (or more frequently if unstable) and report any deterioration in status.

5. Treat hypovolemia if it occurs.

6. Prepare the patient for surgery, if indicated.

7. Maintain the patient on bed rest after the bleeding episode.

8. Additional individualized interventions: _____

_____

NURSING DIAGNOSIS: *Pain related to increased hydrochloric acid secretion or increased spasm, intragastric pressure, and motility of upper GI tract*

Interventions

1. Administer ulcer-healing medications and document their use.

2. Provide bed rest and a quiet environment.

3. Teach and reinforce the role of diet in ulcer healing.

4. Encourage adequate caloric intake from the basic food groups at regular intervals. Encourage frequent small meals.

5. Teach and reinforce required life-style changes.
6. Encourage the patient who smokes to quit.
7. Teach the patient signs and symptoms indicating ulcer recurrence and bleeding.
8. Additional individualized interventions: _____

PATIENT-FAMILY TEACHING CHECKLIST
__ nature and implications of disease
__ pain relief measures
__ all discharge medications' purpose, dosage, administration schedule, and adverse effects requiring medical attention (usual discharge medications include antacids, H_2-receptor antagonists, or both)
__ recommended dietary modifications
__ need for smoking cessation program (if applicable)
__ stress reduction measures
__ signs and symptoms of ulcer recurrence and GI bleeding
__ date, time, and location of follow-up appointment
__ how to contact the doctor

DOCUMENTATION CHECKLIST
__ clinical status on admission
__ significant changes in status
__ pain relief measures
__ nutritional intake and intolerances
__ pertinent diagnostic test findings
__ medication administration
__ patient teaching
__ discharge planning

ASSOCIATED PLANS OF CARE
Esophagitis and Gastroenteritis
Gastrointestinal Hemorrhage
Ineffective Individual Coping
Knowledge Deficit
Pain

Femoral Popliteal Bypass

COLLABORATIVE PROBLEM: *Arterial insufficiency related to arterial graft occlusion, reperfusion injury, or coexisting microangiopathy associated with diabetes or microemboli*
Interventions
1. Assess and document appearance of surgical site.
2. Note the contours of the surgical site and compare with the opposite side.
3. Measure calf circumference hourly for the first 24 hours, then as condition warrants.
4. Position the leg to avoid hyperextension and undue pressure on graft site.
5. Observe for signs and symptoms of fluid volume deficit or hypotension.
6. Administer ordered drugs and monitor for adverse reactions.
7. Observe for signs and symptoms of reperfusion injury.

8. Additional individualized interventions: _____

NURSING DIAGNOSIS: *Impaired skin integrity related to surgical incision and possible preexisting stasis ul-*

Interventions
1. Maintain strict aseptic technique in caring for the surgical wound, drains, and stasis ulcers of the feet and legs.
2. Do not administer injections on the affected side.
3. Assess for signs of infection.
4. Administer antibiotics and observe for adverse reactions.
5. Reposition the patient and perform skin care every 2 hours. Consider using a specialty bed or mattress for the patient with a chronic mobility problem.
6. Monitor and document fluid and food intake.
7. Additional individualized interventions: _____

NURSING DIAGNOSIS: *Impaired physical mobility related to surgery and preexisting disability*
Interventions
1. Before surgery, instruct patient about positioning the affected extremity.
2. After surgery, maintain the patient on bed rest as ordered, usually for 24 to 48 hours. Position the affected joint as ordered.
3. Encourage active or passive range-of-motion exercises of all unaffected joints 3 to 4 times daily.
4. Collaborate with the health care team to design an appropriate rehabilitation program.
5. Additional individualized interventions: _____

NURSING DIAGNOSIS: *Pain associated with the surgical incision*
Interventions
1. See the "Pain" plan, page 69.
2. Identify and document the source and degree of pain, using an analog scale. Instruct the patient to report unrelieved pain.
3. Elevate the affected extremity.
4. Administer pain medication, as necessary, and observe for adverse reactions.
5. Additional individualized interventions: _____

PATIENT-FAMILY TEACHING CHECKLIST
__ medication regimen
__ proper positioning
__ desirable life-style changes, such as smoking cessation
__ rehabilitation regimen
__ date and times of follow-up care
__ symptoms of infection
__ symptoms of arterial insufficiency
__ symptoms requiring medical intervention

CONDENSED PLANS OF CARE

DOCUMENTATION CHECKLIST
___ clinical status on admission
___ significant changes in the preoperative state
___ completion of preoperative checklist
___ preoperative teaching
___ clinical status on admission from postanesthesia unit
___ amount and character of drainage from wounds or drains
___ tube patency
___ pain relief measures
___ activity tolerance
___ nutritional intake
___ elimination status
___ pertinent laboratory finding
___ patient-family teaching
___ discharge planning
___ clinical status upon discharge

ASSOCIATED PLANS OF CARE
Amputation
Pain
Surgical Intervention

Gastrointestinal Hemorrhage

COLLABORATIVE PROBLEM: *High risk for hypovolemic shock related to blood loss*
Interventions
1. See the "Hypovolemic Shock" plan, page 346.
2. Assess the amount of blood loss using the following procedures:
• Maintain accurate intake and output records, including precise measurement and guaiac testing of all vomitus and stools.
• Evaluate vital signs for orthostatic changes every 4 hours, unless the patient is syncopal, frankly hypotensive, or severely tachycardic when supine.
• Evaluate vital signs, hemodynamic pressures, and electrocardiogram (ECG).
• Obtain appropriate laboratory studies, as ordered, including complete blood count, blood urea nitrogen, and creatinine level.
• Assess the patient frequently for clinical signs of hypovolemia.
• Insert and maintain a gastric tube, as ordered, and check drainage for blood.
3. Replace blood loss by:
• establishing and maintaining I.V. access with one or two large-bore cannulas
• rapidly administering I.V. crystalloid solution
• administering and monitoring the response to transfusion of packed red blood cells, fresh frozen plasma, or other blood components as well as volume expanders, as ordered. Prepare the patient for emergency surgery if necessary.

4. Initiate measures to stop bleeding, as ordered, such as:
• maintaining activity restrictions, which usually includes strict bed rest
• performing gastric lavage, usually with room temperature or iced normal saline solution, with or without addition of norepinephrine (Levophed) to the solution; question orders for iced lavage
• administering vasopressin (Pitressin) I.V.
• assisting with insertion, monitoring, and maintaining the placement of a Sengstaken-Blakemore tube or other compression tubes
• preparing the patient with uncontrollable bleeding, if a poor surgical risk, for injection sclerotherapy; after injection, observe for rebleeding, chest pain, fever, and other complications
• preparing the patient for laser therapy, if ordered
• administering vitamin K, (phytonadione [Aqua-MEPHYTON]) I.M., as ordered
• preparing the patient for surgery if bleeding requires more than 2 units of blood per hour to maintain blood pressure, requires more than 6 to 8 units of blood, exceeds more than 2,500 ml in the first 24 hours, or recurs during therapy.
5. Administer medications to control gastric acidity. Monitor gastric aspirate pH and adjust dosage, as ordered, to maintain a pH greater than 4.0. Observe for signs and symptoms of drug interactions and toxicity.
6. Prepare the patient and family for and assist with diagnostic procedures, as ordered, such as endoscopic examination, angiography, or other studies.
7. Additional individualized interventions: _____

_____

NURSING DIAGNOSIS: *High risk for injury: complications related to undetected bleeding, inadequate organ perfusion, accumulation of toxins, electrolyte imbalance, release of procoagulants, or ulcer perforation*
Interventions
1. Continue to perform guaiac tests on all gastric contents and stools at least daily, even after the patient's condition has stabilized.
2. Immediately report and thoroughly investigate any complaint of chest pain.
3. Monitor renal and hepatic function. Note daily serum electrolyte values.
4. Observe for bleeding from other sites.
5. Immediately report any complaint of sudden, severe abdominal pain or rigidity, and prepare the patient for surgery if these occur.
6. Additional individualized interventions: _____

_____

NURSING DIAGNOSIS: *Fear related to sight of blood and distressing physical symptoms*
Interventions
1. Provide care promptly. Avoid expressing dismay or revulsion at the sight of bleeding. Acknowledge the patient's fear.

2. Encourage verbalization of feelings. See the "Ineffective Individual Coping" plan, page 51.
3. Accept expressions of anxiety related to the possibility of death. See the "Dying" plan, page 11.
4. Additional individualized interventions: _____

NURSING DIAGNOSIS: *Knowledge deficit related to potential recurrent bleeding*
Interventions
1. See the "Knowledge Deficit" plan, page 56.
2. Defer detailed teaching until the patient is alert and physiologically stable. Then, as indicated by condition, discuss with the patient:
• precipitating or contributing factors of bleeding episode
• signs and symptoms indicating possible recurrence
• other causes of dark stools
• dietary recommendations.
3. Additional individualized interventions: _____

PATIENT-FAMILY TEACHING CHECKLIST
___ cause and site of bleeding
___ precipitating or contributing factors
___ signs and symptoms indicating possible recurrence of bleeding
___ dietary recommendations, if any

DOCUMENTATION CHECKLIST
___ clinical status on admission
___ significant changes in status
___ pertinent diagnostic test findings
___ bleeding episodes
___ fluid and blood replacement measures
___ intake and output
___ emotional response
___ pharmacologic interventions
___ procedures to stop bleeding
___ patient-family teaching
___ discharge planning

ASSOCIATED PLANS OF CARE
Acute Renal Failure
Disseminated Intravascular Coagulation
Dying
Hypovolemic Shock
Impaired Physical Mobility
Ineffective Individual Coping
Knowledge Deficit
Liver Failure
Nutritional Deficit
Pancreatitis

Hypoglycemia

NURSING DIAGNOSIS: *High risk for injury related to inappropriate exogenous insulin use, lack of food, or excessive exercise*
Interventions
1. Observe for signs and symptoms of hypoglycemia constantly.
2. Document suspected hypoglycemia with bedside glucose fingerstick or serum glucose, following hospital protocol.
3. Treat hypoglycemia promptly, according to protocol.
4. Recheck the glucose level 15 minutes after treatment. Repeat treatment if glucose level remains low.
5. If hypoglycemia occurs frequently, consult the doctor.
6. Additional individualized interventions: _____

NURSING DIAGNOSIS: *Knowledge deficit related to complex disease*
Interventions
1. Once the hypoglycemic episode is over, use it as a learning experience.
2. Review the signs and symptoms of hypoglycemia with the patient and family.
3. Discuss appropriate treatment strategies for hypoglycemia with the patient and family.
4. Review strategies to prevent hypoglycemia with the patient and family.
5. Additional individualized interventions: _____

PATIENT-FAMILY TEACHING CHECKLIST
___ cause and significance of hypoglycemia
___ signs and symptoms
___ preventive measures
___ treatment strategies
___ proper use of insulin or oral agents
___ dietary management
___ exercise and activity plan
___ blood glucose monitoring
___ urine ketone testing (for Type I DM only)
___ chronic complications related to diabetes mellitus
___ learning needs at time of discharge
___ community resources

DOCUMENTATION CHECKLIST
___ clinical status on admission
___ significant changes in status
___ pertinent laboratory and diagnostic test findings
___ I.V. fluid therapy
___ pharmacologic intervention
___ patient-family teaching
___ discharge planning

ASSOCIATED PLANS OF CARE
Diabetic Ketoacidosis
Hyperosmolar Hyperglycemic Nonketotic Syndrome
Hypovolemic Shock
Knowledge Deficit

Hypovolemic Shock

COLLABORATIVE PROBLEM: *Hypovolemic shock related to blood loss, diuresis, dehydration, or third-space fluid shift*
Interventions
1. If the patient has active external bleeding, apply direct, continuous pressure and elevate the area, if possible.
2. Observe for signs and symptoms of fluid loss.
3. Elevate the patient's legs above heart level, unless there is active bleeding from the head and neck or suspected increased intracranial pressure or cardiogenic shock.
4. Obtain initial and serial diagnostic tests.
5. Insert and maintain the following, as ordered:
• two or more large-bore I.V. lines
• indwelling urinary catheter
• central venous pressure (CVP) catheter or pulmonary artery (PA) catheter.
6. Monitor urine output and CVP or pulmonary capillary wedge pressure every 15 minutes to 1 hour.
7. Administer a fluid challenge, if ordered.
8. Administer blood products and crystalloid or colloid I.V. solutions, as ordered.
9. Monitor arterial blood pressure and mean arterial pressure by arterial line or sphygmomanometer.
10. During all fluid administration, monitor the trend of hemodynamic measurements and urine output. Observe for signs of fluid overload.
11. Additional individualized interventions: _____

COLLABORATIVE PROBLEM: *Hypoxemia related to ventilation-perfusion imbalance and diffusion defect*
Interventions
1. Provide standard nursing care related to impaired gas exchange: maintain airway patency; monitor respiratory status; suction as necessary; provide supplemental oxygen, as ordered; and assist with intubation and mechanical ventilation, if indicated.
2. Monitor oxygen saturation through continuous pulse oximetry. Monitor arterial blood gas levels, as ordered—typically, at least every 4 hours.
3. Additional individualized interventions: _____

NURSING DIAGNOSIS: *High risk for injury: complications related to ischemia*
Interventions
1. Prevent paralytic ileus and stress ulcers. Withhold food and fluids; insert a nasogastric tube connected to suction, as ordered; administer cimetidine (Tagamet), ranitidine (Zantac), sucralfate (Carafate), or antacids, as ordered. Monitor bowel sounds.
2. Observe for signs and symptoms of adult respiratory distress syndrome. If present, alert the doctor and document (see the "Adult Respiratory Distress Syndrome" plan, page 193).

3. Observe for signs and symptoms of acute myocardial infarction. See the "Acute Myocardial Infarction—Critical Care Unit Phase" plan, page 268, for more details.
4. Observe for signs and symptoms of disseminated intravascular coagulation. See the "Disseminated Intravascular Coagulation" plan, page 625, for details.
5. Observe for signs and symptoms of acute renal failure. As appropriate, implement measures described in the "Acute Renal Failure" plan, page 548.
6. Observe for signs and symptoms of liver failure. See the "Liver Failure" plan, page 430.
7. Additional individualized interventions: _____

NURSING DIAGNOSIS: *High risk for ineffective individual coping, ineffective family coping, or both related to threat to life*
Interventions
1. Implement measures described in the following plans of care, as appropriate:
• "Ineffective Individual Coping," page 51
• "Ineffective Family Coping," page 47.
2. Additional individualized interventions: _____

PATIENT-FAMILY TEACHING CHECKLIST
__ cause and significance of shock
__ expectations for recovery
__ purpose of monitoring devices
__ rationales for therapeutic interventions

DOCUMENTATION CHECKLIST
__ clinical status on admission
__ significant changes in status
__ pertinent diagnostic test findings
__ care for invasive monitoring lines
__ fluid administration
__ use of inotropes, vasopressors, or other pharmacologic agents
__ measures to support ventilation and oxygenation
__ emotional support
__ patient-family teaching
__ discharge planning

ASSOCIATED PLANS OF CARE
Adult Respiratory Distress Syndrome
Disseminated Intravascular Coagulation
Impaired Physical Mobility
Ineffective Family Coping
Ineffective Individual Coping
Liver Failure
Major Burns
Mechanical Ventilation
Multiple Trauma
Pulmonary Embolism

Hysterectomy

COLLABORATIVE PROBLEM: *High risk for thromboembolic and hemorrhagic complications related to immobility, venous stasis, pelvic congestion, or possible predisposing factors*

Interventions

1. Monitor for signs of bleeding; institute fluid replacement therapy as ordered.
2. Institute measures to prevent and assess for thromboembolic phenomena.
3. Before discharge, instruct the patient to promptly report any bleeding and to avoid heavy lifting, prolonged sitting, and wearing constrictive clothes.
4. Additional individualized interventions: _____

NURSING DIAGNOSIS: *High risk for postoperative infection related to abdominal incision, urinary tract proximity, contamination of peritoneal cavity, hypoventilation, anesthesia, or preoperative infection*

Interventions

1. Monitor for signs and symptoms of peritonitis.
2. Implement standard postoperative nursing measures to prevent or detect infection.
3. Before discharge, teach the patient about signs and symptoms indicating infection.
4. Additional individualized interventions: _____

NURSING DIAGNOSIS: *High risk for urine retention related to decreased bladder and urethral muscle tone from anesthesia and mechanical trauma*

Interventions

1. Monitor for signs of urine retention.
2. Implement measures to deal with retention, if it occurs.
3. Additional individualized interventions: _____

NURSING DIAGNOSIS: *Pain related to abdominal incision and distention*

Interventions

1. Implement measures for pain control.
2. Offer application of heat to the abdomen.
3. Additional individualized interventions: _____

NURSING DIAGNOSIS: *High risk for body-image disturbance related to changes in body appearance and function as a result of surgery*

Interventions

1. Assess the patient's level of understanding regarding hysterectomy and the recovery period.
2. Acknowledge the patient's feelings of loss and dependence and fears of complications.
3. Provide opportunities for the patient to discuss concerns.
4. Encourage the patient to discuss plans for recovery at home.

5. Additional individualized interventions: _____

NURSING DIAGNOSIS: *High risk for sexual dysfunction: decreased libido or dyspareunia related to fatigue, pain, grieving, altered body image, decreased estrogen levels, loss of vaginal sensations, sexual activity restrictions, or concerns about acceptance by spouse or partner*

Interventions

1. Encourage the patient to explore perceptions of how surgery will affect sexual function. Listen sensitively.
2. Discuss the potential impact of surgery on sexuality.
3. Explain that decreased libido and vaginal dryness may result from hormonal loss and that hormonal replacements are available.
4. Suggest ways to ease sexual adjustment during the immediate postoperative period.
5. Provide information and discuss options for conserving the patient's energy and preventing discomfort during return to sexual functioning.
6. Encourage the patient and spouse or partner, if present, to share concerns and feelings with each other.
7. Additional individualized interventions: _____

PATIENT-FAMILY TEACHING CHECKLIST

___ implications of total abdominal hysterectomy
___ all discharge medications' purpose, dosage, administration schedule, and adverse effects requiring medical attention
___ incision care (aseptic technique, dressing changes, irrigations, cleansing procedures, handwashing technique, and proper disposal of soiled dressings)
___ signs and symptoms of possible infection
___ dietary requirements and restrictions, if any
___ activity and exercise restrictions
___ date, time, and location of follow-up appointment
___ how to contact the doctor

DOCUMENTATION CHECKLIST

___ clinical status on admission
___ postoperative clinical assessment
___ significant changes in status
___ appearance of incision and wound drainage
___ I.V. line patency and condition of site
___ assessment of pain and relief measures
___ nutritional intake
___ fluid intake and output
___ patient-family teaching
___ discharge planning

ASSOCIATED PLANS OF CARE

Grieving
Ineffective Individual Coping
Knowledge Deficit
Pain
Surgical Intervention
Thrombophlebitis

Ileal Conduit Urinary Diversion

NURSING DIAGNOSIS: *Knowledge deficit related to an ileal conduit*
Interventions
1. Assess what the patient already knows about the upcoming cystectomy and creation of an ileal conduit, including experience with someone who has an ostomy.
2. Assess the patient's ability to learn.
3. Assess the patient for manual dexterity, sensory deficits, and visual acuity.
4. Inquire about the patient's fluid intake habits.
5. Describe the construction of the conduit, the rationale for bowel preparation, and normal stoma characteristics.
6. Anticipate problems with pouch use, such as tape allergies.
7. Request a doctor's order for an enterostomal (ET) nurse to mark the stoma site before surgery.
8. If the patient is male, discuss what effect the cystectomy may have on sexual functioning.
9. Additional individualized interventions: _____

_____

COLLABORATIVE PROBLEM: *High risk for postoperative peritonitis related to GI or genitourinary anastomosis breakdown or leakage*
Interventions
1. Monitor and document nasogastric (NG) tube patency, NG output, abdominal pain and distention, bowel sounds, and appearance of and drainage from the abdominal incision.
2. Evaluate for signs of GI anastomosis leakage and peritonitis.
3. Monitor for signs of urine leakage.
4. Additional individualized interventions: _____

_____

COLLABORATIVE PROBLEM: *High risk for stomal ischemia and necrosis related to vascular compromise of conduit*
Interventions
1. Apply a disposable transparent urinary pouch, as ordered, and attach the pouch to a bedside drainage bag.
2. Observe the stoma for color changes every 4 hours and as needed.
3. Report color change of stoma (to purple, brown, or black) immediately.
4. Be prepared to differentiate superficial ischemia from necrosis.
5. Additional individualized interventions: _____

_____

COLLABORATIVE PROBLEM: *High risk for stoma retraction and mucocutaneous separation related to peristomal trauma or tension on the intestinal mesentery*
Interventions
1. Apply a pouch with an antireflux valve, as ordered.
2. Use a skin sealant.

3. If mucocutaneous separation occurs, protect the area and take measures to encourage granulation.
4. Additional individualized interventions: _____

_____

NURSING DIAGNOSIS: *Altered urinary elimination related to creation of an ileal conduit*
Interventions
1. Maintain a good pouch seal.
2. Review the construction and function of the conduit.
3. Describe and show normal urine and stoma characteristics.
4. Additional individualized interventions: _____

_____

NURSING DIAGNOSIS: *Body-image disturbance related to urinary diversion*
Interventions
1. Encourage the patient to express feelings.
2. Allow for privacy when teaching ostomy care.
3. Have the patient empty the pouch in the bathroom.
4. Suggest a visit from a United Ostomy Association (UOA) visitor.
5. Show an accepting, tolerant attitude when performing or teaching ostomy care.
6. Additional individualized interventions: _____

_____

NURSING DIAGNOSIS: *Knowledge deficit related to care of the ileal conduit*
Interventions
1. Instruct the patient how to empty the pouch.
2. Demonstrate the use and care of the nighttime bedside drainage bag.
3. Encourage the patient to change the pouch.
4. Teach the patient how to treat minor peristomal skin irritations using karaya powder and a skin sealant.
5. Explain fluid intake requirements and demonstrate pH testing of urine.
6. List recommended ways to control urine odor through diet.
7. Define routine follow-up care, and explain the rationale for it.
8. Address any special concerns the patient has about living with an ostomy.
9. Additional individualized concerns: _____

_____

NURSING DIAGNOSIS: *High risk for sexual dysfunction: male erectile dysfunction related to cystectomy and possible ejaculatory incompetence with prostatectomy*
Interventions
1. Assess the patient's readiness to discuss sexual matters.
2. Describe the separate nerve pathways for sexual excitement, erection, ejaculation, and orgasm. Explain which ones may be affected by surgery and why.

3. If indicated, mention alternatives such as a penile prosthesis or external devices that aid erection. Refer the patient to the urologist or ET nurse for details.
4. Additional individualized interventions: _____

PATIENT-FAMILY TEACHING CHECKLIST
___ extent of tumor and resection
___ nature of urinary diversion and its construction
___ incision care (if not healed)
___ procedure for emptying and changing pouch
___ use and cleaning of bedside drainage system
___ treatment of minor peristomal skin irritations
___ written list of supplies and suppliers, with doctor's prescription to facilitate insurance payment
___ chemotherapy (if needed) and its expected adverse effects
___ availability of support groups such as UOA and the American Cancer Society (list their telephone numbers)
___ amount and types of fluids preferred, along with any dietary considerations, such as avoiding odor-causing foods
___ signs and symptoms to report to the doctor, such as fever, flank pain, or hematuria
___ concerns to report to the ET nurse, such as pouch problems and skin or stoma problems
___ signs and symptoms of urinary tract infection
___ considerations in resuming sexual activity
___ date and time of follow-up appointments
___ how to contact the doctor
___ how to contact the ET nurse

DOCUMENTATION CHECKLIST
___ clinical status on admission
___ significant changes in status
___ pertinent laboratory and diagnostic test findings
___ preoperative marking of stoma site
___ preoperative teaching
___ bowel preparation
___ UOA visitor recommendation (if appropriate)
___ stoma viability
___ mucocutaneous border and sutures
___ urine characteristics
___ patient's response to ostomy
___ fluid intake and output
___ presence of stents
___ GI status
___ incision status
___ patient's progress in learning ostomy care
___ patient-family teaching
___ discharge planning

ASSOCIATED PLANS OF CARE
Grieving
Ineffective Family Coping
Ineffective Individual Coping
Knowledge Deficit
Surgical Intervention

Ineffective Individual Coping

NURSING DIAGNOSIS: *Ineffective individual coping related to perception of a harmful stimulus*
Interventions
1. Form a positive relationship with the patient.
2. Rule out organic causes for behavioral changes.
3. Provide factual information about the illness and treatment plan.
4. With the patient, identify the source of the threat.
5. Help the patient be specific about what seems threatening.
6. With the patient, identify modifiable components of the threat.
7. Help the patient identify personal resources.
8. Identify external resources and make appropriate referrals.
9. Keep pain at a tolerable level.
10. Ensure adequate nutrition and sleep.
11. Control environmental stimuli to reduce stressors and promote rest.
12. Offer alternative strategies to counteract the effects of the threat.
13. Give the patient choices related to care.
14. Provide opportunities for loved ones to interact with the patient in meaningful ways.
15. Assess responses to interventions and collaborate with the doctor if medication is necessary.
16. Additional individual interventions: _____

PATIENT-FAMILY TEACHING CHECKLIST
___ diagnosis, treatment plan, and prognosis
___ expected physiologic responses during recovery
___ community resources appropriate to perceived problems
___ appropriate alternative coping strategies
___ how to contact the doctor

DOCUMENTATION CHECKLIST
___ coping status on admission
___ significant changes in appearance, affect, behavior, and perception
___ psychological responses to hospitalization and interventions
___ significant physiologic stress responses
___ sleep patterns
___ nutritional intake
___ pain control
___ response to caregivers
___ response to interventions designed to increase coping skills
___ suicide risk
___ referrals made
___ patient-family teaching
___ discharge planning

ASSOCIATED PLANS OF CARE
Dying
Grieving
Ineffective Family Coping
Knowledge Deficit
Pain

CONDENSED PLANS OF CARE

Liver Failure

COLLABORATIVE PROBLEM: *Deteriorating neurologic status related to hepatic encephalopathy syndrome*
Interventions
1. Assess neurologic status hourly.
2. Assess for asterixis.
3. Auscultate the chest and assess respiratory rate hourly. Administer oxygen by nasal prongs, as ordered.
4. Stop intake of dietary protein. Also stop administering all drugs containing nitrogen, as ordered.
5. Administer neomycin (Mycifradin) by nasogastric tube, if ordered.
6. Administer lactulose (Cephulac) by nasogastric tube, if ordered. Monitor for diarrhea.
7. Stop any diuretic therapy, as ordered.
8. Administer neutral, acid-free enema solutions, as ordered.
9. Avoid all sedatives metabolized primarily by the liver.
10. Teach the patient and family about necessary interventions, as appropriate.
11. Additional individualized interventions: _____

COLLABORATIVE PROBLEM: *High risk for fever related to liver disease or infection*
Interventions
1. Assess temperature every 4 hours.
2. Observe for cloudy, concentrated urine.
3. Auscultate lung fields at least every 2 hours.
4. Auscultate bowel sounds at least every 4 hours.
5. If infection is diagnosed, assist with treatment, as ordered. If the fever stems solely from liver disease, provide symptomatic care.
6. Additional individualized interventions: _____

COLLABORATIVE PROBLEM: *Fluid and electrolyte imbalance related to ascites*
Interventions
1. Closely monitor fluid and electrolyte status.
2. Percuss and palpate the abdomen every 4 hours.
3. Maintain strict bed rest.
4. Implement dietary restrictions, administer diuretics as ordered, and assist with peritoneovenous (LeVeen) shunt insertion.
5. Teach the patient and family about necessary interventions, as appropriate.
6. Additional individualized interventions: _____

COLLABORATIVE PROBLEM: *High risk for gastrointestinal hemorrhage related to esophageal varices*
Interventions
1. Observe for and report signs of esophageal bleeding. See the "Gastrointestinal Hemorrhage" plan, page 394.
2. Additional individualized interventions: _____

NURSING DIAGNOSIS: *Nutritional deficit related to catabolism from liver disease*
Interventions
1. Implement dietary prescriptions, as ordered.
2. If encephalopathy is present, stop protein intake. Once encephalopathy has subsided, begin protein intake at 20-g/day increments.
3. Emphasize to the patient and family the importance of dietary restriction.
4. Additional individualized interventions: _____

NURSING DIAGNOSIS: *High risk for impaired skin integrity related to jaundice, increased bleeding tendencies, malnutrition, and ascites*
Interventions
1. Monitor skin condition.
2. Monitor prothrombin time, as ordered.
3. Reposition the patient and rub bony prominences every 2 hours. Implement the additional measures in the "Impaired Physical Mobility" plan, page 36, as appropriate.
4. Provide symptomatic treatment for pruritus, as necessary.
5. Additional individualized interventions: _____

PATIENT-FAMILY TEACHING CHECKLIST
___ relationship between alcohol consumption and exacerbation of liver disease
___ cause of changes in neurologic status and relationship to liver disease
___ effects of ascites and methods of treatment
___ importance of diet in liver disease

DOCUMENTATION CHECKLIST
___ clinical status on admission
___ significant changes in status
___ pertinent laboratory and diagnostic test findings
___ weight
___ fluid intake and output measurements
___ fluctuations in fever and associated symptoms
___ skin integrity
___ any signs of GI bleeding
___ patient-family teaching
___ discharge planning

ASSOCIATED PLANS OF CARE
Gastrointestinal Hemorrhage
Impaired Physical Mobility
Nutritional Deficit
Sensory-Perceptual Alteration

Low Back Pain—Conservative Medical Management

NURSING DIAGNOSIS: *Impaired physical mobility related to acute pain and limitations imposed by the therapeutic regimen*
Interventions
1. Maintain strict and complete bed rest for 1 to 6 weeks.
2. Evaluate neurologic function in the lower extremities daily; report new or increasingly abnormal findings to the doctor.
3. Supervise maintenance of body alignment.
4. Administer medications, as ordered, to control pain, decrease inflammation, and reduce muscle spasm, observing for adverse reactions.
5. Assess lung sounds every 8 hours. Supervise pulmonary hygiene measures.
6. Supervise quad sets, calf pumping, and circle motions of the ankle, 10 times each, 4 times daily.
7. Apply antiembolism stockings as ordered, removing them twice daily to provide skin care.
8. Supervise position changes every 2 hours, using the logrolling method.
9. Maintain dietary intake high in bulk, fluids, and fiber and lower than usual in calories while the patient is on bed rest.
10. Coordinate and supervise implementation of a progressive activity schedule.
11. Instruct the patient about movements that may stretch or strain the back.
12. Instruct the patient about the effects of coughing, sneezing, or straining at stool and about appropriate precautionary measures.
13. If ordered, apply pelvic traction.
14. If ordered, apply moist heat.
15. If ordered, teach the proper use and application of a brace or corset.
16. Additional individualized interventions: _____

NURSING DIAGNOSIS: *Altered role performance related to bed rest, effects of medications, prolonged discomfort, and required alterations in activity*
Interventions
1. Include the patient as a participant in care-planning conferences. Allow as many choices as possible within therapeutic guidelines.
2. Discuss positive and negative feelings the patient may experience.
3. Help the patient identify coping resources and refocus negative feelings.
4. Avoid authoritarian attitudes.
5. Refer the patient to the occupational therapy department as appropriate.
6. With the patient, identify strategies to maintain motivation.
7. Additional individualized interventions: _____

NURSING DIAGNOSIS: *Knowledge deficit related to recovery, rehabilitation, and long-term management of low back injury*
Interventions
1. Provide information about the anatomy and physiology of the back.
2. Provide information about needed life-style changes related to sitting, driving, standing and walking, lifting, and exercise.
3. Teach about correct posture, including assessment technique.
4. Discuss the most common causes of low back pain.
5. Discuss how nerve pressure damage may affect the lower extremities' structure and function. Emphasize the importance of reporting ominous changes.
6. Discuss long-term care issues with the family and loved ones.
7. Additional individualized interventions: _____

PATIENT-FAMILY TEACHING CHECKLIST
___ nature of low back injury
___ signs and symptoms indicating delayed healing or reinjury
___ recommended daily exercise program
___ common feelings about life-style changes
___ plan for resuming activity
___ resources for support of life-style modifications
___ role of family members or loved ones in rehabilitation program
___ proper posture, lifting techniques, and positioning to prevent reinjury
___ all discharge medications' purpose, dosage, administration schedule, and adverse effects requiring medical attention (usual discharge medications include analgesics and muscle relaxants)
___ date, time, and location of follow-up appointments
___ how to contact the doctor

DOCUMENTATION CHECKLIST
___ clinical status on admission
___ significant changes in clinical status
___ pertinent diagnostic findings
___ pain relief measures
___ nutritional intake
___ elimination status
___ progressive activity program and progress
___ complications of immobility, if any
___ patient-family teaching
___ discharge planning

ASSOCIATED PLANS OF CARE
Ineffective Individual Coping
Knowledge Deficit
Laminectomy
Pain

CONDENSED PLANS OF CARE

Lung Cancer

COLLABORATIVE PROBLEM: *Hypoxemia related to aberrant cellular growth of lung tissue, bronchial obstruction, increased mucus production, or pleurisy*
Interventions
1. Initiate arterial blood gas measurements and monitor for changes in PO_2, as ordered.
2. Administer humidified oxygen, as ordered.
3. Elevate the head of the bed during dyspneic episodes.
4. Evaluate and document breath sounds, respiratory rate, and chest movements. Observe for dyspnea.
5. During dyspneic episodes, stay with the patient, explain all procedures, and support the patient and family.
6. Encourage the patient to stop or decrease smoking.
7. Teach pursed-lip breathing and relaxation techniques.
8. Teach huff cough or cascade cough.
9. Additional individualized interventions: _____

COLLABORATIVE PROBLEM: *High risk for hemorrhage related to depression of platelet production by chemotherapy*
Interventions
1. Caution the patient to report any bleeding immediately.
2. Initiate and monitor serum platelet counts, as ordered.
3. Caution the patient to use a soft or sponge toothbrush for oral hygiene and to avoid spicy foods.
4. Teach the patient to monitor urine and stools for signs of bleeding and to immediately report any that occur.
5. Instruct the patient to use an electric razor for shaving or, if male, to grow a beard.
6. Administer medications to suppress menses, as ordered.
7. Teach the patient to report any headaches, dizziness, or light-headedness immediately.
8. Avoid I.M. injections. If they are unavoidable, apply pressure for at least 5 minutes after the injection.
9. Avoid administering aspirin or aspirin-containing medications.
10. Apply ice packs to bleeding areas.
11. Administer stool softeners.
12. Additional individualized interventions: _____

NURSING DIAGNOSIS: *Pain associated with involvement of peripheral lung structures, metastasis, or chemotherapy*
Interventions
1. Instruct the patient to report pain or discomfort immediately.
2. Monitor continually for signs of pain or discomfort.
3. Involve the patient in pain-control strategies.
4. Administer pain medication, as needed. Teach the patient or a family member how to administer pain medication after discharge.
5. Additional individualized interventions: _____

NURSING DIAGNOSIS: *High risk for infection related to immunosuppression from chemotherapy and malnutrition*
Interventions
1. Observe strict medical and surgical asepsis.
2. Monitor and record the patient's temperature every 8 hours. Report even slight temperature elevations.
3. Instruct the patient to avoid crowds and persons with infections.
4. Monitor white blood cell counts.
5. Initiate routine cultures.
6. Instruct the female patient to use sanitary napkins instead of tampons.
7. Avoid using indwelling urinary catheters.
8. Additional individualized interventions: _____

NURSING DIAGNOSIS: *High risk for sensory-perceptual alteration related to peripheral neuropathies caused by chemotherapy*
Interventions
1. Assess for, document, and report deficits in neurologic functioning, including paresthesias, abnormal deep tendon reflexes, or foot drop.
2. Discontinue or decrease the chemotherapy dosage, depending on the neuropathies' severity, as ordered.
3. Explain that changes in sensation are related to chemotherapy, and allow the patient to express fears related to this situation.
4. Protect the area of decreased sensory perception from injury: use a bath thermometer; assess the skin every 8 hours for signs of trauma; apply dressings to injured areas; use a night light; and avoid clutter in areas of activity to prevent abrasions, contusions, or falls.
5. Additional individualized interventions: _____

NURSING DIAGNOSIS: *Nutritional deficit related to cachexia associated with tumor growth, anorexia, changes in taste sensation, or stomatitis*
Interventions
1. Estimate required protein needs.
2. Develop diet plans based on calculated dietary needs and the patient's food preferences.
3. Increase dietary protein intake.
4. Provide small, frequent feedings.
5. Document weight weekly.
6. Provide antiemetics as ordered.
7. Assess the oral mucosa for stomatitis daily and document findings.
8. Provide a mild mouthwash with viscous lidocaine before meals.
9. After meals, clean the patient's mouth with a sodium bicarbonate and salt solution, hydrogen peroxide solution, or both.
10. Lubricate lips with petrolatum.
11. Assess oral mucosa for infection daily.
12. Instruct the patient to swish and swallow with yogurt or buttermilk three times a day.

13. Administer oral nystatin, as ordered.
14. Additional individualized interventions: _____

NURSING DIAGNOSIS: *Constipation or diarrhea related to chemotherapy*
Interventions
1. Assess and document bowel elimination pattern on admission.
2. Administer antidiarrheal medication, as ordered.
3. Assess for signs of paralytic ileus. If present, report them to the doctor immediately.
4. Increase dietary fiber intake, provide warm fluids, and promote the optimum amount of exercise to prevent constipation.
5. Administer stool softeners as ordered.
6. Additional individualized interventions: _____

NURSING DIAGNOSIS: *High risk for altered urinary elimination related to possible development of renal toxicity or hemorrhagic cystitis from chemotherapy*
Interventions
1. Assess and document urinary elimination pattern on admission.
2. Force fluids and administer allopurinol (Lopurin) before administering chemotherapeutic agents, as ordered.
3. Alkalinize the patient's urine.
4. Monitor serum creatinine and 24-hour urine creatinine tests, as ordered.
5. Additional individualized interventions: _____

NURSING DIAGNOSIS: *Activity intolerance related to weakness from cachexia, altered protein metabolism, muscle wasting, or hypoxia*
Interventions
1. Determine what activities the patient can tolerate without dyspnea.
2. Instruct the patient to organize activities so that tasks are spaced in manageable units.
3. Teach proper body mechanics to decrease the energy expenditure associated with activities of daily living.
4. Additional individualized interventions: _____

NURSING DIAGNOSIS: *Sleep pattern disturbance related to nocturnal cough*
Interventions
1. Assess and document sleep patterns.
2. Provide assistance with respiratory hygiene during coughing.
3. Instruct the patient to sleep with the head elevated.
4. Exercise caution in administering sedatives and hypnotics.
5. Additional individualized interventions: _____

NURSING DIAGNOSIS: *Self-esteem disturbance related to weight loss, cough, sputum production, hair loss, or role changes*
Interventions
1. Approach the patient with an accepting attitude.
2. Assess and document attitudes and responses related to self-concept and role changes.
3. Encourage the patient and family to share feelings.
4. Help the patient accentuate positive features and minimize evidence of weight loss.
5. Encourage the use of a portable disposal unit for discarding tissues and sputum.
6. Encourage frequent contact with loved ones.
7. Discuss probable hair loss before chemotherapy starts.
8. Remind the patient that hair loss is not permanent.
9. Explain to the patient about scalp tourniquets and scalp hypothermia treatments that may diminish hair loss.
10. Additional individualized interventions: _____

NURSING DIAGNOSIS: *Altered sexuality patterns related to dyspnea and possible sterility*
Interventions
1. Discuss any changes in patterns of sexual expression that have resulted from the diagnosis and treatments.
2. Help the patient and spouse (or partner) discuss their desires for sexual expression and intimacy.
3. Discuss options for sexual expression within the patient's physical limitations.
4. Encourage the use of supplemental oxygen during intercourse.
5. Provide privacy.
6. Explain that reduced sexual responsiveness may result from fatigue or chemotherapy.
7. Explain that chemotherapy may cause sterility.
8. Additional individualized interventions: _____

PATIENT-FAMILY TEACHING CHECKLIST
___ diagnosis
___ effects of chemotherapy
___ prevention, detection, and management of bleeding
___ use of supplemental oxygen
___ smoking cessation
___ breathing exercises
___ all discharge medications' purpose, dose, administration schedule, and adverse effects requiring medical attention; usual discharge medications include analgesics, antiemetics, and stool softeners or antidiarrheals, as appropriate
___ pain relief measures
___ signs of and methods to prevent infection
___ signs of neurologic changes
___ dietary modifications
___ measures to control nausea and vomiting
___ measures to promote normal renal function
___ measures to decrease dyspnea
___ measures to minimize effects of changing body image
___ plans for sexual expression
___ date, time, and location of follow-up appointment
___ how to contact the doctor
___ when to seek emergency medical care
___ community resources

CONDENSED PLANS OF CARE

DOCUMENTATION CHECKLIST
___ clinical status on admission
___ significant changes in status
___ pertinent laboratory and diagnostic test findings
___ response to chemotherapy
___ episodes of dyspnea
___ oxygen therapy
___ bleeding episodes
___ nutritional status
___ bowel elimination
___ urinary elimination
___ activity tolerance
___ sleep patterns
___ patient-family teaching
___ discharge planning

ASSOCIATED PLANS OF CARE
Dying
Grieving
Ineffective Family Coping
Ineffective Individual Coping
Knowledge Deficit
Pain

Mastectomy

COLLABORATIVE PROBLEM: *Lymphedema related to interrupted lymph circulation from surgical axillary node dissection during mastectomy*
Interventions
1. Determine if the patient is to have a radical or modified radical mastectomy.
2. Before surgery, measure and record the circumference of each arm at 2½" (6 cm) above and below the elbow. After surgery, repeat measurement each morning until discharge.
3. Immediately after mastectomy, position the affected arm on a pillow with the elbow higher than the shoulder, and the wrist and hand higher than the elbow.
4. Protect the affected arm from injury.
5. Monitor laboratory data.
6. Inspect the skin for color, translucency, temperature, or breakdown daily.
7. Check peripheral pulses daily.
8. Assess the arm for edema daily by pressing thumb into tissue for 5 to 10 seconds and observing for depression after removing thumb.
9. Administer diuretics and salt-poor albumin, as indicated.
10. Elevate and massage the affected arm daily with lotion, beginning at the wrist and advancing to the shoulder.
11. Administer pain medication 30 to 45 minutes before beginning exercises.
12. Instruct the patient to elevate the affected arm regularly after discharge. Teach appropriate range-of-motion exercises.
13. Refer the patient to Reach for Recovery or a similar support group.

14. Teach the patient and family the signs and symptoms of lymphedema and when it is most likely to occur.
15. Teach the patient how to maintain lymphatic circulation in the affected arm and prevent infection and injury.
16. Additional individualized interventions: _____

NURSING DIAGNOSIS: *Body-image disturbance related to loss of a body part*
Interventions
1. Provide empathetic emotional support; also refer to the "Grieving" plan, page 31.
2. Assess the patient's feelings about the mastectomy.
3. Monitor the patient's comments about and willingness to look at and touch the incision site.
4. Counsel the spouse or partner to hold and touch the patient.
5. Encourage the patient to wear make-up (if appropriate), nightgowns, and soft, front-closing brassieres (if dressings do not interfere).
6. Offer to refer the patient to a mastectomy support group, a member of the clergy, a social worker, or a psychiatric or oncology clinical nurse specialist.
7. Assess the patient's suitability for reconstructive surgery.
8. If reconstruction is an option, support the patient in the decision-making process.
9. If reconstruction is not an option, or will be delayed, provide information about external breast prostheses when the patient asks about them.
10. After reconstruction:
• Assess the incision site.
• Be alert to pallor, cyanosis, coolness, or delayed capillary refill at the surgical site.
• Elevate the head of the bed.
• Monitor the patient's comments and willingness to look at and touch the reconstructed breast.
• Provide psychological support.
• Counsel the patient's spouse or partner about the importance of expressing satisfaction with the reconstructed breast.
• Instruct the patient to begin daily, vigorous massage of the implant or graft 6 weeks after surgery.
• Educate the patient about the value of sharing information about reconstruction with other women.
11. Encourage the patient to talk about sexual concerns.
12. Maintain a hopeful and positive outlook when discussing sexuality. Clarify misconceptions and encourage the patient to talk with members of a mastectomy support group.
13. A few weeks after discharge, make a home call and inquire about the resumption of social activities as well as psychological status. Reintroduce the subject of sexuality and ask about any concerns encountered since surgery.
14. Additional individualized interventions: _____

COLLABORATIVE PROBLEM: *High risk for hypercalcemia related to abnormal calcium transport or skeletal metastases*

Interventions

1. Monitor for hypercalcemia.
2. Monitor blood pressure and heart rate every 2 hours.
3. Auscultate heart sounds and rhythms in four sites and record.
4. Assess electrocardiogram changes.
5. If patient is receiving a digitalis glycoside, measure the apical pulse rate before administering.
6. Assess the patient's level of consciousness every 4 to 8 hours.
7. Document fluid intake and output every 2 hours to monitor fluid balance. Obtain baseline weight on admission.
8. Assess amount and color of urine, and note specific gravity.
9. Assess for flank pain and strain all urine for calculi.
10. Anticipate I.V. administration of saline and a loop diuretic such as furosemide (Lasix).
11. Anticipate administration of calcitonin (Calcimar), glucocorticoids, phosphates, plicamycin (Mithracin), or gallium nitrate (Ganite). Be alert to adverse reactions.
12. Apply an ice collar to the patient's neck if nauseated. Administer an antiemetic, if appropriate.
13. Provide mouth care every 4 hours, after vomiting, and before meals. Clean teeth daily.
14. Auscultate bowel sounds in four quadrants and record changes in pitch and frequency.
15. Teach the patient and family signs and symptoms of hypercalcemia and appropriate interventions.
16. If hypercalcemia does not respond to interventions, alert the family and help them prepare for the patient's death.
17. Additional individualized interventions: _____

PATIENT-FAMILY TEACHING CHECKLIST

___ nature of cancer and implications
___ signs and symptoms of oncologic emergencies
___ importance of support for patient's decision regarding reconstructive surgery
___ signs and symptoms of graft rejection
___ activity recommendations and limitations
___ community or professional resources and support groups
___ need for follow-up appointments
___ need for long-term emotional support as a result of cancer diagnosis

DOCUMENTATION CHECKLIST

___ clinical status on admission
___ presence of adequate support systems
___ activity and exercise tolerance and recommendations
___ patient-family teaching
___ discharge planning

ASSOCIATED PLANS OF CARE
Dying
Grieving
Ineffective Family Coping
Ineffective Individual Coping
Lung Cancer
Pain
Surgical Intervention

Mechanical Ventilation

COLLABORATIVE PROBLEM: *Ineffective alveolar ventilation related to failure to maintain prescribed ventilator settings*

Interventions

1. Confirm orders for mechanical ventilation, particularly:
• ventilator type
• inspiratory mode (control, assist-control, synchronized intermittent mandatory ventilation [SIMV], pressure support)
• expiratory maneuvers (positive end-expiratory pressure [PEEP], continuous positive airway pressure [CPAP]).
2. Collaborate with the respiratory therapist to monitor prescribed settings:
• respiratory rate
• tidal volume
• minute ventilation (MV)
• inspiratory flow rate
• inspiratory-expiratory ratio
• airway pressure
• pressure limit
• sensitivity
• sigh
• alarms and monitors.
3. In collaboration with the respiratory therapist, monitor compliance every 8 hours.
4. Evaluate pulmonary status at least every 2 hours.
5. Additional individualized interventions: _____

COLLABORATIVE PROBLEM: *High risk for hypoxemia related to insufficient oxygen delivery or inadequate PEEP level*

Interventions

1. Compare delivered oxygen percentage to that desired.
2. Be aware if the FIO_2 is greater than 50%.
• With the doctor, consider the risk of oxygen toxicity in relation to the need for oxygen therapy.
• If it is not possible to reduce the oxygen dosage, observe for signs and symptoms of oxygen toxicity.
3. Note PEEP.
• Visually monitor the PEEP level.
• Assist with titration of PEEP.
4. Additional individualized interventions: _____

NURSING DIAGNOSIS: *Ineffective airway clearance related to presence of endotracheal tube, increased secretions, and the underlying disease*
Interventions
1. Provide artificial airway care:
• Support the ventilator tubing.
• Measure cuff pressures at least every 8 hours.
2. Monitor endotracheal tube position.
3. Keep a manual self-inflating bag and mask connected to 100% oxygen at the bedside. If accidental extubation occurs, open the airway and ventilate with the bag and mask. Summon medical assistance.
4. Change the patient's position every 1 to 2 hours. Provide chest physiotherapy as indicated.
5. Suction when needed. Observe these guidelines:
• Hyperoxygenate the patient before, during, and after suctioning.
• If the patient is on PEEP, use a manual self-inflating bag with a PEEP valve or a closed suctioning system.
• Apply suction only while withdrawing the catheter.
• Monitor blood pressure, heart rate, and electrocardiogram (ECG) pattern.
• While suctioning, observe for paroxysmal coughing without deep breaths; remove the catheter if it occurs.
• If the patient reacts adversely to traditional suctioning, consult with the doctor.
6. Additional individualized interventions: _____

COLLABORATIVE PROBLEM: *High risk for injury: complications related to patient deterioration, mechanical breakdown, increased intrathoracic pressure, or bypassed defense mechanisms*
Interventions

ABRUPT RESPIRATORY DISTRESS
1. Keep ventilator alarms turned on at all times.
2. Be familiar with troubleshooting techniques before they are needed.
3. Continually observe whether the patient is breathing in synchrony with the ventilator. If the patient develops sudden respiratory distress or the ventilator fails abruptly, take the following steps:
• Immediately disconnect the ventilator, open the airway if necessary, and ventilate the patient using a manual self-inflating bag and 100% oxygen.
• Once ventilation is established, reevaluate the patient. If the distress has cleared, check the ventilator settings. Obtain arterial blood gas (ABG) levels immediately or evaluate oximetry readings.
• If the distress continues, perform a rapid cardiopulmonary assessment, suction the airway if indicated, or obtain medical assistance.
• Evaluate for signs of tension pneumothorax. If any are present, anticipate immediate chest X-ray, needle thoracentesis, or chest tube insertion.
• If the problem's source cannot be identified and patient panic is suspected, hand-ventilate at a rate faster than the patient's, gradually slow down to the ventilator, and then reconnect the ventilator, coaching the patient to breathe with the ventilator.

• If the problem persists, implement changes in ventilator settings, sedate the patient (usually with morphine sulfate), or paralyze the patient, as ordered. If paralysis is prescribed, be sure that sedation with an amnesic agent also is prescribed.
4. Monitor the patient on PEEP for barotrauma, decreased cardiac output, water retention, and increased intracranial pressure.
5. Additional individualized interventions: _____

DECREASED CARDIAC OUTPUT
1. Monitor the patient for signs and symptoms of decreased cardiac output. Administer I.V. fluid or vasopressors, as ordered.
2. Read pulmonary artery and wedge pressures at the end of expiration.
3. If the patient is on PEEP, consult the doctor about the specific technique for reading wedge pressures. Watch for trends over time.
4. Additional individualized interventions: _____

PULMONARY INFECTION
1. Monitor the humidifier's water level and temperature.
2. Drain condensed fluid in the ventilator tubing into a basin.
3. Observe for signs and symptoms of pulmonary infection.
4. If signs and symptoms of infection are present, consult with the doctor.
5. Additional individualized interventions: _____

GASTROINTESTINAL BLEEDING
1. Insert a nasogastric tube, as ordered.
2. Administer antacids, ranitidine (Zantac), or cimetidine (Tagamet), as ordered.
3. Additional individualized interventions: _____

FLUID RETENTION
1. Monitor for signs and symptoms of fluid retention. If present, consult with the doctor about treatment.
2. Additional individualized interventions: _____

NURSING DIAGNOSIS: *Fear related to inability to speak and dependence on a machine for life support*
Interventions
1. Implement the general measures in the "Ineffective Individual Coping" plan, page 51, as appropriate.
2. Establish a communication method.
3. Reduce the patient's need for communication. Emphasize that a nurse is available immediately if needed.
4. Explain the reason for mechanical ventilation. Stress the temporary nature of ventilation, if applicable.
5. Additional individualized interventions: _____

COLLABORATIVE PROBLEM: *High risk for ineffective weaning related to lack of physiologic or psychological readiness*

Interventions

1. Anticipate weaning when the patient meets weaning criteria.
2. Ascertain that the patient is rested, well nourished, oriented, able to follow commands, and not receiving any respiratory depressants.
3. Explain weaning to the patient and family.
4. Obtain baseline vital signs, ABG values, and pulmonary function measurements. Suction the airway.
5. Implement the weaning method ordered: CPAP, SIMV, T-piece, or pressure support.
6. Monitor the blood pressure, heart rate, pulse oximeter reading, ECG rhythm, respiratory rate, ease of breathing, level of consciousness, and level of fatigue constantly for the first 20 to 30 minutes and every 5 minutes thereafter until weaning is complete.
7. In collaboration with the doctor, terminate weaning if adverse reactions occur.
8. If weaning continues, measure the tidal volume, MV, and ABG values in 20 to 30 minutes.
9. If physiologic parameters indicate weaning is feasible, but the patient resists, consider the possibility of psychological dependence on the ventilator. Consult with the doctor, pulmonary nurse specialist, or psychiatric nurse clinician, as appropriate.
10. Assist with extubation, when ordered.
11. Additional individualized interventions: _____

PATIENT-FAMILY TEACHING CHECKLIST

___ reason for mechanical ventilation
___ communication measures
___ alarms
___ weaning

DOCUMENTATION CHECKLIST

___ clinical status on admission
___ significant changes in status
___ pertinent diagnostic test findings
___ ventilator and patient checks
___ ventilator alarm status
___ airway care
___ measures to prevent or detect and treat complications
___ communication measures
___ emotional support
___ sedative or paralyzing pharmacologic agent, if used
___ weaning
___ patient-family teaching
___ discharge planning

ASSOCIATED PLANS OF CARE

Adult Respiratory Distress Syndrome
Impaired Physical Mobility
Ineffective Individual Coping
Nutritional Deficit
Sensory-Perceptual Alteration

Multiple Sclerosis

NURSING DIAGNOSIS: *Impaired physical mobility related to demyelinization*

Interventions

1. Provide rest and prevent fatigue.
2. Begin a physical therapy program, as ordered.
3. Administer medications as prescribed for pain and muscle spasm, observing precautions.
4. Assess lung sounds at least every 8 hours.
5. Teach the patient the need for mobility aids.
6. Instruct the patient in safety measures.
7. Assess skin and bony prominences for pressure signs.
8. Minimize the cardiovascular effects of immobility.
9. Administer corticosteroids or immunosuppressants, as ordered.
10. Use stress-reduction techniques.
11. Additional individualized interventions: _____

NURSING DIAGNOSIS: *Constipation and altered urinary elimination related to demyelinization*

Interventions

1. Assess and record the patient's present elimination pattern.
2. Evaluate dietary habits.
3. Increase and record fluid intake.
4. Institute and teach a bowel and bladder program.
5. Administer medications as ordered to decrease bowel absorption and reduce bowel spasticity.
6. Prevent exposure to infection.
7. Teach the patient a bowel and bladder program for home use.
8. Additional individualized interventions: _____

NURSING DIAGNOSIS: *High risk for sexual dysfunction related to fatigue, decreased sensation, muscle spasm, or urinary incontinence*

Interventions

1. Assess the effects of multiple sclerosis on the patient's sexual function.
2. Encourage the patient and spouse (or partner) to share sexual concerns. Offer to be available as a resource, or refer the couple to another health professional.
3. Offer specific suggestions for identified problems:
• Initiate sexual activity when energy levels are highest.
• Try different positions.
• Empty the bladder before sexual activity.
• Try oral or manual stimulation.
4. Encourage expressions of mutual affection.
5. Emphasize the importance of discussing birth control and family planning with the doctor.
6. Additional individualized interventions: _____

CONDENSED PLANS OF CARE

NURSING DIAGNOSIS: *Self-esteem disturbance related to progressive, debilitating effects of disease*
Interventions
1. Encourage the patient to participate in all decisions related to care planning. Discourage overdependence on others. Help the patient work toward goals.
2. Facilitate the expression of feelings related to losses. See the "Grieving" and "Ineffective Individual Coping" plans, pages 31 and 51 respectively.
3. Work with the family to promote patient participation in familiar family roles and rituals and to identify new roles.
4. Encourage the patient to touch affected body parts, perform self-lifting activities as much as possible, and participate in grooming.
5. Provide recognition for goals achieved. Acknowledge evidence of inner strengths and growth as well as external achievements.
6. Additional individualized interventions: _____

NURSING DIAGNOSIS: *High risk for ineffective family coping related to progressive, debilitating effects of disease on family members and resultant alteration in role-related behavior patterns*
Interventions
1. Assess the family system.
2. Encourage family members to take turns in the caregiving role, as necessary.
3. Help the family understand and accept mental changes, if present.
4. Promote healthy habits for family members, such as adequate rest, proper dietary intake, and relaxation.
5. Help the family plan changes in the home environment to facilitate care. Refer the family to the social services department.
6. Additional individualized interventions: _____

PATIENT-FAMILY TEACHING CHECKLIST
___ course and nature of multiple sclerosis
___ physical therapy program
___ all discharge medications' purpose, dosage, administration schedule, and adverse effects requiring medical attention (usual discharge medications include corticosteroids, antispasmodics, and stool softeners)
___ mobility aids
___ safety instructions for protection from injury related to sensory deficits
___ information regarding problems associated with immobility
___ stress-reduction techniques
___ community resources
___ recommended therapeutic diet, including selection of foods low in saturated fat
___ bowel and bladder program
___ avoidance of exposure to infection
___ date, time, and location of follow-up appointment
___ how to contact the doctor

DOCUMENTATION CHECKLIST
___ clinical status on admission
___ significant changes in clinical status

___ pertinent laboratory and diagnostic test findings
___ physical therapy program and activity tolerance
___ medication administration
___ nutritional intake
___ fluid intake and output
___ bowel and bladder function
___ patient-family teaching
___ discharge planning

ASSOCIATED PLANS OF CARE
Grieving
Ineffective Family Coping
Ineffective Individual Coping

Myasthenia Gravis

COLLABORATIVE PROBLEM: *Muscle weakness related to reduced number of acetylcholine receptors*
Interventions
1. Administer anticholinesterase medications, as ordered.
2. Keep an emergency airway and suctioning and ventilation equipment nearby. Monitor arterial blood gas levels, as ordered.
3. Keep atropine nearby.
4. Periodically assess muscle strength.
5. Keep a daily log of periods of fatigue and muscle strength.
6. Contact the doctor if the patient states that more or less medication is needed.
7. Administer succinylcholine (Anectine) and pancuronium (Pavulon) with caution, as ordered.
8. Observe for muscle weakness after the administration of aminoglycoside antibiotics or antiarrhythmic medications.
9. Additional individualized interventions: _____

COLLABORATIVE PROBLEM: *High risk for aspiration related to impaired swallowing*
Interventions
1. Plan mealtimes to coincide with peak anticholinesterase effects.
2. Ask the patient for a self-evaluation of swallowing ability, and order foods of appropriate consistency.
3. Provide rest periods during meals.
4. Keep suctioning equipment at the patient's bedside.
5. Teach the patient and family what to do if choking or aspiration occurs.
6. Additional individualized interventions: _____

NURSING DIAGNOSIS: *Activity intolerance related to muscle fatigue*
Interventions
1. Identify sources of excess energy consumption.
2. Space bathing, grooming, and other activities throughout the day.
3. Rearrange the environment to keep frequently used items close by.

4. Plan a rest period before each meal.
5. Additional individualized interventions: _____

NURSING DIAGNOSIS: *Ineffective airway clearance related to decreased inspiratory force and increased secretion production*
Interventions
1. Demonstrate the cascade cough.
2. Encourage the patient not to suppress coughs.
3. Perform chest physiotherapy and suction as needed.
4. Additional individualized interventions: _____

NURSING DIAGNOSIS: *Ineffective breathing pattern related to muscle fatigue*
Interventions
1. Monitor and document respiratory rate and depth every 2 hours.
2. Measure vital capacity, tidal volume, and inspiratory force both before and 1 hour after administration of anticholinesterase medication.
3. Additional individualized interventions: _____

NURSING DIAGNOSIS: *Impaired verbal communication related to fatigue of facial and respiratory muscles*
Interventions
1. Avoid frequent or long conversations with the patient.
2. Provide alternative methods of communication.
3. Additional individualized interventions: _____

NURSING DIAGNOSIS: *Nutritional deficit related to decreased oral intake*
Interventions
1. Perform a nutritional assessment on admission.
2. Provide a balanced diet.
3. Serve the main meal in the morning.
4. Provide liquids in a cup.
5. Have the patient sit erect during meals.
6. Record all food and nutritional supplements consumed. Evaluate calorie, protein, vitamin, and mineral intake.
7. Consult a dietitian.
8. Additional individualized interventions: _____

NURSING DIAGNOSIS: *Knowledge deficit related to required life-style adjustments and new medications*
Interventions
1. Teach the patient and family about the disease and its implications.
2. Instruct about factors that may cause a crisis.
3. Teach the patient and family signs and symptoms of a myasthenic crisis.
4. Teach about medications.

5. Demonstrate how to keep a medication-response log.
6. Provide information about how to obtain a medical alert tag.
7. Teach ways to cope with decreased activity tolerance.
8. Provide the address of the Myasthenia Gravis Foundation.
9. Additional individualized interventions: _____

PATIENT-FAMILY TEACHING CHECKLIST
___ nature of the disease and its implications
___ signs and symptoms of myasthenic and cholinergic crises
___ activity recommendations and limitations
___ airway clearance procedures
___ all discharge medications' purpose, dosage, administration schedule, and adverse effects requiring medical attention (usual discharge medications include anticholinesterases)
___ community resource and support groups
___ how and where to obtain an emergency identification card or bracelet
___ when and how to contact the emergency medical system
___ date, time, and location of follow-up appointments
___ how to contact the doctor

DOCUMENTATION CHECKLIST
___ clinical status on admission
___ significant changes in status
___ responses to medications
___ periods of fatigue or increased weakness
___ swallowing ability
___ respiratory parameters before and after medication administration
___ activity tolerance
___ patient-family teaching
___ discharge planning

ASSOCIATED PLANS OF CARE
Grieving
Ineffective Family Coping
Ineffective Individual Coping
Knowledge Deficit
Total Parenteral Nutrition

Nephrectomy

NURSING DIAGNOSIS: *Knowledge deficit related to perioperative procedures*
Interventions
1. See the "Knowledge Deficit" plan, page 56.
2. See the "Surgical Intervention" plan, page 81.
3. Tell the patient where the incision will be made (flank or abdomen), whether to expect a chest tube or drain, as appropriate, and potential effects of positioning during surgery.
4. Additional individualized interventions: _____

CONDENSED PLANS OF CARE

NURSING DIAGNOSIS: *Pain related to tissue injury, edema, or spasm after surgery*
Interventions
1. See the "Pain" plan, page 69.
2. Teach the patient about postoperative analgesia administration (injection, patient-controlled analgesia pump, or epidural infusion).
3. Additional individualized interventions: _____

COLLABORATIVE PROBLEM: *High risk for fluid and electrolyte imbalance related to decreased renal reserve and third-space fluid shifting immediately after surgery*
Interventions
1. See Appendix C, "Fluid and Electrolyte Imbalances."
2. Preserve and protect remaining kidney: maintain adequate hydration; avoid or minimize use of nephrotoxic agents; and instruct patient about discharge recommendations.
3. Additional individualized interventions: _____

COLLABORATIVE PROBLEM: *High risk for atelectasis related to anesthesia, immobility, pain, presence of chest tube, and location of incision*
Interventions
1. Implement interventions listed under the "High risk for postoperative atelectasis" collaborative problem in the "Surgical Intervention" plan, page 83.
2. Additional individualized interventions: _____

COLLABORATIVE PROBLEM: *High risk for postoperative paralytic ileus or intestinal obstruction related to surgical manipulation, anesthesia, and immobility*
Interventions
1. Implement measures in the "High risk for postoperative paralytic ileus" collaborative problem in the "Surgical Intervention" plan, page 88.
2. Additional individualized interventions: _____

PATIENT-FAMILY TEACHING CHECKLIST
___ plan for resuming normal activity, with restrictions
___ dietary recommendations
___ wound care
___ signs of wound infection or other complications
___ all discharge medications' purpose, dosage, administration, and adverse effects requiring medical attention (discharge medications may include analgesics and antibiotics)
___ necessary home care and referrals for follow-up care
___ when and how to contact the doctor
___ date, time, and place of follow-up appointments

DOCUMENTATION CHECKLIST
___ clinical status on admission
___ preoperative assessment and treatment
___ preoperative teaching and its effectiveness
___ preoperative checklist (usually includes documentation of operative consent, pertinent laboratory test results, skin preparation, voiding on call from the operating room, and removal of nail polish, jewelry, dentures, glasses, hearing aids, and prostheses—check hospital's specific requirements)
___ postoperative assessment and treatment
___ amount and character of drainage on dressing and through drains
___ patency of tubes (I.V., NG tube, urinary catheter, drains)
___ pulmonary hygiene
___ pain relief measures
___ activity tolerance
___ nutritional intake and tolerance
___ fluid intake and output
___ bladder and bowel function
___ pertinent laboratory findings
___ patient-family teaching
___ discharge planning

ASSOCIATED PLANS OF CARE
Knowledge Deficit
Pain
Surgical Intervention

Nutritional Deficit

NURSING DIAGNOSIS: *Nutritional deficit related to difficulty chewing or swallowing, sore throat after endotracheal extubation, or dry mouth*
Interventions
1. Assess and document causes. Initiate referrals as appropriate.
2. Assess level of consciousness and ability to chew and swallow, and check for gag reflex.
3. With the dietitian and as ordered, provide a diet appropriate to the patient's abilities—for example, liquids, soft foods, or food requiring little cutting.
4. If the patient has a sore mouth or throat, obtain an order for viscous lidocaine (Xylocaine).
5. Place the patient sitting upright for meals, with the head flexed forward about 45 degrees, unless contraindicated.
6. Suction food, fluids, or accumulated saliva as needed.
7. Provide assistance, as needed.
8. Document feeding technique and food intake.
9. Additional individualized interventions: _____

NURSING DIAGNOSIS: *Nutritional deficit related to anorexia*
Interventions
1. Assess possible causes of anorexia.
2. Provide as pleasant an eating environment as possible.
3. Before meals, promote rest; administer analgesics or antiemetics, as ordered; avoid painful procedures; and provide oral hygiene.
4. Emphasize the importance of eating.
5. Provide social interaction during meals.
6. Offer small, frequent feedings of highly nutritious foods.
7. Limit fluid intake at mealtimes.

8. If the patient begins to feel nauseated, encourage slow, deep breathing. If vomiting occurs, document the amount and type of emesis. Provide oral hygiene afterward.
9. Praise the patient for signs of increased appetite.
10. Additional individualized interventions: _____

COLLABORATIVE PROBLEM: *Nutritional deficit related to inability to digest nutrients or hypermetabolic state*
Interventions
1. Anticipate the patient's increased nutrient needs. Also observe for signs of inability to absorb nutrients.
2. Obtain a comprehensive nutritional assessment.
3. Assess and document bowel sounds and abdominal distention every 4 hours.
4. Collaborate with nutritional experts to establish nutrient requirements.
5. Provide appropriate nutritional replacements, as ordered:
• enteral feeding
—meal replacements
—nutrient supplements
—defined-formula diets
• parenteral nutrition
—peripheral parenteral nutrition
—central venous nutrition, also known as total parenteral nutrition (TPN).
6. If the patient is receiving tube feedings:
• Check tube placement before each feeding.
• Monitor bowel sounds, bowel movements, abdominal girth, fluid intake and output, and weight.
• Keep the head of the bed elevated during and for 1 hour after feedings.
• Begin with small amounts of dilute solution. Increase the amount and concentration as tolerated.
• Use a continuous enteral pump, as ordered.
7. If the patient is receiving TPN, ensure delivery of the prescribed solutions and monitor for complications.
8. Additional individualized interventions: _____

PATIENT-FAMILY TEACHING CHECKLIST
__ importance of nutrition to recovery
__ rationale for selection of specific nutritional support method

DOCUMENTATION CHECKLIST
__ clinical status on admission
__ significant changes in status
__ pertinent diagnostic test findings
__ specific nutritional support method
__ tolerance of method
__ complications, if any
__ daily nutritional intake
__ medications administered, if any
__ attitude toward eating
__ patient-family teaching
__ discharge planning

ASSOCIATED PLANS OF CARE
See the plan for the specific disorder.

Prostatectomy

COLLABORATIVE PROBLEM: *High risk for hypovolemia related to prostatic or incisional bleeding after surgery*
Interventions
1. Monitor and document the amount of blood collecting on incisional dressings and in the urinary drainage system hourly for the first 12 to 24 hours after surgery, then every 4 hours.
2. Evaluate and document pulse rate, blood pressure, respirations, skin color, and level of consciousness according to unit protocol—typically every 4 hours for 24 hours or until stable, then every 8 hours.
3. Monitor hemoglobin level, hematocrit value, platelet count, and coagulation studies daily. Compare current values with preoperative values. Alert the doctor to abnormal values. Administer blood transfusions as ordered, using universal precautions.
4. Consult the surgeon about applying traction to the catheter or preparing the patient for surgery if bleeding persists.
5. Teach the patient to avoid straining during bowel movements. Avoid using rectal thermometers or tubes or giving enemas.
6. Administer and document stool softeners and laxatives, as ordered.
7. Teach the patient to avoid lifting heavy objects for 6 to 8 weeks after surgery.
8. Additional individualized interventions: _____

NURSING DIAGNOSIS: *High risk for postoperative infection related to preoperative status or urinary catheter or abdominal drain placement*
Interventions
1. Monitor and record vital signs according to unit protocol, typically every 4 hours for 24 hours or until stable, then every 8 hours.
2. Monitor the incision site daily for induration, erythema, and purulent or odorous drainage.
3. Monitor drains and catheters for patency, and irrigate as ordered, using universal precautions.
4. Provide and document meticulous urinary catheter care at least once daily.
5. Administer I.V. fluids as ordered. Beginning on the first postoperative day, encourage oral fluid intake of 8 to 12 8-oz glasses (2,000 to 3,000 ml) daily to maintain a urine output of at least 1,500 ml daily. Record fluid intake and output.
6. Encourage the patient to ambulate the day after surgery.
7. Administer and document prophylactic antibiotics, as ordered.
8. Additional individualized interventions: _____

CONDENSED PLANS OF CARE

NURSING DIAGNOSIS: *Pain related to urethral stricture, catheter obstruction, bladder spasms, or surgical intervention*
Interventions
1. See the "Pain" plan, page 69.
2. Observe for signs of bladder spasms.
3. Irrigate, using universal precautions, and check the urinary catheter and tubing for kinks, blood clots, and mucus plugs, as needed.
4. Assess for incisional pain.
5. For severe or persistent pain, administer analgesics or antispasmodics at the pain's onset. Monitor vital signs and evaluate pain relief.
6. Provide alternative pain relief measures, and teach them to the patient.
7. Additional individualized interventions: _____

NURSING DIAGNOSIS: *High risk for urine retention related to urinary catheter obstruction*
Interventions
1. Monitor and record continuous bladder irrigation, as ordered.
2. If the patient is not on continuous bladder irrigation, irrigate the urinary catheter as needed and ordered.
3. Monitor and document fluid intake and output.
4. Weigh the patient daily.
5. Observe for suprapubic distention and discomfort every 4 hours while the patient is awake.
6. Additional individualized interventions: _____

NURSING DIAGNOSIS: *Urge incontinence related to urinary catheter removal, trauma to the bladder neck, or decrease in detrusor muscle or sphincter tone*
Interventions
1. Before surgery, teach the patient buttock and perineal exercises.
2. Monitor and document the patient's urination pattern after catheter removal.
3. If a suprapubic catheter is present, measure residual volume after each voiding, using universal precautions.
4. Obtain one urine sample with each voiding during the first 24 hours after catheter removal, and note its color, amount, and specific gravity.
5. Provide absorbent incontinence pads. Keep the perineal area clean and dry.
6. Additional individualized interventions: _____

NURSING DIAGNOSIS: *High risk for altered sexuality patterns: decreased libido related to fear of incontinence and decreased self-esteem; infertility related to retrograde ejaculation (from transurethral resection of the prostate or suprapubic prostatectomy); or impotence related to parasympathetic nerve damage (from radical prostatectomy)*
Interventions
1. Teach the patient before surgery, and reinforce after surgery, the expected effects of prostatectomy on sexual functioning. Include the patient's spouse or partner in the discussion.

2. Encourage the patient and spouse or partner to verbalize feelings of loss, grief, anxiety, and fear.
3. Encourage the patient and spouse or partner to discuss feelings about and expectations of the sexual relationship.
4. Provide information about a penile prosthesis, if appropriate.
5. Provide information and refer the patient for sexual counseling, as needed, after surgery.
6. Additional individualized interventions: _____

NURSING DIAGNOSIS: *Self-esteem disturbance related to incontinence, potential impotence, or sexual alterations*
Interventions
1. Encourage the patient to verbalize feelings about postoperative changes in body functioning and how these changes will affect his life-style.
2. Assist the patient in identifying and using effective coping behaviors.
3. Encourage the patient to continue perineal and buttock exercises to decrease incontinence.
4. Compliment the patient on his personal appearance. Instruct his spouse or partner and family to provide compliments and positive feedback to the patient.
5. Encourage the patient to participate in activities of daily living and in decisions affecting his care.
6. Additional individualized interventions: _____

PATIENT-FAMILY TEACHING CHECKLIST
___ surgical outcome and disease
___ all discharge medications' purpose, dosage, administration schedule, and adverse effects requiring medical attention (usual discharge medications include analgesics, antispasmotics if a urinary catheter is present, and antibiotics)
___ urinary catheter care techniques and supplies
___ signs and symptoms indicating obstruction, bleeding, or infection
___ supplies to manage incontinence
___ exercises to regain urinary control
___ common postoperative feelings
___ the appropriate activity level to prevent muscle straining
___ resumption of sexual activity and community resources for sexual counseling
___ community or interagency referral
___ need for consultation with an oncology specialist (if the diagnosis of cancer is confirmed)
___ availability of cancer support groups
___ date, time, and location of follow-up appointment
___ how to contact the doctor

DOCUMENTATION CHECKLIST
___ clinical status on admission
___ significant changes in status after surgery
___ pertinent laboratory and diagnostic test findings
___ episodes of hemorrhage
___ transfusion with blood products
___ infection and treatment
___ fluid intake and output
___ urinary obstruction episodes

___ urine retention
___ urinary incontinence
___ patient-family teaching
___ discharge planning
___ community or interagency referral

ASSOCIATED PLANS OF CARE
Grieving
Ineffective Family Coping
Ineffective Individual Coping
Pain
Surgical Intervention
Thrombophlebitis

Seizures

NURSING DIAGNOSIS: *Ineffective airway clearance related to loss of consciousness, apnea, excessive secretions, jaw clenching, or airway occlusion by tongue or foreign body*
Interventions
1. If an aura or warning phase occurs, clear the patient's mouth of foreign bodies and insert a soft cloth or gauze pad at the corner of the mouth. Never try to force the jaw open or insert an oral airway during the seizure. Maintain an open airway.
2. Suction the oropharynx, as needed. Provide supplemental oxygen by nasal cannula.
3. If seizures are persistent or recur frequently despite drug therapy, notify the doctor immediately. Anticipate the need for endotracheal intubation and mechanical ventilation.
4. After the seizure, insert a nasogastric tube and connect it to low suction, as ordered.
5. Additional individualized interventions: _____

COLLABORATIVE PROBLEM: *High risk for status epilepticus related to inadequate pharmacologic control or misidentification of underlying cause*
Interventions
1. Administer I.V. antiseizure medication, as ordered:
• diazepam (Valium)
• phenobarbital sodium (Luminal) and other barbiturate anticonvulsants
• phenytoin sodium (Dilantin).
2. Consider possible underlying causes, such as:
• head trauma
• electrolyte imbalance
• hypoxia
• hypoglycemia or hyperglycemia
• brain tumors
• infections
• cerebral hemorrhage
• toxins.
3. If seizures are refractory to drug therapy, anticipate possible neuromuscular blockade or general anesthesia, with mechanical ventilation.
4. Additional individualized interventions: _____

NURSING DIAGNOSIS: *High risk for injury: trauma or myoglobinuria related to excessive uncontrolled muscle activity*
Interventions
1. At the seizure's onset, ensure safe patient positioning. Place pillows around the patient and pad the side rails. Do not restrain arms and legs.
2. Stay with the patient during the seizure.
3. After motor activity stops, perform a neurologic evaluation and inspect the oropharynx, tongue, and teeth.
4. Avoid excessive environmental stimulation during the postictal period.
5. If the seizure was prolonged, monitor urine for possible myoglobin content.
6. Additional individualized interventions: _____

NURSING DIAGNOSIS: *Knowledge deficit related to seizure management*
Interventions
1. Assess the patient's and family's current level of understanding.
2. Instruct the patient and family about the disorder and the need to adhere to a medical regimen.
3. Instruct the patient and family about medications and causes of seizures.
4. Additional individualized interventions: _____

PATIENT-FAMILY TEACHING CHECKLIST
___ cause and implications of seizures
___ treatment modalities instituted
___ signs of possible recurrence
___ safety precautions

DOCUMENTATION CHECKLIST
___ clinical status on admission
___ significant changes in status
___ pertinent diagnostic test findings
___ seizure episodes
___ safety precautions instituted
___ pharmacologic interventions
___ patient-family teaching
___ discharge planning

ASSOCIATED PLANS OF CARE
Craniotomy
Drug Overdose
Hypoglycemia
Increased Intracranial Pressure
Mechanical Ventilation
Multiple Trauma
Sensory-Perceptual Alteration

Surgical Intervention

NURSING DIAGNOSIS: *Knowledge deficit: perioperative routines, related to lack of familiarity with hospital procedures*
Interventions
1. See the "Knowledge Deficit" plan, page 56.

2. Instruct the patient in perioperative routines.
3. Additional individualized interventions: _____

COLLABORATIVE PROBLEM: *High risk for postoperative shock related to hemorrhage or hypovolemia*
Interventions
1. Monitor and document vital signs on admission to the nursing unit and every 4 hours. Increase the frequency of monitoring as needed. Report abnormalities.
2. Assess the surgical dressing. Record the date and time of any drainage.
3. Assess the amount and character of drainage from wound-drainage tubes.
4. Reinforce the surgical dressing as needed.
5. Assess the surgical area for swelling or hematoma.
6. Monitor for changes in mental status.
7. Assess and maintain I.V. line patency. Maintain I.V. fluids at the ordered rate.
8. Monitor urine output every hour for 4 hours, then every 4 hours, during the immediate postoperative period. Maintain output at more than 60 ml/hour.
9. Monitor hematocrit and hemoglobin level, as ordered.
10. Monitor fluid intake and output.
11. Additional individualized interventions: _____

NURSING DIAGNOSIS: *Pain related to surgical tissue trauma, positioning, and reflex muscle spasm*
Interventions
1. See the "Pain" plan, page 69.
2. Additional individualized interventions: _____

COLLABORATIVE PROBLEM: *High risk for postoperative atelectasis related to immobility and ciliary depression from anesthesia*
Interventions
1. Assess vital signs according to protocol for the first day after surgery, then every 4 hours. Note the characteristics of respirations.
2. Auscultate breath sounds every 4 hours on the first postoperative day, then once per shift.
3. Instruct and coach the patient in diaphragmatic breathing and chest splinting.
4. Assist the patient in using an incentive spirometer.
5. Help the patient turn every 2 hours unless contraindicated.
6. Help the patient to progressively increase ambulation.
7. Encourage adequate fluid intake.
8. Additional individualized interventions: _____

COLLABORATIVE PROBLEM: *High risk for postoperative thromboembolic phenomena related to immobility, dehydration, and possible fat particle escape or aggregation*
Interventions
1. Instruct and coach the patient to perform leg exercises hourly.

2. Assess twice daily for signs of thrombophlebitis, pulmonary thromboembolism, fat embolism, and peripheral vascular thromboembolism. If present, alert the doctor promptly.
3. Encourage early ambulation after surgery.
4. Avoid using the knee gatch or placing pillows under the patient's knees.
5. Encourage adequate fluid intake.
6. Apply antiembolism stockings, if ordered.
7. Before discharge, teach the patient and family about guidelines for resuming normal activity.
8. Additional individualized interventions: _____

NURSING DIAGNOSIS: *High risk for postoperative injury related to possible changes in mental status caused by anesthesia and analgesia*
Interventions
1. Assess the patient's level of consciousness, orientation, and ability to follow directions every 30 to 60 minutes during the first 8 to 10 hours after surgery.
2. Position the drowsy patient in a side-lying position.
3. Keep side rails up until the patient is awake and alert.
4. Keep the call cord within the patient's reach.
5. Keep the bed in the low position.
6. Monitor postural vital signs and assist with initial postoperative activity.
7. Additional individualized interventions: _____

NURSING DIAGNOSIS: *High risk for infection related to surgical intervention*
Interventions
1. Identify risk factors for surgical wound infection:
• obesity
• extremes of age
• immunosuppression
• poor nutritional status
• diabetes mellitus.
2. Assess the surgical wound and other invasive sites once per shift for evidence of normal healing or healing problems.
3. Determine wound classification: clean, clean-contaminated, contaminated, or dirty.
4. Monitor temperature every 4 hours.
5. Maintain a clean, dry incision.
6. Perform wound care, as ordered, using aseptic technique.
7. Instruct the patient and family in recognizing signs and symptoms of infection.
8. Encourage adequate nutritional intake every shift.
9. Additional individualized interventions: _____

NURSING DIAGNOSIS: *High risk for postoperative urine retention related to neuroendocrine response to stress, anesthesia, and recumbent position*
Interventions
1. Assess for signs of urine retention.
2. Initiate interventions to promote voiding as soon as the patient begins to sense bladder pressure.

3. Provide noninvasive measures to promote voiding.
4. Provide a nonthreatening, supportive atmosphere.
5. Obtain an order for straight catheterization if the patient complains of bladder discomfort or has not voided within 8 hours after surgery.
6. Drain no more than 1,000 ml from the bladder at a time if the patient is catheterized.
7. After catheterization, assess for dysuria, burning, frequency and urgency of urination, and suprapubic discomfort.
8. Additional individualized interventions: _____

COLLABORATIVE PROBLEM: *High risk for postoperative paralytic ileus, abdominal pain, or constipation related to immobility, surgical manipulation, anesthesia, and analgesia*
Interventions
1. Assess the abdomen twice daily.
2. If paralytic ileus occurs, implement treatment, as ordered.
3. Implement comfort measures.
4. Provide a diet appropriate to peristaltic activity. Ensure that peristalsis has returned before progressing from nothing-by-mouth status to liberal fluid and solid food intake.
5. Encourage fluid intake of at least 8 8-oz glasses (2,000 ml) daily, unless contraindicated.
6. Encourage frequent position changes and ambulation.
7. Provide privacy during defecation.
8. Consult with the doctor concerning the use of laxatives, suppositories, or enemas.
9. Additional individualized interventions: _____

COLLABORATIVE PROBLEM: *High risk for malignant hyperthermia related to inherited skeletal muscle disorder, anesthetic agents, and abnormal calcium transport*
Interventions
1. Assess the patient's susceptibility to malignant hyperthermia: personal and family history of malignant hyperthermia and response to anesthesia; history of muscle abnormality (muscular hypertropy or musculoskeletal problems); and young age, male sex.
2. Assess for signs and symptoms of malignant hyperthermia: ventricular arrhythmias (tachycardia, fibrillation); tachypnea; hot, diaphoretic, mottled skin with or without cyanosis; elevated temperature; excessive muscle rigidity; and oliguria or anuria.
3. Monitor vital signs, arterial blood gases, electrolytes, and electrocardiogram (ECG).
4. Alert anesthesiologist or nurse anesthetist to discontinue anesthesia (intraoperatively).
5. Administer dantrolene sodium (Dantrium), as ordered.
6. Administer 100% oxygen.
7. Administer iced I.V. solutions or iced lavages of the stomach, rectum, or bladder; employ hypothermia blanket.
8. Evaluate interventions; repeat regimen as indicated.
9. Before discharge, educate the patient and family about the risk of malignant hyperthermia in future surgical procedures.
10. Additional individualized interventions: _____

COLLABORATIVE PROBLEM: *Nausea or vomiting related to GI distention, rapid position changes, or cortical stimulation of the vomiting center or chemoreceptor trigger zone*
Interventions
1. Prevent GI overdistention.
2. Limit unpleasant sights, smells, and psychic stimuli.
3. Caution the patient to change position slowly.
4. As soon as possible, advance the patient from narcotics to other analgesics (as ordered), then to nonpharmacologic pain control measures.
5. Administer antiemetics, as ordered.
6. Additional individualized interventions: _____

PATIENT-FAMILY TEACHING CHECKLIST
___ plan for resumption of normal activity
___ wound care
___ signs and symptoms of wound infection or other surgical complications
___ all discharge medications' purpose, dosage, administration, and adverse effects requiring medical attention (postoperative patients may be discharged with oral analgesics)
___ when and how to contact the doctor
___ date, time, and location of follow-up appointment with the doctor
___ community resources appropriate for the surgical intervention performed

DOCUMENTATION CHECKLIST
___ clinical status on admission
___ significant changes in preoperative status (level of consciousness, emotional status, baseline physical data)
___ preoperative teaching and its effectiveness
___ preoperative checklist (includes documentation regarding the preoperative consent, urinalysis, complete blood count, 12-lead ECG, chest X-ray, preoperative medication, surgical skin preparation, voiding on call from operating room, and removal of nail polish, jewelry, dentures, glasses, hearing aids, and prostheses)
___ clinical status on admission from the recovery room
___ amount and character of wound drainage (on dressing and through drains)
___ skin condition
___ patency of tubes (I.V., nasogastric, indwelling urinary catheter, drains)
___ pulmonary hygiene measures
___ pain relief measures
___ activity tolerance
___ nutritional intake
___ elimination status (urinary and bowel)
___ pertinent laboratory test findings
___ patient-family teaching
___ discharge planning

ASSOCIATED PLANS OF CARE
Grieving
Impaired Physical Mobility
Ineffective Individual Coping
Knowledge Deficit
Pain
Sensory-Perceptual Alteration

CONDENSED PLANS OF CARE

Total Joint Replacement in a Lower Extremity

COLLABORATIVE PROBLEM: *High risk for postoperative complications (hypovolemic shock, neurovascular damage, or thromboembolic phenomena) related to surgical trauma, bleeding, edema, improper positioning, or immobility*

Interventions

1. For hypovolemic shock, implement these measures:
• See the "Surgical Intervention" plan, page 81.
• Maintain patency of the wound drainage device. Monitor the amount of bleeding.
2. For neurovascular damage, implement these measures:
• Perform neurovascular checks postoperatively every hour for the first 4 hours, then every 2 hours for 12 hours, and then every 4 hours until ambulatory.
• Notify the doctor immediately if signs of impaired neurovascular function occur.
• Maintain positioning as recommended.
• Apply ice packs to the affected joint for 24 to 48 hours after surgery, if ordered.
• Maintain patency of the drainage device.
3. For thromboembolic phenomena, implement these measures:
• Teach the patient about exercises to prevent thromboembolism and encourage their use.
• Monitor for signs of thromboembolism. See the "Surgical Intervention" and "Thrombophlebitis" plans, pages 81 and 361 respectively.
• Apply antiembolism stockings to both legs.
• Monitor for signs of fat embolism daily.
• Administer anticoagulants and monitor clotting studies, as ordered.
4. Additional individualized interventions: _____

NURSING DIAGNOSIS: *Impaired physical mobility related to hip or knee surgery*

Interventions

1. Instruct the patient in the correct postoperative positioning of the affected extremity.
2. Teach the patient how to use the appropriate walking device.
3. Ensure that the patient maintains bed rest for 24 to 72 hours after surgery, as ordered, placing the affected extremity in the prescribed position.
4. Observe for dislocation of a hip prosthesis.
5. Supervise position changes at least every 2 hours.
6. Implement a planned, progressive daily ambulation schedule, as ordered.
7. Ensure that unaffected joints are put through full range-of-motion (ROM) exercises three or four times daily.
8. Help the patient maintain preferred rest and sleep routines.
9. Collaborate with the health care team to design an appropriate rehabilitation plan.
10. Identify, with the patient, the specific methods that will be used to implement the plan.
11. Additional individualized interventions: _____

NURSING DIAGNOSIS: *Impaired skin integrity related to surgery*

Interventions

1. Maintain the patency of the drainage device. Avoid contaminating the drainage port.
2. Do not administer injections in the affected extremity.
3. Assess daily for signs of infection.
4. Additional individualized interventions: _____

PATIENT-FAMILY TEACHING CHECKLIST

___ implications of joint replacement
___ rationale for continued use of antiembolism stockings
___ all discharge medications' purpose, dosage, administration schedule, and adverse effects requiring medical attention (usual discharge medications include analgesics, antibiotics, anti-inflammatories, and anticoagulants)
___ need for laboratory and medical follow-up if discharged on warfarin
___ schedule for progressive ambulation and weight bearing
___ additional activity restrictions
___ signs and symptoms of infection, bleeding, and dislocation
___ use of self-help devices, such as a raised toilet seat
___ appropriate resources for posthospitalization care
___ diet to promote healing
___ wound care
___ date, time, and location of follow-up appointments
___ how to contact the doctor

DOCUMENTATION CHECKLIST

___ clinical status on admission
___ significant changes in status
___ preoperative and postoperative teaching
___ position of affected extremity
___ exercises and range of motion achieved
___ neurovascular checks
___ calf pain
___ wound drainage
___ progressive ambulation
___ pain relief measures
___ patient-family teaching
___ discharge planning and referrals
___ presence or absence of disabling fatigue
___ nutritional intake

ASSOCIATED PLANS OF CARE

Ineffective Individual Coping
Knowledge Deficit
Pain
Surgical Intervention

Total Parenteral Nutrition

NURSING DIAGNOSIS: *High risk for injury related to complications of total parenteral nutrition (TPN) catheter insertion, displacement, use, or removal*
Interventions
1. Observe for signs and symptoms of respiratory distress or shock during insertion of the central venous catheter (CVC).
2. Maintain the patient in Trendelenburg's position during CVC insertion.
3. After CVC insertion, assess for bilateral breath sounds in all lung fields and obtain a chest X-ray.
4. Do not begin administering the TPN solution until the position of the catheter tip is confirmed by chest X-ray.
5. Use locking (Luer-Lok) connections, or tape the connections securely.
6. Before opening the I.V. system to the air, instruct the patient to perform Valsalva's maneuver or clamp the catheter. If the patient is unable to perform Valsalva's maneuver, change the tubing only during exhalation.
7. Observe for signs and symptoms of air emboli. If suspected, place the patient in Trendelenburg's position on the left side, administer oxygen, and notify the doctor immediately.
8. During dressing changes, observe for a suture at the insertion site of a temporary CVC, a suture at the exit site of a permanent CVC, or increased external catheter length.
9. Observe for inability to withdraw blood; complaints of chest pain or burning; leaking fluid; and swelling around the insertion site, shoulder, clavicle, or upper extremity.
10. Observe for visible collateral circulation on the chest wall.
11. When the catheter is being removed, be sure that:
• the patient is supine
• the patient performs Valsalva's maneuver before the catheter is removed
• a completely sealed, airtight dressing is applied over the insertion site after the CVC is discontinued.
12. When the catheter is removed, measure its length and observe for jagged edges.
13. Additional individualized interventions: _____

NURSING DIAGNOSIS: *Nutritional deficit related to inability to ingest nutrients orally or digest them satisfactorily, or increased metabolic need*
Interventions
1. Administer the ordered TPN solution.
2. Infuse TPN solution at a constant rate with an infusion pump.
• Check the volume of solution, flow rate, and patient tolerance every half hour.
• Do not interrupt the flow of TPN solution.
• Do not attempt to "catch up" if the infusion is behind schedule or "slow down" if it is ahead of schedule. Set the I.V. infusion to the ordered rate.
• When discontinuing TPN, decrease the rate to 50 ml/hour for 3 to 4 hours.
3. Ensure that the TPN infusion does not stop suddenly, or take appropriate corrective action:
• For a clotted catheter, hang dextrose 10% in water in another I.V. site to infuse at the ordered TPN rate.
• During cardiopulmonary arrest, stop the TPN infusion and provide a bolus of dextrose 50% in water, as ordered.

4. Monitor fingerstick and laboratory glucose levels, as ordered.
5. Observe for signs and symptoms of hypoglycemia, hyperglycemia, hyperosmolar overload, protein overload, electrolyte imbalances, vitamin deficiencies, or trace mineral deficiencies.
6. Infuse I.V. fat emulsion, as ordered, through one of three infusion methods:
• through a separate I.V.
• through a Y-connector added between the TPN catheter and the I.V. tubing
• as a 3-in-1 solution.
7. If 3-in-1 solution is used, ensure that it is mixed in a ratio of calcium, less than or equal to 15 mEq/liter; phosphorus, less than or equal to 30 mEq/liter; and magnesium, less than or equal to 10 mEq/liter.
8. Check that the infusion pump delivers the correct volume of 3-in-1 solution.
9. Observe for fat separation in the 3-in-1 solution as indicated by a yellow ring around the edges of the solution. Stop the infusion if this occurs, and replace the solution bag with a fresh one.
10. Culture the 3-in-1 solution if the patient develops sepsis.
11. If a separate fat infusion is used, administer slowly over the first 15 to 20 minutes (1 ml/minute for a 10% fat infusion or 0.5 ml/minute for a 20% fat infusion). Observe for adverse reactions; if none occur, increase the rate as ordered.
12. If the fat emulsion is to be infused in a second I.V., infuse it over 4 hours (for a 10% fat emulsion) or 8 hours (for a 20% fat emulsion).
13. Do not use I.V. filters with fat emulsion infusions.
14. Encourage walking or mild exercise to promote nitrogen retention.
15. Weigh the patient at the same time, with the same amount of clothing, and on the same scale daily.
16. When oral intake resumes, initiate a daily calorie count and measure fat intake.
17. Observe for changes in muscle strength and energy level.
18. Additional individualized interventions: _____

NURSING DIAGNOSIS: *High risk for fluid volume excess or deficit related to fluid retention, altered oral intake, or osmotic diuresis*
Interventions
1. See Appendix C, "Fluid and Electrolyte Imbalances."
2. Observe for signs and symptoms of fluid overload.
3. Observe for signs and symptoms of fluid deficit.
4. Assess breath sounds every shift.
5. Record intake and output each shift. Maintain approximate balance.
6. Weigh the patient daily.
7. Additional individualized interventions: _____

NURSING DIAGNOSIS: *Knowledge deficit related to lack of experience with TPN*
Interventions
1. Briefly explain the purpose and method of TPN therapy, including:
• a definition of TPN therapy and the reason for TPN, using terms the patient can understand
• a description of the role of the nutrition support service staff
• a description of the TPN solution
• the procedure for administering TPN solution, including the patient's responsibilities.
2. If the patient is to receive TPN at home, collaborate with the nutritional support team to provide appropriate teaching, including complications.
3. See the "Knowledge Deficit" care plan, page 56.
4. Additional individualized interventions: _____

NURSING DIAGNOSIS: *High risk for infection related to invasive CVC, leukopenia, or damp dressing*
Interventions
1. Follow protocol for dressing changes. Use sterile technique and universal precautions. Apply a clear, completely sealed dressing.
2. Observe the dressing every 8 hours and change it any time it is unsealed or damp.
3. Observe the insertion site every 8 hours for signs of infection. Report any redness, swelling, pain, or purulent drainage.
4. Follow hospital protocol for tubing changes and antibacterial preparation at all connections before changing I.V. tubing.
5. Follow pharmacy or nutrition support services recommendations for I.V. filters.
6. Infuse only TPN solution through the TPN catheter. Do not use the TPN line for injecting medications or withdrawing blood samples.
7. Use only solutions prepared in the pharmacy under a laminar flow hood.
8. Return cloudy or precipitated solution to the pharmacy.
9. Allow each bag or bottle to hang no more than 24 hours.
10. Monitor for signs of infection.
11. Additional individualized interventions: _____

PATIENT-FAMILY TEACHING CHECKLIST
(if the patient is being discharged on home TPN)
__ prevention of complications
__ actions to take if complications occur
__ where and how to obtain supplies
__ catheter site care
__ procedure for TPN administration
__ community resources
__ date, time, and location of follow-up appointment
__ how to contact the doctor

DOCUMENTATION CHECKLIST
__ nutritional status on admission
__ any significant changes in status
__ CVC insertion, including difficulties or complications; length of catheter; position and any change in position; signs of infection, thrombosis, emboli, or other postinsertion complication
__ dressing and tubing changes
__ TPN solution and fat emulsion—for each bag or bottle, record date, time, name of nurse hanging solution; all ingredients in each bag or bottle; and the rate of infusion
__ patient-family teaching
__ discharge planning

ASSOCIATED PLANS OF CARE
Knowledge Deficit
Nutritional Deficit

Appendices and Index

Appendix A: Monitoring Standards

Monitoring of clinical signs and symptoms, laboratory tests, and diagnostic procedures is presented within specific plans of care in this text. This appendix outlines generally accepted standards for implementing selected hemodynamic monitoring techniques for critically ill patients. It should be individualized according to a specific patient's needs and unit protocol. For all monitoring techniques, remember that the trend of values is more significant than isolated readings.

Electrocardiography (ECG) monitoring

- Monitor ECG continuously. Observe for arrhythmias, ST-segment changes, and T-wave abnormalities.
- Monitor in MCL_1 or MCL_6 whenever possible, because they best differentiate ectopy from aberrancy.
- Keep rate alarms on at all times.
- Mount rhythm printouts in the patient's record routinely every 8 hours and as needed for significant arrhythmias.
- Evaluate and document atrial and ventricular rate, rhythm, PR interval, QRS duration, and appearance of P waves, QRS complex, ST segment, and T waves at least once every 8 hours and as needed for significant changes.

Vital sign monitoring

- Monitor apical pulse, blood pressure, and respiratory rate every 15 minutes until stable, then every hour.
- Monitor temperature at least every 4 hours.

Intake and output (I&O) monitoring

- Monitor hourly and 8-hour or 24-hour cumulative intake and output levels.
- Besides standard nursing I&O measures (for example, including gelatin in intake total), record the amount of all I.V. flush solutions administered.
- Measure urine specific gravity hourly or as indicated.
- Measure fingerstick blood glucose levels every 6 hours in diabetic patients, patients on total parenteral nutrition, postoperative cardiac surgery patients, and others, as indicated.

Arterial pressure monitoring

- Monitor arterial pressure continuously in patients with arterial lines.
- Keep pressure alarms on at all times.
- Keep all connections in constant view; the patient can exsanguinate in a matter of minutes if a disconnection occurs.
- Balance and calibrate the transducer according to the manufacturer's directions at least every 8 hours to negate the influence of atmospheric pressure on readings and to confirm the measuring accuracy.
- Use a constant low-flow closed heparinized flush solution to maintain patency.
- Periodically observe for the characteristic arterial waveform on the oscilloscope; investigate damping or abnormal appearance promptly.
- Compare to sphygmomanometer pressure every 8 hours; investigate significant discrepancies between the two.
- Check pulse, skin temperature, and skin color distal to the insertion site at least every 2 hours.

Central venous pressure (CVP) monitoring

- Measure CVP every hour or as needed.
- Before measuring CVP, level the zero point on the manometer with the phlebostatic axis (fourth intercostal space in the midaxillary line).
- Before measuring CVP, confirm catheter patency by observing the manometer fluid level for the characteristic fall and fluctuations with respiration.

Monitoring Standards *(continued)*

Pulmonary artery (PA) monitoring	• Measure systolic, diastolic, and mean pressures every hour or as needed. • Use consistent baseline position for obtaining readings. • Level the transducer's air-fluid interface with the phlebostatic axis. • Follow unit protocol for removing patients from ventilators to record readings. If recording pressures while the patient is on the ventilator, read pressures at end-expiration to minimize respiratory influences on hemodynamic values. Document whether pressures are recorded when the patient is on or off the ventilator. • Balance and calibrate the transducer according to the manufacturer's directions at least every 8 hours to negate the influence of atmospheric pressure on readings and to confirm accuracy of measurement. • Use a constant low-flow closed heparinized flush solution to maintain patency. • Before readings, confirm patency by observing the oscilloscope for characteristic PA waveforms. • Usually, when the above standards are followed, regard a change in values of more than 5 mm Hg as clinically significant.
Pulmonary capillary wedge pressure (PCWP) monitoring	• Measure PCWP every hour or as needed. • To read PCWP, inflate the balloon until the characteristic PCWP waveform appears, using no more than the specified amount of air for that size balloon. After reading the pressure, be sure the balloon is deflated by removing the syringe used for inflation, releasing the lever if used to lock air in the balloon for the reading, and confirming on the oscilloscope the return to the usual PA waveform. • To avoid frequent wedging, which damages the balloon, and to monitor left ventricular filling pressure constantly, consider continuous monitoring of PA diastolic pressure. Verify correlation with PCWP every 4 to 8 hours by confirming that the pressures are within 5 mm Hg of each other.
Cardiac output (CO) monitoring	• Measure CO every hour or as needed. • Obtain at least three readings at a time. Discard any readings that deviate significantly from each other and average the remaining readings. • Use injectate at room temperature. Use iced injectate if room temperature injectate readings consistently deviate more than 15% from each other. • Monitor cardiac index by dividing CO by the patient's body surface area, obtainable from a DuBois nomogram. • Monitor systemic vascular resistance by dividing CO into mean arterial pressure (MAP) minus mean right atrial pressure.
Intracranial pressure (ICP) monitoring	• Monitor ICP continuously in patients with ICP monitoring catheters. • Use a consistent baseline position for obtaining readings, usually a 20- to 30-degree elevation of the head of the bed. • Level the air-fluid interface of the transducer with the reference point for the foramen of Monro, usually considered to be the outer corner of the eye, top of the ear, or the external auditory meatus. • Verify patency of the line by observing the characteristic waveform on the oscilloscope. • Do not read pressures while the patient is moving, coughing, or has the head turned to one side or the other; all will falsely elevate pressures. • Never aspirate an ICP line; doing so may draw brain tissue into the catheter or screw. • Do not flush an ICP line unless specifically ordered to do so by the patient's doctor. • Monitor cerebral perfusion pressure by subtracting ICP from MAP. • Balance and calibrate the transducer at least every 8 hours.

REFERENCES

Daily, E., and Schroeder, J. *Techniques in Bedside Hemodynamic Monitoring,* 4th ed. St. Louis: C.V. Mosby Co., 1989.

Holloway, N., and Gawlinski, A. "Hemodynamic Monitoring," in *Nursing the Critically Ill Adult,* 4th ed. Edited by Holloway, N. Menlo Park, Calif.: Addison-Wesley Publishing Co., 1993.

Nemens E., and Woods, S. "Normal Fluctuations in Pulmonary Artery and Pulmonary Capillary Wedge Pressures in Acutely Ill Patients," *Heart & Lung* 11:393-98, 1982.

Appendix B: Acid-Base Imbalances

Disorder	ABG results	Physiologic basis	Potential causes	Signs and symptoms	Compensatory mechanisms
Respiratory acidosis	↓ pH ↑ $PaCO_2$ Compensatory: ↑ HCO_3^-	Decreased alveolar ventilation, resulting in carbon dioxide retention	Depression of medullary respiratory center from drugs, injury, or disease Pulmonary diseases Inadequate tidal volume (TV) or respiratory rate on ventilator	Decreased mentation, restlessness, combativeness, headache, diaphoresis, anxiety, tachycardia	Renal compensation by HCO_3^- retention, acid elimination, and increased ammonia production
Respiratory alkalosis	↑ pH ↓ $PaCO_2$ Compensatory: ↓ HCO_3^-	Increased alveolar ventilation, resulting in carbon dioxide loss	Hyperventilation from anxiety, pain, excessive TV or respiratory rate on ventilator Respiratory-center stimulation by drugs, injury, or disease Fever or high ambient temperature Sepsis	Increased rate and depth of respirations, "tingling" or numb feeling, lightheadedness or syncope, anxiety	Renal compensation by HCO_3^- elimination, acid retention, and decreased ammonia production
Metabolic acidosis	↓ pH ↓ HCO_3^- Compensatory: ↓ $PaCO_2$	HCO_3^- loss, ↑ acid formation	Diarrhea, diabetes, shock, renal failure, azotemia, small-bowel fistulas	Increased rate and depth of respirations, fatigue, lethargy, acetone odor to breath, unconsciousness	Rapid pulmonary compensation by hyperventilation, renal metabolic compensation (except in renal failure) by HCO_3^- retention, acid elimination, increased ammonia production
Metabolic alkalosis	↑ pH ↑ HCO_3^- Compensatory: ↑ $PaCO_2$	↑ HCO_3^- retention, acids or potassium loss	Vomiting, gastric suctioning, prolonged use of diuretics, excessive HCO_3^- ingestion	Decreased rate and depth of respirations, hypertonicity, twitching to tetanus, seizures, irritability, restlessness, combativeness, unconsciousness	Rapid pulmonary compensation by hypoventilation, renal metabolic compensation by HCO_3^- elimination, acid retention, decreased ammonia production

From: Strange, J. *Shock Trauma Care Plans*. Springhouse, Pa.: Springhouse Corp., 1987, pp 372-73.

Appendix C: Fluid and Electrolyte Imbalances

Causes	Signs and symptoms and laboratory results	Treatment
Hypovolemia Hemorrhage, diabetes insipidus (DI), renal disease, vagal stimulation, drug reactions, hyperosmolar hyperglycemic nonketotic syndrome	Tachycardia, weak pulse, hypotension, oliguria, ↓ central venous pressure (CVP), ↓ level of consciousness (LOC), pallor, ↓ hematocrit and hemoglobin	Correct the cause; administer appropriate I.V. fluids.
Hypervolemia Excessive I.V. fluid administration	Hypertension, edema, bounding pulse, ↑ CVP, pulmonary edema, venous distention, ↓ hemoglobin and hematocrit, ↓ blood urea nitrogen (BUN)	Treat with diuretics, dialysis; no treatment may be needed; prevention is the best treatment.
Intravascular to interstitial shift Hemorrhage, ↓ water intake, concentrated tube feedings, vomiting, diarrhea, burns, prolonged gastric suctioning, soft-tissue injury, intestinal obstruction, fever	Shock state, tachycardia, weak pulse, oliguria, ↓ LOC, dry mucous membranes, ↑ hemoglobin and hematocrit, ↑ BUN, hypotension	Correct the cause; administer appropriate I.V. fluids.
Interstitial to intravascular shift Burns, soft-tissue injury, excessive colloid or hypertonic I.V. administration	Hypertension, bounding pulse, venous distention, ↑ CVP, weakness, ↓ hemoglobin and hematocrit, ↓ BUN, hyponatremia	No treatment is needed except in patients with abnormal heart, liver, or kidney function; they are usually treated with diuretics.
Hyponatremia Excessive sweating or water intake, ↓ salt intake, congestive heart failure (CHF), renal failure, diuretic therapy, freshwater near drowning, vomiting, diarrhea, burns	Confusion, headache, abdominal cramps, apathy, hypotension, weakness, hyperactive reflexes, seizures, oliguria, ↓ serum sodium, ↓ chloride, ↓ urine specific gravity	Decrease water intake or increase sodium intake.
Hypernatremia ↓ water intake, ↑ sodium intake, prolonged watery diarrhea, prolonged hyperventilation, saltwater near drowning, DI	Dehydration; thirst; dry mucous membranes; weakness; fever; warm, flushed skin; muscle pain; ↑ serum sodium level; ↑ serum chloride level; ↑ urine specific gravity	Correct the cause, if possible; restrict sodium intake; increase fluid intake.
Hypokalemia ↓ potassium intake, diuretics, vomiting or diarrhea, burns, CHF, fistulas, colitis, steroids	Diminished reflexes, irregular pulse, thirst, hypotension, electrocardiography (ECG) changes, muscular weakness or irritability, ↓ serum potassium level, ↓ serum chloride level	Increase dietary potassium intake; administer P.O. or I.V. potassium supplements.
Hyperkalemia ↑ potassium intake, burns, soft tissue injury, advanced kidney disease, adrenal insufficiency, hemorrhagic shock, excessive I.V. administration	Irritability, nausea, diarrhea, confusion, flaccid muscles, ECG changes, hypotension, abdominal cramping, ↑ serum potassium level	Decrease intake; treat with dialysis; give a sodium polystyrene sulfonate enema; give sodium bicarbonate, glucose, and insulin together I.V.

continued

APPENDICES

Fluid and Electrolyte Imbalances *(continued)*

Causes	Signs and symptoms and laboratory results	Treatment
Hypocalcemia		
Diarrhea, burns, renal failure, draining wounds, citrated blood administration, acidosis overcorrection, vitamin D deficiency	Carpopedal spasms; tetany; seizures; tingling in fingers, toes, lips; muscle cramps; ECG changes; ↓ serum calcium level	Administer calcium P.O. or I.V.
Hypercalcemia		
Vitamin D overdose, renal disease, excessive antacid use, excessive calcium intake	Pathologic fractures, deep-bone or flank pain, lethargy, nausea, vomiting, ECG changes, osteoporosis, kidney stones, kidney infections, ↑ serum calcium level	Correct the cause; administer disodium phosphate, sodium sulfate, diuretics.
Hypomagnesemia		
Alcohol abuse, vomiting, ↓ intake, malnutrition, diuretics, prolonged GI suctioning, diarrhea, pancreatitis, kidney disease	Tetany, lethargy, nausea, vomiting, tachyarrhythmias, hypotension, confusion, hyperactive reflexes, ↓ serum magnesium level	Increase dietary intake, administer I.V. magnesium.
Hypermagnesemia		
Excessive intake, kidney disease, severe dehydration, repeated magnesium-containing enemas, magnesium antacids in renal failure	Lethargy, flushing, depressed respirations, hypotension, flaccid muscles or paralysis, arrhythmias, ↑ serum magnesium level	Decrease intake; administer I.V. 10% calcium gluconate; treat renal-failure patients with dialysis.

From: Strange, J. *Shock Trauma Care Plans*. Springhouse, Pa.: Springhouse Corp., 1987, pp 374-75.

Appendix D: Nursing Diagnostic Categories Grouped According to Gordon's Functional Health Patterns

This list represents nursing diagnostic categories approved by the North American Nursing Diagnosis Association (NANDA) for clinical use and testing as of summer 1992. Numbers correlate with NANDA's placement of diagnoses under the unitary man schema.

Health perception–health management pattern
1.6.1.	High risk for injury
1.6.1.1.	High risk for suffocation
1.6.1.2.	High risk for poisoning
1.6.1.3.	High risk for trauma
1.6.1.4.	High risk for aspiration
1.6.1.5.	High risk for disuse syndrome
5.2.1.	Ineffective management of therapeutic regimen (individual)*
5.2.1.1.	Noncompliance (specify)
5.4	Health-seeking behaviors (specify)
6.4.2.	Altered health maintenance

Nutritional-metabolic pattern
1.1.2.1.	Altered nutrition: more than body requirements
1.1.2.2.	Altered nutrition: less than body requirements
1.1.2.3.	Altered nutrition: high risk for more than body requirements
1.2.1.1.	High risk for infection
1.2.2.1.	High risk for altered body temperature
1.2.2.2.	Hypothermia
1.2.2.3.	Hyperthermia
1.2.2.4.	Ineffective thermoregulation
1.2.3.1.	Dysreflexia
1.4.1.1.	Altered tissue perfusion (specify type: renal, cerebral, cardiopulmonary, gastrointestinal, peripheral)†
1.4.1.2.1.	Fluid volume excess
1.4.1.2.2.1.	Fluid volume deficit
1.4.1.2.2.2.	High risk for fluid volume deficit
1.4.2.1.	Decreased cardiac output†
1.6.2.	Altered protection
1.6.2.1.	Impaired tissue integrity†
1.6.2.1.1.	Altered oral mucous membrane
1.6.2.1.2.1.	Impaired skin integrity
1.6.2.1.2.2.	High risk for impaired skin integrity
6.5.1.	Feeding self-care deficit
6.5.1.1.	Impaired swallowing
6.5.1.2.	Ineffective breast-feeding
6.5.1.2.1.	Interrupted breast-feeding*
6.5.1.3.	Effective breast-feeding
6.5.1.4.	Ineffective infant feeding pattern*

Elimination pattern
1.3.1.1.	Constipation
1.3.1.1.1.	Perceived constipation
1.3.1.1.2.	Colonic constipation
1.3.1.2.	Diarrhea
1.3.1.3.	Bowel incontinence
1.3.2.	Altered urinary elimination
1.3.2.1.1.	Stress incontinence
1.3.2.1.2.	Reflex incontinence
1.3.2.1.3.	Urge incontinence
1.3.2.1.4.	Functional incontinence
1.3.2.1.5.	Total incontinence
1.3.2.2.	Urinary retention

Activity-exercise pattern
1.5.1.1.	Impaired gas exchange
1.5.1.2.	Ineffective airway clearance
1.5.1.3.	Ineffective breathing pattern
1.5.1.3.1.	Inability to sustain spontaneous ventilation*
1.5.1.3.2.	Dysfunctional ventilatory weaning response*
6.1.1.1.	Impaired physical mobility
6.1.1.1.1.	High risk for peripheral neurovascular dysfunction*
6.1.1.2.	Activity intolerance
6.1.1.2.1.	Fatigue
6.1.1.3.	High risk for activity intolerance
6.3.1.1.	Diversional activity deficit
6.4.1.1.	Impaired home maintenance management
6.5.2.	Bathing or hygiene self-care deficit
6.5.3.	Dressing or grooming self-care deficit
6.5.4.	Toileting self-care deficit
6.6.	Growth and development, altered

Sleep-rest pattern
6.2.1.	Sleep pattern disturbance

Cognitive-perceptual pattern
7.2.	Sensory or perceptual alteration (specify: visual, auditory, kinesthetic, gustatory, tactile, olfactory)
7.2.1.1.	Unilateral neglect
8.1.1.	Knowledge deficit (specify)
8.3.	Thought processes, altered
9.1.1.	Pain
9.1.1.1.	Chronic pain

Self-perception–self-concept pattern
7.1.1.	Body-image disturbance
7.1.2.	Self-esteem disturbance
7.1.2.1.	Chronic low self-esteem
7.1.2.2.	Situational low self-esteem
7.1.3.	Personal identity disturbance
7.3.1.	Hopelessness
7.3.2.	Powerlessness
9.3.1.	Anxiety
9.3.2.	Fear

Role-relationship pattern
2.1.1.1.	Impaired verbal communication
3.1.1.	Impaired social interaction
3.1.2.	Social isolation
3.2.1.	Altered role performance
3.2.1.1.1.	Altered parenting
3.2.1.1.2.	High risk for altered parenting
3.2.2.	Altered family processes
3.2.3.1.	Parental role conflict

continued

Nursing Diagnostic Categories Grouped According to Gordon's Functional Health Patterns *(continued)*

9.2.1.1.	Dysfunctional grieving
9.2.1.2.	Anticipatory grieving
9.2.2.	High risk for violence: self-directed or directed at others
9.4.1.	Caregiver role strain*
9.4.2.	High risk for caregiver role strain*

Sexuality-reproductive pattern
3.2.1.2.1.	Sexual dysfunction
3.3.	Altered sexuality patterns

Coping–stress-tolerance pattern
5.1.1.1.	Ineffective individual coping
5.1.1.1.1.	Impaired adjustment
5.1.1.1.2.	Defensive coping

5.1.1.1.3.	Ineffective denial
5.1.2.1.1.	Ineffective family coping: disabling
5.1.2.1.2.	Ineffective family coping: compromised
5.1.2.2.	Family coping: potential for growth
5.3.1.1.	Decisional conflict (specify)
6.7.	Relocation stress syndrome*
9.2.2.1.	High risk for self-mutilation*
9.2.3.	Post-trauma response
9.2.3.1.	Rape-trauma syndrome
9.2.3.1.1.	Rape-trauma syndrome: compound reaction
9.2.3.1.2.	Rape-trauma syndrome: silent reaction

Value-belief pattern
4.1.1.	Spiritual distress (distress of the human spirit)

* Adopted summer 1992
† The author believes these diagnoses represent renaming of commonly accepted medical terms and recommends that they not be used for nursing diagnoses guiding independent nursing care. Interdependent nursing care related to these problems is included in the collaborative problems in this book and labeled with familiar terms (such as shock and ischemia).

Functional health patterns adapted from Gordon, M. (1991). *Manual of nursing diagnoses.* St. Louis: Mosby-Year Book. Used with permission.

Appendix E: Critical Care Transfer Criteria Guidelines

Although the decision to transfer a patient is a medical one, the critical care nurse often has input in the decision. The following presents general criteria for transfer from a critical care unit to a "stepdown" or medical-surgical unit. Additional disease-specific criteria are presented within the plans in this text. These transfer criteria guidelines should be individualized according to the patient's needs and unit protocol.

General considerations

- No longer requires constant surveillance
- Resuscitation status specified in medical order
- Discharge planning initiated, with assessments made of patient's living arrangements before admission, discharge prognosis, anticipated length of stay, ability to perform activities of daily living, educational goals, family or friend's ability and willingness to assist the patient after discharge, and referrals initiated to appropriate ancillary services

Neurologic system

- Improved or stable level of consciousness and other neurologic vital signs for 12 hours
- Absence of intracranial pressure monitoring line

Pulmonary system

- Pulmonary status stable for 12 hours
- If still requires mechanical ventilation, stable and being transferred to caregivers experienced with this therapy
- PaO_2 greater than 80 mm Hg (except in chronic obstructive pulmonary disease)
- $PaCO_2$ less than 10 mm Hg above patient's normal value

Cardiovascular system

- No longer needs I.V. pharmacologic therapy requiring continuous cardiac monitoring
- Blood pressure within 20 mm Hg of patient's normal value (or otherwise acceptable value) for 12 hours, without I.V. drugs, such as inotropes, vasodilators, or vasoconstrictors; or mechanical assist devices, such as intra-aortic balloon pump
- Absent arterial line and pulmonary artery catheter

Renal system

- Urinary output at least 1 ml/kg/hour, except in chronic renal failure
- If receiving concentrated potassium infusion greater than 20 mEq/hour, transfer to monitored bed

APPENDICES

750

Index

A

Acid-base imbalances, 744t
Acquired immunodeficiency syndrome, 689
 complications of, 602
 and coping, ineffective individual, 605-606
 definition of, 599
 diagnostic criteria for, 600t
 diagnostic studies for, 601-602
 discharge criteria for, 615
 documentation of, 616
 DRG information on, 599
 etiology of, 599
 fluid volume deficit and, 611
 hypoxemia and, 606-607
 infection and, 602, 603t, 604-605
 knowledge deficit and, 613-615
 nursing history for, 599-601
 nutritional deficit and, 610
 and oral mucous membrane, altered, 611-612
 patient-family teaching for, 615
 physical findings for, 601
 and physical mobility, impaired, 609-610
 sensory-perceptual alteration and, 607-608
 sexual dysfunction and, 613
 and skin integrity, impaired, 612
 social isolation and, 608-609
Activities of daily living (ADLs), 26, 282
Acupuncture, 72
Acute myocardial infarction. See Myocardial infarction, acute
Adult respiratory distress syndrome, 696
 complications of, 194
 and coping, ineffective, 197-198
 definition of, 193
 diagnostic studies for, 194
 discharge criteria for, 198
 documentation of, 198
 DRG information on, 193
 etiology of, 193
 hypoxemia and, 194-196
 nursing history for, 193
 patient-family teaching for, 198
 physical findings for, 193-194
AIDS. See Acquired immunodeficiency syndrome
Alzheimer's disease, 697
 and cognitive function, impaired, 93-95
 complications of, 93
 constipation and, 97-98
 and coping, ineffective family, 98
 definition of, 92
 diagnostic studies for, 93
 discharge criteria for, 99
 documentation of, 99
 DRG information on, 92
 etiology of, 92
 nursing history of, 92-93
 nutritional deficit and, 95-96
 patient-family teaching for, 99
 physical findings for, 93
 stages of, 94t
Ambulation, 83, 84, 256
Amputation
 body-image disturbance and, 449-450
 complications of, 445
 definition of, 444
 diagnostic studies for, 444-445
 discharge criteria for, 450

Amputation (continued)
 documentation of, 451
 DRG information on, 444
 hemorrhage and, 445
 infection and, 447
 joint dysfunction and, 448-449
 nursing history for, 444
 pain and, 446-447
 patient-family teaching for, 450
 physical findings for, 444
 and physical mobility, impaired, 448-449
Anemia
 complications of, 619
 definition of, 617
 diagnostic studies for, 618
 discharge criteria for, 624
 documentation of, 624
 DRG information on, 617
 etiology of, 617
 hopelessness and, 623
 hypoxemia and, 619-620
 nursing history for, 617-618
 nutritional deficit and, 620-621
 patient-family teaching for, 624
 physical findings for, 618
 self-care deficit and, 622-623
 and skin integrity, impaired, 622
Aneurysm
 abdominal aortic, repair of, 688
 bleeding and, 264-265
 cardiac decompensation and, 263
 complications of, 262
 definition of, 261
 diagnostic studies for, 261-262
 discharge criteria for, 266
 documentation of, 267
 DRG information on, 261
 hypercapnia and, 264
 hypoxemia and, 264
 knowledge deficit and, 262-263
 nursing history for, 261
 pain and, 266
 patient-family teaching for, 266
 ventricular, 275
Angina pectoris, 698
 activity intolerance and, 295
 arrhythmias and, 294
 definition of, 291
 diagnostic studies for, 292
 discharge criteria for, 297
 documentation of, 297
 DRG information on, 291
 etiology of, 291
 and health maintenance, altered, 295-296
 knowledge deficit and, 296-297
 nursing history for, 291-292
 patient-family teaching for, 297
 physical findings for, 292
Anorexia nervosa and bulimia nervosa
 complications of, 370
 definition of, 367
 diagnostic studies for, 370
 discharge criteria for, 373
 documentation of, 373
 DRG information on, 367
 etiology of, 367
 nursing history for, 368-369
 nutritional deficit and, 370-371
 patient-family teaching for, 373
 physical findings for, 369
 powerlessness and, 371-372
 self-esteem disturbance and, 372-373
Antiembolism hose, 40, 84, 362

Anxiety, 191
Aphasia, 106
Arrhythmias
 cardiac surgery and, 302t
 pacemaker malfunction and, 354-356
 types of, 274
Arterial insufficiency, 342-343
Aseptic technique, 86
Aspiration, 166-167
Asthma
 complications of, 201
 definition of, 199
 diagnostic studies for, 200-201
 discharge criteria for, 204
 documentation of, 204
 DRG information on, 199
 etiology of, 199
 nursing history for, 199-200
 patient-family teaching for, 204
 physical findings for, 200
 pulmonary arrest and, 201-203
 social isolation and, 203
 status asthmaticus and, 201-203
 types of, 199
Atelectasis, 39, 83-84, 259
Autoregulatory mechanisms, 134

B

Back pain, low, 723
 complications of, 460
 definition of, 459
 diagnostic studies for, 460
 discharge criteria for, 465
 documentation of, 465
 DRG information on, 459
 etiology of, 459
 knowledge deficit and, 463-465
 nursing history for, 459-460
 patient-family teaching for, 465
 physical findings for, 460
 and physical mobility, impaired, 460-462
 and role performance, altered, 462-463
Behavior, type A, 289
Bleeding. See Hemorrhage
Blood pressure lability, 320-321
Bowel
 disease, inflammatory
  arrhythmias and, 403
  complications of, 403
  definition of, 401
  diagnostic studies for, 402-403
  discharge criteria for, 409
  documentation of, 410
  DRG information on, 401
  electrolyte depletion and, 403
  etiology of, 401
  fluid volume deficit and, 404
  infection and, 405-406
  nursing history for, 401-402
  nutritional deficit and, 404-405
  pain and, 406
  patient-family teaching for, 410
  physical findings for, 402
  and sexuality patterns, altered, 409
  and skin integrity, impaired, 407-408
  sleep pattern disturbance and, 407
  social isolation and, 408
 elimination pattern, 43, 221
 function, 26
 sounds, 66
Breathing
 deep, 38, 83, 129
 pursed-lip, 216

i refers to an illustration; t, to a table.

INDEX

i refers to an illustration; t, to a table.

i refers to an illustration; t, to a table.

i refers to an illustration; t, to a table.

i refers to an illustration; t, to a table.